Blue Books of Practical Neurology

Movement Disorders 1 and 2 Reissue

Blue Books of Practical Neurology

(Volumes 1–14 published as BIMR Neurology)

Published titles

1. **Clinical Neurophysiology**
   Erik Stålberg and Robert R. Young

2. **Movement Disorders 1**
   C. David Marsden and Stanley Fahn

3. **Cerebral Vascular Disease**
   Michael J. G. Harrison and Mark L. Dyken

4. **Peripheral Nerve Disorders**
   Arthur K. Asbury and R. W. Gilliatt

5. **The Epilepsies**
   Roger J. Porter and Paolo L. Morselli

6. **Multiple Sclerosis**
   W. I. McDonald and Donald H. Silberger

7. **Movement Disorders 2**
   C. David Marsden and Stanley Fahn

8. **Infections of the Nervous System**
   Peter G. E. Kennedy and Richard T. Johnson

9. **The Molecular Biology of Neurological Disease**
   Roger N. Rosenberg and A. E. Harding

10. **Pain Syndromes in Neurology**
    Howard L. Fields

11. **Principles and Practice of Restorative Neurology**
    Robert R. Young and Paul J. Delwaide

12. **Stroke: Populations, Cohorts, and Clinical Trials**
    Jack P. Whisnant

13. **Movement Disorders 3**
    C. David Marsden and Stanley Fahn

14. **Mitochondrial Disorders in Neurology**
    A. H. V. Schapira and S. DiMauro

15. **Peripheral Nerve Disorders 2**
    Arthur K. Asbury and P. K. Thomas

Movement Disorders 1 and 2 Reissue

Edited by

C. David Marsden, FRS, DSc, MB, BS, MRCPsych, FRCP
Professor of Neurology, Institute of Neurology, The National Hospital for Neurology and Neurosurgery, Queen Square, London, UK

and

Stanley Fahn, MD
H Houston Merritt Professor of Neurology, Columbia University College of Physicians and Surgeons, Neurological Institute, New York, USA

Butterworth–Heinemann Ltd
Linacre House, Jordan Hill, Oxford OX2 8DP

A member of the Reed Elsevier plc group

OXFORD LONDON BOSTON
MUNICH NEW DELHI SINGAPORE SYDNEY
TOKYO TORONTO WELLINGTON

Movement Disorders 1 first published 1982
Movement Disorders 2 first published 1987

© Butterworth–Heinemann Ltd 1995

All rights reserved. No part of this publication
may be reproduced in any material form (including
photocopying or storing in any medium by electronic
means and whether or not transiently or incidentally
to some other use of this publication) without the
written permission of the copyright holder except
in accordance with the provisions of the Copyright,
Designs and Patents Act 1988 or under the terms of a
licence issued by the Copyright Licensing Agency Ltd,
90 Tottenham Court Road, London, England W1P 9HE.
Applications for the copyright holder's written permission
to reproduce any part of this publication should be addressed
to the publishers

British Library Cataloguing in Publication Data
A catalogue record for this book is available from the British Library

ISBN 0 7506 2232 6

Printed in Great Britain at the University Press, Cambridge

Blue Books of Practical Neurology

Series Preface

The *Blue Books of Practical Neurology* series is the new name for the *BIMR Neurology* series which was itself the successor to the *Modern Trends in Neurology* series. As before, the volumes are intended for use by physicians who grapple with the problems of neurological disorders on a daily basis, be they neurologists, neurologists in training, or those in related fields such as neurosurgery, internal medicine, psychiatry, and rehabilitation medicine.

Our purpose is to produce monographs on topics in clinical neurology in which progress through research has brought about new concepts of patient management. The subject of each monograph is selected by the Series Editors using two criteria: first, that there has been significant advance in knowledge in that area and, second, that such advances have been incorporated into new ways of managing patients with the disorders in question. This has been the guiding spirit behind each volume, and we expect it to continue. In effect we emphasize research, both in the clinic and in the experimental laboratory, but principally to the extent that it changes our collective attitudes and practices in caring for those who are neurologically afflicted.

C. D. Marsden
A.K. Asbury
Series Editors

Preface to Movement Disorders 1 & 2 Reissue

Many young clinical neurologists and neuroscientists entering the field have purchased *Movement Disorders 3*. They then have asked where they could obtain the first two volumes of *Movement Disorders*, published in 1982 and 1987, both of which have been out of print for some time. Butterworth–Heinemann, encouraged by such demands, have generously agreed to reissue *Movement Disorders 1 and 2*.

The Preface to *Movement Disorders 1* (1982) stated: 'This book is *not* a textbook on movement disorders and does not encompass all that has been written on the subject in recent years. Rather, we have concentrated on a number of topics which, we believe, either have reached a stage that warrants definitive discussion, or are of sufficient practical importance to justify presentation even though, at present, no certain conclusion can be drawn'. This theme was pursued in *Movement Disorders 2* (1987) where we stated: 'So much has happened since then (1982) that we believe a second volume is required to review advances that have occurred in the last five years, and to deal with new topics that were not considered previously'. We followed the same principles in *Movement Disorders 3* (1994). So the three volumes provide a progressive update of major advances in the field over a twelve year period of rapid advance. In addition, the three volumes have covered the major topics in Movement Disorders, so the reader can not only follow the development of facts and theories, but also can dip into individual chapters on most of the major diseases and problems in Movement Disorders.

Once the decision to reissue *Movement Disorders 1 and 2* had been made, a major question was whether to ask the individual authors of their chapters to update or comment on their original writings. At first sight this might have been an attractive option. However, we know how busy we all are! In addition, re-reading the originals led us to conclude that they should stand as they are, for they give a superb flavour of the development of thought on their subjects. Indeed, they provide a glimpse of the contemporary history of Movement Disorders, as the science and practice of the discipline has exploded over this period of time.

Nevertheless, as editors we felt it appropriate to pass some comment on the significance of the originals and on the changes that have occurred since their publication.

Each volume of *Movement Disorders 1–3* has included a number of general chapters reviewing areas that have contributed so much to the field.

In *Movement Disorders 1*, Donald Calne reviewed the topic of dopamine receptors. Of course, this was before the explosion of molecular biology and the cloning of the multiple dopamine receptors now known to exist. Molecular biologists have now cloned five dopamine receptors: (1) with their genes located on different sites in the human genome; (2) with different agonists and antagonists; and (3) with different locations in the brain (Table 1). The importance of the D4 receptor has emerged with the knowledge that clozapine, an effective, non-neuroleptic, antipsychotic drug, acts as an antagonist at this

Preface to Movement Disorders 1 & 2 Reissue

Table 1 Dopamine receptors

Feature	D1	D2	D3	D4	D5
Chromosome	5q31-34	11q22-23	3q13.3	11p	4p16.3
Region	striatum	striatum	accumbens	frontal cx	hypothal
DA Affinity	μmolar	μmolar	nmolar	subμmolar	subμmolar
Agonist	SKF-38393	bromocr.	7-OH-DPAT	?	SKF-38393
Antagonist	SCH-23390	haloper.	UH 232	clozapine	SCH-23390
Adenyl cyclase	stimulates	inhibits	±	inhibits	stimulates

receptor. Nevertheless, the basic concept of the D1 and D2 families of dopamine receptors has proved its worth, and we still struggle to explain their functions and interactions.

Dramatic advances in brain imaging techniques also occurred between *Movement Disorders 1* and *2*. In 1987, Wayne Martin and Donald Calne reviewed the contributions of computed tomography, magnetic resonance imaging and, particularly, positron emission tomography to study blood flow, glucose metabolism and dopamine in the brain. All these modalities had begun to provide novel information in Parkinson's disease, Huntington's disease and dystonia. By 1994, David Brooks could provide an extensive update of a mass of new information on the functional imaging of movement disorders.

A similar remarkable application of the new technologies of molecular genetics was chronicled by Xandra Breakfield and Sue Bressman in 1987, and then by Anita Harding in 1994. In *Movement Disorders 2* (1987), linked markers had been identified for Huntington's disease (chromosome 4), Wilson's disease (chromosome 13) and Lesch-Nyhan syndrome (the X chromosome), amongst the movement disorders, and the search for a dystonic gene was gathering pace. In *Movement Disorders 3* (1994), the Huntington's disease gene had been shown to be an unstable trinucleotide repeat, and one dystonia gene had been mapped by linkage to chromosome 9q32-34 and another to the pericentromeric region of the X chromosome. Even as we write this Preface, new genetic discoveries are hitting the headlines, for example the identification of the gene for dopa responsive dystonia, located at chromosome 14q22. The gene has been identified as being responsible for generating the enzyme GTP cyclohydrolase I, the first enzymatic step for the synthesis of tetrahydrobiopterin, the cofactor for tyrosine hydroxylase activity. The gene for Wilson's disease has been shown to be for copper transport enzyme (Cu-ATPase) located at chromosome 13q14.3, and the gene for dentatorubropallidoluysian atrophy has been shown to be another unstable trinucleotide repeat located at chromosome 12p. Other genetic discoveries recently have identified the genes for paroxysmal ataxia/myokymia located at chromosome 12p13, which is for the potassium channel; for hereditary hyperekplexia located at chromosome 5q for the glycine receptor; and for Unverricht-Lundborg disease located at chromosome 21q22.3.

Of course, many movement disorders are not inherited and the pattern of disease in the community provides important information for formulating and testing aetiological hypotheses on these conditions. In *Movement Disorders 2* the late Bruce Schoenberg reviewed the epidemiology of movement disorders in a benchmark chapter on which new information will be built.

The cause of Parkinson's disease still eludes us. Roger Duvoisin's essay on this topic in 1982 set the scene for the continuing debate between 'nature' and 'nurture'. The studies he reviewed at that time led him to conclude that there was little hereditary contribution to Parkinson's disease. The notion of some environmental factor as the agent responsible for the disease appeared more likely, but none was evident then. The epidemic of encephalitis lethargica in the decade 1916–1926 focused attention on a virus, but Duvoisin could find no evidence for this hypothesis in 1982.

By 1987 the concept of an environmental toxin had been set alight by the recognition of MPTP-induced parkinsonism, and Bill Langston provided a dramatic review of this discovery. Although the first human case was reported in 1979, it was not until 1983 that the offending agent MPTP was clearly identified. It was a tribute to the power and energy of neuroscience that by 1987 Langston was able to lay out the essential details as to how MPTP causes a more-or-less exact replica of Parkinson's disease in man and other primates. The search for some such agent or agents in the environment was now well and truly on. However, by 1994, in *Movement Disorders 3*, Carly Tanner could take a more restrained view of the situation. Despite an extensive epidemiological search, no robust purely environmental cause for Parkinson's disease had been identified. Furthermore, the earlier rejection of genetic contributions to the illness had been called into question, not least by Duvoisin himself. Re-analysis of the evidence, and increasing reports of familial Parkinson's disease had now re-focused attention on an hereditary contribution to the illness. The scenario now was, and still is, one of a complex aetiology involving a genetic predisposition and an environmental exposure to one or perhaps many toxicants. Time will tell if this is correct and where such enquiry will lead. No doubt a further review in some five years will include some fascinating new turns in the saga.

The pathological anatomy and neurochemistry of Parkinson's disease have been recurring themes. In *Movement Disorders 1*, Lysia Forno reviewed the neuropathology of the condition, with an overview of the classical studies and of the Lewy body. The definition of Parkinson's disease, in the absence of knowledge of its causes, still depends heavily on the pathological finding of degeneration of pigmented brainstem neurons, especially those of substantia nigra pars compacta, with Lewy bodies in surviving neurons. Although Lewy bodies are not specific for Parkinson's disease, they are characteristic. However, many other pathological entities may cause parkinsonism in life, a theme expressed by Kurt Jellinger in *Movement Disorders 2*, and by Bill Gibb and Andrew Lees in *Movement Disorders 3*. The latter authors posed the question 'What is Lewy body disease?', emphasising the varied clinical expression of this pathological form of neuronal degeneration, for example clinical Parkinson's disease, diffuse Lewy body disease or Lewy body dementia, and progressive autonomic failure. They also reviewed the vexed contribution of ageing to Parkinson's disease, and the significance of incidental Lewy body degeneration found in increasing frequency in the brains of elderly individuals who exhibit no evidence of parkinsonism in life. On pathological grounds, Gibb and Lees concluded that there is a preclinical phase of Lewy body degeneration of the substantia nigra of some 5–10 years.

Neuropathological studies have found that some 15–20% of those diagnosed as having Parkinson's disease in life, in fact have some other responsible pathology. The alternative parkinsonism–plus syndromes have been reviewed in sequence — multiple system atrophy and autonomic failure by Roger Bannister and the late David Oppenheimer in *Movement Disorders 1*, and by Niall Quinn in *Movement Disorders 3*, the olivopontocerebellar atrophies by Roger Duvoisin and Steele–Richardson–Olszewski disease by Andrew Lees in *Movement Disorders 2*, and corticobasal ganglionic degeneration by Ray Watts, Suzanne Mirra and E.P. Richardson in *Movement Disorders 3*. The distinctive clinical and pathological features of these sporadic parkinson-plus syndromes set them apart from Parkinson's disease. They remain difficult to treat and their cause is quite unknown. In children and young adults Wilson's disease remains a crucial

Preface to Movement Disorders 1 & 2 Reissue

diagnostic challenge for any movement disorder and its management is complex. I. Sternlieb, D.R. Giblin and I.H. Schienberg provided their extensive knowledge of Wilson's disease in *Movement Disorders 2*.

The management of Parkinson's disease itself was a major challenge in 1982 and remains so. Rational therapy depends on an understanding of the pathological neurochemistry and neuropharmacology of the illness. In *Movement Disorders 1*, Oleh Hornykiewicz reviewed the basic changes in brain monoamines in Parkinson's disease, following his fundamental discovery of striatal dopamine deficiency. Urpo Rinne reviewed the alterations in brain neurotransmitter receptors. By 1987 the field had expanded considerably, so Yves Agid, France Javoy-Agid and Merle Ruberg could write a new chapter on brain neurochemistry in Parkinson's disease, incorporating much new information. The significance of changes in cerebral acetylcholine systems in relation to cognitive changes and dementia was now appreciated. Indeed, the crucial importance of cognitive impairment and affective disorders in the overall disability of Parkinson's disease was emphasized by Richard Mayeux in *Movement Disorders 1* and by Richard Brown and CDM in *Movement Disorders 2*. Depression in Parkinson's disease can be treated effectively, but confusional states and dementia remain intractable problems especially in the elderly. Nevertheless there is hope that the newer generation of atypical neuroleptic drugs may prove valuable in this situation.

The other major problem of long-term levodopa therapy for Parkinson's disease is the emergence of fluctuations and dyskinesias, in about 10% of patients per year of treatment. These complications were reviewed by David Parkes, Niall Quinn and CDM, and by SF, in *Movement Disorders 1*. The advent of directly acting dopamine agonists was a major landmark in the development of treatment for Parkinson's disease, and this range of drugs was reviewed by Abe Lieberman and Menek Goldstein in *Movement Disorders 1*. Despite the important contribution of dopamine agonists, however, levodopa still remains the most consistently effective drug treatment for this illness.

The best use of levodopa and the reasons for the emergence of complications in its long-term use depends on a knowledge of its pharmacokinetics and pharmacodynamics, and how these change during chronic therapy. These issues were discussed by Fred Wooten in *Movement Disorders 2*, and by Maral Mouradian and Tom Chase in *Movement Disorders 3*. Despite increasing understanding, however, the exact mechanisms responsible for the development of fluctuations and dyskinesias remain uncertain, and these problems still plague many patients despite optimum drug therapy.

The best strategy for avoiding these problems still is debated. Early use of dopamine agonists rather than levodopa, combinations of low doses of levodopa and dopamine agonists, and the use of the newer delayed-release levodopa preparations with smoother plasma levodopa delivery, all have their advocates. What is needed is hard data from large clinical trials with sufficient numbers of patients to give adequate statistical power to provide clear answers to simple clinical questions. Such trials are in progress throughout the world and it is to be hoped that the next time we return to these vexed issues there will be a shift of emphasis from opinion to solid fact.

Despite the limitations of current syptomatic therapy, there is no doubt that the prognosis and quality of life for those with Parkinson's disease has improved considerably, as reviewed by Gerald Stern in *Movement Disorders 2*. Nevertheless, what is really needed is some means to slow, halt or even reverse the underlying pathology of the illness. The first attempt to treat the basic pathogenesis of Parkinson's disease was the major landmark trial of deprenyl (selegiline) and vitamin E (tocopherol) in *de novo* patients (the DATATOP study from North America). DATATOP showed that: (1) it is possible to carry out a large (over 800 patients) multicentre placebo-controlled

Preface to Movement Disorders 1 & 2 Reissue

double-blind study of potential neuroprotective treatments for Parkinson's disease; (2) that vitamin E (in the doses used) did not have a significant effect; (3) but that deprenyl unequivocally delayed the need for levodopa therapy. It has become clear that deprenyl exerts a modest and long-lasting symptomatic action in Parkinson's disease, which has made it difficult to disentangle any underlying neuroprotective action. The initial experience with deprenyl was reviewed by Merton Sandler and Gerald Stern in *Movement Disorders 1*, and the DATATOP study itself and the whole concept of neuroprotection was surveyed by Ira Shoulson in *Movement Disorders 3*. No doubt the future will bring new innovative methods of altering the underlying progression of Parkinson's disease and other neurodegenerative illnesses.

The continuing problems of symptomatic drug therapy for Parkinson's disease has already led to the cautious reintroduction of novel surgical approaches to treatment. In *Movement Disorders 1*, a number of authors contributed to an overview of surgical treatments for Movement Disorders. Hiroshi Narabayashi gave an account of his extensive and original experience of stereotaxic thalamotomy for tremor in Parkinson's disease and other conditions. It will be necessary to return to this topic in the future with the recent explosion of interest in continuous thalamic stimulation for tremors, and posteroventral pallidotomy for Parkinson's disease. In *Movement Disorders 3*, another topic was aired, namely neural transplantation of dopamine nigral grafts. Katy Steece-Collier and John Sladek provided an overview of the basic neurobiology of brain grafting, while Olle Lindvall surveyed the clinical results obtained up to then in Parkinson's disease. Such dopamine brain grafts are still an experimental form of treatment, but there is now sufficient data to show that the principle of such a revolutionary approach is valid. Time will tell whether such a therapy will play a significant role in the management of Parkinson's disease, but the demonstration that it is possible to repair the damaged human brain by such a means opens a new chapter for neurology in general.

Parkinson's disease and other parkinsonian syndromes account for about half of patients with Movement Disorders. The remainder have excessive abnormal involuntary movements or dyskinesias. The other chapters in *Movement Disorders 1–3* have dealt with these many conditions.

In *Movement Disorders 1*, the various surgical techniques available for the treatment of dystonia (Joe Waltz), spasmodic torticollis (Jeffrey Maccabe and Claude Betrand), blepharospasm (Arthur Battista, and J.F. Talbot, Z. Gregor and Alan Bird), and hemifacial spasm (Peter Jannetta) were all considered. However, the subsequent exploitation of botulinum toxin (reviewed in *Movement Disorders 3* by Paul Greene, SF, Mitchell Brin and Andrew Blitzer) has changed the management of these conditions out of all recognition. The various focal dystonias, and many other focal movement disorders, can now be adequately controlled by repeated injections of botulinum toxin into the affected muscles. Indeed, knowledge of the use of botulinum toxin is now an essential part of the repertoire of the movement disorder doctor.

Dystonia, in its many manifestations, is now usually treatable, as reviewed by SF and CDM in *Movement Disorders 2*. In the same volume, John Rothwell and Jose Obeso reviewed the anatomy and physiology of dystonia, and SF, CDM and Donald Calne surveyed the classification and investigation of dystonia.

Tardive dyskinesias remain a major complication of chronic treatment with dopamine receptor blocking agents. In *Movement Disorders 1*, Angus Mackay reviewed their clinical background, and Chris Goetz and Harold Klawans surveyed the various animal models of tardive syndromes. Much has since been learned about these dyskinesias, but they still are difficult to treat. Hope is pinned on the development of a new generation of selective dopamine receptor blockers which may be designed to avoid tardive dyskinesias and other

Preface to Movement Disorders 1 & 2 Reissue

unwanted extrapyramidal side-effects. If the new understanding of the biology of psychoses, and of dopamine and other neurotransmitters and their receptors, can lead to antipsychotic drugs devoid of extrapyramidal side-effects, the lot of those with schizophrenia and related illnesses will be dramatically improved.

The management of Huntington's disease has been transformed since Ira Shoulson surveyed this issue in *Movement Disorders 1*. The discovery of the gene for Huntington's disease has radically changed diagnosis, genetic counselling and prenatal testing, as described by Anita Harding in *Movement Disorders 3*. As more and more genes responsible for movement disorders yield their secrets to the power of molecular genetics, one can expect similar dramatic changes in the understanding of their causes, improvements in diagnosis, and novel therapies.

Essential tremor is one such common inherited movement disorder which causes much more disability than is generally appreciated. In *Movement Disorders 2*, Bob Lee reviewed the pathophysiology of essential tremor, and Leslie Findley survey the pharmacology and treatment of the condition. Other odd tremors was the subject of a chapter in *Movement Disorders 3* by Lynn Cleeves, Lesley Findley and CDM. Whether the large range of site-specific or task-specific tremors are manifestations of essential tremor or dystonia, or separate entities, will be clarified by discovery of the genes for these conditions.

Gilles de la Tourette's disease is another familial condition but, despite extensive investigation, a simple molecular genetic approach has not yet identified a single linkage. Maybe a more complex multifactorial approach is required. Gilles de la Tourette's syndrome spans both neurology and psychiatry; both aspects were reviewed in *Movement Disorders 2* by Joe Jankovic, and Michael Trimble and Mary Robertson, respectively. Tics and stereotypies are closely related, but stereotypies (reviewed by Joe Jankovic in *Movement Disorders 3*) occur in a wide range of neurobehavioural conditions. Some of the manifestations of epilepsy may mimic a movement disorder, a topic discussed by David Fish and CDM in *Movement Disorders 3*. The latter volume also includes an overview of the paroxysmal dyskinesias by SF, and of startle syndromes by Joe Matsumoto and Mark Hallett. The nosology and pathophysiology of myoclonus were reviewed by CDM, Mark Hallett and SF in *Movement Disorders 1*.

Not all movement disorders are due to brain disease. In *Movement Disorders 3*, CDM surveyed the topic of peripheral movement disorders, including the vexed question of the relationship to trauma. In the same volume Peter Brown dealt with spinal myoclonus, and Philip Thompson clarified the various types of 'stiff people'.

Finally, all movement disorder doctors know that some 1–5% of patients presenting with such conditions will turn out to have psychogenic movement disorder. This difficult but important topic was dealt with by SF in *Movement Disorders 3*.

The trilogy of *Movment Disorders 1–3* more or less completes a cycle of covering the field over a twelve year span, as well as following the burgeoning developments that have occurred in that time period. The decision by Butterworth–Heinemann to reissue *Movement Disorders 1 and 2* provides new readers with the opportunity to follow this existing saga. Those who work in movement disorders have had the privilege to witness and take part in the development of this field of neurology. We, the editors, thank our friends who have written so well in *Movement Disorders 1–3*. We are sure that they will join with us in thanking Butterworth–Heinemann for bringing the first three volumes to fruition, and in thanking all the multitude of patients and their carers for their help and tolerance in attempting to understand and treat their illnesses. There are exciting times ahead and we look forward to the next trilogy!

CDM
SF

Publishers' Note

Movement Disorders 1 and *2* are reissued here in their entirety without addition, deletion or amendment. Each volume carries its original list of contents and contributors, pagination and index.

Butterworths International Medical Reviews

Neurology 2

Movement Disorders

Butterworths International Medical Reviews

Neurology 2

Editorial Board
A. K. Asbury
M. L. Dyken
S. Fahn
R. W. Gilliatt
M. J. G. Harrison
C. D. Marsden
R. J. Porter
E. Stålberg
R. R. Young

Published in this Series
Volume 1 Clinical Neurophysiology
Edited by Erik Stålberg and Robert R. Young

Future volumes to include
Cerebral Vascular Disease
Peripheral Nerves

Butterworths
International
Medical
Reviews

Neurology 2

Movement Disorders

Edited by
C. David Marsden, MSc, MB BS, MRCPsych, FRCP
Professor of Neurology,
University Department of Neurology,
King's College Hospital Medical School and
Institute of Psychiatry; and
Consultant Neurologist,
King's College Hospital and
Bethlem Royal and Maudsley Hospitals,
London, UK

and

Stanley Fahn, MD
H. Houston Merritt Professor of Neurology,
Columbia University College of
 Physicians and Surgeons,
Neurological Institute,
New York,
New York, USA

Butterworth Scientific
London Boston
Sydney Wellington Durban Toronto

All rights reserved. No part of this publication may be reproduced
or transmitted in any form or by any means, including
photocopying and recording, without the written permission of
the copyright holder, application for which should be addressed to
the Publishers. Such written permission must also be obtained
before any part of this publication is stored in a retrieval system of
any nature.

This book is sold subject to the Standard Conditions of Sale of
Net Books and may not be re-sold in the UK below the net price
given by the Publishers in their current price list.

First published 1982

© **Butterworth & Co (Publishers) Ltd. 1981**

British Library Cataloguing in Publication Data
Movement disorders. – (Butterworths
   international medical reviews. Neurology,
   ISSN 0260–0137; 2)
1. Movement disorders
I. Marsden, C. David   II. Fahn, Stanley
616.7'4   RC346

ISBN 0–407–02295–3

Photoset by Butterworths Litho Preparation Department
Printed and bound in England by
Robert Hartnoll Ltd., Bodmin, Cornwall.

Preface

This volume is the second in a new international series of critical reviews of topics in neurology aimed at the fully-fledged clinician and the postgraduate trainee. Movement disorders comprise that group of neurologic dysfunctions in which either a paucity of voluntary movement or excess involuntary movements occur. Parkinsonism is the best known of these conditions and probably accounts for half the population of patients with movement disorders. Basic knowledge about these diseases has increased dramatically in the past decade, and many advances have been made in the treatment of these illnesses. The first half of this volume is devoted to parkinsonism. The second half deals with conditions characterized by abnormal involuntary movements (dyskinesias). A unifying theme in most of these conditions is the central role of the basal ganglia in the pathophysiology of involuntary movements. Thus, discussions on basal ganglia neurotransmitters and their receptors are equally relevant to all the movement disorders.

This book is *not* a textbook on movement disorders and does not encompass all that has been written on this subject in recent years. Rather, we have concentrated on a number of topics which, we believe, either have reached a stage that warrants definitive discussion, or are of sufficient practical importance to justify presentation even though, at present, no certain conclusions can be drawn.

Each half of the book is prefaced by an introductory chapter in which we review briefly other items that may be of practical interest to the reader, and give our reasons for choosing the topics to be discussed in depth. We hope that neurologists-in-training, and those in research or in practice will find this book of value. We believe that its clinical content will help in the often difficult management of patients with movement disorders, while its more scientific sections should aid in understanding of the background of the field.

Having selected the topics to be included, we invited as authors those with particular expertise on these subjects. We are pleased that they presented personal viewpoints since that adds to the strength of this volume. Our editing of all chapters

Preface

makes us share equally with the authors any responsibility for errors, omissions or misinterpretations.

We wish to thank the publishers for inviting us to prepare this volume, the authors for sharing our enthusiasm for the need of this work and for their timely cooperation, and our wives for their patience and understanding.

C. David Marsden
Stanley Fahn

List of Contributors

Roger Bannister, DM, FRCP
Consultant Physician, National Hospital for Nervous Diseases, Queen Square, London; and Consultant Neurologist, St. Mary's Hospital, London, UK

Arthur F. Battista, MD
Professor of Neurosurgery, New York University Medical School, New York, USA

Claude M. Bertrand, CC, MD, FRCS(C)
Professor of Neurosurgery, Université de Montréal; and Honorary Chief of Neurosurgery, Hôpital Notre-Dame, Montréal, Canada

A. C. Bird, MD, FRCS
Professor of Clinical Ophthalmology, Institute of Ophthalmology, London; and Honorary Consultant, Moorfields Eye Hospital, London, UK

Donald B. Calne, DM, FRCP
Professor of Medicine, Division of Neurology, University of British Columbia, Vancouver, Canada

Roger C. Duvoisin, MD
Professor and Chairman, Department of Neurology, College of Medicine and Dentistry of New Jersey, Rutgers Medical School, Piscataway, New Jersey, USA

List of Contributors

Stanley Fahn, MD
H. Houston Merritt Professor of Neurology, Columbia University, New York, New York, USA

Lysia S. Forno, MD
Neuropathologist, Veterans Administration Medical Center, Palo Alto and Professor of Clinical Neuropathology (Pathology), Stanford University School of Medicine, Stanford, California, USA

Christopher G. Goetz, MD
Department of Neurological Sciences, Rush-Presbyterian St. Lukes Medical Center, Chicago, Illinois, USA

Menek Goldstein, PhD
Professor of Neurochemistry, New York University School of Medicine, New York, New York, USA

Z. Gregor, FRCS
Senior Registrar, Department of Clinical Ophthalmology, Institute of Ophthalmology, London, UK

Mark Hallett, MD
Assistant Professor of Neurology, Harvard Medical School, Boston, Massachusetts, USA

Oleh Hornykiewicz, MD
Professor of Biochemical Pharmacology, Institute of Biochemical Pharmacology, University of Vienna, Austria

Peter J. Jannetta, MD
Professor of Neurosurgery and Chairman, Department of Neurosurgery, Health Center, Presbyterian Hospital, Pittsburgh, Pennsylvania, USA

Peter G. Jenner, BPharm, PhD, MPS
Senior Lecturer in Biochemistry, University Department of Neurology, King's College Hospital Medical School and Institute of Psychiatry, London, UK

Harold L. Klawans, MD
Professor of Neurology, Department of Neurological Sciences, Rush-Presbyterian St. Lukes Medical Center, Chicago, Illinois, USA

List of Contributors

Abraham N. Lieberman,, MD
Professor of Neurology, New York University School of Medicine, New York, New York, USA

D. L. McLellan, MA, MB, PhD, MRCP
Senior Lecturer in Neurology, University of Southampton; and Consultant Neurologist, Wessex Neurological Centre, Southampton, UK

J. J. Maccabe, FRCS
Neurological Surgeon, Neurosurgical Unit, The Maudsley Hospital, London, UK

Angus V. P. Mackay, MA, BSc, PhD, MB, ChB, MRCPsych
Physician Superintendent, Argyll and Bute Hospital; and MacIntosh Lecturer in Psychological Medicine, University of Glasgow, UK

C. David Marsden, MSc, MB, FRCP, MRCPsych
Professor of Neurology, University Department of Neurology, King's College Hospital Medical School and Institute of Psychiatry, London, UK

Richard Mayeux, MD
Assistant Professor of Clinical Neurology, Columbia University College of Physicians and Surgeons, Neurological Institute, New York, New York, USA

H. Narabayashi, MD
Professor of Neurology, Juntendo University Hospital, Tokyo; and Director, Neurological Clinic, Naka-Meguro, Tokyo, Japan

David Oppenheimer, DM, FRCPath
University Lecturer and Honorary Consultant in Neuropathology, Radcliffe Infirmary, Oxford, UK

J. D. Parkes, MD, MB, FRCP
Senior Lecturer in Neurology, University Department of Neurology, King's College Hospital Medical School and Institute of Psychiatry, London, UK

N. Quinn, MA, MB, MRCP
Research Registrar, University Department of Neurology, King's College Hospital Medical School and Institute of Psychiatry, London, UK

List of Contributors

U. K. Rinne, MD
Professor, Department of Neurology, University of Turku, Turku, Finland

M. Sandler, MD, FRCP, FRCPath
Professor of Chemical Pathology, Institute of Obstetrics and Gynaecology (University of London); and Consultant Chemical Pathologist, Queen Charlotte's Hospital, London, UK

Ira Shoulson, MD
Associate Professor of Neurology and Medicine; and Assistant Professor of Pharmacology and Toxicology, University of Rochester Medical Center, Rochester, New York, USA

G.M. Stern, MD, FRCP
Consultant Neurologist, University College Hospital, London, UK

J. F. Talbot, MB BS, FRCS
Lecturer in Clinical Ophthalmology, Department of Clinical Ophthalmology, Institute of Ophthalmology, London, UK

Joseph M. Waltz, MD
Director, Department of Neurological Surgery, St. Barnabas Hospital, New York, New York, USA

Contents

1   Problems in Parkinson's disease   1
      C. D. Marsden and Stanley Fahn

2   The cause of Parkinson's disease   8
      Roger C. Duvoisin

3   Pathology of Parkinson's disease   25
      Lysia S. Forno

4   Brain neurotransmitter changes in Parkinson's disease   41
      Oleh Hornykiewicz

5   Brain neurotransmitter receptors in Parkinson's disease   59
      U. K. Rinne

6   Depression and dementia in Parkinson's disease   75
      Richard Mayeux

7   Fluctuations of disability in Parkinson's disease: clinical aspects   96
      C. D. Marsden, J. D. Parkes and N. Quinn

8   Fluctuations of disability in Parkinson's disease: pathophysiological aspects   123
      Stanley Fahn

9   Treatment of advanced Parkinson's disease with dopamine agonists   146
      Abraham N. Lieberman and Menek Goldstein

Contents

10	Deprenyl in Parkinson's disease 166 *M. Sandler and G. M. Stern*	
11	Parkinsonism, system degenerations and autonomic failure 174 *Roger Bannister and David Oppenheimer*	
12	Problems in dyskinesias 191 *C. D. Marsden and Stanley Fahn*	
13	The nosology and pathophysiology of myoclonus 196 *C. D. Marsden, M. Hallett and Stanley Fahn*	
14	Clinical controversies in tardive dyskinesia 249 *Angus V. P. MacKay*	
15	Controversies in animal models of tardive dyskinesia 263 *Christopher G. Goetz and Harold L. Klawans*	
16	Care of patients and families with Huntington's disease 277 *Ira Shoulson*	
17.1	Surgical approaches to the dyskinesias: foreword 291 *C. D. Marsden and Stanley Fahn*	
17.2	Surgical approach to tremor 292 *H. Narabayashi*	
17.3	Surgical approach to dystonia 300 *Joseph M. Waltz*	
17.4	Surgical treatment of spasmodic torticollis 308 *J. J. Maccabe*	
17.5	Peripheral versus central surgical approach for the treatment of spasmodic torticollis 315 *C. Bertrand*	
17.6	Surgical approach to blepharospasm: nerve thermolysis 319 *Arthur F. Battista*	
17.7	The surgical management of essential blepharospasm 322 *J. F. Talbot, Z. Gregor and A. C. Bird*	

17.8 Surgical approach to hemifacial spasm: microvascular decompression   330
Peter J. Jannetta

17.9 Cerebellar and deep brain stimulation in movement disorders   334
D. L. McLellan

17.10 Surgical approaches to the dyskinesias: afterword   345
C. D. Marsden and Stanley Fahn

18.1 Dopamine receptors in movement disorders   348
Donald B. Calne

18.2 Interpretation of radioactive ligand binding to cerebral dopamine receptors   356
Peter G. Jenner and C. D. Marsden

Index   369

1
Problems in Parkinson's disease
C. D. Marsden and Stanley Fahn

INTRODUCTION

The management of Parkinson's disease today is a complex and demanding affair. The individual patient often poses a changing sequence of different problems, each demanding separate attention. There has been a considerable increase in knowledge about all aspects of Parkinson's disease in the last decade. The editors have chosen certain topics for presentation in separate chapters because of their interest and importance to understanding of the disease, and because there is now a substantial body of information to discuss on each of these topics.

Although the cause of Parkinson's disease still is not known, useful, if negative, information has been obtained in the fields of epidemiology, virology and genetics, as is discussed in Chapter 2 by Roger Duvoisin. Any understanding of the etiology of Parkinson's disease must depend upon a thorough knowledge of the pathology of the condition. In Chapters 3, 4 and 5 respectively, Lysia Forno reviews the histopathology; Oleh Hornykiewicz, the changes in neurotransmitter chemistry; and Urpo Rinne, the alterations of receptors in the brain.

The clinical features of Parkinson's disease generally are well-known, but the extent to which intellectual and affective disorders are inherent to the condition is controversial. Richard Mayeux in Chapter 6 reviews the evidence available on these topics, which are increasingly being discussed in the literature.

The routine drug treatment of Parkinson's disease does not require repetition. However, all practitioners are faced with the difficult problem of emergence of fluctuations of response during chronic therapy. In Chapters 7 and 8 the editors discuss and categorize, along with David Parkes and Niall Quinn (Chapter 7), the clinical features and pathophysiology of such fluctuations.

Many new drugs, other than anticholinergics, amantadine, and levodopa preparations, are being tested in Parkinson's disease. New directly-acting dopamine agonists are proving their value when levodopa fails. Bromocriptine is now in routine use in Europe, and newer ergoline derivatives are under extensive clinical trial. The practitioner must find it difficult to assess the relative worth of these different directly-acting agonists; Abe Lieberman and Menek Goldstein survey this field in Chapter 9. Deprenyl is another new drug, on which sufficient experience has been gained in Europe to assess its role, as is discussed in Chapter 10 by Merton Sandler and Gerald Stern.

The many variants of the 'akinetic-rigid syndrome' often cause diagnostic confusion. Roger Bannister and David Oppenheimer discuss the interrelationship of idiopathic orthostatic hypotension, the Shy-Drager syndrome, striatonigral degeneration, and olivopontocerebellar degeneration, and their concept of 'multiple system atrophy', which links these entities, in Chapter 11.

Many other practical problems that face the practitioner in the management of a patient with Parkinson's disease are not discussed, because it is difficult to provide a definitive statement on these matters. To cover these gaps, and to give some guidance on present views, the editors state their own approach to coping with some of these problems.

WHEN SHOULD LEVODOPA TREATMENT BE STARTED?

On theoretical grounds, one could take opposite views on whether to start levodopa treatment at the time of diagnosis. On the one hand, it could be argued that early treatment, by replenishing the missing neurotransmitter, may reverse changes in the postsynaptic dopamine receptors which are responsible for some of the problems in the management of the disease. On the other hand, it has been argued that levodopa itself is toxic. This may come about in one of two ways: saturating the brain with levodopa might lead to the formation of unnatural neurotoxic metabolites such as 6-hydroxydopamine, or could lead to excess formation of naturally-occurring, but neurotoxic intermediaries in the dopaquinone–melanin pathway. There is no convincing human or experimental evidence for any of these suggestions, so we have to turn to the clinical evidence to decide one way or the other.

Unfortunately, this too is controversial. On the one hand, Lesser et al.[3] claim by retrospective analysis of their population of patients that chronic treatment with levodopa is detrimental. They base this conclusion on finding that the level of disability after chronic therapy is related more to the duration of treatment than to the duration of the disease. On the other hand, Markham and Diamond[4] claim exactly the opposite.

Until this dilemma is solved by further studies, the editors advise their patients to delay levodopa therapy until disability warrants it. The judgment as to when that point is reached depends upon the individual patient, his tolerance of the disease, and his individual circumstances and requirements. Until that point is reached, many patients gain benefit from an anticholinergic and/or amantadine.

Another issue may assume importance in the future, namely whether dopamine replacement therapy should be started with levodopa or with a directly-acting dopamine agonist. Whether the latter approach will provide longer and smoother benefit can only be resolved by comparative clinical trials which currently are being undertaken.

MANAGEMENT OF DRUG PROBLEMS

Gastrointestinal upset

Although peripherally-acting dopa decarboxylase inhibitors have markedly reduced the incidence of anorexia, nausea and vomiting provoked by levodopa, this still remains a major problem in a minority of patients. The new formulation of Sinemet (levodopa/carbidopa = 5/1 instead of 10/1) has helped to some extent, but neither this, nor the use of Madopar (levodopa/benserazide) has abolished the problem. Of course, such peripheral decarboxylase inhibitors have no effect on these symptoms when provoked by directly-acting dopamine agonists, such as bromocriptine or pergolide. A new approach to this problem has been the use, in Europe, of peripherally-acting dopamine antagonists, the best of which is domperidone.

Myocardial infarction

A common problem is what to do when a patient with Parkinson's disease has a heart attack. Protection from the peripheral effects of levodopa and dopamine agonists is required after recent myocardial infarction, which predisposes to drug-induced cardiac dysrhythmias. The editors feel that it is safe to continue levodopa, provided that sufficient carbidopa (at least 100 mg/day) is given at the same time. Likewise, domperidone can protect the heart against unwanted effects of dopamine agonists. In countries in which domperidone is not available, it may be more prudent to switch such patients to levodopa/carbidopa. Certainly, the editors believe it is more important to continue some form of dopamine replacement therapy in this situation than to stop it, which causes dramatic and distressing relapse of the parkinsonism.

Accidental sudden withdrawal of levodopa

In the editors' experience, the sudden cessation of levodopa in a patient who has taken the drug for many years may cause a confusing akinetic 'coma-vigil' state, which can easily be reversed by reintroducing levodopa, if necessary, by nasogastric tube. Alternatively, where it is available, an intravenous injection of the water-soluble, fast-acting dopamine agonist, lisuride can be used.

Drug holidays

One of the ploys suggested in recent years to cope with some of the complications of chronic levodopa treatment has been the deliberate withdrawal of levodopa, a so-called 'drug holiday'. The editors will not go into the rationale behind this approach, or into its theoretical implications for the controversy about the cause of loss of efficacy of levodopa therapy. However, they will comment on its practical value. The impression has grown that this is a useful approach for coping with violent fluctuations that may emerge during chronic levodopa treatment. In fact, the published descriptions of this technique referred mainly to its use in patients with loss of response and/or toxic side-effects of chronic levodopa therapy[1,4]. Stopping levodopa in such patients leads to disappearance of mental and dyskinetic complications, with return of the symptoms and signs of Parkinson's disease. When levodopa is reintroduced, a therapeutic response can be achieved, usually at a much lower dosage, often without such toxic complications. However, in the editors' experience, drug holidays do not produce useful lasting benefit in those with severe fluctuations in response to treatment. Although there may be some initial improvement, this soon is lost, and the patient returns to his former state in a matter of weeks or months. Furthermore, the drug holiday itself will have left a profound impact on both the patient and on his physician. During the period of drug withdrawal, the patient will have relapsed back to a state of physical disability due to untreated Parkinson's disease that may come as a complete and devastating surprise. The emotional impact often is profound, the patient and his relatives are severely disturbed and occasionally, disasters occur due mainly to aspiration and deep vein thrombosis. In view of these difficulties and unsatisfactory long-term response, full drug holidays are not recommended.

Recently, Goetz et al.[2] have been evaluating a modified drug holiday, one lasting only for 2 days per week. This approach is usually not accompanied by the disastrous physical and emotional complications seen with the prolonged drug withdrawal. These authors claim that such 'weekend holidays' often, but not always, reduce the toxic complications of levodopa treatment in the subsequent week. How useful this is going to be remains to be established, but it is a maneuver that appears safe and can be undertaken at home.

Psychiatric disturbances

Another common problem for the patient on long-term levodopa therapy is the emergence of a range of mental side-effects. These include a typical toxic confusional state, isolated hallucinosis, delusions, obsessional behavior, global dementia, and psychotic disorders including severe depression and a schizophreniform syndrome. Although many of these conditions can occur in the untreated patient, the first possibility to be considered is that they are a side-effect of drug therapy. Any of the antiparkinsonian drugs may cause a toxic confusional state or hallucinosis. If mild, the first step might be to withdraw amantadine and/or anticholinergics. Recovery may be delayed for days or even weeks. If the disturbance is severe, disrupting family life, or threatening work, it may be necessary to admit the patient to the hospital in order to withdraw all drugs, including levodopa, temporarily.

Commonly, those developing such mental changes already have early or obvious dementia. Reintroduction of levodopa in such patients often causes recurrence of their psychiatric symptoms with little or no improvement in their mobility.

Repeated attempts to introduce a variety of levodopa preparations or dopamine agonists are prevented by such mental complications. A common situation is a patient who is immobile, but rational, or who is mobile, but mad. It may seem illogical, but sometimes the addition of a small dose of a neuroleptic such as thioridazine may allow a compromise between the two extremes.

Not all confusional states, hallucinatory and delusional experiences, or frank dementia are due to drugs in Parkinson's disease. A familiar clinical experience is the patient who has lost benefit of levodopa after chronic therapy, who increasingly becomes confused or demented, and who does not improve mentally or get any worse physically when all drug treatment is stopped. In this situation, thioridazine or a more sedative drug, such as diphenhydramine, may provide some calming benefit.

There is also the problem of a patient in whom chronic levodopa therapy is associated with excessive daytime sleepiness, often accompanied by nocturnal restlessness and noisiness. Of course, this reversal of sleep rhythm is characteristic of many dementing illnesses, and many of these parkinsonian patients show other evidence of dementia. Such daytime sleepiness, however, commonly is a toxic side-effect of levodopa, and can be improved by a reduction of dosage or by 'weekend drug holidays'.

DRUG FAILURES

In some patients, dopamine replacement therapy either never works (primary drug failure), or eventually completely ceases to work (secondary failure).

Primary drug failure

Most patients with Parkinson's disease or postencephalitic parkinsonism show some response to levodopa. The commonest cause for primary drug failure is that the patient has some other disease. Benign essential tremor does not respond to levodopa. Other conditions that may be confused with Parkinson's disease include progressive supranuclear palsy and the various manifestations of multiple system atrophy (see Chapter 11). Perhaps the greatest difficulty occurs in separating Parkinson's disease with dementia from primary dementing illnesses with features of an akinetic-rigid syndrome. The latter include Alzheimer's disease, multi-infarct dementia, normal pressure hydrocephalus and, in a younger age group, the aftermath of severe head injury or anoxic encephalopathy. The best clue for separating Parkinson's disease from these other conditions is the relative timing of onset of the motor disorder and the dementia, but it must be admitted that the diagnosis on occasions can be exceedingly difficulty.

Another problem relates to drug-induced parkinsonism. It is not widely recognized that parkinsonism produced by antipsychotic drugs may persist for as long as 1 to 2 years after stopping the offending agent. Such patients, by virtue of their psychiatric illness, often cannot give an accurate drug history, so may be mistakenly thought to have Parkinson's disease. Contrary to general belief, drug-induced parkinsonism does respond to adequate doses of levodopa, which do not necessarily provoke psychotic disturbances. If there is any question that a patient may be suffering from drug-induced parkinsonism, it is the editors' practice to withdraw levodopa treatment at 6-monthly intervals for 2 years to see if remission has occurred.

There remains a small proportion of patients, who as far as can be ascertained during life have Parkinson's disease, but who do not respond at all to levodopa. Why this should be so is not known, but it is suspected that they will be discovered to have some other pathology.

Secondary drug failure

A large number of patients with Parkinson's disease on chronic levodopa therapy develop fluctuations, as discussed later in this volume, but we are not concerned with this sort of failure of treatment here. The problem at issue is that of the patient who gradually and progressively loses response to treatment which, eventually, seems to be conferring no benefit at all.

A common early symptom heralding this sequence of events is the appearance of unexpected falling. Falls in Parkinson's disease may be due to a number of causes. The patient with sudden transient freezing may trip over his own glued feet. Another cause is the emergence of loss of postural reflexes, such that when the patient turns, arises, or is pushed suddenly, he falls to the ground. Unfortunately, loss of protective reflexes also occurs in Parkinson's disease so that such patients crash to the ground, damaging themselves. The combination of sudden transient freezing with loss of postural and protective reflexes can be disastrous. Many such patients become terrified of falling, and develop secondary psychological disturbances such as agoraphobia and space phobia. Sadly, levodopa has little or no effect on the problem of falling when it is severe.

Another, much less common cause of collapse in Parkinson's disease is postural hypotension, which is discussed in detail in Chapter 11.

The other feature characteristic of the emergence of secondary drug failure is the appearance of intellectual deficit. This problem is discussed at length in Chapter 6 and the contribution of drug toxicity to mental disturbances has been described earlier.

However, it is necessary to mention the practical difficulties imposed by the incontinence that often accompanies these developments at this stage of the illness. Male incontinence is a common problem in Parkinson's disease. Many causes contribute, including prostatic hypertrophy, anticholinergic-induced bladder atony, recurrent bladder infections and perhaps even Parkinson's disease itself by changing external sphincter tone. Levodopa therapy sometimes improves incontinence, but frequently the question of whether or not to undertake prostatectomy arises. In the editors' experience, providing the patient is fit for anesthesia and has clear evidence of prostatic hypertrophy, prostatic resection by the transurethral route may help. A bladder neck resection in the absence of prostatic hypertrophy, unfortunately, often leads to continual dribbling and incontinence. Luckily, incontinence in parkinsonian females is a less frequent occurrence.

Finally, it is worth considering why complete drug failure may occur after a patient has been previously responsive to levodopa. Direct-acting dopamine agonists also appear ineffective in this situation. Such patients fall into two groups. First, there are those who have parkinsonism as a feature of multiple system atrophy. In the early stages of the illness, predominantly presynaptic dopamine neurons have degenerated to produce symptoms of parkinsonism, while the postsynaptic cells containing dopamine receptors are still intact and could respond to levodopa or dopamine agonist therapy. The pathology of these conditions, however, relentlessly progresses so that eventually the postsynaptic cells in the striatum are lost and with them the dopamine receptors. These patients can now no longer respond to dopamine replacement therapy, although there may still be some response to anticholinergic drugs.

The second group consists of patients who do, in fact, have Parkinson's disease, but who eventually fail to respond to therapy. The explanation for this phenomenon is not clear, but it is possible that this group of patients ultimately develop degeneration of dopamine receptors and, hence, cannot respond to levodopa replacement treatment. Biochemical studies reveal that some parkinsonians have decreased numbers of dopamine (and acetylcholine) receptors in the striatum, and this group responds poorly to therapy (*see* Chapter 5). The question as to why some patients with Parkinson's disease, in which the principal pathology is loss of monoamine neurons, would also lose dopamine receptors is not perfectly clear. Perhaps there can be transsynaptic degeneration of the dopamine receptors, or of the striatal neurons on which they lie. This phenomenon might occur in Parkinson's disease secondary to loss of nigrostriatal neurons, by a mechanism that may be analogous to transsynaptic degeneration in the visual pathways. Alternatively, chronic levodopa therapy itself may cause irreversible damage to dopamine receptors, although there is no evidence for this hypothesis.

References

1 DIRENFELD, L. K., FELDMAN, R. G., ALEXANDER, M. P. and KELLY-HAYES, M. Is L-dopa drug holiday useful? *Neurology*, **30**, 785–788 (1980)
2 GOETZ, C. G., TANNER, C., NAUSIEDA, P., WEINER, W. and KLAWANS, H. Modified outpatient drug holiday in the management of parkinsonism. *Neurology*, **31**, 135 (1981)
3 LESSER, R. P., FAHN, S., SNIDER, S. R., COTE, L. J., ISGREEN, W. P. and BARRETT, R. E. Analysis of the clinical problems in parkinsonism and the complications of long-term levodopa therapy. *Neurology*, **29**, 1253–1260 (1979)
4 MARKHAM, C. H. and DIAMOND, S. G. Evidence to support early levodopa therapy in Parkinson disease. *Neurology*, **31**, 125–131 (1981)
5 WEINER, W. J., KOLLER, W. C., PERLIK, S., NAUSIEDA, P. A. and KLAWANS, H. L. Drug holiday and management of Parkinson disease. *Neurology*, **30**, 1257–1261 (1980)

2
The cause of Parkinson's disease
Roger C. Duvoisin

'Parkinson's disease remains so utterly inexplicable .... that we are constantly drawn to it by the lure of the mysterious' .... Brissaud, 1895[6].

INTRODUCTION

In considering the possible cause of Parkinson's disease, one is faced at the outset with doubts regarding its nosologic unity. Is it in fact a disease, a group of similar diseases, or nothing more than a syndrome of diverse etiology? This uncertainty reflects the fact that the definition of Parkinson's disease rests primarily on a combination of clinical and pathological features, none of which is pathognomonic. The clinical features of the disorder are distinctive enough in most cases to permit easy recognition and the postmortem morphologic alterations of the nervous system appear rather characteristic but no clinical or pathological feature is unique to this disorder alone. There is no chemical or serological marker for Parkinson's disease.

Moreover, a small proportion of patients confidently labelled 'Parkinson's disease' in life turn out at postmortem examination, or even on long-term follow-up, to have a distinctive identifiable disorder such as olivopontocerebellar atrophy, striatonigral degeneration, even progressive supranuclear palsy. Clearly these are different diseases. Thus, in fact, the patient population clinically diagnosed as Parkinson's disease includes representatives of several distinct morbid entities.

However, there is a general consensus among many students of parkinsonism that there is a condition which may be termed Parkinson's disease, which may reasonably be held to be a particular morbid entity on combined clinical and pathological grounds and which accounts for the great majority of Parkinson patients currently encountered in neurological practice. It is with this disorder that the chapter is concerned.

GENERAL SPECULATIONS

The etiology of Parkinson's disease is unknown at this time and there is a dearth of sound clues upon which to base reasonable speculations. Its pathology provides few insights into possible etiologic factors. The distribution of the neuronal degeneration is too selective and too widely scattered throughout the neuraxis to permit attribution to a vascular process. The highly selective involvement of certain neuronal populations, notably the pigmented neurons of the brain stem, suggests a metabolic basis for the degeneration. The clinical fact of 'chemical parkinsonism' induced by neuroleptic drugs encourages this view. Many of the neuronal systems affected are catecholamine synthesizing cells, which further points to the possibility that some feature of catecholamine metabolism, perhaps a cytotoxic metabolite, might play a role in the pathogenesis of the observed neuronal degeneration. However, other neuronal systems which are not monaminergic, such as the cranial motor nerve nuclei[17,33], are also affected. Recently attention has been directed to the Alzheimer-type changes seen in the cerebral cortex in some Parkinson's disease patients[26,35]. It is difficult to suggest some unique metabolic feature which might be common to all these neurons and not to others.

The notion of ageing associated with a selective vulnerability of certain neuronal systems, first suggested by Gowers[31] as an explanation of the pathogenesis if not the cause of Parkinson's disease has been repeatedly discussed. At the clinical level, the similarity of the flexed posture, bradykinesia and *marche a petit pas* of senility suggests a common element. The number of substantia nigra neurons is appreciably diminished in Parkinson's disease patients in comparison to age-matched controls[64]. Cell counts have shown evidence of a progressive decrease in the number of neurons in this nucleus with age[40]. Thus it appears reasonable to suggest that some individuals may be born with a lesser number of nigral neurons or suffer some selective insult to the nigra later in life and that, with the normal decline of nigral nerve cells with age, the number may in time fall below a critical value resulting in decompensation of the neuronal system involved and the appearance of parkinsonism. The notion of selective ageing or selective vulnerability clearly implies an inherent and hence genetically determined predisposition. The corollary notion of some injury to the involved neuronal system, implies an environmental factor or factors which might be infectious or toxic, specific or nonspecific. Thus, ultimately, these speculations lead to the two etiologic hypotheses which have long seemed most attractive, first, that Parkinson's disease is a genetic disorder and second, that it is due to viral infection of the nervous system. Both hypotheses could operate together in a multifactorial process. The genetic hypothesis is more easily tested and will be discussed first.

THE ROLE OF HEREDITY

It is a matter of common clinical experience that occasional patients with Parkinson's disease report having one or more similarly affected relatives. Gowers had noted a century ago that 15 percent of his cases of paralysis agitans gave a history of secondary cases in their families[32]. Comparable figures have been noted in more recent clinical surveys[41,49]. The suggestion naturally follows that genetic factors may play a role in the etiology of Parkinson's disease although it is by no means certain that these secondary cases in fact reflect familial concentration. Several reports of affected siblings and pedigrees have been described, such as those of Bell and Clark[3], Allen[1], and Spellman[74] which appear to support that suggestion.

Allen, an early clinical worker in the field of medical genetics, collected 24 kindreds in North Carolina over 40 years ago in which parkinsonism appeared to occur as a dominant disorder. It is difficult to assess the significance of his observations, however, in view of the sparse clinical data provided, the lack of specified diagnostic criteria and atypical features in some cases such as an unusually young age of onset and death from 'the palsy' at an early age. Thus, this report can only be considered of historical interest.

The most recent multiple case family is that reported by Spellman[74] in 1962. The proband had some atypical features including onset before the age of 35 years, emotional lability 'with a tendency to cry easily' and 'inconstant dorsiflexion of the toes bilaterally' on plantar stimulation. One member of the family died at the age of 39 after having been ill for 10 years, another at the age of 42 after having had parkinsonism for 8 years. Clumsiness and 'slight ataxia' were noted in other cases. In view of such atypical features and the evidence of cerebellar involvement, one may reasonably doubt that these patients had Parkinson's disease. Rather, such kindreds probably represent families of olivopontocerebellar atrophy, a condition which sometimes mimics Parkinson's disease and which may occur in either autosomal dominant or recessive hereditary patterns. Possibly some kindreds may represent essential tremor which is clearly a hereditary trait.

The presumed role of heredity in Parkinson's disease received strong support from the large family study carried out by Mjönes[59] in Sweden in the years 1933-44. This was the most extensive and systematic genetic study of parkinsonism done up to that time and it understandably exerted a profound influence on the subject. Mjönes found secondary cases in 38 percent of the families of 250 probands collected from several Swedish clinics and concluded that Parkinson's disease was an autosomal dominant disorder with incomplete penetrance. However, his study may be criticised for several methodological flaws which seriously undermine the conclusions. The probands represented a heterogenous group representing several disorders in addition to Parkinson's disease. Different criteria were employed in diagnosing probands and secondary cases; mere relationship to a proband was itself considered a diagnostic indication for 'without this factor a number of abortive or incipient secondary cases would undoubtedly have been interpreted as, for example, essential tremor'. A large proportion of Mjönes' secondary cases had tremor alone. Whereas 7 percent of the siblings of the 194 probands classified as 'paralysis agitans' by stated criteria were counted as secondary cases, if those who had tremor alone are excluded, the prevalence of secondary cases falls to approximately 3.4 percent of the siblings. Thus it seems very probable that Mjönes appreciably overstated the familial concentration of Parkinson's disease. It is difficult to judge whether the observed prevalence of secondary cases among the proband siblings does in fact represent familial concentration without a control population evaluated in a comparable manner.

In a family study carried out by Duvoisin et al.[13] the prevalence of secondary cases among the adult siblings of 85 index cases was compared to that among the spouses and spouse siblings who served as a control population. All siblings, index cases and spouses were examined by the same team of neurologists following a standardized protocol. The number of secondary cases found among the patients' siblings (4/146) was not significantly greater than that encountered among the spouse siblings (3/145). If we lower the denominator by eliminating siblings under the age of 55, the number becomes 4/62 versus 3/62, respectively. The control population made it possible to make sure that cases of Parkinson's disease were not missed by excluding from the analysis cases with tremor alone. An equal number, 5, of cases of essential tremor were found among the proband siblings and spouse siblings. A significant pitfall was illustrated by one family with several secondary cases. The proband had initially been given the diagnosis of Parkinson's disease by several experienced clinical neurologists, but over the 4-year course of the study, gradually developed signs of cerebellar involvement, optic atrophy and bilateral extensor plantar responses. The diagnosis was then changed to olivopontocerebellar atrophy.

Martin et al.[56] subsequently performed a similar study of 130 patients comparing the prevalence of secondary cases among the proband siblings with that among the spouse siblings. Secondary cases were confirmed by personal examination or by 'communication with a physician'. The prevalence of secondary cases among the proband siblings (16/488) was only slightly greater than that among the spouse siblings (7/450). If one considers only the siblings in the ages at risk, those over the age of 55, these figures are 11/285 (3.9 percent) versus 5/194 (2.6 percent). A weakness of this study is that all siblings were not examined, only those who were reported to be affected. It is possible, therefore, that some secondary cases may have been missed. It is also possible that the secondary cases confirmed 'by communication with a physician' might have had another diagnosis had they been personally examined by the investigators. Even accepting the data as presented, however, the evidence for a role of heredity is negligibly small. Interestingly, the prevalence of secondary cases among proband siblings in these three studies is nearly identical, if one excludes Mjönes' cases with tremor alone. (*Table 2.1*).

Table 2.1 Prevalence of Parkinson's disease among younger siblings compared with that among adult sibs: siblings over 25 and 55 years of age

Study	Number of Probands	Age > 25 years		Age > 55 years	
		Proband/Sibs	Spouse/Sibs	Proband/Sibs	Spouse/Sibs
Mjönes[59]	194	21/674	—	—	—
Duvoisin et al[13]	85	4/146	3/145	4/62	3/62
Martin et al.[56]	130	16/488	7/450	11/285	5/194
Total	409	41/1308 (3.1%)	10/595 (1.7%)	15/347 (4.3%)	8/256 (3.1%)

Martin et al. noted that 15 of their probands gave a history of having an affected parent. These 15 probands had 77 siblings, 10 of whom were affected. The authors culled 11 similar families from Mjönes' report and from this pooled data, using Falconer's method[22] arrived at an estimate of 40 ± 11 percent heritability. So modest a degree of heritability points to an inherited predisposition to the disease which must be multifactorial in etiology; it is too low for a monogenic mendelian transmission.

Kondo et al.[48] more recently conducted a family survey similar in methodology to Mjönes' study, relying on information supplied by the proband and on medical records but avoiding cases who were reported to have tremor alone. They found that 19 percent of the siblings of probands who had an affected parent were also affected and calculated a heritability of 91 percent. One cannot evaluate the accuracy of diagnosis in the probands from the data provided by these authors, but in view of the serious pitfalls encountered in chart studies and the unreliability of anamnestic data for genetic analysis, their conclusions must be regarded with considerable skepticism.

It appears, then, from the best available data that there is very little, if any, familial concentration of Parkinson's disease. The most solid data, that relating to the prevalence of secondary cases among the siblings of probands, provides no evidence for a significant genetic contribution to the etiology of Parkinson's disease. It is only in those families reporting an affected parent that some indication of familial concentration can be found. However, this evidence is weakened by the fact that the allegedly affected parents were not available for examination. This is a serious defect because of the common difficulty in distinguishing essential tremor and because multiple case families may represent olivopontocerebellar atrophy. This entity may be very difficult to distinguish from Parkinson's disease early in its course over a period of several years in the evolution of the disease. Duvoisin et al.[13] noted that in every family in which the proband reported multiple cases 'close examination .... made it apparent that Parkinson's disease was not the correct diagnosis'. Careful examination of the clinical features recorded in some of the multiple case families, such as the family described by Spellman discussed above and including some of Mjönes' families, reveals neurological manifestations that clearly exclude the diagnosis of Parkinson's disease. In the light of these considerations the high estimate of heritability proposed by Kondo et al. seems open to serious doubt and even the lower estimate of Martin et al. may be regarded with some skepticism.

A family study of sufficient magnitude to resolve these issues would be impractical. Because of the relatively advanced age of onset of Parkinson's disease, the children of patients are too young to be at significant risk and the parents are seldom available for examination. In these circumstances, a study of twins as suggested by Kondo et al.[49] seems the most direct and efficient means of pursuing the problem.

Only a few cases of twins have been noted in the extensive literature on the disease dating back more than a century. Gudmundsson[34] briefly noted that one of the 470 cases of parkinsonism he had found in a survey of the Icelandic population had an identical twin; the twin was said to have senile tremor and the pair was considered discordant. Pembrey[66] described another pair of identical twins also discordant for Parkinson's disease. Kissel and André[47] recently reported a third pair of identical twins concordant for a condition termed 'parkinsonism with anosmia'; both twins had an early age of onset of 39 years. Interestingly, even these twin pairs illustrate two of the problems which have confounded genetic studies of Parkinson's disease: the classification of relatives with essential tremor and the presence of atypical features in multiple case families.

To search for clues to possible etiologic factors, as well as to attempt to further define the role of heredity, the author and several collaborators initiated a survey of patients with typical Parkinson's disease who were members of identical twin pairs[12]. Monozygosity was established by appropriate genotyping procedures. Both twins in each pair were personally examined by the investigators. Zero concordance was found in the first 12 consecutively examined twin pairs. The twin study is continuing and at the time of writing 37 monozygotic twin pairs have been examined[78]. Only two pairs have been concordant, giving a concordance rate of 5 percent. So low a concordance rate is remarkable in itself. It is probably identical to the dizygotic concordance. Although data on the dizygotic concordance is not presently available, we may assume that it should be the same as the prevalence among proband siblings of the same age. Taking the combined data from the studies of Duvoisin *et al.* and Martin *et al.* summarised in *Table 2.1*, the author would predict a dizygotic concordance of 4.3 percent. The near identity of dizygotic and monozygotic concordances effectively excludes genetic factors from consideration in the etiology of Parkinson's disease.

ENVIRONMENTAL FACTORS

One must then turn to environmental factors in search of the cause of Parkinson's disease. The low concordance rate among identical twins indicates that such factors are probably not operative in childhood or adolescence during the years the twins are living together, sharing a common environment and exposure to the same infections. Yet the data of the twin study also indicate a long prodromal period dating back at least to young adult life. For example, differences in personality and smoking habits were noted between the probands and their twin.

A negative correlation between smoking and Parkinson's disease has been noted by several investigators[2, 46, 62]. Kessler suggested that nicotine might in some way protect against the development of the disease[46], but the alternate suggestion that the decreased prevalence of smoking marks a behavioral difference, is consistent with the observation that Parkinson patients as a group are less subject to alcoholism[67] and are less adventurous, and appears for this reason to be more plausible. Since smoking habits are generally established in adolescence or early adulthood, it follows that the future Parkinson patient is behaviorally different in some way at this stage in life.

What environmental factors could be operative in late adolescence or early adulthood to initiate the train of events which will eventually result in clinical parkinsonism? It is difficult to identify any contaminant or toxin in our environment. Careful review of clinical accounts of Parkinson's disease a century ago show that little has changed. The symptoms, the age of onset and the rate of progression all seem to be identical to those in patients today. Statistical analyses of Parkinson patients seen in major neurological clinics at the end of the nineteenth century, such as Hart[39] and others[8, 16, 21, 57] reported suggest a prevalence about the same then as today. Analysis of mortality due to paralysis agitans in England and Wales from 1855–1962[14] also suggests a remarkable stability in the disease over at least the last century. What factors in our environment have remained relatively unchanged over this period of time?

The most striking and obvious environmental factor associated with parkinsonism to date has been viral encephalitis, particularly, encephalitis lethargica. Although the distinctive postencephalitic syndrome which developed in its survivors is not Parkinson's disease and is now primarily of historical interest, it gave rise to the idea that Parkinson's disease itself might also be of viral origin. It played so great a role in our thinking on the present subject and was so important a disorder that we cannot avoid discussing encephalitis lethargica in some detail.

Encephalitis lethargica

Encephalitis lethargica occurred chiefly in the decade 1916–26, its incidence declining rapidly thereafter; though sporadic cases may possibly still occur, these must be exceedingly rare[4, 43, 81]. The first cases had been seen a few years earlier[36] but credit for first recognizing the disorder has usually been given to Von Economo[76] and it has consequently been known as Von Economo's encephalitis. The pathological features that were noted on postmortem studies in patients dying in the acute phase leave little doubt that it was a viral encephalitis[37, 50], however, attempts to isolate an infectious agent were unsuccessful. Mild prodromal symptoms suggestive of a respiratory infection were apparently common. There followed an acute or subacute development of hypersomnolence, associated with ocular and bulbar palsies and an akinetic–rigid state. There was a substantial mortality of about 40 percent[15]. A large proportion of survivors recovered with neurological sequelae and those who appeared to have recovered fully were later found to have more subtle sequelae such as neurasthenia and personality changes. Nearly all patients then entered a chronic progressive phase; they were said to have 'chronic encephalitis' or, later, postencephalitic parkinsonism. At least one-third of the survivors were found to have parkinsonian sequelae 3 years after the acute phase and one-half or more after 5 years[38, 63, 65, 83]. Some observers felt that all or nearly all postencephalitics had parkinsonism 'in some degree'[5].

Because the great influenza pandemic of 1918–19 immediately preceded and accompanied the first occurrences of encephalitis lethargica in North America, a more or less direct relationship between the two disorders was suspected. Encephalitis was regarded, along with poliomyelitis, epidemic spinal meningitis and even multiple sclerosis as part of the 'epidemic consitution of influenza'[9]. More specifically, it was postulated that encephalitis lethargica was a sequel of influenza due either to a direct cerebral invasion by the influenza virus or by a modification of the virus, or due to the weakening and predisposition of certain individuals to subsequent infection by the independent etiologic agent of encephalitis lethargica[44]. Whatever merit these postulates had at the time, they were not supported by subsequent experience. Contemporary students of encephalitis such as Flexner[25], McNalty[51], Zinsser[84], Neal[61] and others rejected an etiologic relationship to influenza. Nevertheless, the notion has persisted until recently that the two might yet have been related and even that the flu virus might be a cause of Parkinson's disease. Gamboa et al.[27] reported the apparent detection by immunofluorescence of influenza antigen in postencephalitic brain. However, the findings could have been nonspecific. Martilla et al.[54] and Elizan et al.[19] searched for serological evidence in postencephalitic patients of a relationship to influenza, including swine flu strains which are believed to be very close to the strain responsible for the 1918–19 pandemic; the results were negative.

The postencephalitic Parkinson syndrome which followed encephalitis lethargica was very distinctive in the 1920s. In contrast to Parkinson's disease, it appeared chiefly in the second or third decade of life. Wilson[82] observed that 'in pre-epidemic days juvenile paralysis agitans was an absolute rarity but now is commonplace'. There was a remarkable admixture of features which had not previously been seen in association with parkinsonism: cranial nerve palsies, dystonia, chorea, athetosis, behavioral disturbances and oculogyric crises. Moreover, it was a relatively frequent disorder, numerically more common than Parkinson's disease. Dimsdale's statistical review[11] of the cases of parkinsonism seen in several neurological clinics in London from 1900 to 1942 shows that encephalitis lethargica accounted for as many as two-thirds of the cases of parkinsonism seen in the decade 1920–30.

With the decline of encephalitis lethargica after 1926, the proportion of parkinsonian patients classified as postencephalitic gradually diminished; in Dimsdale's data they comprised about one-half the cases seen in the period 1931–42. Hoehn and Yahr[42] noted that only 12 percent of the Parkinson patients attending a large clinic in New York in the years 1949–64 were postencephalitic. It is a matter of common experience that cases of postencephalitic parkinsonism today are extremely rare; they are all unusually long-term survivors representing the last remnants of the devastation encephalitis lethargica left in its wake.

An analysis of 31 postencephalitic cases seen as recently as the period 1962–64 confirmed that even many years after the epidemic these patients represented a disorder entirely distinct from Parkinson's disease[15]. Interestingly, 27 of the 31 gave a history of an acute episode of encephalitis lethargica. A cluster of similar survivors of encephalitis lethargica were the subjects of Purdon Martin's observations[55] on the postural abnormalities and 'negative' manifestations of parkinsonism. Another cluster of postencephalitics treated with levodopa were vividly described by Sachs[72]. A reading of this material serves to confirm the distinctiveness of the postencephalitic syndrome. This point deserves emphasis because the confusion which surrounded the subject has permitted attempts to lump postencephalitic parkinsonism and Parkinson's disease together into a single common entity.

The cohort hypothesis

It is clear from reviewing medical charts of the 1930s and 1940s that to many physicians the terms 'chronic encephalitis' and 'parkinsonism' become synonymous, and that the nosological distinctions between Parkinson's disease and postencephalitic parkinsonism had become confused. One may readily see in published reports that even straightforward cases of paralysis agitans were erroneously labelled 'post-encephalitic' (see, for example, Keschner and Sloane[45]). In practice, a mere history of the flu sufficed to gain otherwise typical cases of Parkinson's disease, the diagnosis of postencephalitic parkinsonism. In these circumstances, the view that all parkinsonism might be related to encephalitis lethargica becomes possible.

Just such a view was propounded by Poskanzer and Schwab[70]. Their argument was based entirely on an analysis of the age of onset of parkinsonism. They reported that the age of onset in cases observed at the Massachusetts General Hospital in Boston, Mass. had gradually increased from a mean of 32.4 in the period 1920–24 to a mean of 59.4 in the years 1955–59 and suggested that all – or nearly all – cases of parkinsonism extant in 1960 were members of a cohort of survivors of the epidemic of encephalitis lethargica. They further predicted that parkinsonism would largely disappear by the year 1980.

Support for this 'cohort' hypothesis was advanced by Brown and Knox[7] who recognized that two possible explanations of the rise in age of onset after 1920 required consideration: that all cases were postencephalitic, or that two diseases were involved – postencephalitic parkinsonism and Parkinson's disease. They argued that if the two-disease explanation was correct, a substantial decrease in parkinsonism should have occurred since 1921. Because the Registrar-General's mortality data for England and Wales showed no decrease in mortality assigned to paralysis agitans over the period 1920–60, they concluded that the 'cohort' hypothesis must therefore be correct. (Indeed, the detailed analysis of paralysis agitans mortality in England and Wales made by Duvoisin and Schweitzer[14] failed to show a significant change between 1921 and 1965.) However, Brown and Knox overlooked the fact that the Registrar-General assigned deaths due to postencephalitic parkinsonism to encephalitis lethargica, not to paralysis agitans. Paralysis agitans and postencephalitic parkinsonism were explicitly differentiated in the International List of Causes of Death[28], the latter being defined as a sequel of encephalitis lethargica.

The 'cohort' hypothesis provoked considerable interest and debate. Its major criticisms were that it ignored the fact that the age of onset of parkinsonism had been in the sixth decade of life in the nineteenth and twentieth century prior to the epidemic of encephalitis lethargica, that it ignored the extensive evidence documenting the decline of postencephalitic parkinsonism from a prevalence exceeding that of Parkinson's disease in the 1920s to its rarity as a clinical entity by the 1960s and that it overlooked the clinical and pathological evidence that postencephalitic parkinsonism was a distinct entity clearly separate from Parkinson's disease[16]. No attempt was made to explain why the age of onset had dropped suddenly from the sixth to the third decade of life in 1920. In any event, the cohort hypothesis is difficult to apply to the Parkinson population prevalent today, 60 years after the epidemic. Perhaps the most telling criticism of the hypothesis is that Parkinson's disease has not noticeably altered in prevalence or incidence and appears to be just as frequent in 1981 as it was in 1960.

Parkinsonism and other encephalitides

It is understandable, in view of the severe mortality, morbidity and delayed sequelae of encephalitis lethargica, that subsequent epidemics due to other types of encephalitis aroused fear of a comparable train of after effects. Indeed, facial hypomimia, tremor, rigidity, and disturbances of posture and gait reminiscent of Parkinson's disease have been repeatedly described during the acute and convalescent phases of various viral encephalitides. Dickerson et al.[10], for example, noted tremor of the fingers, tongue and eyelid in 90 percent, rigidity in 40 percent, and a mask-like face in 75 percent of 200 patients in the acute phase of Japanese B encephalitis. These manifestations subsided within several weeks. Similar observations have been made in encephalitis due to measles[58], varicella[68], poliovirus[52,79], coxsackie virus[69] and other apparently viral encephalitides[44]. A recent case report describes a transient parkinsonian state alleviated by levodopa therapy in a young woman recovering from western equine encephalitis[73]. Infrequently, the parkinsonian features have been of longer duration. Mulder et al.[60] reported 15 patients who had western equine encephalitis in Colorado in 1955; they found severe sequelae in 6 of 12 adults including 'a clinical syndrome similar to the parkinsonism which followed encephalitis lethargica', but followed the patients for only 6–8 months. Goto et al.[30] noted the persistence of mild static manifestations such as tremor and rigidity in 11.6 percent of 143 unselected survivors of the Japanese B encephalitis epidemic witnessed in Tokyo in 1948.

Only rarely has a chronic progressive Parkinson syndrome been found to follow an encephalitis other than encephalitis lethargica. Finley and his colleagues[23,71] found only 3 cases among 678 patients who had western equine encephalitis in California followed up for 5 years or more. These 3 patients were over 50 years of age and developed a progressive syndrome apparently typical of parkinsonism several years after the acute phase. Although Finley initially thought the parkinsonism in these cases was 'in all probability' encephalitic in etiology, he later concluded that so small a number was not greater than would have been expected by chance[24], given the prevalence of Parkinson's disease indicated by Kurland's epidemiologic survey[49]. A similar case of parkinsonism following coxsackie B meningoencephalitis[77] and another following herpes ophthalmicus have been reported[75]. The scarcity of such reports and the age of the patients render it difficult to consider the reported associations of parkinsonism to preceding viral infections of the central nervous system more than coincidental.

In summary, it appears that a Parkinson syndrome may occur during the acute phase of many viral encephalitides. It is usually mild and transient but may persist for some months into the convalescent phase and, although usually improved, may rarely persist as a permanent static residual. There is no evidence from clinical observation of an association between chronic progressive parkinsonism and any encephalitis other than encephalitis lethargica.

Seroepidemiologic surveys

In some cases of postencephalic parkinsonism manifesting typical sequelae of encephalitis lethargica, such as oculogyric crises, there was no history of an overt episode of encephalitis. Thus, a subclinical episode must be presumed to have occurred. Although, in fact, such instances were unusual, they serve to suggest the possibility that a mild or silent viral infection might result in the subsequent development of parkinsonism. Several seroepidemiological surveys of parkinsonian populations have been carried out looking for evidence of elevated antibody titers to a variety of common viruses.

The suspected association of the 1918–19 flu pandemic to encephalitis lethargica led to recent investigations, searching for serological evidence of influenza antigens. Elizan et al.[19] tested serum and cerebrospinal fluid for antibodies to 12 strains of influenza, and a number of other viruses including herpes simplex, cytomegalovirus, varicella-zoster, measles, rubella, coxsackie, parainfluenza and mumps. The results were negative and these authors concluded that 'none of these viruses are causally associated with Parkinson's disease'. Martilla et al.[53,54] in Finland, similarly found no significant difference in antibody titers to various strains of influenza A in patients with postencephalic parkinsonism or Parkinson's disease as compared with controls. These workers reported an increased titer of complement-fixing antibody to herpes simplex in a survey of 441 cases of Parkinson's disease as compared with normal controls[54], but their data could not be confirmed by Elizan et al.[20] who found similar titers in their patients and in two sets of diseased controls. The discrepancy appears attributable to the low titers in the normal control population employed by the Finnish workers. The selection of controls is difficult with so ubiquitous an infection as herpes simplex.

A study of antibody titers to Murray Valley encephalitis virus in Australia by Eadie[18] failed to reveal a relationship to parkinsonism. More recently Elizan et al.[20] surveyed Parkinson's disease patients in New York City for antibodies to a large number of arboviruses including western equine encephalitis, St. Louis encephalitis, Murray Valley encephalitis and many others, with negative results. As may be seen from a perusal of the list (*Table 2.2*) of viral agents tested for in these seroepidemiological surveys, no evidence has been found to support the association of Parkinson's disease or even postencephalic parkinsonism with any of the viruses which have been suspected at various times as potential etiologic agents.

Serologic studies may, however, fail to show evidence of a defective, incomplete or latent virus. Thus Wetmore et al.[80] pursued the matter further and undertook nucleic acid homology studies in postmortem brain tissue taken from Parkinson's disease patients seeking evidence of nucleic acids complementary to herpes simplex type I DNA and influenza A/NWS RNA. Their results were negative.

In the light of the experience with kuru and Creutzfeld-Jakob disease, it seems plausible to suspect an unconventional viral agent as a possible etiologic factor.

Table 2.2 Viral agents thus far evaluated serologically and excluded as possible etiologic agents of Parkinson's disease. (Data from Elizan *et al.*[19,20], Martilla *et al.*[53,54] and Eadie *et al.*[18])

Virus		Virus
Influenza A	(SW/76/31, SW/76/30, NWS/33, WNS/33, PR/8/34, SW/N-Ir/38, FM/1/47, ERS/1/51, HK/8/60, SW/NJ/8/76, Jap/305/57. Singapore/1/57)	Eastern equine encephalitis Western equine encephalitis Venezuelan equine encephalitis Chikungunya Mayaro
Influenza B	(HK/5/72, GL/1739/54)	Ross River
Parainfluenza 1	(C-35)	Semliki Forest
Coxsackie B-3		Murray Valley encephalitis
Coxsackie B-4		Dengue type 2
Mumps (Enders)		Powassan
Varicella-zoster	(V-Z 10)	Wesselsbron disease
Cytomegalovirus	(AO-169)	Zika Virus
Rubella	(Putman)	US bat salivary gland virus
Measles	(Philadelphia 26)	St. Louis encephalitis
Herpes simlex 1	(McIntyre VR3)	Bussuquara
Herpes simplex 2	(MS)	Batai
Poliovirus type 3		California encephalitis

Attempts to transmit similarly either Parkinson's disease or postencephalitic parkinsonism to the primate, however, have been unsuccessful[29].

The substantial efforts made in recent years to implicate a viral etiology for Parkinson's disease have been to no avail. The hypothesis of a viral cause, however attractive, remains at this time an hypothesis in search of some supportive evidence. It must be candidly admitted that at present, there is no positive evidence of any sort in its favor. The negative results, however, do not necessarily preclude an infectious etiology. Perhaps the wrong viruses have been studied or the sensitivity of the techniques employed were insufficient. Although the list of viruses studied thus far, shown in *Table 2.2*, is an extensive one, many other viruses remain to be considered. Unfortunately, there are few clues available at present to guide the selection of agents to be examined and it is possible that a presently unrecognized virus is involved.

The epidemiological and clinical features of Parkinson's disease suggest several criteria for the selection of candidates for consideration as the possible etiologic agent. First, the virus must be contracted many years, up to three or four decades, prior to the overt onset of extrapyramidal symptoms and would produce at most a nondescript common illness such as a 'cold' or an enteritis, if it produced any symptoms at all. Then the virus must remain quiescent for several decades, producing a gradual degeneration that is highly selective for the neuronal population characteristically affected and sparing glial and other cellular elements. It would differ from the presently known 'slow-virus' diseases which cause a diffuse spongioform encephalopathy or a sclerosing panencephalitis, in producing a much more selective and much more slowly progressive degenerative change. Finally, it must be able to account for the ubiquity and constancy of Parkinson's disease over the past century.

Presumably, a defective, incomplete or unconventional agent could persist in a latent nonreplicating state and cause a premature demise or 'ageing' of the pigmented neurons of the brain stem. Clearly, the search for an agent meeting all these criteria presents formidable obstacles.

SUMMARY AND CONCLUSIONS

The etiology of Parkinson's disease remains an enigma at this time. Speculations on the subject have covered a broad range of possibilities. Two have seemed particularly attractive – heredity and viral infection.

Properly controlled studies on the familial concentration of the disease, notably an ongoing study of twins, appear to have excluded a significant role for heredity.

Thus far, attempts to implicate viral agents have been unsuccessful. Clinical and epidemiological studies appear to have ruled out the arbovirus encephalitogenic agents and a number of other common viruses such as influenza and herpes simplex. However, a viral etiology is not precluded and further research is warranted. Unfortunately, few clues have been forthcoming to guide the search for evidence of viral infection.

References

1 ALLAN, W. Inheritance of the shaking palsy. *Archives of Internal Medicine*, **60**, 424–436 (1927)

2 BAUMAN, R. J., JAMESON, H. D., WEISBERG, L. H., MCKEAN, H. E. and HAACK, D. G. Cigarette smoking and Parkinson's disease. *Neurology*, **30**, 839–843 (1980)

3 BELL, J. and CLARK, A. J. A pedigree of paralysis agitans. *Annals of Eugenics*, **1**, 445–462 (1926)

4 BLATTNER, R. J. Encephalitis lethargica, Type A encephalitis, Von Economo's disease. *Journal of Pediatrics*, **49**, 370–372 (1956)

5 BORTHWICK, G. A. Sequelae of encephalitis lethargica. *Clinical Journal*, **60**, 510–524 (1931)

6 BRISSAUD, E. *Leçons sur les Maladies du Système Nerveux*. Paris, Masson (1895)

7 BROWN, E. L. and KNOX, E. G. Epidemiological approach to Parkinson's disease. *Lancet*, **1**, 974–976 (1972)

8 CHARCOT, J. M. *Leçons sur les Maladies du Système Nerveux Fâites à la Salpêtriére* 4th Edition, Paris, Delahaye and LeCrosnier (1880)

9 CROOKSHANK, F. G. Theory of influenza. In *Influenza: Essays by Several Authors*, edited by F. G. Crookshank, Ch. 16. London, Heineman (1927)

10 DICKERSON, R. B., NEWTON, J. R. and HANSEN, J. E. Diagnosis and immediate prognosis of Japanese B encephalitis. *American Journal of Medicine*, **12**, 277–288 (1952)

11 DIMSDALE, H. Changes in the Parkinsonian syndrome in the twentieth century. *Quarterly Journal of Medicine*, **15**, 155–170 (1946)

12 DUVOISIN, R. C., ELDRIDGE, R., WILLIAMS, A. NUTT, J. and CALNE, D. Twin study of Parkinson disease. *Neurology*, **31**, 77–80 (1981)
13 DUVOISIN, R. C., GEARING, F. R., SCHWEITZER, M. D. and YAHR, M. D. A family study of parkinsonism. In *Progress in Neurogenetics*, edited by A. Barbeau and J. R. Brunette, 492–496. Amsterdam, Excerpta Medica (1969)
14 DUVOISIN, R. C. and SCHWEITZER, M. D. Paralysis agitans mortality in England and Wales, 1855–1862. *British Journal of Preventive and Social Medicine*, **20**, 27–33 (1966)
15 DUVOISIN, R. C. and YAHR, M. D. Encephalitis and parkinsonism. *Archives of Neurology*, **12**, 227–239 (1965)
16 DUVOISIN, R. C., YAHR, M. D., SCHWEITZER, M. D. and MERRITT, H. H. Parkinsonism before and since the epidemic of encephalitis lethargica. *Archives of Neurology*, **9**, 232–236 (1963)
17 EADIE, M. J. The pathology of certain medullary nuclei in parkinsonism. *Brain*, **86**, 781–792 (1962)
18 EADIE, M. J., SUTHERLAND, J. M. and DOHERTY, R. L. Encephalitis in etiology of parkinsonism in Australia. *Archives of Neurology*, **12**, 240–245 (1965)
19 ELIZAN, T. S., MADDEN, D. L., NOBLE, G. R., HERMANN, K. L., GARDINER, J., SCHWARTZ, J., SMITH, H. JR., SEVER, J. and YAHR, M. D. Viral antibodies in serum and CSF of parkinsonian patients and controls. *Archives of Neurology*, **36**, 529–534 (1979)
20 ELIZAN, T. S., SCHWARTZ, J., YAHR, M. D. and CASALS, J. Antibodies against arboviruses in postencephalitic and idiopathic Parkinson's disease. *Archives of Neurology*, **35**, 257–267 (1978)
21 ERB, W. Paralysis Agitans (Parkinsonische Krankheit). In *Die Deutsche Klinik*, edited by E. Leyden and F. Klemperer, **6**, Part 1, 31–50. Berlin, Urban and Schwarzenberg (1901)
22 FALCONER, D. S. The inheritance of liability to certain diseases estimated from the incidence among relatives. *Annals of Human Genetics*, **29**, 51–76 (1965)
23 FINLEY, K. H. Post-encephalitic manifestation of viral encephalitis. In *Viral Encephalitis*, edited by W. S. Field and R. J. Blattner, 69–94. Springfield, C. C. Thomas (1958)
24 FINLEY, K. H. (Personal communication)
25 FLEXNER, S. Obvious and obscure infections of the central nervous system. *Journal of the American Medical Association*, **91**, 21–28 (1928)
26 FORNO, L. S. and ALVORD, E. C. The pathology of parkinsonism. In *Recent Advances in Parkinson's Disease*, edited by E. McDowell and C. Markham, 120–161. Philadelphia, F. A. Davis (1971)
27 GAMBOA, E. T., WOLF, A., YAHR, M. D., HARTER, D. H., DUFFY, P. E., BARDEN, H. and HSU, K. C. Influenza virus antigen in post-encephalitic parkinsonian brain; detection by immunofluorescence. *Archives of Neurology*, **31**, 228–232 (1974)
28 GENERAL REGISTER OFFICE. *Manual of the International List of Causes of Death*. 28–33. London, HMSO (1931)
29 GIBBS, C. J., JR., GAJDUSEK, D. C. Amyotrophic lateral sclerosis. Parkinson's disease and the amyotrophic lateral sclerosis–Parkinsonism–dementia complex of Guan: a review and summary of attempts to demonstrate infection as the etiology. *Journal of Clinical Pathology*, **25** (suppl. 6), 132–140 (1972)

30 GOTO, A. Follow-up study of Japanese B encephalitis. *Psychiatria et Neurologia Japonica*, **64**, 236–266 (1962)
31 GOWERS, W. R. A lecture on abiotrophy. *Lancet*, **1**, 1003–1007 (1902)
32 GOWERS, W. R. *A Manual of Diseases of the Nervous System*, 2nd edition 636–657. Philadelphia, Blakiston (1903)
33 GREENFIELD, J. G. and BOSANQUET, F. The brain stem lesions in parkinsonism. *Journal of Neurology, Neurosurgery and Psychiatry*, **16**, 213–226 (1953)
34 GUDMUNDSSON, K. R. A clinical survey of parkinsonism in Iceland. *Acta Neurologica Scandinavica*, **43** (suppl. 33), 9–61 (1967)
35 HAKIM, A. M. and MATHIESON, G. Dementia in Parkinson disease: a neuropathologic study. *Neurology*, **29**, 1209–1214 (1979)
36 HALL, A. J. *Epidemic Encephalitis*. New York, William Wood (1924)
37 HALLERVORDEN, J.: Zur Pathogenese der post-encephalitischen Parkinsonisms. *Klinische Wochenschrift*, **12**, 692–694 (1933)
38 HARRIS, J. S. and COOPER, H. A. Late results of encephalitis lethargica. *Medical Press and Circular*, **194**, 12–14 (1937)
39 HART, T. S. Paralysis agitans: some clinical observations based on the study of 219 cases seen at the clinic of Professor M. Allen Starr. *Journal of Nervous and Mental Disease*, **31**, 177–178 (1904)
40 HIRAI, S. Aging of the substantia nigra. *Advances in Neurological Sciences*, **12**, 845–849 (1968)
41 HOEHN, M. M. Age distribution of patients with parkinsonism. *Journal of the American Geriatrics Society*, **24**, 79–85 (1976)
42 HOEHN, M. M. and YAHR, M. D. Parkinsonism: onset progression and mortality. *Neurology*, **17**, 427–442 (1967)
43 HUNTER, R. and JONES, M. Acute lethargica-type encephalitis. *Lancet*, **1**, 1023 (1966)
44 ISGREEN, W. P., CHUTORIAN, A. M. and FAHN, S. Sequential parkinsonism and chorea following 'mild' influenza. *Archives of Neurology*, **33**, 384–385 (1976)
45 KESCHNER, M. and SLOANE, P. Encephalitis, idiopathic and arteriosclerotic parkinsonism. *Archives of Neurology and Psychiatry*, **25**, 1011–1041 (1931)
46 KESSLER, I. I. and DIAMOND, K. L. Epidemiological studies of Parkinson's disease: I. Smoking and Parkinson's disease. *American Journal of Epidemiology*, **94**, 16–25 (1971)
47 KISSEL, P., ANDRÉ, J. M. Maladie de Parkinson et anosmie chez deux Jumelles monozygotiques. *Journal of Human Genetics*, **24**, 113–117 (1976)
48 KONDO, K., KURLAND, L. T. and SCHULL, W. J. Parkinson's disease, genetic analysis and evidence of a multifactorial etiology. *Mayo Clinic Proceedings*, **48**, 465–475 (1973)
49 KURLAND, L. T. Epidemiology: incidence, geographic distribution and genetic considerations. In *Pathogenesis and Treatment of Parkinsonism*, edited by W. Fields, 5–49. Springfield, C. C. Thomas (1958)
50 McALPINE, D. The pathology of the parkinsonian syndrome in epidemic encephalitis. *Proceedings of the Royal Society of Medicine*, **19**, 35–45 (1926)
51 McNALTY, A. *Epidemic Diseases of the Central Nervous System*, 11–14. London, Faber and Gwyer (1927)

52 MARINESCO, G. and DRAGANESCO, S. Sur un cas de parkinsonisme infantile au cours de la maladie de Heine-Medin. *Reviews of Neurology*, **50,** 165–168 (1928)
53 MARTILLA, R. J., HALONEN, P. and RINNE, U. K. Influenza virus antibodies in parkinsonism: comparison of postencephalitic and idiopathic Parkinson patients and matched controls. *Archives of Neurology*, **34,** 99–100 (1977)
54 MARTILLA, R. J., AUSTILA, P., NIKESKELAINEN, J. Viral antibodies in the sera from patients with Parkinson's disease. *European Neurology*, **15,** 25–33 (1977)
55 MARTIN, J. P. *The Basal Ganglia and Posture*. Philadelphia, Lippincott (1967)
56 MARTIN, W. E., YOUNG, W. I. and ANDERSON, V. E. Parkinson's disease, a genetic study. *Brain*, **96,** 495–506 (1973)
57 MENDEL, K. *Die Paralysis Agitans*. Berlin, S. Karger (1911)
58 MEYER, B. Encephalitis after measles with severe parkinsonian rigidity: recovery. *British Medical Journal*, **1,** 508 (1943)
59 MJÖNES, H. Paralysis agitans. A clinical and genetic study. *Acta Psychiatrica et Neurologica Sandinavica*, **25** (suppl. 54), 1–195 (1949)
60 MULDER, D. W., PARROTT, M. and THALER, M. Sequelae of Western equine encephalitis. *Neurology*, **1,** 318–327 (1951)
61 NEAL, J. B. *Encephalitis. A Clinical Study*. New York, Grune and Stratton (1942)
62 NEFZEGER, M. D., QUADFASEL, F. A. and KARL, A. A retrospective study of smoking in Parkinson's disease. *American Journal of Epidemiology*, **88,** 149–158 (1968)
63 NIELSEN, J. M. Complications of encephalitis of the Von-Economo Type. *Bulletin of the Los Angeles Neurological Society*, **18,** 84–90 (1953)
64 PAKKENBERG, H. and BRODY, H. The number of nerve cells in the substantia nigra in paralysis agitans. *Acta Neuropathologica*, **5,** 320–324 (1965)
65 PARSONS, A. C. *Report of an Inquiry into the After-histories of Persons Attacked by Encephalitis Lethargica*. London, HMSO (1928)
66 PEMBREY, M. E. Discordant identical twins. II. Parkinsonism. *Practitioner*, **209,** 240–243 (1972)
67 POLLOCK, M. and HORNABROOK, R. W. The prevalence, natural history and dementia of Parkinson's disease. *Brain*, **89,** 429–448 (1966)
68 POSER, C. In discussion on Kurland, L. T. Reference 49 above.
69 POSER, C. M., HUNTLEY, C. J. and POLAND, J. D. Para-encephalitic parkinsonism: report of an acute case due to Coxsackie Virus Type B2 and re-examination of the etiologic concept of postencephalitic parkinsonism. *Acta Neurologica Scandinavica*, **45,** 199–215 (1969)
70 POSKANZER, D. C. and SCHWAB, R. S. Studies in the epidemiology of Parkinson's disease predicting its disappearance as a major clinical entity by 1980. *Transactions of the American Neurological Association*, **86,** 234–245 (1961)
71 RIGGS, N. and FINLEY, K. H. Sequelae of Western encephalitis and St. Louis encephalitis. *California Vector Views*, **7,** 35–111 (1960)
72 SACHS, O. *Awakenings*. London, Duckworth (1973)
73 SCHULTZ, D. R., BARTHAL, J. S. and GARRETT, M. C. Western equine encephalitis with rapid onset of parkinsonism. *Neurology*, **27,** 1095–1097 (1977)
74 SPELLMAN, G. G. Report of familial cases of parkinsonism. *Journal of the American Medical Associatioin*, **179,** 160–162 (1962)

75 STRONG, G. Parkinson's syndrome following severe herpes ophthalmicus. *British Medical Journal*, **1,** 533 (1952)
76 VON ECONOMO, C. *Encephalitis Lethargica; its Sequelae and Treatment.* Translated by K. O. Newman, London, Oxford University Press (1931)
77 WALTERS, J. H. Post-encephalitic Parkinson syndrome after meningoencephalitis due to Coxsackie virus Group B, type 2. *New England Journal of Medicine*, **263,** 744–747 (1960)
78. WARD, C. D., DUVOISIN, R. C., INCE, S. E., NUTT, J. D., ELDRIDGE, R. and CALNE, D. B. Parkinson disease in twins and in a set of quadruplets. (Presented at 33rd Annual Meeting of the American Academy of Neurology, Toronto, Canada, April 1981) *Neurology*, **31,** 110 (1981)
79 WAREMBOURG, H., NIQUET, A., PAUCHANT, M., DUCLOSE, G. Syndrome parkinsonien: sequelle d'une poliomyelite aigue a forme d'encephalite lethargique chez un enfant de 20 mois. *Semaine des Hôpitaux de Paris*, **38,** 2299–2307 (1962)
80 WETMORE, J. G., SCHWARTZ, J. and ELIZAN, T. S. Nucleic acid homology studies of viral nucleic acids in idiopathic Parkinson's disease. *Archives of Neurology*, **36,** 462–498 (1979)
81 WILLIAMS, A., HOUFF, S., LEES, A. and CALNE, D. B. Oligoclonal banding in the cerebrospinal fluid of patients with postencephalitic parkinsonism. *Journal of Neurology, Neurosurgery and Psychiatry*, **42,,** 790–792 (1979)
82 WILSON, S. A. K. *Neurology*, **1,** 115. Baltimore, Williams and Wilkins (1946)
83 ZEIGLER, L. H. Follow-up studies on persons who have had epidemic encephalitis. *Journal of the American Medical Association*, **91,** 138–140 (1928)
84 ZINSSER, H. Present state of knowledge regarding epidemic encephalitis. *Archives of Pathology*, **6,** 271–300 (1928)

3
Pathology of Parkinson's disease
Lysia S. Forno

INTRODUCTION

Neuropathological studies by Tretiakoff, Hassler, Greenfield and others[24, 29, 54] established many years ago the importance of substantia nigra degeneration in Parkinson's disease. The subsequent discovery of dopamine deficiency in parkinsonism[13] and the demonstration of the dopaminergic nigrostriatal pathway[2] further substantiated the belief that the substantia nigra plays a key role in the development of parkinsonism. Contributions from neuropathology to the understanding of parkinsonism since then have been sparse. In this review the current knowledge and recent discoveries will be briefly detailed, and plans for future research will be suggested.

CLASSICAL NEUROPATHOLOGICAL STUDIES

Summary of current knowledge

Briefly stated, what is known about the pathology of parkinsonism is the following. Nerve cells in the substantia nigra degenerate and Lewy bodies are formed in the process. Neuromelanin from the dead or dying nerve cells spills out into the tissue, is taken up by macrophages and is eventually transported away through the bloodstream. We do not know why this happens or how it starts. Because Lewy bodies are formed in the perikaryon we assume that the major changes take place there, rather than in the periphery near or at the axon terminals as in a 'dying-back' process. Is it possible that in some forms of parkinsonism the disease process starts or first becomes manifest in the neostriatum or globus pallidus? This would give the appearance of a supranigral form of parkinsonism and might explain some of the rare cases where no nerve cell degeneration in the substantia nigra can be demonstrated.

We also know that pathological processes are taking place, not only in the substantia nigra and in other pigmented nuclei, such as the locus coeruleus and the dorsal motor vagus nucleus, but in a number of other regions, most frequently in the innominate substance, the hypothalamus, the raphe nuclei of the midbrain and rostral pons, in the sympathetic ganglia, and less often in the spinal cord[4, 20, 23, 36, 41]. Some of these regions are known to contain catecholamine neurons, others are not.

This is the essence of our knowledge about the most common form of parkinsonism, the classical Parkinson's disease of Lewy body type. A few details have been added over the years. Some of the recent studies will be discussed in the following. None of them represents a major breakthrough.

Lewy bodies and Lewy body parkinsonism

Composition and morphology of Lewy bodies

The characteristic intraneuronal inclusions named after Lewy[38] have attracted a great deal of attention. Their light microscopic appearance and staining characteristics have been best described by Greenfield and Bosanquet[24], and their ultrastructure by Duffy and Tennyson[11]. They consist mainly of protein which, in the Lewy

Figure 3.1 Multiple confluent Lewy bodies in a pigmented nerve cell in the substantia nigra. × 5500. Idiopathic parkinsonism

Figure 3.2 Lewy bodies in the locus coeruleus. Idiopathic parkinsonism. Vesicular structures in the core of the Lewy body and radiating filaments. × 36 000. *Inset:* typical small Lewy body. × 5500

bodies in the substantia nigra and locus coeruleus, is present as an electron dense, amorphous core with surrounding radiating filamentous material (*Figures 3.1 and 3.2*), giving them the appearance of sunflowers (*Figure 3.2, inset*). The filaments resemble neurofilaments, but have a more variable diameter. In the substantia nigra and locus coeruleus the Lewy body is often surrounded by neuromelanin granules with no intervening membrane. Dense core vesicles are often present at the periphery. They are rarely present in the numbers reported in one case by Watanabe *et al.*[55]. The core may, instead of dense amorphous material, display circular structures (*Figure 3.2*).

Round or elongated eosinophilic hyaline inclusions have been described in locations outside the pigmented nuclei of the brainstem[31]. Their ultrastructure is much more variable (*Figures 3.3 and 3.4*) and only rarely do they have the radiating filaments of the Lewy bodies in the substantia nigra and locus coeruleus[20, 23, 36]. It may be questioned whether such structures should be called Lewy bodies. Many of these inclusions are located in nerve cell processes, whereas the Lewy body with the radiating filaments is present in the perikaryon of the nerve cell. The terms intraneuritic and perikaryal Lewy bodies, respectively, have been suggested for the two types[23]. The term Lewy bodies for both types appears justified for two reasons: first, because intraneuritic Lewy bodies are only seen in brains with classical perikaryal Lewy bodies in the substantia nigra and locus coeruleus, and second, because Lewy's original description and illustrations[38] include elongated forms in nerve cell processes. Intraneuritic Lewy bodies can also be regarded as a special

28 *Pathology of Parkinson's disease*

Figure 3.3 Intraneuritic Lewy body in the hypothalamus. Idiopathic parkinsonism. Mitochondria and multivesicular bodies are seen along the periphery. × 4500

Figure 3.4 Intraneuritic Lewy body in the stellate ganglion. Idiopathic parkinsonism. Neurofilaments (arrow) have been displaced to the periphery. Dense core vesicles are seen along the border of the inclusion. ×10 000. *Inset*: intraneuritic Lewy body in the stellate ganglion. Idiopathic parkinsonism. The unstained Lewy body (L) is surrounded by positive staining for neurofilaments. Paraffin section. Peroxidase–antiperoxidase stain for neurofilament protein. × 600

form of neuroaxonal dystrophic change[35], although they probably are more common in dendrites than in axons.

The polymorphism of the Lewy bodies and the heterogeneity of the organelles that enter into their composition pose difficulties for chemical characterization. With the immunohistochemical methods now available it may be possible to identify some of the components. If catecholamines or their metabolic products form a part of the Lewy body, it may be possible to demonstrate, within the Lewy inclusion, the enzymes active in the synthesis of amines, such as tyrosine hydroxylase, a marker for catecholamines, or dopamine β-hydroxylase, a marker for noradrenergic and adrenergic neurons. The filamentous material present both in perikaryal and in most intraneuritic Lewy bodies should also be amenable to immunohistochemical characterization. Using the peroxidase–antiperoxidase method of Sternberger[52], tissue with Lewy bodies has been stained for neurofilaments and for the microtubule-associated proteins (Forno and Eng, unpublished observations). With this method, the Lewy bodies are seen as pale, unstained, rounded or elongated structures, rarely surrounded by neurofilament staining (*Figure 3.4, inset*). The peripheral staining corresponds to neurofilaments displaced peripherally as occasionally demonstrated by electron microscopy (*Figure 3.4*). It is suspected that the filamentous material may be a precursor to neurofilaments, but a chemical identification has not been achieved.

Anatomical distribution of Lewy bodies. Other pathological findings in idiopathic parkinsonism of Lewy body type

The presence of Lewy bodies outside of the substantia nigra and locus coeruleus has already been mentioned[4, 20, 36, 41] (*Figures 3.3 and 3.4*). It is not known why certain nerve cell centers are predilection sites, but the distribution is not haphazard, so a systematic involvement appears likely. Certain areas are never involved, for example the cerebellum. The neostriatum and globus pallidus are unusual sites, as are the pontine nuclei and inferior olives, where Lipkin found them in one case[39]. Aminergic systems appear to be most vulnerable to this form of nerve cell degeneration, with serotonergic nuclei such as the dorsal raphe nucleus and superior central nucleus lagging only slightly behind the substantia nigra and locus coeruleus. The sympathetic ganglia are involved in a little over two-thirds of Lewy body parkinsonism cases[20]. For many other predilection sites, e.g. the innominate substance and the posterolateral hypothalamus, the neurotransmitters are still unknown. The cerebral cortex is a rare location for Lewy bodies, but several reports of this finding have appeared[17, 30, 34, 42].

Some of the nuclei where Lewy bodies readily occur also favor the development of neurofibrillary tangles. This is true for the locus coeruleus, the innominate substance, the tuberomammillary nucleus, and the raphe nuclei in the rostral brainstem. The substantia nigra is much less susceptible to neurofibrillary tangle formation with age and in Alzheimer's disease (but *see* pp. 31–32 for certain forms of parkinsonism), and the sympathetic ganglia never display this abnormality. Lewy bodies and neurofibrillary tangles may be present in the same nucleus.

Paired helical filaments, the ultrastructural correlate of the neurofibrillary tangle[56], have been seen within intraneuritic Lewy bodies in the hypothalamus in five cases[23] (and Forno, unpublished observations).

Lewy bodies serve as markers for nerve cell degeneration in areas where such nerve cell loss might otherwise go unnoticed, but nerve cell loss and fibrillary gliosis can be obvious in some nuclei and pathways outside of the pigmented nuclei, e.g. in the innominate substance and ansa peduncularis. The author has not been convinced of any abnormality in the globus pallidus except age-related changes (ferrugination of vessels, status cribrosus), nor of any degeneration in the ansa lenticularis[8]. A slight nerve cell loss in the neostriatum has been reported[3]. It is not obvious in the author's material, but quantitative studies have not been made, and it is indeed remarkable that no trace of the nigrostriatal degeneration is evident. The actual degeneration of this fine-fibered tract in brains from patients with parkinsonism has also not been demonstrated.

Specificity of Lewy bodies for Parkinson's disease

Although Lewy bodies are highly characteristic, they are not pathognomonic for Parkinson's disease. They have been found in 4–6 percent of routine autopsies[17,39], but their occurrence below the age of 60 years is unusual. These incidental cases may represent early undiagnosed, or preclinical parkinsonism. Yahr's observations on the frequently subtle and elusive early symptomatology in Parkinson's disease[58] is consistent with this interpretation. An example of Lewy body formation (in a surgically removed sympathetic ganglion), antedating the onset of parkinsonism, was reported by Stadlan et al.[51]. The rare occurrence of Lewy bodies in postencephalitic parkinsonism[8,39] can be explained by the presence of both postencephalitic and idiopathic parkinsonism in the same patient. Such a coincidence cannot be claimed for a few other conditions where Lewy bodies have been described[23], for example for Hallervorden-Spatz disease[7].

Relationship between Lewy bodies and Alzheimer's disease

The coincidence of Lewy bodies and pathological findings characteristic of Alzheimer's disease was pointed out by Woodard[57]. In his material Lewy bodies were seen in connection with Alzheimer's disease more often than with Parkinson's disease. The author has found some affinity between Alzheimer's disease and Lewy bodies. In 77 cases that fulfilled the criteria for Alzheimer's disease (Forno, unpublished observations) Lewy bodies were present in 11, but 4 of these also had Parkinson's disease. None of the patients with Lewy bodies in this group or in Woodard's series, died before the age of 60 years. Woodard's results, with only 7 parkinsonism patients among his 27 Lewy body cases, do not detract from the importance of Lewy body inclusions in parkinsonism, for he does not mention any parkinsonism patients where they were not found. The findings of Lewy bodies in less than one-tenth of patients with Alzheimer's disease is small in comparison with the near 100 percent correlation in Parkinson's disease.

Perhaps the Lewy body phenomenon can be regarded as a special form of nerve cell degeneration ('Lewy body nerve cell degeneration'[1, 19]) which only gives rise to parkinsonism when the degenerative process involves the substantia nigra severely enough to cause clinically manifest dopamine deficiency. Attempts to establish a genetic factor in Parkinson's disease have not met with success[12, 58], but if we are dealing with Lewy body degeneration which only in a certain percentage of patients results in clinical disease, it would be difficult to make an evaluation of genetic predisposition, since Lewy bodies cannot be demonstrated during life. The Lewy body phenomenon could also be an acquired nerve cell degeneration, due to a virus or to toxic–nutritional or other environmental factors.

The relation between Lewy body nerve cell degeneration and Alzheimer's disease may have some bearing on the question of mental deterioration in Parkinson's disease. Several recent studies[27, 40] have suggested that the intellect is indeed affected in Parkinson's disease. The presence of cortical senile plaques and neurofibrillary tangles in a higher proportion of patients with parkinsonism than in age-matched controls[1, 27] may indicate that Parkinson's and Alzheimer's disease are more closely related than previously thought.

The neurofibrillary tangles. Postencephalitic and other forms of neurofibrillary tangle parkinsonism

Another inclusion, the neurofibrillary tangle, plays a part in the nerve cell degeneration in certain forms of parkinsonism. Since Hallervorden[28] described neurofibrillary tangles in postencephalitic parkinsonism, such tangles in the substantia nigra have come to be regarded as one of the hallmarks of postencephalitic parkinsonism. Typically the tangles are found in connection with a severe diffuse nerve cell loss, contrasting with the focally accentuated nerve cell loss in the midportion of the substantia nigra in idiopathic parkinsonism[16, 24, 29]. The author has examined a number of cases with substantia nigra degeneration and neurofibrillary tangles, but no history of encephalitis lethargica[1, 19]; for such cases the term idiopathic neurofibrillary tangle parkinsonism has been suggested. Documented postencephalitic cases are now becoming increasingly rare in autopsy material; 7 years have elapsed since the last such case was studied in this laboratory. Rare cases are still seen with moderate to severe substantia nigra nerve cell loss and a variable, though usually rather scant, number of neurofibrillary tangles. If neurofibrillary tangles are also present in other cortical and subcortical areas, but senile plaques are few or absent, and if the parkinsonism is of long duration or began at a young age, it appears justified to regard the case as probably postencephalitic. At present, files in this laboratory include 8 postencephalitic and 10 possibly postencephalitic brains. There are 9 other tangle cases with mild substantia nigra degeneration, a few neurofibrillary tangles, mild, often atypical clinical parkinsonism, and a main diagnosis of Alzheimer's disease, usually the senile variant. These figures can be compared with 79 cases of idiopathic parkinsonism of Lewy body type (52 typical cases and 27 cases with very mild clinical symptoms).

Neurofibrillary tangle parkinsonism appears to be a useful pathological classification for a relatively small group (approximately one-fourth) of parkinsonism cases. Within this group the cases with Alzheimer's disease are of least interest. The occurrence of possibly postencephalitic cases suggest either that encephalitis lethargica still occurs, or that a particularly long latency period has followed the subclinical encephalitis before the onset of parkinsonian symptoms. The next few years should make it clear whether postencephalitic and probably postencephalitic cases have truly disappeared.

Two other conditions with parkinsonian symptoms and substantia nigra degeneration with neurofibrillary tangles have not been included in this discussion. One is the Guam parkinsonism–dementia complex where the ultrastructure of the neurofibrillary tangle is the paired helical filament[56] as in Alzheimer's disease and postencephalitic parkinsonism. The other is progressive supranuclear palsy where the neurofibrillary tangles are made up of 16 nm straight tubules[53].

Other forms of parkinsonism

Because the emphasis in this review is on the classical Parkinson's disease, other forms of parkinsonism will only be touched upon. Arteriosclerotic parkinsonism does occur. In the author's material it has been associated with small cystic infarcts (lacunae) in the basal ganglia, and the clinical picture has been slightly atypical or mild, usually with more rigidity than tremor[18]. The disturbance of dopamine metabolism is such cases may be postsynaptic. The role played by massive calcification of the basal ganglia[33] in the pathogenesis of some forms of parkinsonism is uncertain, but pathological processes in the striatum can give rise to parkinsonian symptoms.

APPLICATION OF 'NEWER' METHODS TO THE STUDY OF THE PATHOLOGY OF PARKINSONISM

General remarks. The difficulties in studying structural changes in human degenerative diseases

So far, this review has dealt mainly with 'old' questions and 'old' problems, most of which were being asked even before the levodopa era, and to which classical neuropathological methods have been applied. With much new information now coming in, in neurophysiology, neuropharmacology, neurochemistry and neuroanatomy, we must ask how the new knowledge and the new methods can be applied to the human nervous system and the problems of parkinsonism.

The application of these methods to human brain tissue, especially autopsy tissue, poses special problems. Results are difficult to interpret, and the fear of interpreting postmortem artefacts as important abnormalities holds one back. We must remind ourselves that some of the most important biochemical findings, such as the decreased dopamine content in the striatum and substantia nigra in parkinsonism, came out of studies on human autopsy brain tissue[13]. Many problems cannot be studied adequately in other mammals, since they do not develop true Parkinson's disease. One objection to drawing conclusions from studies on autopsy tissue has been that, at the time the patient dies, the disease has reached an endstage, and only early cases, where death is due to unrelated non-neurological causes, are worth while studying. Such material is, of course, very valuable, but it is incorrect that most cases of progressive neurological disorders such as Parkinson's disease have reached a stationary endstage. There are instead indications that the disease process is still going on. Nerve cells in the substantia nigra, for example, continue to die off, as evidenced by freshly liberated neuromelanin granules deposited in a shape that mirrors the nerve cell they replace. Except for postencephalitic parkinsonism, where the devastation of nerve cells can be almost complete, the nerve cell loss is only moderate, with less than two-thirds of the nerve cells lost[43]. Probably in the course of time, a number of adaptations take place, not only glial scarring (beneficial under some circumstances, harmful in others) but many other changes such as rearrangement of receptors, subtle transsynaptic changes, and perhaps sprouting, either in still healthy nerve cells in the affected nucleus, or from unaffected interconnected or neighboring nuclei. There may also be important changes in the nuclei to which the diseased nerve cell group projects. To recognize such changes we need first more detailed information about the fine structure and connections of the nerve cell centers we are interested in, before we can appreciate the abnormalities. This is where experimental animal studies can guide us.

Methods that may prove useful

The methods to be considered here will be limited to electron microscopy, Golgi silver impregnation, immunohistochemistry and combinations of these methods. Encouraged by finding that synaptic complexes are relatively well preserved in human postmortem brain specimens, preliminary studies have been made of synaptic ultrastructure in the human neostriatum[21], locus coeruleus[22], and substantia nigra (Forno and Norville, unpublished observations). The following main conclusions can be drawn from these studies.

(1) The well known findings by light microscopy can be confirmed and some details can be added, for example in regard to the ultrastructure of Lewy bodies and neurofibrillary tangles, pigment accumulations in cells, gliosis, fiber tracts, and types of nerve cells present.
(2) The synaptic ultrastructure can be compared with normal ultrastructure in the corresponding area in experimental animals. Similarities may be more reliable findings than differences. Certain afferent terminals can perhaps be identified as to their nucleus of origin and their neurotransmitter on the basis of the ultrastructure of the synaptic complex.
(3) A few abnormalities or suspected abnormalities can be detected in brains of patients with parkinsonism or other chronic degenerative diseases.

In the substantia nigra, the author has found rare examples of very fine unmyelinated fibers which may represent axonal sprouts. In the locus coeruleus axosomatic synapses could be seen on nerve cells with Lewy bodies or with neurofibrillary tangles[22]. In the neostriatum of patients with Huntington's disease, nerve terminals were often found to be packed with synaptic vesicles, and in Parkinson's disease examples of similar acumulations in the substantia nigra were seen. Because there is a great normal variation in the vesicle content of individual terminals, the author cannot yet be sure that this is a valid observation, but it could mean that vesicles accumulate in preterminal axons when the postsynaptic elements degenerate[21]. In the locus coeruleus accumulations of large dense core vesicles have been found in Parkinson's and Alzheimer's disease. Such processes can also be found in control material and have been demonstrated in the cat[37], and in the rat[25], but they appear more abundant in Parkinson's and Alzheimer's disease. Again, this relative increase may be related to degeneration of postsynaptic elements. These findings would be of more interest if it could be demonstrated where these terminals were coming from and where on the degenerating nerve cells they have their contact.

The results of electron microscopy studies in human nerve cell nuclei is therefore of value for establishing normal fine structure in nerve cell centers that are involved in parkinsonism and other nervous system degenerative disorders, but they have so far been disappointing in unmasking the degenerative disease process. It may be possible to overcome some of these difficulties by combining electron microscopy with other methods such as Golgi silver impregnation and immunohistochemistry.

Because Golgi impregnation is the method that gives us the most complete picture of the cytoarchitecture of a nerve cell nuclear group[47], this method is particularly well suited for comparative studies of human CNS and other mammalian CNS. It can outline the nerve cell in its entirety, including the dendritic pattern, presence or absence of spines, size and orientation of the dendritic field and often also the course of the axons and the presence of collaterals. Since it is a method that is relatively tolerant of postmortem changes[50], it is well suited for study of human material (*Figures 3.5 and 3.6*). How well will the Golgi method be able to reveal abnormalities in human diseases? The method has only been put to this test to a very limited extent, but in animal studies it has been helpful in demonstrating more nerve cell types than originally thought to be present in the striatum[9], and it has also proved useful for studies of the substantia nigra[15,32] and the locus coeruleus[48]. Recently, the Golgi impregnation method has been combined with electron microscopy, using a gold toning technique[14]. By this method one can examine not only the ultrastructure of a synaptic complex, but also obtain information about where on the soma or dendritic tree it is located. The method has been used by DiFiglia et al.[10] to study the spiny type I and aspiny type I nerve cells in the monkey neostriatum. From their characterization of the spiny type I nerve cells it appears likely that the nerve cell demonstrated in *Figure 3.7* in the putamen (from a patient with parkinsonism) is a spiny type I nerve cell. If all the six or more nerve cell types in the striatum can be characterized in this way we may be able to extrapolate to human studies and established what happens to these nerve cells and their connections in Parkinson's and Huntington's disease. In the

Application of 'newer' methods to the study of the pathology of parkinsonism

substantia nigra it may be possible to demonstrate whether in Parkinson's disease nerve cells that project to limbic areas, are as severely affected as those that project to the neostriatum. Fallon et al.[15] have found distinct differences in cell morphology and in location between nigroneostriatal and mesolimbic dopaminergic nerve cells.

Immunohistochemistry, used for demonstration of catecholaminergic, cholinergic, GABAergic, serotonergic, and peptidergic nerve cells and pathways has become a very valuable tool in experimental animal studies, and is now also getting

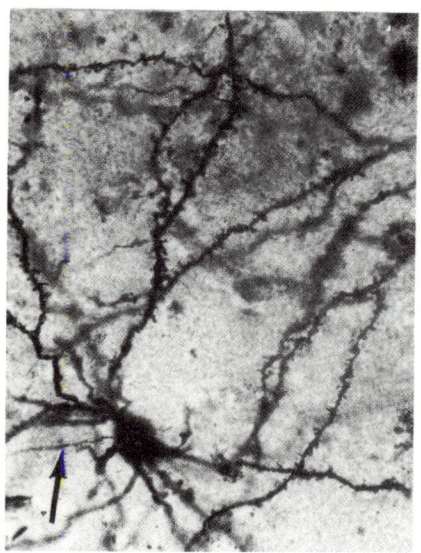

Figure 3.5 Spiny I nerve cell in the putamen from a 48-year-old man without neurological disease. Arrow points to axon. Rapid Golgi method. × 320

Figure 3.6 Spiny nerve cell in the head of the caudate nucleus from a 62-year-old man with Huntington's chorea. Spines appear decreased in number. Rapid Golgi method. × 288

Figure 3.7 Spiny I nerve cell (according to criteria of DiFiglia *et al.*) in putamen in idiopathic parkinsonism. The adjacent axon terminal (arrow) contains floccular material which may represent degenerating synaptic vesicles. × 11 000

increasing use in human material. Pearson[44] has studied tyrosine hydroxylase, a marker for catecholaminergic nerve cells and pathways, in the human brain and compared his results with those obtained with the Falck-Hillarp fluorescence method in rat[6], and Pickel *et al.*[46] have made similar studies in the human fetus. Both Pearson and Pickel *et al.* used the peroxidase–antiperoxidase unlabeled antibody method of Sternberger[52]. This method can be used on formalin fixed material and for some antigens on paraffin embedded tissue, allowing direct comparison with light microscopic findings. How useful these methods will be for demonstration of pathological changes in human degenerative disease is not known as yet, but improved modifications of immunocytochemical methods continue to be achieved. Grzanna and Molliver's elegant study[26] of the noradrenergic system in the rat is a good example. The combinations with electron microscopy[45,49] are also being pursued, and the technical difficulties inherent in such studies will probably be overcome in time.

From what has been said in this section, it will be obvious that the neuropathologist or other neuroscientist who works with human tissue, depends on results from work with experimental animals for help in interpretation of findings. The methods suggested here have had too short a trial period to allow conclusions about what information they will be able to yield.

SUMMARY AND CONCLUSIONS

Although the most characteristic pathological changes in Parkinson's disease – the substantia nigra degeneration, the Lewy bodies and the widespread selective involvement of certain nerve cell centers and pathways – are now reasonably well established, the 'enigma of Parkinsonism'[8] is still very much with us. In this review the two main forms of parkinsonism, one with Lewy bodies and one with neurofibrillary tangles, have been discussed. The Lewy body type is the classical Parkinson's disease, and by far the most common. The neurofibrillary tangle group includes postencephalitic and probably-postencephalitic cases and variants of Alzheimer's disease. It should soon become clear if the postencephalitic and probably-postencephalitic cases will disappear completely. If they do, neurofibrillary tangle parkinsonism will no longer be an important classification.

Brodal[5] has recently lamented that in spite of the increasing knowledge that has accumulated about the neurophysiology, biochemistry and neuroanatomy of the basal ganglia, our understanding of the diseases of the basal ganglia, such as Parkinson's disease and Huntington's chorea, has not progressed much. If we can learn from and compare with results obtained in experimental animals, and if we use electron microscopy, Golgi impregnation studies, immunohistochemistry and combinations of these methods judiciously for studies of the human degenerative diseases, the time may have come for neuropathology to make a small contribution to such better understanding.

References

1 ALVORD, E. C. JR., FORNO, L. S., KUSSKE, J. A., KAUFFMAN, R. J., RHODES, J. S. and GOETOWSKI, CH. R. The pathology of parkinsonism: a comparison of degenerations in cerebral cortex and brainstem. *Advances in Neurology*, **5**, 175–193 (1974)

2 ANDEN, N. E., CARLSSON, A., DAHLSTROM, A., FUXE, K., HILLARP, N. A. and LARSSON, K. Demonstration and mapping out of nigro-neostriatal dopamine neurons. *Life Sciences*, **3**, 523–530 (1964)

3 BERNHEIMER, H., BIRKMAYER, W., HORNYKIEWICZ, O., JELLINGER, K. and SEITELBERGER, F. Brain dopamine and the syndromes of Parkinson and Huntington. Clinical, morphological and neurochemical correlations. *Journal of the Neurological Sciences*, **20**, 415–455 (1973)

4 BETHLEM, J. and JAGER, W. A. DEN HARTOG. The incidence and characteristics of Lewy bodies in idiopathic paralysis agitans (Parkinson's disease). *Journal of Neurology, Neurosurgery and Psychiatry*, **23**, 74–80 (1960)

5 BRODAL, A. *Neurological Anatomy in Relation to Clinical Medicine*, 3rd Edition. Oxford, Oxford University Press (1981)

6 DAHLSTROM, A. and FUXE, K. Evidence for the existence of monoamine-containing neurons in the central nervous system. I. Demonstration of monoamines in the cell bodies of brain stem neurons. *Acta Physiologica Scandinavica*, **62**, Suppl. 232, 1–55 (1964)

7 DEFENDINI, R., MARKESBERY, W. R., MASTRI, A. R. and DUFFY, P. E. Hallervorden-Spatz disease and infantile neuroaxonal dystrophy: ultrastructural observations, anatomical pathology and nosology. *The Journal of the Neurological Sciences*, **20**, 70–83 (1973)

8 DENNY-BROWN, D. *The Basal Ganglia and their Relation to Disorders of Movement*. Oxford, Oxford University Press (1962)

9 DIFIGLIA, M., PASIK, P. and PASIK, T. A Golgi study of neuronal types in the neostriatum in monkeys. *Brain Research*, **114**, 245–256 (1976)

10 DIFIGLIA, M. PASIK, T. and PASIK, P. Ultrastructure of Golgi-impregnated and gold-toned spiny and aspiny neurons in the monkey neostriatum. *Journal of Neurocytology*, **9**, 471–492 (1980)

11 DUFFY, P. E. and TENNYSON, V. M. Phase and electron microscopic observations of Lewy bodies and melanin granules in the substantia nigra and locus caeruleus in Parkinson's disease. *Journal of Neuropathology and Experimental Neurology*, **24**, 398–414 (1965)

12 DUVOISIN, R. C., ELDRIDGE, R., WILLIAMS, A., NUTT, J. and CALNE, D. Twin study of Parkinson disease. *Neurology*, **31**, 77–80 (1981)

13 EHRINGER, H. and HORNYKIEWICZ, O. Verteilung von Noradrenalin und Dopamin (3-Hydroxytyramin) im Gehirn des Menschen und ihr Verhalten bei Erkrankungen des extrapyramidalen Systems. *Klinische Wochenschrift*, **38**, 1236–1239 (1960)

14 FAIREN, A., PETERS, A. and SALDANHA, J. A new procedure for examining Golgi impregnated neurons by light and electron microscopy. *Journal of Neurocytology*, **5**, 311–337 (1977)

15 FALLON, J. H., RILEY, J. N. and MOORE, R. Y. Substantia nigra dopamine neurons: separate populations project to neostriatum and allocortex. *Neuroscience Letters*, **7**, 157–162 (1978)

16 FORNO, L. S. Pathology of Parkinsonism. A preliminary report of 24 cases. *Journal of Neurosurgery*, **24** (Supplement), 266–271 (1966)

17 FORNO, L. S. Concentric hyalin intraneuronal inclusions of Lewy type in the brains of elderly persons (50 incidental cases): relationship to parkinsonism. *Journal of the American Geriatrics Society*, **17**, 557–575 (1969)

18 FORNO, L. S. Pathology of Parkinsonism: nigro-striatal relationships; extranigral lesions; review. In *Proceedings of a Symposium on Parkinsonism*, edited by J. Worm-Petersen and J. Böttcher, 29–48. Denmark, Merck, Sharp and Dohme (1977)

19 FORNO, L. S. and ALVORD, E. C., JR. The pathology of Parkinsonism. Part I. Some new observations and correlations. In *Recent Advances in Parkinson's Disease*, edited by F. McDowell and Ch. Markham. *Contemporary Neurology*, Series No. **8**, 120–130. Philadelphia, F. A. Davis Co. (1971)

20 FORNO, L. S. and NORVILLE, R. L. Ultrastructure of Lewy bodies in the stellate ganglion. *Acta Neuropathologica (Berlin)*, **34**, 183–197 (1976)

21 FORNO, L. S. and NORVILLE, R. L. Ultrastructure of the neostriatum in Huntington's and Parkinson's disease. *Advances in Neurology*, **23**, 123–135 (1979)

22 FORNO, L. S. and NORVILLE, R. L. Synaptic morphology in the human locus ceruleus. *Acta Neuropathologica (Berlin)*, **53**, 7–14 (1981)

23 FORNO, L. S., BARBOUR, P. J. and NORVILLE, R. L. Presenile dementia with Lewy bodies and neurofibrillary tangles. *Archives of Neurology*, **35**, 818–822 (1978)
24 GREENFIELD, J. G. and BOSANQUET, F. D. The brain-stem lesions in parkinsonism. *Journal of Neurology, Neurosurgery and Psychiatry*, **16**, 213–226 (1953)
25 GROVES, P. M. and WILSON, CH. J. Fine structure of rat locus coeruleus. *Journal of Comparative Neurology*, **193**, 841–852 (1980)
26 GRZANNA, R., MOLLIVER, M. E. and COYLE, J. T. Visualization of central noradrenergic neurons in thick sections by the unlabeled antibody method: a transmitter specific Golgi image. *Proceedings of the National Academy of Sciences of the USA*, **75**, 2502–2506 (1978)
27 HAKIM, A. M. and MATHIESON, G. Dementia in Parkinson disease: a neuropathologic study. *Neurology*, **29**, 1209–1214 (1979)
28 HALLERVORDEN, J. Anatomische Untersuchungen zur Pathogenese des postencephalitischen Parkinsonismus. *Deutsche Zeitschrift für Nervenheilkunde*, **136**, 68–77 (1935)
29 HASSLER, R. Zur Pathologie der Paralysis Agitans und des postenzephalitischen Parkinsonismus. *Journal für Psychologie und Neurologie*, **48**, 387–476 (1938)*
30 IKEDA, K., IKEDA, S., YOSHIMURA, T., KATO, H. and NAMBA, M. Idiopathic parkinsonism with Lewy-type inclusions in cerebral cortex: a case report. *Acta Neuropathologica (Berlin)*, **34**, 183–197 (1976)
31 JAGER, W. A. DEN HARTOG and BETHLEM, J. The distribution of Lewy bodies in the central and autonomic nervous system in idiopathic paralysis agitans. *Journal of Neurology, Neurosurgery and Psychiatry*, **23**, 283–290 (1960)
32 JURASKA, J. M., WILSON, C. J. and GROVES, P. M. The substantia nigra in the rat: a Golgi study. *Journal of Comparative Neurology*, **172**, 585–600 (1977)
33 KLAWANS, H. L., LUPTON, M. and SIMON, K. Calcification of the basal ganglia as a cause of levodopa-resistant parkinsonism. *Neurology*, **26**, 221–225 (1976)
34 KOSAKA, K. Lewy bodies in cerebral cortex. Report of three cases. *Acta Neuropathologica (Berlin)*, **42**, 127–134 (1978)
35 LAMPERT, P. A comparative electron microscopic study of reactive, degenerating, regenerating, and dystrophic axons. *Journal of Neuropathology and Experimental Neurology*, **26**, 345–368 (1967)
36 LANGSTON, J. W. and FORNO, L. S. The hypothalamus in Parkinson disease. *Annals of Neurology*, **3**, 129–133 (1978)
37 LEGER, L. Étude ultrastructurale du locus coeruleus du chat. *Thèse de Docteur de Specialité* (3ème cycle), Université Claude Bernard, Lyon-I, Lyon (1973)
38 LEWY, F. H. Paralysis agitans. I. Pathologische Anatomie. In *Handbuch der Neurologie*, edited by M. Lewandowsky, 920–933. Berlin, Springer (1912)
39 LIPKIN, L. E. Cytoplasmic inclusions in ganglion cells associated with parkinsonian states. A neurocellular change studied in 53 cases and 206 controls. *American Journal of Pathology*, **35**, 1117–1133 (1959)
40 MARTTILA, R. J. and RINNE, U. K. Dementia in Parkinson's disease. *Acta Neurologica Scandinavica*, **54**, 431–441 (1976)
41 OHAMA, E. and IKUTA, F. Parkinson's disease; distribution of Lewy bodies and monoamine neuron system. *Acta Neuropathologica (Berlin)*, **34**, 311–319 (1976)

42 OKAZAKI, H., LIPKIN, L. E. and ARONSON, S. M. Diffuse intracytoplasmic ganglionic inclusions (Lewy type) associated with progressive dementia and quadriparesis in flexion. *Journal of Neuropathology and Experimental Neurology*, **20**, 237–244 (1961)

43 PAKKENBERG, H. and BRODY, H. The number of nerve cells in the substantia nigra in paralysis agitans. *Acta Neuropathologica (Berlin)*, **5**, 320–324 (1965)

44 PEARSON, J., GOLDSTEIN, M. and BRANDEIS, L. Tyrosine hydroxylase immunohistochemistry in human brain. *Brain Research*, **165**, 333–337 (1979)

45 PICKEL, V. M., JOH, T. H., REIS, D. J. A serotonergic innervation of noradrenergic neurons in nucleus locus coeruleus: demonstration by immunocytochemical localization of the transmitter specific enzymes tyrosine and tryptophan hydroxylase. *Brain Research*, **131**, 197–214 (1977)

46 PICKEL, V. M., SPECHT, L. A., SUMAL, K. K., JOH, T. H., REIS, D. J. and HERVONEN, A. Immunocytochemical localization of tyrosine hydroxylase in the human fetal nervous system. *Journal of Comparative Neurology*, **194**, 465–474 (1980)

47 PURPURA, D. P. Introduction and perspectives. In *Golgi Centennial Symposium: Perspectives in Neurobiology*, edited by M. Santini, xiii–xvii. New York, Raven Press (1975)

48 RAMON-MOLINER, E. The locus coeruleus of cat. III. Light and electron microscopic studies. *Cell and Tissue Research*, **149**, 205–221 (1974)

49 RIBAK, C. E., VAUGHN, J. E., SAITO, K., BARBER, R. and ROBERTS, E. Immunocytochemical localization of glutamate decarboxylase in rat substantia nigra. *Brain Research*, **116**, 287–298 (1977)

50 SCHEIBEL, M. E., LINDSAY, R. D., TOMIYASU, U. and SCHEIBEL, A. B. Progressive dendritic changes in aging human cortex. *Experimental Neurology*, **47**, 392–403 (1975)

51 STADLAN, E. M., DUVOISIN, R. and YAHR, M. D. The pathology of parkinsonism. *Proceedings of the 5th International Congress of Neuropathology*. Excerpta Medica International Congress Series, **100**, 569–571 (1965)

52 STERNBERGER, L. A. *Immunocytochemistry*, 2nd Edition, New York, John Wiley and Sons (1979)

53 TELLEZ-NAGEL, I. and WISNIEWSKI, H. M. Ultrastructure of neurofibrillary tangles in Steele-Richardson-Olszewski syndrome. *Archives of Neurology*, **29**, 324–327 (1973)

54 TRETIAKOFF, C. Contribution a l'étude de l'anatomie pathologique du locus niger de Soemmering avec quelques deductions relatives à la pathogenie des troubles du tonus musculaire et de la maladie de Parkinson. *Thèse de Paris* (1919)

55 WATANABE, I., VACHAL, E. and TOMITA, T. Dense core vesicles around the Lewy body in incidental Parkinson's disease: an electron microscopic study. *Acta Neuropathologica (Berlin)*, **39**, 173–175 (1977)

56 WISNIEWSKI, H. M., NARANG, H. K. and TERRY, R. D. Neurofibrillary tangles of paired helical filaments. *Journal of the Neurological Sciences*, **27**, 173–181 (1976)

57 WOODARD, J. S. Concentric hyaline inclusion body formation in mental disease: analysis of 27 cases. *Journal of Neuropathology and Experimental Neurology*, **21**, 442–449 (1962)

58 YAHR, M. D. Parkinson's Disease – overview of its current status. *Mount Sinai Journal of Medicine*, **44**, 183–191 (1977)

4
Brain neurotransmitter changes in Parkinson's disease
Oleh Hornykiewicz

NEUROTRANSMITTER SYSTEMS IN THE BASAL GANGLIA

From the clinical point of view, Parkinson's disease has traditionally been regarded as a typical disturbance of the function of the basal ganglia, which comprise the telencephalic subcortical brain centres and associated nuclei, notably the caudate nucleus and putamen (striatum), globus pallidus (pallidum) and substantia nigra.

Recently, the chemical nature of the putative neurotransmitters in several basal ganglia pathways has been elucidated[23, 29, 59] (*Figure 4.1*). It is known that there are at least two chemically distinct types of striatal interneurons: those containing acetylcholine as their putative neurotransmitter and the γ-aminobutyric acid (GABA)-containing interneurons. In addition, GABA seems to be the neurotransmitter in two striatofugal systems and one pallidofugal pathway, viz. a striatonigral, a pallidonigral and a striatopallidal pathway. Other striatal and pallidal output neurons with known putative neurotransmitters include: a striatonigral and a pallidonigral substance P-containing system, and a striatopallidal enkephalin-containing pathway. At least three neurochemically defined inputs to the striatum are known at present: the corticostriatal glutamate pathway; the raphe-striatal 5-hydroxytryptamine system; and the mesotelencephalic (nigrostriatal) dopamine pathway.

Neuropharmacological and clinical observations suggest that in the striatum the dopaminergic input system and the intrinsic cholinergic neurons are functionally interrelated; the proper balance between these two functionally opposing systems seems to be essential for the normal functioning of the striatum as a whole[4, 7, 60]. Increased dopamine function or decreased acetylcholine activity in the striatum has been shown to result in increased locomotion, hyperkinetic behaviour and hypotonia of the skeletal muscles; in contrast, striatal dopamine deficiency and/or cholinergic hyperfunction produce hypokinesia, catalepsy, rigidity of the skeletal muscles and tremor[36]. It seems that in this dopamine–acetylcholine interplay the role of some of the GABA-containing striatonigral projections is to inhibit the activity of the nigrostriatal dopamine neurons[67].

Figure 4.1 Simplified representation of some of the known neurotransmitter systems within the basal ganglia complex. Those neurons (in the striatum and substantia nigra) that are shown to give rise to more than one neurochemically defined (or questionable) pathway have to be visualized as representing distinct and separate neuronal systems. The probable neurophysiological effects of the indicated putative neurotransmitters are: (+) excitatory; (−) inhibitory; (?) = the neurophysiological effect of a putative neurotransmitter, or the origin of the fibre system, not yet established; the interrupted lines are fibre systems whose neurotransmitters are as yet unknown. Abbreviations: ACh = acetylcholine; CTX = cortex cerebri; DA = dopamine; Enk = enkephalin(s); GABA = γ-aminobutyric acid; Glu = glutamic acid; GP 1 = globus pallidus, external part; GP 2 = globus pallidus, internal part; 5-HT = serotonin; LC = locus ceruleus; NA = noradrenaline; RD = dorsal raphe nucleus; RF = reticular formation of the lower brainstem; RN = raphe nuclei; SN_r^c = substantia nigra, compact/reticular zone; SpC = spinal cord; STH = subthalamic nucleus; STR = striatum (caudate + putamen); TH = thalamus.

BASAL GANGLIA DOPAMINE METABOLISM IN PARKINSON'S DISEASE

The most prominent and pathophysiologically important neurochemical change in Parkinson's disease is the severe reduction of all presynaptic neurochemical indices of dopamine neurons in practically all telencephalic areas normally receiving significant dopaminergic innervation (*see* reviews[35, 37-39]). This conspicuous loss of telencephalic dopamine can be directly attributed to the loss of dopamine cell bodies in the substantia nigra and the adjoining areas (paranigral nucleus) of the midbrain tegmentum which is the most characteristic morphological features of Parkinson's disease[32] (*see* Chapter 3). It is now well established that the perikarya located in the zona compacta of the substantia nigra and an area adjacent to the substantia nigra (area A 10 of Dahlström and Fuxe) give rise to a dopamine-containing fibre system densely innervating the striatum, nucleus accumbens, olfactory areas and limbic cortex[30, 62]. *Figure 4.2* shows schematically the mesotelencephalic dopamine system in the human brain, constructed from data obtained in a series of corresponding postmortem studies[12, 13, 25, 28, 34, 53, 68]. The importance of damage to this mesotelencephalic dopamine system for the symptomatology of Parkinson's disease follows from animal experiments showing that elimination of the nigral dopamine input to the basal ganglia (either by lesions or neuroleptic drugs such as reserpine or phenothiazine and butyrophenone derivatives) is very effective is disrupting normal basal ganglia function[42, 78]. As mentioned above, experimentally induced striatal dopamine deficiency leads, both in laboratory animals and man, to symptoms (akinesia, rigidity, tremor) typical of Parkinson's disease[36].

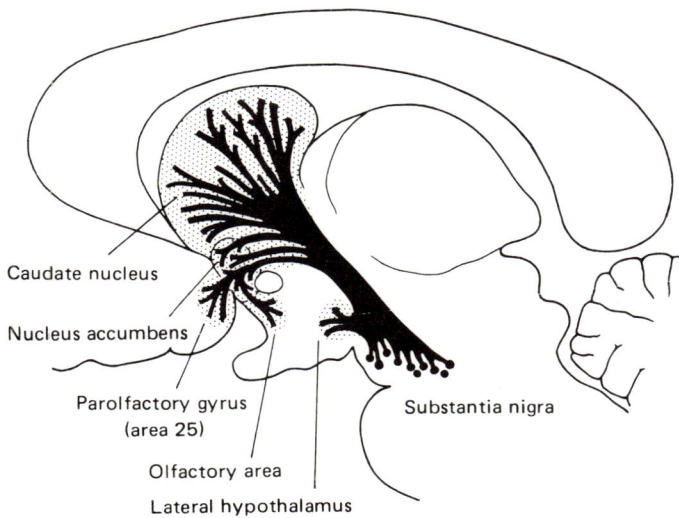

Figure 4.2 Schematic representation of the mesotelencephalitic dopamine system in the human brain, projected into a paramedian sagittal plane. Note that the term 'substantia nigra' includes all dopamine containing mesencephalic cell groups; the term 'caudate nucleus' stands for the striatum (caudate + putamen) and globus pallidus.

Dopamine and homovanillic acid

Striatopallidonigral system

The concentration of dopamine and its main metabolite homovanillic acid is severely reduced in the caudate nucleus, putamen, substantia nigra and globus pallidus of patients with Parkinson's disease[10, 12, 13, 25, 26, 34, 53, 68, 71] (*Table 4.1*). Subnormal striatal dopamine levels have been measured in cases with postencephalitic, idiopathic and arteriosclerotic parkinsonism as well as manganese encephalopathy presenting with parkinsonian symptomatology[13] (*Table 4.2*). This suggests that in principle the reduction of dopamine in the striatum is independent of the aetiology of the parkinsonian condition, the common denominator being the degree of neuronal cell loss in the zona compacta of the substantia nigra. This point is illustrated by the observation (*see Table 4.2*) that in postencephalitic parkinsonism the dopamine depletion is especially severe and of similar magnitude both in the caudate nucleus and putamen; in contrast, in the idiopathic variety the reduction of dopamine is in general less severe, being more marked in putamen than in the caudate nucleus[13, 25]. This difference corresponds to the fact that in general in postencephalitic parkinsonism the nigral cell loss is both severe and diffuse; this is in contrast to the milder and more discrete cell loss in idiopathic parkinsonism affecting predominantly those portions of the substantia nigra, i.e. the caudal,[13, 32] which are known to project preferentially to the putamen[13].

Internal capsule

In addition to the changes in the nuclei of the basal ganglia, the homovanillic acid concentration in the different parts of the internal capsule situated between the substantia nigra and the striatal nuclei is also markedly reduced thus marking the course of the degenerated nigrostriatal pathway[41].

Limbic forebrain regions

Especially noteworthy are the recent observations that apart from the changes in striatal dopamine, in Parkinson's disease there also is a marked reduction of dopamine levels in several limbic forebrain regions, including the nucleus accumbens, the lateral hypothalamus and the cortical region of the parolfactory gyrus (area 25 in Brodmann's classification)[28, 68] (*see Table 4.1*). Significantly, the degree of dopamine loss in these limbic regions is approximately of the same magnitude as in caudate nucleus and putamen.

Quantitative aspects of the disturbed dopamine metabolism

On a quantitative basis, the average reduction in Parkinson's disease of homovanillic acid in the striatal nuclei and limbic forebrain regions is distinctly less severe

Table 4.1 Dopamine (DA), homovanillic acid (HVA), L-tyrosine hydroxylase (TH) and L-dopa decarboxylase (DDC) in discrete brain regions of control and parkinsonian patients*

Brain region	DA (µg/g wet tissue)	HVA (µg/g wet tissue)	TH (nmol CO_2/ 0.5 h/100 mg protein)[53]	DDC (nmol CO_2/ 2 h/100 mg protein)[53]
Putamen[53]				
Controls	5.06 ± 0.39 (17)	4.92 ± 0.32 (16)	17.4 ± 2.4 (3)	431.7 ± 109.1 (13)
Parkinson	0.14 ± 0.13 (3)	0.54 ± 0.13 (3)	3.1 ± 1.2 (3)	32.3 ± 7.1 (13)
Caudate nucleus[53]				
Controls	4.06 ± 0.47 (18)	2.92 ± 0.37 (19)	18.7 ± 2.0 (3)	364.0 ± 95.4 (19)
Parkinson	0.20 ± 0.19 (3)	1.19 ± 0.10 (3)	3.2 ± 0.5 (3)	54.3 ± 14.0 (13)
Globus pallidus				
Controls	0.5 (6)[25]	2.25 (8)[10]	3.5 (1)	22.1 ± 2.7 (9)
Parkinson	0.2 (4)[25]	0.72 (9)[10]	1.7 ± 0.2 (3)	18.0 ± 2.6 (12)
Substantia nigra				
Controls	0.46 (13)[34]	2.32 (7)[10]	17.4 (1)	549.3 ± 293.7 (15)
Parkinson	0.07 (10)[34]	0.41 (9)[10]	6.1 ± 1.5 (3)	21.4 ± 6.0 (10)
Nucleus accumbens[68]				
Controls	3.79 ± 0.82 (8)	4.38 ± 0.64 (8)	–	–
Parkinson	1.61 ± 0.28 (4)	3.13 ± 0.13 (3)	–	–
Lateral hypothalamus[68]				
Controls	0.51 ± 0.08 (4)	1.96 ± 0.28 (3)	–	–
Parkinson	<0.03 (2)	1.03 ± 0.23 (3)	–	–
Parolfactory gyrus[68]				
Controls	0.35 ± 0.09 (4)	0.98 (2)	–	–
Parkinson	0.03 (2)	–	–	–

*All results are expressed as mean ± s.e. (where applicable). Numbers of cases in parentheses. Superscript numbers are references from which data are taken.

Table 4.2 Striatal dopamine (DA) and homovanillic acid (HVA) and diagnostic subgroups of Parkinson's disease

Diagnostic subgroup (no. of cases)	Caudate*		Putamen*	
	DA	HVA	DA	HVA
Aetiological subgroups[13]				
Postencephalitic (6)	2	9	1	9
Idiopathic (13)	16	32	2	21
Arteriosclerotic (5)	32	60	15	44
'Manganese parkinsonism' (1)	13	–	1	–
Hemiparkinsonism (right side (1)[6]				
Right striatum	38	–	25	–
Left striatum	17	–	3	–

*Per cent of control.

than the loss of dopamine (*see Table 4.1*); this is expressed in a marked shift of the molar ratio dopamine:homovanillic acid in favour of the metabolite[10]. A comparable shift of this ratio has been observed in animals with experimental lesions of the substantia nigra[74] or animals treated with dopamine receptor blockers (phenothiazines, butyrophenones)[3, 47], most probably indicating an increased dopamine turnover (synthesis and release) in the functioning dopamine neurons remaining.

Dopamine synthesizing enzymes

The disturbance of dopamine metabolism in Parkinson's disease is accompanied by an analogous reduction of the activity of the synthesizing enzymes tyrosine hydroxylase (tyrosine 3-monooxygenase) and dopa decarboxylase (aromatic L-amino-acid decarboxylase) in the basal ganglia and substantia nigra[51, 53, 64] (*see Table 4.1*). Since in one study[53] the reduction of tyrosine hydroxylase activity in the parkinsonian striatum was less severe than the decrease of dopa decarboxylase activity (*see Table 4.1*), it is possible that in the parkinsonian condition there is an induction of the rate-limiting enzyme, and consequently increased dopamine synthesis rate, in the still-functioning dopamine neurons. Considered together with the shifting of the dopamine:homovanillic acid ratio in favour of the latter, this may indicate an increased turnover of dopamine in the remaining dopamine neurons. (*See below* for the functional significance of this possibility).

COMPENSATORY DOPAMINERGIC CHANGES IN THE PARKINSONIAN STRIATUM

In analogy to the changes known to occur in denervated tissues, the severe dopaminergic denervation of the parkinsonian striatum seems to elicit compensatory mechanisms, both in the remaining dopamine neurons and at the level of the postsynaptic dopamine receptor sites[40].

Presynaptic changes in the remaining dopamine neurons

The presence of an overactivity of the remaining dopamine neurons is indicated by the above-mentioned observation of a shifting of the dopamine:homovanillic acid ratio in favour of the latter as well as the possibility of induction of tyrosine hydroxylase activity. In this respect, the induction of this enzyme activity may be the consequence of the overactivity of the corresponding dopamine neurons resulting in removal of the normally occurring end-product inhibition of this enzyme. The possibility of the remaining dopamine neurons being overactive in Parkinson's disease is supported by a study showing that in rats with partially lesioned substantia nigra there was an increased rate of dopamine formation (from ^{3}H-labelled tyrosine) in the ipsilateral striatum as compared with the striatum contralateral to the lesioned substantia nigra[1]. From the functional point of view, the development of overactivity of remaining neurons in partially denervated tissues represents an attempt to maintain normal function by compensating for the loss of a major part of a given neurotransmitter innervation.

Dopaminergic supersensitivity of the parkinsonian striatum

The existence of supersensitivity of the parkinsonian striatum to dopamine is indicated by clinical observations showing that (1) in contrast to parkinsonian patients, healthy volunteers are comparatively insensitive to central motor effects of dopaminomimetic drugs; (2) parkinsonian patients with more severe akinesia, and consequently higher degrees of striatal dopamine deficiency, responded more sensitively to a test dose of levodopa than less severely affected patients[13] (*Table 4.3*); and (3) in contrast to control subjects, parkinsonian patients easily 'overreact'

Table 4.3 Relationship between striatal dopamine (DA) and homovanillic acid (HVA) in parkinsonism and the severity of akinesia and sensitivity to levodopa (From data of Bernheimer *et al.*[13])

Clinical groupings	Caudate*		Putamen*	
	DA	HVA	DA	HVA
Severity of akinesia				
Mild	0.58 (13)	1.68 (12)	0.44 (13)	1.60 (12)
Marked	0.22 (9)	0.59 (7)	0.05 (9)	0.83 (7)
Sensitivity to i.v. levodopa				
High	0.02 (10)	0.12 (10)	0.01 (10)	0.21 (10)
Low	0.46 (10)	0.95 (10)	0.02 (10)	0.81 (10)
Controls (28)	2.64	3.23	3.44	4.29

*Results are means in µg/g fresh tissue; number of cases in parenthesis.

to dopamine substitution therapy with hyperkinetic (dyskinetic) behaviour which most likely is of striatal origin and responds to dopamine receptor blockade. The basis for this dopaminergic supersensitivity is most probably the fact that the majority of parkinsonian patients not receiving levodopa therapy have increased numbers of postsynaptic dopamine receptors (D-2 receptors, as measured by specific binding of ^{3}H-labelled neuroleptics to striatal membrane preparations) in their caudate nucleus and, more pronounced, in the putamen[48]. In this respect it is important to note that patients on prolonged levodopa regimen did not show this increase[48,70] and may even have a subnormal number of striatal dopamine receptors[69] (*see* Chapter 5).

The development of postsynaptic supersensitivity to dopamine together with the overactivity of the still-preserved neurons which synthesize and release increased amounts of dopamine per unit time, represents an effective compensatory mechanism aimed at a maximum degree of functional utilization of the endogenous dopamine in a condition characterized by a greatly reduced dopaminergic innervation.

In contrast to the striatal dopamine receptors specifically labelled with tritiated neuroleptics (D-2 receptors), the adenylate cyclase-coupled dopamine-sensitive sites (D-1 receptors) seem to be reduced in the parkinsonian striatum. Thus, in a recent study[75], the dopamine-stimulated activity of adenylate cyclase was only 18 per cent of control activity in the caudate nucleus, and 25 per cent of control in the putamen (see Chapter 5).

The functional significance of the disturbance of the adenylate cyclase-coupled dopamine-sensitive sites in the parkinsonian striatum is at present not clear. However, it may be that the opposite behaviour of the D-1 and D-2 sites is in some way related to the possibility of dopamine exerting opposite physiological effects in the striatum. From evidence obtained in behavioural experiments, the existence of separate excitatory and inhibitory striatal dopamine receptors has been proposed[17]; there is also neurophysiological evidence suggesting that the nigrostriatal dopamine fibres may exert either an excitatory[44] of inhibitory[15] influence on the firing rate of single units in the striatum. In view of this evidence it may be hypothesized that the adenylate cyclase-coupled dopamine-sensitive sites in the striatum normally subserve functions whose reduction in Parkinson's disease may be of functional advantage in compensating for the severe dopaminergic disturbance. In this context it is significant that the antiparkinsonian activity of dopamine-substituting agents seems to be mediated exclusively through the D-2 striatal sites[73].

RELATIONSHIP BETWEEN THE STRIATAL AND LIMBIC DOPAMINE DEFICIENCY AND PARKINSONIAN SYMPTOMATOLOGY

By way of simplification it can be said that the striatal and accumbens dopamine systems seem to subserve a 'kinetic' function in the brain. This is shown by a large body of pharmacological evidence indicating that (1) the striatal dopamine is critically involved in a variety of locomotor and stereotyped behaviours[16]; (2) pharmacologically induced changes of the accumbens dopamine are accompanied by marked changes of locomotor behaviour[43, 66].

In view of the ample pharmacological evidence on the 'kinetic' role of the forebrain dopamine, a relationship between its deficiency and some motor deficits in Parkinson's disease is to be expected. In this respect the following observations are especially noteworthy: (1) in a case of hemiparkinsonism the dopamine reduction was more pronounced in the striatum contralateral to the affected side of the body[6] (see Table 4.2); (2) in a clinical–biochemical study correlating the clinical symptoms with the changes in striatal dopamine, the degree of striatal dopamine (and homovanillic acid) deficiency was found to be positively correlated with the severity of akinesia[13] (see Table 4.3); and (3) levodopa, which is converted to dopamine in the brain and other organs, as well as direct-acting dopaminomimetic drugs penetrating the blood–brain barrier (apomorphine, bromocriptine, lisuride), are highly effective in improving the motor deficits, especially akinesia of Parkinson's disease. These observations strongly suggest a direct cause–effect relationship between the striatal dopamine deficiency and the main motor symptoms of Parkinson's disease. Considered together with the wealth of pharmacological evidence bearing on dopamine's role in extrapyramidal motor function, it seems justified to conclude that the deficiency in the striatum and nucleus accumbens is of crucial significance for the clinical manifestation of Parkinson's disease.

Since the disturbance of limbic forebrain mechanisms has been implicated in psychotic behaviour[56], it is possible that the disturbed dopamine metabolism in parkinsonian limbic brain regions, especially the parolfactory gyrus and lateral hypothalamus[68] (*see Table 4.1*), is involved in affective disturbances frequently seen in patients with Parkinson's disease.

STRIATAL DOPAMINE AND THE COMPENSATED AND DECOMPENSATED STAGES OF PARKINSON'S DISEASE

As shown in *Table 4.3* mild, clinically just-detectable symptoms of parkinsonism (especially akinesia) were associated with a disproportionately high degree of striatal dopamine deficiency; in these clinically mild cases the decrease of striatal dopamine exceeded the 80 per cent mark, i.e. only about 20 per cent or less dopamine remaining[13]. From this it may be concluded that smaller degrees of dopamine deficiency will not express themselves in clinically overt symptoms. As pointed out above, in the parkinsonian striatum the remaining presynaptic as well as the postsynaptic dopamine elements undergo biochemical changes aimed at functional compensation of the loss of the majority of dopaminergic innervation. In the beginning stages of Parkinson's disease these homeostatic mechanisms may suffice to fully compensate milder degrees of dopamine deficiency, with the overall result that the condition will remain clinically silent. This is also illustrated by the data obtained in a case of hemiparkinsonism[6] (*see Table 4.2*); although the levels in both striata were subnormal, the reduction of dopamine in the striatum ipsilateral to the side of symptoms apparently was not sufficient in magnitude to produce marked contralateral symptoms. Thus, from a neurochemical point of view, Parkinson's disease can be subdivided into two stages: (1) the compensated, clinically latent stage during which overactivity of the remaining dopamine neurons together with the development of receptor supersensitivity can offset the deterioration of function caused by the continuing decline of striatal dopamine; and (2) the stage of functional decompensation, that is the clinically overt syndrome, which manifests itself only when the degree of neuronal loss and the resulting deficiency exceed the compensatory capacity of the basal ganglia. It is quite probable that in postencephalitic parkinsonism these compensatory changes play an important role for the usually prolonged latency period between the encephalitic event and the manifestation of clinical symptomatology. From the above observations it follows that the main pharmacological feature of specific antiparkinsonian drugs should be the ability to revert the decompensated stage of the striatal dopamine deficiency syndrome to that of functional compensation.

DYSFUNCTION OF NEUROTRANSMITTER SYSTEMS OTHER THAN DOPAMINE

In view of the complex pattern of chemically distinct, but functionally interrelated, neuronal circuits in the basal ganglia (*see Figure 4.1*), it is likely that derangement of any one of these neurotransmitter systems will elicit a 'chain reaction', altering the functional state of other interrelated neuronal systems. Therefore, the severe striatal dopamine dysfunction in Parkinson's disease is likely to upset the neurotransmitter homeostasis within the basal ganglia resulting in changes in interrelated neurostransmitter systems.

Although the severe striatal DA deficiency has to be regarded as the most significant neurochemical alteration in the parkinsonian brain, decreased concentrations of striatal and nigral 5-hydroxytryptamine[11, 71], the GABA-synthesizing enzyme glutamic acid decarboxylase[9, 52, 55, 58, 61, 71], as well as noradrenaline in substantia nigra and nucleus accumbens (and other limbic/hypothalamic regions)[27], have been found in Parkinson's disease (*Table 4.4*). In the substantia nigra and hippocampus the number of specific GABA-binding sites (GABA receptors) was also found to be reduced[54, 72]. Since dopamine seems to exert an inhibitory effect on the striatal cholinergic neurons[8], loss of this dopamine inhibition in Parkinson's

Table 4.4 Noradrenaline (NA), serotonin (5-HT), glutamic acid decarboxylase (GAD) and choline acetyltransferase (CAT) in discrete brain regions of control and parkinsonism patients*

Brain region	NA (μg/g wet tissue)	5-HT (μg/g wet tissue)[11]	GAD (nmol CO_2/h/mg protein)[52]	CAT (pmol/min/mg protein)[55]
Putamen				
Controls	0.10 ± 0.01 (12)[27]	0.32 (6)	622 ± 110 (3)	1656 (3)
Parkinson	0.05 (6)[25]	0.14 (5)	292 (2)	780 (3)
Caudate nucleus				
Controls	0.09 ± 0.01 (11)[27]	0.33 (6)	659 ± 93 (13)	1460 (3)
Parkinson	0.04 (6)[25]	0.12 (5)	321 (2)	694 (3)
Globus pallidus				
Controls	0.06 ± 0.02 (13)[71]	0.23 (6)	553 ± 15 (13)	231 (2)
Parkinson	0.05 ± 0.03 (5)[71]	0.13 (5)	388 (2)	39 (3)
Substantia nigra				
Controls	0.23 ± 0.05 (9)[27]	0.55 (6)	637 ± 149 (13)	63 (6)
Parkinson	0.11 ± 0.03 (3)[27]	0.26 (5)	263 (2)	12 (3)
Nucleus accumbens				
Controls	1.29 ± 0.14 (7)[27]	–	–	–
Parkinson	0.52 ± 0.11 (4)[27]	–	–	–
Hypothalamus				
Controls	1.83 ± 0.25 (4)[27]	0.29 (6)	–	–
Parkinson	0.33 ± 0.09 (4)[27]	0.12 (5)	–	–

*All results are expressed as means ± s.e. (where applicable). Numbers of cases in parentheses. Superscript numbers are references from which data are taken.

disease can be expected to result in a (functional) cholinergic hyperactivity; in this respect, the activity of the acetylcholine synthesizing choline acetyltransferase has been reported to be either unchanged[58] or subnormal[55] (*Table 4.4*).

Serotonin and γ-aminobutyric acid

In respect to 5-hydroxytryptamine and GABA there is evidence to show that both these putative striatal neurotransmitters exert an inhibitory influence on motor behaviour, most probably by inhibiting the activity of the nigrostriatal dopamine system at the level of the substantia nigra[2, 31, 33, 46, 57, 76]. Therefore, neuronal activity of the 5-hydroxytryptamine and GABA systems in the parkinsonian basal ganglia may aggravate the parkinsonian condition by further inhibiting the already largely reduced dopaminergic influence on the striatum. It is therefore possible that the reduction of 5-hydroxytryptamine and glutamic acid decarboxylase is the result of an homeostatic down-regulation of these neuronal systems so as to permit the remaining nigrostriatal dopamine neurons to function at the highest possible level.

Acetylcholine

In contrast to 5-hydroxytryptamine and GABA, the functional consequence of the probable cholinergic hyperactivity in the parkinsonian striatum may be a direct aggravation of the main symptoms of the disease, especially akinesia and rigidity. It is known that cholinergic drugs produce an akinetic-rigid syndrome (catalepsy) in animals[36] and worsen the corresponding symptoms in patients with Parkinson's disease[24]. In this respect, the reported subnormal activity of the acetylcholine synthesizing enzyme choline acetyltransferase in the parkinsonian striatum (*see Table 4.4*) has been interpreted as representing an attempt to reduce this aggravating influence of striatal acetylcholine by reduction of its biosynthesis[50].

Noradrenaline

Especially important is the observation of reduced noradrenaline levels in many forebrain areas of the parkinsonian brain, including dopamine-rich regions such as nucleus accumbens and substantia nigra[27] (*see Table 4.4*). It seems safe to assume that the widespread decrease of brain noradrenaline in Parkinson's disease is the result of degeneration of the neurons in the locus ceruleus[32]. These noradrenaline-containing neurons have been shown to diffusely innervate many parts of the brain[30, 63]; their loss in Parkinson's disease is indicated by a corresponding reduction of noradrenaline levels in the locus coeruleus[27].

The reduction of the coeruleus noradrenaline in Parkinson's disease is important because recent evidence suggests that this subdivision of the noradrenaline fibre system exerts a facilitatory effect on the dopaminergically controlled motor behaviour; this is in contrast to the non-coeruleus noradrenaline fibres which are thought to inhibit the activity of the dopaminergic forebrain mechanisms[22, 45]. The marked reduction of the coeruleus noradrenaline fibre system in Parkinson's disease can, therefore, be expected to aggravate the motor deficits due to dopamine deficiency, because loss of the coeruleus noradrenaline will not only weaken the noradrenaline–dopamine synergy but also tip the balance in favour of a functional predominance of the inhibitory non-coeruleus noradrenaline. It is obvious that these circumstances will play an important role for the clinical effectiveness of dopamine-substituting drug therapy. (Since in Parkinson's disease there is a marked loss of noradrenaline in the hypothalamus[27], parts of the non-coeruleus noradrenaline system also seem to be involved in this disorder; in the rat, the major noradrenaline input to the hypothalamus seems to come from the non-coeruleus cell groups of the pons–medulla region[49, 77].

CLINICAL RELEVANCE OF NEUROTRANSMITTER CHANGES IN PARKINSON'S DISEASE

The direct consequence of the discovery of striatal dopamine deficiency in Parkinson's disease was the introduction of levodopa as the most efficacious antiparkinsonian agent available[5, 14]. This discovery also served as rationale[19] for the later clinical trials leading to the presently used high-dose oral levodopa regimen[18].

The following observations strongly support the view that the levodopa treatment of Parkinson's disease represents a dopamine substitution therapy: (1) as such, levodopa is a pharmacologically inert substance and blockade of its metabolism to dopamine inhibits most of its biological effects; (2) patients receiving prolonged high-dose oral levodopa therapy had higher striatal dopamine and homovanillic acid levels than untreated patients[53, 71] (*Table 4.5*); (3) good responders to levodopa accumulated more dopamine in their striatal nuclei than poor responders[53] (*Table 4.5*); and (4) compounds that act directly on brain dopamine receptors (direct-acting dopaminomimetic agents such as apomorphine, bromocriptine, lisuride and many others) possess antiparkinsonian activity qualitatively

Table 4.5 Levodopa effect on striatal dopamine (DA) and homovanillic acid (HVA) in patients with Parkinson's disease – relationship to therapeutic response (from data of Lloyd et al.[53])

Clinical groupings	Caudate		Putamen	
	DA	HVA	DA	HVA
Untreated (3)	0.20 ± 0.19	1.19 ± 0.10	0.14 ± 0.13	0.54 ± 0.13
Levodopa 2–9 h before death (5)	1.57 ± 0.78	7.67 ± 2.48	1.68 ± 0.68	10.19 ± 3.17
Therapeutic response to levodopa				
Good (3)	1.85	–	1.16	–
Poor (3)	0.22	–	0.05	–

*Results (in µg/g wet weight) are means ± s.e.; number of cases in parenthesis.

identical to that of levodopa. In respect to the last point, it is noteworthy that the antiparkinsonian effects of lisuride are elicited without any significant delay in time when the drug is administered intravenously[65]; this is quite analogous to the prompt effect of intravenously injected levodopa in particularly sensitive (i.e. postencephalitic) cases as reported 20 years ago in one of the original clinical studies[14].

Of particular significance for the clinical effectiveness of levodopa and the direct-acting dopaminomimetic agents, has to be regarded the increased sensitivity of the parkinsonian striatum to dopamine. Most importantly, the supersensitivity of the dopaminergically denervated forebrain structures confers a high degree of regional specificity on the pharmacological effects of dopamine substitution therapy in Parkinson's disease. This most likely is the decisive factor responsible for the specific antiparkinsonian activity of dopaminomimetic drugs, which essentially is confined to the forebrain regions affected in Parkinson's disease, and also may explain the comparative lack of (motor) effects of these drugs in healthy volunteers. The development, in the course of dopamine substitution therapy, of abnormal involuntary movements (dyskinesia), a symptom that also is not readily elicited in normals, may in part have the same pathophysiological basis.

Another clinically highly relevant observation is that chronic levodopa administration abolishes the increased number of striatal dopamine receptors indicating, in functional terms, loss of supersensitivity to dopamine. This loss of dopaminergic supersensitivity during chronic substitution therapy can be expected to have at least two clinically unfavourable consequences: (1) loss of therapeutic potency which is a function of the sensitivity of the parkinsonian striatum to dopamine; and (2) loss of the regional specificity of the dopaminomimetic effect of the antiparkinsonian agents, probably resulting in the emergence of extra-striatal side effects. In addition, the accumulation of dopamine (derived from exogenous sources) in the synaptic area will also tend to reduce the overactivity of the still-functioning dopamine neurons, thus abolishing this functionally important compensatory mechanism. From this point of view, dopamine-substituting agents, especially levodopa, can be regarded as self-limiting drugs[40]. In order to restore the sensitivity of the parkinsonian basal ganglia to dopaminergic stimulation, drug-free intervals (drug holidays) have been suggested[48]. Recent clinical reports seem to confirm the expectation that temporary discontinuation of levodopa therapy in patients with diminishing response, restores the therapeutic efficacy of dopamine-substituting agents[20, 21, 79]. Unfortunately, however, stopping levodopa often causes severe clinical deterioration, which can be both agonizing and dangerous for the patient. Moreover, although there may be initial improvement after reinstituting levodopa, often at a lower dosage, subsequently the patient gradually returns to his former state.

References

1 AGID, Y., JAVOY, F. and GLOWINSKI, J. Hyperactivity of remaining dopaminergic neurones after partial destruction of the nigro-striatal dopaminergic system in the rat. *Nature*, **245**, 150–151 (1973)

2 ANDÉN, N.-E. Inhibition of the turnover of the brain dopamine after treatment with the γ-aminobutyrate: 2-oxyglutarate transaminase inhibitor aminooxyacetic acid. *Archives of Pharmacology*, **283,** 419–424 (1974)

3 ANDÉN, N. E., ROOS, B. E. and WERDINIUS, B. Effects of chlorpromazine, haloperidol and reserpine on the levels of phenolic acids in rabbit corpus striatum. *Life Sciences*, **3,** 149–158 (1964)

4 BARBEAU, A. The pathogenesis of Parkinson's disease. A new hypothesis. *Canadian Medical Association Journal*, **87,** 802–807 (1962)

5 BARBEAU, A., SOURKES, T. L. and MURPHY, G. Les catécholamines dans la maladie de Parkinson. In *Monoamines et Système Nerveux Central*, edited by J. de A-juriaguerra, 247–262. Paris, Georg, Génève and Masson (1962)

6 BAROLIN, G. S., BERNHEIMER, H. and HORNYKIEWICZ, O. Seitenverschiedenes Verhalten des Dopamins (3-Hydroxytyramin) im Gehirn eines Falles von Hemiparkinsonismus. *Schweizer Archiv für Neurologie und Psychiatrie*, **94,** 241–248 (1964)

7 BARTHOLINI, G. Interaction of striatal dopaminergic, cholinergic and GABA-ergic neurons: relation to extrapyramidal function. *Trends in Pharmacological Sciences*, **1,** 138–141 (1980)

8 BARTHOLINI, G., STADLER, H. and LLOYD, K. G. Cholinergic-dopamingergic interrergulations within the extrapyramidal systems. In *Cholinergic Mechanisms*, edited by P. G. Waser, 411–418. New York, Raven Press (1975)

9 BERNHEIMER, H. and HORNYKIEWICZ, O. Das Verhalten einiger Enzyme im Gehirn normaler und Parkinson-kranker Menschen. *Archiv für Experimentelle Pathologie und Pharmakologie*, **243,** 295 (1962)

10 BERNHEIMER, H. and HORNYKIEWICZ, O. Herabgesetzte Konzentration der Homovanillinsäure im Gehirn von Parkinsonkranken Menschen als Ausdruck der Störung des zentralen Dopaminstoffwechsels. *Klinische Wochenschrift*, **43,** 711–715 (1965)

11 BERNHEIMER, H., BIRKMAYER, W. and HORNYKIEWICZ, O. Verteilung des 5-Hydroxytryptamins (Serotonin) im Gehirn des Menschen und sein Verhalten bei Patienten mit Parkinson-Sydrom. *Klinische Wochenschrift*, **39,** 1056–1059 (1961)

12 BERNHEIMER, H., BIRKMAYER, W. and HORNYKIEWICZ, O. Zur Biochemie des Parkinsonsyndroms des Menschen. *Klinische Wochenschrift*, **41,** 564–569 (1963)

13 BERNHEIMER, H., BIRKMAYER, W., HORNYKIEWICZ, O., JELLINGER, K. and SEITELBERGER, F. Brain dopamine and the syndromes of Parkinson and Huntington. *Journal of Neurological Sciences*, **20,** 415–455 (1973)

14 BIRKMAYER, W. and HORNYKIEWICZ, O. Der L-Dioxyphenylalanin (= L-DOPA) – Effekt bei der Parkinson-Akinese. *Wiener Klinische Wochenschrift*, **73,** 787–788 (1961)

15 CONNOR, J. D. Caudate nucleus neurones: correlation of the effects of substantia nigra stimulation with iontophoretic dopamine. *Journal of Physiology*, **208,** 691–706 (1970)

16 COOLS, A. R. *The Caudate Nucleus and Neurochemical Control of Behavior*, Nijmegen, Brakkenstein (1973)

17 COOLS, A. R. and VAN ROSSUM, J. M. Excitation-mediating and inhibition-mediating dopamine-receptors: a new concept towards a better understanding of electrophysiological, biochemical, pharmacological, functional and clinical data. *Psychopharmacologia*, **45,** 243–254 (1976)

18 COTZIAS, G. C., VAN WOERT, M. H. and SCHIFFER, L. M. Aromatic amino acids and modification of parkinsonism. *New England Journal of Medicine*, **276**, 374–379 (1967)

19 COTZIAS, G. C., PAPAVASILIOU, P. S., VAN WOERT, M. H. and SAKAMOTO, A. Melanogenesis and extrapyramidal disease. *Federation Proceedings*, **23**, 713–718 (1964)

20 DIRENFELD, L., SPERO, L., MAROTTA, J. and SEEMAN, P. The L-dopa on-off effect in Parkinson disease: treatment by transient drug withdrawal and dopamine receptor resensitization. *Annals of Neurology*, **4**, 573–575 (1978)

21 DIRENFELD, L. K., FELDMAN, R. G., ALEXANDER, M. P. and KELLY-HAYES, M. Is L-dopa drug holiday useful? *Neurology*, **30**, 785–788 (1980)

22 DONALDSON, I. MacG., DOLPHIN, A. C., JENNER, P., PYCOCK, C. and MARSDEN, C. D. Rotational behaviour produced in rats by unilateral electrolytic lesions of the ascending noradrenergic bundles. *Brain Research*, **138**, 487–509 (1978)

23 DRAY, A. The physiology and pharmacology of mammalian basal ganglia. *Progress in Neurobiology*, **14**, 221–335 (1980)

24 DUVOISIN, R. C. Cholinergic-anticholinergic antagonism in parkinsonism. *Archives of Neurology*, **17**, 124–136 (1967)

25 EHRINGER, H. and HORNYKIEWICZ, O. Verteilung von Noradrenalin und Dopamin (3-Hydroxytyramin) im Gehirn des Menschen und ihr Verhalten bei Erkrankungen des extrapyramidalen Systems. *Klinische Wochenschrift*, **38**, 1238–1239 (1960)

26 FAHN, S., LIBSCH, L. R. and CUTLER, R. W. Monoamines in the human neostriatum. Topographic distribution in normals and in Parkinson's disease and their role in akinesia, chorea and tremor. *Journal of Neurological Sciences*, **14**, 427–455 (1971)

27 FARLEY, I. J. and HORNYKIEWICZ, O. Noradrenaline in subcortical brain regions of patients with Parkinson's disease and control subjects. In *Advances in Parkinsonism*, edited by W. Birkmayer and O. Hornykiewicz, 178–185. Basal, Editiones Roche (1976)

28 FARLEY, I. J., PRICE, K. S. and HORNYKIEWICZ, O. Dopamine in the limbic regions of the human brain: normal and abnormal. *Advances in Biochemical Psychopharmacology*, **16**, 57–64 (1977)

29 FONNUM, F. and WALAAS, I. Localization of neurotransmitter candidates in neostriatum. In *The Neostriatum*, edited by I. Divac and R. G. E. Öberg, 53–69. Oxford, Pergamon Press (1979)

30 FUXE, K., HÖKFELT, T. and UNGERSTEDT, U. Morphological and functional aspects of central monoamine neurons. *International Reviews in Neurobiology*, **13**, 93–126 (1970)

31 GRABOWSKA, M. and MICHALUK, J. On the role of serotonin in apomorphine-induced locomotor stimulation in rats. *Pharmacology, Biochemistry and Behaviour*, **2**, 263–266 (1974)

32 HASSLER, R. Zur Pathologie der Paralysis agitans und des postenzephalitischen Parkinsonismus. *Journal für Psychologie und Neurologie (Leipzig)*, **48**, 387–476 (1938)

33 HOLLISTER, A. S., BREESE, G. R., KUHN, C. M. and COOPER, B. R. An inhibitory role for brain serotonin-containing systems in the locomotor effects of d-amphetamine. *Journal of Pharmacology and Experimental Therapeutics*, **198**, 12–22 (1976)

34 HORNYKIEWICZ, O. Die topische Lokalisation und das Verhalten von Noradrenalin und Dopamin (3-Hydroxytyramin) in der Substantia nigra des normalen und Parkinsonkranken Menschen. *Wiener Klinische Wochenschrift*, **75**, 309–312 (1963)

35 HORNYKIEWICZ, O. Dopamine (3-hydroxytyramine) and brain function. *Pharmacological Reviews*, **18**, 925–962 (1966)

36 HORNYKIEWICZ, O. Biochemical and pharmacological aspects of akinesia. In *Parkinson's Disease*, edited by J. Siegfried, 128–149. Berne, H. Huber (1972)

37 HORNYKIEWICZ, O. Parkinson's disease: from brain homogenate to treatment. *Federation Proceedings*, **32**, 183–190 (1973)

38 HORNYKIEWICZ, O. Dopamine in the basal ganglia: its role and therapeutic implications. *British Medical Bulletin*, **29**, 172–178 (1973)

39 HORNYKIEWICZ, O. Brain dopamine in Parkinson's disease and other neurological disturbances. In *The Neurobiology of Dopamine*, edited by A. S. Horn, J. Korf and B. H. C. Westerink, 633–654 London, Academic Press (1979)

40 HORNYKIEWICZ, O. Compensatory biochemical changes at the striatal dopamine synapse in Parkinson's disease – limitations of L-dopa therapy. *Advances in Neurology*, **24**, 275–281 (1979)

41 HORNYKIEWICZ, O. LISCH, H. J. and SPRINGER, A. Homovanillic acid in different regions of the human brain: attempt at localizing central dopamine fibres. *Brain Research*, **11**, 662–671 (1968)

42 IVERSEN, S. D. Brain dopamine systems and behaviour. In *Handbook of Psychopharmacology*, **8**, edited by L. L. Iversen, S. D. Iversen and S. H. Snyder, 333–384. New York and London, Plenum Publ. Corp. (1977)

43 IVERSEN, S. D. and KOOB, G. F. Behavioral implications of dopaminergic neurons in the mesolimbic system. *Advances in Biochemical Psychopharmacology*, **16**, 209–214 (1977)

44 KITAI, S. T., SUGIMORI, M. and KOCSIS, J. D. Excitatory nature of dopamine in the nigro-caudate pathway. *Experimental Brain Research*, **24**, 351–363 (1976)

45 KOSTOWSKI, W., JERLICZ, M., BIDZINSKI, A. and HAUPTMANN, M. Evidence for existence of two opposite noradrenergic brain systems controlling behavior. *Psychopharmacologia*, **59**, 311–312 (1978)

46 LAHTI, R. A. and LOSEY, E. G. Antagonism of the effects of chlorpromazine and morphine on dopamine metablism by GABA. *Research Communications in Chemical Pathology and Pharmacology*, **7**, 31–40 (1974)

47 LAVERTY, R. and SHARMAN, D. F. The estimation of small quantities of 3,4-dihydroxyphenylethylamine in tissue. *British Journal of Pharmacology*, **24**, 538–548 (1965)

48 LEE, T., SEEMAN, P., RAJPUT, A., FARLEY, I. J. and HORNYKIEWICZ, O. Receptor basis for dopaminergic supersensitivity in Parkinson's disease. *Nature*, **273**, 59–61 (1978)

49 LINDVALL, O. and BJÖRKLUND, A. The organization of the ascending catecholamine neuron systems in the rat brain. *Acta Physiologica Scandinavica*, suppl. **412**, 1–48 (1974)

50 LLOYD, K. G. CNS compensation to dopamine neuron loss in Parkinson's disease. In *Parkinson's Disease*, edited by F. S. Messiha and A. D. Kenny, 255–266. New York, Plenum Press (1977)

51 LLOYD, K. G. and HORNYKIEWICZ, O. Parkinson's disease: activity of L-DOPA decarboxylase in discrete brain regions. *Science*, **170,** 1212–1213 (1970)

52 LLOYD, K. G. and HORNYKIEWICZ, O. L-glutamic acid decarboxylase in Parkinson's disease: effect of L-dopa therapy. *Nature*, **243,** 521–523 (1973)

53 LLOYD, K. G., DAVIDSON, L. and HORNYKIEWICZ, O. The neurochemistry of Parkinson's disease: effect of L-dopa therapy. *Journal of Pharmacology and Experimental Therapeutics*, **195,** 453–464 (1975)

54 LLOYD, K. G., SHEMAN, L. and HORNYKIEWICZ, O. Distribution of high affinity sodium-independent (^{3}H) gamma-aminobutyric acid ([^{3}H]-GABA) binding in the human brain: alterations in Parkinson's disease. *Brain Research*, **127,** 269–278 (1977)

55 LLOYD, K. G., MÖHLER, H., HERTZ, PH. and BARTHOLINI, G. Distribution of choline acetyltransferase and glutamic acid decarboxylase within the substantia nigra and other brain regions from control and parkinsonian patients. *Journal of Neurochemistry*, **25,** 789–795 (1975)

56 MacLEAN, P. The limbic brain in relation to the psychoses. In *Physiological Correlates of Emotion*, edited by P. Black, 129–146. New York, Academic Press (1970)

57 MAJ, J., PAWLOWSKI, L and SARNEK, J. The role of brain 5-hydroxytryptamine in the central action of L-dopa. *Advances in Biochemical Psychopharmacology*, **10,** 253–256 (1974)

58 McGEER, P. L., McGEER, E. G. and FIBIGER, H. C. Glutamic acid decarboxylase and choline acetylase in Huntington's chorea and Parkinson's disease. *Lancet*, **2,** 623–624 (1973)

59 McGEER, P. L., McGEER, E. G. and HATTORI, T. Biochemical interactions in the basal ganglia. *Progress in Brain Research*, **51,** 285–301 (1979)

60 McGEER, P. L., BOULDING, J. E., GIBSON, W. C. and FOULKES, R. G. Drug-induced extrapyramidal reactions. *Journal of the American Medical Assocation*, **177,** 665–670 (1961)

61 McGEER, P. L., McGEER, E. G., WADA, J. A. and JUNG, E. Effects of globus pallidus lesions and Parkinson's disease on brain glutamic acid decarboxylase. *Brain Research*, **32,** 425–431 (1971)

62 MOORE, R. Y. and BLOOM, F. E. Central catecholamine neuron systems: anatomy and physiology of the dopamine systems. *Annual Review of Neurosciences*, **1,** 129–169 (1978)

63 MOORE, R. Y. and BLOOM, F. E. Central catecholamine neuron systems: anatomy and physiology of the norepinephrine and epinephrine systems. *Annual Review of Neurosciences*, **2,** 113–168 (1979)

64 NAGATSU, T., KATO, T., NUMATA (SUDA), Y., IKUTA, K., SANO, M., NAGATSU, I., KONDO, Y., INAGAKI, S. LIZUKA, R., HORI, A. and NARABAYASHI, H. Phenylethanolamine N-methyltransferase and other enzymes of catecholamine metabolism in human brain. *Clinica Chimica Acta*, **75,** 221–232 (1977)

65 PARKES, J. D., SCHACHTER, M., MARSDEN, C. D., SMITH, B. and WILSON, A. Lisuride in Parkinsonism. *Annals of Neurology*, **9,** 48–52 (1981)

66 PIJNENBURG, A. J. J., HONIG, W. M. M., VAN DER HEYDEN, J. A. M. and VAN ROSSUM, J. M. Effects of chemical stimulation of the mesolimbic dopamine system upon locomotor activity. *European Journal of Pharmacology*, **35,** 45–58 (1976)

67 PRECHT, W. and YOSHIDA, M. Blockage of caudate-evoked inhibition of neurons in the substantia nigra by picrotoxin. *Brain Research*, **32**, 229–233 (1971)

68 PRICE, K. S., FARLEY, I. J. and HORNYKIEWICZ, O. Neurochemistry of Parkinson's disease: relation between striatal and limbic dopamine. *Advances in Biochemical Psychopharmacology*, **19**, 293–300 (1978)

69 REISINE, T. D., FIELDS, J. Z., YAMAMURA, H. I., BIRD, E., SPOKES, E., SCHREINER, P. S. and ENNA, S. J. Neurotransmitter receptor alterations in Parkinson's disease *Life Sciences*, **21**, 335–344 (1977)

70 RINNE, U. K., LÖNNBERG, P. and KOSKINEN, V. Dopamine receptors in the parkinsonian brain. In *Abstracts of the 12th CINP Congress*, edited by C. Radouco-Thomas and F. Garcin, 299, Oxford, Pergamon Press (1980)

71 RINNE, U. K., SONNINEN, V., RIEKKINEN, P. and LAAKSONEN, H. Dopaminergic nervous transmission in Parkinson's disease. *Medical Biology*, **52**, 208–217 (1974)

72 RINNE, U. K., KOSKINEN, V., LAAKSONEN, H., LÖNNBERG, P. and SONNINEN, V, GABA receptor binding in the Parkinsonian brain. *Life Sciences*, **22**, 2225–2228 (1978)

73 SCHACHTER, M., BÉDARD, P., DEBONO, A. G., JENNER, P., MARSDEN, C. D., PRICE, P., PARKES, J. D., KENNAN, J., SMITH, B., ROSENTHALER, J., HOROWSKI, R. and DOROW, R. The role of D-1 and D-2 receptors. *Nature*, **286**, 257–259 (1980)

74 SHARMAN, D. F., POIRIER, L. J., MURPHY, G. F. and SOURKES, T. L. Homovanillic acid and dihydroxyphenylacetic acid in the striatum of monkeys with brain lesions. *Canadian Journal of Physiology and Pharmacology*, **45**, 57–62 (1967)

75 SHIBUYA, M. Dopamine-sensitive adenylate cyclase activity in the striatum in Parkinson's disease. *Journal of Neural Transmission*, **44**, 287–295 (1979)

76 TARSY, D., PYCOCK, C., MELDRUM, B. and MARSDEN, C. D. Rotational behaviour induced in rats by intranigral picrotoxin. *Brain Research*, **89**, 160–165 (1975)

77 UNGERSTEDT, U. Use of intracerebral injections of 6-hydroxydopamine as a tool for morphological and functional studies on central catecholamine neurons. In *6-Hydroxydopamine and Catecholamine Neurons*, edited by T. Malmfors and H. Thoenen, 315–322. Amsterdam, North-Holland (1971)

78 UNGERSTEDT, U. Central dopamine mechanisms and unconditioned behaviour. In *The Neurobiology of Dopamine*, edited by A. S. Horn, J. Korf and B. H. C. Westerink, 577–596. London Academic Press (1979)

79 WEINER, W. J., KOLLER, W. C., PERLIK, S., NAUSIEDA, P. A. and KLAWANS, J. L. Drug holiday and management of Parkinson disease. *Neurology*, **30**, 1257–1261 (1980)

5
Brain neurotransmitter receptors in Parkinson's disease

U. K. Rinne

Appreciable advances have taken place during the past 20 years in our knowledge of Parkinson's disease. There is no doubt that progressive loss of dopaminergic substantia nigra neurons and deficiency of dopamine play an essential role in the pathophysiology of the disease. This was first demonstrated by Ehringer and Hornykiewicz[18] and has subsequently been confirmed in a number of other studies showing a decrease of dopamine and its metabolite, homovanillic acid[3, 42, 65, 70, 72, 74], as well as of the enzymes associated with dopamine[41, 43, 50, 66, 78] in the parkinsonian brain. The degree of striatal dopamine deficiency[3], and of decreased tyrosine hydroxylase (tyrosine 3-monooxygenase) activity[66, 78], correlates highly with the severity of the parkinsonian disability. However, other neurons of the extrapyramidal system also may be involved in the pathophysiology of Parkinson's disease, either primarily or as a secondary consequence[2, 4, 44, 50, 51, 62, 65, 66, 73, 74, 76–78]. The present paper is concerned with changes in neurotransmitter receptors in the parkinsonian brain.

DOPAMINE RECEPTORS

According to recent evidence there are multiple receptor mechanisms for dopamine which can be distinguished by physiological, biochemical and pharmacological criteria[12, 26, 28, 29, 89, 90]. At some sites, dopamine receptors are linked with adenylate cyclase and in others not, thus dividing the receptors into two classes, D-1 and D-2 receptors, respectively[29] (see also Chapter 18.1).

Furthermore, both in different animal species and in man, dopamine receptors recently have been demonstrated with a high affinity for ^{3}H-dopamine and dopaminergic agonists but a relatively low affinity for ^{3}H-neuroleptics. It has been suggested that this high affinity binding site for dopamine be referred to as D-3 receptors[39, 93], but it is obvious that this is only the first level of division of dopamine receptors; it is likely that there will be other, different subgroups of dopamine receptors[29]. These D-1, D-2 and D-3 receptors have been demonstrated especially in the striatum, where it has been found that the dopamine receptors involved with motor function are located at least at five different sites[29].

Experimental destruction of the nigrostriatal dopamine pathway in animals is followed by a behavioural supersensitivity and by an increased number of striatal dopamine receptors[14, 53, 91]. Similarly, in addition to the presynaptic loss of nigral dopamine neurons, alterations also have been found in the striatal dopamine receptors in Parkinson's disease. A reduction has been reported of striatal dopamine-sensitive adenylate cyclase activity[86], suggesting the loss of striatal D-1 receptors in Parkinson's disease. In contrast, there seem to be differences in the behaviour of striatal D-2 receptors in Parkinson's disease; either a decreased binding of ^{3}H-spiperone[62, 96], or an increased ^{3}H-haloperidol binding[34] have been reported. However, according to the author's recent studies[78–80], there seem to be at least two subgroups of parkinsonian patients with regard to the number of dopamine receptors.

Table 5.1 Specific ^{3}H-spiperone binding (fmols/mg protein) in parkinsonian and control brains. No levodopa treatment. Mean ± s.e.

Group	No. of patients	Caudate nucleus	Putamen	Pallidum	Receptor density*
Controls					
Without neuroleptics	29	129 ± 10	133 ± 10	30 ± 3	101 ± 14
With neuroleptics	9	293 ± 13	289 ± 22	81 ± 10	306 ± 36
Parkinsonian patients					
Without levodopa					
Subgroup I	5	53 ± 7	52 ± 7	41 ± 12	55 ± 4
Subgroup II	10	173 ± 18	228 ± 25	66 ± 7	205 ± 39
With neuroleptics	7	294 ± 60	339 ± 77	124 ± 38	199 ± 48
Control 1 – Subgroup I		$P<0.001$	$P<0.001$		$P<0.01$
Control 1 – Subgroup II		$P<0.05$	$P<0.01$	$P<0.001$	$P<0.05$
Control 1 – With neuroleptics		$P<0.05$	$P<0.05$	$P<0.05$	
Subgroup I – Subgroup II		$P<0.001$	$P<0.001$		$P<0.01$

*Dopamine-receptor density was assessed as maximum specific ^{3}H-spiperone binding derived from Scatchard analyses
Controls: mean age 66 ± 2 years; causes of death: myocardial infarction (23 cases), pulmonary embolism (11), rupture of the aorta (3), accident (1). *Parkinsonian*: mean age 74 ± 2 years; causes of death: pneumonia (27), myocardial infarction (9), pulmonary embolism (7), ulcerative colitis (1)

In the author's studies the dopamine receptor sites were determined by the specific binding of ^{3}H-spiperone. As shown in *Table 5.1*, most of the parkinsonian patients without levodopa treatment showed an increased binding of ^{3}H-spiperone in the caudate nucleus and putamen. However, in some patients binding was decreased (*Table 5.1*). Scatchard analysis showed that there were corresponding changes in the receptor number, but no change in the mean dissociation constant. An increased number of striatal dopamine receptors was found in parkinsonian patients suffering from psychotic episodes and treated with neuroleptic drugs (*Table 5.1*). Furthermore, changes in the dopamine receptors in the parkinsonian nucleus accumbens were similar to those in the striatum[69].

In contrast to most untreated patients, there was a normal or decreased number of striatal dopamine receptors in parkinsonians treated with levodopa (*Table 5.2*). A corresponding change after levodopa therapy also has been found using the ^{3}H-haloperidol binding technique[34]. These results suggest that levodopa treatment can reverse dopaminergic supersensitivity in the striatum.

Table 5.2 Effect of levodopa treatment on specific ^{3}H-spiperone binding (fmols/mg protein) in parkinsonian and control striatum. Mean ± s.e.

Group	No. of patients	Caudate nucleus	Putamen	Pallidum	Receptor density*
Controls					
Without neuroleptics	29	129 ± 10	133 ± 10	30 ± 3	101 ± 14
With neuroleptics	9	293 ± 13	289 ± 22	81 ± 10	306 ± 36
Parkinsonian patients					
Without levodopa					
Subgroup I	5	67 ± 12	69 ± 12	46 ± 12	53 ± 14
Subgroup II	5	138 ± 25	195 ± 30	39 ± 8	152 ± 34
With neuroleptics	12	263 ± 20	301 ± 24	97 ± 16	276 ± 63
Control 1 – Control 2		$P<0.001$	$P<0.001$	$P<0.001$	$P<0.001$
Control 1 – Subgroup I		$P<0.001$	$P<0.001$		$P<0.05$
Control 1 – With neuroleptics		$P<0.001$	$P<0.001$	$P<0.001$	$P<0.01$
Subgroup I – Subgroup II		$P<0.05$	$P<0.01$		$P<0.05$

* Dopamine-receptor density was assessed as maximum specific ^{3}H-spiperone binding derived from Scatchard analyses

Striatal dopamine receptors seem to respond to treatment with neuroleptic drugs, which caused a great increase in the binding of ^{3}H-spiperone both in parkinsonian patients and 'controls' (*see Tables 5.1 and 5.2*). Similar changes after neuroleptic treatment have been demonstrated in schizophrenic patients[34, 55] and in animals[6, 38, 52]. Therefore in postmortem brain studies of dopamine receptors, it is important to check carefully the possibility of this type of treatment before death.

The significance of alterations of striatal dopamine receptors in the pathophysiology of Parkinson's disease is supported by further analysis of the results of the author's parkinsonian brain studies. There were some important relationships between parkinsonian clinical variables and changes in striatal dopamine receptors. Dyskinesias, daily fluctuations in performance, psychotic episodes, and neuroleptic medication, were especially associated with an increase in the number of striatal dopamine receptors, which may reflect the presence of denervation supersensitivity. On the other hand, the severity of the disease and a deteriorating response to levodopa seemed to be mostly related to a decrease in the number of dopamine receptors in the striatum (*Table 5.3*). This suggests that not only the progressive degeneration of presynaptic nigral dopamine neurons of the substantia nigra, but

Table 5.3 Relationship between clinical variables of the parkinsonian patients and changes in striatal dopamine receptors

	Striatal dopamine receptors	
Variable	Decreased	Increased
Disability of the patients	++	+
Loss of levodopa response	++	+
Dyskinesias	+	++
On–off phenomena	+	++
Psychotic episodes together with neuroleptics	0	++

also a loss of postsynaptic dopamine receptors in the striatum may contribute, at least partly, to the deteriorating response of parkinsonian patients to chronic levodopa treatment.

Long-term follow-up, neuropsychological assessment, mortality and postmortem brain studies indicate that levodopa therapy does not modify the natural course of Parkinson's disease. Levodopa as a replacement therapy merely improves the parkinsonian symptoms; but all the time while the treatment is going on, the underlying pathology of Parkinson's disease causes a progressive loss of substantia nigra neurons. Finally various distressing difficulties arise, such as the loss of benefit, dyskinesias, 'on-off' phenomena, postural instability, psychotic episodes, progressive intellectual deterioration and dementia[66–68]. However, there is an overlap of the dopaminergic innervation in the striatum. Therefore, partial degeneration of the substantia nigra dopamine neurons leads to a greater loss of presynaptic dopamine neurons than of postsynaptic dopamine receptor sites in the striatum. Comparative studies of striatal dopamine concentrations and of dopamine receptors in the postmortem parkinsonian brain show that this is really the case[33,78]. In advanced parkinsonian patients, who have lost the beneficial response to levodopa, there are still enough dopamine receptors in the striatum for drugs stimulating the dopamine receptors directly to improve the parkinsonian disability. Moreover, besides the progression of the underlying pathology of the disease leading to failure of presynaptic nigral neurons to synthesize and store dopamine, changes in the response of striatal dopamine receptors also may be a factor contributing to the mechanisms of daily fluctuations in performance and of other late problems occurring during chronic levodopa therapy[47,67]. Indeed, many recent studies have shown that such agonists are beneficial especially in the treatment of parkinsonian patients with a deteriorating response to levodopa[7,8,13,21,23,27,35–37,56,71,75]. For example, in our long-term follow-up study[67], it was shown that additional bromocriptine therapy had a beneficial effect both on parkinsonian disability and the 'on–off' phenomena of patients with a deteriorating levodopa response. According to pharmacological evidence the antiparkinsonian efficacy of dopaminergic agonists in parkinsonian patients seems to depend on drug interaction primarily with D-2 receptors[82].

CHOLINERGIC RECEPTORS

Studies of enzymes associated with cholinergic neurotransmission[43, 49, 50, 62, 66, 73] have shown that the cholinergic neurons in the extrapyramidal system of the parkinsonian brain are relatively well preserved, although there seems to be some degeneration. Compared with the great degeneration of substantia nigra dopamine neurons, there seems to be an imbalance in the striatal dopaminergic–cholinergic interaction in Parkinson's disease. Indeed, analyses of dopamine and acetylcholinesterase from the same autopsy brain samples showed that cholinergic dominance really is the case in the parkinsonian brain[73].

It has been found that the density of brain muscarinic receptor binding sites decreases with advancing years in old people[95]. However, recent studies also indicate changes in the cholinergic receptors in the parkinsonian brain; these seem to be more specific and not related only to the ageing process. Reisine *et al.*[62] reported an increased muscarinic receptor binding in the putamen but no changes in the caudate nucleus and pallidum of patients with Parkinson's disease. The author's recent studies[79] demonstrated that changes in the cholinergic muscarinic receptors in the parkinsonian striatum were related to changes in the number of dopamine receptors. In a subgroup of parkinsonian patients with a low number of striatal dopamine receptors, the specific binding of ^{3}H-quinuclidinyl benzilate, a marker for cholinergic muscarinic receptors, also was decreased in the caudate nucleus and putamen. On the other hand, high binding was found in the striatum and cerebral cortex of parkinsonian patients with an increased number of striatal dopamine receptors. These changes in cholinergic muscarinic receptors in the parkinsonian patients not on levodopa treatment (*Table 5.4*) seem to be similar to those in patients treated with levodopa (*Table 5.5*).

Table 5.4 Specific binding of ^{3}H-quinuclidinyl benzilate (fmols/mg protein) in parkinsonian and control brains. No levodopa treatment. Mean ± s.e.

Group	No. of patients	Caudate nucleus	Putamen	Pallidum	Frontal cortex
Controls					
Without neuroleptics	18	750 ± 46	704 ± 46	176 ± 21	463 ± 43
With neuroleptics	6	993 ± 69	985 ± 79	221 ± 19	614 ± 59
Parkinsonism					
Subgroup I					
(low binding)	3	385 ± 82	434 ± 113	192 ± 47	321 ± 84
Subgroup II					
(high binding)	6	835 ± 78	885 ± 77	259 ± 31	639 ± 50
With neuroleptics	5	739 ± 92	809 ± 96	191 ± 15	626 ± 82
Control 1 – Control 2		$P<0.01$	$P<0.01$		
Control 1 – Subgroup I		$P<0.01$	$P<0.05$		
Control 1 – Subgroup II				$P<0.05$	$P<0.05$
Subgroup I – Subgroup II		$P<0.01$	$P<0.05$		$P<0.05$

Table 5.5 Specific binding of ^{3}H-quinuclidinyl benzilate (fmols/mg protein) in parkinsonian and control brains. Chronic levodopa treatment. Mean ± s.e.

Group	No. of patients	Caudate nucleus	Putamen	Pallidum	Frontal cortex
Controls					
Without neuroleptics	18	750 ± 46	704 ± 46	176 ± 21	463 ± 43
With neuroleptics	6	993 ± 69	985 ± 79	221 ± 19	614 ± 59
Parkinsonism					
Subgroup I					
(low binding)	1	264	356	–	349
Subgroup II					
(high binding)	3	807 ± 84	774 ± 65	255 ± 75	630 ± 18
With neuroleptics	6	866 ± 77	838 ± 91	251 ± 46	606 ± 57
Control 1 – Subgroup II					$P < 0.01$

An increased number of dopamine receptors induced by treatment with neuroleptics also was associated with an increased binding of ^{3}H-quinuclidinyl benzilate both in parkinsonian patients and controls (*Table 5.4 and 5.5*). This further indicates the close functional interaction of dopamine and cholinergic neurotransmission in the striatum, where the nigrostriatal dopamine neurons exert a tonic inhibition of the striatal cholinergic interneurons[40]. In experimental animals with a pharmacologically induced hyperactivity of dopamine neurons there is also an increase in striatal ^{3}H-quinuclidinyl benzilate binding[57].

γ-AMINOBUTYRIC ACID RECEPTORS

There is neurochemical evidence to indicate a possible extrapyramidal γ-aminobutyric (GABA) neuron abnormality in Parkinson's disease[41, 51, 74, 78].

The possible involvement of GABA neurons in Parkinson's disease has been supported by findings[44, 76] of a decreased GABA receptor binding in the substantia nigra in the parkinsonian brain (*Table 5.6*). It is likely that the GABA receptors in

Table 5.6 Specific receptor binding of ^{3}H-GABA (fmols/mg protein) in parkinsonian and control brains. Mean ± s.e.

Group	No. of patients	Caudate nucleus	Putamen	Pallidum	Substantia nigra	Cerebral cortex	Cerebellar cortex
Controls	11	283 ± 20	245 ± 16	112 ± 22	85 ± 11	787 ± 74	1838 ± 114
Parkinsonian patients							
Without levodopa	7	257 ± 31	226 ± 36	100 ± 17	52 ± 11	619 ± 68	1818 ± 232
With levodopa	5	281 ± 68	243 ± 39	74 ± 14	38 ± 15*	678 ± 130	1570 ± 366
All cases	12	267 ± 32	233 ± 25	89 ± 12	46 ± 9*	644 ± 64	1715 ± 197

* $P < 0.05$ as compared with controls.

the substantia nigra are located on the nigral dopamine neurons, which are greatly decreased in number in Parkinson's disease. However, GABAergic regulation of nigral dopamine neurons also may be carried out by interneuronal connections[10].

In the other brain regions studied, however, there were no changes in GABA receptor binding (*Table 5.6*). A similar finding in the striatum has been also reported by Reisine *et al.*[62]. Correspondingly, experimental lesions of the nigrostriatal pathway in animals have not been followed by alterations of the striatal GABA receptors[63].

SEROTONIN (5-HYDROXYTRYPTAMINE) RECEPTORS

Studies of brain serotonin have offered some evidence of a possible involvement of serotonergic neurons in the neurochemical pathology of Parkinson's disease[2, 4, 20, 65, 74]. Indeed, it has been suggested that serotonergic neurons may contribute functionally to the inhibition of dopamine and noradrenaline systems in the control of motor behaviour[24] and tremor[20].

Although there seems to be some degeneration of presynaptic serotonin neurons in the parkinsonian brain, studies on possible changes in serotonin receptors have yielded differing results. In recent studies[79] there were no changes in the specific binding of ^{3}H-serotonin either in the striatum or in the frontal cortex of patients with Parkinson's disease. Neither did the treatment with levodopa or neuroleptics have any significant effect on ^{3}H-serotonin binding. Serotonin receptors in the limbic cortex of parkinsonian patients, demonstrated with ^{3}H-spiperone binding, did not differ from that in controls[69]. A moderate decrease in serotonin receptors, however, has been reported by Reisine *et al.*[62] in the putamen but not in the caudate nucleus or pallidum of the parkinsonian brain. Furthermore, a decrease of both high and low affinity binding sites, and an increase in the affinity of ^{3}H-serotonin, in the frontal cortex of patients with Parkinson's disease recently has been demonstrated[30].

ENKEPHALIN RECEPTORS

There is recent evidence to indicate that the endogenous enkephalins may act as neurotransmitters or neuromodulators in the extrapyramidal system. Enkephalin-containing neurons have been demonstrated in the striatum of both experimental animals[16, 19, 81, 87] and man[15]. Immunohistochemical studies combined with experimental lesions have demonstrated that enkephalin-like immunoreactive nerve cells are, at least in part, small interneurons within the striatum[11, 25, 83, 84]. Furthermore, the striatum contains relatively high concentrations of opiate receptors[22, 32, 58-60]. It has been found that opiate binding sites in the striatum are reduced by the destruction of the dopaminergic nigrostriatal tract[22, 59, 64]. These findings suggest that some of the striatal opiate receptors are located on dopamine nerve terminals. However, there is experimental evidence[9, 17, 60, 85] to suggest separate pre- and postsynaptic opiate receptors involved in the regulation of the nigrostriatal function. Furthermore, a third population of striatal opiate receptors has been suggested to exist on the terminals of the corticostriatal neurons[11]. There is sufficient evidence, however, to support the concept that endogenous opioid peptides can modulate the activity of the nigrostriatal dopamine neurons[5, 9, 17, 22, 45, 59, 60, 64, 91, 97]. Recently, changes in ^{3}H-naloxone binding[64], and in ^{3}H-leu-enkephalin binding[79], have been found in the parkinsonian striatum, suggesting that endogenous opioid peptides also may be involved in the pathophysiological process of Parkinson's disease, either primarily or as a secondary consequence.

The ^{3}H-naloxone binding was decreased in the parkinsonian caudate nucleus but not in the putamen[64]. In the author's studies [79], the specific binding of ^{3}H-leu-enkephalin was increased in the putamen (*Table 5.7*) as well as in the limbic cortex and hippocampus (*Table 5.8*) of patients with Parkinson's disease. Recent studies

Table 5.7 Specific binding of ^{3}H-leu-enkephalin (fmols/mg protein) in parkinsonian and control brains. Mean <s.e.

Group	Caudate nucleus	Putamen	Nucleus accumbens
Controls	21.4 ± 1.7 (20)	14.8 ± 1.5 (21)	8.9 ± 3.3 (12)
Parkinsonism			
All cases	27.8 ± 2.1 (21)	21.1 ± 1.4 (24)	11.2 ± 1.3 (16)
Without levodopa	25.8 ± 2.9 (10)	21.7 ± 2.1 (12)	10.6 ± 2.0 (7)
With levodopa	30.0 ± 3.1 (11)	20.4 ± 1.9 (12)	11.6 ± 1.7 (9)
Control – all cases	$P<0.05$	$P<0.01$	
Control – without levodopa		$P<0.05$	
Control – with levodopa		$P<0.05$	

Table 5.8 Specific binding of ^{3}H-leu-enkephalin (fmols/mg protein) in parkinsonian and control brains. Mean ± s.e.

Group	Frontal cortex	Limbic cortex	Hippocampus	Amygdala	Hypothalamus
Controls	47.1 ± 4.9 (21)	44.9 ± 4.2 (14)	26.1 ± 2.1 (14)	34.2 ± 4.8 (13)	15.5 ± 2.1 (14)
Parkinsonism					
All cases	60.9 ± 5.4 (24)	68.3 ± 5.4 (18)	39.8 ± 2.5 (17)	42.8 ± 4.8 (16)	18.9 ± 3.0 (17)
Without levodopa	58.7 ± 6.7 (12)	65.0 ± 7.7 (8)	45.8 ± 3.8 (7)	38.4 ± 7.2 (7)	14.1 ± 3.6 (9)
With levodopa	63.2 ± 8.8 (12)	70.9 ± 7.9 (10)	35.6 ± 2.8 (10)	46.2 ± 6.6 (9)	24.3 ± 4.4 (8)
Control – all cases		$P<0.01$	$P<0.001$		
Control – without levodopa		$P<0.05$	$P<0.001$		
Control – with levodopa		$P<0.01$	$P<0.05$		

with ^{3}H-met-enkephalin binding gave similar results (*Tables 5.9 and 5.10*). Treatment with levodopa or neuroleptics did not have any obvious effect on the binding of ^{3}H-leu-enkephalin or ^{3}H-met-enkephalin, except that neuroleptic treatment appeared to increase the binding of ^{3}H-met-enkephalin in the caudate nucleus, putamen and amygdala in non-levodopa treated patients. It is probable that both these ligands bind to the same site, as suggested by Waterfield *et al.*[94]. However, it has been proposed that the two separate types of opiate receptors interact with leu- and met-enkephalins[88].

Table 5.9 Specific binding of ^{3}H-met-enkephalin (fmols/mg protein) in parkinsonian and control brains. Mean ± s.e.

Group	Caudate nucleus	Putamen	Nucleus accumbens
Controls	25.4 ± 3.2 (21)	20.2 ± 2.1 (21)	5.8 ± 0.9 (14)
Parkinsonism			
All cases	38.1 ± 4.4 (21)	28.7 ± 2.3 (21)	12.0 ± 1.3 (13)
Without levodopa	31.8 ± 3.1 (11)	27.1 ± 3.3 (11)	9.2 ± 1.8 (5)
With levodopa	45.2 ± 8.2 (10)	30.3 ± 3.3 (10)	13.7 ± 1.5 (8)
Control – all cases	$P < 0.05$	$P < 0.01$	$P < 0.001$
Control – with levodopa	$P < 0.05$	$P < 0.05$	$P < 0.001$

Table 5.10 Specific binding of ^{3}H-met-enkephalin (fmols/mg protein) in parkinsonian and control brains. Mean ± s.e.

Group	Frontal cortex	Limbic cortex	Hippocampus	Amygdala	Hypothalamus
Controls	36.4 ± 4.9 (21)	36.6 ± 4.0 (18)	17.7 ± 2.0 (17)	27.7 ± 4.0 (18)	13.8 ± 2.2 (17)
Parkinsonism					
All cases	52.7 ± 5.1 (21)	50.9 ± 4.9 (18)	24.4 ± 2.3 (17)	31.1 ± 4.1 (18)	15.7 ± 2.4 (17)
Without levodopa	47.3 ± 5.2 (11)	49.7 ± 5.2 (8)	21.9 ± 3.8 (7)	23.8 ± 2.8 (8)	14.7 ± 2.2 (8)
With levodopa	58.6 ± 8.6 (10)	51.9 ± 8.1 (10)	26.2 ± 2.7 (10)	36.9 ± 6.6 (10)	16.7 ± 4.1 (9)
Control – all cases	$P < 0.05$	$P < 0.05$	$P < 0.05$		
Control – with levodopa	$P < 0.05$		$P < 0.05$		

Recent evidence suggests the existence of a multiple population of opiate receptors in the brain[46,48]. There seem to be at least two types of receptors, of which μ-receptors show a preference for ^{3}H-naloxone and δ-receptors are labelled with enkephalins[31, 46, 88, 92]. Furthermore, it is evident that the two types of opiate receptors mediate different functions[88]. The different results obtained with naloxone and enkephalin binding in the parkinsonian brain, suggest that these two types of opiate receptors are altered differentially in Parkinson's disease. The decrease of naloxone binding in the parkinsonian caudate nucleus[64] suggests that a significant population of opiate receptors is located on the dopamine nerve terminals which degenerate during the course of Parkinson's disease. However, recently it has been demonstrated in rat that, depending on the exact anatomical localization of the lesions causing dopaminergic denervation, there is either a decrease or an increase in opiate receptor binding both in the striatum and amygdala[22]. Using enkephalin-binding techniques in lesioned animals, the same supersensitivity of a population of enkephalin receptors in the nigrostriatal and mesolimbic systems has been demonstrated, as was found in the author's parkinsonian patients. Thus both hypo- and hyperactivity of certain enkephalin-containing neurons in the striatum may be involved in the pathophysiology of Parkinson's disease. Conceivably, manipulation of neuronal systems containing endogenous opiate substances may have clinical applications in Parkinson's disease. However, pilot trials with opiate antagonists have given negative results[1, 54, 61], although this does not prove that endogenous opiate peptides are of no importance in this disease.

Conclusions

(1) In Parkinson's disease there is not only a degeneration of nigrostriatal dopamine neurons but there are also significant changes in striatal dopamine receptors.
(2) There seem to be at least two subgroups of parkinsonian patients with regard to the behaviour of striatal dopamine receptors:
    (a) those with a loss of dopamine receptors;
    (b) those with an increase in the number of dopamine receptors.
(3) Clinically, the patients with a low number of striatal dopamine receptors were more disabled and had lost the beneficial response to levodopa. In contrast, dyskinesias, daily fluctuations in performance and neuroleptic medication, were especially related to an increase of striatal dopamine receptors.
(4) Changes in cholinergic muscarinic receptors in the parkinsonian striatum seem to be related to changes in dopamine receptors suggesting their close functional interaction.
(5) Decreased GABA-receptor binding in the substantia nigra indicates a possible abnormality of extrapyramidal GABA neurons in Parkinson's disease.
(6) In the parkinsonian brain there seem to be increases in the number of enkephalin receptors, both in the striatum and in the mesolimbic system.
(7) There is evidence of multiple receptor disturbances in the parkinsonian brain. Changes in dopamine, cholinergic, GABA and enkephalin receptors indicate the involvement of all these neuronal systems in the pathophysiology of Parkinson's disease, either primarily or as a secondary consequence.

Acknowledgement

The study was supported by a grant from the Sigrid Jusélius Foundation.

References

1. BARBEAU, A., ROY, M., GONCE, M. and LABRECQUE, R. Newer therapeutic approaches in Parkinson's disease. In *Advances in Neurology*, **24,** edited by L. J. Poirier, T. L. Sourkes and P. J. Bédard, 433–450. New York, Raven Press (1979)
2. BERNHEIMER, H., BIRKMAYER, W. and HORNYKIEWICZ, O. Verteilung des 5-Hydroxytryptamins (Serotonin) im Gehirn des Menschen und sein Verhalten bei Patienten mit Parkinson-Syndrom. *Klinische Wochenschrift*, **39,** 1056–1059 (1961)
3. BERNHEIMER, H., BIRKMAYER, W., HORNYKIEWICZ, O., JELLINGER, K. and SEITELBERGER, F. Brain dopamine and the syndromes of Parkinson and Huntington. *Journal of Neurological Sciences*, **20,** 415–455 (1973)
4. BIRKMAYER, W., DANIELCZYK, W., NEUMAYER, E. and RIEDERER, P. Nucleus ruber and L-Dopa psychosis: biochemical post mortem findings. *Journal of Neural Transmission*, **35,** 93–116 (1974)
5. BLOOM, F., SAGAL, D. and LING, N. Endorphins: profound behavioral effects in rats suggest new etiological factors in mental illness. *Science*, **184,** 630–632 (1976)
6. BURT, D. R., CREESE, I. and SNYDER, S. H. Antischizophrenic drugs: chronic treatment elevates dopamine receptor binding in brain. *Science*, **196,** 326–328 (1977)
7. CALNE, D. B., TEYCHENNE, P. F., CLAVERIA, L. E., EASTMAN, R., GREENACRE, J. K. and PETRIE, A. Bromocriptine in parkinsonism. *British Medical Journal*, **4,** 442–444 (1974)
8. CALNE, D. B., PLOTKIN, C., WILLIAMS, A. C., NUTT, J. G., NEOPHYTIDES, A. and TEYCHENNE, P. F. Long-term treatment of parkinsonism with bromocriptine. *Lancet*, **1,** 735–738 (1978)
9. CARENZI, A., FRIGENI, V. and DELLA BELLA, D. Synaptic localization of opiate receptors in rat striatum. *The Endorphins*, **3,** edited by E. Costa and M. Trabucchi, 265–270. New York, Raven Press (1978)
10. CATTABENI, F., MAGGI, A., DEANGELIS, L., BRUNO, F. and RACAGNI, A. A simple approach to study the effect of haloperidol on GABA functional activity in the nigrostriatal system. *Journal of Neurochemistry*, **28,** 1407–1408 (1977)
11. CHILDERS, S. R., COYLE, J. T., SCHWARCZ, R. and SNYDER, S. H. Radioimmunoassay of enkephalins: Levels of methionine- and leucine-enkephalin in morphine-dependent and kainic acid-lesioned rat brains. *Advances in Biochemistry and Psychopharmacology*, **18,** 161–173. New York, Raven Press (1978)
12. COOLS, A. R. and VAN ROSSUM, J. M. Excitation-mediating and inhibition-mediating dopamine-receptors: a new concept towards a better understanding of electrophysiological, biochemical, pharmacological, functional and clinical data. *Psychopharmacologia*, **45,** 243–254 (1976)
13. COTZIAS, G. C., PAPAVASILIOU, P. S., TOLOSA, E. S., MENDEZ, J. S. and BELL-MIDURA, M. Treatment of Parkinson's disease with apomorphines. *New England Journal of Medicine*, **294,** 567–572 (1976)
14. CREESE, F., BURT, D. and SNYDER, S. H. Dopamine receptor binding enhancement accompanies lesion-induced behavioral supersensitivity. *Science*, **197,** 596–598 (1977)
15. CUELLO, A. C. Endogenous opioid peptides in neurons of the human brain. *Lancet*, **1,** 291–293 (1978)

16 CUELLO, A. C. and PAXINOS, G. Evidence for a long Leu-enkephalin striopallidal pathway in rat brain. *Nature*, **271**, 178–180 (1978)
17 DIAMOND, B. I. and BORISON, R. L. Enkephalins and nigrostriatal function. *Neurology*, **28**, 1085–1088 (1978)
18 EHRINGER, H. and HORNYKIEWICZ, O. Verteilung von Noradrenalin und Dopamine (3-Hydroxytyramin) im Gehirn des Menschen und ihr Verhalten bei Erkrankungen des extrapyramidalen Systems. *Klinische Wochenschrift*, **38**, 1236–1239 (1960)
19 ELDE, R., HÖKFELT, T., JOHANSSON, O. and TERENIUS, L. Immunohistochemical studies using antibodies to leucine-enkephalin: Initial observations on the nervous system of the rat. *Neuroscience*, **1**, 349–351 (1976)
20 FAHN, S., LIBSCH, L. R. and CUTLER, R. W. Monoamines in the human neostriatum: Topographic distribution in normals and in Parkinson's disease and their role in akinesia, rigidity, chorea and tremor. *Journal of Neurological Sciences*, **14**, 427–455 (1971)
21 FAHN, S., COTE, L. J., SNIDER, S. R., BATTETT, R. E. and ISGREEN, W. P. The role of bromocriptine in the treatment of parkinsonism. *Neurology*, **29**, 1077–1083 (1979)
22 GARDNER, E. L., ZUKIN, R. S. and MAKMAN, M. H. Modulation of opiate receptor binding in striatum and amygdala by selective mesencephalic lesions. *Brain Research*, **194**, 232–239 (1980)
23 GRÖN, U. Bromocriptine versus placebo in levodopa treated patients with Parkinson's disease. *Acta Neurologica Scandinavica*, **56**, 269–273 (1977)
24 HORNYKIEWICZ, O. Neurohumoral interactions and basal ganglia function and dysfunction. In *The Basal Ganglia*, edited by M. D. Yahr, 269–280. New York, Raven Press (1976)
25 HÖKFELT, T., ELDE, R., JOHANSSON, O., TERENIUS, L. and STEIN, L. The distribution of enkephalin-immunoreactive cell bodies in the rat central nervous system. *Neurosciences Letters*, **5**, 25–31 (1977)
26 IVERSEN, L. L., QUIK, M., EMSON, P. C., DOWLING, J. E. and WATLING, K. J. Further evidence for the existence of multiple receptors for dopamine in the central nervous system. *Advances in Biochemical Psychopharmacology*, **21**, 193–202 (1980)
27 JANSEN, E. N. H. Bromocriptine in levodopa response-losing parkinsonism. *European Neurology*, **17**, 92–99 (1978)
28 KEBABIAN, J. W. Multiple classes of dopamine receptors in mammalian central nervous system: the involvement of dopamine-sensitive adenylyl cyclase. *Life Sciences*, **23**, 479–484 (1978)
29 KEBABIAN, J. W. and CALNE, D. B. Multiple receptors for dopamine. *Nature*, **277**, 93–96 (1979)
30 KIENZL, E., RIEDERER, P. and JELLINGER, K. Transitional states of central serotonin receptors in Parkinson's disease. *Journal of Neural Transmission*, **51**, 113–122 (1981)
31 KOSTERLITZ, H. W., LORD, J. A. H., PATERSON, S. J. and WATERFIELD, A. A. Effects of changes in the structure of enkephalins and of narcotic analgesic drugs on their interactions with μ and β-receptors. *British Journal of Pharmacology*, **68**, 333–342 (1980)

32 KUHAR, M. J., PERT, C. B. and SNYDER, S. H. Regional distribution of opiate receptor binding in monkey and human brain. *Nature*, **245**, 447–451 (1973)
33 LEE, T., SEEMAN, P., RAJPUT, A., FARLEY, I. J. and HORNYKIEWICZ, O. Receptor basis for dopaminergic supersensitivity in Parkinson's disease. *Nature*, **273**, 59–61 (1978)
34 LEE, T., SEEMAN, P., TOURTELLOTTE, W. W., FARLEY, I. J. and HORNYKIEWICZ, O. Binding of ^{3}H-neuroleptics and ^{3}H-apomorphine in schizophrenic brains. *Nature*, **274**, 897–900 (1978)
35 LIEBERMAN, A., ZOLFAGHARI, M., BOAL, D., HASSOURI, H., VOGEL, B., BATTISTA, A., FUXE, K. and GOLDSTEIN, M. The antiparkinsonian efficacy of bromocriptine. *Neurology*, **26**, 405–409 (1976)
36 LIEBERMAN, A., ESTEY, E., KUPERSMITH, M., GOPINATHAN, G. and GOLDSTEIN, M. Treatment of Parkinson's disease with lergotrile mesylate. *Journal of the American Medical Association*, **238**, 2380–2382 (1977)
37 LIEBERMAN, A., DZIATOLOWSKI, M., KUPERSMITH, M., SERBY, M., GOODGOLD, A., KOREIN, J. and GOLDSTEIN, M. Dementia in Parkinson's disease. *Annals of Neurology*, **6**, 355–359 (1979)
38 LIST, S. J. and SEEMAN, P. Dopamine agonists reverse the elevated ^{3}H-neuroleptic binding in neuroleptic-pretreated rats. *Life Sciences*, **24**, 1447–1452 (1979)
39 LIST, S., TITELER, M. and SEEMAN, P. High-affinity ^{3}H-dopamine receptors (D_3 sites) in human and rat brain. *Biochemistry and Pharmacology*, **29**, 1621–1622 (1980)
40 LLOYD, K. G. Chemical neuropathology of the extrapyramidal system. In *Synaptic Constituents in Health and Disease*, edited by M. Brzin, S. Sket and H. Bachelard, 725–740. Oxford, Pergamon Press (1980)
41 LLOYD, K. G. and HORNYKIEWICZ, O. Occurrence and distribution of aromatic L-amino acid (L-Dopa) decarboxylase in the human brain. *Journal of Neurochemistry*, **19**, 1549–1559 (1972)
42 LLOYD, K. G., DAVIDSON, L. and HORNYKIEWICZ, O. Metabolism of levodopa in the human brain. *Advances in Neurology*, **3**, edited by D. B. Calne, 173–188, New York, Raven Press (1973)
43 LLOYD, K. G., DAVIDSON, L. and HORNYKIEWICZ, O. The neurochemistry of Parkinson's disease: Effect of L-dopa therapy. *Journal of Pharmacology and Experimental Therapeutics*, **195**, 453–464 (1975)
44 LLOYD, K. G., SHEMEN, L. and HORNYKIEWICZ, O. Distribution of high affinity sodium-independent (^{3}H)gamma-aminobutyric acid (^{3}H-GABA) binding in the human brain: alterations in Parkinson's disease. *Brain Research*, **127**, 269–278 (1977)
45 LOH, H. H., BRASE, D. A., SAMPATH-KHAHA, S., MIR, J. B. and WAY, E. L. Beta-endorphin in vitro inhibition of striatal dopamine release. *Nature*, **264**, 567–568 (1976)
46 LORD, J. A. H., WATERFIELD, A. A., HUGHES, J. and KOSTERLITZ, H. W. Endogenous opioid peptides: multiple agonists and receptors. *Nature*, **267**, 495–499 (1977)
47 MARSDEN, C. D. 'On–off phenomena' in Parkinson's disease. In *Parkinson's Disease – Current Progress, Problems and Management*, edited by U.K. Rinne, M. Klingler and G. Stamm, 241–254. Amsterdam, Elsevier (1980)
48 MARTIN, W. R., EADES, C. G., THOMPSON, G. A., HUPPLER, R. E. and GILBERT, P. E. The effects of morphine- and nalorphine-like drugs in the nondependent and morphine-dependent chronic spinal dog. *Journal of Pharmacology and Experimental Therapeutics*, **197**, 517–532 (1976)

49 McGEER, P. L. and McGEER, E. G. Cholinergic enzyme systems in Parkinson's disease. *Archives of Neurology*, **25**, 265–268 (1971)

50 McGEER, P. L. and McGEER, E. G. Enzymes associated with the metabolism of catecholamines, acetylcholine and GABA in human controls and patients with Parkinson's disease and Huntington's chorea. *Journal of Neurochemistry*, **26,**, 65–76 (1976)

51 McGEER, P. L., McGEER, E. G. and WADA, J. A. Glutamic acid decarboxylase in Parkinson's disease and epilepsy. *Neurology*, **21**, 1000–1007 (1971)

52 MÜLLER, P. and SEEMAN, P. Brain neurotransmitter receptors after long-term haloperidol: dopamine, acetylcholine, serotonin, alfa-noradrenergic and naloxone receptors. *Life Sciences*, **21**, 1751–1758 (1978)

53 NAGY, J. F., LEE, T., SEEMAN, P. and FIBIGER, H. C. Direct evidence for presynaptic and postsynaptic dopamine receptors in brain. *Nature*, **274**, 278 (1978)

54 NUTT, J. G., ROSIN, A. J., EISLER, T., CALNE, D. B. and CHASE, T. N. Effect of an opiate antagonist on movement disorders. *Archives of Neurology*, **35**, 810–811 (1978)

55 OWEN, F., CROSS, A. J., GROW, T. J., LONGDEN, A., POULTER, M. and RILEY, G. J. Increased dopamine-receptor sensitivity in schizophrenia. *Lancet*, **1**, 223–226 (1978)

56 PARKES, J. D., MARSDEN, C. D. and DONALDSON, I. Bromocriptine treatment in Parkinson's disease. *Journal of Neurology, Neurosurgery and Psychiatry*, **39**, 184–193 (1976)

57 PELHAM, R. W. and MUNSAT, T. L. Identification of direct competition for, and indirect influences on, striatal muscarinic cholinergic receptors: *in vivo* (^{3}H)quinuclidinyl benzilate binding in rats. *Brain Research*, **171**, 473–480 (1979)

58 PERT, C. B., KUHAR, M. J. and SNYDER, S. H. Opiate receptors: Autoradiographic localization in rat brain. *Proceedings of the National Academy of Sciences of the USA*, **73**, 3729–3733 (1976)

59 POLLARD, H., LLORENS-CORTES, C. and SCHWARTZ, J. C. Enkephalin receptors on dopaminergic neurones in rat striatum. *Nature*, **268**, 745–747 (1977)

60 POLLARD, H., LLORENS, C., SCHWARTZ, J. C., GROS, C. and DRAY, F. Localization of opiate receptors and enkephalins in the rat striatum in relationship with the nigrostriatal dopaminergic system: lesion studies. *Brain Research*, **151**, 392–398 (1978)

61 PRICE, P., BAXTER, R. C. H., PARKES, J. D. and MARSDEN, C. D. Opiate antagonists and Parkinson's disease *Archives of Neurology*, **36**, 661 (1979)

62 REISINE, T. D., FIELDS, J. Z., YAMAMURA, H. I., BIRD, E. D., SPOKES, E., SCHREINER, P. S. and ENNA, S. J. Neurotransmitter receptor alterations in Parkinson's disease. *Life Sciences*, **21**, 335–344 (1977)

63 REISINE, T. D., NAGY, J. I., BEAUMONT, K., FIBIGER, H. C. and YAMAMURA, H. I. The localization of receptor binding sites in the substantia nigra and striatum of the rat. *Brain Research*, **177**, 241–252 (1979)

64 REISINE, T. D., ROSSOR, M., SPOKES, E., IVERSEN, L. L. and YAMAMURA, H. I. Alterations in brain opiate receptors in Parkinson's disease. *Brain Research*, **173**, 378–382 (1979)

65 RIEDERER, P. and WUKETICH, ST. Time course of nigrostriatal degeneration in Parkinson's disease. *Journal of Neural Transmission*, **38**, 277–301 (1976)

66 RINNE, U. K. Recent advances in research on Parkinsonism. *Acta Neurologica Scandinavica*, **57**, 77–113 (1978)

67 RINNE, U. K. Recent advances in the treatment of Parkinson's disease. *Acta Neurologica Scandinavica*, **62**, Suppl. 78, 103–121 (1980)

68 RINNE, U. K. Treatment of Parkinson's disease: Problems with a progressing disease. *Journal of Neural Transmission*, **51**, 161–174 (1981)

69 RINNE, U. K. Brain dopamine receptors in Parkinson's disease. In *Neurotransmitter Biochemistry of Human Brain Tissue*, edited by P. Riederer and E. Usdin, 303–317 London, Macmillan (1981)

70 RINNE, U. K. and SONNINEN, V. Brain catecholamines and their metabolites in Parkinsonian patients. Treatments with levodopa alone or combined with a decarboxylase inhibitor. *Archives of Neurology*, **28**, 107–110 (1973)

71 RINNE, U. K. and MARTTILA, R. J. Brain dopamine receptor stimulation and the relief of Parkinsonism. Relationship between bromocriptine and levodopa. *Annals of Neurology*, **4**, 263–267 (1978)

72 RINNE, U. K., SONNINEN, V. and HYYPPÄ, M. Effect of L-dopa on brain monoamines and their metabolites in Parkinson's disease. *Life Sciences*, **10**, 549–557 (1971)

73 RINNE, U., K., RIEKKINEN, P., SONNINEN, V. and LAAKSONEN, H. Brain acetylcholinesterase in Parkinson's disease. *Acta Neurologica Scandinavica*, **49**, 215–226 (1973)

74 RINNE, U. K., SONNINEN, V., RIEKKINEN, P. and LAAKSONEN, H. Postmortem findings in parkinsonian patients treated with L-dopa: Biochemical considerations. In *Currents Concepts in the Treatment of Parkinsonism*, edited by M. D. Yahr, 211–233. New York, Raven Press (1974)

75 RINNE, U. K., MARTTILA, R. J. and SONNINEN, V. Brain dopamine turnover and the relief of Parkinsonism. *Archives of Neurology*, **34**, 626–629 (1977)

76 RINNE, U. K., KOSKINEN, V., LAAKSONEN, H., LÖNNBERG, P. and SONNINEN, V. GABA receptor binding in the parkinsonian brain. *Life Sciences*, **22**, 2225–2228 (1978)

77 RINNE, U. K., KOSKINEN, V., LAAKSONEN, H. and TENOVUO, O. Angiotensin-converting enzyme in the parkinsonian brain. *Annals of Neurology*, **4**, 483 (1978)

78 RINNE, U. K., SONNINEN, V. and LAAKSONEN, H. Responses of brain neurochemistry to levodopa treatment in Parkinson's disease. In *Advances in Neurology*, **24**, edited by L. J. Poirier, T. L. Sourkes and P. J. Bédard, 259–274. New York, Raven Press (1979)

79 RINNE, U. K., KOSKINEN, V. and LÖNNBERG, P. Neurotransmitter receptors in the parkinsonian brain. *Parkinson's Disease – Current Progress, Problems and Management*, edited by U. K. Rinne, M. Klingler and G. Stamm, 93–107. Amsterdam, Elsevier (1980)

80 RINNE, U. K., LÖNNBERG, P. and KOSKINEN, V. Dopamine receptors in the parkinsonian brain. *Journal of Neural Transmission*, **51**, 97–109 (1981)

81 SAR, M., STUMPF, W. E., MILLER, R. J., CHANG, K.-J. and CUATRECASES, P. Immunohistochemical localization of enkephalin in rat brain and spinal cord. *Journal of Comparative Neurology*, **182**, 17–37 (1978)

82 SCHACHTER, M., BÉDARD, P., DEBONO, A. G., JENNER, P., MARSDEN, C. D., PRICE, P., PARKES, J. D., KEENAN, J., SMITH, B., ROSENTHALER, J., HOROWSKI, R. and DOROW, R. The role of D-1 and D-2 receptors. *Nature*, **286**, 157–159 (1981)

83 SCHWARCZ, R., HÖKFELT, T., FUXE, K., JONSSON, G., GOLDSTEIN, M. and TERENIUS, L. Ibotenic acid induced neuronal degeneration: a morphological and neurochemical study. *Experimental Brain Research*, **37**, 199–216 (1973)

84 SCHWARCZ, R., FUXE, K., HÖKFELT, T., TERENIUS, L. and GOLDSTEIN, M. Effects of chronic striatal kainate lesions on some dopaminergic parameters and enkephalin immunoreactive neurons in the basal ganglia. *Journal of Neurochemistry*, **34**, 772–778 (1980)

85 SCHWARTZ, J. C., POLLARD, H., LLORENS, C., MULFROY, B., GROS, C., PHRADELLES, P. and DRAY, F. Endorphins and endorphin receptors in the striatum: relationships with dopaminergic neurons. In *The Endorphins*, **3**, edited by E. Costa and M. Trabucchi, 245–264. New York, Raven Press (1978)

86 SHIBUYA, M. Dopamine-sensitive adenylate cyclase activity in the striatum in Parkinson's disease. *Journal of Neural Transmission*, **44**, 287–295 (1975)

87 SIMANTOV, R., KUHAR, M. J., UHL, G. R. and SNYDER, S. H. Opioid peptide enkephalin: Immunohistochemical mapping in the rat central nervous system. *Proceedings of the National Academy of the USA*, **74**, 2167–2171 (1977)

88 SNYDER, S. H. Brain peptides as neurotransmitters. *Science*, **209**, 976–983 (1980)

89 SPANO, P. F., GOVONI, S. and TRABUCCHI, M. Studies on the pharmacological properties of dopamine receptors in various areas of the central nervous system. *Advances in Biochemical Psychopharmacology*, **19**, 155–165 (1978)

90 SPANO, P. F., MEMO, M., STEFANINI, E., FRESIA, P. and TRABUCCHI, M. Detection of multiple receptors for dopamine. *Advances in Biochemical Psychopharmacology*, **21**, 243–251 (1980)

91 THAL, L., MISHRA, R. K., GARDNER, E. L., HOROWITZ, S. G., VARMUZA, S. and MAKMAN, M. H. Dopamine antagonist binding increases in two behaviorally distinct striatal denervation syndromes. *Brain Research*, **170**, 381–386 (1979)

92 TERENIUS, L. Opiate receptors: problems of definition and characterization. *Advances in Biochemical Psychopharmacology*, **21**, 321–328 (1980)

93 TITELER, M., LIST, S. and SEEMAN, P. High affinity dopamine receptors (D_3) in rat brain. *Communications in Psychopharmacology*, **3**, 411–420 (1979)

94 WATERFIELD, A. A., LESLIE, F. M., LORD, J. A. H., LING, N. and KOSTERLITZ, H. W. Opioid activities of fragments of beta-endorphin and of its leucine[5] analogue. Comparison of the binding properties of methionine- and leucine-enkephalin. *European Journal of Pharmacology*, **58**, 11–18 (1979)

95 WHITE, P., HILEY, C. R., GOODHARDT, M. J., CARRASCO, L. H., KEET, J. P., WILLIAMS, I. E. I. and BOWEN, D. M. Neocortical cholinergic neurons in elderly people. *Lancet*, **1**, 668–671 (1977)

96 WINKLER, M. H., BERL, S., WHETSELL, W. O. and YAHR, M. D. Spiroperidol binding in the human caudate nucleus. *Journal of Neural Transmission*, **16**, 45–51 (1980)

97 ZIEGLGÄNSBERGER, W. and FRY, J. P. Actions of enkephalins on cortical and striatal neurons in naive and morphine tolerant/dependent rats. In *Opiates and Endogenous Opioid Peptides*, edited by H. W. Kosterlitz, 231–238. Amsterdam, Elsevier (1976)

6
Depression and dementia in Parkinson's disease

Richard Mayeux

Depression and dementia constitute two mental symptoms in Parkinson's disease that have been the subject of controversy since the late 19th century. James Parkinson[54] originally suggested that 'the senses and intellects' were not affected in the 'shaking palsy'. However, nearly every subsequent author who wrote about this disease proposed that mental symptoms were part of its complex symptoms. Parkinson may have initiated the eventual controversy since his precarious opening statement was followed by examples of patients he described as 'melancholy', 'dejected', and 'delirious'.

One of the difficulties in reviewing this literature is the extreme variability of definitions used for describing 'mental' changes. At the turn of the century investigators generally did not distinguish depression from intellectual decline and subsequent dementia. In fact, all mental symptoms associated with Parkinson's disease were considered part of a continuum of mental deterioration secondary to the disease process. While this supposition may have been true, it may have also led to indistinct reporting of mental symptomatology rather than the preferred categorization of observed phenomena. While the characteristics, prevalence, and etiology of the various mental disturbances associated with Parkinson's disease remain in question, current investigations suggest that most parkinsonian patients will develop either depression or dementia.

Depression seems to occur most frequently, irrespective of disability. Its basis has been considered reactive by some and endogenous by others. The third edition of the *Diagnostic and Statistical Manual of Mental Disorders (DSM-III)*[22] divides depression into two types of affective disorder: organic affective syndrome and major depressive episode. The organic affective syndrome is characterized by a predominant dysphoric mood over at least a two week period accompanied by at least two of the following symptoms: appetite or weight change, insomnia or hypersomnia, psychomotor agitation or retardation, loss of interest in daily activities, fatigue, feelings of worthlessness, diminished concentration, and recurrent thoughts of death or suicide. No evidence of significant dementia or alteration in consciousness should be present, and the affect must be judged to be related to an underlying disorder. The major depressive episode is distinguished by the absence of a causative or a related 'organic' disorder and includes four of the symptoms described above. Reactive depression is poorly defined but is manifest by clinical features similar to the depressive episode but in response to a critical situation, e.g. death of a loved one, etc. Most investigators have not used such criteria to define depression in Parkinson's disease. It is conceivable that both types of depression occur in Parkinson's disease, particularly if the affective component is out of proportion to the extent of resulting disability. On the other hand, it may be difficult not to consider the disease as a causative or related organic disorder.

Dementia has less frequently been observed in parkinsonian patients, but it tends to parallel disability as well as advancing age. Again, no consistent definition for dementia has been used. DSM-III criteria include loss of intellectual abilities sufficient to impair social or occupational functioning, characterized by memory impairment and at least one of the following symptoms: impairment of abstract thinking or judgement, the presence of aphasia, apraxia, agnosia, or constructional difficulty, and personality change. Consciousness must be intact and the dementia should be judged to be related to an underlying disorder. The absence of depression is crucial as this may also be accompanied by intellectual impairment. Cummings and Benson[17] have used criteria similar to those described above to evaluate dementias in various situations. The definition does not imply an etiology or infer irreversability, thus it is a versatile one. In addition, disorders in which only memory loss or personality change prevail are clearly distinguished. Unfortunately criteria such as these have not always been applied to studies of intellectual disorders in parkinsonian patients.

The purpose of this chapter is to review the literature concerning depression and dementia in Parkinson's disease, and to attempt to clarify some of the controversial issues surrounding the clinical features of these symptoms and their specific relationship to the disease.

DEPRESSION

Prevalence

Depression is frequent in Parkinson's disease, and the reported prevalence varies between 20 percent[55] and 90 percent[50]. This variability most likely relates to the methodology employed as well as the various populations of parkinsonians investigated. Patrick and Levy[55] found 20 percent of their patients to be depressed. In these patients depression was described as a loss of interest accompanied by crying spells, carelessness, and insomnia. The authors concluded that depression was most likely reactive to the disabling nature of the disease since they found that it tended to parallel its severity. Mjones[52] subdivided 'mental changes' into 'reactive' and 'organic'. The reactive type was characterized by a depressive (dysphoric) change during which the patient became irritable, egocentric, discontent, and hypochondrical. When memory became blunted or thought processes became retarded, he referred to this type as an organic change. In this situation decreased concentration and mental fatiguability occurred and the dysphoric symptoms intensified. Mjones found that 40 percent of the patients he examined with 'paralysis agitans' displayed a combination of these symptoms which he observed also to increase with the severity of the disease.

Subsequent investigators began to study larger groups of parkinsonian patients and some compared the incidence of depression to various diseased control groups. Table 6.1 summarizes these investigations. One of the first prospective investigations was by Warburton[72]. In this study, the Maudsley personality inventory was used to examine 140 patients referred for thalamotomy. Using this method,

Table 6.1 Prevalence of depression in Parkinson's disease

Investigator	Year	No. of patients	Controls	No. depressed (%)	Methods	Comments
Patrick and Lewy[55]	1922	100	No	20 (20)	Clinical assessment	Criteria described considered reactive
Mjones[52]	1949	238	No	? (±40)	Clinical assessment	Overlap 'organic and reactive'
Warburton[72]	1967	140	Yes	88 (63)	Maudsley personality inventory	Criteria included fleeting symptoms
Mindham[50]	1970	89	Yes	80 (90)	'Standard diagnoses'	All patients referred for mental illness included postencephalitic and arteriosclerotic cases
Brown and Wilson[13]	1972	111	No	58 (52)	Hamilton depression rating scale	Retrospective chart review included arteriosclerotic and postencephalitic cases
Celesia and Wanamaker[15]	1972	153	No	57 (37)	Modified scale from Warburton	Included fleeting symptoms, and noted less depression in levodopa treated patients
Lieberman et al.[39]	1979	352*	No	107 (30.4)	Clinical inquiry	No criteria stated
Mayeux et al.[47]	1981	55	Yes	26 (47.2)	Clinical inquiry Beck Depression Inventory	Beck score >10 DSM–III criteria in post-test interview

* Nondemented

depression was subdivided into fleeting symptoms, sustained symptoms (lasting weeks to months) resulting in a poor adjustment to illness, and sustained symptoms accompanied by suicidal thoughts or ideation. A group of age and sex matched controls with a variety of medical, surgical, and gynecological disorders were also examined. Depression was found to be more common in the parkinsonian group (56 percent of males, 71 percent of females) than in the control group (23 percent of males, 47 percent of females). Grade 1 depression in this investigation would not have met current DSM-III criteria, however, even if these patients are eliminated from consideration in both groups, the incidence of depression would remain higher in the parkinsonians (parkinsonian males 52 percent, females 60 percent; control males 1 percent, females 11 percent). No relationship to age, duration, or disability from Parkinson's disease could be inferred by Warburton who concluded that depression must be a reactive symptom. In another large prospective investigation Mindham[50] evaluated 89 parkinsonian patients admitted specifically for treatment of 'mental illness'. Using the 'standard diagnoses' described by Cooper[16] he discovered that 90 percent of this group of parkinsonians had prominent affective symptoms. The controls he studied were patients admitted to the same institution and similar diagnostic criteria were applied. Affective symptoms occurred as frequently in the control group. Mindham observed that depression was not always the primary psychiatric diagnosis in the parkinsonian patients, but it was almost always a prominent symptom. The high prevalence of depression in this group of patients has been questioned because the parkinsonian population study was drawn from a mental institution[13]. An additional criticism is that the criteria employed for depression did not require sustained mood change thus including patients with only fleeting symptoms. Nevertheless, the finding did confirm the high frequency of depressive symptoms among parkinsonian patients.

Celesia and Wanamaker[15] prospectively evaluated various psychiatric symptoms in 170 patients. Criteria similar to Warburton's were used to rate depression in their parkinsonian patients. They found 45 percent of their patients to be depressed; however, eliminating grade 1 fleeting, unsustained symptoms this figure would drop to 25 percent. No control group was studied and no relationship to the severity of the disease could be found, however, the authors encountered depression less frequently among levodopa treated patients.

Fifty-two percent of parkinsonian patients were considered depressed, in a retrospective study, by Brown and Wilson[13] who reviewed the records of 111 patients hospitalized over a 15 year period. The Hamilton depression rating scale[32] was used to rate depressive symptoms as absent, mild, moderate, and severe. No patient was considered depressed unless there were clear indications of a prominent affective disorder, such as disturbed appetite or sleep, psychomotor retardation, guilt feelings or suicide thoughts. No control group was evaluated and no relationship to the disease could be established.

Two other investigations have employed depression rating scales and used neurologically impaired patients as controls. Horn[33] studied depression in a group of paraplegics matched for age, sex and socioeconomic status to a group of idiopathic parkinsonians and 'normal' controls. The parkinsonian group emerged more significantly depressed than the two control groups, on the depression scale[21] from the Minnesota Multiphasic personality inventory. Similarly, Robins[63] used the Hamilton depression scale in a prospective study comparing 45 parkinsonians to a similar number of age and sex matched controls with either hemiplegia, spinal cord disease, amputations, or orthopedic conditions. The parkinsonian groups were clearly more depressed than their respective control group. Symptoms such as suicide, psychomotor retardation, and anxiety exemplified the differences in the two groups.

The prevalence of depression appears to be greater in Parkinson's disease than in other chronic disorders, however, Mindham *et al.*[51] have described the difficulty in selecting a suitable control diseased group. Several factors may contribute to mental symptoms in Parkinson's disease, including type of disability, drug therapy, and possibly neurotransmitter abnormalities. These are likely to make the parkinsonian patient very distinct to patients with other neurological diseases, thus contaminating any comparison.

Although no criteria were stated, Lieberman et al.[39] found depression in 30 percent of 352 'nondemented' parkinsonian outpatients interviewed. Mayeux et al.[47] investigated 55 consecutive parkinsonians who were stable and also reputed to be free of dementia. Using the Beck depression index[8] they found significant depression in 47 percent of these patients compared to only 12 percent of a group of spouses. The control group was selected for its similar age, education, and socioeconomic background. In their post-test interview, DSM-III criteria for organic affective disorder were met in nearly all of the depressed patients. A higher mean Beck score was also reported for this group.

Thus, despite the variety of methods described and used in these studies, investigators have consistently shown that between 40 and 50 percent of all patients with Parkinson's disease develop depression at some point during the course of their illness.

Characteristics

The severity of depression in Parkinson's disease has not always been described. In studies where this can be determined, recorded symptoms were usually of mild to moderate intensity[15, 47, 72]. Suicidal thoughts and attempts are not uncommon, but suicide has been rarely documented among parkinsonians[52, 60]. Depression has been reported to be more common among women only in the studies by Warburton[72] and Celesia and Wanamaker[15]. Generally there has not been a correlation between depressive symptoms and the severity of parkinsonism. One investigation did demonstrate a slight, yet significant, relationship between the severity of the disease, as judged by a clinical rating scale of signs and symptoms, and the presence of depression[47]. Most investigators concur that neither the presence nor the intensity of depression can be consistently related to any factor such as age, sex, degree of disability, or type of treatment[33, 47, 63].

Depression may occur even before the onset of overt signs or symptoms of Parkinson's disease. Patrick and Levy[55] reported depressive symptoms in 34 percent of their patients prior to the onset of 'paralysis agitans'. In fact, these authors stated that depression was more frequent prior to, than following, the onset of the disorder. Mindham[50] and Mjones[52] both observed premorbid depression, and 42.6 percent of the depressed parkinsonians studied by Mayeux et al.[47] met criteria for a depressive episode before developing overt symptoms of parkinsonism. These reports lend support to the hypothesis of depression as an endogenous disturbance rather than reactive since no clinical evidence of parkinsonism was present with the onset of the affect change. On the other hand, several authors have observed depression occurring with the onset of, or at least, during the first year of the illness[50, 55]. Thus it seems some patients may experience depression as a reaction to the knowledge of the disease or its disability, however others may develop affective symptoms prior to obvious indications of the disease. Since there is no way to objectively distinguish between reactive or endogenous depression other than by clinical history, it could be concluded that both forms of depression may occur in patients who develop Parkinson's disease.

Mild intellectual impairment has also been observed to accompany depression in some parkinsonians. Lewy[38] first noted this association, and Mjones[52] also commented that impairment of memory and mental 'fatiguability' might occur in association with depression. Lieberman et al.[39] observed that 25 percent of their 'mildly demented' parkinsonians were depressed at the time of the outpatient interview, however, they did not consider depression a prelude to dementia. Brown and Wilson[13] observed depression and dementia to overlap in their study of parkinsonian patients but no correlation or specific details were reported in this study. A correlation between the intensity of depression and the degree of intellectual impairment was found in the study by Mayeux et al.[47]. The graph in Figure 6.1 depicts this relationship. A brief but quantitative neuropsychological measure indicated that as the severity of depression increased deficits in attention, calculation, and recall did as well. This correlation remained significant even when variables such as age, education, and the severity of parkinsonism were eliminated from the analysis. These authors concluded that the relationship between depression and intellectual impairment in Parkinson's disease was an independent one because of the relatively weak relationship of depression to disease severity. These authors also commented that the mean score for the depressed patients was less than one standard deviation from their control group suggesting that the degree of intellectual impairment was mild.

The essential characteristics of depression in parkinsonian patients, e.g. degree of sleep disturbance, appetite change, etc. have not been described in detail. In

Figure 6.1 Correlation between score on Beck depression inventory and the brief neuropsychological measure. ($r = -0.329$, $P = 0.02$)

spite of this, one can assume that these symptoms are present because the depression scales employed in most of these investigations are sensitive measures of these phenomena, particularly those of Beck[8] and Hamilton[32]. Using the current DSM-III criteria for depression, patients who develop Parkinson's disease probably best adhere to an organic affective disorder if the depression occurs during the course of the illness or prior to the development of signs or symptoms of the disease. It would be extremely difficult to consider a major depressive episode in parkinsonian patients since it would be nearly impossible to be certain that the disease was not related to the affective symptoms. Patients who develop depressive symptoms during the first year of the disorder could be depressed as a reaction to the disabling nature of the disease, however, this should resolve as the patients adjust to the disability and treatment.

Treatment

Levodopa has made a significant impact on the inherent symptoms of parkinsonism, but its relationship to depression has remained controversial. Initially levodopa was reported to have a mood elevating effect in depressed parkinsonians[7, 15, 75]. This effect was later attributed to the resolution of the 'reactive' depression associated with the onset of the disease, provided levodopa actually improved the neurological picture. Damasio et al.[18] studied the psychiatric aspects of levodopa in 48 patients. They found that levodopa produced no significant antidepressant effects and might have accounted for reactivation of depression in patients who had a prior psychiatric history. Using an objective depression rating scale, Marsh and Markham[43] followed 27 parkinsonian patients after levodopa therapy was initiated. Fifteen months later, they found no evidence to indicate a significant increase or decrease in the prevalence of depression in their group. Mindham et al.[51] investigated 50 patients with regard to psychiatric symptoms, levodopa, and their relationship to the disability. Almost half of the patients developed depression during the first six months of the study; 12 of these patients had had a prior history of depression. They concluded that levodopa probably caused a re-emergence of pre-existing affective symptoms rather than causing a new illness. In addition, they found that levodopa had little, if any, antidepressant actions in their patients even if the physical signs improved.

A remarkable report has suggested that levodopa may have provoked or at least contributed to the eventual suicide of a parkinsonian patient[60]. In this patient a prior history of depression was mentioned, beginning with the onset of the disease. In spite of the neurological improvement with levodopa, the patient's emotional state deteriorated and he eventually took his life. Thus it appears that levodopa may transiently relieve depressive symptoms in some patients particularly if they are reactive to the initial disability, on the other hand, levodopa is more likely to reactivate depression in those patients with a premorbid history or have no demonstrable effect.

Several investigators have commented on the favorable response to tricyclic antidepressants in depressed parkinsonians[13, 15, 18]. Three major tricyclic antidepressants have been studied: imipramine[68], desipramine[35], and nortriptyline[5].

Imipramine and desipramine have been found to be effective in placebo controlled trials. The effects of these two agents appears to be similar and this might be expected since desipramine is a major metabolite of imipramine. Strang[68] and Laitinen[35] found that these agents act to reduce depression and fatigue in parkinsonian patients. During the brief test period reported in both studies (approximately one month) signs and symptoms of parkinsonism also improved, particularly rigidity and akinesia. Anderson et al.[5] studied the effect of nortriptyline in depressed parkinsonians. While the mean depression score was significantly reduced in this study, no change in posture, gait, tremor or akinesia was observed. These authors concluded that this was a true antidepressant effect and not due to the weak dopaminergic effect of this antidepressant. The demonstrated effectiveness of these agents is probably also independent of their weak anticholinergic effect. There has been minimal central anticholinergic activity demonstrated with these antidepressants[61]. Damasio et al.[18] demonstrated that levodopa and tricyclic antidepressants can be used simultaneously and without difficulty. In their study, favorable results were also reported with amitriptyline, however, this tricyclic has not been studied in a controlled method in parkinsonians. Successful improvement in depression may be realized with tricyclic antidepressants as indicated by these reports. Unfortunately, until studies evaluate the long term effectiveness of these agents their position in the treatment of Parkinson's disease remains unsolved.

Lebenshon and Jenkins[36] used electroconvulsive therapy (ECT) for depression in two parkinsonian patients who were resistant to more conventional therapies. Surprisingly, improvement in bradykinesia and rigidity, as well as mood occurred. Two other patients have been described in whom mood and parkinsonism improved following ECT[6, 77]. Mood elevation was reported to occur before neurological improvement in both studies, and only a few treatments were required. Both authors reported their benefit to be temporary, and both have attributed the result to the reputed alteration on catecholamine and indolamine receptors induced by ECT. While the consistency of these observations needs to be evaluated, there may be a place for ECT in depressed parkinsonian patients who are otherwise unresponsive to tricyclic antidepressants or other forms of therapy.

DEMENTIA

Prevalence

Only a few studies have examined the prevalence of dementia among patients with Parkinson's disease [15, 38, 39, 44, 57]. Interpretation of this literature is quite difficult because of the failure, in most studies, to clearly define dementia and the inclusion of 'arteriosclerotic' parkinsonism. The latter entity most likely represent a form of vascular dementia due to multiple infarcts. Nevertheless, intellectual deterioration has consistently been observed in patients suffering from Parkinson's disease. Lewy[38] observed mental disturbances in 64 percent of the patients he examined and in most this was considered a true dementia characterized by impairment of memory and slowed cognitive ability. Mjones'[52] overlap of reactive and organic mental changes in 40 percent of his patients may have included some patients with significant dementia. Pollack and Hornabrook[57] specifically addressed this issue in their survey of parkinsonism in New Zealand. Twenty percent of the patients examined in this study were found to have 'mental deterioration' of a significant proportion as to make the individual fully dependent on the family or on state aid. Unfortunately, details of the mental state examination are not described and the majority of demented patients evaluated were those associated with arteriosclerosis.

Celesia and Wanamaker[15] graded dementia into three types. Grade 1 was mild slowing manifested by defective abstract reasoning, concept formation, and calculation ability. Visuospatial impairment and apathy were also noted. Grade 2 was characterized by a more general impairment of cognition with disturbance in memory, while grade 3 indicated severe impairment in all intellectual activities. Sixty-one of 153 (40 percent) patients with idiopathic Parkinson's disease were found to be demented. Over half of this group were considered moderately to severely impaired. In a similar study the prevalence of dementia was found to be 29 percent by Martilla and Rinne[44] in southwest Finland. Among 444 patients with Parkinson's disease, 128 were considered demented by criteria similar to those described above. When arteriosclerosis was clinically evident by their clinical examination the frequency of dementia significantly increased. Less than half (39 percent) of the demented patients were significantly impaired (grade 2 or 3). Lieberman et al.[39] used similar criteria and found that one-third of their large outpatient population with Parkinson's disease were demented, however, severity was not determined. The results of each of these investigations are listed in Table

Table 6.2 Prevalence of dementia in Parkinson's disease

Investigator	Year	No. of patients studied	No. with dementia (%)	Comments
Lewy[38]	1923	70	?54 (77)	All mental disturbance, some 'true dementias', criteria not described
Mjones[52]	1949	238	?(40)	Included all mental disturbances, some with dementia, criteria not described
Pollack and Hornabrook[57]	1966	131	26 (20)	Included arteriosclerotic patients, methods of neuropshychological assessment not described, no criteria stated
Celesia and Wanamaker[15]	1972	153*	61 (40)	Total 170 patients seen, distinguished postencephalitic arteriosclerotic, toxic forms, criteria described. DSM–III met
Martilla and Rinne[44]	1976	444	128 (29)	Included 124 patients with clinical arteriosclerosis of whom 56.4% were demented (methods and criteria same as Celesia and Wanamaker)
Lieberman et al.[39]	1979	520	168 (32)	Criteria and methods well described, dementia meets DSM–III criteria

* Idiopathic

6.2. The incidence of demented parkinsonians among the general population is difficult to ascertain from these studies. Boller et al.[10] who studied neuropathological specimens, found the occurrence of dementia in parkinsonism to be six times greater than that of an age matched population, and Lieberman et al.[39] has suggested a 10-fold greater incidence.

Characteristics

Most investigators have not attempted to characterize the clinical features of dementia in patients with Parkinson's disease. Conversely, there are numerous reports describing defects in certain mental activities in parkinsonian patients, who are either not considered demented by the authors or the issue was not addressed in the report. In the epidemiological studies reviewed above dementia was usually judged on an ordinate scale from mild to severe impairment. In most circumstances DSM-III criteria for dementia would have been met, particularly when moderate to severe impairment was found such as in the study of Celesia and Wanamaker[15].

Certain deficits in intellectual function tend to highlight the parkinsonian patient. The most clear example of this is the high frequency of perceptual motor, or visuospatial impairment. This has been reported so frequently in association with parkinsonism that it may not be an indication of dementia, particularly when this is the only demonstrable impairment. DeLancy Horne[20] found parkinsonians were unable to correctly identify complex visual stimuli particularly after a brief delay. Map or route walking was defective in a group of parkinsonians studied by Bowen et al.[12]. Loranger et al.[40] found marked deficits in their parkinsonian patients in tasks such as digit span, block design, picture arrangements, and object assembly from the Wechsler adult intelligence scale. Investigators have also found that parkinsonians have difficulty solving problems that require sequential mental activity[70], and that depend on judgement of visual perception[19]. These deficits are most often indicated on standard neuropsychological measures that include visual memory[76]. In all of these studies, parkinsonian patients were compared to controls who performed significantly better. Flowers [24, 25] found defective tracing of visual stimuli and inability to predict movements on spatial tasks among parkinsonians. Mayeux et al.[48] re-examined this issue comparing the performance of age matched controls to that of parkinsonians on tracing tasks. In this study the patient's simple hand tracing was interrupted by hesitations and inability to maintain stimulus boundaries. This deficit was not considered to be related to the motor disability, however, failure to complete line drawings of cubes or angles tended to parallel overall intellectual ability. The authors concluded that these deficits might represent a perceptual defect because of the correlation with general neurophysical measures. There was no particular relationship to signs or symptoms of parkinsonism and similar distortions were not noted among controls. In contrast, Mortimer et al.[53] found a particularly strong association between the severity of motor symptoms of parkinsonism and the degree of impairment on visuospatial tasks, particularly block design and digit symbol.

Most of the tasks described above require a sequence of mental activities, for example, with digit span backwards a series of numbers must be mentally retained and then read in reverse. Similarly, to complete a constructional task, a plan or sequence of movements must be generated by the patient before the task can be attempted. The basal ganglia are considered to participate in, and even regulate some complex sequential motor activities, as well as some complex intellectual activities[1, 12, 14, 65, 71]. It is possible that these deficits could be related to degenerative changes within the basal ganglia of patients with Parkinson's disease.

Another example of unusual deficits in intellectual activity among parkinsonians has been presented by Wilson et al.[73] who found slowed short-term memory. Overall accuracy of memory was the same as in age matched controls in this study, but scanning of elements presumably held in short term memory was significantly slowed for the parkinsonian patients. The authors did not consider this deficit as a result of bradykinesia concomitant dementia, or slowed reaction time, but rather as an alteration produced by the diseased basal ganglia. Matison et al.[45] described a form of anomia or word finding disturbance among parkinsonian patients that they

Table 6.3 Forms of intellectual dysfunction observed in parkinsonism

Investigator	Year	No. of patients	Impaired intellectual activity
Talland[70]	1962	45	Problem solving, requiring sequencing
DeLancy Horne[20]	1971	11	Delayed visual recognition
Bowen, Hoehn, Yahr[12]	1972	47	Spatial orientation (route-walking)
Lorranger et al.[40]	1972	63	Perceptual-motor tasks from WAIS
Danta[19]	1975	66	Visual vertical/horizontal judgement
Yahr and Proctor-Brown[76]	1975	86	Recall, visual reproduction, digit span
Flowers[24]	1978	15	Tracking or wave forms
Flowers[25]	1978	10	Predictive hand movements for tracking
Wilson et al.[73]	1980	20	Short term memory scanning
Mayeux et al.[47]	1981	55	Digit span, recall, visuospatial
Mortimer et al.[53]	1981	60	Visuospatial perception
Matison et al.[45]	1981	22	Tip-of-the-tongue phenomenon (anomia)
Mayeux et al.[48]	1981	17	Visual tracing of lines and forms

WAIS = Wechster Adult Intelligence Scale.

considered unrelated to dementia. The parkinsonians were unable to name pictured items as well as controls and their ability to generate word lists of items within a specific category was impaired. In contrast, the estimate of their patients lexicons were considered normal and no clinical evidence for dementia could be found.

These reports suggest that many parkinsonians develop a disturbance in visuospatial discrimination, and less frequently in certain memory or language skills. These deficits by their unique nature, and when present alone, probably do not warrant a diagnosis of dementia. *Table 6.3* summarizes the unique nature of these intellectual deficits in parkinsonian patients.

Relationship of dementia to the disease

Many investigations of Parkinson's disease have indicated a close relationship between the extent of disability and the severity of the disease to a decline or impairment of intellectual activity[15, 39, 44, 47, 52] (refer to *Table 6.4*). Mjones[52] commented on a 'certain parallelism' between motor and intellectual deficits suggesting that as the severity of motor deficits increased in 'paralysis agitans' the degree of mental symptoms also increased. Celesia and Wanamaker[15] also noted

Table 6.4 Relationship between intellectual impairment and parkinsonism

Investigator	Year	No. of patients	Factors related to intellectual dysfunction
Garron et al.[27]	1972	47	Age, degree of disability, particularly akinesia
Lorranger et al.[40]	1972	63	Severity of clinical symptoms and functional disability
Celesia and Wanamaker[15]	1972	153	Age, duration of illness, degree of motor disability
Martilla and Rinne[44]	1976	444	Age, hypokinesia, rigidity
Lieberman et al.[39]	1979	520	Late age of onset, severity of disease
Matthews and Haaland[46]	1979	42	Duration of illness
Mayeux et al.[47]	1981	55	Age, education, depression, severity of parkinsonism
Mortimer et al.[53]	1981	60	Bradykinesia

that the severity, as well as the frequency, of dementia increased with disability as measured by the Columbia University disability scale. Garron et al.[27] specifically noted a correlation between intellectual impairment and bradykinesia as did Loranger et al.[40]. Mayeux et al.[47] also observed the relationship between the severity of parkinsonism and deficits on neuropsychological measures in patients who were not considered clinically demented by DSM-III criteria. This relationship is observed in *Figure 6.2* below.

Duration of illness has been implicated as a factor in subsequent deterioration of perceptual motor skills in parkinsonian patients[46] and in the development of dementia[15] but this is an inconsistent association. Increasing age has also been associated with intellectual impairment in several studies[15, 39, 47]. In each of these investigations dementia was more frequently observed in patients who develop the disease later in life. Lieberman et al.[39] found that demented parkinsonian patients were an average of 5 years older than nondemented parkinsonians, developed the signs and symptoms of the disease later in life, had a brief duration of illness, but were less likely to respond favorably to levodopa. This led to the hypothesis that two separate forms of parkinsonism might exist: a motor disorder, typically in younger patients with the usual progression of the illness and therapeutic response; and a motor-'cognitive' disorder, occurring in older patients with a more fulminant course and poor response to therapy. Earlier, Garron et al.[27] had noted the association between delayed onset of parkinsonism, akinesia, and intellectual deterioration. Similarly Sroka et al.[67] have subdivided parkinsonian patients into typical and atypical; the latter characterized arbitrarily as a dysfunction including brain stem or cerebellar signs, as well as an unusual evolution of the disease. In the

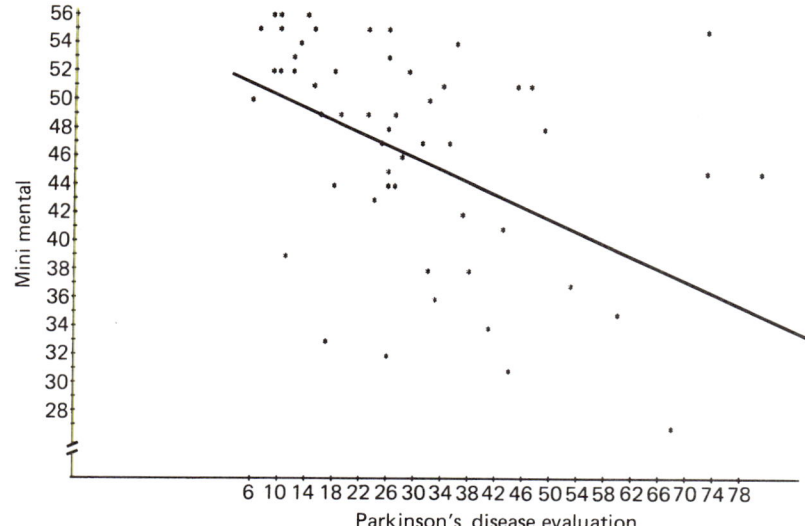

Figure 6.2 Correlation between severity of Parkinson's disease and the brief neuropsychological measure. (r = −0.426, P = 0.002)

atypical group, 'organic mental syndrome', i.e. permanent changes in cognition, abstraction, reasoning and judgement in memory was present in 68 percent compared to 15 percent of 'typical' parkinsonians. While age was similar in both groups duration of illness was significantly less for those patients with atypical Parkinson's disease and dementia.

Etiology

The cause of dementia has not been firmly established in Parkinson's disease. Neuropathological studies lack clinical correlation, and clinical studies often speculate on possible explanatory lesions. As a result two views exist. Several investigators have suggested that dementia is related to the neuropathological findings consistent with Alzheimer's disease[4, 10, 28, 19]. Others argue that the clinical characteristics of Parkinson's disease are unique to that of Alzheimer's disease and therefore attribute dementia to the degeneration within the basal ganglia[2, 3, 49].

Alvord et al.[4] observed two distinct patterns of degenerative changes in the brains of patients with Parkinson's disease: a 'Lewy body' type in which the degree of clinical parkinsonism correlated with the degree of neuronal loss in substantia nigra and the degree of dementia with cortical degeneration. The other, 'Alzheimer's tangle' type, in which the degree of dementia and cortical degeneration were parallel, but the degree of parkinsonism was not necessarily associated with neuronal loss in substantia nigra. This form probably included postencephalitic cases and variants of senile dementia. These correlations were done retrospectively and dementia was graded on an ordinate scale from 0 to 4+. The authors only suggested, but were not certain, that dementia was related to the presence of Alzheimer's tangles; no statistical correlation was reported.

Hakim and Mathieson[29] retrospectively studied 34 consecutive cases who met neuropathological criteria for Parkinson's disease. A similar number of age and sex matched controls were studied for the presence of senile plaques, neurofibrillary tangles, and granulovascular degeneration in the hippocampus and for neocortical neuronal loss. Clinical records were reviewed to determine the presence of intellectual decline. Fifty-six percent of the patients had evidence of either memory loss, confusion, or 'florid' dementia. Virtually all of the parkinsonian's brains, however, had histologic evidence of Alzheimer's disease by their criteria. Careful clinicopathological correlation with dementia was lacking, but in spite of this the authors concluded that dementia in Parkinson's disease was the result with these concomitant findings of Alzheimer's disease. In a similar postmortem study, Boller et al.[10] found clinical documentation of severe dementia in 9 of 29 parkinsonian patients. Manifestations included inattention, impairments in memory, calculations, constructions, digit span, and abstraction. All 9 of these patients had a quantitative predominance of histological changes suggestive of Alzheimer's disease. In 7 less impaired patients with poor memory and slowed responses, a less clear-cut relationship was established. In this study a significant relationship was established between the severity in intellectual impairment and the presence of senile plaques and neurofibrillary tangles.

Clinical stigmata of Alzheimer's disease usually have been found to correlate with quantitative measures of plaques, tangles, and other degenerative changes[9]. Similar correlations have been found to exist for cholinergic activity in the brains of patients dying of Alzheimer's disease[56]. The investigation of cholinergic activity in the brains of demented parkinsonians might confirm or deny the coincidence of these two degenerative diseases since there is a less than precise relationship between the presence of histologic changes of Alzheimer's disease and dementia in parkinsonism. Levels of choline acetyltransferase and cholinesterase have been measured in several regions of brain, including hippocampus, in 5 patients with Parkinson's disease, but the levels were found to be no different from that of a control group of a similar age[42]. The presence of dementia was not considered in this report, and until a histochemical analysis of demented parkinsonians is carried out, the coexistence of Parkinson's disease and Alzheimer's disease remains less than definitive.

Radiological studies have also tried to address the issue of dementia in Parkinson's disease by searching for radiographic evidence of neuronal degeneration. Selby[66] found that cortical atrophy on pneumoencephalogram was present in 57 percent of parkinsonian patients while ventricular enlargement was found in 30 percent. This was strikingly different from controls who underwent pneumoencephalography. While no correlation between decline in intellectual function and cerebral atrophy was found, a statistically significant relationship between ventricular dilation and impaired mental function existed. The exact nature of this impairment was not described. Sroka et al.[67], who as previously noted separated parkinsonism into typical and atypical forms, noted that no patient with a normal computed tomogram of the brain had evidence of dementia by their criteria. While all their parkinsonians with dementia had abnormal scans, ventricular enlargement again correlated better with intellectual decline than did cortical atrophy. Two-thirds of the 'atypical' parkinsonians with dementia they reported had enlarged ventricles. Computed tomographic evidence of atrophy has only weakly implicated impaired mental function in studies of other forms of dementia, particularly Alzheimer's disease[23] and Sroka et al.[67] generally concurred with this view in their parkinsonian patients. In spite of this, the dementia in the atypical parkinsonian patients was discussed with the view that coincident Alzheimer's disease might explain the intellectual dysfunction.

The alternative hypothesis used to explain dementia in Parkinson's disease has been based on the concept of 'subcortical dementia'[2, 3, 49]. Investigators have attributed dementia in Parkinson's disease to basal ganglia or 'subcortical' dysfunction rather than cerebral degeneration[2, 3, 44, 47, 49]. This concept is based on the premise that the aphasia, apraxia, and agnosia observed in Alzheimer's disease is not consistently observed in all demented parkinsonian patients. While this concept may be true, only a few studies have contrasted the clinical manifestations of dementia in these two disorders[26, 49]. In the study by Mayeux et al.[49] patients with dementia of the Alzheimer type (based on clinical criteria) and patients with Parkinson's disease were staged into three groups by appropriate disability rating scales. Patients then completed a similar brief neuropsychological measure. Significant differences emerged in their overall intellectual ability; at every stage the parkinsonian patients were less impaired. In fact, the most severely disabled parkinsonian had a higher overall neuropsychological score than did the least disabled patient with Alzheimer's disease. Other factors such as duration of illness and age tended to parallel the disability rating. Remarkably, memory impairment and disordered visuospatial ability deteriorated through stages in both groups, however, language was remarkably preserved in the parkinsonian patients.

These types of differences have been the basis of the argument that dementia in Parkinson's disease is not related to cortical neuronal degeneration and concomitant Alzheimer disease. Investigators have generally concluded that basal ganglia degeneration underlies the disorder of mentation in parkinsonism. Lending support to this view is the remarkably consistent correlation between the severity of parkinsonism and the presence of intellectual impairment. Thus basal ganglia dysfunction must be considered, at least in part, as a cause of dementia in Parkinson's disease.

Recently Javoy-Agid and Agid[34] have added to the controversy by their finding of decreased dopamine in neurons in cortical projection areas receiving input from mesencephalic dopamine containing neurons. The authors suggested that this deficiency may play a role in certain aspects of mental impairment associated with parkinsonism, particularly akinesia and its relationship to cognition as well as psychopathology. Alterations in mesocortical and mesolimbic[58] systems may contribute to the observed relationship between movement and neuropsychological disorders of parkinsonism. Needless to say, this attractive hypothesis also deserves further investigation.

Levodopa and dementia

As with depression, levodopa has played a controversial role with regard to dementia. The presence of dementia in Parkinson's disease has been considered a key factor limiting levodopa therapy[37, 64]. Loranger et al.[40] had initially reported improvement on perceptual motor tasks of the Wechsler adult intelligence scale in their patients following one year of levodopa therapy. There was little to no correlation between improvement in motor signs of parkinsonism and change in dementia. Some of these patients were retested on an average of 2–3 years later and a similar set of psychological measures then indicated a decline in function to pretreatment levels[41]. The authors concluded that the decline in mental function following the initial improvement was due to 'cortical atrophy', i.e. the progressive nature of the disease. Halgin et al.[30] reported nearly the same observations. Similar neuropsychological measures were used and they followed patients for 2- and 4-year periods. Thus it appears that intellectual function may improve briefly following the initiation of levodopa, but this positive effect has been consistently found to be a brief one[11, 30, 31, 41, 59, 62, 69]. In each of these reports, investigators have attributed resurgence of intellectual decline to the disease rather than to levodopa.

In severely demented parkinsonian patients, levodopa has been found to be associated with extremely undesirable effects. Excitement, hyperkinesia, somnolence, and akinesia were frequently observed by Sacks et al.[64]. Hallucinations and depression were also more prevalent in the demented parkinsonians. Sweet et al.[69] have found that dementia improved slightly during the first 6 months of levodopa therapy but the occurrence of agitation, hallucinations, and delusions increased remarkably in demented patients. Levodopa may have also contributed in some way to a permanent dementia in a patient with Parkinson's disease[74].

Conclusions

There is little doubt that depression and dementia constitute two important problems in patients with Parkinson's disease. Clinicians can expect to encounter one or the other of these problems in the course of a patient's illness. While manifestations of these symptoms have been somewhat elucidated, their etiology and treatment remain an enigma. Continued advances in the treatment of the inherent motor disability of Parkinson's disease have largely been based on morphological and biochemical studies. Similar basic studies are lacking in the analysis of depression and dementia. For example, comparison of catecholamine and indolamine metabolism in depressed and nondepressed parkinsonians might help to unravel the question of depression as an endogenous or reactive symptom. Histochemical studies, along with careful clinical correlation, such as those performed in Alzheimer's disease might also reveal a clue regarding the role of Alzheimer tangles and cortical atrophy in the dementia of Parkinson's disease.

Further investigation of the mesocortical and mesolimbic pathways could contribute to our understanding of both the affective and intellectual changes. Certainly until these investigations are completed the controversy surrounding the cause and treatment of depression and dementia will persist.

References

1 AJURIAGUERRA, J. De. The concept of akinesia. *Psychological Medicine*, **5**, 129–137 (1975)
2 ALBERT, M. L., FELDMAN, R. G. and WILLIS, A. L. The subcortical dementia of progressive supranuclear palsy. *Journal of Neurology, Neurosurgery and Psychiatry*, **38**, 121–130 (1974)
3 ALBERT, M. L. Subcortical dementia. In *Alzheimer's Disease: Senile Dementia and Related Disorders*, 173–180. New York, Raven Press (1978)
4 ALVORD, E. C., FORNO, L. S., KUSSKE, J. A., KAUFFMAN, R. J., RHODES, J. S. and GOETOWSKI, C. R. The pathology of parkinsonism: a comparison of degenerations in cerebral cortex and brain stem. *Advances in Neurology*, **5**, 175–193 (1974)
5 ANDERSEN, J., AABRO, E., GULMANN, N., HJELMSTED, A. and PEDERSEN. H. E. Antidepressive treatment of Parkinson's disease. *Acta Neurologica Scandinavia*, **62**, 210–219 (1980)
6 ASNIS, G. Parkinson's disease, depression and ECT: a review and case study. *American Journal of Psychiatry*, **134**, 191–195 (1977)
7 BARBEAU, A. L-Dopa therapy in Parkinson's disease: a critical review of nine years experience. *Journal of Canadian Medical Association*, **101**, 791–800 (1969)
8 BECK, A. T. In *Depression*, 333–338. University of Pennsylvania Press, Philadelphia, (1967)
9 BLESSED, G., TOMLINSON, B. E. and ROTH, M. The association between quantitative measures of dementia and senile changes in the cerebral grey matter of elderly subjects. *British Journal of Psychiatry*, **114**, 797–811 (1968)
10 BOLLER, F., MIZUTANI, R., ROESSMANN, U. and GAMBETTI, P. Parkinson's disease, dementia, and Alzheimer's disease: clinicopathological correlations. *Annals of Neurology*, **7**, 329–335 (1980)
11 BOTEZ, M. I. and BARBEAU, A. Neuropsychological findings in Parkinson's disease: a comparison between various tests during long-term levodopa therapy. *International Journal of Neurology*, **10**, 222–232 (1975)
12 BOWEN, F. P., HOEHN, M. M. and YAHR, M.D. Parkinsonism: alterations in spatial orientation as determined by a route-walking test. *Neuropsychologica*, **10**, 335–361 (1972)
13 BROWN, G. L. and WILSON, W. P. Parkinsonism and depression. *Southern Medical Journal*, **65**, 540–545 (1972)
14 BUCHWALD, N. A., HULL, C. D., LEVINE, M. S. and VILLABLANCA, J. The basal ganglia and the regulation of response and cognitive sets. *Growth and Development of the Brain*, 171–189. New York, Raven Press (1975)
15 CELESIA, G. G. and WANAMAKER, W. M. Psychiatric disturbances in Parkinson's disease. *Diseases of the Nervous System*, **33**, 577–583 (1972)

16 COOPER, J. E. Diagnostic change in a longitudinal study of psychiatric patients. *British Journal of Psychiatry*, **113**, 129–142 (1967)
17 CUMMINGS, J., BENSON, D. F. and LOVERME, S. Reversible dementia. *Journal of the American Medical Association*, **243**, 2434–2439 (1980)
18 DAMASIO, A. R., LOBO-ANTUNES, J. and MACEDO, C. Psychiatric aspects in parkinsonism treated with L-dopa. *Journal of Neurology, Neurosurgery, and Psychiatry*, **34**, 502–507 (1971)
19 DANTA, G. and HILTON, R. C. Judgement of the visual, vertical and horizontal in patients with parkinsonism. *Neurology*, **25**, 43–47 (1975)
20 DELANCY HORNE, D. Performance on delayed response tasks by patients with parkinsonism. *Journal of Neurology, Neurosurgery, and Psychiatry*, **34**, 192–194 (1971)
21 DEMPSY, P. An unidimensional depression scale for the MMPI. *Journal of Consulting Psychology*, **28**, 364–370 (1964)
22 *Diagnostic and Statistical Manual of Mental Disorders*. Third Edition. Washington, DC, American Psychiatric Association (1980)
23 EARNEST, M. P., HEATON, R. K., WILKINSON, W. E. and MANKE, W. F. Cortical atrophy, ventricular enlargement and intellectual impairment in the aged. *Neurology*, **29**, 1138–1143 (1979)
24 FLOWERS, K. Some frequency response characteristics of parkinsonism on pursuit tracking. *Brain*, **101**, 19–34 (1978)
25 FLOWERS, K. Lack of prediction in the motor behaviour of parkinsonism. *Brain*, **101**, 35–52 (1978)
26 GAINOTTI, G., CALTAGIRONE, C., MASULLO, C. and MICHELLI, G. Patterns of neuropsychologic impairment in various diagnostic groups of dementia. *Aging*, **13**, 245–250. New York, Raven Press (1980)
27 GARRON, D. C., KLAWANS, H. L. and NARIN, F. Intellectual functioning of persons with idiopathic parkinsonism. *Journal of Nervous and Mental Disease*, **154**, 445–452 (1972)
28 HAKIM, A. M. and MATHIESON, G. Basis of dementia in Parkinson's disease. *Lancet*, **2**, 729 (1978)
29 HAKIM, A. M. and MATHIESON, G. Dementia in Parkinson disease: a neuropathologic study. *Neurology*, **29**, 1209–1214 (1979)
30 HALGIN, R., RIKLIN, M. and MISIAK, H. Levodopa, parkinsonism, and recent memory. *Journal of Nervous and Mental Disease*, **164**, 268–272 (1977)
31 HAMEL, A. R. and RIKLIN, M. Cognitive and perceptual effects of long range L-dopa therapy in parkinsonism. *Journal of Clinical Psychology*, **31**, 321–333 (1975)
32 HAMILTON, M. A rating scale for depression. *Journal of Neurology, Neurosurgery and Psychiatry*, **23**, 56–61 (1960)
33 HORN, S. Some psychological factors in parkinsonism. *Journal of Neurology, Neurosurgery and Psychiatry*, **37**, 27–31 (1974)
34 JAVOY-AGID, F. and AGID, Y. Is the mesocortical dopaminergic system involved in Parkinson's disease? *Neurology*, **30**, 1326–1330 (1980)
35 LAITINEN, L. Desipramine in treatment of Parkinson's disease. *Acta Neurologica Scandinavia*, **45**, 109–113 (1969)

36 LEBENSOHN, Z. and JENKINS, R. B. Improvement of parkinsonism in depressed patients treated with ECT. *American Journal of Psychiatry*, **132**, 283–285 (1975)

37 LESSER, R. P., FAHN, S., SNIDER, S. R., COTE, L. J., ISGREEN, W. P. and BARRETT, R. E. Analysis of the clinical problems in parkinsonism and the complications of long-term levodopa therapy. *Neurology*, **29**, 1253–1260 (1979)

38 LEWY, F. H. *Die Lehre Von Tonus und der bewegung zugleich systematiche Untersuchinger sur Klinik, Physiologie, Pathologie und Pathogenese der Paralysis Agitans.* Berlin, Springer (1923)

39 LIEBERMAN, A., DZIATOLOWSKI, M., COOPERSMITH, M., CERB, M., GOODGOLD, A., LOREIN, J. and GOLDSTEIN, M. Dementia in Parkinson's disease. *Annals of Neurology*, **6**, 355–359 (1979)

40 LORANGER, A. W., GOODELL, H., McDOWELL, F. H., LEE, J. E. and SWEET, R. D. Intellectual impairment in Parkinson's syndrome. *Brain*, **95**, 405–412 (1972)

41 LORANGER, A. W., GOODELL, H., LEE, J. E. and McDOWELL, F. Levodopa treatment of Parkinson's syndrome. *Archives of General Psychiatry*, **26**, 163–168 (1972)

42 McGEER, P. L. and McGEER, E. G. Cholinergic enzyme systems in Parkinson's disease. *Archives of Neurology*, **25**, 265–268 (1971)

43 MARSH, G. G. and MARKHAM, C. H. Does Levodopa alter depression and psychopathology in parkinsonism patients? *Journal of Neurology, Neurosurgery and Psychiatry*, **36**, 925–935 (1973)

44 MARTTILA, R. J. and RINNE, U. K. Dementia in Parkinson's disease. *Acta Neurologica Scandinavia*, **54**, 431–441 (1976)

45 MATISON, R., MAYEUX, R., ROSEN, J. and FAHN, S. Tip-of-the-tongue anomia in Parkinson's disease. *Neurology*, **31**, p. 102 (1981)

46 MATTHEWS, C. G. and HAALAND, K. Y. The effect of symptom duration on cognitive and motor performance in parkinsonism. *Neurology*, **29**, 951–956 (1979)

47 MAYEUX, R., STERN, Y, ROSON, J. and LEVENTHAL, J. Depression, intellectual impairment, and Parkinson's disease. *Neurology*, **31**, 645–650 (1981)

48 MAYEUX, R., STERN, Y. and ROSEN, J. Visuospatial function in Parkinson's disease. *Neurology*, **31**, p. 61 (1981)

49 MAYEUX, R., STERN, Y., ROSEN, J. and BENSON, D. F. Subcortical dementia: a recognizable clinical syndrome. *Annals of Neurology*, **10**, 100–101 (1981)

50 MINDHAM, R. H. S. Psychiatric syndromes in parkinsonism. *Journal of Neurology, Neurosurgery and Psychiatry*, **30**, 88–191 (1970)

51 MINDHAM, R. H. S., MARSDEN, C. D. and PARKES, J. D. Psychiatric symptoms during L-dopa therapy for Parkinson's disease and their relationship to physical disability. *Psychological Medicine*, **6**, 23–33 (1976)

52 MJONES, H. Paralysis agitans. *Acta Psychiatrica et Neurologica*, **54**, suppl., 1–195, (1949)

53 MORTIMER, J. A., PIROZZOLO, F. J., HANSCH, E. C. and WEBSTER, D. D. Relation of motor symptoms to intellectual deficits in Parkinson's disease. *Neurology*, **31**, p. 61 (1981)

54 PARKINSON, J. An essay of the shaking palsy, 1817. *Medical Classics*, **2**, 964–997 (1938)

55 PATRICK, H. T. and LEVY, D. M. Parkinson's disease: a clinical study of 146 cases. *Archives of Neurology and Psychiatry*, **7**, 711–720 (1922)

56 PERRY, E. K. The cholinergic system in old age and Alzheimer's disease. *Age and Aging*, **9**, 1–8 (1980)
57 POLLOCK, M. and HORNABROOK, R. W. The prevalence, natural history and dementia of Parkinson's disease. *Brain*, **89**, 429–448 (1966)
58 PRICE, K. S., FARLEY, I. J. and HORNYKIEWICZ, O. Neurochemistry of Parkinson's disease: relation between striatal and limbic dopamine. *Advances in Biochemical Psychopharmacology*, **19**, 293–300 (1978)
59 RADBILL, R., ROSENBERG, G. and SCHWARTZ, A. Effects of levodopa therapy in Parkinson's disease. II. Measurement of behavioral changes. *Canadian Medical Journal*, **111**, 1218–1222 (1974)
60 RAFT, D., NEWMAN, M. and SPENCER, R. Suicide on L-dopa. *Southern Medical Journal*, **65**, p. 312 (1972)
61 REHAVI, M., MAAGANI, S. and SOKOLOVSKY, M. Tricyclic antidepressants as antimuscarinic drugs: *in vivo* and *in vitro* studies. *Biochemical Pharmacology*, **26**, 1559–1567 (1977)
62 RIKLAN, M., WHELIHAN, W. and CULLINAN, T. Levodopa and psychometric test performance in parkinsonism–five years later. *Neurology*, **26**, 173–179 (1976)
63 ROBINS, A. H. Depression in patients with parkinsonism. *British Journal of Psychiatry*, **128**, 141–145 (1976)
64 SACKS, O. W., KROHL, M. S., MESSELOFF, C. R. and SCHWARTZ, W. F. Effects of levodopa in parkinsonian patients with dementia. *Neurology*, **22**, 615–619 (1972)
65 SCHWAB, S., CHAFETZ, M. E. and WALKER, S. Control of two simultaneous voluntary acts in normals and in parkinsonism. *Archives of Neurology and Psychiatry*, **75**, 591–598 (1954)
66 SELBY, G. Cerebral atrophy in parkinsonism. *Journal of the Neurological Sciences*, **6**, 517–559 (1968)
67 SROKA, H., ELIZAN, T. S., YAHR, M. D., BURGER, A. and MENDAZU, M. R. Organic mental syndrome and confusional states in Parkinson's disease. *Archives of Neurology*, **38**, 339–342 (1981)
68 STRANG, R. R. Imipramine in treatment of parkinsonism: a double-blind placebo study. *British Journal of Medicine*, **2**, 33–34 (1965)
69 SWEET, R. D., McDOWELL, F. H., FEIGENSON, J. S., LORANGER, A. W. and GODELL, H. Mental symptoms in Parkinson's disease during chronic treatment with levodopa. *Neurology*, **26**, 305–310 (1976)
70 TALLAND, G. A. Cognitive function in Parkinson's disease. *Journal of Nervous and Mental Diseases*, **135**, 196–205 (1962)
71 TEUBER, H. and PROCTOR, F. Some effects of basal ganglia lesions in subhuman primates and man. *Neuropsychologica*, **2**, 85–93 (1964)
72 WARBURTON, J. W. Depressive symptoms in parkinsonian patients referred for thalamotomy, *Journal of Neurology, Neurosurgery, and Psychiatry*, **30**, 368–370 (1967)
73 WILSON, R. S., KASZNIAK, A. W., KLAWANS, H. L. and GARRON, D. C. High Speed memory scanning in parkinsonism. *Cortex*, **16**, 67–72 (1980)
74 WOLF, S. M. and DAVIS, R. L. Permanent dementia in idiopathic parkinsonism treated with Levodopa. *Archives of Neurology*, **29**, 276–278 (1973)

75 YAHR, M. D., DUVOISIN, R. S., SCHEAR, M. J., BARRETT, R. E. and HOEHN, M. M. Treatment of parkinsonism with levodopa. *Archives of Neurology*, **21,** 343–354 (1969)

76 YAHR, M. D. and PROCTOR-BROWN, F. Intellectual deficits in parkinsonism. *International Journal of Neurology*, **10,** 280–281 (1975)

77 YUDOFSKY, S. C. Parkinson's disease, depression, and electroconvulsive therapy: a clinical and neurobiologic synthesis. *Comprehensive Psychiatry*, **20,** 579–581 (1979)

7
Fluctuations of disability in Parkinson's disease – clinical aspects
C. D. Marsden, J. D. Parkes and N. Quinn

INTRODUCTION

Sudden, extreme and occasionally unpredictable changes in disability are a characteristic feature of untreated and treated Parkinson's disease[2, 11, 22, 25, 27, 47, 48, 51, 52]. These response variations or 'swings' are a prominent feature of the untreated disease, where they take the form of freezing and paradoxic kinesis, but have been greatly accentuated by the introduction of levodopa. All types of response variations increase in frequency and severity with progression of the disease and duration of therapy. The clinical presentation of different types of response swings will be the subject of this chapter. The possible mechanisms of such fluctuations will be the subject of Chapter 8, but this chapter will highlight some important pathophysiological concepts.

Three basic factors, the stage of disease, changes in environment and drug therapy, appear to be responsible for response swings in parkinsonism. The primary lesion causing parkinsonism appears to be loss of dopaminergic neurons throughout the brain leading to failure of dopamine synthesis. Changes in environment, the mood, the degree of motor effort, sleep and fatigue will all profoundly modify the appearance of parkinsonism. The addition of drug treatment to this already brittle setting often results in a completely unstable response.

Response variation in parkinsonism follows three different time scales: *short-term*, with variations occurring over seconds or minutes, *medium-term* with variation over several hours and *long-term* with improvement or deterioration over a few days. Because they are seen in the untreated disease, short duration response swings are felt to be mainly due to the disease itself, whilst some of the medium- and long-term variations may be caused by treatment. Short-term variation is exemplified by freezing episodes of sudden onset and equally rapid recovery and medium-term fluctuations by the rapid response to anti-parkinsonian drugs; an underlying long duration response often becomes evident only when levodopa is discontinued after years of treatment and the patient deteriorates over a few days, with marked worsening of existing symptoms, to sometimes become totally disabled, bedridden and unable to feed or dress.

Parkinsonism usually is a slow progressive disorder, the course from onset to death averaging 11 years in the era before levodopa[16]. However, levodopa therapy has now restored life expectancy towards normal. The response to treatment in parkinsonism usually is reasonably stable for the first 2 to 5 years of levodopa therapy. Subsequently, over 50 per cent of subjects develop increasingly frequent and severe abnormal movements, severe 'on–off' response fluctuation and often distressing delirium[48, 49].

CLASSIFICATION OF RESPONSE SWINGS

A standard nomenclature for the different kinds of response swings seen in parkinsonism is essential for a better understanding of the disease. The authors discussed some of the problems involved in classification in 1976[25]. Further experience has not caused great modification to the scheme proposed although it has allowed for some refinement of details:

(1) Variation due to underlying Parkinson's disease
    (a) Freezing
    (b) Emotion and awareness
    (c) Sleep and sleep benefit
    (d) Fatigue and neurasthenia
(2) Variation due to treatment
    (a) Medium duration response
    (b) Long duration response
    (c) End-of-dose deterioration ('wearing off')
    (d) Drug-resistant 'off periods'
    (e) Complicated end-of-dose effect
    (f) Random oscillations ('yo-yo')
    (g) 'Resistant fluctuations'
(3) Dyskinesias in untreated patients
    (a) Dystonia
    (b) Chorea
(4) Dyskinesias in treated patients
    (a) Peak dose
    (b) Diphasic
    (c) Early morning dystonia
    (d) Myoclonus

It is usually possible to distinguish response swings due to the basic pathophysiology of parkinsonism from those induced by drug treatment although it must be admitted that this is sometimes difficult or impossible in the late stage of disease when neurasthenia, freezing, peak-dose effects and abnormal movements may all occur in the same patient over a short period.

Variation due to underlying disease

Freezing

The slowness and stiffness of Parkinson's disease are capable of modification with surprising ease. 'The characteristic slow, short, shuffling steps of the patient can be overcome when, with the support of another person, arm linked within his own, he can be persuaded to stride out boldly, often to his own astonishment. A parkinsonian friend told me he could walk more quickly over the stones of a rocky sea beach than on the flat, probably as he was compelled to lengthen his stride'.[53]

In normal subjects, any loss of equilibrium when moving suddenly is usually corrected rapidly. However, parkinsonians are remarkable in their loss of righting reactions, not only when standing but also when they are sitting; the slightest push will make a patient fall backwards. Amongst those less affected, lateral equilibrium may be preserved and many patients can stand briefly on one foot[27].

Freezing of gait may be due to fear of falling or to a disturbance of the control of posture. Martin[27] suggested that the major difficulty lay in compensating for anteroposterior movements of the centre of gravity so that to move either forwards or backwards placed the patient in immediate danger of falling. However, many patients with parkinsonism are unable to sway or rock their body from side to side in order to take the weight off the foot so that it can be raised. This is the explanation of the symptom usually known as 'the foot sticking to the floor' or start hesitation. It is difficult to separate start hesitation from freezing episodes occurring during active movement, or even from extreme degrees of fatigue resulting in apparent sudden paralysis, for all may occur in the same patient.

Freezing episodes are unusual in the first years of parkinsonism although a small number of patients actually experience a single freezing episode as their first symptom. Such episodes become increasingly common, however, with the progression of disease and with the development of postural deformities and other gait disturbances such as anteropulsion, retropulsion or lateropulsion[32]. Freezing episodes most commonly involve walking, but rapid fatigue, start hesitation or freezing may also occur whilst writing, talking, dressing or attempting to turn in bed. Freezing usually involves one specific motor activity whilst other motor skills may be retained. The patient, unable to walk on the level, may negotiate stairs and can usually still talk. Despite a severe degree of immobility, the patient who is frozen to the floor usually retains postural tone and is rigid rather than atonic. Falls during freezing occur because the feet stick while walking yet the centre of gravity continues to progress, and they occur more often during attempts to turn than when the patient is frozen in other circumstances.

Freezing episodes may first appear after the start of levodopa treatment and be wrongly attributed to an adverse effect of this drug rather than to the progression of the underlying parkinsonism. When freezing accompanies moderate degrees of disability, levodopa initially will usually cause at least some improvement in the frequency of such episodes.

Paradoxic kinesis

The converse of freezing, paradoxic kinesis, usually occurs under the influence of strong emotion, stress or fear. The enfeebled and immobile victim is suddenly able to walk or even run, although only for a brief period after which he or she sinks exhausted[12, 17, 33]. Despite the effect of emotion, or sudden change in alertness, the patient with paradoxic kinesis can rarely respond so well to the dictates of the will, although a degree of motivation may profoundly influence the parkinsonian's ability to move[21].

Emotion and awareness

Sleep, changes in alertness and emotional factors have considerable effects on mobility in parkinsonism[44]. The first appearance of symptoms of parkinsonism, and in particular tremor, at a time of stress, shock or bereavement has always been recognized and these factors profoundly modify the subsequent course of disease[3, 4, 44]. Purvis Stewart[47] recounted the classic example of a patient whose severe parkinsonian tremor first developed one day after visiting a menagerie where a lion escaped from its cage. In addition to this obvious provocation of tremor and to a lesser extent stiffness by anxiety, the amplitude of parkinsonian tremor may vary six- or sevenfold over a short period without obvious change in awareness or emotion[1]. The mechanism underlying emotional precipitation of parkinsonian and other tremors has been widely investigated and appears to be partly peripheral in origin[10, 24].

Increase in parkinsonian rigidity and tremor caused by contralateral movement or reinforcement is a well-known phenomenon. Movement of the opposite limbs increases rigidity rather than tremor[28] whilst mental stress usually results in an increase in both tremor and rigidity. However, in subjects treated with levodopa we have observed repeatedly that motor effort, but not mental stress, will cause an increase in the severity of dyskinesias.

Sleep and sleep benefit

Parkinsonian tremor, rigidity and cogwheel phenomena usually disappear during sleep although a minor degree of tremor may persist during slow-wave sleep[5, 13, 46]. During the day the degree of akinesia varies in relation to the level of activation[39], and functional capacity may decline particularly in the afternoon or evening. Some patients who are disabled by severe tremor for much of the day are free from tremor for the first hour after waking. Sleep benefit[22] with little disability at the start of the day but subsequent severe disablement is conspicuous in up to 20 per cent of all subjects and dramatic in a few patients, particularly those with moderately severe disease and with a fluctuant response to levodopa. Sleep benefit may be seen in both untreated and treated patients, and is possibly related to central accumulation and storage of dopamine. This hypothesis accords well with

Figure 7.1 Early morning benefit. This patient profits from his early morning benefit to prepare himself for the day and awaits his first dose-related 'on' period before breakfasting. In this and subsequent figures, disability is depicted on the ordinate, from normal on the top to severely disabled on the bottom

the experience of one of our patients (*Figure 7.1*) who experiences striking early morning benefit unless he has previously awoken, fully mobile, in the middle of the preceding night, in which case early morning benefit does not occur.

Fatigue and neurasthenia

'A parkinsonian once claimed – I could hit anyone hard with the right hand several times quickly but I couldn't keep it up. Dynamometer records made by myself in unilateral and bilateral cases disclose this reduction of strength unmistakably'[53]. Schwab[43] used a bulb ergometer to assess this aspect of parkinsonian disability which, like many of the phenomena described in this chapter, is most common and disabling in patients with moderate to severe degrees of parkinsonism. Fatigue increases in severity with the advance of the disease and is shown in many ways: writing deteriorates, becomes smaller and illegible; speech becomes less distinct, more monotonous and then unintelligible; walking becomes more hesitant, faltering and slow, and the usual natural progression of parkinsonism may be seen in microcosm over a brief period of a few seconds or minutes. Fatigue may be exceptionally prominent in the postencephalitic form of illness[41], but if sought for can usually be identified in most subjects. Indeed, fatigue appears to be an essential part of akinesia. The first appearance of fatigue is often subtle with difficulty in maintaining two voluntary motor activities at the same time[42] (*Figure 7.2*) whereas one movement alone may not tire. Similarly, different activities using the same muscles but different motor programmes may be differentially affected.

Figure 7.2 Difficulty in maintaining two simultaneous voluntary motor acts. The bulb ergogram of a parkinsonian patient's non-dominant hand exercised alone, is represented at *top right*. He is then instructed to draw the six lines shown at *bottom left* with his dominant hand. A normal subject can accomplish this task in 5 s, with a normal simultaneous ergogram from the non-dominant hand. This patient, however, completes the figure in 17 s, with infrequent and low amplitude squeezes of the bulb (*bottom right*) occurring only during the pauses between drawing of the six constituent lines. (From Schwab et al.[42], courtesy of the Editor and Publishers, *Archives of Neurology and Psychiatry*, **72**, 591–598, copyright © 1954, American Medical Association)

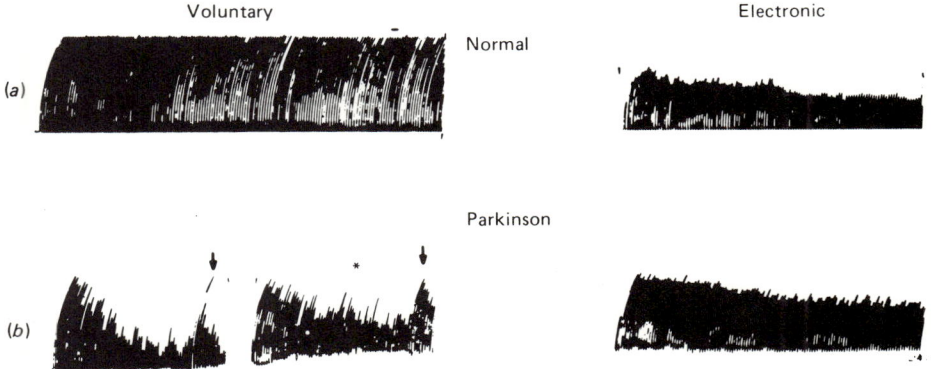

Figure 7.3 Parkinsonian fatigue – voluntary and electronic ergograms. (*a, left*): Normal voluntary ergogram obtained against a resistance of 280 g (10 oz). The subject is not fatigued and is able to do this amount of work indefinitely. Amplitude is evenly sustained. (*a, right*): Stimulation of the same muscle produces the electronic ergogram, which shows little fatigue. (*b, left*): Voluntary ergogram of a patient with Parkinson's disease showing the fatigue curve for a 280 g weight. At the arrow, the patient is urged to make a vigorous squeeze, which he does with normal amplitude. To the right of this curve, under the asterisk, is a repeat ergogram with a 112 g (4 oz) weight, showing little change from reducing the work done. (*b, right*): Electronic ergogram in the same limb, a normal curve showing about three times the work done as the voluntary ergogram. (From Schwab et al.[43], courtesy of the Editors and Publishers, *Neurology (Minneapolis)*

Although Schwab[43] likened parkinsonian fatigue to that seen in myasthenia, there are important differences. Unlike the myasthenic, the parkinsonian can briefly overcome severe fatigue by an effort of will; also, despite the onset of apparent paralysis with fatigue in parkinsonism, peripheral nerve stimulation provokes a normal motor response[43] (*Figure 7.3*). The diurnal fluctuation of parkinsonism is seldom as pronounced as in myasthenia. However, both in parkinsonism and myasthenia the onset of fatigue and recovery with rest have a comparable time course, with diminution in the power of contraction after a few seconds of sustained effort.

Levodopa usually improves parkinsonian fatigue to approximately the same extent as akinesia. As with other aspects of disability, fatigue usually recurs after some years of treatment and then contributes to the development of response swings.

Fatigue over a longer time course, with prostration and lack of vital force amounting to neurasthenia, is another aspect of parkinsonian exhaustion. Tiredness with fatigue and reluctance of motor effort usually improves after a brief rest period and may dramatically respond to levodopa.

Variation due to treatment

Most treatment for Parkinson's disease ultimately produces some degree of response fluctuation; the beneficial response 'swings', or varies, from 'all' to 'none', or from 'on' to 'off'. Many of these response variations are dose-related and dependent on drug pharmacokinetics. However, dose-unrelated and often unpredictable response swings become increasingly common during long-term levodopa therapy. It is sometimes difficult to separate unpredictable response swings of this nature from the effects of fatigue, emotion and other non drug-related factors.

The different kinds of drug-related response swings in parkinsonism have been discussed in detail by Barbeau[2], Fahn[11], Shoulson et al.[45], Tolosa et al.[51], Marsden and Parkes[25], Muenter et al.[30] and Marsden[22]. During the last decade it has become apparent that the late development of response swings occurs after 2 to 5 years of therapy in approximately 50 per cent of all subjects treated with levodopa, and quantitative methods to assess the frequency and severity of response swings have become of great importance[26].

Medium duration response

In the first months or years of its use levodopa produces improvement for several hours after a single dose. This medium duration response, which is equivalent to the 'short duration improvement' of Muenter[30, 31], varies with changes in plasma dopa and dopamine levels, with sudden clinical improvement taking place 15 min–1 h after an oral dose, followed by the gradual reappearance of rigidity, tremor and akinesia 3–4 h later.

Long duration response

Most parkinsonians also obtain long duration improvement from their treatment in the form of a 'plateau' upon which medium-term responses are superimposed. This prolonged benefit often is not evident and may only be appreciated when anticholinergics, amantadine, levodopa or bromocriptine are discontinued and the patient, after an initial deterioration, again markedly worsens 2 to 7 days later (*Figure 7.4*). This late deterioration is presumed to result either from gradual elimination of parent drug and its metabolites from the body, or from gradual changes in receptor sensitivity. Similarly, at the start of treatment with constant doses of amantadine, levodopa or bromocriptine it can take 4 to 7 days to achieve a steady plasma level[34, 36], while full therapeutic benefit may take even longer to appear.

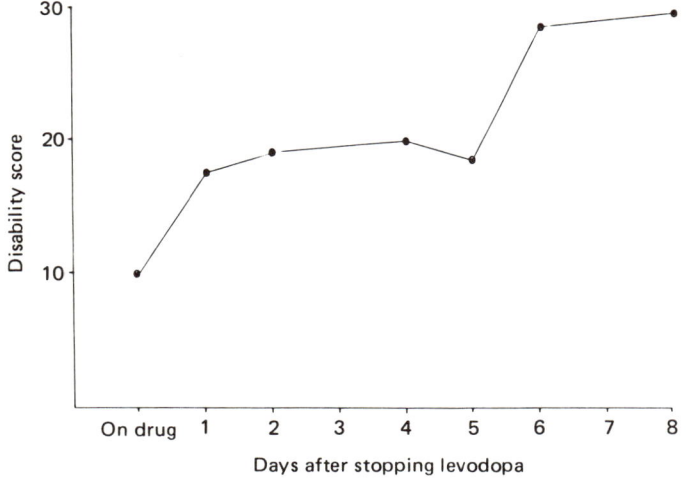

Figure 7.4 Late deterioration after withdrawal of levodopa. This patient showed a moderate deterioration during the first 2 days of levodopa withdrawal, followed by a more severe, late deterioration after 6 days

This long duration response may mislead in two ways. Firstly, in patients with medium-term response swings superimposed upon long duration improvement, the disability during the 'off' period is usually much less severe than that evident in the untreated state, leading to an underestimate of the severity of the underlying disease. However, it should be stressed that for a minority of patients the 'off' period is a positive phenomenon causing physical disability and mental anguish that can greatly exceed that resulting from a longer period of drug withdrawal. A second problem is that patients who do not display medium duration response after many years of treatment may be incorrectly suspected of no longer 'responding' to levodopa until the drug is stopped.

End-of-dose deterioration ('wearing off')

The combination of medium and long duration responses to levodopa initially produces a smooth, stable clinical effect (*Figure 7.5*). The patient's function is maintained more or less constant throughout the day. However, as time passes this continuous benefit begins to fragment, the duration of action of each separate levodopa dose appearing to shorten from 4 to 3, 2, or even less hours (*Figure 7.6*). In other words, it tends to approach the time course of short duration responses which are probably related to the severity of the underlying disease. The reason for this decline is not entirely obvious[15, 23]. There is no known change in the metabolism of levodopa with the progression of treatment. The authors have

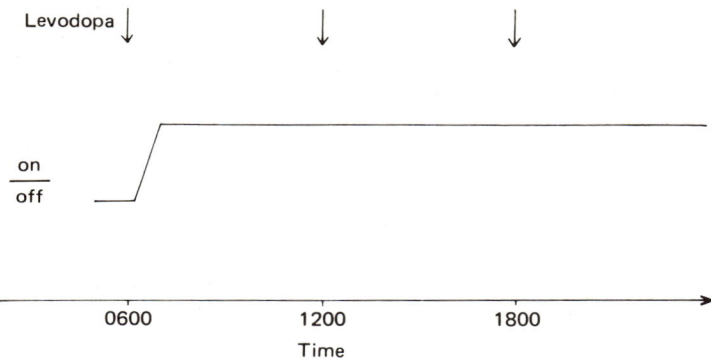

Figure 7.5 Smooth response. Increasing early morning akinesia may be an early sign of impending end-of-dose deterioration

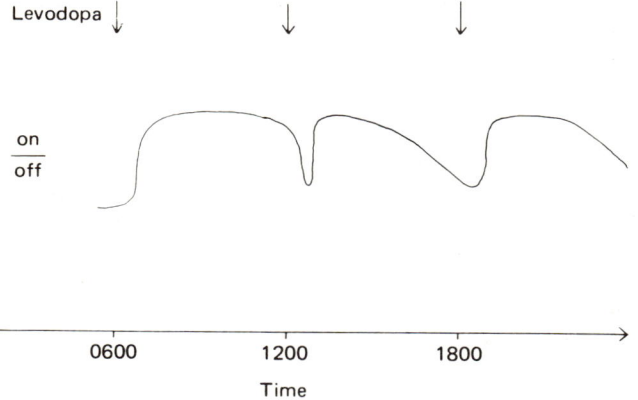

Figure 7.6 End-of-dose deterioration. At the end of the first cycle, the patient 'turns off' shortly after the second dose of levodopa. A number of patients are led to believe erroneously that the taking of the second dose is responsible for this, whereas it is usually due to the 'wearing off' of the first dose before the second has time to act

concluded that progression of the disease with gradual loss of the ability of the brain to synthesize and store dopamine rather than any change in the pharmacokinetic handling of levodopa during long-term therapy is likely to be responsible for this phenomenon[22].

Dose-related response variations may be avoided, at least to some extent, by giving levodopa in small but frequent (2-hourly) doses, which usually results in fairly steady plasma dopa levels[9]. In patients with a stable response to levodopa, plasma dopa levels may show less variation during the day than in patients with marked response fluctuation[35]. When plasma levodopa levels are kept constant by continuous intravenous infusion of levodopa, the clinical response is said to be steady rather than fluctuant[45]. Dose-related response fluctuation over a short time course thus largely may be due to changes in availability of dopamine in the brain itself; other factors appear to be of minor importance. Changes in growth hormone and prolactin release as a consequence of dopamine stimulation of hypothalamic and pituitary endocrine systems do not seem to influence the clinical response[35]. However, changes in the concentration of the dietary amino acids leucine, isoleucine and valine, which compete with levodopa for entry to the brain, occurring as a result of high protein intake interfere to some extent with the response to levodopa[2].

The time course of the medium duration response to dopamine-like drugs, and also the time course of behavioural events attributed to dopamine receptor stimulation, follows drug plasma levels (*Table 7.2*). However, both the initial onset and the peak response are usually delayed and occur 15–30 min after the initial increase and peak plasma drug level respectively are achieved.

Table 7.1 Duration of drug-related response in parkinsonism

	Medium duration response (hours)	Peak plasma level (hours)	Peak clinical response (hours)	Long-term response (days)*
Benzhexol 2 mg p.o.	1–6	–	2–4	2–4
Amantadine 100 mg p.o.	1–8	2–8[34]	2–4	2–4
Levodopa 500 mg p.o.	1–5	1–3[40]	1.5–3	1–7
Bromocriptine 25 mg p.o.	1–6	0.5–3[9]	1.5–3.5	Uncertain
Pergolide 4 mg p.o.	1.5–8	–	2–5	Uncertain
Lisuride 1 mg p.o.	1–3	0.5–2.5[38]	1–2	Uncertain

Data from the King's College Hospital Parkinson's Disease Clinic. Superscript numbers indicate references from which other data are taken
*Period of delayed response assessed on drug withdrawal from long-term treatment

Progression of the underlying disease may cause loss of response to many antiparkinsonian drugs, but true pharmacological tolerance is less common. Tolerance often develops to the emetic action of levodopa after two or three months of treatment but not to the antiparkinsonian response. In contrast, tolerance to the antiparkinsonian action of some apomorphine derivatives may develop in a matter of weeks. Amantadine loses its initial effect in approximately 15–25 per cent of all subjects after some 6–8 weeks of treatment. Tolerance is not a problem with other antiparkinsonian drugs including anticholinergics and bromocriptine.

Drug-resistant 'off periods'

As duration of disease and treatment increases some patients develop 'off' periods which occur at a particular time of day, most commonly late afternoon or evening (*Figure 7.7*), and which are not altered either by attempts to forestall their

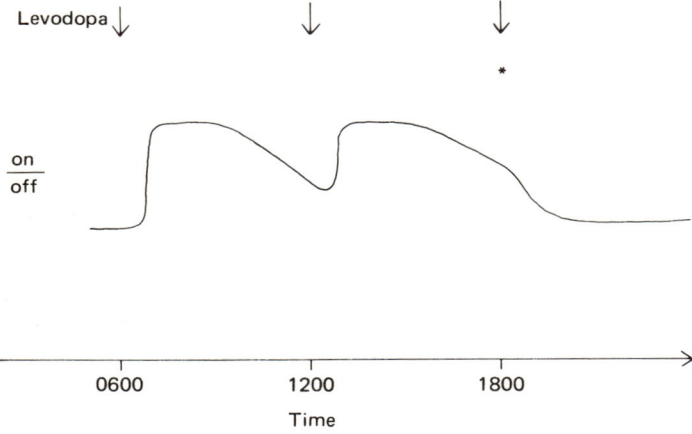

Figure 7.7 End-of-dose deterioration plus drug-resistant 'off' period. The third dose of levodopa (*) has no effect. Addition of, or replacement by, bromocriptine, lisuride or pergolide may not significantly alter this 'off' period

occurrence by increasing or altering the timing of the preceding dose of levodopa, or by adding other dopamine agonists[8]. It is not known whether this is due to receptor refractoriness increasing throughout the day, to competitive blocking by accumulated drug metabolites or to other unknown factors.

Complicated end-of-dose effect

As response fluctuations become more complex, it is increasingly difficult for the physician to determine what is happening to the patient. In this situation the chances of helping the patient through rational adjustment of his therapy are directly proportional to the ability of the physician to recognize the phenomenon the patient may describe, to the time he can spend taking detailed timetables of daily events and, probably equally or even more important, to the intelligence of the patient or spouse and the extent to which they have been educated about the

Classification of response swings 107

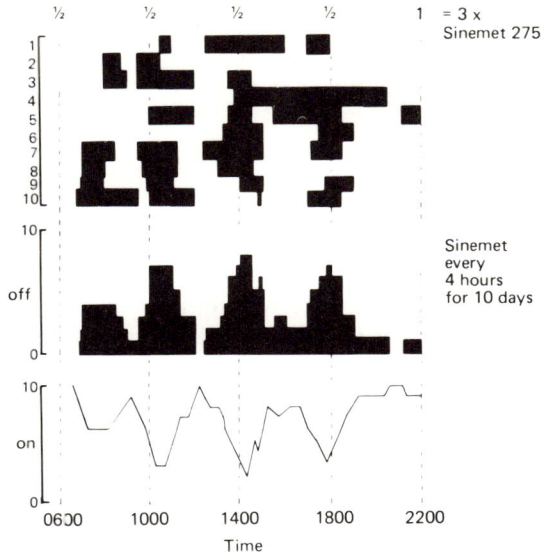

Figure 7.8a Cumulative 'on–off' chart; complicated end-of-dose deterioration. During the first 10 days of in-patient observation 'off' periods (*top*) were unpredictable for any single day. For example, none of the times of 'off' periods on day 1 overlapped with those on day 2. However, when the total number of days 'off' out of a maximum of 10 are summated for each 15 min period of the day (*centre*) it becomes clear that 'off' periods are not randomly distributed, but are grouped around each dosage time, with 'on' periods (*bottom*) peaking in interdose periods

Figure 7.8b Cumulative 'on–off' chart; complicated end-of-dose deterioration. The interdose interval was shortened by 30 min from that in *Figure 7.8a* and the 6-day cumulative chart drawn up, which suggested that the underlying response pattern was still end-of-dose deterioration. (Interestingly, the addition of metoclopramide 10 mg three times a day abolished all 'on' periods for 36 h until after it was discontinued)

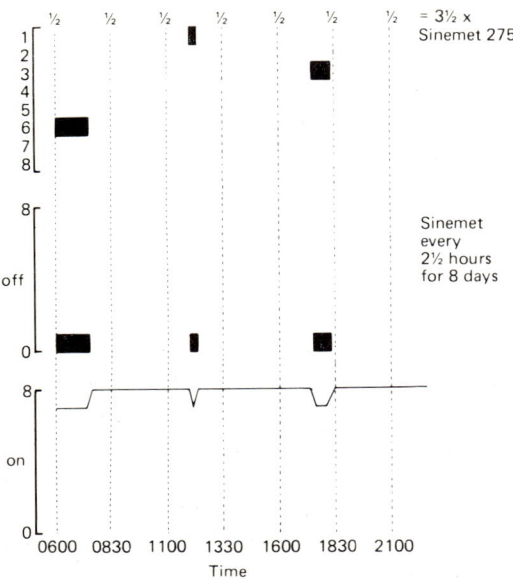

Figure 7.8c Cumulative 'on–off' chart; complicated end-of-dose deterioration. A further shortening of interdose periods to 2½ h resulted in an almost continuous response to Sinemet over the next 8 days of observation prior to discharge, although total daily dosage had increased by only half a tablet compared to the admission dose

disease. The problem of assessment of 'on' and 'off' periods is compounded by the fact that a patient may have one mobile, choreic limb while at the same time presenting a rigid, tremulous, akinetic extremity elsewhere. The authors have found that for patients themselves the single most discriminant test for 'on' versus 'off' is the ability to sustain rapid, large-amplitude alternating finger movements.

Relying on the history of many patients often leads to largely random modification of treatment in the out-patient department. The only way of analyzing the problem effectively often lies in in-patient or day-patient observation. The authors have adopted two techniques to clarify response patterns. The first is overnight discontinuation of treatment followed by a single dose of levodopa, a levodopa test in which the patient is observed continuously through one full cycle of the drug's action. This gives information on morning and peak dose disability, and on latency to and duration of clinical effect, and also helps to distinguish between 'off' period, diphasic and peak dose dyskinesias (*see below*). This procedure, however, has only limited relevance to the effects of cumulative, overlapping doses of levodopa. The second technique is the cumulative 'on–off' chart. *Figure 7.8* shows an example of the use of this technique. Unfortunately, since the underlying disease is progressing all the time, treatment modifications based on such analyses may have to be revised after only a few months.

Random oscillations ('yo-yo')

Drug-resistant 'off' periods, complicated end-of-dose effects and additional short freezing episodes together account for the development of apparently random oscillations in many patients. The existence of 'yo-yo-ing' independent of these factors is unusual, for with extended observation and careful analysis the contributing factors often can be separately recognized, despite the patient's history of apparently random oscillations.

'Resistant fluctuators'

The aim of any classification of response swings must be to develop a rationale for better management of patients. Often, in the first instance, this entails changing the size and frequency of levodopa dosage. When this approach no longer helps, one turns to other drugs either because of their longer duration of action or because they possess direct dopamine receptor stimulating properties. Although such manoeuvres may be successful in a number of patients, there remains a 'hard core', approximately 10–15 per cent of all patients in the authors' experience, who continue to have severe response swings (*Figure 7.9*) despite the use of levodopa in different formulations, bromocriptine, deprenyl, lisuride or pergolide, either alone or in differing combinations. It is this group, 'resistant fluctuators', who present the most difficult therapeutic challenge of all.

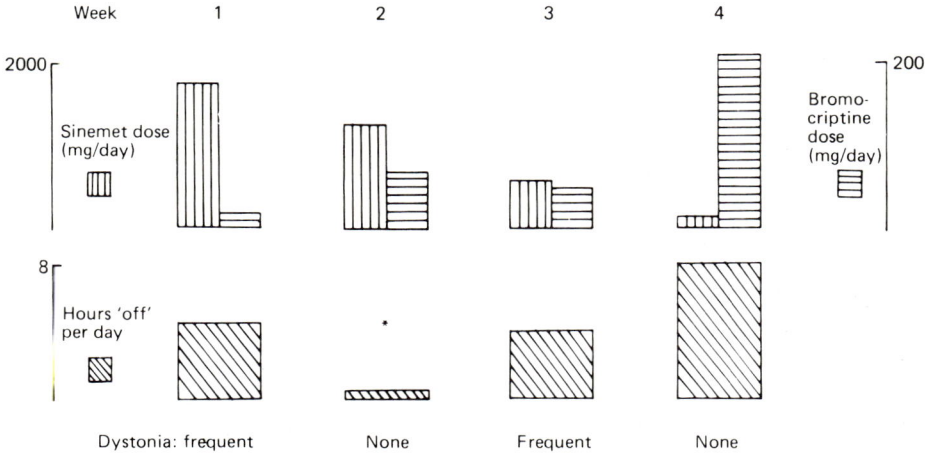

* Severe exhausting chorea

Figure 7.9 'Resistant fluctuator'. This subject (*see also Figures 7.15 and 7.16*), who had previously tried bromocriptine, deprenyl and diprobutine in addition to Sinemet, illustrates some of the problems faced by the group of 'resistant fluctuators'. Mean daily dosages of Sinemet and bromocriptine and mean number of hours 'off' per day over four 7-day periods during a 7-week admission are shown. The patient faces the impossible choice between being 'on' almost continuously but with disabling chorea (week 2), 'off' for 4–5 hours a day but with morning and evening dystonia (weeks 1 and 3), or 'off' for 8 hours a day without dystonia (week 4)

DYSKINESIAS

Dyskinesias in untreated patients

Dystonia

Dystonia occurs in untreated as well as treated parkinsonian subjects. Charcot[6] described in Parkinson's disease the typical aspect of the hand and foot which he likened to that of arthritis. Initially, deformity may be intermittent although eventually it becomes fixed, usually without any X-ray evidence of gross arthritis. The characteristic hand posture is one of slight ulnar deviation with some 40 to 70 degrees of flexion of the metacarpophalangeal joints and hyperextension of interphalangeal joints; the foot becomes painful and cramped, with clawing of the toes which curl under the ball of the foot. The foot is generally held inverted so that the patient takes festinant steps on the outer border of the dystonic foot, which can be very painful and troublesome[14]. Approximately a quarter to a third of patients managed before the levodopa era may have developed hand and foot dystonia eventually. In some cases foot dystonia was an early rather than late symptom, as in the six subjects described by Stewart[47] who initially complained of spontaneous strong flexion and curling of the toes when walking which was accompanied by hyperextension of the hallux and usually recovered after one or two minutes. This posture often caused the patient to catch his foot on any little unevenness of the ground. Before the levodopa era, it was recognized that inversion or pronation of the foot might either first appear following thalamotomy for Parkinson's disease[54] or occasionally be relieved by the operation[14].

Chorea

It is not certain whether chorea ever occurred in untreated patients with idiopathic Parkinson's disease as opposed to postencephalitic parkinsonism. However, Martin[27] described involuntary tongue protrusion in patients with apparent idiopathic parkinsonism who were engrossed in watching horseracing or wrestling; it also occurred whilst dozing or when inattentive.

The authors have seen three patients with idiopathic Parkinson's disease, treated with anticholinergics but not with levodopa or other dopamine agonists, who had typical orobuccolingual dyskinesia. Another patient, receiving no treatment at all, developed a typical orofacial dyskinesia on performing alternating finger movements.

Dyskinesias in treated patients

Drug-related dyskinesias interfere with the smooth control of symptoms of parkinsonism. As with 'on–off' response variations, they become more severe and disabling with progression of both treatment and disease.

Peak dose dyskinesias

In most cases, at least during the initial period of treatment, levodopa dyskinesias occur at the same time as the greatest degree of clinical improvement and are predominantly choreic in nature (*Figure 7.10*). They occur at times when plasma dopa levels are high or above a certain critical concentration in individual patients[30], and are almost always increased in severity if the size of individual doses of levodopa is increased. However, the nature and severity of dyskinesias in different subjects varies considerably; approximately 10–20 per cent of subjects

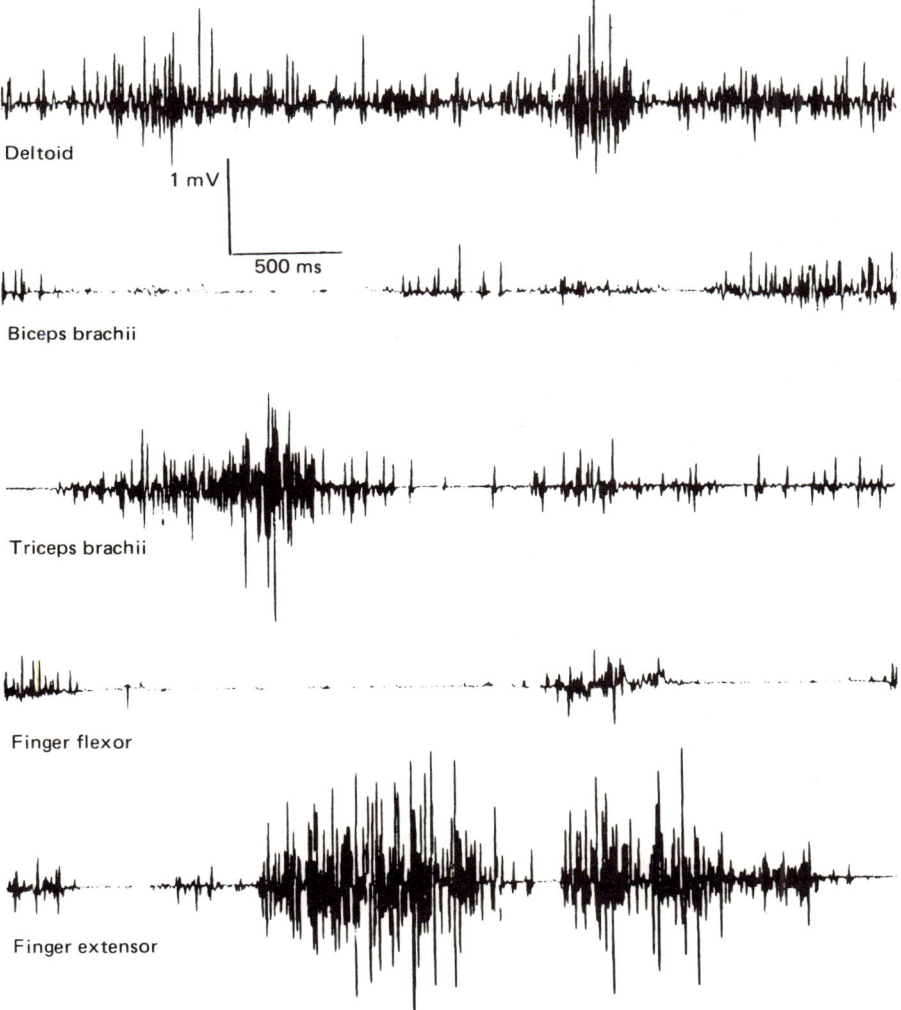

Figure 7.10 Drug-induced chorea. Frequent randomly occurring short (200 ms) bursts of EMG activity with occasional co-contraction occurring during peak-dose chorea. (Obeso, Rothwell, Quinn and Marsden, unpublished observations)

Figure 7.11 Drug-induced dystonia. EMG tracing shows co-contraction with prolonged burst of activity in antagonist pair occurring during peak-dose dystonia. The characteristic hand postures illustrated were exhibited by the same patient as shown in *Figure 7.14*, and occurred both during his episodes of diphasic dyskinesia and also as a peak-dose phenomenon. (Obeso, Rothwell, Quinn and Marsden, unpublished observations)

Figure 7.12 Timing of dyskinesias. Schematic representation of types of peak dose and diphasic dyskinesias

who respond to levodopa do not develop involuntary movements. Orofacial dyskinesia is often the first involuntary movement to appear, and when it occurs alone is more frequently seen in old rather than young patients. Peak dose dyskinesias may be predominantly dystonic in nature (*Figure 7.11*) in perhaps 10–15 per cent of patients[37]. During initial levodopa treatment, peak dose dyskinesias may be apparent only at the time of maximum action of the drug (*Figure 7.12*), gradually increasing and then waning slowly. Often, however, with the passage of time this phase expands to fill the whole of the 'on' period, the severity of the dyskinesias varying little throughout. This 'square wave' response (*Figure 7.12*) usually accompanies the development of sudden 'on–off' switches.

Peak dose akinesia[7], in which the patient may be immobile or speechless at the time levodopa would be expected to produce greatest therapeutic benefit, may be due in some cases to dystonia, particularly involving the mouth, tongue and larynx rather than more florid chorea.

Diphasic dyskinesias

Less common than peak dose dyskinesias are diphasic dyskinesias[30], which affect predominantly young patients with an earlier age of onset of the disease than average; patients with previous thalamotomy, though in a minority, may be more prone to this problem. This group comprises 5–10 per cent of all patients treated with levodopa, and up to 20–25 per cent of those with prominent drug-induced abnormal involuntary movements[20].

Figure 7.13 Diphasic dyskinesia. Repetitive flexion/extension movements of the right knee and toes, with periodic inversion of the foot occurring exclusively at onset and end of action of dose. Peak dose abnormal movements were restricted to mobile dystonia of the trunk and neck. The skin changes are due to psoriasis, not to amantadine!

Figure 7.14 Diphasic dyskinesia. Disabling flailing movements of the left leg make walking impossible for 10–15 min at the beginning and end of the drug's action. Peak dose dyskinesias are mobile, dystonic, of moderate severity, but not greatly disabling. The patient lives alone and still goes out to work

After a single dose of levodopa in such patients, the first sign of effect is heralded by the appearance of dyskinesias (*Figure 7.12*), which may occur before any therapeutic response is obvious. These dyskinesias most commonly affect the legs and are greater on the side more affected by the disease. There may be choreic 'twiddling' movements (*Figure 7.13*), rhythmic alternating kicking at a slow frequency, or sometimes violent flailing of the limbs (*Figure 7.14*) amounting to hemiballism or biballism, which can be particularly explosive and distressing[22]. On occasion these movements may be mistaken for convulsions. Some patients learn to anticipate such severe dyskinesias and retire to bed, lie on a mattress on the floor or arrange to be tied down by their spouse. Ten to twenty per cent of patients have fixed dystonia (*Figure 7.15*), which involves prolonged bizarre spasms of muscle contraction distorting posture into grotesque positions. Approximately 50 per cent of such episodes are extremely painful and may be accompanied by mental anguish, hypertension, tachycardia, mydriasis, flushing and profuse sweating. Two of the authors' patients have died during such florid dystonic diphasic dyskinesias.

The initial bout of dyskinesia is followed by a phase of improvement, either without dyskinesia or, more commonly, with a milder dyskinesia of a different variety. The end of the period of therapeutic benefit is announced by an abrupt return of involuntary movements, usually of longer duration, which resolve as the patient reverts to parkinsonian immobility. In contrast to peak dose dyskinesia, this situation sometimes may be improved rather than worsened by an *increase*, not a reduction, in levodopa dosage[20], but the success of this manoeuvre depends on the nature and severity of any coexisting peak dose dyskinesias in these subjects.

Not all patients have diphasic dyskinesias both at the commencement and at the end of action of single levodopa dose. Some may have involuntary movements only as the effect of therapy begins, others only as it wears off. Even with an increase in daytime dosage, such patients may remain at risk of dyskinesias in the early morning and late at night, when levodopa levels are passing through a critical level, but the onset of sleep may effectively protect against the late night variety. Nor are these dyskinesias exclusively related to treatment with levodopa, for they have

Figure 7.15 Diphasic dystonia. Agonizing, painful dystonia with marked anxiety and autonomic changes. Episodes, which usually last one hour, often occur either before the first or after the last Sinemet dose of the day. Single doses of Sinemet or lisuride aborted the dystonia and turned the patient 'on', but the dystonia returned after a couple of hours if no further doses were given. (The same patient as *Figure 7.9 and 7.16*)

been observed after single doses of bromocriptine 22.5 mg and apomorphine 2 mg[19] and also, by the authors, after a single intravenous injection of lisuride 0.15 mg.

Early morning dystonia

Melamed[29] described early morning dystonia as a late side-effect of levodopa therapy. In the authors' experience, this dystonia (*Figure 7.16*) occurs when the patient is akinetic and rigid and without other dyskinesias after first waking, before

Figure 7.16 Early morning dystonia. The subject in *Figure 7.15*, when he did not develop the full-blown picture illustrated, would nevertheless regularly develop fixed, painful dystonia confined to the legs in the early morning. The classical foot posture of early morning foot dystonia is shown well in this photograph, although most cases are unilateral and for some reason only occur on weight-bearing or attempting to walk

the first daily dose of levodopa is taken, and slowly subsides over 1–2 h even if the first dose of levodopa is withheld. In the four patients reported by Melamed, and in the authors' own patients with this problem, the abnormal posture was first detected 2–6 years after starting levodopa and completely disappeared several days following levodopa withdrawal, only to recur several days after its readministration; all four had other adverse reactions to levodopa with severe 'on–off' phenomena and declining effect. The dystonic foot posture is usually unilateral and occurs most frequently on the side with the major parkinsonian signs. Although levodopa appears to precipitate early morning dystonia, paradoxically this may also be relieved or forestalled by the first daily dose of levodopa (*Figure 7.17*) and also, more rapidly, by intravenous injection of lisuride. In some patients baclofen (Lioresal) 5–40 mg daily, but not diazepam, has been claimed to abolish such dystonic foot postures[29].

Figure 7.17 Early morning dystonia (indicated by hatched bars). This patient's early morning dystonia regularly occurred just after taking his first levodopa dose at breakfast. It would last 20 min, and resolved before he turned 'on' (*top*). When he omitted his morning levodopa the dystonia still occurred, but was more severe and lasted 3 h (*centre*). He now takes his first dose of levodopa very early, in bed, and is free of dystonia on rising

Figure 7.18 Drug-induced myoclonus. Illustrated is an EMG tracing from a patient who, rather unusually, developed myoclonus as a peak-dose effect. It shows randomly occurring short bursts of activity with cocontraction. (Obeso, Rothwell, Quinn and Marsden, unpublished observations)

It seems, therefore, that early morning dystonia may be provoked by a critical low level of dopamine receptor stimulation and may disappear with a rise or fall from this level. The occurrence of early morning dystonia in some patients who at other times report early morning benefit, and its similarity in timing, raises the intriguing possibility that there may be a common mechanism underlying both phenomena.

Myoclonus

Levodopa-induced myoclonus[18] (*Figure 7.18*) is quite different from other levodopa dyskinesias, involving different muscles and with a different character and timing. Involuntary myoclonic jerks most often involve the legs and are most frequent during sleep[50]. They appear to be directly related to the daily dosage and period of levodopa treatment but also occur in untreated subjects. Klawans *et al.*[18] reported that levodopa caused a nocturnal myoclonus which responded in a dramatic way to the administration of methysergide 2 mg nightly. Nocturnal myoclonus is a non-specific syndrome that occurs in many different disorders[50], and its exact relationship to parkinsonism and levodopa treatment remains uncertain.

CONCLUSION

Parkinson's disease, although in most respects a chronic, progressive disorder, can also be seen as a paroxysmal condition. The untreated patient may have brief episodes of sudden mobility (paradoxic kinesis) or akinesia (freezing), although the latter are uncommon and usually do not occur in the initial 2–5 years of levodopa treatment. However, in the later stages of the disease, often following prolonged levodopa therapy, freezing episodes become more frequent and more severe.

Many aspects of parkinsonian disability, other than freezing, improve during the initial period of levodopa treatment. However, as the disease continues there is a continuing loss of dopamine neurons. In consequence, the initial smooth response to therapy may become fragmented after several years. Most commonly the following sequence of events is observed. Initially, morning pre-dose akinesia increases, to be followed by noticeable 'wearing-off' of the effect of other daily doses leading to immobility just after, or before, the subsequent dose. These fluctuations are dose-related and usually can be diminished by giving levodopa more often, in smaller amounts. Moreover, their impact on the patient's life is not disastrous, principally because they are predictable.

As the severity and complexity of the 'on–off' phenomena increase, patients develop fluctuations which are more sudden, of greater magnitude and frequency, and which are above all unpredictable. At this stage, short freezing episodes lasting seconds or minutes, together with longer 'off' periods lasting minutes or hours, may severely restrict the patient's life even though his 'on' period disability may have changed little since the early days of treatment. On retrospective and averaged analysis, some of these fluctuations can be seen to bear an overall relationship with time of dosage, and the patients can be helped by manipulating their drug regime.

Other 'off' periods, however, may be resistant both to an increase in the preceding dose of levodopa and to the use of other dopamine agonist drugs even though some occur regularly at a particular time of day. The end point of this continuum is characterized by a totally unpredictable response to timing, dose and plasma levels of drugs ('yo-yoing'). Although the use of long-acting dopamine agonist drugs (bromocriptine, pergolide) may help some patients, other 'resistant fluctuators' improve only transiently, if at all.

Dyskinesias, in the form of dystonia or orofacial dyskinesia, occur in untreated patients but are uncommon and are not a major cause of response fluctuations in these subjects. However, dyskinesias occur in 60–80 per cent of patients receiving levodopa, and, as with other types of response fluctuation, increase in frequency and severity with progression of disease and duration of treatment. Of all treatment side effects it is these abnormal movements which most commonly limit the dosage of levodopa. Whilst they occur most commonly at peak dose, when they are choreic or dystonic in appearance, certain dyskinesias may be provoked by intermediate or low levels of dopaminergic stimulation. Thus, the treatment for episodes of chorea, dystonia or ballism occurring at the onset and end of action of a dose may consist of an increase rather than a decrease in drug dosage, and early morning dystonia may be helped by taking the first daily dose of levodopa on waking, or by adding night-time doses of longer-acting agonist drugs.

The successful management of the more advanced stages of the 'on–off' phenomenon demands great attention to detail in the examination and above all the history of the patient. Where the conventional clinic consultation is inadequate for these purposes, day-patient or in-patient observation may be particularly helpful. However, whilst encouraging improvements often result from rearrangement of existing treatment, even without recourse to additional drugs, these are all too often only temporary; the relationship between treatment and stage of disease is constantly changing. Although much can be gained from accurate assessment of individual patients, it is of crucial importance to discover the mechanisms underlying response fluctuations so as to be able to design more effective therapy for the 'resistant fluctuator'.

References

1 ACKMANN, J. J., SANCES, A., LARSON, S. J., and BAKER, J. B. Quantitative evaluation of long-term Parkinson tremor. *IEEE Transactions in Biomedical Engineering*, **24,** 49–56 (1977)

2 BARBEAU, A. Long-term side effects of levodopa. *Lancet,* **1,** 395 (1971)

3 BIGNE, J. and LAPUERTA, L. Sobre la influencia de las emociones en el sindrome parkinsoniano. *Revista Clinica Espanola*, **83,** 289–291 (1961)

4 BOMAN, K. Effect of emotional stress on spasticity and rigidity. *Scandinavian Journal of Clinical and Laboratory Investigation*, Suppl 108, **23,** 63 (1969)

5 BROUGHTON, R., TASSINARI, C. A., ROGER, J., GASTAUT, H. and POIRE, R. A polygraphic study of abnormal movements during different stages of sleep. *Canadian Medical Association Journal*, **97,** 243–244 (1967)

6 CHARCOT, J. M. In *Lectures on the Diseases of the Nervous System*, 141. London, New Sydenham Society (1877)
7 CLAVERIA, L. E., CALNE, D. B. and ALLEN, J. G. 'On–off' phenomena related to high plasma levodopa. *British Medical Journal*, **2**, 641–643 (1973)
8 DeBONO, A., DONALDSON, I., MARSDEN, C. D., and PARKES, J. D. Bromocriptine in parkinsonism. *Lancet*, **2**, 987–988 (1975)
9 DeBONO, A. G., JENNER, P., MARSDEN, C. D., PARKES, J. D., TARSY, D. and WALTERS, J. Plasma dopa levels and growth hormone response to levodopa in parkinsonism. *Journal of Neurology, Neurosurgery and Psychiatry*, **40**, 162–167 (1977)
10 DINSDALE, H. B., VALBERG, L. S., LANGWORTH, E. P., FRANSMAN, S. L., SIMURDA, M. A. and IRVINE, R. F. Peripheral mechanisms producing and modifying tremor. *Journal, Canadian Medical Association*, **97**, 242 (1967)
11 FAHN, S. 'On–off' phenomenon with levodopa therapy in parkinsonism. *Neurology (Minneapolis)*, **24**, 431–441 (1974)
12 FROMENT, J. and GARDERE, H. Paradoxic parkinsonian kinesis, striatal paradoxes and disturbances of the function of stabilisation. *Archives of Neurology and Psychiatry*, **15**, 820–821 (1926)
13 FROMENT, J. and GARDERE, H. Parkinsonian rigidity and cogwheel phenomenon disappear during repose. Their dystatic character. *Archives of Neurology and Psychiatry*, **15**, 820 (1926)
14 GORTVAI, P. Deformities of the hands and feet in parkinsonism and their reversibility by operation. *Journal of Neurology, Neurosurgery and Psychiatry*, **26**, 33–36 (1963)
15 HEFTI, F. and MELAMED, E. L-dopa's mechanism of action in Parkinson's disease. *Trends in NeuroSciences*, **3**, 229–231 (1980)
16 HOEHN, M. M. and YAHR, M. D. Parkinsonism: onset, progression and mortality. *Neurology (Minneapolis)*, **17**, 427–442 (1967)
17 JARKOWSKI, J. *Kinesie Paradoxale des Parkinsoniens*. Paris, Masson (1925)
18 KLAWANS, H. L., GOETZ, C. and BERGEN, D. Levodopa-induced myoclonus. *Archives of Neurology (Chicago)*, **32**, 331–334 (1975)
19 LHERMITTE, F., AGID, Y., FEUERSTEIN, C., SERRE, F., SIGNORET, J. L., STUDLER, J. M. and BENNET, A. M. Mouvements anormaux provoques par la L-dopa dans la maladie de Parkinson: Corrélation avec les concentrations plasmatiques de dopa et de O-méthyl-dopa. *Revue Neurologique*, **133**, 445–454 (1977)
20 LHERMITTE, F., AGID, Y. and SIGNORET, J. L. Onset and end-of-dose Levodopa-induced dyskinesias. *Archives of Neurology (Chicago)*, **35**, 261–263 (1978)
21 MANDELL, A. J., MARKHAM, C. H., TALLMAN, F. F. and MANDELL, M. P. Motivation and ability to move. *American Journal of Psychiatry*, **119**, 544–549 (1962)
22 MARSDEN, C. D. 'On–off' phenomenon in Parkinson's disease. In *Parkinson's Disease – Current Progress, Problems and Management*, edited by Rinne, U.K., Klinger, M., Stamm, G. 241–254. Amsterdam, Elsevier/ North Holland (1980)
23 MARSDEN, C. D. and JENNER, P. L-dopa's action in Parkinson's disease. *Trends in NeuroSciences*, **4**, 148–150 (1981)
24 MARSDEN, C. D. and OWEN, D. A. L. Mechanisms underlying emotional variation in parkinsonian tremor. *Neurology (Minneapolis)*, **17**, 711–715 (1967)

25 MARSDEN, C. D. and PARKES, J. D. 'On–off' effects in patients with Parkinson's disease on chronic levodopa therapy. *Lancet*, **1,** 292–295 (1976)

26 MARSDEN, C. D. and SCHACHTER, M. Assessment of extrapyramidal disorders. *British Journal of Clinical Pharmacology*, **11,** 129–151 (1981)

27 MARTIN, J. P., HURWITZ, L. J. and FINLAYSON, M. H. The negative symptoms of basal ganglia disease; a survey of 130 post-encephalitic cases II. *Lancet*, **2,** 62–66 (1962)

28 MATSUMOTO, K., ROSSMANN, F., LIN, T. H. and COOPER, I. S. Studies on induced exacerbation of parkinsonian rigidity: the effect of contralateral voluntary activity. *Journal of Neurology, Neurosurgery and Psychiatry*, **26,** 27–32 (1963)

29 MELAMED, E. Early-morning dystonia: a late side effect of long term levodopa therapy in Parkinson's disease. *Archives of Neurology (Chicago)*, **36,** 308–310 (1979)

30 MUENTER, M. D., SHARPLESS, N. S., TYCE, G. M. and DARLEY, F. L. Patterns of dystonia ('I-D-I' and 'D-I-D') in response to L-dopa therapy for Parkinson's disease. *Mayo Clinic Proceedings*, **52,** 163–174 (1977)

31 MUENTER, M. D., TYCE, G. M. L-dopa therapy of Parkinson's disease: plasma L-dopa concentration, therapeutic response and side effects. *Mayo Clinic Proceedings*, **46,** 231–239 (1971)

32 NOICA, D. Le phénomène d'antéropulsion, de rétropulsion et de latéropulsion chez les malades atteints de parkinsonisme. *Revue Neurologique*, **2,** 112–115 (1929)

33 NOICA, D. Sur la kynesic paradoxale. *Revue Neurologique*, **2,** 657–662 (1931)

34 PACIFICI, G. M., NARDINI, M., FERRARI, P., LATINI, R., FIESCHI, C. and MORSELLI, P. L. Effect of amantadine on drug-induced parkinsonism: relationship between plasma levels and effects. *British Journal of Clinical Pharmacology*, **3,** 883–889 (1976)

35 PAPAVASILIOU, P. S., McDOWELL, F.H., WANG, Y. Y., ROSAL, V. and MILLER S. T. Plasma DOPA and growth hormone in parkinsonism: oscillations in symptoms. *Neurology (Minneapolis)*, **29,** 194–200 (1979)

36 PARKES, J. D. Bromocriptine. *New England Journal of Medicine*, **301,** 873–878 (1979)

37 PARKES, J. D., BEDARD, P. and MARSDEN, C. D. Chorea and torsion in parkinsonism. *Lancet*, **2,** 155 (1976)

38 PARKES, J. D., SCHACHTER, M., MARSDEN, C. D., SMITH, B. and WILSON, A. Lisuride in Parkinsonism. *Annals of Neurology*, **9,** 48–52 (1981)

39 PLOSKI, H. A., LEVITA, E. and RIKLAN, M. Impairment of voluntary movement in Parkinson's disease in relation to activation level, autonomic malfunction and postural rigidity. *Psychosomatic Medicine*, **28,** 70–77 (1966)

40 ROSSOR, M. N., WATKINS, J., BROWN, M. J., REID, J. L. and DOLLERY, C. T. Plasma levodopa, dopamine and therapeutic response following levodopa therapy of Parkinsonian patients. *Journal of the Neurological Sciences*, **46,** 3, 385–392 (1980)

41 SAINTON, P. and SCHULMANN, E. Le parkinsonisme variable dans l'encéphalite épidémique; parkinsonisme de fatigue et crises parkinsoniennes. *Revue Neurologique*, **37,** 1066–1070 (1921)

42 SCHWAB, R. S., CHAFETZ, M. E. and WALKER, S. Control of two simultaneous voluntary motor acts in normals and in Parkinsonism. *Archives of Neurology and Psychiatry*, **72,** 591–598 (1954)

43 SCHWAB, R. S., ENGLAND, A. C. and PETERSON, E. Akinesia in Parkinson's disease. *Neurology (Minneapolis)*, **9,** 65–72 (1959)
44 SCHWAB, R. S. and ZIEPER, I. Effects of mood, motivation, stress and alertness on the performance in Parkinson's disease. *Psychiatria et Neurologia*, **150,** 345–357 (1965)
45 SHOULSON, I., GLAUBIGER, G. A. and CHASE, T. N. On–off response. Clinical and biochemical correlations during oral and intravenous levodopa administration in Parkinsonian patients. *Neurology (Minneapolis)*, **25,** 1144–1148 (1975)
46 STERN, M., ROFFWARG, H. and DUVOISIN, R. The Parkinsonian tremor in sleep. *Journal of Nervous and Mental Diseases*, **147,** 202–210 (1968)
47 STEWART, PURVES. Paralysis agitans; with an account of a new symptom. *Lancet*, **2,** 1258–1260 (1898)
48 SWEET, R. D. and McDOWELL, F. H. Plasma concentrations and the 'on–off' effect after chronic treatment of Parkinson's disease. *Neurology (Minneapolis)*, **24,** 953–956 (1974)
49 SWEET, R. D., McDOWELL, F. H., FEIGENSON, J. S., LORANGER, A. W. and GODELL, H. Mental symptoms in Parkinson's disease during chronic treatment with levodopa. *Neurology (Minneapolis)*, **26,** 305–310 (1976)
50 SYMONDS, C. P. Nocturnal myoclonus. *Journal of Neurology, Neurosurgery and Psychiatry*, **16,** 166–171 (1953)
51 TOLOSA, E. S., MARTIN, W. E., COHEN, H. P. and JACOBSON, R.L. Patterns of clinical response and plasma dopa levels in Parkinson's disease. *Neurology (Minneapolis)*, **25,** 177–183 (1975)
52 WILSON, S. A. K. *Modern Problems in Neurology*, 157–159. New York, William Wood and Co. (1929)
53 WILSON, S. A. K. In *Neurology*, edited by A. Ninian Bruce, 929. London, Butterworth (1954)
54 ZOLL, J. G. Inversion or pronation of the foot following thalamotomy for Parkinson's disease. *Applied Neurophysiology*, **41,** 232–236 (1978)

8
Fluctuations of disability in Parkinson's disease: pathophysiology

Stanley Fahn

INTRODUCTION

Clinical fluctuations in the response to dopamine replacement therapy is one of the major burdens to the patient with Parkinson's disease (and to his conscientious physician). A patient who may have a superb response from medication ('on' phase) may become immobile ('off' phase) either suddenly or gradually. The 'on' phases indicate that the striatal dopamine receptors are capable of responding to the medication and, therefore, the patient would be able to function nearly normally. The prospect of such benefit from medication, however, is negated by the occurrence of the 'off' phenomenon, which then represents a tragedy for such a patient. The existence of these fluctuations frequently makes the patient unemployable or unable to travel outside the home independently. Probably nowhere else in medicine are such 'on–off' phenomena from medication so prevalent and so vicious. Unfortunately, treatment for this problem has been unsatisfactory. Perhaps a better understanding of the pathophysiology of the clinical fluctuations from levodopa would lead to better therapy. The purpose of this chapter is to explain, on the basis of available data, the pathophysiological mechanisms for the different types of clinical fluctuations. It should be understood by the reader that the data on this subject are limited. The author, therefore, also presents personal working hypotheses that help him to understand what may be happening to the patient, which in turn suggest clinical approaches on how to help him,

The previous chapter by Marsden, Parkes and Quinn outlines their clinical classification of fluctuations in parkinsonism, both those due to the disease and those due to medications. For the sake of the reader, their classification is followed in this discussion of the pathophysiology of fluctuations. However, it is reorganized slightly and the disease-related fluctuations and dykinesias are grouped together, as are the drug-related fluctuations and dyskinesias, as follows:

(1) Disease-related
   (a) Fluctuations
      (i) Freezing
      (ii) Paradoxic kinesis
      (iii) Emotion and awareness
      (iv) Sleep and sleep-benefit
      (v) Fatigue and neurasthenia
   (b) Dyskinesias
      (i) Dystonia
      (ii) Chorea

(2) Treatment-related
   (a) Fluctuations
      (i) Medium duration response
      (ii) Long duration response
      (iii) End-of-dose deterioration ('wearing-off')
      (iv) Drug resistant 'off periods'
      (v) Complicated end-of-dose effect
      (vi) Random oscillations
      (vii) 'Resistant fluctuators'
   (b) Dyskinesias
      (i) Peak dose dyskinesias
      (ii) Diphasic dyskinesias
      (iii) Early morning dystonia
      (iv) Myoclonus

This list represents a reorganization of the one on p. 97. The reader is directed to Chapter 7 for detailed clinical descriptions of the phenomena to be discussed here. At the end of this chapter an alternative classification of the drug-induced fluctuations and dyskinesias based on pathophysiology rather than on clinical features are presented. It is hoped that the pathophysiological classification will help the reader by suggesting rational approaches to treatment, based on the hypothetical mechanisms proposed.

PATHOPHYSIOLOGY OF PARKINSONIAN SYMPTOMS

To understand the pathophysiology of symptoms due to Parkinson's disease, one must keep in mind the neurochemical changes found in this condition. Hornykiewicz (Chapter 4) reviews the changes in neurotransmitters; in summary, the primary changes seem to be reductions in monoamine levels, particularly dopamine. Rinne (Chapter 5) describes the changes in neurotransmitter receptors, but these appear to be secondary either to altered transmitter availability or to chronic medication. The uneven reduction of dopamine in the striatum in Parkinson's disease has been interpreted to indicate that the reduction of monoamines in the brain is secondary to degeneration of monoamine neurons, rather than representing a metabolic defect in synthesis, storage, or uptake of the monoamines[26]. Of course, the etiology of the progressive loss of these monoamines neurons is not understood, although hypotheses have been suggested (*see* Chapter 2).

Monoamines are reduced not only in the striatum but also in other areas of brain. For example, dopamine is deficient in the mesolimbic and mesocortical pathways[32], and norepinephrine is likewise reduced in nerve terminals throughout the brain derived from cells originating in the locus ceruleus (*see* Chapter 4). It seems reasonable, *a priori,* that symptoms in Parkinson's disease can be directly attributed to the degree of loss of monoamine and their deficient neurotransmitters. Although reduced norepinephrine and serotonin undoubtedly are responsible for some of the symptoms encountered, as yet we cannot correlate specific symptoms with these neurotransmitter deficiencies with any degree of certainty[26]. On the other hand, a strong case can be made for relating many symptoms, such as bradykinesia, rigidity, and tremor, to striatal dopamine deficiency[25]. This evidence is listed here.

(1) In the brain, dopamine is highly concentrated within the basal ganglia, particularly the striatum, whereas serotonin is more uniformly and widely distributed, and norepinephrine is barely detected in the striatum and is most concentrated in the limbic system[19].
(2) The most profound reduction of any neurotransmitter is that of dopamine (*see* Chapter 4).
(3) In a patient with hemiparkinsonism, the reduction of dopamine was more pronounced in the striatum contralateral to the side of symptoms, and serotonin was essentially normal[4].
(4) In the straitum, the reduction of dopamine and its major metabolite, homovanillic acid, parallels the degree of cell loss in the substantia nigra[30].
(5) Treatment of Parkinson's disease with monoamine oxidase inhibitors results in little clinical improvement. Postmortem determinations of the monoamines in the brains of three patients treated prior to death with these agents revealed increases of norepinephrine and serotonin to above normal levels, but essentially no reversal of the reduced dopamine level[30].
(6) Reserpine depletes the brain of its three monoamines and produces a parkinson-like effect of hypokinesia and rigidity. The clinical effect can be reversed in animals[10] and in man[14] with levodopa. The serotonin precursor, 5-hydroxytrytophan, has no effect[10]. Although levodopa is the precursor to both dopamine and norepinephrine, the injection of levodopa results in a marked increase of dopamine in the brain of both normal and reserpinized animals, but only a small increase in the level of norepinephrine[8]. Furthermore, restoring the brain level of norepinephrine to normal without changing the dopamine concentration in the reserpinized animal by using dihydroxyphenylserine does not reverse the reserpine effect[13].
(7) Administration of levodopa can reverse most manifestations of parkinsonism, particularly bradykinesia and rigidity[2, 12, 31, 66].
(8) The bradykinesia which occurs in animals from chemical stimulation of the caudate nucleus can be alleviated by intracaudate injection of levodopa[57].

(9) Phenothiazines and butyrophenones given in high dosage produce a syndrome resembling parkinsonism, consisting of bradykinesia, rigidity, tremor, masked facies, and shuffling gait. These drugs block the postsynaptic dopaminergic receptor[9].
(10) Parkinsonism is a rare complication of α-methyldopa therapy for hypertension[29, 58]. It is believed thats its metabolite, α-methyldopamine, acts as a false transmitter and competes with dopamine at the receptor or storage sites.

There is recent evidence presented by Narabayashi and his colleages[47] that norepinephrine deficiency may be responsible for the symptoms of sudden transient freezing and start-hesitation. These investigators treated parkinsonian patients with the norepinephrine precursor, L-threo-dihydroxyphenylserine (DOPS), and found that these particular gait symptoms could be relieved by this agent, whereas levodpa had no effect.

DISEASE-RELATED FLUCTUATIONS

Freezing

Freezing when walking presents in several forms: *start-hesitation, sudden transient freezing* while walking, and *terminal-hesitation*. Because of their association with each other and their clinical similarity in that the patients' feet seem 'glued to the ground', it seems reasonable to assume that these phenomena share a common mechanism. Visual or auditory stimuli can overcome a freezing episode, whereas fear of falling and attempting to accomplish 'two things at the same time' accentuate it. Levodopa may provide some relief in the early stages of the disease, but tends to aggravate freezing as the illness progresses[1, 23]. Hence, a reduction of levodopa may provide some lessening of the problem. Narabayashi's experience with DOPS[47] in which this norepinephrine precursor can eliminate the symptoms of freezing would indicate that freezing is related to norepinephrine deficiency, probably within the accumbens, since this neurotransmitter is virtually absent from the striatum (*see* Chapter 4). To explain how levodopa can aggravate this clinical problem, one can postulate that the excess dopamine formed serves as a false transmitter in norepinephrine nerve terminals.

Paradoxic kinesis

The mechanism of paradoxic kinesis is unclear. If it is the opposite of freezing, one may assume that the influence of strong emotion and stress, which can cause a brief burst of movement, is able to produce a sudden release of norepinephrine from remaining nerve terminals. But how this would come about is not known. Another possible mechanism is that the basal ganglia neuronal circuitry is bypassed in these periods, and the intact corticospinal tract is activated directly by reticulocortical (including norepinephrine) pathways.

Emotion and awareness

In Chapter 7, Marsden *et al.* suggest that emotional stress exacerbates parkinsonian symptoms, in part, by a peripheral mechanism. This author favors a central mechanism. It is reasonable to consider that emotional stress, being centrally derived, probably in the limbic system, may exert some inhibitory effect on dopaminergic nigral neurons by central pathways connecting the limbic system with the basal ganglia.

Sleep and sleep-benefit

In general, movement disorders associated with basal ganglia pathology disappear during sleep. It seems reasonable to suggest that during sleep, motor physiology bypasses the basal ganglia. Hence, the abnormal basal ganglia would not exert any influence during sleep. It is suggested in Chapter 7 that enrichment of dopamine stores may occur during sleep, which could explain why an occasional patient performs best upon arising.

Fatigue and neurasthenia

Fatigue, decreasing amplitude with rapid successive movements, and neurasthenia can all be considered part of the bradykinesia spectrum. Therefore, these are symptoms of the disease, and would appear to be related to striatal dopamine deficiency, as described above for bradykinesia.

DISEASE-RELATED DYSKINESIAS

Dystonia

Dystonic fixed postures, such as neck and trunk flexion, and also posturing of the hands (flexion at the metacarpal-phalangeal joints and extension at the interphalangeal joints) are common features in Parkinson's disease. Dystonia of the feet usually begins intermittently with curling or extension of the toes, and later may become fixed. The mechanism of dystonia is is not understood. Hyperactivity of the cholinergic system in the striatum is one possible explanation, based on two pieces of information. Anticholinergic agents can reduce dystonia[21,36], and antipsychotic drugs, which can induce acute dystonia, may act by blocking dopamine receptors, thereby causing disinhibition of acetylcholine neurons in the striatum. In Parkinson's disease, it would seem that chronic cholingeric disinhibition is the result of dopamine deficiency. Perhaps this plays a role in parkinsonian dystonia.

Chorea

Choreic movements in untreated patients do not appear to be part of Parkinson's disease. Since oral dyskinesias can occur spontaneously in the elderly, the presence of mouthing movements in untreated patients can be considered as a feature of this phenomenon. It should be recalled that edentulousness, as well as anticholinergic drugs, has been associated with oral dyskinesias[6, 24, 59].

TREATMENT-RELATED FLUCTUATIONS

Medium duration response

This phenomenon was probably first described by Muenter and Tyce in 1971[46], who referred to it as short duration improvement. This is a fundamental pharmacokinetic response and probably serves as the basis for the type of clinical fluctuation known as the 'wearing-off' phenomenon ('end-of-dose deterioration'), which will be discussed later. In the medium duration response, clinical benefit occurs when the plasma concentration of levodopa is high, and loss of benefit accompanies the falling plasma level. Clinical response lags approximately half an hour behind the

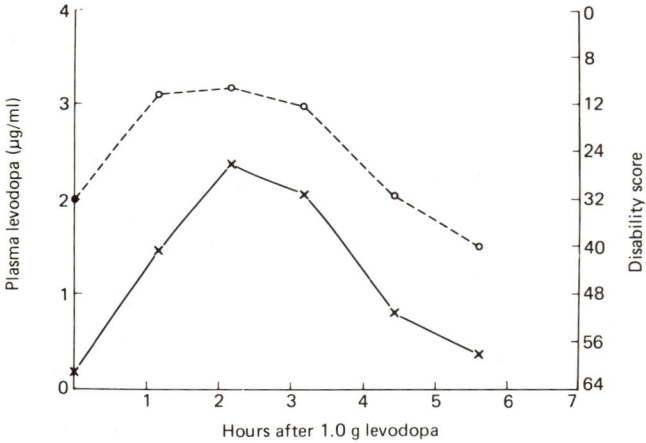

Figure 8.1 Medium duration response to levodopa. Interrupted line represents disability score and solid line, the plasma level of levodopa following the initial dose after an overnight fast. The two lines tend to parallel each other. (From Muenter and Tyce[46], courtesy of the Mayo Foundation)

plasma level (*Figure 8.1*). This dependence on the availability of plasma levodopa indicates that there are inadequate reserves of brain dopamine. A possible explanation for this will be discussed in the next section in comparison with the long duration response.

Long duration response

Many Parkinsonian patients can maintain the clinical benefit derived from a single dose of levodopa for many hours, even though the plasma level of levodopa has

Figure 8.2 Long duration response to levodopa. Interrupted line represents disability score and solid line, the plasma level of levodopa following the initial dose after an overnight fast. Note the sustained improvement although the plasma level of levodopa has fallen. (From Muenter and Tyce[46], courtesy of the Mayo Foundation)

fallen (*Figure 8.2*). In fact such patients, if on chronic levodopa therapy, can retain the clinical benefit for 3–5 days if levodopa is suddenly discontinued. One may conclude that there is a reservoir of dopamine in the striatum, either in remaining dopaminergic nerve terminals or nondopaminergic neurons[41]. As these stores are slowly depleted, symptoms of parkinsonism return.

In contrast, medium duration response would seem to represent inadequate storage sites for dopamine, so that the striatum is continually dependent on a supply of dopamine precursor via the circulation. Marsden and Parkes[39] suggest that as the disease progresses, the loss of more dopamine terminals leads to loss of storage capacity for dopamine. Duration of therapy with levodopa may play a role in inducing the medium duration response because (1) this response is usually not encountered in the first year or two of levodopa therapy, (2) it becomes more common with duration of treatment[3], and (3) because the long duration can be seen in patients with advanced disease[46]. How could levodopa, itself, induce the medium duration response? It is possible that a metabolite of dopamine is toxic to the nerve terminals.

'Wearing-off' phenomenon (end-of-dose deterioration)

The 'wearing-off' phenomenon can be best understood by realizing that it represents a series of medium duration responses with sequential doses of levodopa. After each dose, the benefit slowly 'wears-off' within 1–3 hours. The benefit from levodopa parallels the plasma levels, and the plasma half-life of levodopa is very short in most patients studied (*Figure 8.3*). If the plasma level can be maintained, the 'wearing-off' phenomenon is eliminated (*Figure 8.4*).

130 *Fluctuations of disability in Parkinson's disease: pathophysiology*

Figure 8.3 Averaged plasma levels of levodopa (*lower curve*) and clinical responses (*upper curve*) in seven patients measured throughout the day with repeated doses of levodopa given at regular intervals, indicated by the arrows. (From Shoulson et al.[56], courtesy of the Editor and Publishers, *Neurology*)

Figure 8.4 Smooth plasma levels of levodopa (*lower curve*) and clinical response (*upper curve*) during intravenous infusion of levodopa. Results are the average from five patients. (From Shoulson et al.[56], courtesy of the Editor and Publishers, *Neurology*)

It should be pointed out to the reader that many authors fail to distinguish between the gradual 'wearing-off' phenomenon and the more sudden and random 'on-off' effect. Both types have been referred to as the 'on-off' phenomenon, which appears to be used as a synonym for clinical fluctuations. In order to understand the pathophysiology of the various types of clinical fluctuations, they should not be lumped together, but rather should be considered as separate entities, as is being done in this chapter. The term 'on-off' phenomenon should be reserved for the phenomenon for which the term was coined, a sudden and dramatic change of clinical motility.

Patients with the 'wearing-off' phenomenon require doses of levodopa at closer intervals. Some of these patients can not remain free from parkinsonism throughout the night unless they take additional levodopa during the nighttime hours. When severe, the 'wearing-off' phenomenon renders these patients essentially 'dopa-dependent' and they cannot be without frequent administrations of the medication.

Drug resistant 'off' periods

Many patients report that they respond best to the first dose of levodopa in the morning, and become more resistant later in the day. It is not clear whether there is some central pharmacodynamic problem with the dopamine receptors or a peripheral pharmacokinetic problem. It is common for the plasma levels of levodopa to reach the higher peaks with the first dose of the day and lower peaks with each subsequent dose (*see Figures 8.3 and 8.5*). This phenomenon is not

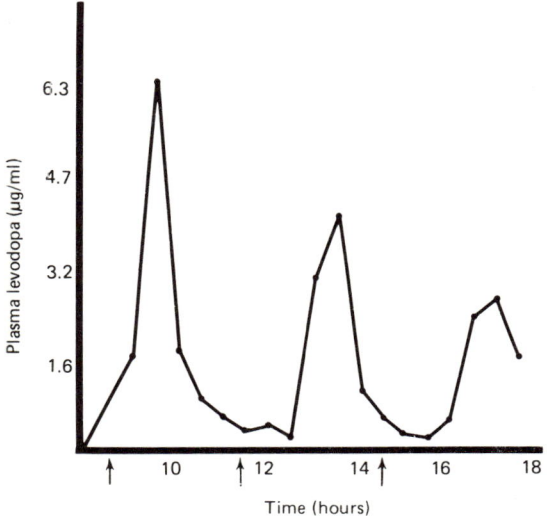

Figure 8.5 Variable plasma levels of levodopa depending on the order of dose. The most rapid rise and fall and also the highest peak of plasma dopa occurred with the first dose in the day after an overnight fast. Subsequent doses showed progressively lower peaks and more delayed rise and falls in the plasma levels. Levodopa 1000 mg was given at the times indicated by the arrows. The patient remained fasting throughout the study except for intake of water.

understood, but may relate to intestinal absorption of levodopa, and its occurrence may be a factor in the varying responses to different doses of levodopa throughout the day.

Complicated end-of-dose effect

The author agrees with Marsden and his colleagues (Chapter 7) that detailed mapping of the patient's mobility throughout the day is the best way to determine if there is any pattern of the 'off' periods in relationship with dosing. Usually one can decide if a patient has the pharmacokinetic problem of 'wearing-off' phenomenon or the pharmacodynamic one of random, sudden 'on–off'. It is not uncommon that patients have both phenomena.

Random oscillations ('on–off' phenomenon)

Sudden 'off' periods that occur in the 'on-off' effect seem to appear unrelated to dosing. Furthermore, they can end abruptly with a sudden 'on' period without the administration of another dose of levodopa. Fahn[18] studied serial plasma levels of levodopa and its metabolites in patients with the sudden 'on–off' phenomenon and observed that the 'off' periods developed only during the falling phase of plasma levodopa. The plasma levels could be low or high, i.e. at the beginning or end of the declining phase. Fahn suggested that the sudden 'off' episode may be the result of sudden desensitization block of dopamine receptors, due to some conformational change of the receptor protein. This block could be overcome by supplying more levodopa, creating a rising phase and higher levels in plasma and therefore higher brain levels of dopamine. As these levels fall, inadequate amounts are present to activate the desensitized receptor or maintain the receptor in the active conformational form, and the 'off' effect suddenly appears.

Other hypotheses have been advanced to explain the 'on–off' phenomenon: decreased bioavailability in plasma due to amino acid competition for intestinal transport of levodopa[11]; competition with amino acids for transport into brain; formation of dopa metabolites that act as false transmitters[54] or as competitors against dopamine for receptors; or a central noradrenergic mechanism[56]. In the author's opinion, a sudden desensitization of dopamine receptors due to conformational change (hence, a pharmacodynamic problem) as the result of chronic bombardment by dopamine seems to be the most satisfactory explanation[18], because the other hypothesis cannot explain the long latency of approximately 2 years before the 'on–off' phenomenon appears. The receptor desensitization hypothesis also is compatible with the observation that the receptors had been excessively bombarded by dopamine because these patients had previously experienced considerable choreic movements, indicating excess dopamine at receptors. In addition, this hypothesis is supported by the observation that the 'on–off' phenomenon persists even when levodopa is replaced by direct-acting dopamine agonists. Desensitization block has been observed at cholinergic and GABAergic receptors with chronic administration of acetylcholine and GABA, respectively[34, 48]. These observations suggest that the phenomenon of desensitization of neurotransmitter receptors may be a universal phenomenon.

Several laboratories have investigated the problem of the 'on–off' phenomenon. Sweet and McDowell[60] measured plasma levels of dopa in 10 patients, but only during periods when the patient was 'on' or 'off' and not serially. A low-protein diet elevated the plasma levels of levodopa and resulted in a lessening of the 'on–off' in 3 of 11 patients. Interestingly, they found that the average plasma level during the 'off' phase in the presence of a low-protein diet was higher than the average plasma level during the 'on' phase with a normal diet. Since 8 of 11 patients continued to have 'on–off' effects in the presence of a low-protein diet, and since these patients also had higher levels when 'on' and lower levels when 'off', this would suggest that the 'off' effect may be occurring during the declining plasma slope of levodopa even with the low-protein diet.

Mena and Cotzias[42] studied the influence of a low-protein diet on clinical responsiveness to levodopa. Plasma levels of levodopa were not determined. Lowering protein intake resulted in less severe clinical oscillations in some of their patients. The two patients with the most severe clinical fluctuations were not benefitted by a low-protein diet.

Tolosa et al.[61] measured hourly plasma levels of levodopa in three patients with a smooth clinical response, 11 patients with clinical fluctuations, and three with no clinical benefit from levodopa. The first group had low plasma levels all day without any sharp rise in concentration even after ingestion of levodopa. The absence of peaks and valleys of plasma dopa in smooth reponders needs to be replicated. The second group of patients consisted of a mixture of those patients who had a sudden rise and fall in plasma levels after each dose, and those who failed to show any rise in the plasma levodopa level after some doses. The author sees this as a problem of delayed gastric emptying (*see below*). The third group (non-responders) did have elevation of levodopa in plasma. Tolosa and colleagues concluded that these patients had end-stage disease with severe nigrostriatal neuronal loss and therefore were unable to respond. The intactness of dopamine receptors by administration of dopamine agonists was not tested in this study. It is difficult to understand why loss of nerve terminals should lead to nonresponsiveness as long as levodopa can be converted to dopamine in the striatum[41], and direct testing of the intactness of the dopamine receptors is necessary before any conclusion can be reached regarding non-responders.

The patients studied by Shoulson et al.[56] probably had the 'wearing-off' phenomenon (Shoulson, personal communication), and illustrations from this study are discussed above (*see Figures 8.3 and 8.4*).

Chapter 7 refers to random oscillations as the 'yo-yo' effect, whereas in this chapter they are referred to as the 'on–off' effect. Instead, the term 'yo-yo' is used to represent patients with a combination of peak dose dyskinesia and the 'wearing-off' phenomenon. Such patients switch from dyskinesia to 'off' and then back again with each dose of levodopa. It is also likely that extreme sensitivity of the dopamine receptors is a factor to account for the rapid onset dyskinesia after each dose.

'Resistant fluctuators'

This clinical category by Marsden *et al.* (Chapter 7) is theoretically compatible with any of the other categories, since it is a term applied to any patient who is difficult to treat. In terms of the author's own day-to-day experience, most patients in this group are those with the 'on–off' phenomenon (random oscillators).

TREATMENT-RELATED DYSKINESIAS

Peak dose dyskinesias

This form of dyskinesia is easiest to understand. It correlates with high plasma levels of levodopa, and therefore suggests that striatal dopamine levels are excessively high. Too much dopaminergic activity in the striatum leads to choreic dyskinesias, since chorea appears to be the obverse of bradykinesia. It is more difficult to explain peak dose dystonia since the mechanism of dystonia is less well understood. As discussed above, it is suggested that excessive striatal cholinergic activity may be a mechanism for dystonia, but it is difficult to explain how high striatal dopamine levels would lead to hypercholinergic activity; the opposite would be predicted. It seems that in levodopa-induced dystonia this type of dyskinesia may represent a more severe form of chorea. In other words, temporarily sustained postural changes (dystonia) may not be specific for only one pathophysiological explanation but rather may represent different striatal mechanisms.

Diphasic dyskinesias

Described by Muenter *et al.*[45] in 1977 as the 'D-I-D' (dyskinesia-improvement-dyskinesia) phenomenon, this uncommon pattern is poorly understood. Although Lhermitte *et al.*[38] believed that increasing the dosage of levodopa will lessen the dyskinesia, the author's own experience does not agree with this concept. He has found that higher dosages simply convert a patient with diphasic dyskinesia into one with peak dose or constant dyskinesia. Lowering the dosage reduces the dyskinesia, but also the improvement phase. Why dykinesia should appear when the plasma levels are rising and falling, but not when they are at their peak, is not easy to explain. In this condition, there is apparently a differential sensitivity to dopamine by at least two dopamine receptors. We know that more than one type of receptor exists (*see* Chapters 18.1 and 18.2). Perhaps the more sensitive receptor, when activated at a lower brain concentration of dopamine, induces dyskinesia. When the other receptor is activated at a higher concentration of dopamine, the dyskinesia is suppressed and only the benefit (absence of bradykinesia) is seen. Whether such a scheme of interactions by dopamine receptors exists is not known, but it seems reasonable to hypothesize its existence in order to explain the phenomenon of diphasic dyskinesia.

Early morning dystonia

This form of dyskinesia occurs when plasma levels of levodopa are very low. Hence, little brain dopamine should be available to activate dopamine receptors. Its prevention by nighttime dosing with levodopa or by utilizing pergolide (as seen in one of the author's patients) supports the notion that the dystonia is a 'rebound' phenomenon of too little dopamine to activate the dopamine receptors. The patient is usually more disabled with painful dystonia than with concurrent parkinsonism. Some unusual property of the dopamine receptor may also play a role in this phenomenon in order to explain the dystonic manifestation rather than simple exacerbation of other parkinsonian symptoms, although some increase of parkinsonism does accompany the appearance of dystonia.

Myoclonus

Myoclonus from levodopa is usually associated with signs of levodopa toxicity such as alteration of the sleep–wake cycle, hallucinations, and confusion. Hence, myoclonus appears to represent a central toxic state, but probably in cortical or other brain sites rather than in striatum.

PATHOPHYSIOLOGIC CLASSIFICATION OF TREATMENT-RELATED FLUCTUATIONS AND DYSKINESIAS

The preceding sections of this chapter were organized to enable the reader to understand the pathophysiological mechanisms of the various categories of problems listed in Chapter 7 by Marsden, Parkes and Quinn. In the sections that follow this topic has been reorganized along pathophysiological grounds, and at the same time, several other clinical problems have been introduced that can be interpreted using similar pathophysiological mechanisms. It is usually possible on clinical grounds to categorize the various levodopa-induced adverse effects as either a pharmacokinetic problem, a pharmacodynamic problem, or a combination of the two.

Pharmacokinetic problems

The pharmacokinetic problems (*Table 8.1*) relate to the bioavailability of levodopa. The goal of levodopa administration is to provide an adequate amount of dopamine to the receptors in the striatum. *Figure 8.6* illustrates the steps along this route and the steps that can interfere with the maintenance of brain dopamine concentrations. After levodopa is ingested, it must pass into the small intestine by the process of gastric emptying. Next, levodopa must be absorbed into the circulation before it is metabolized by gut enzymes and flora. From plasma levodopa it is transported into the brain, in part, by the L-neutral amino acid transport system[63]. A similar

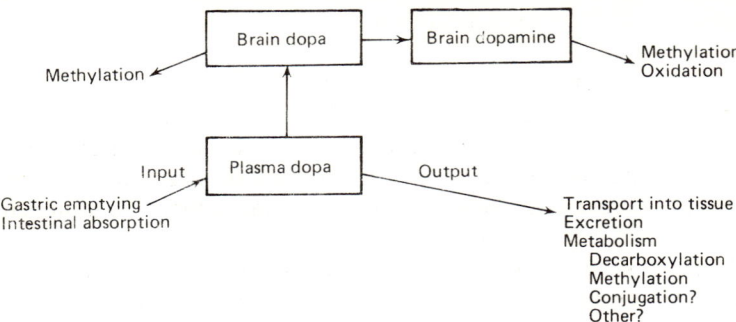

Figure 8.6 Diagram illustrating the steps along the route from oral administration of levodopa to its conversion to brain dopamine, and of the steps that can prevent the maintenance of constant brain dopamine levels.

transport system is utilized in the transport of levodopa across the intestinal mucosa[62] and across the erythrocyte membrane[28], although nonsaturable passive diffusion also occurs. Aside from uptake of circulating levodopa into other tissues, it can also disappear peripherally by being metabolized by dopa decarboxylase and catechol-O-methyltransferase (COMT). These factors all contribute to the short half-life of plasma levodopa. Within brain, COMT can metabolize both levodopa and dopamine, and monomine oxidase inactivates dopamine (*Figure 8.6*).

The following clinical problems are related to pharmacokinetic mechanisms (*Table 8.1*).

'Wearing-off' phenomenon (end-of-dose deterioration)

As discussed in detail above, this problem correlates with plasma levels of levodopa and, by shortening the intervals between doses, can be minimized. Another approach is to utilize direct-acting dopamine agonists that have a longer biological half-life.

Table 8.1 Pharmacokinetic problems with levodopa therapy

Symptom	Mechanism	Treatment
'Wearing-off' phenomenon (End-of-dose deterioration)	Short plasma half-life with inadequate stores of dopamine	(1) Shorter intervals between doses (2) Long acting agonists
Failure to respond to each dose	Delayed gastric emptying	Dissolve levodopa before ingestion
Peak dose dyskinesia	High peak plasma levels	Reduce individual dosages
Reduced response if levodopa is ingested after high protein meals	Transport competes with amino acids	Determine optimum meals
Dyskinesia without benefit	3-O-Methyldopa	Direct agonists
Decreased benefit	3-O-Methyldopa	Direct agonists
Decreased benefit	Pyridoxine	Reduce pyridoxine

Failure to respond to individual doses of levodopa

Despite a shortening of the intervals of levodopa dosing, many patients develop a problem whereby they fail to respond to occasional doses of levodopa, as a result of delayed gastric emptying[20,52]. Plasma levels of levodopa fail to rise whenever this occurs, (as observed, for example, by Tolosa et al.[61] in some of their patients with fluctuations). The author found that levodopa tablets remain along the stomach wall in this situation. Rivera-Calimlim et al.[52] recommended utilizing antacids to overcome the problem, but such an approach was not helpful in this author's hands, and he found dissolving or suspending the levodopa preparation in water or other liquids aided the passage of levodopa into the small intestine and allowed the patient to respond to each dose of medication.

Peak dose dyskinesia

Peak dose dyskinesia has been discussed in an earlier section of this chapter. It is listed again here to place it within the pathophysiological classification. Reducing the individual dosage of medication should avoid the problem, but if the therapeutic index is low, the patient may have an inadequate response from a lower dosage.

Response varies in relationship to meals

Many patients report a slower and reduced response to levodopa if the medication is ingested after a meal, especially if the meal was high in protein. In part this is due to delayed gastric emptying. In contrast, an enhanced response is seen when levodopa is taken on an empty stomach. Another mechanism that plays a role after a high-protein meal is the competition of levodopa with other amino acids for absorption from the intestine into the circulation[40]. Treatment needs to be individualized because a slower rate of absorption of levodopa is an advantage to those who tend to become toxic from the medication. For such patients, it is better to take levodopa immediately after a meal. For those patients with insufficient response, it is preferable to take levodopa on an empty stomach.

Competition with 3-O-methyldopa

Although various metabolites of levodopa have been considered at one time or another as a possible source for some of the clinical problems seen with chronic levodopa therapy, the only one implicated by fairly reasonable evidence is 3-O-methyldopa (OMD). This compound is the major accumulated metabolite of levodopa because of its long biological half-life (approximately 12 hours)[5,35]. With levodopa therapy for parkinsonism the concentration of OMD is greater than that of dopa in both plasma and cerebrospinal fluid[18,44,55].

Muenter et al.[44] showed that there was an inverse relationship between fasting OMD levels in plasma and the degree of improvement with levodopa therapy. They then administered OMD to patients receiving levodopa for parkinsonism and found that the response to levodopa diminished in direct proportion to the dosage of OMD with its resulting elevation of the concentration of OMD in plasma[43]. Other workers found increased plasma levels of OMD in patients with involuntary movements and with clinical fluctuations[27, 53].

Wade and Katzman[64] showed that OMD inhibited uptake of dopa into the brain when both compounds were injected simultaneously into the carotid artery. Recently, it was found that the presence of high plasma levels of OMD in rat interferes with striatal uptake and utilization of levodopa[50]. Although not proven, it seems reasonable to consider that the high levels of OMD could contribute to decreased efficacy of levodopa, dyskinesia without adequate benefit[53], and perhaps even some 'off' periods. Utilization of direct-acting dopamine agonists, or the development of a safe and effective COMT inhibitor should circumvent any problems due to OMD.

Loss of efficacy in the presence of pyridoxine

Pyridoxine has been shown to antagonize the clinical effectiveness of levodopa[17], but only in the absence of carbidopa[16, 18, 33, 49]. Plasma levels of dopa are reduced in the presence of chronic pyridoxine administration[17, 37]. It is believed that since pyridoxine is a cofactor for dopa decarboxylase activity, high levels of this vitamin enhance peripheral decarboxylation. Avoiding excess pyridoxine or utilizing a peripheral decarboxylase inhibitor, such as carbidopa, are effective means of treating this problem.

Pharmacodynamic problems

The term pharmacodynamic problem refers to the effect of dopa or dopamine at the molecular level on either dopamine receptors and/or nerve terminals (*Table 8.2*).

Gastrointestinal upset

Nausea, vomiting and anorexia are common accompaniments of levodopa administration. These symptoms are believed to be due to activation of the dopamine receptors in the area postrema. Although part of the central nervous system, the area postrema lies outside the blood-brain barrier. Therefore, the dopamine receptors in this vomiting center can be considered 'peripheral' receptors. Utilizing a peripheral decarboxylase inhibitor (e.g. carbidopa) to prevent formation of peripheral dopamine, or employing a peripherally acting dopamine receptor antagonist (e.g. domperidone)[7], can reduce or eliminate this problem.

Table 8.2 Pharmacodynamic problems with levodopa therapy

Symptom	Mechanism	Treatment
Gastrointestinal upset	Activation of dopamine receptors in area postrema	(1) Carbidopa (2) Domperidone
Confusion, drowsiness, hallucinations, myoclonus, altered sleep–wake cycle, postural hypotension	Activation of non-striatal dopamine receptors	(1) Reduce dosage (2) Drug holiday
Loss of efficacy	Steady desensitization of dopamine receptors	(1) Drug holidays (2) Try directs agonists
Increased parkinsonism	As above	Reduce dosage
Sudden 'on–off' phenomenon	Transient desensitization block	Difficult
Diphasic dyskinesias	Differential sensitivity of at least two receptors	Try direct agonists
Dyskinesia plus parkinsonism	Somatotopic differential sensitivity of receptors	Difficult

Central adverse effects, other than dyskinesias and fluctuations

The activation of central nervous system dopamine receptors outside the striatum probably accounts for a large number of central adverse effects seen with levodopa therapy. Dopamine receptors are in limbic structures, frontal cortex, and in hypothalamus. It seems reasonable to assume that these non-striatal dopamine receptors, when excessively activated, could account for the toxic symptoms of confusion, delusions, hallucinations, drowsiness, myoclonus, altered sleep-wake cycle, and postural hypotension. So far, the only effective approach has been to reduce the dosage of levodopa or utilize drug holidays.

Loss of efficacy

It is well recognized that patients tend to respond less well with continuing levodopa therapy. One factor to account for this is that Parkinson's disease is a progressive disorder and there is continuing loss of dopaminergic neurons, although how this could lead to a loss of responsiveness to levodopa is not clear. A controversial point is whether chronic levodopa therapy can also lead to a loss of efficacy (see Chapter 1). Rinne et al.[51] have shown that some patients develop desensitization of striatal dopamine receptors with chronic levodopa therapy. These patients have a poorer response to treatment. Also supporting this concept is the restoration of efficacy following a drug holiday[15,65]. Another symptom that may be related to the desensitization of dopamine receptors is the occasional problem of increased parkinsonism as a sign of toxicity[22]. A reduction of dosage restores clinical improvement.

Sudden 'on–off' effect (random oscillations)

This phenomenon has already been discussed in detail. Transient, conformational desensitization of the dopamine receptors as a consequence of chronic exposure to high levels dopamine was proposed as the possible mechanism. For the author, this problem has not satisfactorily been solved by the use of direct-acting dopamine agonists or by altering the timing of the dosages of levodopa. It remains a major problem.

Diphasic dyskinesia

The differential sensitivity of more than one dopamine receptor has already been suggested as the mechanism of this symptom. If levodopa dosage is kept high to avoid the problem, the patient tends to become toxic or develop peak dose dyskinesia. Lowering the dosage eliminates diphasic dyskinesia at the expense of increased parkinsonism. Direct-acting agonists may prove useful for this condition.

Simultaneous dyskinesia and parkinsonism

In addition to temporally related dyskinesias (e.g. peak dose and diphasic), many patients develop dyskinesia in one part of the body, while another part remains parkinsonian. In other words, these patients fail to obtain a somatotopically uniform response to levodopa. Usually the face area is more sensitive and the leg area less sensitive. This leads to a clinical picture of facial dyskinesia when the legs become mobile and no facial dyskinesia when the legs are immobile. Differential sensitivity of dopamine receptors in different somatotopic sites in the striatum probably accounts for the problem. Treatment is difficult and the patient usually must accept either dyskinesia with less parkinsonism or more parkinsonism to avoid the dyskinesia.

Probable combined pharmacokinetic and pharmacodynamic problems

Early morning dystonia

This problem was discussed in the previous section. Early morning dystonia occurs with low plasma levels of levodopa, and is an unusual response to inadequate dopamine receptor activity. Treatment by nighttime administration of levodopa may be helpful, as may be long-acting direct-acting agonists (*Table 8.3*).

Table 8.3 Combined pharmacokinetic and pharmacodynamic problems with levodopa therapy

Symptom	Mechanism	Treatment
Early morning dystonia	(1) Low plasma level (2) Unusual receptor response	(1) Nighttime levodopa (2) Direct dopamine agonists
'Yo-yo-ing'	(1) Extreme receptor sensitivity (2) Short plasma half-life	Try direct dopamine agonists

'Yo-yo-ing'

As discussed above, the use of this term in this chapter refers to patients with swings from the 'off' state to dyskinesia and back again. These patients usually obtain an enhanced response to a dose of levodopa, producing dyskinesia when the bradykinesia disappears. One patient described it as follows: 'It's like being on the express train going through a local station', where the local station represents the ideal state of normal mobility without dyskinesia. It has already been suggested that this phenomenon may be due to enhanced receptor sensitivity (a pharmacodynamic problem) and the 'wearing-off' effect from a short plasma half-life of levodopa (a pharmacokinetic problem). Treatment is difficult. Keeping the dosage of levodopa low with parkinsonian symptoms but avoiding severely uncomfortable dyskinesia may be a better alternative than excessive swings in performance. The direct-acting agonists may prove helpful in some patients.

CONCLUSION

In this chapter the possible pathophysiological mechanisms of the dyskinesias and fluctuations, described clinically by Marsden, Parkes and Quinn in Chapter 7, have been discussed. A pathophysiological classification of treatment-induced problems was suggested. These were divided into pharmacokinetic problems, pharmacodynamic problems, and a combination of the two. At our present stage of therapeutic manipulations, pharmacokinetic problems are more easily treated than the other two categories.

References

1 AMBANI, L. M. and VAN WOERT, M. H. Start hesitation: Side effect of long-term levodopa therapy. *New England Journal of Medicine*, **288**, 1113–1115 (1973)

2 BARBEAU, A. L-dopa therapy in Parkinson's disease: A critical review of nine years' experience. *Journal, Canadian Medical Association*, **101**, 794–800 (1969)

3 BARBEAU, A. High-level levodopa therapy in severely akinetic parkinsonian patients: twelve years later. In *Parkinson's Disease: Current Progress, Problems and Management*, edited by U. K. Rinne, M. Klingler and G. Stamm, 229–239. Amsterdam, Elsevier/North-Holland Biomedical Press (1980)

4 BAROLIN, G. S., BERNHEIMER, H. and HORNYKIEWICZ, O. Seitenverschiedenes Verhalten des Dopamins (3-Hydroxytyramin) im Gehirn eines Falles von Hemiparkinsonismus. *Schweizer Archiv für Neurologie und Psychiatrie*, **94**, 241–248 (1964)

5 BARTHOLINI, G., KURUMA, I. and PLETSCHER, A. Distribution and metabolism of L-3-O-methyldopa in rats. *British Journal of Pharmacology*, **40**, 461–467 (1970)

6 BIRKET-SMITH, E. Abnormal involuntary movements in relation to anticholinergics and levodopa therapy. *Acta Neurologica Scandinavia*, **52**, 158–160 (1975)

7 BOGAERTS, M., BRAEMS, M. and MARTENS, C. Domperidone in the prevention of L-dopa induced nausea. *Postgraduate Medical Journal*, **55** *(Suppl, 1)*, 51–52 (1979)

8 CARLSSON, A. The occurrence, distribution and physiological role of catecholamines in the nervous system. *Pharmacological Reviews*, **11**, 490–493 (1959)
9 CARLSSON, A. Mechanism of action of neuroleptic drugs. In *Psychopharmacology: A Generation of Progress*, edited by M. A. Lipton, A. DiMascio and K. F. Killam, 1057–1070. New York, Raven Press (1978)
10 CARLSSON, A., LINDQVIST, M. and MAGNUSSON, T. 3,4-Dihydroxyphenylalanine and 5-hydroxytryptophan as reserpine antagonists. *Nature*, **180**, 1200 (1957)
11 COTZIAS, G. C., MENA, I. and PAPAVASILIOU, P. S. Overview of present treatment of parkinsonism with L-dopa. *Advances in Neurology*, **2**, 265–277 (1973)
12 COTZIAS, G. C., PAPAVASILIOU, P. S. and GELLENE, R. Modification of parkinsonism – chronic treatment with L-dopa. *New England Journal of Medicine*, **280**, 337–345 (1969)
13 CREVELING, C. R., DALY, J., TOKUYAMA, T. and WITCOP, B. The combined use of α-methyltyrosine and threo-dihydroxyphenylserine selective reduction of dopamine levels in the central nervous system. *Biochemical Pharmacology*, **17**, 65–70 (1968)
14 DEGWITZ, R., FROWEIN, R., KULENKAMPFF, C. and MOHS, U. Über die Wirksungen des L-dopa beim Menschen und deren Beeinflussung durch Reserpin, Chlorpromazin, Iproniazid und Vitamin B6. *Klinische Wochenschrift*, **38**, 120–123 (1960)
15 DIRENFELD, L. K., FELDMAN, R. G., ALEXANDER, M. P. and KELLY-HAYES, M. Is L-dopa drug holiday useful? *Neurology*, **30**, 785–788 (1980)
16 DUVOISIN, R. C. Pyridoxine as an adjunct in the treatment of parkinsonism. *Advances in Neurology*, **2**, 229–247 (1973)
17 DUVOISIN, R. C., YAHR, M. D. and COTE, L. J. Pyridoxine reversal of L-dopa effect in parkinsonism. *Transactions of the American Neurological Association*, **94**, 81–84 (1969)
18 FAHN, S. 'On–off' phenomenon with levodopa therapy in parkinsonism: clinical and pharmacologic correlations and the effect of intramuscular pyridoxine. *Neurology*, **24**, 431–441 (1974)
19 FAHN, S. Biochemistry of the basal ganglia. *Advances in Neurology*, **14**, 59–88 (1976)
20 FAHN, S. Episodic failure of absorption of levodopa: a factor in the control of clinical fluctuations in the treatment of parkinsonism. *Neurology*, **27**, 390 (1977)
21 FAHN, S. Treatment of dystonia with high dosage anticholinergic medication. *Neurology*, **29**, 605 (1979)
22 FAHN, S. and BARRETT, R. E. Increase of parkinsonian symptoms as a manifestation of levodopa toxicity. *Advances in Neurology*, **24**, 451–459 (1979)
23 FAHN, S., COTE, L. J., SNIDER, S. R., BARRETT, R. E. and ISGREEN, W. P. Role of bromocriptine in the treatment of parkinsonism. *Neurology*, **29**, 1077–1083 (1979)
24 FAHN, S. and DAVID, E. Oral-facial-lingual dykinesia due to anticholinergic medication. *Transactions of the American Neurological Association*, **97**, 277–279 (1972)
25 FAHN, S. and DUFFY, P. Parkinson's disease. In *Scientific Approaches to Clinical Neurology*, edited by E. S. Goldensohn and S. Appel, 1119–1158. Philadelphia, Lea and Febiger (1977)

26 FAHN, S., LIBSCH, L. B. and CUTLER, R. W. Monoamines in the human neostriatum: topographic distribution in normals and in Parkinson's disease and their role in akinesia, rigidity, chorea, and tremor, *Journal of the Neurological Sciences*, **14**, 427–455 (1971)

27 FEUERSTEIN, C., TANCHE, M., SERRE, F., GAVEND, M., PELLAT, J. and PERRRET, J. Does O-methyldopa play a role in levodopa-induced dyskinesias? *Acta Neurologica Scandinavia*, **56**, 79–82 (1977)

28 FLOUD, A. and FAHN, S. L-Dopa (L-3,4-dihydroxyphenylalanine) uptake by human red blood cells. *Biochimica et Biophysical Acta*, **645**, 165–169 (1981)

29 GRODEN, B. M. Parkinsonism occurring with methyldopa treatment. *British Medical Journal*, **1**, 1001 (1963)

30 HORNYKIEWICZ, O. Metabolism of brain dopamine in human parkinsonism. In *Biochemistry and Pharmacology of the Basal Ganglia*, edited by E. Costa, L. J. Cote and M. D. Yahr, 171–185. New York, Raven Press (1966)

31 HORNYKIEWICZ, O. Dopamine (3-hydroxytyramine) and brain function. *Pharmacological Reviews*, **18**, 925–964 (1966)

32 JAVOY-AGID, F. and AGID, Y. Is the mesocortical dopaminergic system involved in Parkinson disease? *Neurology*, **30**, 1326–1330 (1980)

33 KLAWANS, H. L., RINGEL, S. P. and SHENKER, M. Failure of vitamin B6 to reverse the L-dopa effect in patients on a dopa decarboxylase inhibitor. *Journal of Neurology, Neurosurgery and Psychiatry*, **34**, 682–686 (1971)

34 KRNJEVIC, K. Inhibitory action of GABA and GABA-mimetics on vertebrate neurones. In *GABA in Nervous System Function*, edited by E. Roberts, T. N. Chase and D. B. Tower, 269–281, New York, Raven Press (1976)

35 KURUMA, I., BARTHOLINI, G. and PLETSCHER, A. L-dopa induced accumulation of 3-O-methyldopa in brain and heart. *European Journal of Pharmacology*, **10**, 189–192 (1970)

36 LAL, S., HOYTE, K., KIELY, M. E., SOURKES, T. L., BAXTER, D. W., MISSALA, K. and ANDERMANN, F. Neuropharmacological investigation and treatment of spasmodic torticollis. *Advances in Neurology*, **24**, 335–351 (1979)

37 LEON, A., SPIEGEL, H. E., THOMAS, G. and ABRAMS, W. B. Pyridoxine antagonism of levodopa in parkinsonism. *Journal of the American Medical Association*, **218**, 1924–1927 (1971)

38 LHERMITTE, F., AGID, Y. and SIGNORET, J. L. Onset and end-of-dose levodopa-induced dyskinesias. *Archives of Neurology*, **35**, 261–262 (1978)

39 MARSDEN, C. D. and PARKES, J. D. 'On–off' effects in patients with Parkinson's disease on chronic levodopa therapy. *Lancet*, **1**, 292–295 (1976)

40 McDOWELL, F. H. and SWEET, R. D. The 'on–off' phenomenon. In *Advances in Parkinsonism*, edited by W. Birkmayer and O. Hornykiewicz, 603–612, Basle, Editiones Roche (1976)

41 MELAMED, E., HEFTI, F. and WURTMAN, R. J. Nonaminergic striatal neurons convert exogenous L-dopa to dopamine in parkinsonism. *Annals of Neurology*, **8**, 558–563 (1980)

42 MENA, I. and COTZIAS, G. C. Protein intake and treatment of Parkinson's disease with levodopa. *New England Journal of Medicine*, **292**, 181–184 (1975)

43 MUENTER, M. D., DiNAPOLI, R. P., SHARPLESS, N. S. and TYCE, G. M. 3-O-Methyldopa, L-dopa and trihexyphenidyl in the treatment of Parkinson's disease. *Mayo Clinic Proceedings*, **48,** 173–183 (1973)

44 MUENTER, M. D., SHARPLESS, N. S. and TYCE, G. M. Plasma 3-O-methyldopa in L-dopa therapy of Parkinson's disease. *Mayo Clinic Proceedings*, **47,** 389–395 (1972)

45 MUENTER, M. D., SHARPLESS, N. S., TYCE, G. M. and DARLEY, F. L. Patterns of dystonia ('I-D-I' and 'D-I-D') in response to L-dopa therapy of Parkinson's disease. *Mayo Clinic Proceedings*, **52,** 163–174 (1977)

46 MUENTER, M. D. and TYCE, G. M. L-dopa therapy of Parkinson's disease: Plasma L-dopa concentration, therapeutic response, and side effects. *Mayo Clinic Proceedings*, **46,** 231–239 (1971)

47 NARABAYASHI, H. Presented at the XII World Congress of Neurology, Kyoto, Japan (1981)

48 NASTUK, W. L. Activation and inactivation of muscle postjunctional receptors. *Federation Proceedings*, **26,** 1639–1646 (1967)

49 PAPAVASILIOU, P. S., COTZIAS, G. C., DUBY, S. E., STECK, A. J., FEHLING, C., and BELL, M. A. Levodopa in parkinsonism: potentiation of central effects with a peripheral inhibitor. *New England Journal of Medicine*, **286,** 8–14 (1972)

50 RECHES, A. and FAHN, S. O-Methyldopa interferes with striatal utilization of levodopa. *Annals of Neurology*, **10,** 94–95 (1981)

51 RINNE, U. K., KOSKINEN, V. and LONNBERG, P. Neurotransmitter receptors in the parkinsonian brain. In *Parkinson's Disease: Current Progress, Problems and Management*, edited by U. K. Rinne, M. Klingler and G. Stamm, 93–107. Amsterdam, Elsevier/North-Holland Biomedical Press (1980)

52 RIVERA-CALIMLIM, L., DUJOVNE, C. A., MORGAN, J. P., LASAGNA, L. and BIANCHINE, J. R. L-Dopa treatment failure: explanation and correction. *British Medical Journal*, **4,** 93–94 (1970)

53 RIVERA-CALIMLIM, L., TANDON, D., ANDERSON, F. and JOYNT, R. The clinical picture and plasma levodopa metabolite profile of parkinsonism nonresponders. Treatment with levodopa and decarboxylase inhibitor. *Archives of Neurology*, **34,** 228–232 (1977)

54 SANDLER, M. The dopa effect: Possible significance of transamination and tetrahydroisoquinoline formation. *Advances in Neurology*, **2,** 255–264 (1973)

55 SHARPLESS, N. S. and McCANN, D. S. Dopa and 3-O-methyldopa in cerebrospinal fluid of parkinsonism patients during treatment with oral L-dopa. *Clinica Chimica Acta*, **31,** 155–169 (1971)

56 SHOULSON, I., GLAUBIGER, G. A. and CHASE, T. N. 'On–off' response: Clinical and biochemical correlations during oral and intravenous levodopa administration in parkinsonian patients. *Neurology*, **25,** 1144–1148 (1975)

57 SPIEGEL, E. A., SZEKELY, E. G. and ZIVANOVIC, D. Striatal bradykinesia alleviated by intracaudate injection of L-dopa. *Experientia*, **25,** 39–40 (1968)

58 STRANG, R. R. Parkinsonism occurring during methyldopa therapy. *Journal Canadian Medical Association*, **95,** 928–929 (1966)

59 SUTCHER, H. D., UNDERWOOD, R. B., BEATTY, R. A. and SUGAR, O. Orofacial dyskinesia. A dental dimension. *Journal of the American Medical Association*, **216,** 1459–1463 (1971)

60 SWEET, R. D. and McDOWELL, F. H. Plasma dopa concentrations and the 'on–off' effect after chronic treatment of Parkinson's disease. *Neurology*, **24,** 953–956 (1974)
61 TOLOSA, E. S., MARTIN, W. E., COHEN, J. P. and JACOBSON, R. L. Patterns of clinical response and plasma dopa levels in Parkinson's disease. *Neurology*, **25,** 177–183 (1975)
62 WADE, D. N., MEARRICK, P. T. and MORRIS, J. Active transport of L-dopa in the intestine. *Nature*, **242,** 463–465 (1973)
63 WADE, L. A. and KATZMAN, R. Synthetic amino acids and the nature of L-dopa transport at the blood-brain barrier. *Journal of Neurochemistry*, **25,** 837–842 (1975)
64 WADE, L. A. and KATZMAN, R. 3-O-Methyldopa uptake and inhibition of L-dopa at the blood brain barrier, *Life Sciences*, **17,** 131–136 (1975)
65 WEINER, W. J., KOLLER, W. C., PERLIK, S., NAUSIEDA, P. A. and KLAWANS, H. L. Drug holiday and management of Parkinson disease. *Neurology*, **30,** 1257–1261 (1980)
66 YAHR, M. D., DUVOISIN, R. C., SCHEAR, M. J., BARRETT, R. E. and HOEHN, M. M. Treatment of parkinsonism with levodopa. *Archives of Neurology*, **21,** 343–354 (1969)

9
Treatment of advanced Parkinson's disease with dopamine agonists
Abraham N. Lieberman and Menek Goldstein

RATIONALE FOR USE OF DIRECT DOPAMINE AGONISTS

Declining efficacy of levodopa

The response to levodopa in patients with Parkinson's disease diminishes considerably after a few years of treatment. Several theories have been advanced to explain this diminished response.

The decreased efficacy of levodopa has been related mainly to disease progression because most patients are, after several years treatment, worse than they were before beginning treatment[41, 59, 60]. The mechanisms underlying disease progression are not yet known. Initially, it was thought that compensation for the striatal dopamine deficiency is achieved through increased conversion of levodopa to dopamine by the remaining nigrostriatal neurons and by the development of supersensitivity of the postsynaptic receptors[1, 2, 13, 21, 31, 32, 42, 81] (*see* Chapter 4). Compensation may also be achieved through the conversion of levodopa to dopamine in striatal interneurons, which under ordinary circumstances do not synthesize dopamine[61, 62]. It may be that levodopa no longer compensates for the dopamine deficiency as Parkinson's disease progresses because the remaining neurons are too few in number to generate enough dopamine to stimulate the striatum. The benefit that many patients derive from dopamine agonists which bypass the degenerating presynaptic neurons and stimulate the postsynaptic dopamine receptors directly supports this hypothesis. However, it has been argued that severely incapacitated patients (with excessive degeneration of nigrostriatal neurons), in particular those with postencephalitic parkinsonism, respond as well as moderately incapacitated patients (with less excessive degeneration of nigrostriatal neurons). It is noteworthy that while many severely disabled patients respond to levodopa, their response is of shorter duration than that of less disabled patients. It is conceivable that the favorable response to levodopa of severely disabled patients is related more to supersensitivity of the postsynaptic receptors than to dopamine synthesis, and that this supersensitivity disappears quickly.

Emergence of fluctuations

Associated with the diminished response to levodopa are 'on–off' phenomena, and associated with the 'on–off' phenomena are dyskinesias (*see* Chapter 7).

On the assumption that the oscillations, in part, are related to inadequate delivery of dopamine to postsynaptic receptors due to erratic availability of dopa to the presynaptic neurons, several approaches have been taken to augment the delivery of dopa to the CNS. These have included prescribing a low-protein diet to maximize the amount of dopa absorbed through the gastrointestinal tract and entering through the blood–brain barrier[63], increasing the dose of levodopa, increasing the frequency of administration of levodopa (to an hourly basis in some patients), giving levodopa only on 'demand' (i.e. when the patient begins to go 'off'), giving levodopa parenterally[75], varying the ratio of levodopa to carbidopa from between 10:1 to 1:1, using a different decarboxylase inhibitor (benserazide)[48]. Another approach has been to add drugs which augment the activity of levodopa or lessen its adverse reactions. These drugs include amantadine, anticholinergic agents, tricyclic antidepressants, type B monoamine oxidase inhibitors (deprenyl)[4,17], lithium, GABAergic agents (valproate, diazepam)[70], serotonergic agents (tryptophan, 5-hydroxytryptophan[9,64], methysergide, clonazepam), dopamine-blocking agents (haloperidol, pimozide, thioridazine) cyclic AMP phosphodiesterase inhibitors[23], baclofen[44], catechol-O-methyl-transferase inhibitors[18], 3-methyldopa[5] and dopamine β-hydroxylase inhibitors (fusaric acid)[8]. The complexity of the levodopa dosing schedules and the variety of adjuvant agents employed attest to the failure of these approaches. Still another approach has been to consider the oscillations solely as a consequence of chronic levodopa administration and to recommend a period of drug abstinence or 'holiday'. However, the authors' experience with 20 patients undergoing drug holidays has been less favorable, with the holidays resulting in variable and inconsistent benefit of relatively short duration.

Based on the limitations of all of the above approaches, the authors postulated the following to explain the 'on–off' phenomena. With advancing Parkinson's disease there is a decrease in the number of presynaptic dopaminergic nigrostriatal neurons and of their nerve terminals. Since the principal means of inactivation of the newly generated dopamine in the synaptic cleft is re-uptake by the presynaptic nerve terminals, a decrease in the number of these terminals may lead to excessive concentrations of dopamine at the receptor site. This may result in a desensitization block analogous to the cholinergic crisis of myasthenia gravis[19]. In this scheme, 'on' periods result from activation of receptors by a specific concentration of dopamine and 'off' periods result from failure of the receptors to be activated. Two mechanisms may be responsible for the failure of receptors to be activated. In one mechanism, failure of receptor activation may occur because of insufficient concentrations of dopamine in the synaptic cleft. In the second mechanism, failure of receptor activation may occur because of an excessive concentration of dopamine in the synaptic cleft resulting in desensitization blockade. Such a scheme could explain the two major types of 'on–off' phenomena encountered clinically. In the first, 'off' periods occur several hours after the last dose of levodopa, unaccompanied by dyskinesias, and usually benefited by the next dose of levodopa. This type of 'off' effect is related to a decreased or falling plasma levodopa concentration, and presumably to a decreased or falling dopamine concentration in the synaptic cleft. The second type 'off' periods occur in no fixed relationship to the last dose of levodopa, and have even been, at times, related to high plasma levodopa concentrations (*see* Chapter 8).

All these complex effects of levodopa which may be responsible for the emergence of fluctuations in clinical response might be avoided by the use of directly acting dopamine agonists.

Other possible advantages of dopamine agonists

It now is realized that there is more than one type of dopamine receptor in the brain (*see* Chapters 5, 18.1 and 18.2). Which of the various dopamine receptors are involved in the therapeutic response to levodopa is not known. Indeed, individual receptor types might be concerned with specific therapeutic actions or unwanted effects. Directly acting dopamine agonists conceivably could be directed towards specific dopamine receptors, in contrast to the rather 'blunderbuss' action of levodopa. Another advantage of such drugs may be a longer duration of action compared to levodopa, which might provide a smoother, more sustained therapeutic response.

SELECTION OF DOPAMINE AGONISTS

Given the complexities underlying the diminished response to levodopa and the associated 'on–off' phenomena, the most successful means of treating both of these states, in the authors' experience, has been through augmenting the activity of the dopaminergic system with drugs that bypass the degenerating presynaptic nigrostriatal neurons and stimulate the postsynaptic receptors directly (*Figure 9.1 and Table 9.1*). Fundamental to the development of these drugs was the establishment of experimental animal models of Parkinson's disease: rats with nigrostriatal lesions and monkeys with ventral tegmental mesencephalic lesions[68]. The antiparkinsonian effects observed in the animal models have, with few exceptions, been duplicated in man. With the animal models a large number of compounds can be tested to see which ones are most effective and which induce the fewest dyskinesias. Such screening is essential, as only a few of the many active compounds can be tested in man. As an example, lergotrile was first shown to have anti-parkinsonian activity in the animal models before it was tested in man[56]. After a long (and expensive) clinical trial, the drug was found to be hepatotoxic in approximately 25 per cent of patients. Several congeners of lergotrile were available, but not all of them could be subjected to the same kind of clinical trial. It was reasoned that the cyano group at the eighth position of the ergoline molecule and the halogen were likely to be responsible for the hepatotoxicity. Compounds without these moieties were tested in the animal models to see if they had anti-parkinsonian activity. Three compounds with alkyl chains at the N6 position of the ergoline molecule were found to have such activity. A clinical trial involving all three compounds was again impractical. It was then discovered that the antiparkinsonian activity of these three compounds correlated with the length of the alkyl side chain at the N6 position, and that the propyl compound was more potent and longer acting than the ethyl or methyl compound[25, 26]. Pergolide (N6-propylergoline) was subsequently tested in man and found to be an effective antiparkinsonian drug[49]. Observations in the animal models coupled with *in vitro*

Figure 9.1 Structures of certain dopamine agonists employed to treat Parkinson's disease

experiments using striatal membranes have further broadened our understanding of the basic mechanisms involved in how these drugs work. These studies have enabled the authors to determine that some agonists require presynaptic dopamine while others do not. Thus, the activity of bromocriptine may be blocked by pretreatment with α-methyl paratyrosine, which inhibits dopamine synthesis[38]. Because the activity of bromocriptine is dependent on presynaptic dopamine synthesis and stores, bromocriptine may not be effective in some severely disabled patients with depleted stores. In contrast, the activity of lisuride, a semisynthetic ergoline, is independent of presynaptic dopamine synthesis and stores, and thus lisuride may be more effective in severely disabled patients than bromocriptine[33, 34]. These studies also reveal that some agonists behave differently at low than at

Table 9.1 Comparison of dopamine agonists (DA)

Drug	Monkeys: intraperitoneal dose (mg/kg)	Monkeys: tremor stopped (hours)	Human oral dose to acheive peak level(mg)	Human peak level (ng)	Human time to peak (hours)	Human $T_{1/2}$ (hours)	DA receptor predominantly stimulated	Human daily dose (mg)
Carbidopa + levodopa	$\frac{10}{100}$	0.5–2	$\frac{25}{250}$	2.2^M $(1-3)^R$	1.5 (1–3)	2.0 (0.5–2.0)	D-1 Cyclase linked	$\frac{100}{1000}$
Benserazide + levodopa			$\frac{50}{200}$	3.4 (1–5)	1.1 (0.5–2.0)	1.5 (0.5–1.0)	D-1 Cyclase linked	$\frac{200}{800}$
Bromocriptine	5	2–6	5.0	2.3	1.2 (0.5–1.5)	6.0*	D-2 Non-cyclase linked	45 (15–100)
Lergotrile	5	2–6					D-2 Non-cyclase linked	50 (20–100)
Lisuride	0.5	2–6	0.3	0.25	1.0	2.0*	D-2 Non-cyclase linked	2.5 (1–5)
Pergolide	0.5	12–24	0.14	0.18	2.0 (1.0–3.0)	24.0 (15–42)*	D-1 Cyclase linked	2.5 (1–5)

All values are mean values; ranges are in parentheses.
*$T_{1/2}$ for bromocriptine, lisuride and pergolide refers to total radioactivity which includes that of the parent drug and of its metabolites.

high concentrations. Thus, in low doses, bromocriptine stimulates the presynaptic (auto) receptors and, through feedback inhibition, decreases dopamine synthesis. This has been the basis for using bromocriptine to treat patients with Huntington's disease, a condition characterized by a relative excess of dopaminergic activity[58]. At high doses, bromocriptine stimulates the postsynaptic striatal receptors. This, of course, is the basis for its use in Parkinson's disease. These studies have also shown that the various agonists have different affinities for both the agonist and the antagonist binding sites on the postsynaptic striatal membranes. Thus, pergolide, unlike bromocriptine or lergotrile, has a higher affinity for dopamine agonist binding sites than for dopamine antagonist binding sites[28]. Moreover, guanine nucleotides which reduce the binding affinity of dopamine agonists, but not antagonists, inhibit the binding of pergolide but not that of the other ergots; and thermal exposure of striatal membranes results in differential destruction of dopamine agonist but not antagonist binding sites, and reduces the binding of pergolide but not bromocriptine or lergotrile. Lastly, it has been shown that the ergots act on different dopamine receptors. Thus, pergolide may be referred to as a 'cyclase linked' drug because, like dopamine, it predominantly stimulates the adenylate cyclase linked receptors[28], whereas lisuride, bromocriptine and lergotrile may be referred to as 'non-cyclase linked' drugs because they predominantly stimulate the non-adenylate cyclase linked receptors[74,76].

CLINICAL STUDIES OF DOPAMINE AGONISTS

Non-ergolines

Apomorphine was the first agonist to be used in man. Apomorphine administered intravenously improved many parkinsonian symptoms, including some which were no longer satisfactorily responding to levodopa[15]. However, the benefits were short-lived and the method of administration was impractical for use in a chronic condition. Apomorphine administered orally also had an anti-parkinsonian effect but resulted in azotemia that could only be reversed by discontinuing the drug[12]. Apomorphine was abandoned as a treatment for Parkinson's disease and a congener, *N-propyl-noraporphine*, was tested[12,65]. Cotzias et al.[12] showed that N-propyl-noraporphine in slowly increasing doses induced significant improvement in 24 patients with Parkinson's disease who had previously been treated with levodopa. Dyskinesias and 'on–off' phenomena, which were present with levodopa, were not abolished by N-propyl-noraporphine. The major limitation of N-propyl-noraporphine, like that of apomorphine, was azotemia. This could not be circumvented without reducing the drug's anti-parkinsonian effect. Tachyphylaxsis to the anti-parkinsonian effect of N-propyl-noraporphine developed within 3 weeks and studies with the drug were abandoned.
    The next agonist to be studied was *piribidel* (Trivastal, ET 495). This drug was found to be effective in relieving tremor in monkeys, and was subsequently tested in man[24]. The anti-parkinsonian efficacy of piribidel in man was less than that of

levodopa, while adverse reactions, dyskinesias and mental changes were as prominent as with levodopa. The discrepancy between the relatively good anti-parkinsonian activity of piribidel when administered parenterally to the monkey and the more modest anti-parkinsonian activity when administered orally to man has been related to the higher doses of piribidel that could be given parenterally. Some of the studies with piribidel are summarized below.

Chase et al.[10] conducted a single-blind crossover trial of piribidel in 16 patients with Parkinson's disease. At maximum dose levels, overall improvement in parkinsonian signs averaged 30 percent. Anti-parkinsonian efficacy was judged to be approximately half that of levodopa. Adverse effects included mental changes and dyskinesia. Vakil et al.[82], although unable to demonstrate a significant improvement in any individual clinical feature of Parkinson's disease, obtained the impression that tremor responded best. The improvement in tremor was especially prominent in a few patients. Similar results were noted by Sweet et al.[77] in 20 patients. The authors found piribidel effective in relieving tremor in three of eight patients[57]. Dyskinesias occurred in three other patients none of whom experienced relief of tremor. Mental changes occurred in two patients.

Another agonist, an isoquinoline derivative, *R084650*, was studied in 37 patients with persistent symptoms despite levodopa treatment; it was found to be only slightly more effective than a placebo[3,69].

Ergolines

The most effective dopamine agonists are the ergot alkaloids. The first ergot compound to be used successfully was *bromocriptine*, an ergoline polypeptide, derived from plant alkaloids. Bromocriptine was shown to inhibit prolactin secretion by interfering with hypophyseal dopaminergic neurons[11], and because such drugs are usually also striatal dopamine agonists, bromocriptine was successfully tested first in the animal models and then in man[6]. Bromocriptine is particularly useful in many patients who cannot tolerate levodopa or whose response to levodopa has diminished, and for a time, it was the only consistently effective drug for these patients. However, at the doses necessary to achieve an anti-parkinsonian effect adverse reactions, predominantly mental changes, frequently developed. Other, less commonly encountered reactions were orthostatic hypotension, erythromelalgia and fluid retention. Although bromocriptine by itself induces less dyskinesias than levodopa, the combination of bromocriptine and levodopa sometimes results in severer dyskinesias than either drug alone. Bromocriptine's half-life (6–8 h) is considerably longer than that of levodopa (2–4 h), and it was thought that it would be particularly effective in patients with oscillations in performance. Although most investigators found this to be so, some did not. Bromocriptine is also effective in newly diagnosed patients who have never been treated with levodopa. Although these patients did not develop 'on–off' phenomena or dyskinesias, drug trials were abandoned because bromocriptine in the doses necessary to achieve an anti-parkinsonian effect comparable to that of levodopa is more expensive than levodopa. While tolerance to the anti-parkinsonian effects of bromocriptine developed, this did not occur in some patients for at least 2 years. Such 'longevity' compares favorably with the anticholinergic drugs and levodopa. Several papers on bromocriptine are summarized below.

Calne et al.[7] reported 92 patients who had been treated with bromocriptine for up to 30 months of whom 48 (52 percent) continue to benefit. In those treated originally with levodopa, addition of bromocriptine allowed a mean 41 percent reduction in the dose of levodopa. The largest group of patients to benefit from bromocriptine entered the study because of excessive dyskinesias or 'on–off' phenomena induced by levodopa. In 40 patients (43 percent) bromocriptine was stopped because of adverse reactions, absence of therapeutic response or non-compliance with the protocol. The main problems were psychiatric disturbances (eight patients) and erythromelalgia (seven patients). These adverse effects occurred on high dosages (66–150 mg). The authors administered bromocriptine to 106 patients with advanced Parkinson's disease and increasing disability despite optimal treatment with levodopa[55], including 51 patients with the 'on–off' effect. Upon addition of bromocriptine to levodopa, 55 patients (52 percent) had at least a one-stage decrease in disease severity (51 patients had 'on–off' effect). Of these 55 patients, (24 percent) experienced a decrease in disease severity in their 'on' period, and 19 in both 'on' and 'off' periods. Mean dose of bromocriptine was 51 mg, permitting a 26 percent reduction in the dose of levodopa. Bromocriptine was discontinued in 54 of 106 patients (51 percent) because of adverse effects including mental changes (29 patients) and increased involuntary movements (11 patients). All adverse effects were reversible. Fahn et al.[20] treated 53 patients with bromocriptine. These patients had either intractable symptoms despite optimum levodopa therapy or adverse effects from levodopa, limiting its usefulness. All were initially maintained on optimal levodopa therapy. Nineteen patients (36 percent) had sustained improvement on doses of bromocriptine that ranged from 5 to 90 mg. Improvement occurred in all categories of clinical problems, including some patients who has lost benefit from levodopa therapy. A high incidence of adverse effects (70 percent) limited the drug's usefulness. Parkes et al.[66] treated 37 patients with bromocriptine at dosages of 2.5–300 mg daily. Bromocriptine alone or combined with levodopa caused a reduction in disability of up to 30 percent in 11 patients who were treated for one year. Tolerance did not develop during this period. Bromocriptine was of no value in six patients who had previously not responded or had lost their response to levodopa. It resulted in improvement in oscillations in performance in four of five patients. Bromocriptine was felt to be less potent than levodopa and to cause more hallucinations and less emesis.

Rascol et al.[71] used bromocriptine 15–75 mg alone or with levodopa for 5 to 29 months in 44 patients. Used as a sole therapeutic agent it was found excellent in 12 patients who had not received levodopa. Anti-parkinsonian activity was judged to be comparable to that achieved with levodopa. Oscillations in performance did not occur with bromocriptine alone. Among patients whose response to levodopa had decreased, bromocriptine produced a further improvement (if mental changes did not occur). In patients with dementia, bromocriptine was not useful. Bromocriptine did not improve the 'on–off' effects but reduced some of the side-effects of levodopa, particularly dyskinesia. Lees et al.[43] administered bromocriptine to 86 patients. Eight of 30 patients with mild disease, who had never been treated with levodopa, were treated with bromocriptine and showed sustained benefit for 2 years, without 'on–off' effects or dyskinesias. Thirty-three patients with residual disabilities despite maximum tolerated doses of levodopa were also given bromocriptine. Although benefit accrued in some, treatment was abandoned because of unacceptable side-effects in many, and there was no improvement in the 11 with severe 'on–off' disability, Only two of 23 patients unable to tolerate or respond to levodopa responded to bromocriptine. Although it was found that benefit from 70 mg of bromocriptine was comparable to that from 750 mg of levodopa with carbidopa, bromocriptine was thought to offer no advantage to the majority of patients receiving levodopa. Godwin-Austin and Smith[22] compared the effects of bromocriptine with levodopa in 18 patients with Parkinson's disease. Although there were wide individual differences in response to the two drugs, there was no significant difference between therapeutic effects. Bromocriptine was comparable to levodopa in some patients. Side-effects were more common with bromocriptine but were similar to those caused by levodopa. Kartzinel and Calne[39] studied nine patients with 'on–off' phenomena on levodopa. Although oscillation in performance still occurred when levodopa was replaced with bromocriptine, they were significantly reduced in frequency. The authors also studied the long-term efficacy of bromocriptine in 28 patients with Parkinson's disease, all of whom were treated for at least 2 years (mean 2.8 years, range 2–5 years)[54]. All of the patients had first been treated with levodopa alone or combined with carbidopa. Bromocriptine 56 mg, when added to levodopa, resulted in at least a one-stage improvement in 21 of the 28 patients (75 percent). After 2 years, however, only 5 of the 21 patients (24 percent) maintained this degree of improvement.

The next agonist to be studied was *lergotrile*, a semisynthetic ergoline that was effective in 11 of 20 patients who were showing signs of disease progression on levodopa[47]. Among these patients there was a significant reduction in rigidity, tremor, bradykinesia, gait disturbance and total score when lergotrile was added to levodopa. Mean daily dose of lergotrile was 52 mg; the dose of levodopa was reduced by 15 percent. Dyskinesias were less prominent with the combination of levodopa and lergotrile than with levodopa alone, while mental changes and orthostasis were more prominent. Elevations in serum transaminase levels were noted in three patients. Lergotrile was subsequently administered to 53 patients with advanced Parkinson's disease who had increasing disability despite optimal treatment with levodopa/carbidopa[52]. Thirty-nine patients (74 percent) demonstrated significantly decreased rigidity, tremor, bradykinesia, gait disturbance and total score without increased dyskinesia. Twenty-one of the 53 patients (40 percent) improved by at least one-stage. Twenty-three patients had had 'on–off' phenomena, and in 13 of these oscillations decreased. The mean daily dose of lergotrile was 49 mg, permitting a 10 percent reduction in the dose of levodopa. Lergotrile was discontinued in 33 of 53 patients (62 percent) because of adverse effects, including hepatotoxicity (11 patients), mental changes (12 patients) and orthostatic hypotension (8 patients). In a third study, Klawans et al.[40] administered lergotrile to 25 patients with Parkinson's disease. Of six patients not receiving levodopa, five showed definite improvement in parkinsonian symptoms. Lergotrile was more effective in relieving 'on-off' problems than in reversing loss of levodopa efficacy. In a fourth study, increased serum activities of serum glutamate-oxalacetate transaminase (SGOT) and serum glutamate-pyruvate transaminase (SGPT) occurred in 12 of 19 patients with Parkinson's disease when they were treated with lergotrile (50–150 mg)[78]. Hepatocellular injury was confirmed by microscopic examination of liver biopsies obtained from three of these patients. Light microscopy revealed features of mild acute hepatocellular injury, and electronmicroscopy showed proliferation of the smooth endoplastic reticulum and apparently unique mitocondrial changes in hepatocytes. Although lergotrile had a definite antiparkinsonian effect, the incidence of adverse effects, particularly hepatotoxicity, doomed it.

Bromocriptine and lergotrile were compared in two studies. In a study by the authors, bromocriptine and lergotrile were administered at different times to 81 patients with advanced Parkinson's disease and increasing disability despite optimal treatment with levodopa[53]. Sixty-six patients were treated with bromocriptine and 53 patients with lergotrile. Thirty-eight patients were, at different times, treated with both drugs. Both groups had decreased rigidity, tremor, bradykinesia, gait disturbance, total score and stage upon addition of bromocriptine or lergotrile to levodopa. Twenty-five patients (39 percent) improved by at least one-stage on bromocriptine and 21 (40 percent) improved by at least one-stage on lergotrile. Nineteen of 27 patients with 'on-off' effects improved on bromocriptine, while 13 of 21 patients with 'on-off' effects improved on lergotrile. The number of hours 'on' increased by 85 percent, from 6 to 11, on bromocriptine or lergotrile. The mean dose of bromocriptine was 47 mg, and the mean dose of lergotrile 49 mg. Bromocriptine was discontinued in 29 of 66 patients (44 percent) because of adverse effects and lergotrile was discontinued in 33 of 53 patients (62 percent) because of adverse effects. While the results of treament with bromocriptine or lergotrile were comparable, there were differences among individual patients, with some improving more on bromocriptine and others more on lergotrile. Bromocriptine and lergotrile were also compared by Teychenne et al.[79]. Both drugs were combined with levodopa. There was a similar, but not identical profile of response. Initially, lergotrile tended to induce more orthostasis while bromocriptine caused more dyskinesia. Neurological deficits improved with increasing dosages of each drug up to 150 mg. However, efficacy often declined, and adverse effects were more common with dosages greater than 100 mg/day. In general, the best overall therapeutic results with bromocriptine and lergotrile were obtained in the dose range of 50–100 mg daily for each. It was concluded that bromocriptine and lergotrile were similar in their therapeutic properties and that they are comparable in efficacy to levodopa.

Since bromocriptine and lergotrile are dopamine agonists, the question arises why, if progressive loss of nigrostriatal neurons is responsible for the increasing Parkinson's disease, responses are not obtained in all patients able to tolerate the drugs? One explanation is that in such patients there are changes in the striatum which make them incapable of responding to an agonist[72,73] (*see* Chapter 5). Another explanation is that bromocriptine and lergotrile are mixed agonists and antagonists[27]. At the presynaptic (auto) receptor both drugs behave like agonists, inhibiting synaptosomal tyrosine hydroxylase, and also like antagonists, reversing the apomorphine-induced inhibition of synaptosomal tryosine hydroxylase. At the postsynaptic receptor both drugs behave like agonists, displacing bound ^{3}H-dopamine from striatal membranes, and also like antagonists, displacing bound ^{3}H-haloperidol from striatal membranes. The finding of mixed agonist–antagonist properties at both pre- and postsynaptic receptors suggested that more effective agonists may achieve better therapeutic responses.

A third ergot alkaloid, *CF 257397*, which was effective in the animal models of Parkinson's disease, was subsequently investigated in man[80]. However, during treatment, severe clinical deterioration characterized by worsening rigidity, bradykinesia, dysphagia and dysphonia developed in some patients and the drug was stopped. It was suggested that (in man) CF 257397 might undergo conversion to an antagonist metabolite that in turn might result in worsening Parkinson's disease. It is possible that this metabolite is present only in man, which would explain the discrepancy between the animal and human studies.

Pergolide is a new semisynthetic ergot alkaloid that is more potent and longer acting than the previously tested ergots in the animal models of Parkinson's disease[45,46]. Pergolide, on a milligram per milligram basis, is 10 times more potent and four times longer acting than bromocriptine or lergotrile in relieving parkinsonian symptoms in the experimental models. The greater potency and duration of activity or pergolide, a congener of lergotrile, is attributed to increased length of the alkyl side chain at the N6 position of the ergoline molecule.

In the first clinical study in Parkinson's disease, pergolide was investigated in 13 patients with advanced disease and oscillations in performance[49]. In all nine patients who completed the trial, pergolide alone (two patients) or combined with levodopa (seven patients) had a marked anti-parkinsonian effect. There was a reduction in rigidity, bradykinesia, gait disorder and in total disability score. Pergolide had a marked effect in all of the patients with 'on–off' phenomena resulting in an increase in the duration of the time patients were 'on'. The number of hours the patients were 'on' increased by 200 percent, from 3.8 to 11.4. In three patients oscillations disappeared completely. The mean daily dose of pergolide was 2.4 mg.

Pergolide was subsequently investigated in a total of 40 patients. For the group as a whole, there was a decrease in disability in both the 'on' and the 'off' period. Among individual patients, 26 improved by at least one stage in their 'on' period (65 percent), and 14 (35 percent) improved by at least one stage in their 'off' period. The 31 patients with 'on–off' phenomena showed an improvement in the number of hours in which they were 'on' and mobile. In nine patients 'on–off' phenomena disappeared completely. Improvement with pergolide began within the first week of treatment on as little as 0.4 mg/day. The mean daily dose was 2.4 mg (range 0.1–10.0 mg). The mean duration of treatment was 6 months, with a range of 2 to 20 months. In some patients the effects of pergolide and levodopa were thought to be synergistic.

Pergolide was discontinued in three patients because of ventricular ectopy. This requires additional comment. Because of the occurrence of asymptomatic ventricular ectopy in 2 of 20 normal individuals in a preliminary dose-ranging study in which the subjects underwent continuous Holter monitoring[45], all 13 participants in the first clinical trial also underwent continuous Holter monitoring for 1–5 days before starting the drug (as a baseline) and during the entire dose-ranging portion of the study (mean duration 6 weeks, range 2–10 weeks)[49]. Seven of the patients developed, on one occasion during the 2 to 10 weeks of monitoring, an asymptomatic ventricular arrhythmia. This consisted of a couplet (four patients), a salvo (two patients) and multifocal premature ventricular contractions (PVCs) (one patient). These rhythms were unassociated with an increase in PVCs. An eighth patient in the second study developed an increase in PVCs. Because of a lack of experience with the drug, pergolide was discontinued in three patients with heart disease who developed the ectopic rhythms at below 1 mg. Pergolide was continued in the others, including three patients with heart disease who developed the ectopic rhythms above 1 mg. Twenty months later, these patients are asymptomatic with unremarkable repeat Holter monitoring. The significance of these ectopic rhythms is not clear because the Holter tapes obtained during the treatment period of 2 to 10 weeks covered a longer period and sampled more heart beats than the pretreatment tapes (1–5 days). Moreover, in addition to pergolide, all but one of the patients who developed ectopic rhythms also received levodopa. Eight patients experienced orthostatic hypotension (two with syncope) immediately upon the addition of pergolide 0.1 mg to levodopa. All eight patients had experienced similar changes on levodopa alone. The orthostasis could be eliminated by reducing or eliminating levodopa. Only two of the eight patients could not eventually be continued on pergolide. Two patients were excluded from the study because of mental changes and one patient because of an increase in choreoathetosis. Although choreoathetosis was less on treatment with pergolide alone than on levodopa alone, on combined treatment choreoathetosis increased. Two patients developed increased SGOT and SGPT activities without clinical symptoms within 1 to 3 months of starting pergolide. The drug was discontinued in both patients, who also had a prior history of hepatotoxicity on other drugs. None of the seven patients in the study who had previously experienced hepatotoxicity on lergotrile experienced it on pergolide.

Pergolide and bromocriptine were compared in 25 patients who had been once treated with both drugs. Twenty-four of the patients had 'on–off' phenomena. At the time bromocriptine was added to levodopa the mean age of the patients was 62 years, duration of disease was 9 years and duration of levodopa treatment 6 years. During treatment with bromocriptine, the disability score as measured in the 'on' period decreased by 34 percent, from 29 to 19, and 11 patients (44 percent) improved by at least one stage. Disability as measured in the 'off' period decreased by 26 percent, from 66 to 44. The number of hours in which patients were 'on' increased by 62 percent, from 7 to 11.5. All of these changes were significant. Bromocriptine had to be discontinued in nine patients (36 percent) because of adverse reactions (eight because of mental changes). In the remaining 16 patients, bromocriptine was eventually discontinued because of diminished efficacy. Mean dose of bromocriptine was 60 mg (range 10–100 mg), duration of treatment was 23 months (range 2–65 months). At the time of treatment with pergolide, the patients were older (65 years), had had the disease longer (12.7 years), and were more disabled. Nonetheless, for the group as a whole, the disability score as measured in the 'on' period decreased by 40 percent, from 44 to 26, and 14 patients (56 percent) improved by at least one stage. Disability as measured in the 'off' period decreased by 25 percent, from 69 to 53. The number of hours in which the patients were 'on' increased by 224 percent, from 3.4 to 11 hours. All of these changes were significant. The mean dose of pergolide was 2.1 mg (range 0.1–10.0 mg). Although the authors' study did not compare bromocriptine and pergolide directly, they consider pergolide to be more potent because of its effect at a more advanced stage of the disease.

Another new semisynthetic ergot alkaloid that is effective in experimental models of Parkinson's disease is *lisuride* hydrogen maleate[33, 34, 35, 36]. Lisuride is 10 to 20 times more potent on a milligram per milligram basis than bromocriptine or lergotrile. Its duration of activity is shorter than that of bromocriptine. Its effects are independent of presynaptic dopamine synthesis or stores. Lisuride is also a central serotonin agonist. Lisuride was evaluated in 10 patients with moderately advanced Parkinson's disease whose response to levodopa had diminished[50]. In the group of 10 patients there was a reduction in disability when levodopa was replaced with lisuride. The mean dose of lisuride was 3.6 mg/day. Among the ten patients, four were better on lisuride than on levodopa. A decline in efficacy was noted in all patients on lisuride alone after a mean of 3.9 months.

Lisuride was combined with levodopa in 20 patients with more advanced Parkinson's disease, 14 of whom had 'on–off' phenomena[51]. For the group of 20 patients as a whole, there was a noticeable decrease in disability as measured in both the 'on' and the 'off' periods. Seventeen patients (85 percent) improved by at least one stage. Lisuride combined with levodopa resulted in a more than twofold increase (108 percent) in the time in which patients were 'on', from 4.6 to 9.6 hours. In some patients the effects of lisuride and levodopa appeared to be synergistic. Similar results have been obtained by others[29].

Adverse effects necessitating dicontinuation of lisuride in the entire group of 30 patients included toxic psychoses in nine patients, an increase in choroeoathetosis in two patients and digital vasospasm in one patient (this patient had also experienced similar changes on bromocriptine and lergotrile). All of the adverse effects were reversible within a few days of discontinuing lisuride. Two other patients experienced orthostatic hypotension shortly after starting lisuride, but this did not require discontinuing the drug. Four patients experienced fluid retention with weight gains of between 5 and 15 pounds. Two of these patients, both with heart disease, developed mild congestive failure. All patients responded to diuretics and in all lisuride was continued.

Lisuride and bromocriptine were compared in 18 patients who had once been treated with both drugs. Fourteen of the patients had 'on–off' phenomena. At the time of treatment with bromocriptine, the patients were on average 3 years younger and had less advanced disease. On bromocriptine, disability as measured in the 'on' period decreased by 31 percent, from 32 to 22, and nine patients (50 percent) improved by at least one stage. Disability as measured in the 'off' period decreased by 24 percent, from 63 to 48, and two patients experienced at least a one stage improvement. The mean number of hours in which they were 'on' increased by 76 percent, from 6.8 to 12 hours. All of these changes were significant. Mean dose of bromocriptine was 55 mg. On lisuride, disability as measured in the 'on' period decreased by 28 percent, from 46 to 33, and nine patients (50 percent) improved by at least one stage. Disability as measured in the 'off' period decreased by 13 percent, from 72 to 63, and three patients improved by at least one stage. The number of hours 'on' increased by 127 percent, from 4.4 to 10.0 hours. All of these changes were significant. Mean dose of lisuride was 2.5 mg. It is concluded that lisuride is more potent than bromocriptine because of its effect at a more advanced stage of the disease.

In 17 patients who were treated with both drugs, *pergolide and lisuride* were compared. All 17 patients had 'on–off' phenomena. Ages of the patients and disease severity were comparable in the two groups at the time of treatment with each drug. On pergolide, disability as measured in the 'on' period decreased by 41 percent, from 48 to 28, and ten patients (59 percent) improved by at least one stage. Disability as measured in the 'off' period decreased by 17 percent, from 71 to 59, and five patients (29 percent) improved by at least one stage in the 'off' period. The number of hours 'on' increased by 200 percent, from 3.7 to 11.2. All of these changes were significant. Mean dose of pergolide was 2.2 mg. On lisuride, disability as measured in the 'on' period decreased by 29 percent, from 48 to 34, and seven patients (41 percent) improved by at least one stage. Disability as measured in the 'off' period decreased by 17 percent, from 71 to 59, and two patients (12 percent) improved by at least one stage in the 'off' period. The number of hours 'on' increased by 102 percent, from 4.1 to 8.3 hours. All of these changes were significant. The mean dose of lisuride was 2.8 mg. Decreases in disability in both 'on' and 'off' periods were comparable for pergolide and lisuride. There was a greater improvement in the number of hours in which patients were 'on' with pergolide.

Adverse effects of pergolide (mental changes, orthostasis) were comparable to those of levodopa and differed from those of lisuride, bromocriptine and lergotrile; the latter three drugs produced mental changes in more patients. The cardiac effects of these drugs cannot be compared because only with pergolide was there such a long period of Holter monitoring.

CONCLUSIONS

The differential anti-parkinsonian effects of these drugs and the differential spectrum of adverse reactions may reflect the differences in the ability of these drugs to stimulate the different dopamine receptors. Pergolide and dopamine predominantly stimulate the adenylate cyclase linked receptors ('cyclase linked' drugs), whereas lisuride, bromocriptine and lergotrile predominantly stimulate the non-adenylate cyclase linked receptors ('non-cyclase linked' drugs). The similarity of adverse mental changes arising from treatment with lisuride, bromocriptine and lisuride implies that stimulation of the non-adenylate cyclase linked receptors (which are on the axons of a descending corticostriatal tract) may be more involved in these reactions than stimulations of the cyclase linked receptors (which are on striatal interneurons).

The availability of drugs which preferentially activate one or another class of dopaminergic receptors opens up several new therapeutic strategies. One strategy would be to withhold levodopa from newly diagnosed parkinsonian patients on the assumption that the diminished respose to levodopa, which ensues with treatment, is more a consequence of treatment than of disease progression. This strategy has until now been feasible only in minimally disabled patients because it has not been possible to withhold levodopa from the more disabled patients. The introduction of drugs such as bromocriptine, pergolide and lisuride may make it possible to withhold levodopa from all newly diagnosed patients with Parkinson's disease and treat them with one of these agonists. When the response to one agonist decreases, the patient could be changed to another, or another could be added. Once the response to the second or third agonist diminishes, the patient could be treated with levodopa. A second strategy would be to discontinue levodopa in patients whose response to it is just beginning to decrease and treat them with bromocriptine, pergolide or lisuride. When these patients begin to show a decreased reponse to one agonist they could be changed to another. Once they begin to show a decreased response to the second or third agonist, they could, after having had a protracted 'levodopa holiday', be treated with levodopa again. A third strategy would consist of treating either newly diagnosed patients or those whose response to levodopa is beginning to decrease with a combination of an agonist and levodopa. The agonist and levodopa, when combined, could be given in lower doses than if they were administered alone. Treatment with a lower dose of each drug might delay the development of tachyphylaxsis to both drugs. Finally, combining a long-acting with a short-acting and/or a 'cyclase linked' drug with a 'non-cyclase linked' drug might result in synergistic effects. Such synergistic effects have already been noted when levodopa (a short-acting 'cyclase linked' drug) is combined with pergolide (a long-acting 'cyclase linked' drug), or when levodopa (a short-acting 'cyclase linked') is combined with lisuride (a short-acting 'non-cyclase linked' drug). Even more effective combinations might consist of combining pergolide (long-acting 'cyclase linked') with lisuride (short-acting 'non-cyclase linked'); pergolide with bromocriptine or lisuride with bromocriptine.

References

1 AGID, Y., JAVOY, F. and GLOWINSKI, J. Hyperactivity of remaining neurones after partial destruction of the nigro-striatal dopaminergic system in the rat. *Nature (London)*, **245**, 150–151 (1973)

2 AGID, Y., JAVOY, F. and GLOWINSKI, J. Chemical or electrolytic lesions of the substantia nigra: early effects on neostriatal dopamine metabolism. *Brain Research*, **74**, 41–49 (1974)

3 BIRKET-SMITH, E., BOTTCHER, J. and DUPONT, E. Dopaminergic agonist RO 8-4650 in Parkinson's disease. 1. Patients treated with dopa. *Acta Neurologica Scandinavia*, **58**, 74–76 (1978)

4 BIRKMAYER, W., RIEDERER, P., YOUDIM, M. B. H. Potentiation of antikinetic effect after L-dopa treatment by an inhibitor of MAO-B, deprenil. *Journal of Neural Transmissions*, **36**, 303–326 (1975)

5 CALNE, D. B., REID, J. L. and VAKIL, S. D. Parkinsonism treated with 3-0-methyldopa. *Clinical Pharmacology and Therapeutics*, **14**, 386–389 (1973)

6 CALNE, D. B., TEYCHENNE, P. F., CLAVERIA, L. E. Bromocriptine in parkinsonism. *British Medical Journal*, **4**, 442–444 (1974)

7 CALNE, D. B., WILLIAMS, A. C. and NEOPHYTIDES, A. Long-term treatment of parkinsonism with bromocriptine. *Lancet*, **i**, 735–738 (1978)

8 CHASE, T. N. Fusaric acid in Parkinson's disease. *Neurology*, **24**, 637–639 (1974)

9 CHASE, T. N., Ng, L. K. Y. and WATANABE, A. M. Parkinson's disease modification by 5-hydroxytryptophan. *Neurology (Minneapolis)*, **22**, 479–484 (1972)

10 CHASE, T. N., WOODS, A. C. and GLAUBIGER, G. A. Parkinson's disease treated with a suspected dopamine receptor agonist. *Archives of Neurology (Chicago)*, **30**, 383–386 (1974)

11 CORRODI, H., FUXE, K. and HOKFELT, T. Effect of ergot drugs on central catecholamine neurons: evidence for a stimulation of central dopamine neurons. *Journal of Pharmacy and Pharmacology*, **25**, 409–411 (1973)

12 COTZIAS, G. C., PAPAVASILIOU, P. S. and TOLOSA, E. S. Treatment of Parkinson's disease with aporphines: possible role of growth hormone. *New England Journal of Medicine*, **294**, 567–572 (1976)

13 DAVIDSON, L., LLOYD, K. and DANKOVA, J. L-Dopa treatment in Parkinson's disease: effect on dopamine and related substances in discrete brain regions. *Experientia (Basel)*, **27**, 1048–1049 (1971)

14 DEN HARTOG JAGER, W. A. and BETHLEM, J. The distribution of lewly bodies in the central and autonomic nervous system in idiopathic paralysis agitans. *Journal of Neurology, Neurosurgery and Psychiatry*, **23**, 283–289 (1960)

15 DUBY, S. E., COTZIAS, G. C. and PAPAVASILIOU, P. S. Injected apomorphine and orally administered levodopa in parkinsonism. *Archives of Neurology (Chicago)*, **27**, 474–480 (1972)

16 EADIE, M. J. The pathology of certain medullary nuclei in parkinsonism. *Brain*, **86**, 781–792 (1963)

17 EISLER, T., TERAVAINEN, H., NELSON, R. Deprenyl in Parkinson disease. *Neurology*, **31**, 19–23 (1981)

18 ERICSSON, A. D. Potentiation of the L-dopa: effect in man by the use of catechol-O-methyltransferase inhibitors. *Journal of the Neurological Sciences*, **14**, 193–197 (1971)

19 FAHN, S. 'On–off' phenomenon with levodopa therapy in parkinsonism. *Neurology (Minneapolis)*, **24**, 431–441 (1974)

20 FAHN, S., COTE, L. J. and SNIDER, S. The role of bromocriptine in the treatment of parkinsonism. *Neurology (Minneapolis)*, **29**, 1077–1083 (1979)

21 FELTZ, P. and de CHAMPLAIN, J. Enhanced sensitivity of caudate neurons to microiontopheretic injections of dopamine in 6-hydroxydopamine treated cats. *Brain Research*, **43**, 601–605 (1972)

22 GODWIN-AUSTIN, R. B. and SMITH, N. J. Comparison of the effects of bromocriptine and levodopa in Parkinson's disease. *Journal of Neurology, Neurosurgery and Psychiatry*, **40**, 479–482 (1977)

23 GODWIN-AUSTIN, R. B., TWOMEY, J. A., HANKS, G. Oxpentifylline in Parkinson's disease. *Journal of Neurology, Neurosurgery and Psychiatry*, **43**, 360–364 (1980)
24 GOLDSTEIN, M., BATTISTA, A. F., OHMOTO, T. *et al.* Tremor and involuntary movements in monkeys: effect of L-dopa and of a dopamine receptor stimulating agent. *Science*, **179**, 816–817 (1973)
25 GOLDSTEIN, M., LEW, J. Y. and ENGEL, J. The dopaminephilic properties of ergoline derivatives. In *Dopaminergic Ergot Derivatives and Motor Function*, edited by K. Fux and D. B. Calne, 253–260. Oxford, Pergamon Press (1979)
26 GOLDSTEIN, M., LEW, J. Y. and SAUTER, A. The affinities of ergot compounds for dopamine agonist and dopamine antagonist receptor sites. In *Ergot Compounds and Brain Function: Neuroendocrine and Neuropsychiatric Aspects,* edited by D. Calne, M. Goldstein, A. Lieberman, M. Thorner, 75–82, New York, Raven Press (1980)
27 GOLDSTEIN, M., LEW, J. Y., NAKAMURA, S. Dopaminephilic properties of ergot alkaloids. *Federation Proceedings*, **37**, 2202–2205 (1978)
28 GOLDSTEIN, M., LIEBERMAN, A. N., LEW, J. Y. The interactions of pergolide with central dopaminergic receptors. *Proceedings of the National Academy of Sciences*, **77**, 3725–3728 (1980)
29 GOPINATHAN, G., TERAVAINEN, H., DAMBROSIA, J. Studies on Parkinson disease II: evaluation of lisuride as a therapeutic agent (abstract). *Neurology*, **30**, 366 (1980)
30 HAKIM, A. and MATHIESON, G. Dementia in Parkinson's disease: a neuropathologic study. *Neurology (Minneapolis)*, **29**, 1209–1214 (1979)
31 HEFTI, F., MELAMED, E., and WURTMAN, R. J. Partial lesions of the dopaminergic nigrostriatal system in rat brain: biochemical characterization. *Brain Research*, **195**, 123–137 (1980)
32 HORNYKIEWICZ, O. The mechanisms of action of L-dopa in Parkinson's disease. *Life Science*, **15**, 1249–1259 (1974)
33 HOROWSKI, R. Differences in the dopaminergic effects of the ergot derivatives bromocriptine, lisuride and LSD as compared with apomorphine. *European Journal of Pharmacology*, **51**, 157–166 (1978)
34 HOROWSKI, R. Hypothermic action of lisuride in rats and differences to bromocriptine in the antagonistic effect of neuroleptics. *Naunyn-Schmiedeberg's Archiv für Experimentelle Pathologie and Pharmakologie*, **306**, 147–151 (1979)
35 HOROWSKI, R. and WACHTEL, H. Direct dopaminergic action of lisuride hydrogen maleate, an ergot derivative, in mice. *European Journal of Pharmacology*, **36**, 373–383 (1976)
36 HOROWSKI, R. and WACHTEL, H. Pharmacologic effects of lisuride in rodents mediated by dopaminergic receptor: mechanism of action and influence of chronic treatment with lisuride. In *Ergot Compounds and Brain Function: Neuroendocrine and Neuropsychiatric Aspects*, edited by D. Calne, M. Goldstein, A. Lieberman and M. Thorner, 237–252. New York, Raven Press (1980)
37 HUNTER, K. R., SHAW, K.M. and LAWRENCE, D. R. Sustained levodopa therapy in parkinsonism. *Lancet*, **2**, 929–931 (1973)
38 JOHNSON, A. M., LOEW, D. M. and VIGOURET, J. M. Stimulant properties of bromocriptine on central dopamine receptors in comparison to apomorphine, amphetamine and L-dopa. *British Journal of Pharmacology*, **56**, 59–68 (1976)

39 KARTZINEL, R. and CALNE, D. B. Studies with bromocriptine, part I. 'On-off' phenomena. *Neurology (Minneapolis)*, **26**, 508–510 (1976)
40 KLAWANS, H. L., GOETZ, C. G. and VOLKMAN, P. Lergotrile in the treatment of parkinsonism. *Neurology (Minneapolis)*, **28**, 699–702 (1978)
41 LANGRALL, H. M. and JOSEPH, C. Evaluation of safety and efficacy of levodopa in Parkinson's disease and syndrome. *Neurology (Minneapolis)*, **22**, 3–16 (1972)
42 LEE, T., SEEMAN, P. and RAJOUT, A. Receptor basis for dopaminergic supersensitivity in Parkinson's disease. *Nature (London)*, **273**, 59–61 (1978)
43 LEES, A. J., HADDAD, S. and SHAW, K. M. Bromocriptine in parkinsonism: a long-term study. *Archives of Neurology (Chicago)*, **35**, 503–505 (1978)
44 LEES, A. J., SHAW, K. M., and STERN, G. M. Baclofen in Parkinson's disease. *Journal of Neurology, Neurosurgery and Psychiatry*, **41**, 707–708 (1978)
45 LEMBERGER, L. and CRABTREE, R. E. Pharmacologic effects in man of a potent long-acting dopamine receptor agonist. *Science*, **205**, 1151–1153 (1979)
46 LEMBERGER, L., CRABTREE, R. E. and CALLAGHAN, J. T. Pergolide: clinical pharmacologic effects of a potent, long-acting dopamine receptor agonist. *Clinical Pharmacology and Therapeutics*, **27**, 642–651 (1980)
47 LIEBERMAN, A. N., ESTEY, E. and KUPERSMITH, M. Treatment of Parkinson's disease with lergotrile mesylate. *Journal of the American Medical Association*, **238**, 2380–2382 (1977)
48 LIEBERMAN, A. N., ESTEY, E. and GOPINATHAN, A. Comparative effectiveness of two extracerebral dopa decarboxylase inhibitors in Parkinson's disease. *Neurology (Minneapolis)*, **28**, 964–968 (1978)
49 LIEBERMAN, A. N., GOLDSTEIN, M., LEIBOWITZ, M. Treatment of advanced Parkinson's disease with pergolide. *Neurology*, **31**, 675–682 (1981)
50 LIEBERMAN, A. N., GOLDSTEIN, M., NEOPHYTIDES, A. Lisuride in Parkinson's disease: efficacy of lisuride compared to levodopa. *Neurology*, **31**, 961–965 (1981)
51 LIEBERMAN, A. N., GOLDSTEIN, M. and LEIBOWITZ, M. Lisuride combined with levodopa in advanced Parkinson's disease. *Neurology*, **31**, 1466–1469 (1981)
52 LIEBERMAN, A. N., GOPINATHAN, G. and ESTEY, E. Lergotrile in Parkinson's disease: further studies. *Neurology (Minneapolis)*, **29**, 267–272 (1979)
53 LIEBERMAN, A. N., KUPERSMITH, M. and CASSON, I. Bromocriptine and lergotrile: comparative efficacy in Parkinson's disease. *Advances in Neurology*, **24**, 461–473. New York, Raven Press (1979)
54 LIEBERMAN, A. N., KUPERSMITH, M. and NEOPHYTIDES, A. Long-term efficacy of bromocriptine in Parkinson's disease. *Neurology (Minneapolis)*, **30**, 518–523 (1980)
55 LIEBERMAN, A. N., KUPERSMITH, M. and NEOPHYTIDES, A. Bromocriptine in Parkinson's disease: report on 106 patients treated for up to 5 years. In *Ergot Compounds and Brain Function: Neuroendocrine and Neuropsychiatric Aspects*, edited by D. Calne, M. Goldstein, A. Lieberman and M. Thorner, 245–253. New York, Raven Press (1980)
56 LIEBERMAN, A. N., MIYAMOTO, T. and BATTISTA, A. Studies on the anti-parkinsonian efficacy of lergotrile. *Neurology*, **25**, 459–462 (1975)
57 LIEBERMAN, A. N., SHOPSIN, B. and LeBRUN, Y. Studies on piribidel in parkinsonism. *Advances in Neurology*, **9**, 399–407 (1975)

58 LOEB, C., ROCCATAGLIATA, G., ALBANO, C. Bromocriptine and dopaminergic function in Huntingdon disease. *Neurology*, **29**, 730–734 (1979)

59 LUDIN, H. P. and BASS-VERRY, F. Study of deterioration in long-term treatment of parkinsonism with L-dopa plus decarboxylase inhibitor. *Journal of Neural Transmission*, **38**, 249–258 (1976)

60 MARSDEN, C. D. and PARKES, J. C. Success and problems of long-term levodopa therapy in Parkinson's disease. *Lancet*, **i**, 345–349 (1977)

61 MELAMED, E., HEFTI, F. and WURTMAN, R. J. Nonaminergic striatal neurons convert exogenous L-dopa to dopamine in parkinsonism. *Animals of Neurology*, **8**, 558–563 (1980)

62 MELAMED, E., HEFTI, F. and WURTMAN, R. J. Diminished decarboxylation of L-dopa in rat striatum after intrastriatal injections of kainic acid. *Neuropharmacology*, **19**, 409–411 (1980)

63 MENA, J. and COTZIAS, G. C. Protein intake and treatment of Parkinson's disease with levodopa. *New England Journal of Medicine*, **292**, 181–184 (1975)

64 MENA, J., COURT, J. and FUENZALIDA, S. Modification of chronic manganese poisoning treatment with L-dopa or 5-OH tryptophan. *New England Journal of Medicine*, **282**, 5–10 (1970)

65 PAPAVASILIOU, P. S., COTZIAS, G. C. and ROSAL, V. L. F. Treatment of parkinsonism with N-n-propyl norapomorphine and levodopa (with or without carbidopa). *Archives of Neurology (Chicago)*, **35**, 787–791 (1978)

66 PARKES, J. D., MARSDEN, C. D. and DONALDSON, I. Bromocriptine treatment in Parkinson's disease. *Journal of Neurology, Neurosurgery and Psychiatry*, **39**, 184–193 (1976)

67 PARKES, J. D., SCHACHTER, M. and MARSDEN, C. D. Lisuride in parkinsonism. *Annals of Neurology*, **9**, 48–52 (1981)

68 POIRIER, L. J. and SOURKES, T. L. Influence of the substantia nigra on the catecholamine content of the striatum. *Brain*, **88**, 181–192 (1965)

69 PRESTHUS, J., ANHERHUS, J. and BUREN, A. Dopaminergic agonist Ro 8-4650 in Parkinson's disease 2. Patients not treated with dopa. *Acta Neurologica Scandinavia*, **58**, 77–79 (1978)

70 PRICE, P. A., PARKES, J. D. and MARSDEN, C. D. Sodium valproate in the treatment of levodopa-induced dyskinesia. *Journal of Neurology, Neurosurgery and Psychiatry*, **41**, 702–706 (1978)

71 RASCOL, A., GIRWAUD, B. and MONTALBAN, J. L. Long-term treatment of Parkinson's disease with bromocriptine. *Journal of Neurology, Neurosurgery and Psychiatry*, **42**, 143–150 (1979)

72 REISINE, T. D., FIELDS, J. Z., YAMAMURA, H. I. Neurotransmitter receptor alterations in Parkinson's disease. *Life Sciences*, **21**, 335–344 (1977)

73 RINNE, U. K., KOSKINEN, K. and LONNBERG, P. Neurotransmitter receptors in the parkinsonian brain. In *Parkinson's Disease: Current Progress, Problems and Management*, 93–107. Amsterdam, Elsevier/North Holland Biomedical Press (1980)

74 ROSENFELD, M. R., MAKMAN, M. H. and AHN, H. S. Selective influence of ergot alkaloids on cortical and straital dopaminergic and serotonergic receptors. In *Advances in Biochemical Psychopharmacology*, **23**, edited by D. Calne, M. Goldstein, A. Lieberman and M. Thorner, 83–93. New York, Raven Press (1980)

75 SHOULSON, I., GLAUBIGER, A. and CHASE, T. N. 'On–off response' clinical and biochemical correlations during oral and intravenous levodopa administration in parkinsonian patients. *Neurology (Minneapolis)*, **25**, 1140–1148 (1975)

76 SPANO, P. F., SANTANI, L. and MEMO, M. Interactions of dopaminergic ergot derivatives with cyclic nucleotide system. In *Advances in Biochemical Psychopharmacology*, **23**, edited by D. Calne, M. Goldstein, A. Lieberman and M. Thorner, 95–101. New York, Raven Press (1980)

77 SWEET, R. O., WARTERLAIN, C. G. and McDOWELL, F. H. Piribidel, a dopamine agonist in Parkinson's disease. *Clinical Pharmacology and Therapeutics*, **16**, 1077–1082 (1974)

78 TEYCHENNE, P. F., JONES, E. A., ISHAK, K. G. and CALNE, D. B. Hepatocellular injury with distinctive mitochondrial changes induced by lergotrile mesylate: a dopaminergic ergot derivative. *Gastroenterology*, **76**, 575–583 (1979)

79 TEYCHENNE, P. F., PFEIFFER, R. F. and BERN, S. M. Comparison between lergotrile and bromocriptine. *Annals of Neurology*, **3**, 319–324 (1978)

80 TEYCHENNE, P. F., PFEIFFER, R. F., BERN, S. M. and CALNE, D. B. Experiences with a new ergoline (CF 25-397) in parkinsonism. *Neurology*, **27**, 1140–1143*(1977)

81 UNGERSTEDT, U. Post-synaptic supersensitivity after 6-hydroxy-dopamine induced degeneration of the nigro-striatal dopamine system. *Acta Physiologica Scandinavia*, **367**, (Suppl.), 69–93 (1971)

82 VAKIL, S. D., CALNE, D. B. and REID, J. L. Pyridyl-piperonyl-piperazine (ET 495) in parkinsonism. *Advances in Neurology*, **3**, 121–125 (1973)

10
Deprenyl in Parkinson's disease
M. Sandler and G. M. Stern

CLINICAL CONSIDERATIONS

Following the seminal observation that the substantia nigra and corpus striatum in parkinsonian brains are deficient in dopamine[7], attempts were promptly made to inhibit degradation of this neurotransmitter in the hope of prolonging the effects of endogenous and exogenous dopamine. Thus, in 1962, Birkmayer and Hornykiewicz[2] described the effect of combining levodopa medication with the then available inhibitors of monoamine oxidase (MAO). Improvement was described as 'satisfying', but the emergence of intolerable side effects, such as toxic delirium and marked enhancement of drug-induced involuntary movements, led to the temporary abandonment of this form of adjuvant therapy. These authors did not encounter potentially catastrophic hypertension, but others[12] have since been able to demonstrate that this was more than a theoretical hazard. Even when the combination of levodopa plus the MAO inhibitor tranylcypromine was employed together with a peripheral decarboxylase inhibitor, in an attempt to limit dopamine generation to the brain, breakthrough hypertension was still observed[28].

Recent advances in knowledge concerning MAO and its inhibitors (*see* Costa and Sandler[5], Singer *et al.*[25] and Wolstenholme and Knight [32] and an appreciation that the enzyme exists in two forms, A and B, with different substrate specificities[13], provoked a renaissance of interest in selective MAO inhibition. Prompted by Knoll's[14] demonstration of the specific MAO B inhibitory properties of (−)-deprenyl, Birkmayer *et al.*[4] were able to show that deprenyl together with levodopa and a peripheral decarboxylase inhibitor could produce an enhanced antikinetic effect and a smoothing out of certain on–off oscillations. Intravenous administration of deprenyl 10 mg during the off phase provoked spectacular improvement – 30 minutes after the injection hitherto immobile patients were able to walk, with general improvement in all movements, and when deprenyl 10 mg was given intramuscularly, the onset of kinetic improvement occurred later but lasted for as long as four days. In an open study, Birkmayer *et al.*[4] then proceeded to give deprenyl 10 mg thrice daily to patients taking their usual dose of levodopa and a peripheral decarboxylase inhibitor. Average disability scores of 64 were reduced to

37 and it was again possible to demonstrate that single oral doses, although less dramatic than intramuscular administration, had a longer beneficial effect, lasting up to 2 days. Nocturnal medication caused agitation, insomnia, hyperkinesia and, in a few patients, orthostatic hypotension. The authors were able to observe sustained benefit for as long as 7 months but questioned whether this improvement would be enduring; they also wondered whether long-term combined therapy could prolong the period of effective control of parkinsonian disabilities and perhaps favourably influence the progressive degeneration of dopaminergic neurons. In 1977, Birkmayer et al.[3] were able to present the results of an open trial of prolonged (−)-deprenyl therapy in 223 patients. The addition of (−)-deprenyl to conventional therapy resulted in a statistically significant reduction in functional disability and this response was independent of the duration of previous levodopa treatment.

In a double-blind crossover trial in 41 patients receiving maximum tolerated doses of levodopa alone or in combination with carbidopa[16], (−)-deprenyl 10 mg daily prolonged the benefits of levodopa and was helpful in about half the patients who had experienced episodes of end-of-dose akinesia or wearing-off effect of the previous oral dose. Improvement was also marked in those patients troubled by nocturnal and early morning akinesia. Particular attention was paid to the responses in those who were distressed by severe, unpredictable on–off disabilities and rapid oscillations of motor performance unrelated to the timing of oral medication; in these patients, no definite improvement was found. A daily dose of (−)-deprenyl 10 mg made a mean reduction of 200 mg levodopa possible. Drug-induced dyskinesias were unacceptably aggravated in 14 patients and, for this reason, deprenyl was withdrawn.

In the following year, Birkmayer[1] described the results of (−)-deprenyl therapy in 90 patients observed for over two years and compared them with results in a similar group of patients receiving conventional medication. He found a greater improvement in the group taking (−)-deprenyl, which also permitted a lower dose of levodopa to be administered with consequently fewer recorded side-effects.

Rinne et al.[20], in 1978, reported their experience in 47 patients with Parkinson's disease on long-term levodopa therapy with and without on–off changes and described a significant reduction in on–off disabilities in 68 per cent; but their overall impression was that the degree of improvement was mostly in the moderate or minimal range and none of their patients showed a dramatic response. Peak dose dyskinesia was aggravated in about half of them, but despite this the authors concurred that deprenyl was a valuable adjuvant, at least for certain patients experiencing complications of chronic levodopa therapy.

A recent double blind crossover trail against placebo[24] further confirmed that deprenyl can prolong the action of levodopa; it produced an objective improvement in mobility in five of ten patients with dose-related response swing and subjective improvement in a further four. In another group of seven patients with random fluctuations in symptoms, only two noted subjective improvement and there was an apparent increase in the severity of response in five. It was again shown that deprenyl exacerbated any tendency to levodopa-induced dyskinesia but had no serious side-effects.

Cutting across the findings in all the earlier trials are those of Eisler et al.[8] who, in a double blind study of (−)-deprenyl in patients with Parkinson's disease, were unable to demonstrate advantage over placebo. Furthermore, they found the side-effects, including the exacerbation of on–off effect, unacceptable and considered that any minor benefit from the therapy might be due simply to its mood elevating effect. Even so, the general concordance in these several trials featuring differing disability patterns, groups of patients and rating scales, leaves us with little doubt that (−)-deprenyl has some adjuvant effect in the treatment of Parkinson's disease. It permits a smoother response with a decreased amount of levodopa, and in about half the patients who are troubled by true end-of-dose akinesia, worthwhile benefit can be demonstrated. Furthermore, in experienced hands, (−)-deprenyl is safe, devoid of a 'cheese reaction' and relatively free of side-effects at a daily dose of 10–20 mg.

The one dissenting voice, that of Eisler et al.[8] in the trial mentioned above, presents findings so different from other published studies as to be puzzling. The adverse reactions reported by these authors, in particular elevation of mood and insomnia, conflict with the present authors' experience to such an extent as to raise the possibility that the (−)-deprenyl they used might have been contaminated with (+)-deprenyl, which has a much greater amphetamine-like effect[18].

Many theoretical questions concerning the role of selective MAO inhibitors in the management of Parkinson's disease remain to be investigated, but there are two important practical problems to be resolved concerning efficacy. Are the beneficial effects sustained? Will patients who are treated with 'triple therapy' throughout the course of their illness enjoy a more benign course with a more prolonged period of effective control of symptoms and fewer late complications? The answers to these questions must await more ready availability of the drug.

BIOCHEMICAL CONSIDERATIONS

The earliest clinical publications[29, 30] on deprenyl, administered at that time for the treatment of depressive illness, employed a racemic mixture of the drug. In fact, (−)-deprenyl is known to have greater MAO inhibitory ability than the (+)-form, which has therefore been employed in subsequent investigations. (−)-Deprenyl (*Figure 10.1*) is a 'suicide' inhibitor of MAO B; it is itself metabolized by the enzyme to form a product which combines irreversibly – and lethally – with the active centre of the enzyme (for review see Singer et al.[25]). In man, the drug is converted almost quantitatively to a mixture of methamphetamine and amphetamine[18] (*Figure 10.1*). Whilst the optical rotation of these metabolites has yet to be studied, the relative absence of amphetamine-like effects, in contradistinction to the sequence of events following administration of the (+)-form, points to the probability of these metabolites also having the (−)-configuration of the parent compound. The (−)-isomers are known to have substantially less 'amphetamine-like' pharmacological actions that the (+)-forms[18].

(−)-Deprenyl is an extremely powerful MAO B inhibitor and a daily dose of 10 mg is easily sufficient to provide complete inhibition of platelet MAO[9] (*Figure*

10.2). It should be noted that platelet MAO is solely of the B variety[6]. A convenient test for the degree of MAO B inhibition *in vivo* is provided by measuring the urinary excretion of phenylethylamine, a relatively specific substrate for this form of the enzyme. Its output rises inversely with the remaining whole-body activity[9] (*Figure 10.2*).

When Birkmayer *et al.*[4] first found (−)-deprenyl to be a helpful adjuvant to levodopa in the treatment of parkinsonism, their observation appeared to conflict

Figure 10.1 The structural formulae of (*a*) deprenyl, (*b*) methamphetamine and (*c*) amphetamine. (From Reynolds *et al.*[18], courtesy of the Editor and Publishers, *British Journal of Clinical Pharmacology*)

Figure 10.2 Typical changes in platelet monoamine oxidase (MAO) activity (interrupted line) and free urinary phenylethylamine (PEA) output (solid line) in normal volunteer receiving (−)-deprenyl. (From Elsworth *et al.*[9], courtesy of the Editor and Publishers, *Psychopharmacology*)

with what was then known about dopamine metabolism. The work of Waldmeier et al.[31] had indicated that, in the brain, dopamine is metabolized by MAO A whereas at selective inhibitory concentrations (−)-deprenyl is an MAO B inhibitor. This problem was resolved by Glover et al.[10, 11] who pointed out that the studies of Waldmeier and his colleagues were performed in the rat: in *human* brain, dopamine is predominantly metabolized by MAO B.

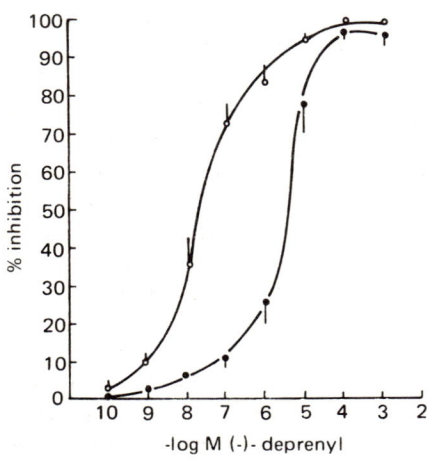

Figure 10.3 Selective inhibitions by (−)-deprenyl of phenylethylamine (○) and 5-hydroxytryptamine (●) oxidation in human striatum. Results represent mean ± s.e. from separate determinations on homogenates of striatum from 6 individuals. (From Glover et al.[10], courtesy of the Editor and Publishers, *Journal of Neural Transmission*)

A daily dose of (−)-deprenyl 10 mg is commonly employed clinically. It is interesting to note that this dose, if dissolved in total body water, gives an approximate concentration of 10^{-6}M, which is optimal for selectivity in the human brain[10] (*Figure 10.2*). Such a concentration *in vitro* provides 95 per cent inhibition of MAO B, with only some 10–15 per cent of MAO A being inhibited. Even so, under a chronic dosage schedule, one might expect MAO A to be irreversibly inhibited more rapidly than it is regenerated so that an end result over a period of time might be total inhibition of MAO A as well as MAO B. For obvious reasons, direct observations on this point in man are few although some rather exiguous observations of Riederer et al.[19] suggest that a small amount of MAO A activity may survive under chronic drug regimens of this kind. The point awaits resolution. It is of more than academic importance, for it may well shed light on the mechanism of clinical benefit which follows the use of some MAO inhibitors, but not (−)-deprenyl[17], in depressive illness (for extended discussion see Sandler[22]) and also provide information as to why (−)-deprenyl, uniquely among MAO inhibitors employed clinically, is quite free from the 'cheese effect'.

As is well known, the 'cheese effect' is an episode of hypertension which follows the ingestion of tyramine or other indirectly acting sympathomimetic amine in an individual who has been treated with an MAO inhibitor; it is commonly explained in terms of a sudden release from its stores of noradrenaline which is able to escape into the circulation because of inhibition of the enzyme which normally inactivates it. All the MAO inhibitors which have been employed clinically – including iproniazid, isocarboxazid, phenelzine, tranylcypromine in particular, and the selective MAO A inhibitor clorgyline – have been associated with this sometimes fatal drug effect. Why (−)-deprenyl should be exempt from this adverse reaction is a matter of some controversy. Knoll[14] has explained it in terms of the known high MAO A activity of the gut mucosa[9,27] which acts as an enzymatic barrier to the passage of tyramine into the circulation. Chronic (−)-deprenyl dosage, however, seems likely to provide a particularly high local concentration of the drug in the gut lumen so that mucosal MAO A is likely to be inactivated relatively rapidly. Yet even prolonged (−)-deprenyl treatment is associated with freedom from the 'cheese effect'[9] so that some other mechanism must be sought. The fact that (−)-deprenyl possesses some degree of amine uptake inhibiting ability[14] again hardly provides a satisfactory explanation, for tranylcypromine, with its profound 'cheese effect' potential, is also a strong inhibitor of monoamine re-uptake.

Very recently, Sandler et al.[23] have performed some experiments in the pig which may help to shed further light on the problem. This animal was chosen because tyramine, in all tissues other than the gut wall (which contains significant MAO A activity), appears to be wholly metabolized by MAO B. Thus, an MAO A inhibitor such as clorgyline, given in selective inhibitory dosage, would not be expected to be associated with a 'cheese effect' whereas the reverse would be predicted from the interaction of tyramine and an MAO B inhibitor. When these authors pretreated groups of pigs with clorgyline and (−)-deprenyl, respectively, and compared them with untreated controls, they found low and high degrees of tissue MAO inhibition when the animals were subsequently sacrificed. However, the clorgyline-treated animals showed a typical hypertensive response when challenged with intravenous tyramine (to bypass the gut) whereas deprenyl-treated pigs were, paradoxically, quite free of such an effect. Thus, it would appear that the administration of an 'orthodox' MAO inhibitor is associated with two separate, and perhaps distinct, pharmacological reactions: MAO inhibition proper and a facilitated release of noradrenaline from its binding sites. The data are interpreted as pointing to a facilitated release with 'orthodox' inhibitors rather than its retardation with deprenyl because intravenous tyramine challenge in man after administration of doses of deprenyl somewhat larger than the 10–20 mg usually employed have resulted in a modest hypertensive response[17].

If it be accepted that MAO inhibition and facilitated noradrenaline release are separate and distinct, the occasional association of certain non-MAO inhibiting compounds, e.g. isoniazid[21,26] and indomethacin[15], with a 'cheese effect' only then begins to make sense. Whether the further conceptual leap[22], that the central counterpart of the 'cheese effect' might conceivably be necessary for the lightening of affect associated with MAO inhibition is interesting but still lacks experimental verification. Such considerations, however, are beyond the scope of this chapter.

References

1 BIRKMAYER, W. Long-term treatment with L-deprenyl. *Journal of Neural Transmission*, **43**, 239–244 (1978)

2 BIRKMAYER, W. and HORNYKIEWICZ, O. Der L-Dioxyphenylalanin (= DOPA) Effekt beim Parkinson-Syndrom des Menschen: Zur Pathogenese und Behandlung der

Parkinson-Akinese. *Archiv für Psychiatrie und Nervenkrankheiten*, **203,** 560–574 (1962)

3 BIRKMAYER, W., RIEDERER, P., AMBROZI, L. and YOUDIM, M. B. H. Implications of combined treatment with Madopar and L-deprenyl in Parkinson's disease. *Lancet*, **2,** 439–443 (1977)

4 BIRKMAYER, W., RIEDERER, P., YOUDIM, M. B. H. and LINAUER, W. The potentiation of the anti-akinetic effect after L-DOPA treatment by an inhibitor of MAO-B, deprenyl. *Journal of Neural Transmission*, **36,** 303–326 (1975)

5 COSTA, E. and SANDLER, M. (Editors) *Monoamine Oxidases – New Vistas.* New York, Raven Press (1972)

6 DONNELLY, C. H. and MURPHY, D. L. Substrate- and inhibitor-related characteristics of human platelet MAO *Biochemical Pharmacology*, **26,** 853–858 (1977)

7 EHRINGER, H. and HORNYKIEWICZ, O. Verteilung von Noradrenalin und Dopamin (3-Hydroxytyramin) im Gehirn des Menschen und ihr Verhalten bei Erkrankungen des extrapyramidalen Systems. *Klinische Wochenschrift*, **38,** 1236–1239 (1960)

8 EISLER, T., TERÄVÄINEN, H., NELSON, R., KREBS, H., WEISE, V., LAKE, C. R., EBERT, M. H., WHETZEL, N., MURPHY, D. L., KOPIN, I. J. and CALNE, D. B. Deprenyl in Parkinson's disease. *Neurology*, **31,** 19–23 (1981)

9 ELSWORTH, J. D., GLOVER, V., REYNOLDS, G. P., SANDLER, M., LEES, A. J., PHUAPRADIT, P., SHAW, K. M., STERN, G. M. and KUMAR, P. Deprenyl administration in man: a selective monoamine oxidase B inhibitor without the 'cheese effect'. *Psychopharmacology*, **57,** 33–38 (1978)

10 GLOVER, V., ELSWORTH, J. D. and SANDLER, M. Dopamine oxidation and its inhibition by (−)-deprenyl in man. *Journal of Neural Transmission*, Suppl. 16, 163–172 (1980)

11 GLOVER, V., SANDLER, M., OWEN, F. and RILEY, G. J. Dopamine is a monoamine oxidase B substrate in man. *Nature (London)*, **265,** 80–81 (1977)

12 HUNTER, K. R., BOAKES, A. J., LAURENCE, D. R. and STERN, G. M. Monoamine oxidase inhibitors. *British Medical Journal*, **3,** 388 (1970)

13 JOHNSTON, J. P. Some observations upon a new inhibitor of monoamine oxidase in brain tissue. *Biochemical Pharmacology*, **17,** 1285–1297 (1968)

14 KNOLL, J. Analysis of the pharmacological effects of selective monoamine oxidase inhibitors. In *Monoamine Oxidase and its Inhibition*, edited by G. E. W. Wolstenholme and J. Knight, 135–155. Amsterdam, Elsevier (1976)

15 LEE, K. Y., BEILIN, J. L. and VANDONGEN, R. Severe hypertension after ingestion of an appetite suppressant (phenylpropanolamine) with indomethacin. *Lancet*, **1,** 1110–1111 (1979)

16 LEES, A. J., SHAW, K. M., KOHOUT, L. J., STERN, G. M., ELSWORTH, J. D., SANDLER, M. and YOUDIM, M. B. H. Deprenyl in Parkinson's disease. *Lancet*, **2,** 791–796 (1977)

17 MENDIS, N., PARE, C. M. B., SANDLER, M., GLOVER, V. and STERN, G. M. Is the failure of (−)-deprenyl, a selective monoamine oxidase B inhibitor, to alleviate depression related to freedom from the 'cheese effect'? *Psychopharmacology*, **73,** 87–90 (1981)

18 REYNOLDS, G. P., ELSWORTH, J. D., BLAU, K., SANDLER, M., LEES, A. J. and STERN, G. M. Deprenyl is metabolized to methamphetamine and amphetamine in man. *British Journal of Clinical Pharmacology*, **6,** 542–544 (1978)

19 RIEDERER, P., YOUDIM, M. B. H., BIRKMAYER, W. and JELLINGER, K. Monoamine oxidase activity during (−)-deprenyl therapy: human brain post-mortem studies. In *Dopamine*, (edited by P. J. Roberts, G. N. Woodruff and L. L. Iversen, 377–382. New York, Raven Press (1978)

20 RINNE, U. K., SIIRTOLA, T. and SONNINEN, V. L-Deprenyl treatment of on-off phenomena in Parkinson's disease. *Journal of Neural Transmission*, **43**, 253–262 (1978)

21 ROBINSON, D. S., LOVENBERG, W., KEISER, G. and SJOERDSMA, A. Effect of drugs on human blood platelets and plasma amine oxidase activity *in vitro* and *in vivo*. *Biochemical Pharmacology*, **17**, 109–119 (1968)

22 SANDLER, M. Monoamine oxidase inhibitor efficacy in depression and the cheese effect. *Psychological Medicine* **11**, 455–458 (1981)

23 SANDLER, M., GLOVER, V., ASHFORD, A. and ESMAIL, A. The inhibition of tyramine oxidation and the tyramine hypertensive response ('cheese effect') may be independent phenomena. *Journal of Neural Transmission*, **48**, 241–247 (1980)

24 SCHACHTER, M., MARSDEN, C. D., PARKES, J. D., JENNER, P. and TESTA, B. Deprenyl in the management of response fluctuations in patients with Parkinson's disease on L-DOPA. *Journal of Neurology, Neurosurgery and Psychiatry*, **43**, 1016–1021 (1980)

25 SINGER, T. P., VON KORFF, R. W. and MURPHY, D. L. (Editors) *Monoamine Oxidase: Structure, Function and Altered Functions*. New York, Academic Press (1979)

26 SMITH, C. K. and DURACK, D. T. Isoniazid and reaction to cheese. *Annals of Internal Medicine*, **88**, 520–521 (1978)

27 SQUIRES, R. F. Multiple forms of monoamine oxidase in intact mitochondria as characterized by selective inhibitors and thermal stability; a comparison of eight mammalian species. In *Monoamine Oxidases: New Vistas*, edited by E. Costa and M. Sandler, 335–370. New York, Raven (1972)

28 TEYCHENNE, P. F., CALNE, D. B., LEWIS, P. J. and FINDLEY, L. J. Interactions of levodopa with inhibitors of monoamine oxidase and L-aromatic amino acid decarboxylase. *Clinical Pharmacology and Therapeutics*, **18**, 273–277 (1975)

29 TRINGER, L., HAITS, G. and VARGA, E. The effect of (−)-phenylisopropylmethylpropinylamine HCl in depression. In *Society of Pharmacology of Hungary Fifth Conference on Hungarian Therapeutics*, edited by G. P. Leszkowsky, 111–114. Budapest, Hungarian Academy of Sciences (1971)

30 VARGA, E. and TRINGER, L. Clinical trial of a new type of promptly acting psycho-energetic agent (phenyl-isopropylmethyl-propinylamine-HCl, E-250). *Acta Medica Academiae Scientiarum Hungaricae*, **23**, 289–295 (1967)

31 WALDMEIER, P. C., DELINI-STULA, A. and MAITRE, L. Preferential deamination of dopamine by an A type monoamine oxidase in rat brain. *Naunyn-Schmiedeberg's Archives of Pharmacology*, **292**, 9–14 (1976)

32 WOLSTENHOLME, G. E. W. and KNIGHT, J. (Editors) *Monoamine Oxidase and its Inhibition*, Amsterdam, Elsevier-Excerpta Medica-North Holland (1976)

11
Parkinsonism, system degenerations and autonomic failure

Roger Bannister and David Oppenheimer

The clinical syndrome of parkinsonism occurs in several different conditions, of which the commonest is, of course, Parkinson's disease (synonyms: paralysis agitans, idiopathic parkinsonism). A much rarer condition, giving rise to a clinical picture which may be almost indistinguishable from Parkinson's disease, is *striatonigral degeneration*, described in 1961[4] and 1964[5] by Adams *et al.* and reviewed more recently by Adams[3], Takei and Mirra[39], and Borit *et al.*[13]. The lesions in this disease may be more or less confined to the striatum (particularly the putamen) and substantia nigra; but in some cases they are more widespread and may be combined with those of olivopontocerebellar atrophy. The occurrence of clinical parkinsonism, and of degenerative changes in the putamen and substantia nigra, in some cases of olivopontocerebellar atrophy had been recognized for many years before striatonigral degeneration was described as a separate entity; and there are strong arguments, both clinical and pathological, for including these two conditions under the single heading of *multiple system atrophy* – a term applicable to cases in which a limited number of nervous structures (including striatum, pigmented nuclei, pontine nuclei, inferior olives and cerebellar Purkinje cells) are at risk. Individual cases of multiple system atrophy suffer damage in a selection of these structures, the selection differing from case to case[31]. The label *striatonigral degeneration* may be retained for cases in which the striatum and pigmented nuclei are mainly affected.

Whatever their clinical resemblances, Parkinson's disease and striatonigral degeneration differ in their histopathology. In both conditions, the pigmented nuclei are affected; but there, as a rule, the similarity ends. The cytoplasmic inclusions (so-called Lewy bodies) which are characteristic of Parkinson's disease (*Figure 11.1*) are not found in striatonigral degeneration; and the striatal atrophy seen in the latter (*Figure 11.2*) is not a feature of Parkinson's disease. On present evidence it would be unreasonable to regard these two diseases as different parts of a single spectrum or, in other words, to treat Parkinson's disease as a variety of

Figure 11.1 Parkinson's disease. Lewy inclusion body in pigmented neuron in locus coeruleus. The cell nucleus is out of the plane of focus. The dark granules are neuromelanin. Lendrum's phloxine-tartrazine, × 1700

Figure 11.2 (*a*) Normal basal ganglia, anterior thalamic level. (*b*) Basal ganglia in a case of striatonigral degeneration. The putamen is grossly shrunken, and the myelinated bundles have disappeared. Myelin stains

multiple system atrophy. There is, however, an extra feature occurring in a minority of cases of both conditions which may suggest a common aetiological factor; that is, a progressive failure of autonomic functions, associated, in nearly every case coming to autopsy, with loss of preganglionic autonomic cells. When, as most commonly occurs, autonomic failure is associated with parkinsonism and other neurological disturbances, the usual clinical diagnosis of *Shy-Drager syndrome*, though many such cases have little in common with the clinical state described by Shy and Drager[36] in 1960:

> The full syndrome comprises the following features: orthostatic hypotension, urinary and rectal incontinence, loss of sweating, iris atrophy, external ocular palsies, rigidity, tremor, loss of associated movements, impotence, the findings of an atonic bladder and loss of the rectal sphincter tone, fasciculations, wasting of distal muscles, evidence of a neuropathic lesion in the electromyogram that suggests involvement of the anterior horn cells, and the finding of a neuropathic lesion in the muscle biopsy. The age of onset is usually in the fifth to the seventh decade of life. The disorder appears to be more frequent in the male. Any of the above signs or symptoms may be the presenting ones, and the hypotension may be a relatively late finding. The duration of the illness ... shows the disorder to be of relatively slow progression.

As with parkinsonism, autonomic failure may occur in a number of unrelated conditions[22]. After eliminating such diseases as diabetic and other peripheral neuropathies, tabes dorsalis and cerebral vascular disease, in all of which orthostatic hypotension and other autonomic disturbances may occur, we are left with a residue of cases in which autonomic failure appears to result from a primary – i.e. unexplained – selective neuronal degeneration. Unfortunately there is at present no generally accepted nomenclature for cases of this type. One common practice is to group together all cases of 'primary' autonomic failure under the heading of 'Shy-Drager syndrome' or that of 'idiopathic orthostatic hypotension'; but there are serious objections to both these usages. A patient suffering from incontinence and orthostatic hypotension, with no other neurological disorders, can hardly be said to exhibit the Shy-Drager syndrome. The term 'idiopathic orthostatic hypotension' is even more objectionable, as it stresses a single feature of autonomic failure and ignores the concomitant neurological disturbances. The word 'idiopathic', though almost meaningless, vaguely implies that the disease is a definite entity (as it does in the term 'idiopathic parkinsonism'). For reasons which they hope will soon be apparent, the authors regard progressive autonomic failure as an expression of neuronal decay which may occur in more than one type of degenerative disease of the nervous system.

CLINICAL FEATURES OF PROGRESSIVE AUTONOMIC FAILURE

A convenient clinical classification is as follows:

(1) Patients with 'pure' autonomic failure, without associated neurological disorders

(2) Patients with progressive autonomic failure associated with parkinsonism
(3) Patients with progressive autonomic failure and a variety of neurological disturbances (commonly but not always including parkinsonism) – i.e. patients with the Shy-Drager syndrome

The particular autonomic functions affected vary from case to case but are similar in these three groups. The patients are middle-aged or elderly, and males are affected about twice as often as females. Occasionally there is a family history of a similar disorder[26]. In men, impotence and loss of libido are commonly the first symptoms. Disturbances of micturition (particularly incontinence) are common early symptoms in both sexes, and in men have often been diagnosed as evidence of prostatism. Indeed, many patients have undergone prostate operations which have not led to clinical improvement. Patients living in hot climates may complain of an inability to sweat. The most dramatic symptom, however, and the commonest reason for seeking medical advice, is postural dizziness, or even fainting, on standing erect.

The postural attacks may be 'drop' attacks resembling sudden brainstem vascular dysfunction, but more commonly there is a gradual fading of consciousness over half a minute or so while the patient is standing or walking. A transient neckache radiating to the occipital region of the skull and shoulders often precedes actual loss of consciousness. Sometimes there are transient visual disturbances, scotomata, positive hallucinations or tunnel vision, suggesting occipital lobe ischaemia. The patient may then fall to his knees. Experience teaches him that after lying flat, recovery and loss of all symptoms, including the neckache, will occur within few minutes. The recovery from such transient neurological symptoms is usually complete, and (possibly because many patients have virtually continuous cerebral vasodilatation due to years of postural hypotension) occlusive cerebrovascular incidents are rare. The attack differs from normal fainting in that the patient cannot sweat and there is no vagal cardiac slowing. The disease is likely to be progressive for 5 or more years before significant incapacity occurs. Some rarer non-neurological presentations occur. A few patients, if treated by bed rest for hypotensive symptoms, develop persistent recumbent hypertension, mainly due to loss of baroreflexes, of such severity that they may develop papilloedema with retinal haemorrhages.

The neurological, as opposed to the cardiovascular, features are equally insidious. The commonest early features are an extrapyramidal disorder in which rigidity is more obvious than akinesia or tremor. The diagnosis is sometimes dramatically revealed when a mild postural hypotension becomes severe on treatment with levodopa, or when there is an unexpected lack of response to levodopa in what appears at first to be a case of Parkinson's disease. In some patients a cerebellar tremor, often with a marked truncal component, is an early sign of cerebellar system involvement. (It may be noted in passing that Shy and Drager[36] did not include cerebellar disturbances in the account, quoted above, of the syndrome bearing their name.) The extrapyramidal disorder may progress and additional features may emerge, including pyramidal signs, muscle wasting, pupillary inequalities and respiratory abnormalities including sleep apnoea and laryngeal stridor. The order of development of neurological symptoms is variable. Recently the authors have seen for the first time patients in whom laryngeal stridor was the first presenting symptom.

PHYSIOLOGICAL INVESTIGATION

In progressive autonomic failure the homeostatic control of blood pressure is disturbed by lesions at several levels from the hypothalamus to the periphery (*Figure 11.3*). In cybernetic terms the baroreceptors, as feedback transducers, do not produce the required change in the effectors, the resistance vessels, the heart and the kidneys. This causes both a change in the 'set point' pressure and an instability in the response to various stresses. Defects in the cardiovascular reflexes

Figure 11.3 Diagram of main pathways involved in neural control of blood pressure. LC = locus coeruleus; NTS = nucleus tractus solitarius; NA = nucleus ambiguus; ILC = intermediolateral column. (From Bannister[6], courtesy of the Editor and Publishers, *Lancet*)

affect short-term adjustment, but the long-term compensatory changes of blood volume, which are more difficult to study, are equally important.

When, on standing, a fall in systolic blood pressure of more than 20 mmHg is found in a patient with symptoms, further investigation is justified, and a battery of tests is now available. Radial or brachial artery catheterization will show precisely the extent of postural fall and the fluctuations with various manoeuvres. On tilt, the blood pressure falls owing to lack of constriction in resistance and capacity vessels in muscles and in the splanchnic area; but inappropriate active vasodilation may also occur[1]. There is also a lack of the overshoot in phase IV of the Valsalva manoeuvre which normally occurs as a result of reflex peripheral vasoconstriction (*Figures 11.4 and 11.5*). The instability of blood pressure in autonomic failure is

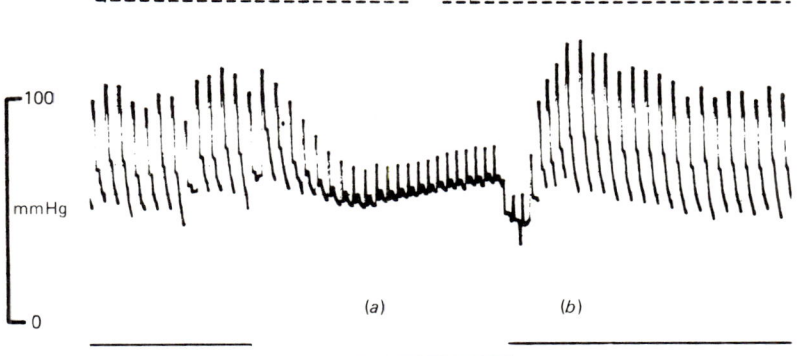

Figure 11.4 Valsalva manoeuvre in a patient with normal baroreceptor reflexes showing (*a*) halting of fall of pulse pressure with tachycardia in phase II; (*b*) 'overshoot' of systolic and diastolic pressures and bradycardia in phase IV. *Upper trace*: time in seconds; *middle trace*: arterial pressure; *lower trace*: time marker for Valsalva manoeuvre. (From Bannister et al.[9], courtesy of the Editor and Publishers, *Brain*)

Figure 11.5 Valsalva manoeuvre showing very abnormal response in chronic autonomic failure showing (*a*) continuing fall of pulse pressure throughout phase II; (*b*) 'blocked' response with slow mechanical recovery in phase IV without evidence of 'overshoot' or bradycardia. (From Bannister et al.[9], courtesy of the Editor and Publishers, *Brain*)

due partly to lack of baroreflex control, but probably also to supersensitivity of partially denervated vessels to the transmitter noradrenaline. This may cause recumbent hypertension, leading to hypertensive retinopathy or even cerebral haemorrhage. Investigation of cardiac function[29] has shown that in autonomic failure cardiac output falls on head-up tilt, as venous pressure is reduced due to pooling of blood in the legs, resembling the response in the Starling isolated heart-lung experimental preparation.

Cardiovascular reflexes, like somatic reflexes, have afferent, central and efferent connections, and the next stage in the investigation of postural hypotension and a blocked Valsalva manoeuvre is to try to show whether the lesion is afferent or efferent. If the vasoconstrictor response to stress (a reflex arising from the hypothalamus) is lost, as it is in almost all cases of progressive autonomic failure, then the lesion is presumed to be efferent. There is no simple way of testing the afferent pathway in the presence of an efferent lesion. Recently refined techniques of investigation have been used, combining lower-body suction to simulate the effect of posture, with neck pressure to 'unload' the carotid baroreceptors and so isolate the contribution of other afferents, including those from low-pressure areas[2]. Further evidence of the lack of sympathetic activity has also been provided by accurate assay of plasma noradrenaline, which is low in patients with autonomic failure and fails to rise on standing[9]. There is some uncertainty whether patients with 'pure' autonomic failure always have a lower resting plasma noradrenaline than patients with multiple system atrophy[44].

A major difficulty has been to decide whether the sympathetic efferent lesion is preganglionic or postganglionic, or both. This is of practical importance because it affects the degree of denervation supersensitivity and the response to pressor drugs. Following complete experimental postganglionic sympathetic denervation, supersensitivity of vessels to the transmitter noradrenaline occurs, with loss of the response to tyramine. Tyramine acts by releasing noradrenaline from the cytoplasmic pool but not the granular pool, which is released by the nerve impulses[7]. All patients with progressive autonomic failure show some supersensitivity to intravenous noradrenaline, and there is evidence that this is greater in 'pure' autonomic failure than in the Shy-Drager syndrome[7]. A small response to intravenous tyramine usually occurs in patients with autonomic failure, but little noradrenaline is released because the plasma noradrenaline fails to rise. In cases of 'pure' autonomic failure it has been shown that there is no response to tyramine given as an intra-arterial infusion, and this is strong evidence of a postganglionic lesion[24]. Recently it has been shown that α- and β- receptor binding on platelets and lymphocytes is defective in autonomic failure[17], and there may be similar changes in α- and β-receptors in the myocardial and limb blood vessels.

Such studies in cases of chronic autonomic failure have provided good evidence of an efferent sympathetic lesion which is more preganglionic in the Shy-Drager syndrome and more postganglionic in 'pure' autonomic failure. This sympathetic efferent lesion, affecting resistance and capacity vessels and the heart, is usually more severe than the vagal lesion, shown by lack of sinus arrhythmia. This makes an interesting contrast with diabetic autonomic neuropathy, in which the vagal efferent lesion is usually more severe than the sympathetic efferent lesion[10, 18].

PATHOLOGY

At the time of writing, the European and American literature contains detailed reports on the CNS histology in some 42 cases of progressive autonomic failure. With very few exceptions, these reports indicate a natural division of cases into two distinct groups. In the first group there are eight males and two females, with a mean age at death of 72 years. Five of these ten patients suffered from clinical parkinsonism and showed histological changes characteristic of Parkinson's disease – loss of pigmented cells from the substantia nigra, and Lewy inclusion bodies. All ten had Lewy bodies in characteristic sites. Nine showed loss of cells from the lateral horns of the thoracic cord. In the tenth, the cord was not examined. Loss of cells from the dorsal vagal nuclei was noted in six cases. In one case there was cell loss from the inferior olives, but in the other nine no lesions were found in the striatum or in the cerebellar system. Two of these cases (cases 6 and 8 of Oppenheimer[32]) had presented clinically as 'pure' autonomic failure, with no other neurological disturbance.

The second group consists of 32 patients, 19 male and 13 female, with a mean age at death of 58 years; that is, 14 years less than in the first group. The average estimated duration of the disease was not very different: 6.2 years for the first group and 5.5 years for the second; in other words, the age at onset was on average considerably lower in the second group. Clinically, all 32 patients had suffered from neurological disorders other than autonomic failure – most commonly parkinsonism, which was present in 24, and ataxia, present in at least 17.

Pathologically, this group consists of cases of multiple system atrophy, with lesions in a selection of the following structures: striatum, substantia nigra, locus coeruleus, pontine nuclei, inferior olives, cerebellar Purkinje cells, vestibular and dorsal vagal nuclei, pyramidal tracts, anterior horn cells and intermediolateral cell columns. The substantia nigra had been affected in every case, and the striatum in all but three; in other words, 29 of the patients were affected by striatonigral degeneration. All but six showed cell loss in those parts of the cerebellar system commonly affected in olivopontocerebellar atrophy. Lewy inclusion bodies on the other hand have been observed in only one case belonging to this group[40].

A feature common to both groups is a loss of preganglionic sympathetic cells (intermediolateral column cells) from the thoracic cord (*Figure 11.6*). In most cases, loss of these cells has been reported in general terms, without quantitative assessment of their numbers; but in two cases reported by Sung et al.[38] and in 21 cases examined by Oppenheimer[32], systematic cell counts have been carried out, with controls. Results in these two studies are in good agreement. In Oppenheimer's series (5 in group 1, 16 in group 2) loss of lateral horn cells ranged from 40 per cent to about 90 per cent, the mean loss being about 70 per cent. Similar counts in three cases of Parkinson's disease without clinical signs of autonomic disturbance showed no difference from controls; but in three cases of multiple system atrophy without clinical autonomic failure the counts showed loss of about half the lateral horn cells. For various reasons, similar counting procedures have not so far been carried out on the preganglionic cells of the parasympathetic system; but cell loss in the dorsal vagal nuclei has been reported in 6 of 10

Figure 11.6 Spinal cord, midthoracic region, showing (a) normal population of nerve cells in the lateral horns (arrows) (b) loss of these cells in a case of Shy-Drager syndrome. Klüver-Barrera stain, × 40

cases in group 1, and in 22 of 32 cases in group 2. Much less is known about the sacral parasympathetic outflow, but Sung et al.[38] have reported cell loss from what they consider to be the relevant part of the sacral grey matter in four cases of multiple system atrophy with autonomic failure. The region in question comprises the sacral intermediolateral column and 'Onuf's nucleus' – a group of cells described by Onufrowicz in 1900[30].

Lesions in autonomic ganglia have been looked for in some 30 cases and reported as present in seven of these. For the most part these reports are of 'mild to moderate' loss of sympathetic ganglion cells and scattered residual nodules of Nageotte, with no mention of control studies on elderly subjects not suffering from autonomic disturbances. Hyaline eosinophilic inclusion bodies, resembling those described by Jager and Bethlem[21] in Parkinson's disease, have been observed in four cases; but the only convincing account of serious damage in sympathetic ganglia is that of Rajput and Rozdilsky[34]. Their case 6 had a combination of Parkinson's disease and autonomic failure; sympathetic ganglia showed severe cell loss and cellular degeneration, and numerous eosinophilic inclusion bodies. Changes in parasympathetic ganglia or visceral nerve plexuses have not, as far as is known, been reported. The authors' own observations on the innervation of gut and bladder, on cardiac and other peripheral ganglia and on sweat glands in the skin have disclosed no significant changes. On the other hand, degenerative changes in somatic motor and sensory nerves have frequently been observed.

Laryngeal stridor has already been mentioned as a not infrequent component of the Shy-Drager syndrome. In such cases, there is clinical evidence of selective paralysis of vocal cord abduction, and in three cases post-mortem examination has shown selective atrophy of the posterior crico-arytenoid muscles[8]. The main histological changes in all three cases were those of a myopathy; in one of them, there were also changes suggestive of partial denervation. Quantitative studies of the nuclei ambigui in two of these cases were inconclusive.

To summarize the histological findings in cases of progressive autonomic failure, the common finding is a severe loss of preganglionic sympathetic cells from the lateral horns of the thoracic cord. For the rest, the cases fall into one of two groups, the first showing changes in substantia nigra, locus coeruleus and dorsal vagal nuclei resembling those of Parkinson's disease, the second showing various combinations of lesions in structures which are at risk in multiple system atrophy, the most constant of these being cell loss and gliosis in the substantia nigra and putamen. Autopsied cases of clinically 'pure' autonomic failure, in the authors' experience, fall into the first group; but it must be remembered that in many patients with the Shy-Drager syndrome the autonomic disturbances are the first to appear; in other words, the patients at an early stage of the disease are cases of 'pure' autonomic failure.

NEUROCHEMISTRY

Information on neurochemical changes in these conditions is still rather fragmentary, and the interpretation of the available data is made difficult by disagreements on classification. For example, many authors make no distinction between 'idiopathic orthostatic hypotension' and Shy-Drager syndrome, whereas Kontos et al.[24] reported differences in response to infusions of tyramine and noradrenaline between patients with the Shy-Drager syndrome on the one hand and those with idiopathic orthostatic hypotension (i.e. clinically 'pure' autonomic failure) on the other. In contrast in 1976 Black and Petito[12] published their postmortem biochemical findings in three cases of what they describe as a 'rare but clinically well-defined degenerative neurological disease, idiopathic orthostatic hypotension (IOH), the Shy-Drager syndrome'. From their rather scanty histological descriptions it seems that two of their cases showed Lewy inclusion bodies in pigmented nuclei, whereas only the third case showed cell loss from the substantia nigra and putamen. It is likely that Black and Petito were dealing with cases of two different diseases, only one of which could properly be labelled 'Shy-Drager syndrome'. A different classification was proposed in 1977 by Ziegler et al.[44], who divided cases of primary orthostatic hypotension into a group with CNS disturbances (Shy-Drager syndrome) and a group with lesions mainly in peripheral nerves. They found normal resting levels of plasma noradrenaline in the first group and low levels in the second. In both groups, the level failed to rise on exertion. Both groups had low resting levels of plasma dopamine-β-hydroxylase, the enzyme concerned with the conversion of dopamine to noradrenaline. These authors give no indication of the nature of the pathological process, or processes, in the second group.

In 1979 Spokes et al.[37] reported the neurochemical findings in the brains of four cases of histologically verified multiple system atrophy with autonomic failure. They found significantly reduced levels of both dopamine and noradrenaline in various sites, in particular in the striatum, nucleus accumbens, substantia nigra and locus coeruleus. Dopamine levels in the striatum and substantia nigra were similar to those found in cases of Parkinson's disease[11,27], but the deficiency in noradrenaline was more marked in the cases of multiple system atrophy than that found in Parkinson's disease[19]. There was also a marked loss of tyrosine hydroxylase (the rate-limiting enzyme in catecholamine synthesis) in the hypothalamus and anterior perforated substance, which had not been recorded for Parkinson's disease. Estimations of two other enzymes – glutamic acid decarboxylase and choline acetyltransferase – did not yield clear-cut results. In a companion paper by Quik et al.[33] a comparison was made between these same four cases, eight cases of Parkinson's disease and 18 normal controls in respect of dopamine receptor sites in the striatum, substantia nigra and frontal cortex. Loss of binding sites in the substantia nigra was found both in Parkinson's disease and in the cases of multiple system atrophy, whereas loss in the dentate nucleus was greater in striatonigral degeneration.

Studies of this kind, using 'normal' controls, leave many important questions unanswered, in particular whether the observed chemical abnormalities are characteristic of autonomic failure, of striatonigral degeneration or of olivopontocerebellar atrophy. It is worth remarking that of the four cases studied by Spokes et al.[37] all had autonomic failure, and all had the former, but only three cases had the latter condition. Choline acetyltransferase levels were found to be reduced in most of the areas examined but were relatively high in pons, cerebellum and red nucleus in the one patient who did not have olivopontocerebellar atrophy. The significance of results of this kind cannot be fully assessed until parallel investigations are carried out on cases of (1) 'pure' autonomic failure (2) progressive autonomic failure associated with Parkinson's disease and (3) multiple system atrophy without evidence of autonomic failure. So far, very few such investigations have been carried out. As a case of 'pure' autonomic failure case A (and perhaps case C) of Black and Petito[12] may serve as an example, with their case B (seemingly a case of striatonigral degeneration) as a foil. Their figures show relatively high levels of tyrosine hydroxylase activity in the substantia nigra and caudate nucleus in cases A and C, but no detectable activity in case B. To the best of the authors' knowledge, there have been no chemical observations in cases with autonomic failure associated with Parkinson's disease; but there is at least one report[35] on the brain chemistry in a case of striatonigral degeneration with severe parkinsonism but no overt autonomic disturbance. The main abnormal finding was a virtual absence of dopamine and of homovanillic acid from the striatum and globus pallidus.

There seem to be no published reports on the neurochemistry of the lateral horns of the spinal cord in cases of progressive autonomic failure, or any convincing account relating chemical and histological changes in autonomic ganglia to those in the brain and spinal cord. Without more information on these matters, speculation on the specific defects in autonomic failure (as opposed to those of Parkinson's disease, striatonigral degeneration and olivopontocerebellar atrophy) is gravely hampered.

TREATMENT OF POSTURAL HYPOTENSION

Treatment of postural hypotension due to autonomic failure is fraught with difficulties. First, it is important not to be overconcerned about low standing blood pressure if the patient is without symptoms. Patients can sometimes tolerate a standing systolic pressure as low as 70 mmHg without a fall of cerebral blood flow because their capacity for cerebral autoregulation is better than normal[41]. If the standing pressure is raised, for example by pressor drugs, the patient may develop recumbent hypertension and may, as a result of a reactive increase of cerebrovascular resistance, develop cerebral ischaemic symptoms on standing despite the higher standing systolic pressure. A second principle is that though the loss of baroreflexes determines the initial response to standing, it is the volume control, determined by low-pressure receptors and the kidney, which is more important though less well understood[42]. Most patients with autonomic failure can still release renin, but have defects of renal preservation of sodium when recumbent and are sensitive to sodium depletion. Head-up body tilt at night often improves postural hypotension by reducing renal arterial pressure, promoting renin release and increasing blood volume. Some patients with incapacitating symptoms while on pressor drugs have been maintained satisfactorily for years solely by head-up tilt at night. The volume of blood pooling in the lower part of the body may be reduced by elastic stockings or by the inflatable antigravity suit worn by aviators; this treatment, however, will reduce the valuable myogenic response to stretch which is present even in partially denervated vessels. It is therefore logically unsound though sometimes necessary as a temporary expedient.

The ideal of treatment with drugs is to produce selective vasoconstriction on standing, resembling the effect of release of noradrenaline by normal sympathetic efferent activity. Fludrocortisone approaches closest to this. In a dose of 0.1 mg daily, which does not cause fluid retention, fludrocortisone enhances supersensitivity to intravenous noradrenaline and improves standing blood pressure[16]. In larger doses it also increases blood volume. Indomethacin, the prostaglandin inhibitor, has been reported to improve postural hypotension[23], but in other studies it has not increased standing pressure despite an increase in sensitivity to infused noradrenaline[14]. Monoamine oxidase inhibitors and tyramine have been recommended[28], but these may cause potentially dangerous recumbent hypertension[15]. Propranolol and pindolol have recently been tried, with some reports of improvement, on the ground that a β-adrenoreceptor blocking drug might reduce any tendency to vasodilatation and that the added agonist effect of pindolol might also enhance constriction. It must be stressed that studies on the action of drugs in the treatment of postural hypotension require rigorous control, which has been lacking in many published reports. Meanwhile the search is continuing for more effective drugs, acting centrally or peripherally, which will promote selective vasoconstriction on standing.

TREATMENT OF OTHER SYMPTOMS

If the patient has autonomic failure with parkinsonism, the extrapyramidal signs may benefit from levodopa, but the response is unlikely to be as complete as in the uncomplicated case of Parkinson's disease, and in any case, levodopa is likely to aggravate the postural hypotension. There have been hardly any reports of sustained improvement of the extrapyramidal syndrome of multiple system atrophy, and there has been similar lack of response to bromocriptine, which helps some patients with Parkinson's disease[43]. A recent study has investigated the effect of lisuride, an antagonist of 5-hydroxytryptamine with dopamine-receptor stimulating properties[25]. In animals it increases brain dopamine and reduces brain dopamine turnover. It differs from bromocriptine in that its effects are not abolished by inhibition of tyrosine hydroxylase. Lisuride probably acts as a direct pre- and postsynaptic agonist. Unfortunately not only did the patients fail to show any improvement in their extrapyramidal syndrome, but the drug caused severe hallucinations, though these were reversible on withdrawing the drug. The hallucinations were of a particularly unpleasant character. Hallucinations may occur in patients with Parkinson's disease on treatment with levodopa or bromocriptine, or occasionally in patients with multiple system atrophy. However, the particularly potent hallucinatory effects of lisuride might be the result of its structural similarity to LSD. Clearly there is a lack of correspondence between the effects of different drugs in multiple system atrophy. If, in a patient with this condition, the striatal postsynaptic receptors are damaged, there are often other central defects which determine unusual drug responses. The search for better drugs must continue.

Some patients develop laryngeal stridor and sleep apnoea. The laryngeal stridor is due to selective abductor paralysis and usually requires treatment by tracheostomy[8]. In some the central disturbance of respiratory control and sleep apnoea[20] may be the effective cause of death. Alternatively, the denervation supersensitivity of sympathetic α- and β-receptors of the heart may render patients more liable to cardiac arrhythmia, from which they may die. The evidence of such supersensitivity comes in part from the increased responsiveness to isoprenaline (isoproterenol), and indirectly from increased β-receptor binding on lymphocytes[17], though there is as yet no proof that β-receptors are similarly affected in blood vessels or the myocardium. Though patients with pure autonomic failure may remain stable for years, patients with the Shy-Drager syndrome at present rarely survive longer than 5 years from diagnosis.

CONCLUSIONS

In the authors' view, progressive autonomic failure occurs as an additional feature in two distinct, well recognised types of primary degenerative disease, namely Parkinson's disease and multiple system atrophy. Cases of clinically pure autonomic failure examined at autopsy show *either* Lewy inclusion bodies, linking these cases to Parkinson's disease, *or* minor changes of multiple system atrophy. The evidence for this view comes mainly from the accumulation of histological findings over the past 20 years. The contrary view – that progressive autonomic failure, or idiopathic orthostatic hypotension, or the Shy-Drager syndrome, constitutes a separate neuropathological entity – seems to the authors to ignore this evidence. Unnecessary confusion also results when one group of writers uses the term 'idiopathic orthostatic hypotension' or 'IOH' as a synonym for the Shy-Drager syndrome while another group uses the same term exclusively for cases of 'pure' autonomic failure. The remedy for this confusion would be to drop the use of the term 'idiopathic orthostatic hypotension' altogether. These points of nomenclature are stressed not from pedantry, but because it is important when assessing the effects of treatment – in particular, treatment with drugs – to have a clear idea of what disease one is treating. This is especially so when two different diseases with similar clinical manifestations, for instance Parkinson's disease and striatonigral degeneration, are being investigated. A similar caution is necessary if one is pursuing biochemical or physiological studies during life or after death on series of cases of autonomic failure. If valid comparisons are to be made, like must be grouped with like. For this, accurate diagnosis is essential.

References

[1] ABBOUD, F. M. and ECKSTEIN, J. W. Active reflex vasodilatation in man. *Federation Proceedings*, **25**, 1612–1617 (1966)

2 ABBOUD, F. M., ECKBERG, D. L., JOHANNSEN, U. J. and MARK, A. L. Carotid and cardiopulmonary baroreceptor control of splanchnic and forearm vascular resistance during venous pooling in man. *Journal of Physiology (London)*, **286**, 173–184 (1979)

3 ADAMS, R. D. The striatonigral degenerations. *Handbook of Clinical Neurology*, edited by P. J. Vinken and G. W. Bruyn, vol. 6, chapter 26, 694–702. Amsterdam, North Holland Publishing Company (1968)

4 ADAMS, R. D., VAN BOGAERT, L. and VAN DER EECKEN, H. Dégénerescences nigrostriées et cérébello-nigro-striées. *Psychiatrica et Neurologia (Basel)*, **142**, 219 (1961)

5 ADAMS, R. D., VAN BOGAERT, L. and VAN DER EECKEN, H. Striato-nigral degeneration. *Journal of Neuropathology and Experimental Neurology*, **23**, 584–608 (1964)

6 BANNISTER, R. Chronic autonomic failure with postural hypotension. *Lancet*, **2**, 404–406 (1979)

7 BANNISTER, R., DAVIES, I. B., HOLLY, E., ROSENTHAL, T. and SEVER, P. Defective cardiovascular reflexes and supersensitivity to sympathomimetic drugs in autonomic failure. *Brain*, **102**, 163–176 (1979)

8 BANNISTER, R., GIBSON, M., MICHAELS, L. and OPPENHEIMER, D. R. Laryngeal paralysis in multiple system atrophy. *Brain*, **104**, 351–386 (1981)

9 BANNISTER, R., SEVER, P. and GROSS, M. Cardiovascular reflexes and biochemical responses in progressive autonomic failure. *Brain*, **100**, 327–334 (1977)

10 BENNETT, R., HOSKING, D. J. and HAMPTON, J. R. Cardiovascular control in diabetes mellitus. *British Medical Journal*, **2**, 585–587 (1975)

11 BERNHEIMER, H., BIRKMAYER, W., HORNYKIEWICZ, P., JELLINGER, K. and SEITELBERGER, F. Brain dopamine and the syndromes of Parkinson and Huntington: clinical morphological and neurochemical correlations. *Journal of the Neurological Sciences*, **20**, 415–455 (1973)

12 BLACK, I. B. and PETITO, C. K. Catecholamine enzymes in the degenerative neurological disease idiopathic orthostatic hypotension. *Science*, **192**, 910–912 (1976)

13 BORIT, A., RUBINSTEIN, L. J. and URICH, H. The striatonigral degenerations: putaminal pigments and nosology. *Brain*, **98**, 101–112 (1975)

14 DAVIES, B., BANNISTER, R., HENSBY, C. and SEVER, P. The pressor actions of noradrenaline and angiotensin II in chronic autonomic failure treated with indomethacin. *British Journal of Clinical Pharmacology*, **10**, 223–229 (1980)

15 DAVIES, I. B., BANNISTER, R. and SEVER, P. Pressor amines and monoamine oxidase inhibitors for treatment of postural hypotension in autonomic failure. Limitations and hazards. *Lancet*, **1**, 172–175 (1978)

16 DAVIES, B., BANNISTER, R., SEVER, P. and WILCOX, C. The pressor actions of noradrenaline, angiotensin II and saralasin in chronic autonomic failure treated with fludrocortisone. *British Journal of Clinical Pharmacology*, **8**, 253–260 (1979)

17 DAVIES, I. B., MATHIAS, C. J., SUDERA, D., LETHBRIDGE, K., BANNISTER, R. BOYLSTON, A. and SEVER, P. Characterisation of alpha and beta adrenergic receptors in denervation supersensitivity in man. *Clinical Science and Molecular Medicine*, **59**, 6P (1980)

18 EWING, D. J. Cardiovascular reflexes and autonomic neuropathy. *Clinical Science and Molecular Medicine*, **55**, 321–327 (1978)

19 FARLEY, I. J. and HORNYKIEWICZ, O. Noradrenaline in subcortical brain regions of patients with Parkinson's disease and control subjects. In *Advances in Parkinsonism – Biochemistry, Physiology, Treatment*, edited by W. Birkmayer and O. Hornykiewicz, 178–185. Basel, Editions Roche (1977)

20 GUILLEMINAULT, C., TILKIAN, A., LEHRMAN, K., FORNO, L. and DEMENT, W. C. Sleep apnoea syndrome: states of sleep and autonomic dysfunction. *Journal of Neurology, Neurosurgery and Psychiatry*, **40**, 718–725 (1977)

21 JAGER, W. A. DEN H. and BETHLEM, J. The distribution of Lewy bodies in the central and autonomic nervous systems in idiopathic paralysis agitans. *Journal of Neurology, Neurosurgery and Psychiatry*, **23**, 283–290 (1960)

22 JOHNSON, R. H. and SPALDING, J. M. K. *Disorders of the Autonomic Nervous System.* Oxford, Blackwell, (1974)

23 KOCHAR, M. S. and ITSKOVITZ, H. D. Treatment of idiopathic orthostatic hypotension (Shy-Drager syndrome) with indomethacin. *Lancet*, **1**, 1011–1014 (1978)

24 KONTOS, H. A., RICHARDSON, D. W. and NORVELL, J. E. Norepinephrine depletion in idiopathic orthostatic hypotension. *Annals of Internal Medicine*, **82**, 336–341 (1975)

25 LEES, A. J. and BANNISTER, R. The use of Lisuride in the treatment of multiple system atrophy with autonomic failure (Shy-Drager syndrome). *Journal of Neurology, Neurosurgery and Psychiatry*, **44**, 347–351 (1981)

26 LEWIS, P. Familial orthostatic hypotension. *Brain*, **87**, 719–728 (1964)

27 LLOYD, K. G., DAVIDSON, L. and HORNYKIEWICZ, O. The neurochemistry of Parkinson's disease – effect of L-dopa therapy. *Journal of Pharmacology and Experimental Therapeutics*, **195**, 453–464 (1975)

28 NANDA, R. N., JOHNSON, R. H. and KEOGH, H. J. Treatment of neurogenic orthostatic hypotension with a monoamine oxidase inhibitor and tyramine. *Lancet*, **2**, 1164–1167 (1976)

29 NIARCHOS, A. P., MAGRINI, F., TARAZI, R. C. and BRAVO, E. L. Mechanisms of spontaneous supine blood pressure variations in chronic autonomic insufficiency. *American Journal of Medicine*, **65**, 547–552 (1978)

30 ONUFROWICZ, B. On the arrangement and function of the cell groups of the sacral region of the spinal cord in man. *Archives of Neurology and Psychopathology*, **3**, 387–412 (1900)

31 OPPENHEIMER, D. R. Diseases of the basal ganglia, cerebellum and motor neurons. In *Greenfield's Neuropathology*, 3rd edition, edited by W. Blackwood and J. A. N. Corsellis, Ch. 14. London, Arnold (1976)

32 OPPENHEIMER, D. R. Lateral horn cells in progressive autonomic failure. *Journal of the Neurological Sciences*, **46**, 393–404 (1980)

33 QUIK, M., SPOKES, E. G., MACKAY, A. V. P. and BANNISTER, R. Alterations in (3H) spiperone binding in human caudate nucleus, substantia nigra and frontal cortex in the Shy-Drager syndrome and Parkinson's disease. *Journal of the Neurological Sciences*, **43**, 429–437 (1979)

34 RAJPUT, A. H. and ROZDILSKY, B. Dysautonomia in Parkinsonism: a clinicopathological study. *Journal of Neurology, Neurosurgery and Psychiatry*, **39**, 1092–1100 (1976)

35 SHARPE, J. A., REWCASTLE, N. B., LLOYD, K. G., HORNYKIEWICZ, O., HILL, M. and TASKER, R. R. Striatonigral degeneration: response to Levodopa therapy with pathological and neurochemical correlation. *Journal of the Neurological Sciences*, **19**, 275–286 (1973)

36 SHY, G. M. and DRAGER, G. A. A neurological syndrome associated with orthostatic hypotension. *Archives of Neurology (Chicago)*, **2**, 511–527 (1960)

37 SPOKES, E. G., BANNISTER, R. and OPPENHEIMER, D. R. Multiple system atrophy with autonomic failure; clinical, histological and neurochemical observations on four cases. *Journal of the Neurological Sciences*, **43**, 59–82 (1979)

38 SUNG, J. H., MASTRI, A. R. and SEGAL, E. Pathology of Shy-Drager syndrome. *Journal of Neuropathology and Experimental Neurology*, **38**, 353–368 (1979)

39 TAKEI, Y. and MIRRA, S. S. Striatonigral degeneration: a form of multiple system atrophy with clinical Parkinsonism. In *Progress in Neuropathology*, edited by H. M. Zimmerman, Vol 2, 217–251. New York, Grune and Stratton, (1973)

40 THAPEDI, I. M. ASHENHURST, E. M. and ROZDILSKY, B. Shy-Drager syndrome: report of an autopsied case. *Neurology*, **21**, 26–32 (1971)

41 THOMAS, D. J. and BANNISTER, R. Preservation of autoregulation of cerebral blood flow in autonomic failure. *Journal of the Neurological Sciences*, **44**, 205–212 (1981)

42 WILCOX, C. S., AMINOFF, M. J. and SLATER, J. D. H. Sodium homeostasis in patients with autonomic failure. *Clinical Science and Molecular Medicine*, **53**, 321–328 (1977)

43 WILLIAMS, A. C., NUTT, J., LAKE, R., PFEIFFER, R., TEYCHENNE, P. E., EBERT, M. and CALNE, D. B. Actions of bromocriptine in the Shy-Drager and Steele-Richardson-Olszewski syndromes. In *Dopaminergic Ergots and Motor Control*. New York, Raven Press (1978)

44 ZIEGLER, M. G., LAKE, C. R. and KOPIN, I. J. The sympathetic nervous system defect in primary orthostatic hypotension. *New England Journal of Medicine*, **296**, 293–297 (1977)

12
Problems in dyskinesias
C. D. Marsden and Stanley Fahn

INTRODUCTION

It was more difficult to choose appropriate topics amongst diseases characterized by abnormal involuntary movements. There have been a number of published proceedings of the first major international symposia on certain dyskinesias. Thus, the reader is referred to *Advances in Neurology*, Vol. 1 (1972), and Vol. 23 (1979) for excellent reviews of the 'state of the art' on most aspects of Huntington's disease; to *Advances in Neurology*, Vol. 14 (1976) for torsion dystonia; and to *Advances in Neurology* (in press), for Gilles de la Tourette's syndrome. One group of dyskinesias not covered in these publications, and which provokes many diagnostic and nosologic difficulties, is the myoclonias. Accordingly, the editors have devoted Chapter 13, with Mark Hallett, to the clinical features of these disorders.

Although much has been written about Huntington's disease, there is no extensive account of the practical management of this disorder, which is considered here by Ira Shoulson (Chapter 16). Drug-induced tardive dyskinesias have gained increasing attention in recent years, so Angus Mackay was asked to provide a critical review of controversial clinical matters on this topic in Chapter 14, and Christopher Goetz and Harold Klawans to discuss experimental studies in the field in Chapter 15.

One of the more difficult decisions facing the physician looking after patients with dyskinesias is when to consider the various surgical approaches that have been used to treat these conditions. Accordingly, in Chapter 17, the editors asked a panel of expert neurosurgeons to describe briefly the approaches they apply to specific problems: Hirotaro Narabayashi on tremor, Joseph Waltz on dystonia, Claude Bertrand and Jeffrey Maccabe on different approaches to torticollis, Alan Bird and Arthur Battista on different approaches to blepharospasm, and Peter Jannetta on hemifacial spasm. They also asked Lindsay McClellan to review critically the possible role of brain stimulation in the management of dyskinesias.

Finally, the editors have written a brief 'afterword' in which they describe their practice of referral for surgery for these conditions.

This has left many topics in dyskinesias untouched. In what follows in this chapter, they discuss briefly a number of items in which advances have occurred recently, or which pose particular problems to the practitioner.

DRUG TREATMENT OF BENIGN ESSENTIAL TREMOR

Most patients discover that alcohol is the most potent way to control benign essential tremor, but this can no longer be prescribed in the National Health Service of the United Kingdom nor, it is believed, in France. Simple sedatives generally do not help, and cause drowsiness. A proportion of patients gain benefit from β-adrenergic antagonists, such as propranolol, but the degree of improvement usually is not dramatic. There seems to be no clear relation between plasma propranolol level and therapeutic response, and benefit, if it is going to be achieved, will be obtained with dosages of up to 240 mg daily.

In fact, because of their extensive use in cardiology, a wide range of β-blockers is now available. Some, such as metoprolol, are cardioselective, acting mainly upon $β_1$-adrenergic receptors, so do not affect airway resistance. Such cardioselective β-blockers have been used safely in some patients with bronchitis or asthma, and have been reported to relieve tremor. From this observation, some workers have concluded that the benefits from propranolol are due to blockade of $β_1$-receptors. However, the doses used often have been greater than required to achieve cardioselectivity, and other studies have now shown that cardioselective β-blockers are less effective than drugs blocking $β_1$- and $β_2$-receptors. For example, both atenolol and metoprolol produce less benefit than propranolol in double-blind trials. Another related issue is whether the benefical effect of β-antagonists is due to a peripheral or central action. Propranolol enters the brain, and produces side-effects such as hallucinations and vivid dreams. However, other β-blockers which have difficulty entering the central nervous system, such as sotolol, which also is a $β_1$- and $β_2$-antagonist, are equally as effective as propranolol. The provisional conclusion from studies such as these is that peripheral $β_2$-blockade is the important action responsible for control of tremor, but further investigations using the increasing range of β-blockers available are to be expected.

Another question to consider is why only some patients with essential tremor respond to β-blockade. It is the belief of one of the editors (CDM) that this nosological entity includes at least two subtypes. On the one hand there is the patient with mild to moderate exaggeration of physiological postural tremor (usually in the frequency of 8–12 Hz), which is more of a social inconvenience and distress than a physical disability. On the other hand, there are patients with more marked and disabling tremor, usually at a slower frequency of 5–7 Hz. The former enhanced physiological tremor is reduced by propranolol, but the latter often is not.

Recently, there has been a report that primidone may help some patients with essential tremor, and it is worthwhile remembering that amobarbital (amylobarbitone, Amytal) was used frequently prior to the advent of β-blockers. Whether this benefit is due to the phenobarbitone to which primidone is metabolized, or to the parent drug and its other metabolites is not known. Further assessment of this approach is required, but for patients who fail to respond to a β-blocker, a trial of primidone may be worthwhile. However, unfortunately, all too often none of these treatments really produce as much effect as alcohol. Wise advice as how to use spirits or wine prior to social or professional events may be the best counsel. Nevertheless, the risks of alcohol addiction should not be underestimated, particularly in those dependent on fine manual skills for employment, such as the microsurgeon or dentist.

THE MANAGEMENT OF TICS

Much has been written about the beneficial effects of haloperidol in the treatment of tics, such as occur in Gilles de la Tourette's syndrome. In fact, equal benefit can be obtained from a range of other antipsychotic drugs, such as pimozide. The real question is whether or not to use such powerful drugs at all.

Gilles de la Tourette's syndrome and other tic disorders begin in childhood. Many are life-long, so to commence treatment with haloperidol or another neuroleptic carries the risk of inducing a tardive dyskinesia. Both the editors have experience of this iatrogenic complication. They try, if possible, to persuade patients with mild tics and their families to avoid any drug treatment. If therapy is required, a behavioral approach is sometimes worthwhile before considering medication. If a drug is needed, the general approach is to start with agents least likely to cause permanent side-effects. The editors begin treatment with a benzodiazepine, such as clonazepam; then may try clonidine, either singly or in combination; only if these fail do they turn to antipsychotics. It must be emphasized, also, that psychotherapeutic support is an essential component in the management of the social and school problems posed by symptoms of Gilles de la Tourette's syndrome.

DIAGNOSIS AND TREATMENT OF DYSTONIA

Dystonia frequently is misdiagnosed as hysterical or as some other movement disorder. The former can only be avoided by being aware of the many and varied manifestations of the disease, and by following the general principle that, despite the teachings of Charcot, hysterical movement disorders are exceedingly rare. It is much more common to misdiagnose a case as hysterical through ignorance than to miss the diagnosis of hysteria. The latter often is considered because of the bizarre nature of the initial symptoms of the disease, which commonly take the form of an action dystonia affecting one movement but not another. For example, a child may develop a dystonic foot when walking forwards, but not backwards, on running or sitting. Dystonia appears to distort motor programs for certain acts, rather than individual movements; muscles can be employed normally to carry out a movement in one setting, for example, to dorsiflex the foot when walking backwards or running, but not when the same movement is required for the critically involved motor program of walking forwards. Once this fact is realized, the peculiar circumstances in which dystonia occurs become diagnostic of the disorder, rather than a source of confusion.

Misdiagnosis of dystonia as other movement disorders commonly occurs because too much attention is paid to the accompanying features of the illness than to the underlying dystonia itself. Thus, myoclonus and tremor commonly occur in dystonia, but the obvious coexistence of dystonic spasms and postures establish the diagnosis despite these other types of abnormal involuntary movements. A patient with spasmodic torticollis, for example, has torticollis even though the neck may exhibit myoclonic jerks or tremor. Furthermore, dystonic spasms can be rapid, leading to a misdiagnosis of chorea unless it is recognized that the former follow a repetitive pattern, rather than the random, continous and flowing movements of chorea.

The treatment of dystonia is not an easy task. At least 50 percent of patients do not gain useful benefit from drug therapy, and even in those who do respond, it may be difficult to discover the most effective agent. The editors' practice is first to review the need for drug treatment at all. Many patients with the isolated focal forms of dystonia, such as torticollis or writer's cramp, may be happier to live with their disability, if mild, rather than go through the tedium and side-effects of multiple drug trials, once the options are explained to them. If drugs are indicated, they start with an anticholinergic, such as trihexyphenidyl (benzhexol) or ethopropazine. The trick in the use of these agents is to gradually build up the dose, as dictated by side-effects, to the maximum that the patient can tolerate. Children may be able to take as much as 80 mg/day of trihexyphenidyl, providing it is introduced slowly enough. Adults are far less tolerant, usually because of mental effects. The next best group of drugs for ameliorating dystonic spasms is the benzodiazepines, such as diazepam. Again, patients with dystonia can tolerate very large amounts of such a drug, for example, up to 80 mg of diazepam daily, without drowsiness. Although other drugs are employed to treat dystonia, the majority of patients end up on a combination of an anticholinergic and a benzodiazepine.

A few patients have been reported to respond to carbamazepine in moderate dosage (300 mg daily), and there are descriptions of occasional responses to levodopa preparations, usually in small doses. However, whether such patients are all suffering from a recognized variant of the syndrome of torsion dystonia (dystonia with marked diurnal fluctuation), is open to question. Nevertheless, in patients with severe dystonia, the editors would try both carbamazepine and levodopa/carbidopa at some stage in their illness. Despite fears to the contrary, they have never seen any persistent deterioration after levodopa.

Antipsychotic drugs such as a phenothiazine, haloperidol, or pimozide also are sometimes used to treat dystonia. The same considerations about the risks of producing a tardive dyskinesia apply in this disease as in tics. Indeed, the editors have both seen this to occur. This makes them reluctant to employ such drugs unless disability is so severe that it becomes essential. Even so, given alone, they are not particularly effective agents. Frequently, it is necessary to give them in dosages that cause an unacceptable degree of parkinsonism. In that event, additiion of an anticholinergic may help if the patient is not already on one. However, often the sufferer is either disabled by his dystonia, or by the drug-induced parkinsonism, and it is impossible to strike the balance between the two.

Another drug that has been available in Europe for a decade is tetrabenazine, which is a short acting analog of reserpine with fewer peripheral side-effects. Tetrabenazine certainly may help some patients with dystonia (in doses up to 300 mg daily), but frequently causes unacceptable side-effects in the form of parkinsonism, akathisia and, most seriously, a delayed depression.

In general, chair- or bed-bound children with dystonia do not gain useful benefit from antipsychotic drugs or tetrabenazine. However, adults, particularly those with severe disabling axial dystonia, may be helped and one editor (CDM) uses a combination of pimozide, tetrabenazine and an anticholinergic to maintain mobility in such individuals. Alternatively, SF might refer such a patient for cervical cord stimulation (*see* Chapter 17.3).

With regard to that group of conditions known as the adult-onset focal dystonias, drug treatment also is unsatisfactory. Some patients with Meige's syndrome (blepharospasm and oromandibular dystonia, or the cranial dystonia syndrome) may respond to treatment with a variety of agents, including baclofen in high dosage (up to 120 mg daily, built up slowly), clonazepam, an antipsychotic such as perphenazine or pimozide, tetrabenazine, or ethopropazine. It is worthwhile trying each of these drugs in sequence, although it must be admitted that a proportion of patients gain no useful benefit from any of them. The same range of drugs can be used in patients with spasmodic torticollis, but most are not helped. Few patients with dystonic writer's cramp need to take or tolerate such drugs; they are better off learning to write with the opposite hand or to use a dictaphone.

The role of surgical treatment of the various forms is discussed in Chapter 17.

13
The nosology and pathophysiology of myoclonus
C. D. Marsden, M. Hallett and Stanley Fahn

'The word "myoclonus" has been abused almost as much as "spasm" . . . Though extensive, . . . [the literature on myoclonus] does not satisfy, many reports being ambiguous or meagre.'

INTRODUCTION

These words of Kinnier Wilson[190] are almost as true now as they were when written in 1940. Of all the movement disorders, myoclonus is the most difficult to encapsulate into any simple framework. The purpose here is to review the information that is available on the clinical manifestations of myoclonus, the diseases that cause the syndrome, and such pathophysiology as is known. Treatment will not be discussed in detail.

One of the reasons why myoclonus has proved so difficult to grasp is that there have been numerous historical descriptions of the disorder in diseases whose pathology was not known at the time. Many were given flamboyant names like 'electric chorea' or 'saltatoric spasm'. One of the aims of this chapter is to review such reports critically and to suggest discarding all those that do not fit with modern experience, thereby reducing the concept of myoclonus to manageable proportions.

Definition

The first necessity is to define the term 'myoclonus'. Literally speaking, it means 'a quick movement of muscle'. It is used here to describe muscle jerks due to brief muscle contractions similar to those produced by electric shocks to a peripheral motor nerve. The second characteristic of the authors' definition of myoclonus is that it arises in the central nervous system. Earlier writers had extended the term to encompass muscle jerks due not only to diseases of the central nervous system but also to muscle twitching resulting from peripheral injuries; these would now be called fasciculations and not be included in the author's definition of myoclonus. This definition now becomes *muscle jerking, irregular or rhythmic, arising in the central nervous system*.

Sudden, brief movements may be produced not only by the positive muscle contractions of myoclonus but also by sudden, brief lapses of muscle contraction that are characteristic of *asterixis*. The lapses of posture that consitute asterixis may be looked upon as negative myoclonus. In fact, there is an association between myoclonus and many metabolic encephalopathies, such as hepatic or renal failure. This association has a physiological basis; Marsden *et al.*[123], in studies on the effects of electrical stimulation of the human motor cortex through the scalp, have observed typical asterixis. Strong shocks cause brief muscle contractions typical of myoclonic jerks, each contraction being followed by a silent period. Weak shocks may only cause inhibition of muscle contraction, the silent period being accompanied by a postural lapse identical to that seen in asterixis. In other words, activity in the motor cortex may either cause muscle contraction or asterixis.

Distinction from other dyskinesias

Myoclonus, as defined above, must be distinguished from other dyskinesias. Muscle jerks also occur in the syndromes of tics, chorea and dystonia, and rhythmic muscle contraction is characteristic of tremor. Myoclonus is distinguished from *tics* because the latter can be controlled by an effort of will, at least temporarily, whereas myoclonus cannot. In addition, in contrast to myoclonus, many tics characteristically are complex movements which are accompanied by a conscious urge to move and by relief after the tic has occurred. Unfortunately, the separation of different movement disorders is not always as easy as this, and it may be impossible clinically to distinguish simple tics from isolated myoclonic jerks.

Many of the individual movements of *chorea* also resemble myoclonic jerks. But the characteristic feature of chorea is that these movements continue in a constant flow, randomly distributed over the body, with each involved muscle jerking randomly in time. It is therefore impossible to know where or when to expect the next twitch. Many types of myoclonus are characterized by distinctive and repetitive patterns of muscle jerking which affect the same muscle groups time and time again, sometimes even rhythmically. In other types of myoclonus, the muscle jerking may be chaotic but without the characteristic continuous flow of movements that is so distinctive of chorea.

The distinction of myoclonus from *dystonia* is usually obvious; myoclonic jerks are brief contractions while dystonic spasms are prolonged and distort the body into characteristic dystonic postures. Difficulty arises because myoclonus and dystonia may coexist in the same patient. In this case, the authors include the patient in the category of dystonia rather than myoclonus. In other words, the presence of dystonia takes precedence. Some patients with dystonia, however, have such obvious and severe myoclonic jerking as to warrant the distinction of 'myoclonic dystonia'.

When myoclonus is rhythmic, it becomes important to distinguish it from *tremor*. The characteristic feature of the latter is that the movement is sinusoidal. Rhythmic myoclonus is more like a 'square wave', with an interval between each movement. It is worthwhile emphasizing that rhythmic myoclonus is usually due to co-contraction of muscles despite the subject's attempting to relax, whereas the rest tremor of Parkinson's disease and some forms of essential tremor are due to alternating contractions of agonists and antagonists. This is one example of where electrophysiological analysis of myoclonus may help in diagnosis, as is discussed later in this chapter.

THE HISTORY OF MYOCLONUS

The history of myoclonus is intertwined with that of epilepsy and most movement disorders (*Table 13.1*), and it is necessary to review a great deal of the history of neurology in order to understand how the various terms arose.

Epilepsy has been known since ancient times. It is not exactly clear when it first became apparent that patients with epilepsy could have occasional single jerks that were not directly connected with their seizures. Many different aspects of the disease were accurately described in the 19th century, and the jerks seen in epileptic patients were mentioned. In 1861, Reynolds[149] discussed the 'clonic spasm' of epileptics and described this as a common interictal phenomenon. Single or repetitive jerks as a manifestation of epilepsy were also recognized at about this time. In 1841 West[188] described what is now known as infantile spasms[89] and about half a century later, Kozhevnikov[99] described *epilepsia partialis continua*. All four reported patients had seizure disorders with associated periods of continuous repetitive clonic movements which sometimes progressed to a full seizure. Kozhevnikov believed that this repetitive clonus was a cortical phenomenon because of additional clinical signs of a hemiplegia, which he associated with damage to the cerebral cortex. It is of some interest to note that his 'report' is really only the abstract of a meeting and that it also included some of the discussion that followed his oral presentation. Many other physicians in the audience apparently had seen similar cases, and there were numerous subsequent reports by a variety of authors describing jerks as either ictal or interictal phenomena. In 1928, Muskens[133] stated that myoclonus was a 'fragment of epilepsy', and two years later, Hodskins and Yakovlev[79] noted the high incidence of jerking in patients with epilepsy. In 1945, Lennox[109] considered myoclonus part of the 'petit mal triad' and, ever since, jerks which might be called myoclonus have been recognized as a part of the syndrome of epilepsy.

Chorea is another movement disorder which has a very long history. The term chorea means dance and was applied initially to epidemics of dancing mania in the Middle Ages, in which large numbers of people danced together for days until they collapsed from exhaustion. Many such dances were described, but the most renowned was that of St Vitus, chorea Sancti Viti. As early as 1686, Sydenham[169] used this term to describe rheumatic chorea, and, since then the term has had a more specific meaning. About 200 years later, Huntington[83] described hereditary chorea and suggested that this movement disorder was identical to that described by Sydenham. However, the involuntary movements in these two conditions probably are not the same (this is only one example of how confusion can arise when superficially similar movements are given the same name).

The first possible description of an involuntary movement disorder which, in retrospect, might be called myoclonic was that of Dubini[37] in 1846. The condition

Table 13.1 History of myoclonus

Date	Author	Terminology	Reference
Ancient		Association with epilepsy	
(1686	Sydenham	Rheumatic chorea)	169
(1817	Parkinson	Paralysis agitans)	140
1822	Pritchard	Convulsive tremor	145
1841	West	Infantile spasms	188
1846	Dubini	Electric chorea	37
1861	Henoch	Electric chorea	75
1861	Reynolds	Clonic spasm in epilepsy	149
1862	Politzer	Palatal nystagmus	144
(1871	Hammond	Athetosis)	70
(1872	Huntington	Hereditary chorea)	83
(1878	Beard	Jumpers of Maine)	6
1880	Bergeron (Berland)	Electric chorea	7
1881	Friedreich	Paramyoclonus multiplex	44
1883	Lowenfeld	'Myoklonus'	117
(1885	Gilles de la Tourette	Tics with vocalization)	52
1890	Morvan	Fibrillary chorea	132
1891	Unverricht	Familial myoclonic epilepsy	176
1895	Koshewnikow	Epilepsia partialis continua	99
(1895	Schultze	'Myokymia')	154
1899	Rabot	Non-progressive myoclonic epilepsy	146
1903	Lundborg	Familial progressive myoclonic epilepsy	120
1911	Lafora and Glueck	Familial progressive myoclonic encephalopathy with inclusion bodies	105
1913	Sioli	Progressive myoclonic encephalopathy with lipoid inclusions	160
1919	Lhermitte	Segmental skeletal myoclonus	111
1920	Creutzfeldt	Spongiform encephalopathy	28
1921	Jakob		87
1921	Ramsay Hunt	Dyssynergia cerebellaris myoclonica	82
1928	Muskens	'A fragment of epilepsy'	133
1930	Hodskins and Yakovlev	Myoclonus in epilepsy, and sympathomatic myoclonus in myoclonic encephalopathies	79
1933	Lindenmulder	Familial essential myoclonus	115
1934	Dawson	Subacute sclerosing panencephalitis	30
(1938	Denny-Brown and Pennypacker	Fasciculation)	36
1938	Grinker	Epileptic discharges in the EEG	55
1945	Lennox	Myoclonic absences	109
1947	Dawson	Giant somato-sensory evoked potentials in myoclonus	31
1960	Lennox	Myoclonic-astatic epilepsy	110
1963	Lance and Adams	Post-hypoxic action myoclonus	107
1967	Halliday	Physiology of myoclonus	65
1971	Aicardi and Chevrie	Cryptogenic myoclonic epilepsy	2
1977	Lombroso and Fejerman	Benign infantile myoclonus	116

he described has sometimes been called spasmus Dubini, but Dubini himself called it *'electric chorea'*. The use of the term chorea should not come as a surprise since it was the only type of involuntary movement known at that time. Dubini described 38 cases of an acute febrile illness which included spasms of the neck and back with involuntary jerking movements. In retrospect, the illness was almost certainly an infection, perhaps meningitis or encephalitis, and the movements may well have been terminal convulsions, for about 90 per cent of the patients died. However, Dubini's description of involuntary movements was important to the concepts of the time. Recognition of quick involuntary movements in patients with infectious disease of the brain continued over the years. Such movements were described in diphtheria by Remak[148] (1881); in encephalitis by Walsh[186] (1920), Reimold[147] (1925) and Von Economo[185] (1929); in the disease described by Creutzfeld[28] (1920) and Jakob[87] (1921); and in subacute sclerosing panencephalitis (SSPE) by Dawson[30] (1934).

Another group of cases were classified under the term electric chorea during the mid-19th century. Henoch[75] described 30 otherwise normal children aged 9–15 years who had a chronic disorder characterized by multifocal repetitive (3–6 per min) sudden jerks, particularly of the neck and shoulders. Hennig[74] gave the name electric chorea to the cases described by Henoch. In 1880, Berland[7] described patients seen by his teacher, Bergeron, with a disorder of multifocal rapid muscle twitches which affected children between the ages of 7 and 14 years. The disorder, however, differed from that described by Henoch, for it was transient. Nevertheless, people tended to use the term electric chorea for both these disorders and to consider them the same disease. Although Bonduelle[10] has said that he finds this entity useful, most clinicians probably have never seen a case. It would seem that today many of these patients would be described as exhibiting tics (these will be discussed later). However, the definition of electric chorea became controversial: some writers compared the disorder to that which will subsequently be described as paramyoclonus multiplex. Confusion continued to grow and in 1907 Gowers described electric chorea as 'a peculiar malady that is met with chiefly in Lombardy and some adjacent parts of Italy'[54]. The authors believe that the term electric chorea is best not used.

Another disorder of quick involuntary movements, although distinct from that which would today be called myoclonus, was described in 1880 by Beard as the 'jumping Frenchman of Maine'[6]. Other apparently similar disorders were described, including Miryachit by Hammond[71]. Perhaps the cases of saltatoric spasm, which is a jumping movement of the legs which occurs only when standing (described by Bamberger[5] in 1859), were similar to such jumpers. The syndrome of excessive startle or *hyperekplexia* has been described by many others[50, 165, 167].

The term myoclonus was first used in a case report by Friedreich in 1881, when he described the syndrome of *paramyoclonus multiplex*[44]. The origin of the term is clear: *clonus* refers to a quick movement, *myo* to muscle, *para* to symmetrical (such as in paraplegia) and *multiplex* to the fact that there are multiple sites. The important point is that Friedreich wished to distinguish this type of involuntary movement, which he believed to originate in the spinal cord, from 'clonic spasm', which was thought at that time to come from the brain. Friedreich's patient was a comb-maker 50 years of age who was admitted to hospital with pneumonia but who also described a 5-year history of muscle jerking which was not sufficiently severe to prevent him from following his trade. The jerks affected virtually all muscles of the body except the face and occurred in different muscles at different times, i.e. the disorder was multifocal and not generalized. The jerks occurred frequently (10 to 50 per min) and were more prominent when the patient was at rest; they were accentuated by tactile or stretch stimuli and disappeared with voluntary movement and sleep. Intelligence was unaffected, there was no history of epilepsy and no family history, and there were no other significant neurological deficits. The disorder began after a fright. The patient died 5 years later and examination of the muscles and spinal cord at autopsy was said to be normal[153].

Following Friedreich's case report, there were a flurry of additional reports allegedly, but often inaccurately, describing similar patients. Lowenfeld[117] described a case in 1883 and thought the disorder should be termed simply 'myoklonus'. Seeligmüller[155] described another patient in 1886 and suggested that the disorder be called 'myoclonie'. His patient was a man of 24 years with multifocal body jerks who had developed involuntary movements and vocalizations at the age of 5 years, and had recently worsened in association with anxiety; he was successfully treated with galvanic current. Obviously this would now be called a case of the tic of Gilles de la Tourette. In 1891, Unverricht reviewed the literature, which then contained 40 case reports of paramyoclonus multiplex[176]. He rejected at least four fifths of them, ascribing the aetiology of the involuntary movement to other causes. Nevertheless, it became clear that there was a disorder of multifocal jerking without any other significant abnormality of the nervous system, perhaps best called *essential myoclonus*, and in 1933 Lindenmulder[115] described the first family with essential myoclonus.

Another series of case reports which had at one time been related to paramyoclonus multiplex were categorized as '*fibrillary chorea*'. In the 19th century, all small muscle twitches were referred to as fibrillations. The distinction between fibrillation and fasciculation was not made until the report of Denny-Brown and Pennypacker in 1938[36]. It is not clear when fibrillations themselves were first described, but their existence was certainly known at the time of the reports by Duchenne[38] and Aran[4] of progressive muscular atrophy in the middle of the 19th century, and that by Charcot[23] in 1869 of amyotrophic lateral sclerosis. In 1888, Kny[96] reported several cases under the name of 'myoclonus fibularis multiplex'. He seems to have been making an analogy to Freidreich's case, while noting that the myoclonic contractions were perhaps smaller in magnitude. Review of the original description in translation by Wilson suggests that he was describing amyotrophic lateral sclerosis; Kny may not have been aware of Charcot's earlier description. In 1890, Morvan[132] described five cases of 'fibrillary chorea'. These patients developed an acute illness, often progressing to death, which was characterized by muscle twitching, weakness, fatigue, sweating, fever and coma. The clinical description evokes a picture of some metabolic or toxic insult, perhaps uraemia. Schultze later introduced the term 'myokymia'[154] to describe a generalized rippling of muscles which presumably was due to frequent fasciculations. These patients were soon related to the cases of Kny and Morvan and, as noted above, to paramyoclonus multiplex. Schultze's cases now probably would be regarded as examples of Issacs' syndrome[84] or a similar disorder of continuous muscle activity. Although Bonduelle has suggested that this still is a useful category of myoclonus[10], there seems to be little substantial evidence for this.

Another disorder which used to be equated with paramyoclonus multiplex was *convulsive tremor*. The notion of convulsive tremor was discussed most extensively by Hammond[69,71] in the latter half of the last century. The original cases had been described by Pritchard[145], but seem to have been forgotten until Hammond described his own patients. Hammond, however did not accept most of Pritchard's cases as clear examples of convulsive tremor. The pure disorder apparently was characterized by the paroxysmal onset of severe generalized tremor which might be accompanied by sweating and fever and would last only for minutes. Hammond was at pains to separate it from epilepsy because of the lack of loss of consciousness. His descriptions seem quite different from those of Friedreich and others, yet Hammond[71] stressed that his cases of convulsive tremor were identical to those described under the rubric of paramyoclonus multiplex. The entity of convulsive tremor does not seem to be useful.

It is important to clarify the use of the term 'tic'. Apparently the word had been widely used in France for some centuries to describe habitual unpleasing gestures. The term preferred in England had been habit spasm, and that used in the United States was habit chorea[131]. A generalized tic disorder was first described in 1825 by Itard[85]. It was, however, the careful and complete description of Gilles de la Tourette in 1885 that established tic as a specific neurological disorder[52]. It is of some interest to note that he used the term 'tic convulsif' for his cases, relating this type of tic to epilepsy. In 1902, Meige and Feindel reviewed the entire subject of tic, defining the term as it is used today[129]. These authors suggested that adjectives such as 'convulsive' to describe the tic were not helpful.

Another seminal series of cases was described by Unverricht in 1891, who reported a family of two boys and eight girls half of whom were affected by myoclonic jerks and epilepsy with onset between the ages of 9 and 15 years[176]. Subsequently, the same author described a family of five children, three of whom were affected by jerks and epilepsy beginning between the ages of 13 and 15 years[177]. None of these patients with *familial myoclonic epilepsy* was demented. While the syndrome worsened with time, there was no rapid progression and the disorder was not fatal. In 1899, Rabot[146] also described a family with jerks and myoclonus in which the disorder clearly was not progressive. Lundborg[120] produced an important review of the literature and a classification of myoclonus in 1903. One class was symptomatic myoclonus, of which Dubini's disease was an obvious example. A second was that of essential myoclonus for which Friedreich had clearly described the first example. The third class was familial myoclonic epilepsy; this was divided into two groups, the non-progressive group of Rabot and the slowly progressive group described by Unverricht. Lundborg himself described 18 cases of myoclonus from 10 families in a peasant community in Sweden. Their illness was characterized by onset in late childhood or adolescence, no other neurological deficits besides myoclonus and epilepsy, long survival, and no progressive dementia. Siblings only were affected, and consanguinity was evident, suggesting autosomal recessive inheritance.

In 1911, Lafora and Glueck[105] described a boy aged 17 years, four of whose 14 brothers had died in infancy, who at the age of 14 had developed epilepsy followed by myoclonic jerking, rapidly progressive dementia, spasticity and visual disturbance. He died 22 months after the onset of the illness and, at autopsy, amyloid inclusion bodies were found throughout the nervous system. Despite the obvious difference between Lafora body disease, which became established as due to an autosomal recessive inheritance, and the familial myoclonic epilepsy of Unverricht and Lundborg, the two became equated and confused. In 1913, Sioli[160] described a case of rapidly progressive myoclonus, epilepsy and dementia with lipoid rather than amyloid inclusions, and this formed a second pathological substrate for this familial syndrome.

Another influential observation was that of Ramsay Hunt, who used the term *dyssynergia cerebellaris myoclonica* to describe six cases of myoclonus, four of whom also had epilepsy, in combination with a cerebellar tremor[82]; two of these patients had Friedreich's ataxia, but the pathology in the others was not known. Subsequently numerous similar cases of familial muscle jerking and epilepsy[137, 72, 184, 100, 101] associated with a variety of other progressive neurological abnormalities were described under the broad categories of 'storage diseases' or 'spinocerebellar degenerations'. It is important to separate these from cases of *essential myclonus* which, although familial, produces no epilepsy or other neurological abnormality. In addition, it is important to distinguish this syndrome, which could be called *symptomatic myoclonus* from the first entity reviewed above, which might be called *epileptic myoclonus*, even if the physiology of some of the myoclonic jerks may occasionally be similar.

Another important cause of symptomatic myoclonus was reported in 1963 by Lance and Adams[107], who described for the first time myoclonus resulting from an episode of cerebral hypoxia. One of the interesting features of this 'post-hypoxia myoclonus' was the worsening of jerking with voluntary action, which they called 'action myoclonus'. The same phenomenon had been described earlier by Wohlfart and Hook[191] in a case of familial myoclonic epilepsy, and subsequently has been reported in a number of other conditions.

Another disorder commonly included under the rubric of myoclonus, which can, however, usually be separated from the arrhythmic muscle jerks discussed so far, is that of rhythmic *segmental myoclonus*, in which the affected groups of muscles undergo rhythmical repetitive contractions, often continuing during sleep, at a rate of one to three per second. This disorder was first described in relation to rhythmical movements of the palate, and was called 'palatal nystagmus'; subsequently, however, the word nystagmus was rejected because of its association with the eyes. The original descriptions were those of Politzer[144], Kupper[104], Spencer[163] and Klien[95]. Later, Guillain and Mollaret described many cases with pathology[57, 58]. It soon become apparent, however, that palatal myoclonus often included other muscles in the body, and that, at times, such muscles could be affected even without the palate. Several further descriptions of segmental skeletal myoclonus followed these original reports[60, 111, 141].

Finally, myoclonus in normal subjects is a well recognized phenomenon. Jerking at night can be a normal physiological process and occurs in most people when first falling asleep; it also may occur when waking and at similar times during naps in the day ('hypnic jerks')[138]. Such *physiological myoclonus* has almost certainly been known for centuries, although perhaps it was described for the first time in print by DeLisi in 1932[34]. Symonds[170] reviewed the topic of 'nocturnal myoclonus', noting that jerking occurs in normal people and that patients with epilepsy often have an increased incidence of myoclonic jerks when falling asleep or when arising. He also noted that nocturnal myoclonus can be an independent abnormal phenomenon.

CLASSIFICATION OF MYOCLONUS

It is suggested that the classification of myoclonus should be approached in the same way as that of epilepsy. In neither disorder does a single classification suffice. Both myoclonus and epilepsy can be divided according to clinical type, aetiology, pathophysiology, and perhaps even anatomical, pharmacological and biochemical pathology. At present there is no great overlap between these different classifications for either myoclonus or epilepsy, but increased understanding should improve the situation.

The classification of myoclonus according to clinical type is based on two distinguishing features: (1) the myoclonus may be *arrythmic* or *rhythmic*, and (2) it may be *generalised* or *focal*. However, these clinical distinctions do not provide a useful separation between different aetiological and pathological entities; most cases of myoclonus may produce focal or generalized muscle jerks, or both, and many different conditions may cause irregular or rhythmical myoclonus.

The classification of myoclonus adopted here is based on aetiology. The major aetiological categories are physiological myoclonus, essential myoclonus, epileptic myoclonus and symptomatic myoclonus.

(1) *Physiological myoclonus* (normal subjects)
   (a) Sleep jerks (hypnic jerks)
   (b) Anxiety-induced
   (c) Exercise-induced
   (d) Hiccough
(2) *Essential myoclonus* (no other neurological deficit)
   (a) Familial essential myoclonus
   (b) Sporadic essential myoclonus
   (c) Periodic movements of sleep (nocturnal myoclonus)
(3) *Epileptic myoclonus* (seizures dominate and no encephalopathy, at least initially)
   (a) Fragments of epilepsy
      Isolated epileptic myoclonic jerks
      Epilepsia partialis continua
      Idiopathic stimulus-sensitive myoclonus
      Photosensitive myoclonus
      Myoclonic absences in petit mal

(b) Childhood myoclonic epilepsies
   Benign myoclonus of infancy
   Infantile spasms
   Myoclonic astatic epilepsy (Lennox-Gastaut)
   Cryptogenic myoclonic epilepsy (Aicardi)
(c) Benign familial myoclonic epilepsy (Rabot)
(4) *Symptomatic myoclonus* (progressive or static encephalopathy dominates)
   (a) Storage disease
      Lafora body disease
      Lipidoses, e.g. GM2 gangliosidosis (Tay-Sachs)
      Ceroid-lipofuscinosis (Batten)
      Sialidosis ('cherry-red spot')
   (b) Spinocerebellar degenerations
      Baltic myoclonus
      Ramsay Hunt syndrome
      Friedreich's ataxia
      Ataxia telangiectasia
   (c) Basal ganglia degenerations
      Wilson's disease
      Torsion dystonia
      Hallervorden-Spatz disease
      Progressive supranuclear palsy
      Huntington's disease
   (d) Dementias
      Creutzfeldt-Jakob disease
      Alzheimer's disease
   (e) Viral encephalopathies
      Subacute sclerosing panencephalitis
      Encephalitis lethargica
      Arbo virus encephalitis
      Herpes simplex encephalitis
      Post-infectious encephalitis
      Infantile polymyoclonus (neuroblastoma)
   (f) Metabolic encephalopathies
      Hepatic failure
      Renal failure
      Dialysis syndrome
      Hyponatraemia
      Hypoglycaemia
      Non-ketotic hyperglycaemia
   (g) Toxic encephalopathies
      Bismuth
      Heavy metal poisons
      Methyl bromide
      Drugs

(h) Physical encephalopathies
   Post-hypoxia (Lance-Adams)
   Post-traumatic
   Heat stroke
   Electric shock
   Decompression injury
(i) Focal CNS damage
   Post-stroke
   Post-thalamotomy
   Tumour
   Trauma

Physiological myoclonus occurs in normal people when falling asleep or waking (hypnic jerks), or when anxious; it also includes hiccough.

Essential myoclonus is abnormal, but its pathology is unknown. It may occur in patients with no other neurological abnormalities, as in hereditary essential myoclonus, or in those whose only other deficit is sleep disturbance, as in true nocturnal myoclonus. Both these entities will be discussed later.

Epileptic myoclonus occurs in patients whose main complaint is one of epilepsy but who also have myoclonus. They do not have obvious evidence of other cerebral disease, at least initially. This category of myoclonus will be discussed in detail later. As knowledge increases, many of these patients may well be identified as cases of symptomatic myoclonus.

Symptomatic myoclonus occurs as part of an obviously more widespread encephalopathy. Such patients may or may not have epilepsy as well; many do. However, both their epilepsy and their myoclonus are secondary to a known pathology, which may cause a *progressive myoclonic encephalopathy*, as in lipid storage diseases or spinocerebellar degenerations, or a *static myoclonic encephalopathy*, as after cerebral hypoxia or trauma. Many other groups of diseases are included in this category and it is important to recognize that they may cause obvious myoclonus, but it is not necessary to describe them in detail here. Discussion will be limited to a number of conditions in which myoclonus is a dominant or presenting feature; these include the Ramsay Hunt syndrome, the

Table 13.2 Incidence and natural history of myoclonus in 94 patients seen at the Mayo Clinic between 1945 and 1956

Category	Number	Dead (%)	Worse (%)	Same (%)	Better (%)
Essential myoclonus	19	7	0	71	22
Epileptic myoclonus	45	3	3	19	75
Symptomatic myoclonus	30	33	43	20	3

Data from Aigner and Mulder[3], who excluded patients with palatal myoclonus. Their groups I and IV are combined in this table and represent our category 'symptomatic myoclonus'. Their groups II and III represent our categories 'epileptic myoclonus' and 'essential myoclonus' respectively.

disease described by Unverricht and Lundborg, post-hypoxic myoclonus, palatal myoclonus and related syndromes, and spinal segmental myoclonus. *Table 13.2* gives some indication of the relative frequency of myclonus.

A number of conditions which are sometimes included in the rubric of myoclonus are better considered separately. Startle syndromes in particular, such as familial and sporadic hyperekplexias, including the 'jumpers of Maine'[165], are more conveniently dealt with amongst the group of paroxysmal movement disorders. These include paroxysmal kinesogenic choreoathetosis and paroxysmal dystonic choreoathetosis. They will not be discussed further; nor will the various types of myoclonus or opsoclonus that are confined to the eyes.

CLINICAL FEATURES OF CERTAIN TYPES OF MYOCLONUS
Essential myoclonus

As discussed earlier, Friedreich was probably the first to describe a sporadic example of this condition, which he called 'paramyoclonus multiplex'[44]. A number of cases that conform to the typical picture of the disease have been described since then, many with other affected family members. Aigner and Mulder[3] drew attention to the benign nature of essential myoclonus, which separated the condition from most of the other types they encountered.

Daube and Peters[29] described 12 typical cases in two families in which the condition was inherited as an autosomal dominant trait. Chaotic, arrhythmic jerks of the arms, neck, trunk and legs began between the ages of 1 and 20 years and persisted throughout life. The jerks were absent or reduced at rest and were increased on action. Despite their frequency and widespread distribution, the jerks were of relatively small amplitude and so produced remarkably little disability over many years. Otherwise the patients were normal; there was no other neurological deficit, intellect was normal, epilepsy did not occur and the EEG was unremarkable.

Mahloudji and Pikielny[122a] described another family of six affected members in two generations and reviewed the other families described in the literature up to that time[8, 29, 51, 115]. Lindenmulder[115] drew up the following criteria for the diagnosis of benign hereditary or familial essential myoclonus: (1) onset in the first or second decade of life; (2) males and females equally affected; (3) a benign course, often variable but compatible with active life of normal span; (4) dominant inheritance with variable severity; (5) absence of seizures, dementia, gross ataxia and other neurological deficits, and (6) a normal EEG. Other characteristics noted included a predeliction for the face, trunk and the proximal muscles of the limbs; the myoclonus could be generalized, confined to one side or even be segmental; it was absent during sleep and was aggravated by emotional stress.

Korten *et al.*[98] decribed another family in which 12 members were affected over two generations. Their report was of particular interest for two reasons. First, there was a remarkable association between typical essential tremor and myoclonus in this family; four of the patients with myoclonus also had essential tremor and seven other members of the family had benign essential tremor only. The authors concluded that 'there is an intrinsic relationship between essential tremor and essential myoclonus'. Their conclusion was supported by the observation that both the tremor and the myoclonus were improved by alcohol in this family; this had also been reported in another family with hereditary essential myoclonus[63]. Second, the myoclonus varied considerably from time to time; 'periods of virtually rhythmic discharges alternated with phases of asynchronous, dysrhythmic myoclonus complexes, alternating with bilateral synchronous complexes'[48]. Fahn and Singh[42] drew attention to another clinical manifestation of essential myoclonus, which they called 'oscillatory myoclonus', i.e. a tendency in some patients for the jerks to occur in bursts, often triggered by a movement but then settling down.

So far, attention has been directed towards familial examples of essential myoclonus, but in the authors' experience (more than 10 sporadic cases, but only two families), sporadic cases conforming in all respects to criteria for diagnosis are much more common.

Periodic movements in sleep (*nocturnal myoclonus*) can be considered as a type of essential myoclonus because it is non-progressive and is not associated with other neurological pathology. It should not be confused with sleep jerks (hypnic jerks), which are sudden and singular myoclonic jerks that occur on falling asleep[138], and are generalized (if the individual is lying down) or segmental, involving the neck (if sitting upright). In the authors' classification hypnic jerks are placed with physiological myoclonus.

In contrast to hypnic jerks, nocturnal myoclonus is characterized by repetitive jerking of the legs during sleep. First described by Symonds[170], this disorder was reviewed recently by Coleman *et al.*[25]. The periodic movements involve the legs and may be synchronous or asynchronous in the two limbs. The jerks occur during non-REM sleep approximately every 30 s and last 1.5–2.5 s. A bout can last several hours. Coleman and his colleagues recorded such nocturnal myoclonus in 53 (13 per cent) of 409 patients with sleep disorders. It was found in patients with excessive daytime drowsiness as well as in those with insomnia. They concluded that nocturnal myoclonus itself does not produce sleep disturbance but rather that these leg jerks appear in individuals with a chronic disturbance of daily sleep–waking patterns. Treatment of nocturnal myoclonus has not been satisfactory.

A variant of this syndrome occurs in individuals who also have symptoms of the restless leg syndrome. Boghen and Peyronnard[9] described a family with this combination of symptoms, in whom it was inherited as an autosomal dominant trait. It is likely that sporadic cases also exist but, judged by the paucity of such case reports, their numbers are few.

Epileptic myoclonus

Myoclonus often coexists with epilepsy; indeed, many forms of myoclonus may arise as the consequence of isolated spike discharges in motor cortex, which may be considered a fragment of epilepsy. It has been emphasized earlier that myoclonus and epilepsy may occur in certain symptomatic myoclonias as part of an encephalopathy of known pathology. Such pathology may be progressive, as in certain neuronal storage diseases, in which case the illness might be termed progressive myoclonic encephalopathy. Alternatively, the pathology may be static, as after cerebral hypoxia or trauma, when the condition may be called static myoclonic encephalopahy. Neither progressive nor static myoclonic encephalopathies will be considered here. Epileptic myoclonus occurs in certain syndromes in which epilepsy is the dominant feature. Epileptic myoclonus may be generalized, as in the common myoclonic epilepsies of childhood, or focal, as in epilepsia partialis continua.

The problem of generalized epileptic myoclonus is much commoner in children and adolescents than in adults. Terminology is very confused. The following practical classification according to age at onset of myoclonic jerks is based on that by Aicardi[1].

(1) First year of life
   (a) Benign myoclonus of infancy
   (b) Infantile spasms
   (c) (Cryptogenic myoclonic epilepsy)
(2) Second to sixth year of life
   (a) Myoclonic astatic epilepsy (Lennox-Gastaut)
   (b) Cryptogenic myoclonic epilepsy (Aicardi)
   (c) Intermediate forms
(3) Older children and adolescents
   (a) Photosensitive epileptic myoclonus
   (b) Myoclonic absences
   (c) Primary generalized epilepsy

Many of the conditions listed are well-known and need not be considered in detail. Some, however, are less recognized and require further description.

Little needs to be said about *infantile spasms*. The common flexor (and rare extensor) myoclonic jerks are quite distinctive, the EEG is characteristic and the generally poor prognosis for mental development is established. Spasms nearly always start before 9 months of age, and always before 1 year. Lombroso and Fejerman[116] noted that in some babies with repetitive jerks which look like infantile spasms the EEG may be normal and the course of the illness benign. They suggested the term *benign myoclonus of early infancy* for this condition to distinguish such babies from those in whom myoclonus is symptomatic of an underlying perinatal cerebral pathology, such as that due to congenital malformation, haemorrhage or anoxia, all of which may provoke an *infantile myoclonic encephalopathy*. The onset of typical spasms after the age of 1 year indicates *myoclonic astatic epilepsy*, which has become known as the Lennox-Gastaut syndrome.

Lennox[110] originally described cessation of motion as 'akinetic', loss of posture as 'astatic', and loss of tone as 'atonic'. He described a typical patient as 'an overactive child having myoclonic jerks, drop seizures and periods of brief immobility (such as accompany a slow spike wave discharge), together with progressive mental decay. The only other finding that might be added to this excellent description is one of frequent facial and dental injuries which these children sustain and which Lennox himself recognized. The attacks are very frequent and may occur in the form of massive jerks causing a fall, sudden collapse of muscular tone also causing a fall, less severe head-nods or sagging at the knees, 'absence' attacks with blinking of the eyes, and tonic-clonic fits, commonly at night. The children may go into 'absence' status. Their attacks are very resistant to drug therapy and most patients are or become mentally retarded. Unfortunately, the fact that such children also have brief periods of immobility resembling the typical 'absence' of true petit mal led some authors to add the term 'petit mal' to 'myoclonic astatic', particularly since atypical slow spike wave discharged were found in the EEG of such children. Gastaut et al.[49] then described 'childhood epileptic encephalopathy with diffuse slow spike waves (otherwise known as "petit mal variant" or Lennox syndrome)', and Niedermeyer[134] suggested the name 'Lennox-Gastaut syndrome'. Unfortunately, however, the use of this term was gradually extended to include all forms of epilepsy with generalized slow (2 per second) spike wave EEG discharges, which are associated with atonic absences, myoclonic jerks and tonic seizures, especially at night. Such children, who present usually in the second to sixth year of life, 'are of major important to paediatricians; . . . [they] frequently fall during the day and wear helmets to protect their heads, . . . [and] are so resistant to conventional anticonvulsant drugs'[1]. The inclusion of all such children in a single diagnostic category, the Lennox-Gastaut syndrome, led to clinical confusion. While a large proportion of those conforming to the broad criteria for the Lennox-Gastaut syndrome were or became mentally retarded, many such children developed normally. Aicardi and Chevrie[2] were able to identify a group of young children with the following characteristics: '(1) massive myoclonic jerks as the only or main seizure type; (2) bursts of bilateral irregular spike-waves at a rhythm of 2.5 per second or more accompanying the myoclonias; (3) no signs of organic brain damage antecedent to the first seizure; (4) absence of tonic seizures during both wakefulness and sleep (the latter is difficult to ascertain in every patient)'[1]. These patients were said to exhibit *cryptogenic myoclonic epilepsy*. Their first seizure occurred between 3 months and 9 years of age, usually around 2 years; myoclonus appeared around 2½ to 3 years of age and slow spike wave discharges in the EEG usually around 4 years of age. As in the syndrome described by Lennox, presenting features were falls, head-nods and tonic fits; but whereas most children with Lennox's syndrome continued to have fits and over 90 per cent developed mental retardation, in close to 50 per cent of those with cryptogenic myoclonic epilepsy the seizures ceased and over a third remained mentally normal. Because of these prognostic differences it seems practical and sensible to make a distinction between myoclonic astatic epilepsy, the term preferred by the authors for the Lennox-Gastaut syndrome, and cryptogenic myoclonic epilepsy. However, the distinction is not clear-cut, and transitional forms between the two entities are often encountered.

Epileptic myoclonus with onset in childhood after the age of about six years or in adolescence is generally of less serious import. A small proportion of those with petit mal and typical spike wave discharges at a frequency of three per second may have *myoclonic absences*. During such attacks the child may jerk rhythmically (three times a second), each jerk being related to the spike of a spike-and-wave complex; as the attack proceeds, the arms may flex and rise, but consciousness returns as soon as the attack ceases[173]. *Photosensitive myoclonic epilepsy* is elicited by intermittent photic stimulation which provokes generalized spike wave or polyspike-wave discharges at the rate of three per second, which also occur spontaneously in the resting EEG. Such paroxysms are accompanied by either brief absences or absence attacks with eyelid myoclonia resembling rapid blinking and upward deviation of the eyes; in this respect the condition differs from the typical absence attack of petit mal, in which the eyelids flutter and the eyes stare straight ahead. Alternatively, such spontaneous or photically induced paroxysms may be associated with myoclonic jerking of the arms[90, 91].

Many older children and adolescents presenting with idiopathic generalized, often nocturnal, tonic seizures may also describe myoclonus. The latter commonly occurs at breakfast time, within half an hour or waking, and is limited to the arms, hence the colloquial description 'the flying saucer syndrome'. Such early morning myoclonus commonly precedes daytime seizures. The EEG may show generalized spike wave or polyspike wave discharges but these are not due to photosensitivity; often, however, the EEG is normal. Such morning myoclonus tends to improve with maturity along with improvement of the generalized seizures. In a proportion of adults with epilepsy, however, morning myoclonic jerks continue to be a problem. It is this type of myoclonus that has been noted so frequently as an interictal phenomenon in idiopathic primary generalized epilepsy[133, 149, 171]; myoclonic jerks occur in about a quarter of such patients, usually between grand mal episodes, but often prefacing these major attacks.

An indication of the frequency of the different types of epileptic myoclonus in relation to that of symptomatic myoclonus is given in *Table 13.3*; the data are based on the experience of Aicardi with 145 such children seen over 10 years[1]. The relatively low incidence of myoclonus associated with primary generalized epilepsy reflects that author's great expertise in the field, but the relative frequency of cryptogenic myoclonic epilepsy, and of unclassifiable types, is notable.

Table 13.3 Frequency of different types of myoclonus, both epileptic and symptomatic, amongst 145 children with prominent myoclonus and epilepsy (From Aicardi[1], courtesy of the Editor and Publishers, *Research and Clinical Forums*)

	Number	Mean age at first fit
Epileptic myoclonus		
Myoclonic astatic epilepsy	19	3.1 years
Cryptogenic myoclonic epilepsy	55	2.8 years
Intermediate or unclassified forms	31	4.5 years
Primary generalized epilepsy	8	>10 years
Symptomatic myoclonus		
Progressive myoclonic encephalopathies	11	4.7 years
Static myoclonic encephalopathies	21	1.9 years
Total	145	

Amongst the epileptic myoclonias, *epilepsia partialis continua* must also be considered. First described by Kozhevnikov in 1895[99], this form of epileptic myoclonus has subsequently been described in may different conditions. Kozhevnikov himself suggested that the condition could be due to focal cortical encephalitis, a hypothesis that received confirmation from the study of serial cortical biopsy specimens some 30 years later[139]. It is now known that it can occur with abscess, granuloma, tumour, trauma, demyelination, haemorrhage or infarction affecting not only the cerebral cortex but also subcortical areas alone or in combination[93, 103, 174]. The syndrome has been defined as 'regular or irregular clonic muscular twitches affecting a limited part of the body, occurring for a minimum of one hour, and recurring at intervals of no more than ten seconds'[174]. The extent of the repetitive twitching may vary from movements of a single muscle group to jerking of the whole of one side of the body. As in the case of focal epilepsy, the hand is affected most frequently. Jerking may occur once every several seconds or be almost continuous. The frequency, distribution and intensity of epilepsia partialis continua vary from moment to moment and from day to day. Sometimes the repetitive jerks spread to cause a typical Jacksonian motor seizure, which may become generalized to produce a grand mal fit. Epilepsia partialis continua may continue for a few hours, or may persist for weeks, months or even years. Most patients also exhibit neurological signs appropriate to the pathological cause of the condition. Usually these include a degree of muscle weakness and hyperreflexia in the affected segments. The surface EEG usually is abnormal, but occasionally electrocorticography may be required to detect the discharge over the motor cortex that is responsible for the myoclonus. Surface EEG abnormalities consist equally of focal slow waves or spike/sharp waves. Radiological studies, including computerized axial tomography (CT scan), usually establish the nature and location of the responsible lesion, but in some patients this remains a mystery. Treatment is frequently difficult. Although the condition often remits spontaneously, the outcome cannot be predicted, and the response to anticonvulsant drugs usually is unsatisfactory. Occasionally it may prove necessary to resort to surgical excision to provide relief.

Familial progressive myoclonus epilepsy, described by Unverricht[176, 177] and Lundborg[120], has been considered to be the typical familial epileptic myoclonus, but as indicated earlier, great confusion has surrounded this entity. Unverricht originally described eight patients in two families who developed grand mal fits between the ages of 9 and 15 years; myoclonus developed later. Lundborg described 18 patients from 10 families in Sweden with a similar disease; however, his patients went on to develop ataxia and a degree of dementia. Definitive pathology was not available to either of these authors so that when Lafora and Glueck[105] described the presence of inclusion bodies in similar cases, it was assumed that all patients with progressive myoclonus epilepsy might have such pathology. Subsequently it was discovered that this syndrome might be produced by a number of different pathologies[126, 187]. Watson and Denny-Brown[187], from their own experience and from a review of the literature, were able to conclude that progressive myoclonus epilepsy was not a disease in its own right but a symptom complex that could be produced by a variety of diffuse neuronal insults to the central nervous system. It is now realized that these include (1) Lafora body disease, (2) lipoid storage diseases such as GM2 gangliosidosis (of which Tay-Sachs disease is the archetype) and (3) cerebellar degenerations, typically characterized by loss of Purkinje cells. The type of familial epileptic myoclonus described in Scandinavia by Unverricht and Lundborg, and recently christened 'Baltic myoclonus' by Eldridge et al.[39], falls into the latter category. There have been several other reports of this disorder[72,184], the most recent being that of Koskiniemi et al.[100,101] who reviewed the clinical picture and progression of the disease in 93 cases in Finland. The condition was familial in 25 out of 67 kinships, the pattern of inheritance suggesting an autosomal recessive trait. Although the illness began with myoclonus or epilepsy in roughly equal proportions, nearly all patients subsequently developed cerebellar ataxia, and about a quarter developed spasticity, intellect was not greatly affected. A thorough neuropathological study was made in one of these cases, and some material was available in five others. The most striking finding was loss of Purkinje cells without evidence of any inclusion bodies or other storage material. In their review of Baltic myoclonus, Eldridge et al.[39] also reported a discrete loss of Purkinje cells without inclusion bodies in those cases where pathology was available. In the light of this evidence, it would seem that the 'familial myoclonus epilepsy' described by Unverricht and Lundborg should properly be included amongst the symptomatic myoclonias, in particular in the category of symptomatic myoclonias associated with degeneration of the cerebellum, as in the Ramsay Hunt syndrome. However, there may be a very rare category of benign non-progressive epileptic myoclonus without cerebellar ataxia or dementia, as described by Rabot[146], which could properly be included amongst the epileptic myoclonias. As yet the authors have not encountered an example.

Symptomatic myoclonus

Spinocerebellar degenerations

BALTIC MYOCLONUS
The reasons for including progressive familial myoclonus here have been outlined above. Patients present with myoclonus and/or epilepsy between the ages of about 7 and 12 years[39,100,101]. The myoclonus typically is provoked by external stimuli such as light, noise or touch, and occurs on attempted movement. The fits usually are of grand mal type, but drop attacks and absences also occur. The EEG shows generalized spike and wave paroxysms and obvious photosensitivity. As the disease progresses, ataxia of gait, intention tremor and dysarthria inevitably develop, and in about a quarter of patients spasticity develops with hyperactivity of tendon reflexes. The physical disabilities lead to social isolation and educational impoverishment so that the sufferers tend to be emotionally immature and intellectually deprived, but they do not become frankly demented. In the final stages of the illness the patients are bedridden, with such severe action and stimulus-sensitive myoclonus that they are unable to care for themselves; speech is severely dysarthric

and swallowing may be difficult. Death may occur between 5 and 20 years after the onset of the illness. The most striking pathological change on thorough neuropathological examination is loss of Purkinje cells in the cerebellum. In cases where family history was available, the disease was confined to siblings and consanguinity occurred in some families; autosomal recessive inheritance therefore seems likely.

RAMSAY HUNT SYNDROME
In contrast to Baltic myoclonus, in which cerebellar ataxia develops after the myoclonus and fits and in which loss of Purkinje cell is found at autopsy, myoclonus may also develop in association with a known spinocerebellar degeneration with a different pathology.

In 1921, Ramsay Hunt, described six patients with cerebellar ataxia and myoclonus under the term 'dyssynergia cerebellaris myoclonica'[82]. These patients differed from others which he had reported under the term 'dyssynergia cerebellaris progressiva'[81], because they had myoclonus as well as cerebellar tremor. In spite of these differences Ramsay Hunt considered these patients as one group because they had the combination of two disorders, myoclonic epilepsy and cerebellar degeneration. Hence, from the outset this disorder was defined as a syndrome rather than a specific clinical entity, although this fact has tended to be forgotten by many authors.

Four of Ramsay Hunt's patients were sporadic cases, without pathology, which he believed to be mixtures of dyssynergia cerebellaris progressiva and the myoclonic epilepsy of Unverricht. The other two patients were twins with a syndrome of Friedreich's ataxia associated with myoclonic epilepsy. A similar case had been seen by Boschi in 1913[11]. All of the patients had a slowly progressive severe, coarse intention tremor and independent myoclonus of the limbs which was also brought out by voluntary movement. Although the patients were said to have had myoclonic epilepsy, in two of the six cases there was no history of fits. One of the patients with Friedreich's ataxia died and findings at autopsy were those of typical Friedreich's ataxia with marked atrophy of the dentate nucleus. This was the only post-mortem examination available to Ramsay Hunt in all of his cases of dyssynergia cerebellaris progressiva and dyssynergia cerebellaris myoclonica: he speculated that the atrophy of the dentate nucleus was responsible for the severe intention tremor of the limbs in both disorders, and possibly also for the myoclonus.

A number of other cases with similar clinical features have been reported over the years, and a general clinical picture emerges. The initial symptoms occur in the first or second decade of life and are slowly progressive. The first manifestations are those of intention tremor and dysarthria; myoclonus usually is a later feature, and progressive ataxia develops. Epilepsy, while common, is not always present. The myoclonus may be present at rest but often appears, or is made worse, by attempted action, and can be quite violent; it can throw patients to the floor from a sitting position. The myoclonus is also said to be able to move the arm in the opposite direction to that which is desired, a phenomenon called 'myoclonies oppositionistes'. The combination of such severe action myoclonus and ataxia may eventually cause great disability.

Wohlfart and Hook[191], in a report of 10 cases, for the first time emphasized the fact that the myoclonus was brought out prominently by intention, and coined the term 'action myoclonias'. They noted that it was difficult to separate coarse cerebellar tremors from myoclonus, an important fact to be kept in mind when reading the literature critically. Other clinical features have been associated with the myoclonus and cerebellar ataxia in some of the cases, including a mitochondrial myopathy[46], polyneuropathy and pes cavus[66], peroneal muscular atrophy[162], and deafness[128]. Numerous families have been reported with this combination of cerebellar degeneration and myoclonic epilepsy; the genetic trait seems to be autosomal dominant in some[51, 86, 102] and autosomal recessive in others[128, 136, 193].

Post-mortem examinations have not provided a consistent pathology. Many patients have not had lesions of the dentate nucleus[13, 171], and there can be lesions of the dentate without myoclonus[10]. Christophe and Gruner[24] have noted the confusing situation in which patients with myoclonic epilepsy, but no clinical evidence of a cerebellar degeneration, can show the pathological changes of Friedreich's ataxia at autopsy. To add to the confusion, cerebellar signs may be present in patients with epilepsy of any type[79], and this, of course, also makes clinical classification difficult.

Post-hypoxic myoclonus

The syndrome of post-hypoxic myoclonus was first described in detail by Lance and Adams in 1963[107], and is often called the Lance-Adams syndrome; other cases, however, had been reported earlier[27, 48, 73, 168, 179]. Lance and Adams described four patients with chronic 'intention' or 'action' myoclonus resulting from a period of hypoxia. One of their patients had suffered the syndrome for 8 years. Myoclonic jerks occurred in isolation or in a repetitive pattern, and were induced by attempts at voluntary movements or by some types of sensory stimuli. The authors noted that the term 'action myoclonia' had been used by Wohlfart and Hook[191] to describe the myoclonus in some patients with the Ramsay Hunt syndrome.

The action myoclonus in these post-hypoxic patients was associated with a cerebellar abnormality, as evidenced by the presence of dysarthria, gait ataxia and intention tremor, which the authors felt they could separate from the action myoclonus itself. Their patients also experienced occasional grand mal seizures.

The myoclonic jerks were associated with a brief electromyographic discharge and were usually followed by a silent period or pause in the continuing electromyographic activity. The pauses were felt to be as significant features as the myoclonic jerks themselves and were felt to be responsible for postural lapses, including falling when attempting to walk. The myoclonic jerks were associated with spikes in the electroencephalogram, and the silent periods with slow waves which followed the spikes. Often, in a repetitive series of myoclonic jerks, the jerks grew progressively larger, with a corresponding increase in the amplitude of the EEG spikes, and this was termed an 'augmenting series'.

The authors speculated that the physiology of the myoclonus might be related to an abnormal discharge arising in thalamus or the dentatothalamic pathway because of the similarity of the augmenting series of myoclonic jerks to the 'augmenting response' which can be obtained by stimulation of the thalamus. This theory has not been supported by subsequent observations which have shown that thalamotomy does not benefit patients with this syndrome[40]; stereotaxic recordings have demonstrated that activity in the thalamus follows discharges in the motor cortex and that stimulation of the thalamus does not cause the myoclonus[113].

Fahn[40] reviewed the clinical features of 57 cases of chronic post-hypoxic myoclonus which had been reported in the literature up till that time, and reported two additional cases. The period of anoxia which preceded the development of the syndrome lasted from 1 to 16 days. The patients usually had seizures and myoclonus in the acute stage, but this was not necessarily witnessed by the observer. Affected muscles included those of the face, which interfered with speech, and of the pharynx, which might interfere with swallowing. No spontaneous remissions of the chronic disorder have been reported, and in one case the syndrome appears to have lasted for at least 44 years. In one of the new cases reported by Fahn, there was diurnal fluctuation in the intensity of the myoclonus.

Chronic myoclonus with clinical features similar to those of chronic post-hypoxic myoclonus can also be seen after heat trauma[20, 183] and heat stroke (unpublished observations).

The syndrome of chronic post-hypoxic myoclonus should be differentiated from the myoclonus which can appear as the acute effect of cerebral hypoxia when the patient is in, or recovering from, coma. This type of myoclonus, which is frequently transient, has not been studied in as much detail as the chronic post-hypoxic myoclonus. It is often generalized and rhythmic, or at least pseudoperiodic[14, 168, 192], and can also be stimulus-sensitive[135]. Obviously, the feature of production by intention cannot be assessed since the patients are in coma or are uncooperative at this stage of their recovery.

Following the demonstration of successful therapy of this syndrome with 5-hydroxytryptophan (5-HTP)[112, 114], there has been considerable interest in the analysis of serotonin (5-HT) metabolism in this disorder. Reduction in cerebrospinal fluid levels of 5-hydroxyindoleacetic acid (5-HIAA), the principal metabolite of serotonin, in patients with this condition was originally described by Guilleminault et al.[61], and similar observations were made by Chadwick et al.[20], Van Woert et al.[182] and Richardson et al.[150]. Successful therapy with 5-HTP or clonazepam leads to elevation of the concentration of 5-HIAA in cerebrospinal fluid.

There have been several reports of pathological examinations of the brain in patients demonstrating the syndrome of post-hypoxic myoclonus. Castaigne et al.[16] emphasized changes in the subthalamic nucleus, the thalamus and the tegmentum of the brain stem. The case reported by Richardson et al.[150] showed neuronal loss and increase of astrocytes in the midbrain periaqueductal grey region and the dorsolateral grey of the tegmentum. Cooper et al.[26] reported some pathological changes in the dentate nucleus in a cerebellar biopsy from a patient with post-hypoxic myoclonus, but neither Castaigne et al. nor Richardson et al. found significant pathology in the dentate. Chadwick et al.[21] reported two cases with widespread damage similar to that seen in the large number of reported cases with post-hypoxic encephalopathy without the feature of post-hypoxic myoclonus. The latter authors also studied the levels of 5-HT and 5-HIAA in cortex and striatum, but no abnormal changes were identified. In addition, they looked for selective damage of the serotonin-containing nerve cells in the dorsal raphe of the brain stem but could find none.

The exciting feature about post-hypoxic myoclonus has been its positive reponse to medical therapy. Lance and Adams[107] originally noted that the myoclonus could be suppressed with high doses of barbiturates, but the patients were made too sleepy for this regimen to be useful. Diazepam also gave some benefit, but the response was still incomplete[106]. Dramatically successful therapy with 5-HTP was first reported by Lhermitte et al.[112, 114] and subsequently confirmed by many other investigators[18, 19, 20, 32, 33, 61, 180, 181, 182,]. Van Woert and Sethy[180] and Chadwick et al.[18] suggested using the levorotatory form of 5-HTP together with carbidopa in order to prevent the extracerebral metabolism of 5-HTP to 5-HT, thereby reducing some of the peripheral side effects of the treatment. Subsequently, other drugs have been reported to be of value in some cases, including carbamazepine[78], levodopa[130], clonazepam[12, 19, 20, 53], valproate[40], and oestrogens[40].

Focal and segmental myoclonus

Focal and segmental myoclonias deserve special consideration because they present as unique clinical syndromes, different in many ways from generalized myoclonias, irrespective of their aetiology. Also, they shed some light on anatomical localization. The focal and segmental myoclonias can present either as rhythmic or arrhythmic jerks and, as a general rule, they fall in the realm of symptomatic myoclonus. Whether they can ever be the initial or sole feature of essential myoclonus will be discussed later.

Undoubtedly, the best known of the focal and segmental myoclonias is *palatal myoclonus*. Described more than 100 years ago, its early history was reviewed by Guillain[56], and its anatomical pathology by Guillain et al.[57, 58, 59]. Throughout its long history there have been repeated discussions on the proper terminology of this condition, i.e. whether it is a true myoclonus, a type of tremor, or even a form of nystagmus. Guillain himself dismissed any relationship with nystagmus, the term used by Spencer[163] in 1886. The characteristics of the muscle jerks and the fact that synchronous contractions occur elsewhere, for example in the ocular and limb muscles[172], establish the disorder as one of myoclonus.

Guillain[56], almost 50 years ago, pointed out the following characteristics of the condition: (1) palatal myoclonus may be bilateral or unilateral; (2) the contractions are synchronous and rhythmic; (3) they may be associated with contractions of external ocular muscles, and those of larynx, neck, diaphragm, trunk and limbs; (4) the contractions occur at an average rate of 120–130 per minute, with a range of 80–180 per minute; (5) they do not cease during sleep; (6) they disappear after damage to the corticobulbar or corticospinal motoneuron pathways; (7) there is hypertrophic degeneration of the contralateral inferior olive.

Recently, Jacobs et al.[88] described two exceptions to this general clinical concept of palatal myoclonus: one of their patients had absence of myoclonus during sleep and another lost the palatal myoclonus after 2 years' duration, without recurrence over the next 5 years. The antecedent history of these two patients, however, was exceptional; the first patient was 19 years of age, with onset of palatal myoclonus after head trauma; the second patient, a girl, was 7 years old at the time of onset, which was 18 months after an ill-defined infectious illness.

Palatal myoclonus is one of the commonest types of specific myoclonic syndromes encountered in neurological practice. In the series of 67 patients with myoclonus of various types seen at Johns Hopkins Hospital, palatal myoclonus accounted for 10[168]. Only acute generalized myoclonus from encephalitis (14 cases) was more common.

The cause of most cases of palatal myoclonus is cerebrovascular disease. Of the ten cases in the series by Swanson *et al.*, seven were the result of a brainstem stroke[168]. The other three cases included one each of multiple sclerosis and encephalitis, and one of unknown aetiology. In the series of 17 cases of palatal myoclonus reported by Herrmann and Brown[77], seven were the result of brainstem infarction and four others had brainstem tumours. The remaining six cases consisted of one each of the following: brainstem trauma, multiple sclerosis, obstructive hydrocephalus, association with hereditary tremor, idiopathic olivary degeneration, and one of unknown cause. Recently, a patient with palatal myoclonus associated with dialysis encephalopathy has been reported[164].

The pathological lesion responsible for palatal myoclonus has been claimed to be in the so-called Guillain-Mollaret triangle, an area including the red nucleus, the inferior olivary nucleus, the dentate nucleus and their connecting pathways, particularly the central tegmental tract and the dentato-olivary pathway. Lapresle[108] pointed out that a lesion of the dentato-olivary pathway causes transsynaptic hypertrophic degeneration of the olives, a phenomenon well described by many workers. He reviewed studies of others and his own, indicating that this pathway travels from the dentate nucleus through the superior cerebellar peduncle, decussating to the opposite side, and then along the internal and dorsal surface of the red nucleus to merge with the central tegmental tract at that level and to eventually innervate the inferior olivary nucleus. This view fits with the observations of Jellinger[92], who reported 29 cases of hypertrophy of the inferior olives seen at autopsy. Except for one case, all were associated with a lesion of the dentato-olivary pathway. Of interest clinically was the fact that palatal myoclonus had been described in only two patients in this series.

In their review of the literature, Matsuo and Ajax[127] reported a median interval between the precipitating cause and the time that palatal myoclonus was recognized of between 10 and 11 months. Based on this finding they proposed that development of denervation supersensitivity in the inferior olives, with subsequent spontaneous rhythmic firing of these neurons, causes palatal myoclonus. It is difficult to understand how the concept of supersensitivity is compatible with olivary hypertrophic degeneration seen on pathological examination. Furthermore, it is to be anticipated that denervation supersensitivity, analogous to that proposed in the striatum in Parkinson's disease, would be most compatible with decreased function due to absence of the neurotransmitter. Increased firing rates could occur only from facilitatory afferents not affected by the primary lesion, and not from increased function of the supersensitive receptors. In fact, supersensitive receptors reflect decreased receptor activation, which is why they become supersensitive in the first place. It is therefore difficult to understand how supersensitivity itself can have any bearing on the phenomenon of palatal myoclonus, even if supersensitive receptors do develop in this disorder.

At least two patients with palatal myoclonus have responded to treatment with 5-hydroxytryptophan, the precursor of serotonin[121, 189] but the relationship to involvement of serotonergic pathways is not clear. There has also been one report of a patient with palatal myoclonus responding to carbamazepine[152].

Rhythmical myoclonus in the segmental region of the head and neck has been described in some cases in which palatal myoclonus was absent. Denny-Brown[35] mentioned a case of 'bulbar myoclonus' in a patient with Creutzfeldt-Jakob disease, Troupin and Kamm[175] described a patient who developed transient lingual myoclonus following head trauma and Fahn and Singh[41] described a patient with rhythmical myoclonic contractions (at a frequency of two per second) of the neck, arms and upper torso. This young man had a lifelong porencephalic cyst of the left hemisphere. The myoclonus was completely controlled with 5-hydroxytryptophan.

Focal and segmental myoclonus, both rhythmic and arrhythmic, occurs in other somatotopic areas besides the head and neck. Segmental myoclonus from spinal cord pathology has been well described in man. Of the 67 cases reported by Swanson et al.[168], seven had *spinal myoclonus*; there were two cases with involvement of one arm, one with arm plus abdomen, two with one leg, and two with both legs.

With lesions in the spinal cord, rhythmic segmental myoclonus is more common than the arrhythmic type. Recent examples of rhythmic spinal myoclonus have been reported following infection[76, 80, 161], degenerative disease of the cord[80, 159], tumour[47], myelopathy from cervical osteoarthritis[80] and demyelinating disease[97]. Arrhythmic myoclonus has been seen with infection[15], motor neuron disease[43] and following spinal anaesthesia[45].

Experimentally, rhythmical myoclonus has been produced in animals. Luttrell and Bang[119] caused both generalized and segmental rhythmical myoclonus in cats and kittens inoculated with Newcastle disease virus. Application of penicillin to spinal cord of rats and cats also has caused the development of segmental myoclonus[94, 118]. Although the myoclonus was not absolutely rhythmical, contractions occurred frequently at intervals of 2 to 20 seconds.

The presence of rhythmicity of focal and segmental myoclonus in man may be important in terms of aetiology. Rhythmic focal and segmental myoclonus always seems to be associated with structural pathology. Although the arrhythmic, chaotic type can also be the result of structural pathology, in some cases arrhythmic segmental myoclonus may represent a non-generalized form of essential myoclonus. One of the authors has seen several patients with arrhythmic focal and segmental myoclonus in whom no other neurological findings and no laboratory abnormalities were present. There was no antecedent history of possible injury to the spinal cord, and no progression of myoclonic symptoms. These patients showed a dramatic response to clonazepam therapy. At the moment, it seems reasonable to consider the possibility of essential myoclonus in such patients.

PATHOPHYSIOLOGY OF MYOCLONUS

In discussing the classification of myoclonus, it was pointed out that aetiology and pathophysiology often do not coincide. However, there are striking differences between the pathophysiology of essential myoclonus, many forms of epileptic myoclonus and symptomatic myoclonus, all of which must be considered separately. Surprisingly little is known about physiological myoclonus, which will not be discussed further. (The review presented here is based on a lecture[122b] given to the British branch of the International League Against Epilepsy in Oxford, November 1979, and published in full elsewhere. The authors are grateful to the Editor and Publishers of *Research and Clinical Forums* for permission to reproduce freely from that work.)

In his seminal review of 1967, Halliday[65] divided myoclonus into three major categories on the grounds of their electrophysiological correlates: pyramidal, extrapyramidal and segmental myoclonus.

Pyramidal myoclonus consisted of jerking due to a brief burst of action potentials in the electromyogram (EMG) from the active muscles, usually associated with some cortical event related in time to the discharge in the muscle. Because of the very short interval (about 15–40 ms) between the discharge in the EEG and the EMG burst in the jerking muscle Halliday[65, 66] considered that the myoclonus was due to a discharge in the cerebral cortex being propagated by pyramidal pathways to muscle, resulting in fast pyramidal myoclonus.

He contrasted this with the second type, *extrapyramidal myoclonus*, in which the cortical events were sometimes less obvious. The critical feature was the prolonged duration of the muscle EMG burst causing this type of myoclonic jerk. An example of extrapyramidal myoclonus occurs in subacute sclerosing panencephalitis (SSPE), where the actual jerks are appreciably long on clinical observation – the 'hung-up' myoclonic jerk of SSPE. *Figure 13.1* shows the prolonged EMG activity occurring in the right sternomastoid muscle associated with a cortical event in the EEG of a patient with SSPE. In view of the long duration of the EMG burst, and the fact that the cortical event was not invariably time-locked to the muscle event, Halliday considered that this might be myoclonus arising in some extrapyramidal site, hence the term extrapyramidal myoclonus. At that time, he also included under this heading a number of other forms of muscle jerking with prolonged bursts of action potentials in the EMG. However, most of these have now been discarded, for they are examples of extrapyramidal basal ganglia movement disorders, not myoclonus.

The third type of myoclonus described by Halliday, *segmental myoclonus*, was local myoclonus arising as a result of damage to the spinal cord or brainstem, such as the repetitive myoclonic jerking which can occur in one arm or leg as a result of spinal cord trauma, cord tumours or even virus infections. A similar event can occur in brainstem innervated muscles. *Figure 13.2* shows an example of segmental myoclonus affecting one lower limb as a result of spinal cord disease.

Figure 13.1 Electroencephalogram and electromyogram (EMG) from a 15-year-old patient with subacute sclerosing panencephalitis. The polyphasic slow-wave complexes, repeated every 10–14 s, are associated with a slow torticollic-like movement. In the three individual complexes shown at a higher speed (*bottom*), the onset of the EMG burst can be seen to precede the cortical discharge. The muscle discharges were limited to the right side of the body at this stage. (From Halliday[66], courtesy of the Publishers, *Modern Trends in Neurology*)

Figure 13.2 Electromyograms from muscles of the right lower limb in a 3-year-old girl operated on 3 years previously for a spinal deformity. Synchronous burst discharges can be seen in the EMG of quadriceps femoris (*channel 1*) and biceps femoris (*channel 2*) with a duration of 1–1.5 s and a frequency between 32 and 37 per min. The surface electrodes placed over tibialis anterior (*channel 3*) and gastrocnemius (*channel 4*) show the same bursts at very much smaller amplitude. Time trace in seconds. Calibration 500 μV. (From Halliday[68], courtesy of the Publishers, *Myoclonic Seizures*)

Table 13.4 Electrophysiological types of myoclonus (From Halliday[66])

	'Pyramidal' myoclonus	'Extrapyramidal' myoclonus	'Segmental' myoclonus (spinal or bulbar)
Electromyogram	Very brief, irregular, assymmetric discharges. May occur in trains showing recruitment. Jerks very variable in severity and distribution	Jerks associated with slow bursts of action potentials, often showing waxing and waning	Often symmetrical and rhythmical bilateral jerking between 20 and 130/min. Predominantly flexor, and confined to the affected segments of the brainstem or cord. Each jerk is associated with a brief burst of action potentials.
Electroencephalogram	Muscle jerks may accurately follow, with short and constant latencies, (a) bilateral polyspike and slow-wave complexes (b) diffuse cortical spiking (c) a contralateral Rolandic spike focus (d) a fast focal Rolandic 'after-discharge'	Muscle jerks may be associated with (a) polyphasic slow-wave complexes or (b) cortical slow-waves, or (c) be without EEG correlate (commonest)	No EEG correlates

Table 13.5 Electrophysiological classification of myoclonus used in this chapter

	Essential myoclonus	Epileptic myoclonus	Symptomatic myoclonus
Cortical myoclonus			
Cortical reflex myoclonus	0	+/−	+
Spontaneous cortical myoclonus	0	+	+
Epilepsia partialis continua	0	+	+
Subcortical myoclonus			
Reticular reflex myoclonus	0	?	+
Spontaneous reticular myoclonus	0	?	+
Cortically-triggered reticular myoclonus	0	?	?
Other subcortical myoclonus (e.g. thalamus)	0	?	?
Ballistic movement overflow myoclonus	+	0	+/−
Brainstem or spinal cord segmental myclonus	+/−	0	+

0 = Thought not to occur; +/− = sometimes occurs; + = commonly occurs; ? = not known

The distinctive features of the different types of myoclonus described by Halliday are shown in *Table 13.4*.

However, the authors' experience has led them to reconsider this physiological division of myoclonus. They believe that it is possible to distinguish the different types of myoclonus by neurophysiological criteria, as shown in *Table 13.5*.

Cortical myoclonus

The characteristic of cortical myoclonus is that the muscle jerk is generated by a discharge arising in the cerebral cortex. Such a cortical discharge may be triggered by some external stimulus as in *cortical reflex myoclonus*, may occur spontaneously as in *spontaneous cortical myoclonus*, or it may occur repetitively as in *epilepsia partialis continua*. The relation between these events and with epilepsy, is illustrated in *Figure 13.3*.

Figure 13.3 Relation of myoclonus to epilepsy

Electrophysiological studies of epilepsy suggest a series of events. The interictal spike discharge is the surface representation of a cellular paroxysmal depolarization shift, believed from experimental work to represent a giant excitatory postsynaptic potential. This spike discharge can become repetitive, and rhythmical local repetitive interictal spikes can then spread from the areas in which they arise to become generalized. If the spontaneous interictal spike happens to be in the motor cortex the opposite face, arm or leg would jerk (interictal spikes occurring in other parts of the brain present another problem). Repetitive interictal spikes result in epilepsia partialis continua. If these spread to involve neighbouring areas, a Jacksonian fit occurs, which, if it becomes generalized, causes a grand mal fit.

Cortical reflex myoclonus

The authors originally studied this form of stimulus-sensitive myoclonus in detail in patients with post-hypoxic action myoclonus[20]. Its characteristics are: (1) the electromyogram (EMG) correlate consists of a short 10–30 ms burst of activity; (2) the resulting myoclonic jerk normally is confined to one part of the body, i.e. it is

Figure 13.4 Electromyographic activity of a myoclonic jerk produced by a tap to the toes of patient D. B. The monosynaptic reflex is followed by a focal myoclonic response in tibialis anterior more than soleus (From Hallett *et al.*[64], courtesy of the Editor and Publishers, *Neurology*)

focal; (3) the jerks are triggered by peripheral sensory stimuli, which may be touch or stretch of muscle, or both, or by voluntary action (action myoclonus); (4) a brief positive–negative transient in the EEG precedes the muscle jerk by a short interval (about 15–30 ms for the arm, 25–40 ms for the leg); (5) muscles are activated in a sequence passing down the brainstem and spinal cord.

Figure 13.4 illustrates a tendon tap delivered to the toe of the right foot in a patient with post-hypoxic action myoclonus, which provokes a muscle jerk in only that part of the body where the stimulus occurs. A tap to one leg will make that leg jerk but not the rest of the body, showing that cortical reflex myoclonus is focal and is produced by simuli such as touch or tap. In such a patient, a tap to the jaw causes

Figure 13.5 Electromyographic activity of a myoclonic jerk produced by a tap to the jaw of patient D. B. The monosynaptic reflex is followed by the myoclonic response in orbicularis oris and stenocleidomastoid, but it may run into the myoclonic response in masseter. (From Hallett *et al.*[64], courtesy of the Editor and Publishers, *Neurology*)

a brisk jaw jerk, and the subsequent myoclonic burst travels down the brainstem, as can be seen by looking at the EMG of muscles innervated by different bulbar nerves (*Figure 13.5*).

There is a cortical correlate of this type of myoclonus, although it is quite subtle. Examination of the EEG in a patient with post-hypoxic cortical reflex myoclonus *Figure 13.6* shows no obvious EEG spike discharges in relation to the repetitive jerks, but slower waves are evident over the contralateral arm area (RA). If the EMG spikes are used as a trigger to back-average the EEG in order to time-lock the EEG to the muscle jerks, a different picture is obtained. As can be seen in *Figure 13.7*, there is a negative-going transient event preceding the muscle jerk by about 20 ms. In this way it is possible a back-average a cortical event from jerks occurring spontaneously, or from jerks occurring in response to a tendon tap or a

Figure 13.6 EMG–EEG correlation in action-induced myoclonic jerking in patient E. A. Electroencephalographic recordings are referential to an Fz reference and the electromyogram is from left finger extensors. (From Hallett et al.[64], courtesy of the Editor and Publisher, *Neurology*)

Figure 13.7 Averaged electroencephalographic activity in relation to action-induced myoclonic jerks in patient E. A. The records are the averages of 16 individual events aligned with the onset of the myoclonic jerk (arrow). Electroencephalographic recordings are referential to an Fz reference and the electromyogram is from right finger extensors. A vertical line is drawn through a 'negative-going' transient recorded from over the left motor cortex preceding the jerk. (From Hallett et al.[64], courtesy of the Editor and Publishers, *Neurology*)

peripheral muscle stimulus. Each time a small negative-going transient, focally related in the opposite motor cortex, appears about 20 ms before the focal muscle jerk. The authors believe this to be the cortical correlate of focal cortical reflex myoclonus.

Shibasaki et al.[156, 157], working on other forms of myoclonus, have used the same back-averaging techniques to examine EEG–EMG relationships in other types of myoclonias. *Figure 13.8* shows a sensory-evoked potential in a patient with a progressive myoclonic encephalopathy produced by a peripheral nerve stimulus which generated a late myoclonic response, and the cortical potential associated with a spontaneous myoclonic jerk. A 'negative-going' spike preceded the spontaneous myoclonic jerk by about 20 ms and resembled the N33 component of the sensory-evoked potential. By using the back-averaging technique, these authors were able to pick out such a cortical correlate in all seven patients with progressive myoclonic encephalopathy, but in none of the other patients studied (*Table 13.6*). This phenomenon of cortical reflex myoclonus therefore is not peculiar to post-anoxic action myoclonus but occurs also in progressive myoclonic encephalopathies and in a number of other diffuse degenerative disease. The many other reports of a similar mechanism occurring in variety of pathological conditions have been reviewed elsewhere[64].

The phenomenon of cortical reflex myoclonus was of considerable interest to the authors because 10 years ago Marsden *et al.*, in work on the function of the human

Figure 13.8 Sensory-evoked potential (SEP, *left*) and averaged EEG in the spontaneous myoclonic jerk (*right*) obtained by jerk-locked averaging in a male, aged 17 years with progressive myoclonic epilepsy. The wave form of the N33 component of the high amplitude SEP and that of the myoclonus-related spike resemble each other quite well. Moreover, the time interval from the early positive peak of the SEP to the late muscle (C) reflex was 14 ms (*x*) and that from the onset of the cortical spike to the myoclonic discharge 12 ms (*y*). R.PR indicates that recordings of the EEG were from the head sensory area of the right parietal cortex. (From Shibasaki *et al.*[157], courtesy of the Editor and Publishers, *Brain*)

Table 13.6 Myoclonus-related cortical activities shown by jerk-locked averaging (From Shibasaki et al.[157], courtesy of the Editor and Publishers, *Brain*)

	Number of cases	Spike	Sharp wave	Interval (EEG–EMG)
Progressive myoclonic encephalopathies	7	7	0	7–15 ms
Subacute spongiform encephalopathy	2	0	2	50–280 ms
Midbrain infarction	1	0	0	
Essential myoclonus	3	0	0	
Others	2	0	1	100 ms

stretch reflex, observed that as far as the human hand is concerned the stretch mechanism does not operate at the classical spinal stretch reflex latency[123, 124, 125] but at a much longer delay; further evidence led the authors to the conclusion that this delay indicated the existence of a transcortical stretch reflex mechanism for the human hand, a mechanism predicted by Phillips in 1969[143]. There is now a wealth of evidence from both human and animal studies for the existence of a projection of muscle spindles directly to the sensorimotor cortex in the brain. With regard to the human hand, this mechanism overrides the local classical Sherringtonian spinal stretch reflex. A further interesting aspect of this transcortical stretch reflex mechanism is that there is a powerful cutaneous input summating on the same cortical motor neurones. Taking this into account, it is possible to build up a picture of how a skin stimulus, a muscle stretch stimulus, or even voluntary action will provoke a cortical myoclonic discharge. The recordings of muscle spindle afferents by Vallbo[178] have shown how spindles discharge during voluntary muscle contraction in accordance with the principles of α–γ coactivation. Dawson[31] observed that such patients frequently have giant cortical action potentials in response to peripheral stimuli (*see also* Halliday[67]), illustrating that the cortex becomes oversensitive to peripheral stimulation. The resulting cortical discharge travels rapidly along fast-conducting 'pyramidal' pathways to produce the characteristic myoclonus.

Dawson was the first to describe a patient with stimulus-sensitive cortical reflex myoclonus[31], but since then there have been many reports of such cases[64, 123, 151, 157, 166]. In the majority of these patients, cortical sensory-evoked potentials were greatly enlarged, often unilaterally if the myoclonus was unilateral. The exact reason for both the giant evoked potentials and the stimulus-sensitive cortical reflex myoclonus in these cases is not clear. Many patients did not have evident cortical pathology. Indeed, where the pathology was known, it frequently involved the cerebellum[123], as in the original case described by Dawson. It may be that this type of myoclonus arises as a result of loss of inhibitory cerebellar influence on motor cortical function, leading to pathological facilitation of long-loop transcortical stretch and/or cutaneous reflexes[122b, 123].

Spontaneous cortical myoclonus

The authors have recently observed patients with muscle jerks whose duration, distribution and latency to cortical events all correspond to those seen in cortical reflex myoclonus, but in whom such jerks occur spontaneously. Indeed, such spontaneous jerks occur in many patients with cortical reflex myoclonus, but they may occur in isolation. Frequently such patients have some form of progressive or static myoclonic encephalopathy, but sometimes the pathology and cause are unknown. For example, in two patients with histologically proven Creutzfeldt-Jakob disease, Shibasaki *et al.* has recently demonstrated by back-averaging the existence of a cortical discharge preceding, and time-locked to, their spontaneous myoclonic jerking[158]. In the first patient there was no obvious EEG activity related to the jerks, but back-averaging revealed a sharp wave with onset about 50–85 ms prior to the onset of the EMG of the myoclonus. In the second patient the EEG did show a periodic discharge associated with the repetitive myoclonic jerks, but back-averaging was necessary to reveal the exact relation of these events; a diffuse surface-negative shift began some 300 ms before the EMG event; 60 ms prior to the EMG onset there was an abrupt sharp negative wave distributed focally over the contralateral motor area.

The motor pathways employed to conduct the discharges responsible for such spontaneous cortical myoclonus may be either the fast-conducting 'pyramidal' corticomotoneuron system or more slowly conducting pathways traversing the brainstem, perhaps via the red nucleus or other portions of the reticular formation. In the former case, the EMG burst is short and the interval between the cortical EEG event and the EMG activity is fixed and short; in the latter, the EMG activity may be prolonged and the latency between EEG and EMG is long and variable. Halliday's 'pyramidal myoclonus' would have included both cortical reflex myoclonus and fast spontaneous cortical myoclonus, while his 'extrapyramidal myoclonus' would have included slow spontaneous cortical myoclonus.

In generalized epileptic myoclonus, such as infantile spasms, myoclonic astatic epilepsy and cryptogenic myoclonic epilepsy, the relation of the myoclonic jerking to the spike wave or polyspike wave complexes seen in the EEG can be complicated. Such EEG events may occur with no evident myoclonus, suggesting that the EEG discharges are not necessarily invading the motor cortex output neurons. Myoclonic jerks may appear to follow the spike or spike wave complexes, but exact latency measurements are difficult to obtain, and it is not clear whether fast-conducting 'pyramidal' or slow-conducting brainstem pathways are involved. Indeed, the massive and prolonged myoclonic jerks and spasms of all these conditions may be associated only with EEG silencing or flattening, or with low amplitude fast activity; sometimes the surface EEG remains unchanged during such spasms. In addition, the bursts of generalized spike wave or polyspike wave discharge that do occur in these conditions tend to last for many seconds or even minutes, and occur throughout the surface EEG. At present it is not possible to decide where in the brain such widespread EEG paroxysms arise, or what their relation is to the myoclonus that occurs in these conditions. In general, the weight of evidence of lack of any focal EEG correlate and of any time-locked constant relationship between EEG and EMG events, and their complete independence on occasion, all point to a subcortical origin of such myoclonus. The authors tentatively ascribe it to some spontaneous brainstem or thalamic origin (*see below*).

Epilepsia partialis continua

Cortical reflex myoclonus and spontaneous cortical myoclonus are of great interest in relation to epilepsy, particularly to the phenomenon of epilepsia partialis continua. In this condition, repetitive clonic muscular twitching occurs in a specific part of the body for days or weeks. In such patients, there is normally clear evidence of a cortical discharge preceding, and tightly time-locked to, the repetitive EMG discharges. Back-averaging again demonstrates a clear-cut cortical spike. For example, *Figure 13.9* shows one such patient, described by Thomas *et al.*[174] with focal epilepsia partialis continua of the left hand, associated with a right motor cortex spike discharge time-locked to the event. In a number of patients with this syndrome, removal of the affected area of the motor cortex has abolished the subsequent jerking[103].

It is important to note that the cortical discharges that precede focal epilepsia partialis continua, or indeed cortical myoclonus of any type, may not be evident in the simple surface EEG. In some such cases, back-averaging of EEG events using the EMG of the myoclonus to trigger the averager, may reveal the focal EEG abnormality responsible for the myoclonus. However, in some cases even back-averaging the surface EEG will not disclose the cortical event, which is only evident at electrocorticography. Indeed, it is quite possible that even recordings from the surface of the exposed motor cortex, on occasion, may not detect abnormal discharges arising in, and confined to, the large Betz cells of layer V, which give rise to the fast-conducting 'pyramidal' pathway.

Subcortical myoclonus

As in the case of cortical myoclonus, myoclonus arising in some subcortical site may be triggered by peripheral stimuli or may arise spontaneously.

Reticular reflex myoclonus

This type of myoclonus was first identified by Hallett *et al.* in a patient with post-hypoxic action myoclonus[62], but the authors now believe it to occur in many other conditions. It is distinguished by the following characteristics: (1) the EMG correlate is a brief burst lasting 10–30 ms; (2) the resulting myoclonic jerk occurs throughout the body, i.e. it is generalized; (3) the jerks can be triggered by peripheral sensory stimuli such as touch or muscle stretch, or by voluntary action; (4) the cortical EEG correlate, if present, is not time-locked to the EMG event; (5) muscles are activated up the brainstem and down the spinal cord.

Figure 13.9 Electroencephalogram of a male patient, aged 25 years, with epilepsia partialis continua of left arm. Muscle activity is recorded by surface leads on left arm (channel 7). Focal short-duration spikes preceding each jerk arise from right Rolandic region, are equipotential in electrodes 4 and 6, and are seen best in channels 2 and 6. Note also that a longer-duration sharp wave in the electroencephalogram follows each muscle contraction in electrodes 4 and 6 over right Rolandic region (seen best in channels 2 and 4) and, to lesser degree, in electrodes 3 and 5 from Rolandic region (visible only occasionally in channels 1 and 3). (From Thomas *et al.*[174], courtesy of the editor and Publishers, *Archives of Neurology*)

Clinical features of certain types of myoclonus 233

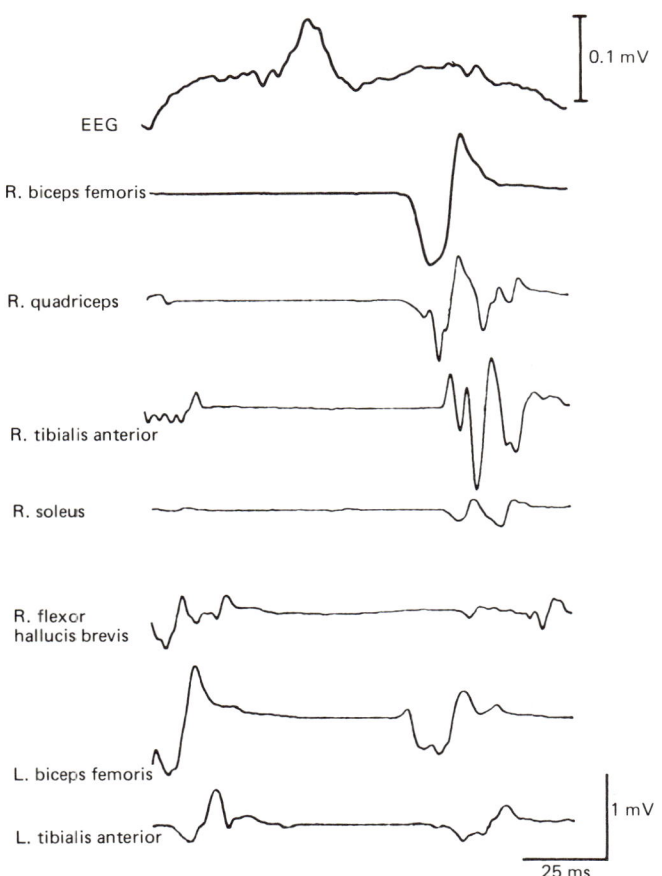

Figure 13.10 Electrical events of a myoclonic jerk evoked by a sharp tap on the undersurface of the right toes. The electroencephalogram is recorded from an electrode 1 cm to the left and 2 cm behind the vertex and referred to a midfrontal electrode (a positive deflection is downward). The upper voltage calibration marker refers to the EEG while the lower marker refers to all of the EMG records of the muscles indicated. (From Hallett *et al.*[62], courtesy of the Editor and Publishers, *Journal of Neurology, Neurosurgery and Psychiatry*)

Figure 13.10 illustrates the characteristic findings in a patient with post-hypoxic myoclonus, and shows EMG records of right and left leg muscles in response to a tendon tap to the toes of the right foot. The tap provoked a small monosynaptic burst in the toe muscles, followed by a widespread myoclonic jerk affecting the whole of the right leg together with the left leg. In other words, a single stimulus put into one leg provoked a generalized myoclonic burst affecting the whole body. The EMG of this myoclonic discharge was a very short burst of activity, lasting no more than 10–30 ms. Another feature of this form of myoclonus is that an associated cortical event in the EEG is evident. As seen from *Figure 13.10*, the tendon tap was associated with a large discharge over the cerebral cortex, recorded from the surface EEG. The discharge was widespread, affecting both hemispheres

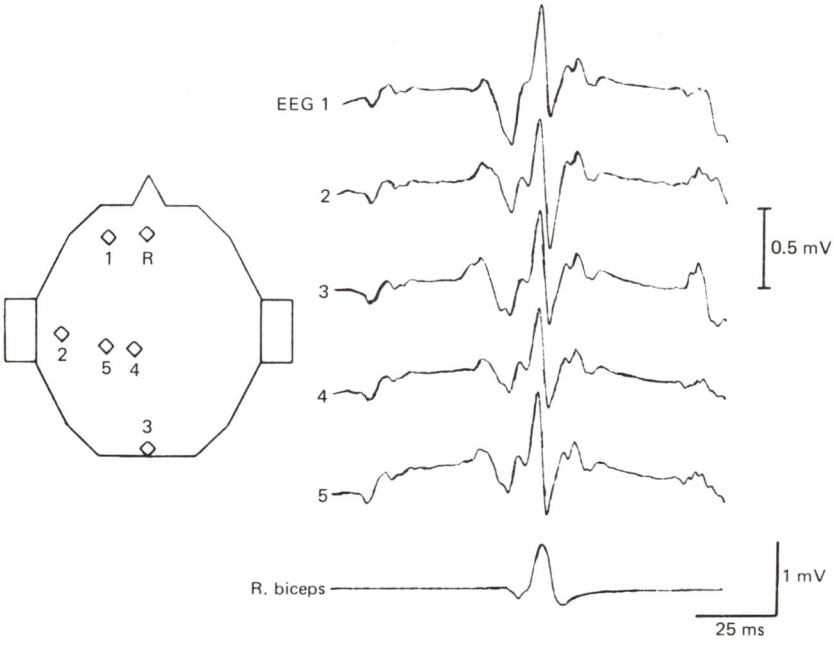

Figure 13.11 Electroencephalographic correlate of a spontaneous myoclonic jerk. The electroencephalogram is sampled from five widely separate sites in the left hemisphere, as indicated in the diagram, and referred to a midfrontal electrode (R) (a positive deflection is downward). Activity in the right biceps is taken as a marker of the myoclonic jerk. It is apparent that the electrocortical spike activity is widespread. The upper voltage calibration marker refers to the EEG record. (From Hallett *et al.*[62], courtesy of the Editor and Publishers, *Journal of Neurology, Neurosurgery and Psychiatry*)

front and back (*Figure 13.11*). The important finding was that the EEG discharge did not preface the earliest muscle event, which occurred in those muscles innervated by the lower brainstem nuclei. EMG activity in these muscles was evident before anything could be recorded in the surface EEG (*Figure 13.12*). In other words the discharge travelled up the brainstem to the cortex. From these findings we concluded that this form of myoclonus originated within the brainstem itself, propagating a wave up to the brain and down to the muscles to produce muscle jerks. *Figure 13.13*, which illustrates the relationship between the cerebral event recorded in the EEG and the EMG of the muscle jerking, confirms this conclusion. Examination of single records of the EEG/EMG relationship showed large EEG spike discharges associated with the EMG events occurring in the muscle. However, if the EMG event was used as a trigger to back-average a series of such myoclonic jerks, the relationship disappeared and it became apparent that the cortical event was not time-locked to the events in the muscle. This suggests that it was not the cortical event which drove the muscle to contract, but a secondary phenomenon related to a discharge which, the authors argue, was occurring in the reticular formation in the brainstem. They define this as a form of reticular reflex myoclonus. Chadwick, who collaborated in these studies, has

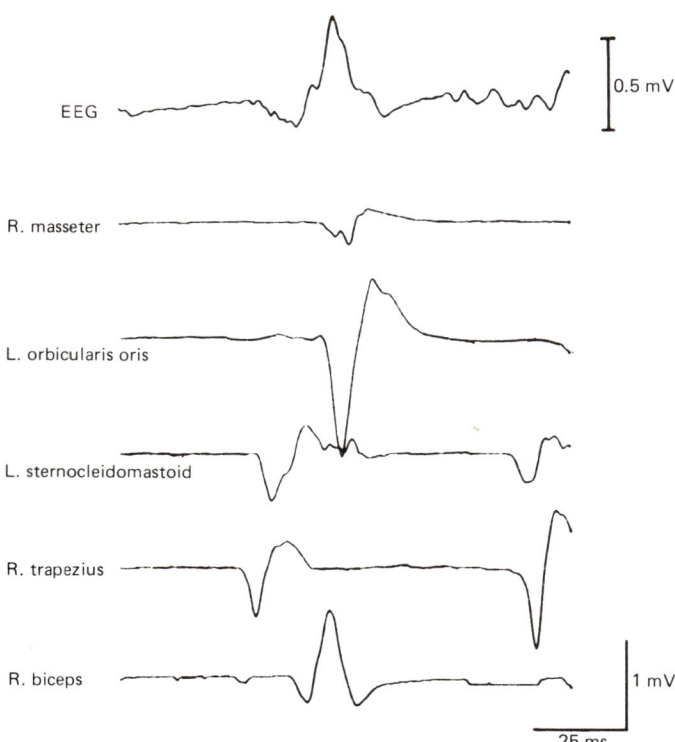

Figure 13.12 Electrical record of spontaneous myoclonic jerk including activity in cranial nerve muscles. The electroencephalographic recording (EEG) is from a point 1 cm to the left and 2 cm behind the vertex referred to a midfrontal electrode (a positive deflection is downward). Note the activation of the cranial nerves up the brainstem and the onset of activity in trapezius before that in the EEG. The upper voltage calibration refers to the EEG record and the lower voltage calibration to all of the EMG records. (From Hallett et al.[62], courtesy of the Editor and Publishers, *Journal of Neurology, Neurosurgery and Psychiatry*)

Figure 13.13 The EEG–EMG correlation of the myoclonus. In each part of the diagram the electroencephalogram is recorded from the vertex referred to the left ear (a positive deflection is downward) and the electromyogram (EMG) is from the left sternocleidomastoid muscle. (*a*) shows the events in a single spontaneous jerk. (*b*) is the average of 84 spontaneous jerks with the averaging being triggered on the occurrence of the EMG event. Since the EEG record in (*b*) shows essentially no activity, the timing of the EEG spike seen in (*a*) must vary considerably with respect to the EMG jerk. (From Hallett et al.[62], courtesy of the Editor and Publishers, *Journal of Neurology, Neurosurgery and Psychiatry*)

described a similar phenomenon in patients with uraemia[22] and the authors have seen examples of this form of myoclonus both in uraemia and in hyponatraemia. They believe that this myoclonus arising from discharge in the brainstem may be one of the commonest forms of symptomatic metabolic myoclonus.

Experimentally, this is the type of myoclonus that Zuckerman and Glaser described with urea infusions in the cat[194]. By careful electrophysiological depth-electrode recordings, they established this to be generated from discharges in the nucleus gigantocellularis medullaris. It is also related to the experimental myoclonus produced in the cat by focal injection of cobalt into the brain stem[17]. Therefore, both clinical and experimental evidence exists to suggest that this is a fundamental form of myoclonus arising from a brainstem discharge, and causing muscle jerking below and widespread cortical events above.

Spontaneous reticular myoclonus

Many of the patients with post-hypoxic or metabolic myoclonus also exhibit spontaneous jerks, as do uraemic animals. In the latter, such spontaneous jerks also arise from the nucleus gigantocellularis medullaris of the brainstem, and the authors therefore believe that spontaneous reticular myoclonus may occur in these and other conditions.

Cortically triggered reticular myoclonus

It must be pointed out that both cortical reflex and reticular reflex myoclonus, and spontaneous cortical and spontaneous reticular myoclonus, may occur in the same patient, as in some of the authors' cases of post-hypoxic or metabolic myoclonus.

It also seems highly probably that a cortical discharge might provoke a brainstem reticular discharge which would cause a generalized myoclonic jerk. However, the authors have not yet encountered a convincing example of this pathophysiological mechanism.

Other subcortical myoclonus

The probable subcortical origins of generalized epileptic myoclonus with 3-per-second, or slow spike wave, or polywave discharges already have been discussed, although the exact site of origin of the myoclonus cannot be decided at present.

The myoclonus of subacute sclerosing panencephalitis also probably originates from a subcortical site because (1) the prolonged EMG bursts (about 500 ms) often precede the EEG correlate (*see Figure 13.1*), and (2) jerking may continue even when the periodic EMG discharges have ceased to be apparent[142].

The origins of familial essential myoclonus may also be subcortical. Hallett *et al.*[63] and Shibasaki *et al.*[158] were unable to find any EEG correlate of this myoclonus even with back-averaging techniques. In the two familial cases studied by Hallett *et al.*, the myoclonus was found to be provoked, at least in part, by

Figure 13.14 Electromyographic (EMG) activity in various muscles for patient M. W. when attempting left thumb flexion. The task was a 20 degree flexion against a force of 0.07 N·m. When a myoclonic jerk occurred, as in both (a) and (b), there was widespread activation of many muscles approximately synchronous with the appropriate activity, with similar burst length and preservation of the reciprocal organization of agonists and antagonists. In (a) muscles of the opposite arm were activated, while in (b) muscles of the ipsilateral leg and those supplied by the cranial nerves were activated. Voltage calibration is 1 mV for left flexor pollicis longus (FPL) in (a) and (b), 0.25 mV for the other EMG records in (a) and 0.12 mV for the other EMG records in (b). Time calibration is 100 ms. FF = finger flexors, FE = finger extensors, B = biceps, T = triceps, BF = biceps femoris, TA = tibialis anterior, SO = soleus, S = sternocleidomastoid and OO = orbicularis oculi. (From Hallett et al.[63], courtesy of the Editor and Publishers, *Brain*)

voluntary action. When these patients attempted to execute a simple motor task, they initiated the correct EMG activity in the agonist and antagonist muscles. In a fast ballistic movement, for example, they activated the agonist first, which then silenced while the antagonist fired, and then fired again – the typical triphasic pattern of ballistic movement EMG firing. However, these patients could not confine such activity to the muscles required to execute the act. EMG activity, in typical triphasic pattern, spilt over into other remote and unnecessary muscles. Thus, a simple fast flexion of the left thumb might provoke contraction of the muscles of the opposite right arm and even of the legs (*Figure 13.14*). The essential abnormailty seemed to be an inability to confine the activity required to execute a ballistic movement to the appropriate muscles, and the authors therefore called this type of abnormaility 'ballistic movement overflow myoclonus'. The parts of the brain responsible for deciding which muscles are required to carry out a willed movement are not known, so that the likely site of the physiological derangements causing ballistic movement overflow myoclonus in hereditary myoclonus cannot be decided.

Finally, by definition, segmental myoclonus arises subcortically, either in the brainstem/cerebellum, as in the case of palatal myoclonus, or in the cord, as in spinal myoclonus. The reasons why rhythmic repetitive discharges, usually persisting during sleep, occur with such pathology are unknown. Characteristically, the EMGs of affected muscles show co-contraction of agonists and antagonists rather than reciprocal inhibition, and activity in flexor muscles predominates. Some disturbance of normal inhibitory interneuronal function in cord or brainstem seems likely to be responsible.

CONCLUSION

Despite considerable experimental and clinical neurophysiological study, understanding of the pathophysiology of the many varieties of myoclonus encountered in clinical practice is not complete. Careful investigation of each patient commonly reveals unsuspected and little understood abnormalities that cannot be explained by the mechanisms reviewed here. No doubt further observations using new techniques will lead to considerable revision of the scheme put forward here, which should be regarded as a tentative working approach to the physiological understanding and study of the myoclonias.

References

1 AICARDI, J. Myoclonic epilepsies. *Research and Clinical Forums*, **2**, 47–55 (1980)
2 AICARDI, J. and CHEVRIE, J. J. Myoclonic epilepsies of childhood. *Neuropaediatrie*, **3**, 177–190 (1971)
3 AIGNER, B. R. and MULDER, D. W. Myoclonus. Clinical significance and an approach to classification. *Archives of Neurology*, **2**, 600–615 (1960)
4 ARAN, F. A. Recherches sur une maladie non encore décrite du système musculaire (atrophie musculair progressive). *Archives Générales de Médecine*, **24:4**, 172–214 (1850)
5 BAMBERGER (1859), quoted in reference 54
6 BEARD, G. M. Remarks on 'Jumpers or Jumping Frenchmen'. *Journal of Nervous and Mental Diseases*, **5**, 526 (1878)
7 BERLAND (1880), quoted in reference 190
8 BIEMOND, A. Paramyoclonus multiplex (Friedreich). *Psychiatria, Neurologia, Neurochirurgia*, **66**, 270–276 (1963)
9 BOGHEN, D. and PEYRONNARD, J.-M. Myoclonus in familial restless legs syndrome. *Archives of Neurology*, **33**, 368–370 (1976)
10 BONDUELLE, M. The myoclonias. In *Handbook of Clinical Neurology, Vol. 6*, edited by P. J. Vinken and G. W. Bruyn, 761–781. Amsterdam, North Holland Publishing Co. (1968)

11 BOSCHI, G. Ataxie héréditaire avec paramyoclonus multiplex: type Unverricht. *Journal de Neurologie*, **18**, 141–150 (1913)
12 BOUDOURESQUES, J., ROGER, J., KHALIL, R., VIGOUROUX, R. A., GOSSETT, A., PELLISTER, J. F. and TASSINARI, C. A. A propos de 2 observations du syndrome de Lance and Adams. Effet thérapeutique du Ro–05–4023. *Revue Neurologique*, **15**, 306–307 (1971)
13 BRADSHAW, J. A study of myoclonus. *Brain*, **77**, 138–157 (1954)
14 BUTENUTH, J. and KUBICKI, S. Über die proghostische Bedeutung bestimmter Formen der Myockonien und korrespondierender EEG–Muster nach Hypoxien. *Zeitschrift für Electroencephalographie und Electromyographie*, **2**, 78–83 (1971)
15 CAMPBELL, A. M. G. and GARLAND, H. Subacute myoclonic spinal neuronitis. *Journal of Neurology, Neurosurgery and Psychiatry*, **19**, 268–274 (1956)
16 CASTAIGNE, P., CAMBIER, J., ESCOUROLLE, R., CATHALA, H. P. and LECASBLE, R. Observation anatomo-clinique d'un syndrome myoclonique post-anoxique. *Société Française de Neurologie* (Séance du 4 Juillet 1964), 60–73 Paris, Société Française de Neurologie (1964)
17 CESA-BIANCHI, M. G., MANCIA, M. and MUTANI, R. Experimental epilepsy induced by cobalt powder in lower brain-stem and thalamic structures. *Electroencephalography and Clinical Neurophysiology*, **22**, 525–536 (1967)
18 CHADWICK, D., REYNOLDS, E. H. and MARSDEN, C. D. Relief of action myoclonus by 5-hydroxytryptophan. *Lancet*, **2**, 111–112 (1974)
19 CHADWICK, D., HARRIS, R., JENNER, P., REYNOLDS, E. H. and MARSDEN, C. D. Manipulation of brain serotonin in the treatment of myoclonus. *Lancet*, **2**, 434–435 (1975)
20 CHADWICK, D., HALLETT, M., HARRIS, R., JENNER, P., REYNOLDS, E. H. and MARSDEN, C. D. Clinical, biochemical and physiological factors distinguishing myoclonus responsive to 5-hydroxytryptophan, tryptophan plus a monoamine oxidase inhibitor and clonazepam. *Brain*, **100**, 455–487 (1977)
21 CHADWICK, D., HALLETT, M., JENNER, P. and MARSDEN, C. D. Serotonin and action myoclonus – a review. In *Neurotransmitter Systems and Their Clinical Disorders*, edited by N. J. Legg, 151–165 London, Academic Press (1978)
22 CHADWICK, D. and FRENCH, A. T. Uraemic myoclonus: an example of reticular reflex myoclonus. *Journal of Neurology, Neurosurgery and Psychiatry*, **42**, 52–55 (1979)
23 CHARCOT, J. M. and JOFFROY, A. Deux cas d'atrophie musculaire progressive avec lésions de la substance grise et des faisceaux antéro-latéraux de la moelle épinière. *Archives de Physiologie et Normale Pathologie*, **2**, 744 (1869)
24 CHRISTOPHE, J. and GRUNER, J. La dyssynergie cérébelleuse myoclonique de Ramsay Hunt. Etude anatomique d'un cas. *Revue Neurologique*, **95**, 297–309 (1956)
25 COLEMAN, R. M., POLLAK, C. P. and WEITZMAN, E. D. Periodic movements in sleep (nocturnal myoclonus): relation to sleep disorders. *Annals of Neurology*, **8**, 416–421 (1980)
26 COOPER, I. S., AMIN, I., RIKLAN, M., WALTZ, J. M. and POON, T. P. Chronic cerebellar stimulation in epilepsy. Clinical and anatomical studies. *Archives of Neurology*, **33**, 559–570 (1970)

27 COURVILLE, C. B. *Untoward Effects of Nitrous Oxide Anaesthesia.* Pacific Press Publishing Association, Mountain View, California (1939)
28 CREUTZFELDT, H. G. Über eine eigenartige herdfömige Erkrankung des Zentralnervensystems. *Zeitschrift für die gesamte Neurologie und Psychiatrie*, **57**, 1–18 (1920)
29 DAUBE, J. and PETERS, H. A. Hereditary essential myoclonus. *Archives of Neurology (Chicago)*, **15**, 587–594 (1966)
30 DAWSON, J. R. Cellular inclusions in cerebral lesions of epidemic encephalitis (second report). *Archives of Neurology and Psychiatry*, **31**, 685–700 (1934)
31 DAWSON, G. D. Investigations on a patient subject to myoclonic seizures after sensory stimulation. *Journal of Neurology, Neurosurgery and Psychiatry*, **10**, 141–162 (1947)
32 DeLEAN, J. Action myoclonus and serotonergic activity. *New England Journal of Medicine*, **296**, 1414–1415 (1977)
33 DeLEAN, J. RICHARDSON, J. C. and HORNYKIEWICZ, O. Beneficial effects of serotonin precursors in postanoxic action myoclonus. *Neurology*, **26**, 863–868 (1976)
34 De LISI, L. Sudi un fenomeno motorio constante del sonno normale: le mioclonie ipniche fisiologiche. *Revista di Pathologia Nervosa e Mentale*, **39**, 481–496 (1932)
35 DENNY-BROWN, D. Discussion. *Transactions of the American Neurological Association*, **8**, 62–63 (1956)
36 DENNY-BROWN, D. and PENNYBACKER, J. B. Fibrillations and fasiculations in voluntary muscle. *Brain*, **61**, 311–334 (1938)
37 DUBINI, A. Primi cenni sulla corea electria. *Annals of the University of Medicine (Milano)*, **117**, 1–5 (1846), quoted in reference 155
38 DUCHENNE DE BOULOGNE, G. B. A. Recherches faites à l'aide du galvanisme sur l'état de la contractilité et de la sensibilité électro-musculaires dans les paralysies des membres supérieurs. *Compte Rendue de l'Academie des Sciences*, **29**, 667 (1849)
39 ELDRIDGE, R., IIVANAINEN, M., STERN, R. and KORBER, R. Baltic myoclonus epilepsy: a treatable, inherited disorder distinct from Lafora disease. *Neurology*, **31**, 67–68 (1981)
40 FAHN, S. Posthypoxic action myoclonus: review of the literature and report of two new cases with response to valproate and estrogen. In *Advances in Neurology*, Vol. 26, 49–84, edited by S. Fahn, J. N. Davis and L. P. Rowland, New York, Raven Press (1979)
41 FAHN, S. and SINGH, N. Segmental tremor vs. rhythmical myoclonus; successful treatment with serotonin precursors. *Neurology*, **30**, 383–384 (1980)
42 FAHN, S. and SINGH, N. An oscillating form of essential myoclonus. *Neurology*, **31**, 80 (1981)
43 FRENKEN, C. W. G. M., KORTEN, J. J., GABREELS, R. J. M. and JOOSTEN, E. M. E. Spinal myoclonus. *Clinical Neurology and Neurosurgery*, **1**, 44–53 (1974)
44 FRIEDREICH, N. Neuropathologische Beobachtung beim paramyokonus multiplex. *Virchows Archiv für Pathologische Anatomie und Physiologie und für Klinische Medizin*, **86**, 421–434 (1881)
45 FOX, E. J., VILLANUEVA, R. and SCHUTTA, H. S. Myoclonus following spinal anesthesia. *Neurology*, **29**, 379–380 (1979)

46 FUKUHARA, N., TOKIGUCHI, S., SHIRAKAWA, K. and TSUBAKI, T. Myoclonus epilepsy associated with ragged-red fibres (mitochondrial abnormalities). Disease entity or a syndrome? *Journal of the Neurological Sciences*, **47**, 117–133 (1980)

47 GARCIN, R., RONDOT, P. and GUIOT, G. Rhythmic myoclonus of the right arm as the presenting symptom of a cervical cord tumour. *Brain*, **91**, 75–84 (1968)

48 GASTAUT, H. and REYMOND, A. Étude électroencéphalographique des myoclonies. *Revue Neurologique*, **85**, 596–609 (1952)

49 GASTAUT, H., ROGER, J., SOULAYROL, R., TASSARINI, C. A., REGIS, H., DRAVET, C., BERNARD, R., PINSARD, N. and SAINT-JEAN, M. Childhood epileptic encephalopathy with diffuse slow spike waves (otherwise known as 'petit mal variant' or Lennox syndrome), *Epilepsia*, **7**, 139–179 (1966)

50 GASTAUT, H. and VILLENEUVE, A. The startle disease or hyperekplexia. *Journal of the Neurological Sciences*, **5**, 523–542 (1967)

51 GILBERT, G. J., McENTEE, E. J. and GLASER, G. H. Familial myoclonus and ataxia. Pathophysiologic implications. *Neurology*, **13**, 365–372 (1963)

52 GILLES DE LA TOURETTE, G. Étude sur une affection nerveuse caractérisée par de l'incoordination motrice accompagnée d'echolalie et de coprolalie. *Archives de Neurologie (Paris)*, **9**, 19–42, 159–200 (1885)

53 GOLDBERG, M. A. and DORMAN, J. D. Intention myoclonus: successful treatment with clonazepam. *Neurology*, **26**, 24–26 (1976)

54 GOWERS, W. R. *A Manual of Disease of the Nervous System*, 2nd edition, Vol. 2. Philadelphia, Blakiston's (1907)

55 GRINKER, R. R., SEROTA, H. and STEIN, S. L. Myoclonic epilepsy. *Archives of Neurology and Psychiatry*, **40**, 968–980 (1938)

56 GUILLAIN, G. The syndrome of synchronous and rhythmic palato-pharyngo-laryngo-oculo-diaphragmatic myoclonus. *Proceedings of the Royal Society of Medicine*, **31**, 1030–1038 (1938)

57 GUILLAIN, G. and MOLLARET, P. Deux cas de myoclonies synchrones et rythmées vélo-pharyngo-laryngo-oculo-diaphragmatiques. Le problème anatomique et physio-pathologique de ce syndrom. *Revue Neurologique*, **2**, 545–566 (1931)

58 GUILLAIN, G. and MOLLARET, P. Nouvelle contribution a l'étude des myoclonies vélo-pharyngo-laryngo-diaphragmatiques. *Révue Neurologique*, **2**, 249–264 (1932)

59 GUILLAIN, G., MOLLARET, P. and BERTRAND, I. Sur la lésion responsable du syndrome myoclonique du tronc cérébral. Étude anatomique d'un cas demonstratif sans lésions focales. *Revue Neurologique*, **2**, 666–674 (1933)

60 GUILLAIN, G., BERTRAND, I. and LEREBOULLET, J. Myoclonies arythmiques unilatérales des membres par lésion due noyau dentelé du cervelet. *Revue Neurologique*, **2**, 73–78 (1934)

61 GUILLEMINAULT, C., THARP, B. R. and COUSIN, D. HVA and 5-HIAA CSF measurements and 5-HTP trials in some patients with involuntary movements. *Journal of the Neurological Sciences*, **18**, 435–441 (1973)

62 HALLETT, M., CHADWICK, D., ADAM, J. and MARSDEN, C. D. Reticular reflex myoclonus: a physiological type of human post-hypoxic myoclonus. *Journal of Neurology, Neurosurgery and Psychiatry*, **40**, 253–264 (1977)

63 HALLETT, M., CHADWICK, D. and MARSDEN, C. D. Ballistic movement overflow myoclonus. A form of essential myoclonus. *Brain*, **100**, 299–312 (1977)

64 HALLETT, M., CHADWICK, D. and MARSDEN, C. D. Cortical reflex myoclonus. *Neurology*, **29**, 1107–1125 (1979)

65 HALLIDAY, A. M. The electrophysiological study of myoclonus in man. *Brain*, **90**, 241–284 (1967)

66 HALLIDAY, A. M. The clinical incidence of myoclonus. In *Modern Trends in Neurology*, edited by D. Williams, Vol. 4, 69–105. London, Butterworths (1967)

67 HALLIDAY, A. M. Cerebral evoked potentials in familial progressive myoclonic epilepsy. *Journal of the Royal College of Physicians*, **1**, 123–134 (1967)

68 HALLIDAY, A. M. The neurophysiology of myoclonic jerking – a reappraisal. In *Myoclonic Seizures*, edited by M. H. Charlton 1–29. Amsterdam, Excerpta Medica (1975)

69 HAMMOND, W. H. On convulsive tremor. *New York Journal of Medicine*, **5**, 185–198 (1867)

70 HAMMOND, W. A. *Treatise on Diseases of the Nervous System*. New York, Appleton (1871)

71 HAMMOND, W. A. *Diseases of the Nervous System* New York, Appleton (1892)

72 HARENKO, A. and TOIVAKKA, E. I. Myoclonic epilepsy (Unverricht-Lundborg) in Finland. *Acta Neurologica Scandinavica*, **37**, 282–296 (1961)

73 HASSLER, R. Clinical and anatomical findings in stereotactic pain operations on the thalamus. *Archiv für Psychiatrie und Nervenkrankheiten*, **200**, 93–122 (1959)

74 HENNIG (1864), Traite des maladies des enfants, quoted in reference 190

75 HENOCH (1861), quoted in reference 190

76 HENRY, P., VITAL, C., MAMO, H., BARAT, P., DJINDJIAN, R. and LOISEAU, P. Myoclonies rythmées, bilatérales, synchrones, d'évolution ascendante. Lésions inflammatoires de la moelle et du tronc cerebral. *Revue Neurologique*, **128**, 105–115 (1973)

77 HERRMANN, C. Jr. and BROWN, J. W. Palatal myoclonus: a reappraisal. *Journal of the Neurological Sciences*, **5**, 473–492 (1967)

78 HIROSE, G., SINGER, P. and BASS, N. H. Successful treatment of posthypoxic action myoclonus with carbamazepine. *Journal of the Americal Medical Association*, **219**, 1432–1433 (1971)

79 HODSKINS, M. B. and YAKOVLEV, P. I. Anatomico-clinical observation on myoclonus in epileptics and on related symptom complexes. *American Journal of Psychiatry*, **9**, 827–848 (1930)

80 HOEHN, M. M. and CHERINGTON, M. Spinal myoclonus. *Neurology*, **27**, 942–946 (1977)

81 HUNT, J. R. Dyssynergia cerebellaris progressiva: a chronic progressive form of cerebellar tremor. *Brain*, **37**, 247–268 (1914)

82 HUNT, J. R. Dyssynergia cerebellaris myoclonica – primary atrophy of the dentate system: a contribution to the pathology and symptomatology of the cerebellum. *Brain*, **44**, 490–538 (1921)

83 HUNTINGTON, G. On chorea. *The Medical and Surgical Reporter*, **26**, 317–321 (1872)

84 ISSACS, H. A syndrome of continuous muscle fibre activity. *Journal of Neurology, Neurosurgery and Psychiatry*, **24,** 319–325 (1961)
85 ITARD, J. M. G. Mémoire sur quelques fonctions involontaires des appareils de la locomotion, de la préhension et de la voix. *Archives Générales de Médecine*, **8,** 403 (1825)
86 JACOBS, J. Myoclonus and ataxia occurring in a family. *Journal of Neurology, Neurosurgery and Psychiatry*, **28,** 272–275 (1965)
87 JAKOB, A. Über eigenartige Erkrankungen des Zentralnervensystems mit bemerkenswerten anatomischen Befunden (spastische Pseudosklerose, Encephalomyelopathie mit disseminierten Degenerationsherden). *Zeitschrift für die Gesamte Neurologie und Psychiatrie*, **64,** 147–228 (1921)
88 JACOBS, L., NEWMAN, R. P. and BOZIAN, D. Disappearing palatal myoclonus. *Neurology*, **31,** 748–751 (1981)
89 JEAVONS, P. M. and BOWER, B. D. Infantile spasms. *Clinics in Developmental Medicine*, No. 15 London, Heinemann (1964)
90 JEAVONS, P. M. Nosological problems of myoclonic epilepsies in childhood and adolescence. *Developmental Medicine and Child Neurology*, **19,** 3–8 (1977)
91 JEAVONS, P. M. and HARDING, G. F. A. *Photosensitive epilepsy: a review of the literature and a study of 460 patients.* London, Heinemann (1975)
92 JELLINGER, K. Hypertrophy of the inferior olives. Report on 29 cases. *Zeitschrift für Neurologie*, **205,** 153–174 (1973)
93 JUUL-JENSEN, P. and DENNY-BROWN, D. Epilepsia partialis continua. *Archives of Neurology*, **15,** 563–578 (1966)
94 KAO, L. I. and CRILL, W. E. Penicillin-induced segmental myoclonus. I. Motor responses and intracellular recording from motoneurons. *Archives of Neurology*, **26,** 156–161 (1972)
95 KLIEN, H. Zur Pathologie der kontinuierlichen rhythmischen Krämpfe der Schlingmusculatur. *Neurologie Zentralblatt*, **26,** 245–254 (1907)
96 KNY, E. Über ein dem Paramyoclonus Multiplex (Friedreich) nahestehendes Krankheitsbild. *Archives für Psychiatrie und Nervenkrankheiten*, **19,** 577–590 (1888)
97 KOIKE, H. and YODHINO, Y. Spinal myoclonus with dermal and retinal changes affected by myelitis. *Archives of Neurology*, **34,** 383–385 (1977)
98 KORTEN, J. J., NOTERMANS, S. L. H., FRENKEN, C. W. G. M., GABREELS, F. J. M. and JOOSTEN, E. M. G. Familial essential myoclonus. *Brain*, **97,** 131–138 (1974)
99 KOZHEVNIKOV, A. Y. Eine besondere Form von corticaler Epilepsie. *Neurologisches Zentralblatt*, **14,** 47–48 (1895)
100 KOSKINIEMI, M., DONNER, M., MAJURI, H., HALTIA, M. and NORIO, R. Progressive myoclonus epilepsy. A clinical and histopathological study. *Acta Neurologica Scandanavica*, **50,** 307–332 (1974)
101 KOSKINIEMI, M., TOIVAKKA, E. and DONNER, M. Progressive myoclonus epilepsy. Electroencephalographical findings. *Acta Neurological Scandinavica*,, **50,** 333–359 (1974)
102 KREINDLER, A., CRIGHEL, E. and POILICI, I. Clinical electroencephalographic investigations in myoclonic cerebellar dyssynergia. *Journal of Neurology, Neurosurgery and Psychiatry*, **22,** 232–237 (1959)

103 KUGELBERG, E. and WIDEN, L. Epilepsia partialis continua. *Electroencephalography and Clinical Neurophysiology*, **6,** 503–506 (1954)

104 KUPPER. Über klonische Krämpfe der Schingmuskulatur. *Archiv für Ohrenheilkunde*, **1,** 296–297 (1873)

105 LAFORA, G. and GLUECK, B. Beitrag zur Histopathologie der Myokonischen Epilepsie. *Zeitschrift für die gesamte Neurologie und Psychiatrie*, **6,** 1–16 (1911)

106 LANCE, J. W. Myoclonic jerks and falls: aetiology, classification and treatment. *Medical Journal of Australia*, **1,** 113–120 (1968)

107 LANCE, J. W. and ADAMS, R. D. The syndrome of intention or action myoclonus as a sequel to hypoxic encephalopathy. *Brain*, **86,** 111–136 (1963)

108 LAPRESLE, J. Rhythmic palatal myoclonus and the dentato-olivary pathway. *Journal of Neurology*, **220,** 223–230 (1979)

109 LENNOX, W. G. The petit mal epilepsies. *Journal of the American Medical Association*, **129,** 1069–1074 (1945)

110 LENNOX, W. G. *Epilepsy and Related Disorders*. Boston, Little, Brown (1960)

111 LHERMITTE (1919) La section totale de la moelle dorsale, cited in reference 47

112 LHERMITTE, F., PETERFALVI, M., MARTEAU, R., GAZENGEL, J. and SERDARA, M. Analyse pharmacologique d'un cas de myoclonus d'intention et d'action postanoxique. *Revue Neurologique*, **124,** 21–31 (1971)

113 LHERMITTE, F., TALAIRACH, J., BUSER, P., GAUTIER, J. -C., BANCAUDE, J., GRAS, R. and TRUELLE, J. -L. Myoclonies d'intention et d'action post-anoxique. Étude stéréotatique et destruction du noyau ventral lateral du thalamus. *Revue Neurologique*, **124,** 5–20 (1971)

114 LHERMITTE, F., MARTEAU, R. and DEGOS, C. -F. Analyse pharmacologique d'un nouveau cas de myoclonies d'intention et d'action post-anoxiques. *Revue Neurologique*, **126,** 107–114 (1972)

115 LINDENMULDER, F. G. Familial myoclonus occurring in three successive generations. *Journal of Nervous and Mental Disease*, **77,** 489–491 (1933)

116 LOMBROSO, C. T. and FEJERMAN, N. Benign myoclonus of early infancy. *Annals of Neurology*, **1,** 138–143 (1977)

117 LOWENFELD (1883), quoted in reference 155

118 LOTHMAN, E. W. and SOMJEN, G. G. Motor and electrical signs of epileptiform activity induced by penicillin in the spinal cord of decapitated cats. *Electroencephalography and Clinical Neurophysiology*, **41,** 237–252 (1976)

119 LUTTRELL, C. N. and BANG, F. B. Newcastle disease encephalomyelitis in cats. I. Clinical and pathological features. *Archives of Neurology*, **79,** 647–657 (1958)

120 LUNDBORG, H. *Die progressive Myoklonus-Epilepsie*. Uppsala, Almqvist and Wiksell (1903)

121 MAGNUSSEN, E., DUPONT, A. and DE FINE OLIVARIUS, B. Palatal myoclonus treated with 5-hydroxytryptophan and a decarboxylase inhibitor. *Acta Neurologica Scandanavica*, **55,** 251–253 (1977)

122a MAHLOUDJI, M. and PIKIELNY, R. T. Hereditary essential myoclonus. *Brain*, **90,** 669–674 (1967)

122b MARSDEN, C. D. The physiology of myoclonus and its relation to epilepsy. *Research and Clinical Forums*, **2,** 31–45 (1980)

123 MARSDEN, C. D., MERTON, P. A. and MORTON, H. B. Is the human stretch reflex cortical rather than spinal. *Lancet*, **1**, 759–761 (1973)
124 MARSDEN, C. D., MERTON, P. A. and MORTON, H. B. Servo-action in the human thumb. *Journal of Physiology*, **257**, 1–44 (1976)
125 MARSDEN, C. D., MERTON, P. A., MORTON, H. B., ADAM, J. E. R. and HALLETT, M. Automatic and voluntary responses to muscle stretch in man. In *Progress in Clinical Neurophysiology*, edited by J. E. Desmedt, **4**, 167–177. Basel, Karger (1978)
126 MATTHEWS, W. B. HOWELL, D. A. and STEVENS, D. L. Progressive myoclonus epilepsy without Lafora bodies. *Journal of Neurology, Neurosurgery and Psychiatry*, **32**, 116–122 (1969)
127 MATSUO, F. and AJAX, E. T. Palatal myoclonus and denervation supersensitivity in the central nervous system. *Annals of Neurology*, **5**, 72–78 (1979)
128 MAY, D. L. and WHITE, H. H. Familial myoclonus, cerebellar ataxia and deafness. *Archives of Neurology*, **19**, 331–338 (1968)
129 MEIGE, H. and FEINDEL, E. *Der Tic*. Berlin, Deuticke (1903)
130 MINOLI, G. and TREDICI, G. Levodopa in treatment of myoclonus. *Lancet*, **2**, 472 (1974)
131 MITCHELL, S. quoted in reference 54
132 MORVAN, A. M. De la chorée fibrillaire. *Gazette hebdomadaire de Medecine et de Chirurgie*, **27**, 173–176, 187–189, 200–202 (1890)
133 MUSKENS, L. J. J. *Epilepsy: comparative pathogenesis, symptoms, treatment*. New York, William Wood (1928)
134 NIEDERMEYER, E. The Lennox-Gastaut syndrome: a severe type of childhood epilepsy. *Deutsche Zeitschrift für Nervenheilkunde*, **195**, 263–282 (1969)
135 NIEDERMEYER, E., BAUER, G., BURNITE, R. and REICHENBACK, D. Selective stimulus-sensitive myoclonus in acute cerebral anoxia. A case report. *Archives of Neurology*, **34**, 365–368 (1977)
136 NOAD, K. B. and LANCE, W. J. Familial myoclonic epilepsy and its association with cerebellar disturbance. *Brain*, **83**, 618–629 (1960)
137 NOVELETTO, A. Problèmes actuels de la myoclonie-épilepsie progressive de Unverricht-Lundborg. Révue bibliographique et critique. *Encéphale*, **47**, 223–252 (1958)
138 OSWALD, I. Sudden bodily jerks on falling asleep. *Brain*, **82**, 92–103 (1959)
139 OMOROKOW, L. Die Kojewnikoffsche Epilepsie in Siberien. *Zeitschrift für die Gesamte Neurologie und Psychiatrie*, **107**, 487–496 (1927)
140 PARKINSON, J. *An essay on the shaking palsy*. London, Sherwood, Neely and Jones (1817)
141 PATRIKIOS, M. J. Sur un cas d'automatisme moteur particulier des membres supérieurs après traumatisme de la moelle cervicale. *Révue neurologique*, **69**, 179–188 (1938)
142 PETSCHE, H., SCHINKO, H. and SEITELBERGER, F. Neuropathological studies on van Bogaert's subacute sclerosing leucoencephalitis. In *Encephalitides*, edited by L. van Bogaert *et al.*, 353–385. Amsterdam, Elsevier (1961)
143 PHILLIPS, C. G. Motor apparatus of the baboon's hand. *Proceedings of the Royal Society* (Series B), **173**, 141–174 (1969)
144 POLITZER (1862), Wien Medizinhalle quoted in reference 56

145 PRITCHARD (1822), quoted in reference 69

146 RABOT, L. *La Myoclonie Épileptique*. Thèse, Paris (1899)

147 REIMOLD, W. Über die myoklonische Form der Encephalitis. *Zeitschrift für die Gesamte Neurologie und Psychiatrie*, **95**, 21–36 (1925)

148 REMAK, E. Discussion. *Berliner klinische Wochenschrift*, **15**, 289–292 (1881), quoted in reference 155

149 REYNOLDS, J. R. *Epilepsy: its symptoms, treatment and relation to other convulsive diseases*. London, John Churchill (1861)

150 RICHARDSON, J. C., REWCASTLE, N. B. and DeLEAN, J. Hypoxic myoclonus: clinical and pathological observations. In *Physiological Aspects of Clinical Neurology*, edited by F. Clifford Rose. Oxford, Blackwell (1977)

151 ROSEŃ, I., FEHLING, C. and SEDGWICK, M. Focal reflex epilepsy with myoclonus. Electrophysiological investigation and therapeutic directions. *Electroencephalography and clinical Neurophysiology*, **42**, 95–106 (1977)

152 SAKAI, T., SHIRAISHI, S. and MURAKIAMI, S. Palatal myoclonus responding to carbamazepine. *Annals of Neurology*, **9**, 199–200 (1981)

153 SCHULTZE (1886), quoted in reference 190

154 SCHULTZE, F. R. Beiträge zur Muskelpathologie. Myokymie (Muskelwogen), besonder an den Unterestremitäten. *Deutsche Zeitschrift für Nervenheilkunde*, **6**, 65–76, 167–168 (1895)

155 SEELIGMÜLLER, A. Ein Fall von Paramyoklonus multiplex (Freidreich) (Myoclonia congenita). *Deutsche Medizinische Wochenschift*, **12**, 405–408 (1886)

156 SHIBASAKI, H. and KUROIWA, Y. Electroencephalographic correlates of myoclonus. *Electroëncephalography and Clinical Neurophysiology*, **39**, 455–463 (1975)

157 SHIBASAKI, H., YAMASHITA, Y. and KUROIWA, Y. Electroencephalographic studies of myoclonus. Myoclonus-related cortical spikes and high amplitude somatosensory evoked potentials. *Brain*, **101**, 447–460 (1978)

158 SHIBASAKI, H., MOTOMURA, S., YAMASHITA, Y., SHII, H. and KUROIWA, Y. Periodic synchronous discharge and myoclonus in Creutzfeldt-Jakob disease: diagnostic application of jerk-locked averaging method. *Annals of Neurology*, **9**, 150–156 (1981)

159 SHIVPOUE, E. and TEASDALL, R. D. Spinal myoclonus with vacuolar degeneration of anterior horn cells. *Archives of Neurology*, **37**, 451–453 (1980)

160 SIOLI, F. Über den histologischen Befund bei familiärer Myoklonus-Epilepsie. *Archiv für Psychiatrie und Nervenkrankheiten*, **51**, 30–39 (1913)

161 SILFVERSKIOLD, B. P. Rhythmic myoclonus in three girls. *Acta Neurologica Scandinavica*, **38**, 45–59 (1962)

162 SMITH, N. J., ESPIR, M. L. E. and MATTHEWS, W. B. Familial myoclonic epilepsy with ataxia and neuropathy with additional features of Friedreich's ataxia and peroneal muscular atrophy. *Brain*, **101**, 461–472 (1978)

163 SPENCER, H. R. Pharyngeal and laryngeal 'nystagmus'. *Lancet*, **2**, 702–704 (1886)

164 SNIDER, W. D., DeMARIA, A. A. and MANN, J. D. Diazepam and dialysis encephalopathy. *Neurology*, **29**, 414–415 (1979)

165 STEVENS, H. 'Jumping Frenchmen of Maine'. *Archives of Neurology* (Chicago), **12**, 311–314 (1965)

166 SUTTON, G. G. and MAYER, R. F. Focal reflex myoclonus. *Journal of Neurology, Neurosurgery and Psychiatry*, **37**, 207–217 (1974)

167 SUHREN, O., BRUYN, G. W. and TUYNMAN, J. A. Hyperexplexia. A hereditary startle syndrome. *Journal of the Neurological Sciences*, **3**, 577–605 (1966)

168 SWANSON, P. D., LUTTRELL, C. N. and MAGLADERY, J. W. Myoclonus – a report of 67 cases and review of the literature. *Medicine*, **41**, 339–356 (1962)

169 SYDENHAM, T. Schedula monitoria de novae febris ingressu. Londini, G. Kettilby (1686)

170 SYMONDS, C. P. Nocturnal myoclonus. *Journal of Neurology, Neurosurgery and Psychiatry*, **16**, 166–171 (1953)

171 SYMONDS, C. Myoclonus. *Medical Journal of Australia*, **41**, 765–768 (1954)

172 TAHMOUSH, A. J., BROOKS, J. E. and KELTNER, J. L. Palatal myoclonus associated with abnormal ocular and extremity movements: a polygraphic study. *Archives of Neurology*, **27**, 431–440 (1972)

173 TASSARINI, C. A., LYAGOUBI, S., SANTOS, V., GANBARELLI, F., ROGER, J., DRAVET, C. and GASTAUT, H. Étude des décharges de pointes-ondes chez l'homme. II. Les aspects cliniques et électroencéphalographiques des absences myocloniques. *Revue neurologique*, **121**, 379–383 (1969)

174 THOMAS, J. E., REGAN, R. J. and KLASS, D. W. Epilepsia partialis continua. *Archives of Neurology*, **34**, 266–275 (1977)

175 TROUPIN, A. S. and KAMM, R. F. Lingual myoclonus. Case report and review. *Diseases of the Nervous System*, **55**, 378–380 (1974)

176 UNVERRICHT, H. *Die Myoklonie*. Leipzig und Wien, Franz Deuticke (1891)

177 UNVERRICHT, H. Über familiäre Myoklonie. *Deutsche Zeitschrift für nervenheilkunde*, **7**, 32–67 (1895)

178 VALLBO, A. B. Muscle spindle response at the onset of isometric voluntary contractions in man. Time difference between fusimotor and skeletomotor effects. *Journal of Physiology*, **218**, 405–431 (1971)

179 VAN BOGAERT, L., RADERMECKER, J. and TITECA, J. Les syndromes myocloniques. *Folia Psychiatrica, Neurologica et Neurochirurgica Neerlandica*, **53**, 650–690 (1950)

180 VAN WOERT, M. H. and SETHY, V. H. Treatment of postanoxic intention myoclonus. *Lancet*, **1**, 1285 (1974)

181 VAN WOERT, M. H. and SETHY, V. H. Therapy of intention myclonus with L-5-hydroxytryptophan and a peripheral decarboxylase inhibitor MK 486. *Neurology*, **25**, 135–140 (1975)

182 VAN WOERT, M. H., ROSENBAUM, D., HOWIESON, J. and BOWERS, M. B. Long-term treatment of myoclonus and other neurologic disorders with L-5-hydroxytryptophan and carbidopa. *New England Journal of Medicine*, **296**, 70–75 (1977)

183 VAN WOERT, M. H. and HWANG, E. C. Myoclonus: biochemical and pharmacological approaches. In *Clinical Neuropharmacology*, Vol. 3. edited by H. L. Klawans. New York, Raven Press (1978)

184 VOGEL, F., HAFNER, H. and DIEBOLD, K. Zur Genetik der Progressiven Myoklonus-epilepsien. *Human Genetiks*, **1**, 437–475 (1965)

185 VON ECONOMO, C. Die Encephalitis lethargica, ihre Nachkrankheiten und ihre Behandlung. Berlin und Wien, Urban und Schwarzenberg (1929)

186 WALSHE, F. M. R. On the symptom complexes of lethargic encephalitis with special reference to involuntary muscular contractions. *Brain*, **43**, 197–219 (1920)

187 WATSON, C. W. and DENNY-BROWN, D. Myoclonus epilepsy as a symptom of diffuse neuronal disease. *Archives of Neurology and Psychiatry*, **70**, 151–168 (1953)

188 WEST, W. J. On a peculiar form of infantile convulsants. *Lancet*, **1**, 724–725 (1841)

189 WILLIAMS, A., GOODENBERGER, D. and CALNE, D. B. Palatal myoclonus following herpes zoster ameliorated by 5-hydroxytryptophan and carbidopa. *Neurology*, **28**, 358–359 (1978)

190 WILSON, S. A. K. *Neurology*, edited by A. N. Bruce. Baltimore, Williams and Wilkins (1940)

191 WOHLFAHRT, G. and HOOK, O. A clinical analysis of myoclonic epilepsy (Unverricht-Lundborg), myoclonic cerebellar dyssynergia (Hunt) and hepatolenticular degeneration (Wilson). *Acta Psychiatrica et Neurologica Scandinavica*, **26**, 219–245 (1951)

192 WOLF, P. Periodic synchronous and stereotyped myoclonus with postanoxic coma. *Journal of Neurology*, **215**, 39–47 (1977)

193 ZIEGLER, D. K., VAN SPEYBROECH, N. W. and SEITZ, E. F. Myoclonic epilepsia partialis continua and Friedreich's ataxia. *Archives of Neurology*, **31**, 308–311 (1974)

194 ZUCKERMAN, E. G. and GLASER, G. H. Urea-induced myoclonic seizures. *Archives of Neurology*, **27**, 14–28 (1972)

14
Clinical controversies in tardive dyskinesia
Angus V. P. Mackay

In the years since the introduction of chlorpromazine in 1953, and of its diverse descendents such as the butyrophenones and thioxanthenes, no serious competitor has emerged to challenge the usefulness of the dopamine antagonist in the management of acute schizophrenic illness and psychotic agitation. While the pharmacodynamic property of dopamine antagonism appears to confer antipsychotic power, it also exacts a price in the form of undesirable neurological effects. Hence the term neuroleptic is often applied to this chemically heterogeneous group of antipsychotic drugs whose pharmacological properties coincide only in the ability to diminish central dopamine transmission. Most of the neurological effects which are recognized early in the course of neuroleptic treatment (acute dystonias, parkinsonism and akathisia) are reversible and may be managed by the temporary addition of an anticholinergic drug. However, within the past 10 years the realization has spread that certain other neurological effects, sometimes irreversible, can develop over a time scale of years. These reactions are referred to as the tardive (late and gradual in appearance) dyskinesias.

The clinical identity, significance and management of this group of neurological phenomena have been the subject of some contention. It is the purpose of this section to focus upon controversial issues at the clinical level and, while in most instances failing to provide clear solutions, at least to try to define the important questions.

JUST CRAZY MOVEMENTS IN CRAZY PEOPLE?

The question as to whether these abnormal movements reflect endogenous brain dysfunction or iatrogenic disorder has been in the air since the neuroleptic-associated dyskinesias were first described[44]. For the purpose of this question the term tardive dyskinesia will be restricted to mean only the commonest manifestation, the orofacial or the buccolinguo-masticatory (BLM) triad[50]. The following statements appear to be true and non-contentious:

(1) Drug-naive patients with a psychiatric diagnosis of schizophrenic illness sometimes show abnormal stereotyped and repetitive movements[32, 35].
(2) Orofacial dyskinesia may occur in individuals who are not schizophrenic and who have never been exposed to neuroleptic drugs[26].

What is the relationship of these dyskinesias to those occurring in association with chronic neuroleptic therapy?

While we no longer have access to the large populations of drug-naive patients described in such rich detail by Emil Kraepelin[32] and Eugen Bleuler[4], examination of their clinical descriptions suggests that most of these abnormal hyperkinesias were phenomenologically different from what might today be described as tardive dyskinesia. Descriptions of schizophrenic stereotypy vary from simple and isolated tics to patterns of behaviour far more complex than involuntary hyperkinetic dyskinesia[35]. These complex motor patterns were felt by Bleuler to hold meaning for the patient and, where orginally semi-purposeful, would disintegrate into abbreviated and distorted stereotypies with the passage of time[4, 45]. Although certain abnormal facial movements described in the old literature appear to have resembled orofacial dyskinesia, the majority could be regarded as tic-like disturbances whose repetitive, stereotyped quality would differentiate them from chorea, athetosis or dystonia. Kraepelin[32] described an 'athetoid ataxia' which consisted of athetoid movements of the face and fingers in schizophrenic patients, but Bleuler was quite clear in his view that true choreo-athetosis was extremely rare in uncomplicated schizophrenic illness[4]. This latter view is supported by more recent studies which have found that chorea or athetosis is indeed very rare in chronic psychiatric populations uncontaminated by neuroleptic therapy, and certainly of a prevalence much lower than current estimates of dyskinesia in neuroleptic-treated patients[38, 47]. So while it would seem that psychotic patients do move in odd ways, the modern epidemic of orofacial dyskinesia cannot be explained on that basis. Furthermore, if neuroleptic treatment is taken as the defining characteristic, the buccolinguo-masticatory (BLM) triad is found regardless of medical diagnosis[9, 20, 31].

The influence of age on involuntary movements is potent (*Figure 14.1*). Not only is there clearly an increased predisposition to drug-associated orofacial dyskinesia in elderly patients[36], but cephalic dyskinesia, which is phenomenologically indistinguishable from tardive dyskinesia, is seen in the elderly non-psychotic individual who has never been given an antipsychotic drug. This syndrome is quite common and would fall within the category of early senile chorea, presumed to be a reflection of spontaneous degeneration of the corpus striatum[51]. Involuntary orofacial dyskinesia may, of course, represent one aspect of several well defined neurological conditions such as Huntington's disease and Wilson's disease (*see Figure 14.1*). As Baldessarini has put it, 'persistent dyskinesias represent a syndrome or reaction pattern and not necessarily a single disease, they can occur in association with senility and many other overt or presumed states of organic CNS disease[2].

The essential concept which on present evidence appears to be valid is that, all other things being equal, the *probability* of orofacial dyskinesia is greatly increased in the presence of neuroleptic therapy. Whether or not neuroleptics can be said confidently to be the 'cause' of dyskinesia is largely rhetorical. Neuroleptic drugs

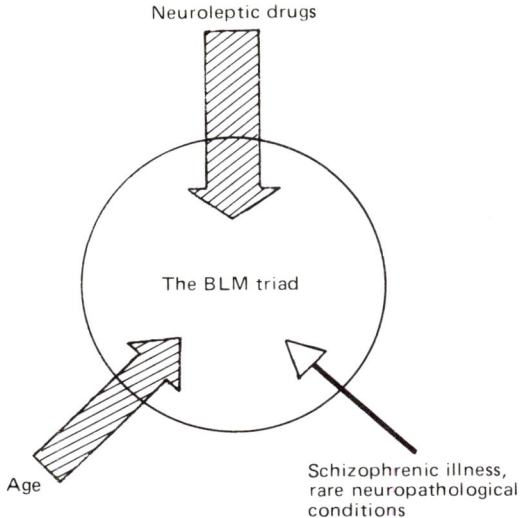

Figure 14.1 Factors associated with the buccolinguo-masticatory (BLM) triad

are associated with the syndrome and act to potentiate any pathophysiological process whose expression is cephalic dyskinesia. In many cases it seems fair to assume that dyskinesia would never have been expressed but for neuroleptic exposure, in others it might have occurred anyway with advancing age.

THE EXTENT OF THE SYNDROME

One approach to drawing up the boundaries of tardive dyskinesia is to subtract from the total of neurological phenomena associated with neuroleptic treatment those syndromes with relatively clear diagnostic boundaries (parkinsonism, acute dystonias) and then to consider what remains. Two questions then deserve attention. Firstly, is there one neurological syndrome left or several? Secondly, is late onset a reliable defining characteristic?

Let us first consider the phenomena. Involuntary hyperkinesia appears to be the most general characteristic, but within this broad category a wide variety of phenomena exist. These include orofacial dyskinesia, chorea (quasi-purposeful, non-repetitive, jerky movements), athetosis (slow, sinuous, writhing movements), dystonia (abnormal degree of fixity of any attitude owing to sustained muscle contraction), hemiballismus (continual, wild, flail-like movements of an arm), tics (repetitive paroxysms of muscle contraction) and various other abnormal postures[35]. Tremor is not a characteristic of this group of phenomena.

Orofacial dyskinesia, or the buccolinguo-masticatory syndrome[17, 19], is the best known and prevalent feature and represents the core of any definition of tardive dyskinesia. It consists of rhythmical involuntary movements of the tongue, face, mouth or jaw (e.g. protrusion of the tongue, puffing of the cheeks, puckering of the mouth and chewing motions)[43]. In elderly individuals, orofacial dyskinesia is usually the first and most prominent of the drug-associated hyperkinesias. It is often associated with choreiform movements of the extremities and distal athetosis[35]. Abnormalities of gait and trunk posture are frequent and include lordosis, rocking and swaying, shifting weight, shoulder-shrugging and rotatory pelvic movements[35]. Complex quasi-purposeful hyperkinesias are to be distinguished from the voluntary fidgitiness associated with akathisia, in which the pivotal diagnostic feature is not a sign but the symptom of inner restlessness[36].

In young individuals axial dystonia may dominate the clinical picture and in children a syndrome has been reported which comprises predominantly chorea of the extremities, athetosis, myoclonus and hemiballismus[35].

Crane has proposed that all neuroleptic-induced side effects of the CNS be referred to as encephalopathies[11], but in a later classification he reserves this term for syndromes which mimic naturally occurring diseases[12]. This classification contains 11 subsyndromes, of which one is tardive dyskinesia. In the classification proposed in 1976 the term tardive dyskinesia is confined to dyskinesias which persist in the face of drug withdrawal[11], but in the most recent classification it is clear that all late onset dyskinesias, reversible and irreversible, are considered as tardive dyskinesia[13]. While providing an impressive and comprehensive catalogue of drug-induced extrapyramidal syndromes, detailed phenomenological categorizations such as these do relatively little to delineate any more clearly the boundaries of tardive dyskinesia. For example, severe dyskinetic syndromes resembling Huntington's disease are classified separately as 'chemical encephalopathies' and hypotonia is designated as a discrete category[13], whereas it is not clear that any qualitative phenomenological or pharmacological distinction from tardive dyskinesia exists.

One recent suggestion has the virtues of parsimony and of clinical usefulness. It is that all drug-induced motor disorders are classified on the basis of phenomenological and temporal criteria, supplemented by pharmacological criteria[13]. Thus tardive dyskinesia would apply to hyperkinetic and dystonic disorders which are relatively late in appearance, tend to persist after drug withdrawal and tend to respond unfavourably to neuroleptic withdrawal and anticholinergic medication.[13].

Dystonia seems to be a source of particular confusion. It is a disorder of muscle tone expressed as postural abnormality, intermittent contractile spasms and complex action dystonias where purposeful movememts are deformed. Most authors agree that axial dystonia (usually lordosis and neck flexion) can sometimes occur relatively late in association with neuroleptic treatment, that it is commonest in patients under the age of 50 and that it may coexist with hyperkinesias such as the BLM triad and distal choreo-athetosis. It is to be distinguished from the so-called acute dystonias[36] on the basis of time-course relative to drug exposure, association with late onset hyperkinesia, moderate persistence after drug withdrawal and relative lack of response to anticholinergic drugs.

An appealingly objective approach has been the application of multivariate analysis to all observable motor abnormalities in patients receiving neuroleptic drugs in the hope that discrete phenomenological clusters would emerge[14, 29, 30].

Kidger et al.[30] examined 182 medicated psychiatric patients and 85 non-medicated non-psychiatric controls. Principal component analysis of abnormal movement at eight anatomical sites revealed three major components: a cephalic dyskinesia (component I), an axial and limb dyskinesia (component II), and a third component incorporating high frequency tremor of the lips and hands. The latter component undoubtedly corresponds to parkinsonian tremor and it was concluded that the other two (cephalic and axial/peripheral dyskinesia) represent central and peripheral subsyndromes of tardive dyskinesia. This is largely in agreement with previous work, but Kidger et al. took care to make the important distinction between peripheral dyskinesia and akathisia, an essentially subjective phenomenon. By making systematic enquires about feelings of inner restlessness they could conclude that there was no special relationship between akathisia and peripheral dyskinesias (component II). The relationship of akathisia to extrapyramidal disorder in general seems to require systematic investigation.

Multivariate analysis, then, defines two clusters of phenomena which might legitimately be considered as subsyndromes of tardive dyskinesia – a cephalic dyskinesia and a trunk/limb dyskinesia. Application of the principle of supplementary pharmacological definition tends to confirm the existence of these two subsyndromes of tardive dyskinesia. The cephalic subsyndrome tends to behave typically, namely to worsen with anticholinergic medication and to improve with further neuroleptic challenge. The peripheral dyskinesia on the other hand tends to behave like parkinsonism – improving with anticholinergics and worsening with neuroleptics. The pharmacological characteristics of late onset axial dystonia are not clear but, unlike the acute varieties, there seems to be no immediate beneficial response to anticholinergic medication[13].

It would thus seem that drug-induced disorders of movement and posture, other than the acute dystonias and variants of parkinsonism (including akathisia), cannot be classed as a single syndrome on either phenomenological or pharmacological grounds. While varying degrees of coexistence are observed, the head and neck hyperkinesias, the limb and trunk hyperkinesias, and the rarer axial dystonias deserve recognition as individual entities. Compression into a unitary tardive dyskinesia syndrome may result in aetiopathological confusion and dilution of overall therapeutic response in drug trials.

Dyskinesia may appear as an intercurrent disorder in the course of neuroleptic therapy or may appear for the first time only after reduction or withdrawal of neuroleptic therapy. There seems little justification for regarding the 'withdrawal emergent' dyskinesias as in any way fundamentally different, either phenomenologically or pharmacologically, from those which appear during uninterrupted treatment. The only qualified distinction would be that withdrawal emergent dyskinesias seem to occur more frequently in young people[13] and may be more readily reversible.

There is no doubt that tardive dyskinesias usually occur after exposure to neuroleptic drugs for periods much longer than those preceding the onset of the acute dystonias and parkinsonism, and therefore the term 'tardive' appears justifiable as descriptive of the majority of cases encountered. While most cases appear after at least 2 years of neuroleptic treatment[10], tardive dyskinesia is not uncommonly detectable after 6 months, and cases appearing after even briefer exposures have been reported[28, 42]. Therefore, late onset cannot and should not be taken as an essential diagnostic criterion. Not only would it prove an unreliable criterion but, more importantly, there is good reason to encourage early recognition of the syndrome since the quicker the neuroleptic is withdrawn the better the chance of eventual recovery[25, 42].

'Persistent' is another potentially misleading adjective commonly applied to this group of dyskinesias. It appears to mean different things to different authors but has been used most commonly to imply irreversibility in the face of drug withdrawal. This is certainly quite variable; a substantial proportion (up to 50 per cent) of patients will probably recover after cessation of neuroleptic treatment[36]. What distinguishes the tardive dyskinesias from other neuroleptic-induced neurological disorders in this respect is that recovery, like emergence, is often very slow. Reversal can still be hoped for after months or years, and probably should not be formally assessed after drug-free periods of less than 3 years[36]. Studies in which reversibility has been assessed over periods of only a few months have undoubtedly led to an inflated impression of permanence.

WHO IS MOST AT RISK?

A wide range of variables related to the patient and to his drug history has been examined with a view to identifying factors which clearly increase the probability of tardive dyskinesia[36]. Of the many patient variables investigated for an association with point prevalence, age is the only one upon which the published literature agrees[36]. The influence of age is not merely a reflection of the duration of neuroleptic treatment but appears to denote a particular vulnerability of the ageing brain.

Individual susceptibility to neuroleptic drugs is strikingly variable; a typical syndrome sometimes develops in young patients after modest exposure for only a few months[28]. Attempts have been made to identify some electroencephalographic correlate of susceptibility, perhaps a reflection of minimal brain dysfunction[28], but no clear relationship has so far emerged. If the stimulus to the development of tardive dyskinesia is a chronic reduction in dopamine transmission then any condition associated with impaired central dopamine transmission would be expected to carry the risk of dyskinesia. In respect of the clear influence of age, neuroleptic drugs might be exaggerating the effects of a natural degenerative process in the extrapyramidal system[30, 46]. It has also been suggested that patients with non-schizophrenic psychoses, affective in particular, might constitute a high-risk group[28]. Although the evidence for that is anecdotal, a background of temporary reductions in catecholamine transmission associated with depressive illness might co-operate with pharmacological antagonism at dopamine receptors in provoking postsynaptic receptor proliferation.

In view of the aetiopathological implication of neuroleptic drugs in tardive dyskinesia it is rather surprising that neither dosage nor length of neuroleptic exposure has been shown to relate clearly to the risk of tardive dyskinesia. As Kane *et al.* have put it, 'it may be that the lack of evidence for such intuitive relationships is merely a methodological problem, given the difficulties involved in retrospective data analyses'[28]. The precise dating of the onset of tardive dyskinesia requires not only the recognition of the syndrome but also the clear recording of this in case notes – requirements all too rarely met in long-stay psychiatric wards. For different reasons, it has so far proved impossible to compile a 'league table' of risk according to type of neuroleptic. Patients tend to be switched from one drug to another over the years and at any one time a patient is often receiving a neuroleptic cocktail. All that can be concluded at present is that any patient exposed to chronic inhibition of central dopamine systems runs the risk of contracting tardive dyskinesia.

It should be pointed out, however, that dopamine 'antagonists' acting presynaptically to inhibit storage of neurotransmitter, such as reserpine and tetrabenazine, do not appear to cause tardive dyskinesias[35]. There have been occasional reports of tardive dyskinesias appearing in patients on reserpine, but most were also taking, or had taken, postsynaptic neuroleptic agents. In any case, considering the widespread and prolonged use of reserpine to treat hypertension, the rare incidence of an oral dyskinesia on reserpine alone is not greater than might be expected to occur knowing the existence of spontaneous dyskinesias of this type. This observation is of importance, for it provides the rationale for using such presynaptically acting dopamine antagonists to treat tardive dyskinesia, and it may have significance for the pathophysiology of the condition.

If chronic neuroleptic therapy is associated with tardive dyskinesia then common sense might predict that frequent interruptions to drug therapy might protect against the occurrence of tardive dyskinesia. Some evidence does exist to support this hypothesis[27], but the effect of drug holidays on the reversibility of established tardive dyskinesia is in fact counterintuitive. In a comparison of 12 cases of reversible tardive dyskinesia with nine cases of irreversible tardive dyskinesia Jeste *et al.*[25] found that the one factor which discriminated best between these groups was the number of drug-free intervals (assessed retrospectively) of at least 3 months duration. In this study it was those patients who had experienced a greater number of prolonged 'drug holidays' who were liable to have irreversible dyskinesia, a finding which supports the earlier observation of Degwitz[16]. This is a most significant and disturbing finding in view of the increasingly popular strategy of drug holidays. The findings of Jeste *et al.* require urgent confirmation, preferably through prospective study.

NEUROCHEMICAL IMBALANCE OR DEGENERATIVE DISEASE?

Most attention has so far been directed at neurochemical indices of dysfunction in neuroleptic-treated patients displaying tardive dyskinesia, despite the fact that simple neurochemical models cannot readily explain irreversible dyskinesia or the obvious predilection for the oral musculature. The less tardive and more rapidly reversible dyskinesias such as the withdrawal emergent dyskinesias might seem to be candidates for a underlying abnormality which is largely neurochemical. For obvious reasons, the focus of most attention has been the striatal dopamine system.

Evidence cited in support of a relative dopaminergic overactivity model is pharmacological; the dyskinesia usually worsens in the face of neuroleptic withdrawal or dopamine potentiation[48] and usually improves if dopamine systems are inhibited. Yet there is no direct clinical biochemical evidence for generalized central dopamine overactivity in tardive dyskinesia. Investigations of dopamine metabolite concentrations in lumbar CSF of patients with tardive dyskinesia have failed to reveal consistent abnormality[15, 21, 39, 40], making it unlikely that disturbance of presynaptic release of dopamine contributes much to the clinical picture. There is unhappily no simple clinical test of dopamine receptor function in the basal ganglia. The only central dopamine receptor system whose activity can be readily monitored is the tubero-infundibular system in which dopamine receptor activity is related to circulating prolactin concentrations. While the reaction of dopamine receptors in the pituitary to chronic neuroleptic exposure might be different from those in the brain, the observation of prolactin levels, and their response to dopamine receptor mediated pharmacological challenge, offers a safe and easy way of assessing one species of dopamine receptor in patients with tardive dyskinesia. Studies of the sensitivity of tubero-infundibular dopamine receptors in this way have failed to establish evidence of dopamine receptor supersensitivity in patients with tardive dyskinesia[18]; indeed one study has reported subsensitivity to dopaminergic stimulation by agents such as levodopa and apomorphine[49].

An imbalance between neurotransmitter systems in which dopamine is strategic need not, of course, be reflected as gross abnormality of the dopamine systems *per se*. It seems likely that functionally important interactions take place between dopamine, acetylcholine and γ-amino-*n*-butyric acid (GABA) in the maintenance of extrapyramidal homeostasis, but clinical access to cholinergic and GABAergic transmission is even more problematic than to dopamine. So while both intuition and pharmacological experience would predict some abnormality in transmitter function in the basal ganglia, no direct clinical evidence is yet available which points to any particular neurotransmitter system as being primarily disturbed in tardive dyskinesia.

It seems likely that the reversible dyskinesias are incipient forms of irreversible dyskinesia and that they will convert into permanent dyskinesia with the passage of time and continued neuroleptic exposure[13, 25]. Irreversibility and increased susceptibility with age tend to imply structural degeneration of brain tissue. Central dopamine transmission declines with age[5], probably reflecting loss of nigrostriatal dopaminergic neurons[37], and the ageing process also affects cholinergic and GABAergic transmission in the extrapyramidal system[3]. Localized neuronal degeneration may be accelerated by hypoxia, which is likewise associated with age[3]. Hypoxic changes mainly affect diencephalic structures such as the basal ganglia, and the ventrolateral segment of the corpus striatum seems particularly vulnerable due to a tenuous vascular supply (Lyon, personal communication quoted by Gerlach and Faurbye[23]). In the context of tardive dyskinesia, it may be highly significant that the ventrolateral striatum is concerned with the innervation of oral musculature. A plausible and parsimonious hypothesis would be that while pharmacological insult to the basal ganglia can be corrected in the young brain in which high levels of neuronal resistance and redundancy still exist, in the ageing brain the capacity to react against sustained imbalance is impaired due to neuronal degeneration and loss of 'buffer capacity'[22] in the system. The effects of chronic neuroleptic exposure would interact with natural degeneration, perhaps to potentiate impairment of dopaminergic transmission[30], and this pathological interaction might be most readily evident in those susceptible areas of the basal ganglia which are concerned with the control of oral movements.

The question arises whether nigrostriatal degeneration is more evident in the brains of patients suffering from tardive dyskinesia or in controls matched for age and psychiatric diagnosis. During life, the computerized axial tomographic X-ray scan (CAT scan) offers a non-invasive technique for the identification of gross structural abnormality in the brain. A recent CAT study[18] of 50 long-stay psychiatric patients found slight but statistically significant differences between dyskinetic and non-dyskinetic patients in one measure of ventricular dilatation. This was a relatively young group of patients (average age 48 years) and it is unclear whether or not the dyskinesia was at an irreversible stage.

The most direct approach to this question in human brain is neuropathological study but, rather surprisingly, no properly controlled study has so far been reported (for review see Jellinger[24]). In 1968, Hunter et al.[23] described non-specific postmortem changes in two patients with tardive dyskinesia, and myelin degeneration in a third. Faurbye[19] found evidence of caudate atrophy in 13 of 15 cases of tardive dyskinesia in an open study. In a non-blind controlled study reported in 1970, Christensen et al.[6] found evidence of ventricular dilatation, cortical atrophy, degeneration of the substantia nigra and midbrain gliosis in the majority of 28 patients with tardive dyskinesia. This study, however, suffered from inadequate matching of dyskinetic and control cases according to age, sex and duration of neuroleptic therapy. Several groups of workers have investigated various neurochemical variables in postmortem brain tissue from patients dying with a hospital diagnosis of schizophrenic illness. The most consistent abnormality detected is an increased density of dopamine receptors in dopamine-rich areas such as caudate nucleus. The vast majority of cases in any series appear to have been exposed to neuroleptic medication, and some recent results suggest that the dopamine receptor abnormalities detected in postmortem schizophrenic brain tissue might all be due to medication[34]. It has not been possible to identify with any certainty from case notes which of the schizophrenic cases coming to postmortem biochemical assay had suffered from tardive dyskinesia and therefore a correlation of dyskinesia with dopamine receptor proliferation has so far been impossible.

Retrospective postmortem studies of this sort encounter serious pitfalls. The validity of a case note entry of tardive dyskinesia must be open to serious question and many cases must die without any mention of abnormal movements in the case notes. The only reliable approach must be a prospective postmortem study in which cases of moderate to severe tardive dyskinesia are identified and rated by generally accepted criteria and closely matched with non-dyskinetic controls (with particular attention to age, psychiatric diagnosis and medication). A large cohort must be identified and followed until death, when brain tissue can be used for detailed neuropathological and neurochemical investigation (including receptor ligand binding studies). Only then can the relative importance of neurochemical abnormality and structural degeneration be properly assessed. A multicentre Medical Research Council investigation embodying this approach is currently being mounted in the UK.

At present, then, the question of subtle neurochemical imbalance versus gross degeneration must await definitive study. The question is not merely academic. It has direct bearing on the understanding of the aetiopathological processes and therefore on approaches to treatment and prevention.

DOES TARDIVE DYSKINESIA MATTER?

'Beware Freedom Drugs, say Doctors'. Thus proclaimed the headline of a recent article dealing with tardive dyskinesia which appeared in a national newspaper[41]. Public awareness of the price paid by patients for long-term neuroleptic treatment is rightly growing. The impetus has come mainly from American sources and a spur appears to have been the spectre of litigation. External pressures apart, how does a doctor weigh the price against the benefit when prescribing for chronic psychotic morbidity?

Most clinicians would agree that no justifiable case exists for prolonged neuroleptic medication (for periods of more than 6 months) in illnesses other than schizophrenia and, to a lesser extent, intractable affective psychosis. Chronic schizophrenic illness carries a poor prognosis and there is no doubt that prolonged neuroleptic treatment reduces the probability of relapse into florid psychosis. However, there is no evidence that the suppression of florid psychotic episodes affects the long-term course and eventual outcome of the schizophrenias[7], and the case for neuroleptic medication in the treatment of the 'negative' features of the schizophrenic defect state is by no means clear[33]. For some schizophrenic patients occasional relapses into florid psychosis may not matter greatly, particularly for those who are long-stay hospital in-patients. For them, brief pharmacotherapeutic reaction to each florid exacerbation may be sufficient. For others, perhaps with a family and steady employment, a relapse can have serious and far-reaching consequences and here prophylactic medication becomes an important aspect of management. Generalization is impossible but it is fair to say that chronic neuroleptic therapy is often clinically indicated, and a reasonable set of guidelines governing the decision to use long-term neuroleptic therapy has been drawn up by an American psychiatric task force.[50]

On the other side of the coin, tardive dyskinesia assumes major importance, mainly because it can be irreversible, is essentially untreatable and its mechanism is obscure. Any iatrogenic disorder with these qualities rightly deserves serious attention. However, it must be said that for most patients with tardive dyskinesia the distress is more often in the eyes of the beholder than in the patient. Patients are rarely aware of their dyskinesia and even more rarely complain of it. This of course may partly be a reflection of schizophrenic indifference or of institutionalization, but it also seems to hold true for out-patients in psychiatric remission. It is uncommon for the dyskinesia to be of sufficient severity or distribution to be seriously disruptive to everyday function, and threat to life due to disorders of respiration or swallowing is extremely rare. Nonetheless, the management of chronic schizophrenic illness may be seriously hampered by obvious and often embarrassing involuntary movements. The patient undergoing rehabilitation who is being reintroduced into the community has sufficient stigmata to overcome without the added drawback of abnormal movements to attract attention and immediately label the individual as odd. So tardive dyskinesia does matter, whether or not the patient complains.

It is for the patient in the community that the risks and benefits are most significant. The consequences of a florid relapse can be very damaging and the disadvantages of dyskinesia can likewise be damaging. The clinical art is to identify whether the patient will benefit from prolonged neuroleptic treatment, and, if so, to use the neuroleptic in as sparing a way as possible, thus approaching an optimum risk to benefit ratio.

References

1 ASNIS, G. M., SACHAR, E. J., LANGER, G., HALPEN, F. S. and FINK, M. Normal prolactin responses in tardive dyskinesia. *Psychopharmacology*, **66**, 247–250 (1979)
2 BALDESSARINI, R. Tardive Dyskinesia: An evaluation of the etiologic association with neuroleptic therapy. *Canadian Psychiatric Association Journal*, **19**, 551–554 (1974)
3 BARBEAU, A. Ageing and the extrapyramidal system. *Journal of the American Geriatric Society*, **21**, 145–149 (1973)
4 BLEULER, E. *Dementia praecox or the Group of Schizophrenias*. Vienna (Translated by J. Zinkin, 1950). New York, International Press (1911)
5 CARLSSON, A. and WINDBLAD, B. Influence of age and time interval between death and autopsy on dopamine and 3-methoxytyramine levels in human basal ganglia. *Journal of Neural Transmission*, **38**, 271–276 (1976)
6 CHRISTENSEN, E., MOLLER, J. E. and FAURBYE, A. Neuropathological investigation of 28 brains from patients with dyskinesia. *Acta Psychiatrica Scandinavica*, **46**, 14–23 (1970)
7 CIOMPI, L. The natural history of schizophrenia in the long term. *British Journal of Psychiatry*, **136**, 413–420 (1980)
8 COHEN, K. L., COOPER, R. A. and ALTSHUL, S. Prolactin levels in tardive dyskinesia. *New England Journal of Medicine*, **300**, 46 (1979)
9 CRANE, G. E. Dyskinesia and neuroleptics. *Archives of General Psychiatry*, **19**, 700–703 (1968)
10 CRANE, G. E. Persistent dyskinesia. *British Journal of Psychiatry*, **122**, 395–405 (1973)
11 CRANE, G. E. Risks of long-term therapy with neuroleptic drugs. In *Antipsychotic Drugs: Pharmacodynamics and Pharmacokinetics*, **25**, edited by Sedvall, Uvnas and Zotterman, Wenner-Gren, 411–419. Oxford, Pergamon Press (1976)

12 CRANE, G. E. Tardive dyskinesia and related neurologic disorders. In *Handbook of Psychopharmacology*, **10,** edited by L. L. Iversen, S. D. Iversen and S. H. Snyder, 165–196. New York, Plenum Press (1978)

13 CRANE, G. E. A classification of the neurological effects of neuroleptic drugs. In *Tardive Dyskinesia Research and Treatment*, edited by W. E. Fann, R. C. Smith, J. M. Davis and E. F. Domino, 187–191. New York, Spectrum Publications Inc. (1980)

14 CRANE, G. E., NARANJO, E. R. and CHASE, C. Motor disorders induced by neuroleptics – a proposed new classification. *Archives of General Psychiatry*, **23,** 179–184 (1971)

15 CURZON, G. Involuntary movements other than parkinsonism: biochemical aspects. *Proceedings of the Royal Society of Medicine*, **66,** 873–877 (1973)

16 DEGKWITZ, R. Extrapyramidal motor disorders following long-term treatment with neuroleptic drugs. In *Psychotropic Drugs and Dysfunction of the Basal Ganglia*, edited by G. E. Crane and R. Gardner, Jr. Washington DC, US Government Printing Office Public Health Service Publication No. 1938 (1969)

17 DELWAIDE, P. J. and DESSEILLES, M. Spontaneous bucco-lingual-facial dyskinesia in the elderly. *Acta Neurologica Scandinavica*, **56,** 256–262 (1977)

18 FAMUIWA, O. O., ECCLESTON, P., DONALDSON, A. A. and GARSIDE, R. F. Tardive dyskinesia and dementia. *British Journal of Psychiatry*, **135,** 500–504 (1974)

19 FAURBYE, A., RASCH, P. J., PETERSON, P. D., BRANDBORG, G. and PAKKENBERG, H. Neurological symptoms in pharmacotherapy of psychosis. *Acta Psychiatrica Scandinavica*, **40,** 10–27 (1964)

20 GERLACH, J. Tardive dyskinesia. *Danish Medical Bulletin*, **46,** 209–245 (1979)

21 GERLACH, J., THORSEN, K. and FOG, R. Extrapyramidal reactions and amine metabolites in cerebrospinal fluid during haloperidol and clozapine treatment of schizophrenic patients. *Psychopharmacologia*, *(Berlin)*, **40,** 341–350 (1975)

22 GERLACH, J. and FAURBYE, A. Pathophysiological aspects of reversible and irreversible tardive dyskinesia. In *Tardive Dyskinesia Research and Treatment*, edited by W. E. Fann, R. C. Smith, J. M. Davis and E. F. Domino, 355–363. New York, Spectrum Publications Inc (1980)

23 HUNTER, R., BLACKWOOD, W., SMITH, M. and CUMMINGS, J. Neuropathological findings in three cases of persistent dyskinesia following phenothiazine medication. *Journal of Neurological Sciences*, **7,** 263–273 (1968)

24 JELLINGER, K. Neuropathologic findings after neuroleptic long-term therapy. In *Neurotoxicology*, edited by L. Roizin, H. Shiraki and N. Grćević. New York, Raven Press (1977)

25 JESTE, D. V., POTKIN, S. G., SINHA, S., FEDER, S. and WYATT, R. J. Tardive dyskinesia – reversible and persistent. *Archives of General Psychiatry*, **36,** 585–590 (1979)

26 JONES, M. and HUNTER, R. Abnormal movements in patients with chronic psychiatric illness. In *Psychotropic Drugs and Dysfunction of the Basal Ganglia*, edited by G. E. Grane and R. Gardner, Jr., 53–65. Washington DC, US Government Printing Office, Public Health Service Publication No. 1938 (1969)

27 JUS, A., PINEAU, R., LACHANCE, R., PERCHAT, G., JUS, K., PIRES, P. and VILLENEUVE, R. Epidemiology of tardive dyskinesia, Part II. *Diseases of the Nervous System*, **37,** 257–261 (1976)

28 KANE, J., STRUVE, F. A., WEINHOLD, P. and WOERNER, M. Strategy for the study of patients at high risk for tardive dyskinesia. *American Journal of Psychiatry*, **137**, 1265–1267 (1980)
29 KENNEDY, P. F., HERSHON, H. I. and McGUIRE, R. J. Extrapyramidal disorders after prolonged phenothiazine therapy. *British Journal of Psychiatry*, **118**, 509–518 (1971)
30 KIDGER, T., BARNES, T. R. E., TRAUER, T. and TAYLOR, P. J. Sub-syndromes of tardive dyskinesia. *Psychological Medicine*, **10**, 513–520 (1980)
31 KLAWANS. H. L., BERGEN, D., BRUYN, G. W. and POULSON. G. W. Neuroleptic-induced tardive dyskinesias in nonpsychotic patients. *Archives of Neurology*, **30**, 338–339 (1974)
32 KRAEPLIN. E. *Dementia praecox and paraphrenia.* Edinburgh, Livingston (1919)
33 MACKAY, A. V. P. Positive and negative schizophrenic symptoms and the role of dopamine. *British Journal of Psychiatry*, **137**, 379–386 (1980)
34 MACKAY, A. V. P., BIRD, E. D., SPOKES, E. G., ROSSOR. M., IVERSEN. L. L., CREESE, I. and SNYDER, S. H. Dopamine receptors and schizophrenia: drug effect or illness? *Lancet*, **2**, 915–916 (1980)
35 MARSDEN, C. D., TARSY, D. and BALDESSARINI R. J. Spontaneous and drug-induced movement disorders in psychotic patients. In *Psychiatric Aspects of Neurological Disease*, edited by D. F. Benson and D. Blumer. New York, Grune and Stratton (1975)
36 MARSDEN, C. D., MINDHAM, R. H. S. and MACKAY, A. V. P. Extrapyramidal movement disorders produced by antipsychotic drugs. In *The Pharmacology and Treatment of Schizophrenia*, edited by P. B. Bradley and S. R. Hirsch. Oxford University Press (in press)
37 McGEER, P. L., McGEER, E. G. and SUZUKI, J. S. Ageing and extrapyramidal function. *Archives of Neurology*, **34**, 33–35 (1977)
38 METTLER, F. A. and CRANDELL, A. Neurologic disorders in psychiatric institutions. *Journal of Nervous and Mental Diseases*, **128**, 148–159 (1959)
39 NAGAO, T., OHSHIMO, T., MITSUNOBU, K., SATO, M. and OTSUKI, S. Cerebrospinal fluid monoamine metabolites and cyclic nucleotides in chronic schizophrenic patients with tardive dyskinesia or drug-induced tremor. *Biological Psychiatry*, **14**, 509–523 (1979)
40 PIND, K. and FAURBYE, A. Concentration of homovanillic acid and 5-hydroxyindoleacetic acid in the cerebrospinal fluid after treatment with probenecid in patients with drug-induced tardive dyskinesia. *Acta Psychiatrica Scandinavica*, **46**, 323–326 (1970)
41 PYE, M. and POTTER, E. Beware freedom drugs, say doctors. *Sunday Times*, 26th October (1980)
42 QUITKIN, F., RIFKIN, A., GOCHFELD, L. and KLEIN, D. F. Tardive dyskinesia – are first signs reversible? *American Journal of Psychiatry*, **134**, 84–87 (1977)
43 SCHIELE, B. C., GALLANT, D., SIMPSON, G., GARDNER, E. A., COLE, J., CRANE, G., CHASE, T., AYD, F., LEVINE, J. and OCHOTA, L. Neurological syndromes associated with antipsychotic drug use. *Archives of General Psychiatry*, **28**, 463–467 (1973)
44 SIGWALD, J., BOUTTIER, D. and COURVOISIER, S. Les accidents neurologiques des médications neuroleptiques. *Revue Neurologique*, **100**, 553–595 (1959)

45 SLATER, E. and ROTH. M. *Clinical Psychiatry*, 3rd edition. London, Baillieré, Tindall and Cassell (1972)
46 SMITH, J. M. and BALDESSARINI, R. J. Changes in prevalence, severity and recovery in tardive dyskinesia with age. *Archives of General Psychiatry*, **37,** 1368–1373 (1980)
47 SMITH, J. M., KUCHARSKI, L. T., EBLEN, C., KNUTSEN, E. and LUNN, C. An assessment of tardive dyskinesia in schizophrenic out-patients. *Psychopharmacologia (Berlin)*, **64,** 99–104 (1979)
48 SMITH, R. C., TAMMINGA, C. and DAVIS, J. Effects of apomorphine and amphetamine on tardive dyskinesia. In *Tardive Dyskinesia Research and Treatment*, edited by W. E. Fann, R. C. Smith, J. M. Davis and E. F. Domino, 333–334. New York, Spectrum Publications Inc. (1980)
49 TAMMINGA, C. A., SMITH, R. C., PANDEY, G. DAVIS, J. M. and FROHMAN, L. A. A neuroendocrine study of supersensitivity in tardive dyskinesia. In *Tardive Dyskinesia Research and Treatment*, edited by W. E. Fann, R. C. Smith, J. M. Davis and E. F. Domino, 345–354. New York, Spectrum Publications Inc. (1980)
50 Task Force on Late Neurological Effects of Antipsychotic Drugs. Tardive dyskinesia: Summary of a Task Force Report of the American Psychiatric Association. *American Journal of Psychiatry*, **137,** 1163–1172 (1980)
51 WEINER, W. J. and KLAWANS, H. L. Lingual-facial-buccal movements in the elderly, II. Pathogenesis and relationship to senile chorea. *Journal of the American Geriatric Society*, **21,** 318–320 (1973)

15
Controversies in animal models of tardive dyskinesia
Christopher G. Goetz and Harold L. Klawans

Although the pathologic sequence of changes underlying the development of tardive dyskinesia remains unknown, the similarity of the abnormal movements to other forms of chorea suggests an analogous physiologic basis. A number of clinical and pharmacologic observations have helped to clarify the pathophysiology of the movements seen in tardive dyskinesia and suggest etiologic as well as therapeutic implications. In summary, there is substantial evidence that tardive dyskinesias are caused by chronic dopamine receptor site blockade, and that the pathophysiology of the disorder is due to the resultant receptor site supersensitivity.

Experimental studies in animals have clarified some issues but have also introduced new questions and heightened controversies. In an attempt to present a coherent and comprehensive approach to the entire question of animal models of tardive dyskinesia, the authors have divided the available material into three sections. The first deals with controversies as to the relevance of animal models to tardive dyskinesia, with particular attention to behavioral, biochemical and neuropathologic studies. The second section discusses the use of animal models to study risk factors in tardive dyskinesia, and the third section is devoted to controversies over prevention and treatment.

PRIMATE AND RODENT MODELS

All animal models involve the prolonged administration of neuroleptic drugs. Two major experimental models exist for tardive dyskinesia, one produced mostly in primates, the other in a variety of rodent species. Long-term administration of neuroleptic agents to primates elicits actual abnormal movements whereas in rodents it does not.

Dr Goetz is the recipient of the NINCDS Teacher/Investigator Award

Primates

Gunne and Bárány[16], Deneau and Crane[10] and Messiha[26] have described primates that, like man, developed spontaneous buccolingual dyskinesia after prolonged neuroleptic treatment. Their model has several distinct and positive features. First, the movements described are similar in many ways to those seen in humans with tardive dyskinesia. Furthermore, as the animals studied are relatively close to man in evolutionary terms, similar pathophysiologic mechanisms can at least be inferred. Finally, long-term administration of the moderate to high doses of drug required to produce such movements in primates mimics the disorder in humans.

There are, however, several serious problems with the primate model. First, the movements are only transient, often appearing to increase with each new dose of neuroleptic. They also may be decreased by anticholinergic drugs, a pattern not seen in tardive dyskinesia in man. In the study by Gunne and Bárány[16], all dyskinetic monkeys had coincident parkinsonism and/or dystonic signs. After administration of the neuroleptic, a dystonic reaction replaced the ambient buccolingual movements for 4 hours, and as dystonia abated the dyskinesia returned. This pattern does not resemble the behavior of patients with tardive dyskinesia.

Rodents

Clow et al. described spontaneous mouthing movements in rats after 12 months of trifluoperazine or thioridazine administration[7]. These movements, however, resolved after drug withdrawal, a pattern not always typical of tardive dyskinesia in man. Iversen et al.[18] also reported spontaneous oral movements in rats similarly treated for several months, but these movements were tremulous and may have represented parkinsonian features. Rodent models of spontaneous movements induced by neuroleptics are relatively inexpensive, but they have not yet been studied in detail.

A more commonly used animal model for tardive dyskinesia is one which measures the effect of long-term neuroleptic administration on the subsequent response to a challenging dose of either amphetamine or apomorphine. Stereotypies induced by amphetamine and apomorphine are two closely related behaviors that correlate with enhanced dopaminergic activity in the striatum[31]. Amphetamine acts primarily as an indirect agonist to release presynaptic stores of dopamine, and apomorphine acts as a direct agonist to stimulate the postsynaptic dopamine receptors[14]. When either of these agents is administered to guinea pigs, characteristic gnawing, mouthing stereotypy develops that correlates with increased dopaminergic striatal activity. In order to reproduce the pharmacologic setting of tardive dyskinesia the authors examined the threshold for dopaminergic stereotypies before and after long-term exposure to neuroleptics.

In the initial behavioral studies, two groups of guinea pigs were given daily subcutaneous injections of chlorpromazine (5 mg/kg for 3 weeks in one group, 10 mg/kg for 4 weeks in the other). Beginning 4 days after the last injection of chlorpromazine, amphetamine or apomorphine was given to the two groups of animals[30]. It was found that doses of amphetamine which were too small to produce stereotyped behavior in control animals were effective in producing such behavior in the animals pretreated with chlorpromazine. The animals were evaluated weekly for 4 weeks, and it was found that the alteration in threshold for stereotyped behavior persisted. This implies that neuroleptic pretreatment in some way altered the sensitivity of the dopaminergic receptors in the striatum to the dopamine released by the amphetamine. An alternative explanation may be that the absolute amount of dopamine available to act at the striatum is increased as a result of pretreatment with chlorpromazine. It is known that chlorpromazine increases the synthesis and turnover of striatal dopamine by a feedback mechanism. However, two studies[15, 29] have shown that the concentration of dopamine in the brain after chronic neuroleptic therapy is not elevated. Therefore, it is unlikely that amphetamine releases increased amounts of dopamine in animals pretreated with chlorpromazine.

The studies in which apomorphine was given to animals pretreated with chlorpromazine also demonstrated a persistent decrease in the threshold for apomorphine-induced stereotyped behavior. Since apomorphine acts directly at dopaminergic receptor sites in the striatum, these results support the hypothesis of a postsynaptic neuroleptic-induced alteration in sensititivity to dopaminergic agents.

It appears from this initial study that pretreatment with neuroleptic agents altered the sensitivity or the threshold of the dopaminergic receptors to dopamine and hence altered the threshold for the production of stereotyped behavior. Likewise, the striatal dopaminergic receptors in patients undergoing neuroleptic therapy may be altered in such a way that, upon termination of therapy, normal amounts of dopamine may trigger an abnormal response.

Since this original description of chlorpromazine-induced behavioral supersensitivity, other investigators[4, 13, 25, 33] have reported similar findings with other neuroleptic agents in a variety of experimental animals. In addition to showing supersensitivity to amphetamine and apomorphine, animals show heightened responses to methylphenidate[6], another indirect dopamine agonist, after prolonged exposure to neuroleptics. These studies all indicate that long-term administration of antipsychotic drugs followed by drug withdrawal produces a behavioral state of increased responsiveness to dopamine agonists which is consistent with the development of supersensitivity that lasts for at least several weeks.

In further studies with this model of neuroleptic-induced supersensitivity, the authors sought biochemical evidence of this behavioral change. Burt et al.[3] assayed receptor binding with the dopamine antagonist [^{3}H]haloperidol and found an increase in the number of dopamine receptor sites after long-term treatment with haloperidol followed by a short period of drug withdrawal. Hitri et al.[17] used [^{3}H]dopamine to determine if there is an alteration in dopamine receptor binding in the striatum and nucleus accumbens after long-term treatment with haloperidol and subsequent drug withdrawal in rats. Haloperidol pretreatment resulted in a 60 percent increase in binding sites and a ninefold increase in the affinity constant in the caudate putamen, whereas there was no effect in the nucleus accumbens (*Table 15.1*).

Table 15.1 Effect of chronic haloperidol pretreatment on dopamine receptor site binding

	Caudate putamen		Nucleus accumbens	
	n (pmol/g brain)	Ka (mol/l)	n (pmol/g brain)	Ka (mol/l)
Control	90	7×10^7	152	8×10^7
Haloperidol pretreatment	151	64×10^7	171	11×10^7

n = number of binding sites; Ka = affinity constant, see Hitri et al.[17] for details. Animals were treated with intraperitoneal haloperidol 0.5 mg/kg daily for 14 days and were sacrificed 7 days after withdrawal of the drug

Studies using different ligands have produced generally similar changes in striatal dopamine receptors. Muller and Seeman[27] reported a 77 percent increase in [^{3}H]apomorphine binding and a 34 percent increase in [^{3}H]haloperidol binding in the rat striatum after neuroleptic exposure. Clow et al.[8] reported increased striatal affinity without increased receptor numbers using [^{3}H]spiperone in rats treated with trifluoperazine for 6 months. Friedhoff et al.[12] have also reported increases in binding. Although the physiologic significance of changes in receptor numbers versus changes in receptor affinity has yet to be determined, these results are all direct biochemical evidence for the existence of supersensitive dopaminergic function in the rat striatum after prolonged haloperidol pretreatment. As such, they support the behavioral studies and suggest that long-term treatment with neuroleptic agents enhances dopaminergic striatal responsiveness.

Although studies of dopamine receptor binding in the striatum are generally consistent with one another regardless of ligand or neuroleptic used, this is not the case for binding results in the mesolimbic system. The authors' studies demonstrated that prolonged administration of haloperidol did not alter [^{3}H]dopamine binding in the nucleus accumbens, which is consistent with the observation that tardive dyskinesia occurs without alteration of the underlying psychiatric state for which the patient is receiving neuroleptic treatment. It has been suggested that dopamine acting at dopamine receptors in limbic systems plays a major role in the pathophysiology of schizophrenia[20]. If this is true then neuroleptic-induced alterations in dopamine receptor binding should worsen schizophrenia. The fact that these characteristics were unchanged in the nucleus accumbens may explain why the development of tardive dyskinesia is not related to any worsening of the underlying schizophrenia and is consistent with the hypothesis that these receptors play the major role in the pathophysiology of schizophrenia. However, Muller and Seeman[27] found that mesolimbic [^{3}H]haloperidol binding increased by 34 percent and [^{3}H]apomorphine binding increased by 77 percent after long-term exposure to neuroleptics. These discrepancies remain unexplained.

This animal model, which involves long-term treatment of rodents with neuroleptics and the subsequent neuropathologic, behavioral or biochemical analysis (usually with the aid of dopamine agonists) of the dopaminergic system, has been the major behavioral model for the study of tardive dyskinesia. In spite of its wide use, however, this model has several important limitations. First, the animals do not develop spontaneous involuntary movements, as seen in humans, but demonstrate an altered threshold, with a subsequent abnormal response, to another exogenous agent.

A second limitation of this model is its course. Altered dopaminergic sensititivity can be induced in rodents after 3 weeks. This rapid alteration does not correlate well with the more prolonged exposure necessary in humans. Although a rodent's life span is shorter than man's, the short absolute time required for the changes observed suggests that a different mechanism may be active. Linked to the above limitation is the natural history of the animal's supersensitivity. In the rodent studies, while supersensitivity persists for some time after cessation of neuroleptic exposure, it eventually completely resolves.

In one experiment, animals treated with haloperidol for 3 weeks became supersensitive to apomorphine and remained so for 3 additional weeks after cessation of the neuroleptic. After 6 weeks however, animals were no longer supersensitive to apomorphine, and the binding increases seen originally were returning towards normal values[34]. Although the duration of supersensitivity is, in absolute terms, rather short (3 weeks), it is the same as that of the original exposure to neuroleptics. By extrapolation to man, where neuroleptic exposure must be prolonged to induce tardive dyskinesia with regularity, reversibility may require a drug-free period close to or equal to that of the original neuroleptic exposure. This question has not been specifically addressed and hence the degree to which this time factor is a limitation to the animal model of tardive dyskinesia remains unclear.

In humans, tardive dyskinesia may clearly persist long after cessation of neuroleptic administration. This potential discrepancy between human and animal data may limit the use of the animal model, especially if it is used to evaluate treatments for tardive dyskinesia. Since supersensitivity in the animal tends to resolve spontaneously, abatement coincident with pharmacologic manipulation cannot necessarily be interpreted as evidence for drug activity.

A final characteristic of the model that is in conflict with current understanding of the epidemiology of tardive dyskinesia is that animal supersensitivity is a population event occurring in 100 percent of animals appropriately treated. In man, the occurrence of tardive dyskinesia is not universal, and patients generally exposed to similar prolonged treatment with high doses of neuroleptics do not necessarily develop involuntary movements. Even if they do, the degree and anatomic distribution of such movements may differ dramatically among patients. The current model produces an all-or-nothing effect, where animals either become supersensitive or remain unaffected. More careful behavior rating reports and sequential studies of behavioral and biochemical changes may reduce this limitation.

Neuropathology

Although no consistent neuropathologic changes have been seen in patients with tardive dyskinesia, Fog and Pakkenberg[11] reported that animals treated chronically with moderate doses of perphenazine showed a 20 percent cell loss from basal ganglia regions. A higher dose for shorter periods did not induce the cell degeneration. A further study, examining the ventrolateral and dorsomedial striatum separately, demonstrated that the cell loss induced by neuroleptic administration appeared only in the ventrolateral region, suggesting for the first time a highly specific locus for alterations[28].

Heavy metals

Another area of research pertinent to the pathophysiology of tardive dyskinesia is that of heavy metal toxicity. Since chronic manganese poisoning causes extrapyramidal dysfunction in man, Weiner et al.[35] studied the effect of prolonged exposure to neuroleptics on manganese levels in basal ganglia in guinea pigs. They demonstrated significant increases in manganese in the caudate nucleus and cerebellar hemisphere, but no change in manganese in the frontal cortex, after long-term administration of neuroleptics. Bird et al.[1] found a similar accumulation of manganese in the basal ganglia of monkeys after exposure to neuroleptics. If such accumulation plays a role in the pathophysiology or pathogenesis of dopaminergic supersensitivity in animals, and by extrapolation to tardive dyskinesia in man, metal chelation therapy administered with neuroleptics might help to prevent or reverse tardive dyskinesia. This question has not been specifically studied.

RISK FACTORS

Despite its limitations the amphetamine-apomorphine threshold model remains the major experimental means of studying dopaminergic mechanisms that may relate to tardive dyskinesia. The same animal model has been used to study possible risk factors that may increase the likelihood of developing dopaminergic supersensitivity and, by extrapolation to man, the likelihood of developing tardive dyskinesia.

Three questions arise regarding risk factors in the development of dopaminergic supersensitivity: (1) Is there a relationship between the daily neuroleptic dose and the degree of eventual supersensitivity? (2) Do equipotent antipsychotic doses of different neuroleptics differ in their ability to elicit supersensitivity? (3) Does duration of neuroleptic exposure play a significant role in the development of dopaminergic supersensitivity? If the model is an accurate one of tardive dyskinesia in humans, the answers to these questions have not only theoretical importance, but also very practical implications as to which neuroleptic classes, doses and lengths of treatment are safest in regard to the prevention of tardive dyskinesia.

In order to answer these questions, different doses of four neuroleptics (chlorpromazine, prochlorperazine, thioridazine and trifluoperazine) were given to groups of guinea pigs or rats for 3 weeks and the degree of behavioral supersensitivity was evaluated using the dopamine agonist apomorphine. The resulting dose responses are shown in *Figure 15.1*. Chlorpromazine, prochlorperazine and trifluoperazine showed a definite dose effect, with larger doses causing greater

Figure 15.1 Behavioral supersensitivity scores to challenge dose of apomorphine after 3 weeks of daily neuroleptic treatment with 4 different drugs. The daily intraperitoneal doses of each neuroleptic are shown in mg/kg. Animals were tested to apomorphine 0.2 mg/kg 4 days after drug withdrawal. NS = normal saline

supersensitivity[22]. At low doses, no supersensitivity was seen. Thioridazine induced no supersensitivity at the doses studied. These results suggest that exposure dose is a risk factor in the development of dopaminergic striatal supersensitivity for at least some drugs. If used as a model for tardive dyskinesia in humans, the model suggests that keeping the daily neuroleptic dose as low as possible may decrease the incidence of the disorder, and that very low doses may not be associated with any risk of supersensitivity. The same data are plotted in *Figure 15.2* after converting specific doses of neuroleptic (mg/kg) to chlorpromazine equivalents. This method allows a comparison of behavioral effects, in this case supersensitivity, caused by different neuroleptics with the milligram doses controlled for comparable antipsychotic potency. The graph demonstrates that at equivalent antipsychotic doses, some drugs appear more likely to induce behavioral supersensitivity than others. However, the direct extrapolation of these data to human incidence of tardive dyskinesia has not been confirmed. Such human studies are difficult to perform, since patients commonly receive many different neuroleptic agents over several years.

A similar study, investigating the biochemical aspects of stereotyped behavior, compared receptor site changes in animals receiving chronic haloperidol or clozapine. The latter neuroleptic has been associated with a low incidence of early onset extrapyramidal complications as well as tardive dyskinesia. The biochemical effects in brain that may correlate with the clinically observed differences in extrapyramidal dysfunction between the two drugs have been studied by Kobayashi et al.[24]. Using similar techniques to those already described, caudate dopamine receptor changes were assayed after prolonged treatment with haloperidol or clozapine. Treatment with haloperidol led to an increase in the number of striatal receptors, while treatment with clozapine did not alter striatal dopamine binding.

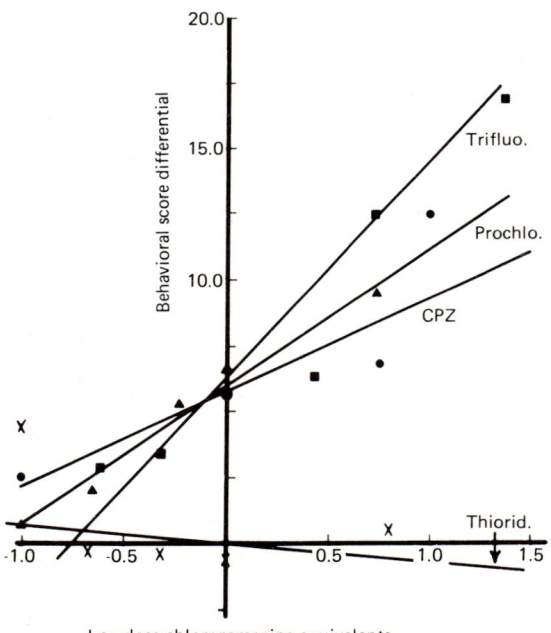

Figure 15.2 Behavioral score differentials from *Figure 15.1* compared to log-dose of the neuroleptics administered, all transformed to chlorpromazine equivalents. TRIFLUO = trifluoperazine; PROCHLO = prochlorperazine; CPZ = chlorpromazine; THIORID = thioridazine.

Striatal muscarinic receptors and γ-amino-*n*-butyric acid (GABA) binding were unaltered by long-term administration of haloperidol and of clozapine. These data demonstrate that a drug known to be associated with a high incidence of early extrapyramidal side effects and also with the development of tardive dyskinesia induces an increase in the dopamine receptor site population in the striatum, while a drug without these effects does not cause these changes. The results are consistent with the behavioral and biochemical data presented earlier and suggest that drug–induced alterations in striatal dopaminergic function may underly and be an accurate measure of the degree of developing dopaminergic supersensitivity.

Prolonged continuous neuroleptic therapy has been suggested as a possible risk factor for tardive dyskinesia. In order to test the influence of duration of therapy in the model for tardive dyskinesia, the authors studied the development of apomorphine-induced stereotypy after different periods of neuroleptic exposure[23]. Male albino rats were given daily injections of one of three different doses of chlorpromazine (0.5, 2.5 or 5 mg/kg) for 3, 6 or 9 consecutive weeks. These doses were chosen because previous work had shown that increased daily doses over 3 weeks increase subsequent stereotypic behavior. Following each pretreatment, the behavioral response to apomorphine was assessed. For the groups receiving 2.5 and 5.0 mg/kg the degree of stereotypic behavior induced by apomorphine increased in direct proportion to the duration of treatment. For the group receiving 0.5 mg/kg no such relationship was found. These results suggest that both dosage and duration of therapy are risk factors for subsequent supersensitivity. The effect of prolonged but intermittently interrupted administration of neuroleptics on the eventual development of dopaminergic supersensitivity has not yet been studied.

Epidemiologic studies of tardive dyskinesia have shown that the prevalence of abnormal involuntary movements increases with age. Most animal studies of the behavioral or biochemical effects of neuroleptic exposure, however, use young animals. To assess the influence of age on the development of dopaminergic supersensitivity, Smith and Leelavathi[32] compared the threshold to amphetamine, apomorphine and methylphenidate stereotypy after neuroleptic treatment in animals of different ages. After a single dose of a dopaminergic agent, older rats showed a higher stereotypic score than younger rats. After continuous prolonged neuroleptic treatment, older rats showed the highest absolute stereotypic scores, although the greatest degree of change occurred in the young and middle-aged animals.

Although there is no behavioral correlate in man for acute dopaminergic stereotypy, two observations are pertinent. First, animals at all ages show a progressive increase in dopaminergic sensitivity after exposure to neuroleptic drugs a phenomenon also seen in man. Second, older animals appear to be more sensitive acutely as well as chronically, and at any one time are more likely to show the heightened dopaminergic response. A repeat study using apomorphine doses that are subthreshold in all animals in the acute experiment might prove more useful for assessing the relative likelihood of developing dopaminergic sensitivity after chronic neuroleptic exposure in young and old animals separately.

Females have also been reported to have a higher incidence of tardive dyskinesia. The role of sex hormones relative to this model has not been investigated but deserves attention.

TREATMENT

Anticholinergic drugs will exacerbate pre-existing tardive dyskinesia. It has been suggested that exposure to anticholinergic drugs early in the course of neuroleptic treatment may increase the relative risk of developing tardive dyskinesia later[9,19]. To test this hypothesis experimentally, Borison and Diamond[2] treated animals for 3 weeks either with haloperidol alone or with haloperidol and benztropine, an anticholinergic agent. After drug withdrawal, animals who had received haloperidol alone showed the expected supersensitivity to subsequent challenge with apomorphine. The animals treated also with the anticholinergic were markedly more sensitive to apomorphine, showing intense and higher order stereotypic behavior. These results support the hypothesis that long-term exposure to anticholinergics may be potentially dangerous in patients receiving neuroleptic agents.

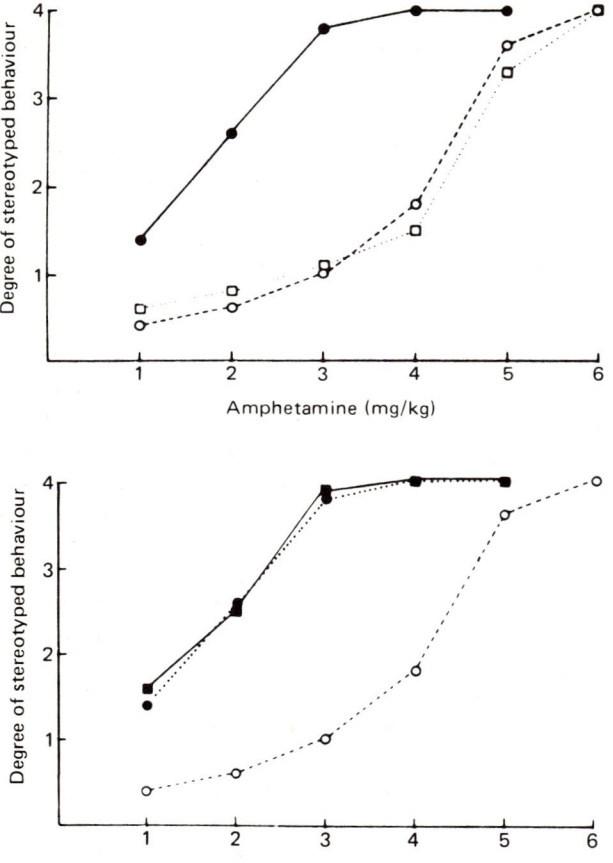

Figure 15.3 Effect of concurrent lithium and haloperidol vs haloperidol treatment on subsequent development of amphetamine stereotyped behavior (*top*). Lithium is effective in preventing supersensitivity when given concurrently, but ineffective if given after chronic haloperidol treatment. (*bottom*). Animals were treated with intraperitoneal haloperidol 0.5 mg/kg per day for 21 days, alone (●) or with a diet containing 2.79% LiCl (□) (*top*), and were challenged with a range of intraperitoneal doses of amphetamine 7 days after drug withdrawal. Alternatively, lithium diet (■) was administered for 7 days after haloperidol was stopped (*bottom*), prior to amphetamine challenge. (○) Control

The effect of lithium carbonate on the development of dopaminergic supersensitivity has also been studied[21]. *Figure 15.3* demonstrates that animals treated for prolonged periods with lithium and haloperidol do not develop the sensitivity to amphetamine seen after long-term administration of haloperidol alone. This effect is seen only when lithium is given concurrently with haloperidol, and there is no effect on stereotypy if lithium is given after pretreatment with haloperidol. These results suggest that prophylactic treatment with concomitant lithium can prevent the development of dopaminergic supersensitivity in animals. It may be possible that, in humans, lithium may be of value in the prevention of tardive dyskinesia, although probably not in the treatment of such disorders once manifested. The mechanism of this effect, be it peripheral or central, has not yet been clarified.

Friedhoff et al.[12] have addressed the question of reversing dopaminergic supersensitivity from another perspective. In rats, they induced supersensitivity with haloperidol, as measured by a reduced threshold to apomorphine. The sensitivity was reversed by subsequent treatment with levodopa/carbidopa. These studies suggest that dopaminergic receptor mechanisms are malleable and that subsensitivity may be produced by agents that augment dopaminergic function. Since levodopa induces chorea in patients with Parkinson's disease its administration to patients with tardive dyskinesia may be controversial. The animal studies, however, suggest that precursors, or agonist therapy, could reverse the supersensitivity induced by neuroleptics.

Christensen and Møllier Nielsen[5] administered apomorphine with neuroleptics to mice and demonstrated that the addition of apomorphine prevented the development of neuroleptic-induced behavioral dopaminergic supersensitivity. Whether the combination of agonist and antagonist is simply equivalent to a lower antagonist dose or whether the apomorphine has a distinct selective pharmacologic activity relative to the pathophysiology of dopaminergic supersensitivity has yet to be determined. In a similar experiment Borison and Diamond[2] treated rats with amantadine and neuroleptics. They also demonstrated that animals who received both drugs did not show subsequent supersensitivity to apomorphine compared to animals treated with neuroleptics alone. The fact that dopaminergic behavioral supersensitivity induced with a neuroleptic can be prevented by either apomorphine or amantadine, both drugs that affect the dopaminergic system differently, suggests that their action is one of neuroleptic antagonism as opposed to a specific pharmacologic effect. The practical application of these data to the prevention of tardive dyskinesia in humans may be limited, since the addition of a dopaminergic agent to the treatment of an actively hallucinating schizophrenic patient might be considered hazardous even if he is receiving coincident neuroleptic therapy.

Future perspectives

Until an inexpensive and accurate model of tardive dyskinesia is developed, all behavioral studies will be of limited usefulness. The model described by Clow et al.[7] is perhaps the most promising, although the expense and time required for such long-term investigations may prohibit its extensive use. Nevertheless, since neuroleptics are rarely administered for short periods, studies of the effects of long-term exposure will necessarily become the rule for the future. More extensive analysis of various risk factors may help in the prevention of tardive dyskinesia and in the early identification of those subjects who must be most carefully followed. Finally, an understanding of the pathophysiology of tardive dyskinesia may lead to the eventual development of neuroleptic agents that will not induce the striatal dopaminergic supersensitivity which appears to be the hallmark of the condition. In this way, future physicians may avoid the induction of an iatrogenic disorder that can be not only cosmetically embarrassing, but also dangerous and, in some cases, life threatening.

References

1 BIRD, E. D., COLLINS, G. H., DODSON, M. H. and GRANT, L. G. The effect of phenothiazines on the manganese concentration in the basal ganglia of sub-human primates. In *Progress in Neuro-Genetics*, **1**, (Proceedings of the 2nd International Congress in Neuro-Genetics and Neuro-Ophthalmology, Montreal). Amsterdam, Excerpta Medica (1967)

2 BORISON, R. L. and DIAMOND, B. I. Anticholinergics promote neuroleptic-induced tardive dyskinesia. In *Long Term Effects of Neuroleptics, Advances in Biochemical Psychopharmacology*, **24**, edited by F. Cattabeni, G. Racagni, P. F. Spano and E. Costa, 359–362. New York, Raven Press (1980)

3 BURT, D. R., CREESE, I. and SNYDER, S. H. Antischizophrenic drugs: chronic treatment elevates dopamine receptor binding in brain. *Science*, **196**, 326–328 (1977)

4 CARLSON, K. R. Tardive dyskinesia resulting from chronic narcotic treatment. In *Tardive Diskinesia*, edited by W. E. Fann, R. C. Smith, J. M. Davis and E. F. Domino, 27–34. New York, S.P. Medical and Scientific Books (1980)

5 CHRISTENSEN, A. V. and MØLLIER NIELSEN, I. Dopaminergic supersensitivity. Influence of dopamine agonists and drugs used for the treatment of tardive dyskinesia. In *Long Term Effects of Neuroleptics, Advances in Biochemical Psychopharmacology*, **24**, edited by F. Cattabeni, G. Racagni, P. F. Spano and E. Costa, 341–350. New York, Raven Press

6 CHRISTENSEN, A. V. and MØLLIER NIELSEN, I. On the supersensitivity of DA-receptors after single and repeated administration of neuroleptics. In *Tardive Diskinesia*, edited by W. E. Fann, R. C. Smith, J. M. Davis and E. F. Domino, 35–50. New York, S.P. Medical and Scientific Books (1980)

7 CLOW, A. T., JENNER, P. and MARSDEN, C. D. Changes in cerebral dopamine function induced by a year's administration of trifluoperazine or thioridazine and their subsequent withdrawal. In *Long Term Effects of Neuroleptics, Advances in Biochemical Psychopharmacology*, **24**, 335–340. New York, Raven Press (1980)

8 CLOW, A. T., JENNER, P. and MARSDEN, C. D. An experimental model of tardive dyskinesia. *Life Sciences*, **23**, 421–424 (1978)

9 CRANE, G. E. Factors pre-disposing to drug-induced neurological side effects. In *Advances in Biochemical Psychopharmacology*, **9**, edited by E. Costa, 242–251. New York, Raven Press (1974)

10 DENEAU, G. A. and CRANE, G. E. Dyskinesia in Rhesus monkeys tested with high doses of chlorpromazine. In *Psychotropic Drugs and Dysfunction of the Basal Ganglia*, edited by G. E. Crane and J. R. Gardner, Jr., 12–14. Washington, DC, US Public Health Service Publication No. 1938 (1969)

11 FOG, R. and PAKKENBERG, H. Anatomical and metabolic changes after long and short term treatment with perphenazine in rats. In *Tardive Diskinesia*, edited by W. E. Fann, R. C. Smith, J. M. Davis and E. F. Domino, 89–94. New York, S.P Medical and Scientific Books (1980)

12 FRIEDHOFF, A. J., ROSENGARTEN, H. and BONNET, K. Receptor cell sensitivity modification as a model for pathogenesis and treatment of tardive dyskinesia. *Psychopharmacology Bulletin*, **14**, 77–79 (1978)

13 GIANUTSOS, G., DRAWBAUGH, R. B., HYNES, M. D. and LAL, H. Behavioral evidence for dopaminergic supersensitivity after chronic haloperidol. *Life Sciences*, **14**, 887 (1974)

14 GLOWINSKI, J. Effects of amphetamine on various aspects of catecholamine metabolism in the central nervous system of the rat. In *Amphetamines and Related Compounds*, edited by E. Costa and S. Garattini, 301–317. New York, Raven Press (1970)

15 GULDBERG, H. C. and YATES, C. M. Effects of chlorpromazine on the metabolism of catecholamines in dog brain. *British Journal of Pharmacology*, **36**, 535–537 (1969)

16 GUNNE, L. M. and BÁRÁNY, S. A primate model for tardive dyskinesia. In *Tardive Dyskinesia*, edited by W. E. Fann, R. C. Smith, J. M. Davis and E. F. Domino, 1–12. New York, S.P. Medical and Scientific Books (1980)

17 HITRI, A., WEINER, W. J., BORISON, R. L., DIAMOND, B. I., NAUSIEDA, P. A. and KLAWANS, H. L. Dopamine binding following prolonged haloperidol pretreatment. *Annals of Neurology*, **3**, 134–140 (1978)

18 IVERSEN, S. D., HOWELLS, R. B. and HUGHES, R. P. The behavioral consequences of long term treatment with neuroleptic drugs. In *Long Term Effects of Neuroleptics, Advances in Biochemical Psychopharmacology*, **24**, edited by F. Cattabeni, G. Racagni, P. F. Spano, and E. Costa, 305–314. New York, Raven Press (1980)

19 KLAWANS, H. L. *The Pharmacology of Extrapyramidal Movement Disorders*. Basel, S. Karger (1973)

20 KLAWANS, H. L., GOETZ, C. and WESTHEIMER, R. The pharmacology of schizophrenia. In *Clinical Neuropharmacology*, **1**, edited by H. L. Klawans, 1–28. New York, Raven Press (1975)

21 KLAWANS, H. L., WEINER, W. J. and NAUSIEDA, P. A. Effect of lithium on an animal model of tardive dyskinesia. *Progress in Neuropsychopharmacology*, **1**, 53–60 (1976)

22 KLAWANS, H. L., CARVEY, P., NAUSIEDA, P. A., GOETZ, C. G. and WEINER, W. J. Effect of dose and type of neuroleptic in an animal model of tardive dyskinesia. *Neurology*, **30**, 383 (1980)

23 KLAWANS, H. L., NAUSIEDA, P. A., GOETZ, C. G., CARVEY, P. and WEINER, W. J. Effect of duration of neuroleptic therapy in an animal model of tardive dyskinesia. *Neurology*, **31**, (4, Part 2) 103 (1981)

24 KOBAYASHI, R. M., FIELDS, J. Z., HRUSKA, R. E., BEAUMONT, K. and YAMAMURA, H. I. Brain neurotransmitter receptors and chronic antipsychotic drug treatment: A model for tardive dyskinesia. In *Animal Models in Psychiatry and Neurology*, edited by J. Hanin and E. Usdin, 405–411. Oxford, Pergamon (1977)

25 LAL, H., GIANUTSOS, G. Alterations in neuropharmacology of apomorphine by chronic treatment with haloperidol. In *Tardive Diskinesia*, edited by W. E. Fann, R. C. Smith, J. M. Davis and E. F. Domino, 35–50. New York, S.P. Medical and Scientific Books (1980)

26 MESSIHA, F. S. Biochemical studies after chronic administration of neuroleptics to monkeys. In *Tardive Diskinesia*, edited by W. E. Fann, R. C. Smith, J. M. Davis and E. F. Domino. New York, S.P. Medical and Scientific Books (1980)

27 MULLER, P. and SEEMAN, P. Effects of long term neuroleptic treatment of neurotransmitter receptors: relation to tardive dyskinesia. In *Tardive Diskinesia*, edited by W. E. Fann, J. M. Davis and E. F. Domino, 115–126. New York, S.P. Medical and Scientific Books (1980)

28 NEILSON, E. B. and LYON, M. Evidence for cell loss in corpus striatum after long term treatment with a neuroleptic drug (flupenthixol) in rats. *Psychopharmacology*, **14**, 34–36 (1978)

29 NYBACK, H. and SEDVALL, G. Effect of chlorpromazine on accumulation and disappearance of catecholamines formed from tyrosine C-14 in brain. *Journal of Pharmacology and Experimental Therapeutics*, **162**, 294–298 (1968)

30 RUBOVITS, R., PATEL, B. C. and KLAWANS, H. L. Effect of prolonged chlorpromazine pretreatment on the threshold for amphetamine-induced stereotypy: a model for tardive dyskinesias. *Advances in Neurology*, **1**, 671–675 (1973)

31 SCHEEL-KRUGER, J. Comparative studies of various amphetamine analogs demonstrating different interactions with the metabolism of the catecholamines in the brain. *European Journal of Pharmacology*, **19**, 47–49 (1971)

32 SMITH, R. C. and LEELAVATHI, D. E. Behavioral and biochemical effects of chronic neuroleptic drugs: interaction with age. In *Tardive Diskinesia*, edited by W. E. Fann, R. C. Smith, J. M. Davis and E. F. Domino, 65–88. New York, S.P. Medical and Scientific Books (1980)

33 TARSY, D. and BALDESSARINI, R. J. Pharmacologically-induced behavioral supersensitivity to apomorpine. *Nature* (New Biology), **245**, 262 (1973)

34 WEINER, W. J., CARVEY, P., HITRI, A., NAUSIEDA, P. A. and KLAWANS, H. L. The time course of haloperidol-induced dopamine receptor site supersensitivity in guinea pigs. In *Fourth International Catecholamine Symposium*, edited by E. Usdin 704–706. New York, Pergamon Press (1979)

35 WEINER, W. J., NAUSIEDA, P. A. and KLAWANS, H. L. Regional brain manganese levels in an animal model of tardive dyskinesia. In *Tardive Diskinesia*, edited by W. E. Fann, R. C. Smith, J. M. Davis, and E. F. Domino, 159–164. New York, S.P. Medical and Scientific Books (1980)

16
Care of patients and families with Huntington's disease

Ira Shoulson

INTRODUCTION

Patients with Huntington's disease experience immense disability resulting from motor, intellectual and pyschological disturbances. Clinical decline is related to progressive neuronal degeneration in the basal ganglia and to a lesser extent in cerebral cortex, cerebellum and limbic structures. Because of the hereditary nature of Huntington's disease, the family must shoulder burdens which endure beyond the life of the patient. Guidelines for clinical care remain sparse despite the magnitude of illness and the investigative attention accorded to the genetic and neuropathologic aspects of the disease.

This discussion will consider broad aspects of clinical care of Huntington's disease, including early diagnosis, genetic counseling, chronic care and pharmacotherapy. The perspective is based on an assessment of 130 patients with Huntington's disease and their families (78 apparently unrelated kindreds) who were evaluated in the University of Rochester Hungtington Disease Clinic between 1977 and 1981. All had family histories confirmatory of the disease. At the time of initial evaluation, patients were systematically rated in terms of clinical features, functional capacity and corresponding stage of illness[38, 40, 42, 43].

Several aspects of functional capacity were assessed and rated on a scale ranging from 3 to 0.

(A) Engagement in occupation
    3 – *usual level*: full-time employment, actual or potential (e.g. job offer or qualified), with normal work expectations and satisfactory performance.
    2 – *lower level*: full or part-time employment, actual or potential, with a lower than usual expectation or performance relative to patient's training and education.
    1 – *marginal level*: part-time, voluntary or salaried employment, actual or potential, with lower expectation and less than satisfactory work performance.
    0 – *unable*: totally unable to engage in voluntary or salaried employment.

(B) Capacity to handle financial affairs
   3 – *full*: normal capacity to handle personal and family finances (income tax, balancing checkbook, paying bills, budgeting, shopping).
   2 – *requires slight assistance*: mildly impaired ability to handle financial affairs such that accustomed routine responsibilities require organization and assistance from family member or financial advisor.
   1 – *requires major assistance*: moderately impaired ability to handle financial affairs such that patient comprehends nature and purpose of routine financial procedures and is competent to handle funds but requires major assistance in the performance of these tasks.
   0 – *unable*: patient is unable to comprehend the financial process and is unable to perform tasks related to routine financial procedures.
(C) Capacity to manage domestic responsibilities
   2 – *full*: no impairment in performance of routine domestic tasks (cleaning, laundering, dishwashing, table setting, recipes, answering mail, civic responsibilities).
   1 – *impaired*: moderate impairment in performance of routine domestic tasks such that patient requires some assistance in carrying out these tasks.
   0 – *unable*: marked impairment in function with marginal performance requiring major assistance.
(D) Capacity to perform activities of daily living
   3 – *full*: complete independence in eating, dressing and bathing activities.
   2 – *mildly impaired*: somewhat labored performance in eating (avoids certain foods which cause chewing/swallowing problems), in dressing (difficulty in fine tasks only, e.g. buttoning, tying shoes), in bathing (difficulty in fine performance only, e.g. brushing teeth); requires only slight assistance.
   1 – *moderately impaired*: substantial difficulty in eating (swallows only liquid or soft foods and requires considerable assistance), in dressing (performs only gross dressing activities and requires assistance with everything else) and in bathing (performs only gross bathing tasks, otherwise requiring assistance).
   0 – *severely impaired*: indicates patient requires total care in activities of daily living.
(E) Care can be provided
   2 – *home*: patient living at home and family readily able to meet care needs.
   1 – *home or extended care facility*: patient may be living at home but care needs would be better provided at an extended care facility.
   0 – *total care facility only*: patient requires full-time skilled nursing care.

The total score is then calculated. Stage I is equal to a score of 11–13; stage II to a score of 7–10; III to a score of 3–6; IV, 1–2, and V, 0.

In this sample of patients, the scores for total functional capacity corresponded in a broad fashion to the duration of illness estimated at the time of initial evaluation (*Figure 16.1*). The male predominance (1.5:1.0) of this cohort was due largely to the high ascertainment from regional Veteran's Administration facilities. Eighty-two patients were seen in follow-up evaluation during the 4-year observation period.

Figure 16.1 Distribution of all patients at the time of initial evaluation according to stage of disability and estimated duration of symptoms. Bars represent standard deviation

EARLY DIAGNOSIS

Huntington's disease is foremost a hereditary disorder wherein the central nervous system bears the overwhelming burden of genetic expression. The HD gene is fully expressed in the heterozygote state, but clinical features rarely become manifest before the reproductive years of life. The mutation rate for the *de novo* appearance of Huntington's disease is exceedingly low and probably negligible. Despite considerable investigative effort to detect the presymptomatic HD gene carrier, the diagnosis of the disease rests exclusively on clinical analysis.

Disordered movement, dementia and psychiatric disturbances are the cardinal clinical features of Huntington's disease. Any one of these features may mark the onset of clinical expression[11, 33, 50]. Irrespective of presenting symptom, the movement disorder constitutes the most distinctive element in diagnostic analysis and, coupled with the hereditary nature of Huntington's disease, affords a relatively high degree of diagnostic precision.

Chorea was predictably found to be the predominant movement disorder in patients with adult-onset Huntington's disease, especially in the initial stages of illness (*see Figure 16.2*). Minimally disabled patients typically manifested fleeting movements of the extremities or grimacing tics involving the face, lips and eyelids. Most patients and family members were unaware of these movements. In the earliest stages (I and II), dystonia and parkinsonism were rarely encountered in the adult-onset patient. But choreic movements seemed to evolve gradually into a choreoathetotic pattern. With advancing disability (stages III and IV), dystonia and parkinsonism were observed more frequently as the predominant disorders of movement. However, a sizable proportion of adult patients had prevailing choreic features in all stages of illness. A consistent pattern of movement disorder was not found in those kindreds where more than one individual was affected with Huntington's disease. It is unclear whether the pattern of predominant movement disorder was related to underlying pathologic alterations or to modification by neuroleptic therapy. Regardless, the clinician should be prepared to encounter prevailing dystonic or parkinsonian features in the adult patient with more advanced disability. Nine patients with onset of illness before the age of 20 were characteristically found to be hypokinetic and rigid with mild to moderate dystonic features and occasional signs of cerebellar dysfunction. This pattern of juvenile Huntington's disease was present in all stages of illness.

Voluntary saccadic eye movements and optokinetic nystagmus were measured clinically at the time of initial evaluation. Sluggish horizontal saccades and disordered optokinetic mystagmus were detected infrequently in stage I, but the occurrence of eye movement abnormalities increased precipitously with advancing disability and paralleled the rising prevalence of dystonic and parkinsonian features (*Figure 16.2*). These observations support the quantitative findings of Avanzini et al.[1].

Figure 16.2 Distribution of predominant motor features and occurrence of eye movement abnormalities according to stage of disability. Patients with juvenile onset (under 20 years old) are excluded. E = eye movement abnormalities; C = chorea; D = dystonia; P = parkinsonism

The family history was eminently pivotal in the diagnostic evaluation. When a family history of Huntington's disease could be firmly established, the presence of a choreic, dystonic or parkinsonian movement disorder helped to confirm the diagnosis in the propositus. In many instances, however, there was a positive family history of movement disorder or dementia which could not be established conclusively as Huntington's disease. In this setting, other hereditary disorders prompted consideration in differential diagnosis:

Hereditary ataxias (spinocerebellar degeneration)
Familial chorea without dementia[3, 10, 14, 19]
Familial chorea with acanthocytosis and peripheral neuropathy[4, 21]
Familial chorea and myoclonus[47]
Familial paroxysmal dystonic choreoathetosis[24]
Wilson's disease
Joseph's disease[37]

The dominantly inherited ataxias, especially those associated with choreic features and sluggish eye movements often posed difficulty in early diagnosis. A variety of familial choreic syndromes have recently been described, but most have their clinical onset in childhood and are not likely to be confused with juvenile Huntington's disease. Wilson's disease merits emphasis because of the critical implications for therapy. In view of these important considerations in differential diagnosis, it is recommended the patients suspected of having Huntington's disease be evaluated by a neurologist who is skilled in the examination of movement disorders and hereditary disease.

When a hereditary pattern cannot be established, the differential diagnosis is broadened to include drug-induced, metabolic, immunologic, hematologic, infectious and congenital causes[41]. In the author's Huntington disease clinic, tardive dyskinesia has been the most troublesome consideration in the diagnostic evaluation. This possibility was especially confounding because patients with tardive dyskinesia may often have choreic features in the extremities, sluggish eye movements, disordered gait and a family history of psychotic illness[6]. The foregoing concerns underscore the necessity to avoid neuroleptic therapy in persons at risk for Huntington's disease.

Because computed tomography (CT) is frequently normal in the early stages of the disease[31, 44], this tool is not sufficiently sensitive for early detection. With advancing disability (stages III and IV), there is greater likelihood of discerning caudate atrophy on CT scan. However, the isolated finding of caudate atrophy is not specific for the diagnosis[44].

Early diagnosis of Huntington's disease would be revolutionized by the development of an accurate test to detect the presymptomatic gene carrier[22, 35]. Although linkage analysis in patients with Huntington's disease has thus far failed to establish close phenotypic associations[34], the elaboration of new chromosome markers will increase the likelihood of early recognition of the heterozygote state[30]. More direct examination of the genotype, using techniques such as recombinant DNA analysis[17], holds promise of improving early detection. With the prospect of eventually having reliable test for early detection, the role of genetic counseling assumes added importance in the care of patients and families with Huntington's disease.

GENETIC COUNSELING

Several problems are relatively unique to genetic counseling in Huntington's disease. The delayed onset of symptoms and signs complicates the explanation of clinical issues and the understanding of genetic risk. The fact that there is no reliable method of presymptomatic detection may undercut the potential effectiveness of counseling efforts. Dementia and psychiatric disturbances in affected family members impair comprehension, emotional response and planning capacity. The prospect that a reliable early detection test will be developed while therapy remains palliative may create a state of cognitive dissonance.

While there is no clear-cut evidence that counseling reduces the size of the Huntington's disease gene pool, there is compelling logic to adopt some type of genetic information program in the setting of clinical care. It is obviously difficult to gather concensus or formulate guidelines for genetic counseling in Huntington's disease. Through the experience in the Rochester Huntington's Disease Clinic the author has managed to establish some premises for counseling.

(1) Genetic counseling is considered an integral part of ongoing clinical care. As expressed by Harper[20], 'Ignorance or inadequate information has, on balance, produced more problems than has knowledge of the disorder (HD) and its genetic risk'.
(2) The entire family, not just the propositus, deserves the offer of genetic counseling.
(3) Information provided in genetic counseling must be sufficiently clear, accurate and complete to serve as the basis for reproductive planning.
(4) Counseling should be non-directive and present the options available to the counselee regarding reproduction. Strong admonitions against having children are often counterproductive. When the counselor appears heavyhanded, the patient and family may feel isolated or abandoned. The final choices should be made by the individual counselee in accordance with his or her own value system.
(5) Genetic counseling should ideally include the provision of information regarding the clinical disorder and genetic risk, an evaluation of learning and attitudes, and a measure of reproductive outcomes.

Family members express some common concerns at the time of initial evaluation. They desire a frank explanation of the clinical features of Huntington's disease, including the nature and course of disability. They are initially shocked by the prospect that other family members might develop the disease, but they also want to know what can be done to lessen this risk in the family.

Counseling procedures in the author's clinic are designed to address these concerns. After assessing the informant's knowledge of Huntington's disease, the clinical features of the disorder are explained. This is usually done in relationship to the illness of the propositus. The counselor indicates that the disease progresses steadily but that the rate of decline varies considerably from one patient to another. Its hereditary nature is explained in relationship to the family's own pedigree. The fundamentals of mendelian genetics (concepts of dominance, penetrance and mutation) are usually found to be too complex for the average counselee to comprehend. However, the concept of a 50:50 chance of developing (or not developing) the disease seems to be well understood. Finally, reproductive planning and options are considered. These procedures are repeated at each follow-up evaluation.

An assessment of learning is usually accomplished in a casual manner by asking counselees to summarize their understanding of the clinical and genetic aspects of their illness. Misconceptions are commonly encountered in this phase of counseling. Many families adhere to the notion that Huntington's disease skips generations or has a peculiar predilection for one sex. Some families believe that if results from poor upbringing or particular social circumstances. These and other misconceptions are discussed in a frank but supportive manner.

Attitudes regarding genetic counseling have been explored by several investigators. Stern and Eldridge[46] have examined the reactions of US families to the medical, social and genetic implications of Huntington's disease. More than half of their respondents expressed a desire to modify family size, but this attitude was more commonly shared by affected rather than at-risk adults. Most indicated that they would avail themselves of a reliable screening test. Those interested in counseling preferred a supportive source of information rather than a threatening source. This preference may account for the commonly expressed opinion that lay organizations set up to deal with the problems of Huntington's disease were a better source of information than were medical specialists or genetic counselors. Barette and Marsden[2] have assessed how family members in the UK were first informed about the disease and what effects hereditary aspects had upon them and their children. The hospital consultant was found to be the major source of diagnostic information. Failure to establish the family history was cited as the most common cause of delay in diagnosis. Only 7 percent of respondents preferred not to know the facts of the disease, while 69 percent wished that they had known earlier. The vast majority of the sample claimed they would take some kind of measure to limit reproduction and that they would welcome a reliable predictive test if it were available.

It is unclear to what extent attitudes can be modified as a result of genetic counseling or whether changed attitudes are translated into changed reproductive behavior. Harper et al.[20] are presently attempting to evaluate the efficacy of genetic counseling in terms of reproductive outcome. They have undertaken a prospective study to measure birthrate and size of the Huntington's disease gene pool in a relatively stable cohort in the UK. Their findings will help to serve as the basis for long-term prevention of the disease.

Improved understanding of the disease and its genetic risks has in a sense created a new type of patient, the individual 'at risk'. The person with knowledge that he or she is at risk bears psychosocial burdens in addition to the genetic risks. There is a higher prevalence of neuropsychiatric disorders in this population, suggesting that at-risk status *per se* may predispose to psychological disturbances[23]. Wexler[48] has found that at-risk individuals develop untoward reactions to the prospect of developing Huntington's disease. 'Symptom searching' is a frequent phenomenon in this genetically vulnerable population. They experience overwhelming grief for the affected parent, occasional anger because of not having been sufficiently informed prior to having children, or depression regarding the prospect of lingering

284 Care of patients and families with Huntington's disease

uncertainty. The person at risk for Huntington's disease should appropriately be welcomed and integrated into the clinical care program for patient and family.

The role of the genetic counselor can be fulfilled by one of many care providers. In the author's clinic, the neurologist serves a dual role as genetic counselor and care provider. In order settings, genetic counseling is more naturally directed by a genetic specialist, psychiatrist, social worker, nurse or family physician. All who provide counseling and care for the patient and family need to anticipate the impact of predictive tests. Once a reliable measure is developed, the administration and interpretation of such a test will depend largely on the preparation and skill of clinicians.

CHRONIC CARE

Patients with Huntington's disease suffer a progressive loss of functional capacity. The disorder is not characterized by remissions or exacerbations of illness. Decline is steady, but the pace of functional incapacity varies and cannot be accurately predicted in a given patient at the time of initial evaluation. In our cohort, however, patients with major psychotic or depressive disturbances and those with clinical onset before the age of 30 seemed to decline at a faster rate. Through follow-up examinations the author has been able to establish a general pattern of functional decline in Huntington's disease[40]. This profile has helped to better anticipate care needs and assist in long-term planning (*Figure 16.3*).

Figure 16.3 Profile of functional decline in Huntington's disease

Initially, the symptomatic person experiences a loss of gainful skills in the capacity as worker or manager of the household. Work performance becomes unsatisfactory and of lowered expectation. Full-time employment often turns into part-time or voluntary work. The capacity to handle financial affairs becomes impaired so that accustomed tasks require the assistance of others. The loss of gainful skills necessitates early financial planning with the prospect of further decline. Families are routinely evaluated by a social worker who is well acquainted with the psychosocial consequences of the disease. They are advised to formulate short-term and long-term financial plans based on the background of the patient (e.g. veteran, pensioner, early retiree) and resources of the family. The patient and family are frequently urged to seek legal or financial advice about estate planning, early retirement, disability and insurance.

With progression of the disease, domestic skills begin to wane and additional support is needed at home. Patients require assistance in managing their finances (shopping, budgeting, paying bills, taxes) and performing normal household duties (cleaning, laundering, preparing meals). The family usually bears the direct burden resulting from loss of domestic skills. When it is not possible for the family to assume these roles, efforts are made to organize community health services and voluntary agencies to help maintain family integrity.

Eventually, self-care skills begin to deteriorate. As the motor features become more disabling, independence can no longer be maintained in regard to ambulation and activities of daily living (eating, dressing, bathing). A considerable amount of support is required at this advanced stage of disability, especially when speech, swallowing and bladder/bowel functions are involved. Housekeeping aides and visiting nurses may provide valuable assistance in maintaining the patient at home as part of the family structure. As the mobile resources of the community become more limited, the patient may well require chronic care outside the home. In this event, a variety of options should be considered, including extended care or domiciliary facilities, chronic-care infirmaries, Veteran's hospitals and nursing homes. Chronic care at a psychiatric center may be needed for patients with an unremitting psychotic disturbance. Unfortunately, resources are invariably sparse and often inadequate for meeting care requirements in the advanced stages of disability. There has been no systematic appraisal of available care resources and how they might be best applied to the needs of patients with Huntington's disease and their families.

The spouse and children (at-risk individuals), and the family at large, also deserve support in a chronic care program. The spouse has unique problems, neither being affected nor at risk to develop the disease[18]. He or she initially reacts with disbelief or denial of illness, but may become resentful or hostile as the reality of progression and threat of transmission to children take form. The unique concerns of the individual at risk have been noted in the foregoing section. As a collective unit, the family is encouraged to be assertive, independent and resourceful in coping with the inevitable burdens of the illness. We and others[25,50] have found that a combined family approach is the most useful and efficient for genetic counseling and the provision of chronic care.

Lay and voluntary organizations set up to help those with Huntington's disease serve an invaluable role in the chronic care of patient and family. Despite fiscal constraints, these groups have managed to coalesce diverse interests into substantive support for education, research and clinical care. They provide a unique resource which is not available within the structure of traditional health care.

Patients are strongly urged to contact their local lay organization and to become active in its support.

While this perspective of chronic care may seem overly pessimistic, there seems little to be gained by denying the inevitable and progressive disability of the disease. Studies are needed to define the nature and temporal course of disability more accurately. These findings would help to improve anticipation and planning for chronic care in Huntington's disease and other degenerative disorders. Systematic appraisal of the natural course of the illness will also help provide a more meaningful reference point for assessing the impact of therapeutic interventions.

PHARMACOTHERAPY

Rational strategies of neurotransmitter replacement have characterized recent approaches to the experimental therapeutics of Huntington's disease[39]. Although these efforts have produced few substantive gains, more promising strategies have been generated. Current drug therapies are aimed at the amelioration of symptoms and specifically of the motor and psychiatric disturbances. Unfortunately, symptomatic pharmcotherapy is usually short-lived and of palliative consequence. There is also potential for adverse drug effects, and the possibility cannot be excluded that symptomatic therapies might hasten the decline of the disease[40]. The clinician is accordingly advised to use sparingly the available symptomatic drugs and to administer them at minimum therapeutic dosage.

Drugs which reduce nigrostriatal neurotransmission, either by depleting presynaptic dopamine or by blocking postsynaptic dopaminergic receptors, have been found to be the most effective agents for reducing the intensity of chorea. Reserpine and tetrabenazine act primarily at the presynaptic level. These drugs exert potent antichoreic effects, but their use is often associated with disturbing features of parkinsonism, akathisia, depression and psychomotor retardation[45]. Tetrabenzine seems to be much better tolerated than reserpine and is relatively devoid of hypotensive effects. Frequent dose adjustments to minimize adverse effects and occasionally short-lived antichoreic effects are the major drawbacks of tetrabenazine therapy. In the US tetrabenazine is available only at a few research centers.

Despite the widespread use of antipsychotic drugs in Huntington's disease[36], there have been few controlled studies examining their efficacy[13]. The antipsychotic drugs acting primarily to block postsynaptic dopaminergic receptors (butyrophenones, phenothiazines, thioxanthenes) produce antichoreic effects which are often of temporary benefit and associated with adverse effects. Some patients respond better to one class of neuroleptic drug than another, but the response cannot be predicted in advance of therapy. Administration of antipsychotic drugs to patients with Huntington's disease may be associated with parkinsonism and the real risk of developing superimposed tardive dyskinesia.

The benzodiazepines may provide modest antichoreic effects, but this is usually accomplished at the expense of excessive sedation and depression. Patients who manifest a predominance of parkinsonian features may benefit from antiparkinsonian agents including levodopa, amantadine, dopamine agonists and anticholinergics. The use of these drugs requires frequent dose adjustment and careful clinical monitoring. There are no effective agents for symptomatic relief of dystonic or cerebellar features which may develop in some patients with Huntington's disease.

The general experience in the Rochester clinic indicates that symptomatic drugs should be reserved for patients with disabling chorea. It has been found that drug-induced parkinsonism in patients with advanced disease may seriously impair speech and swallowing and predispose to aspiration pneumonia[45]. Patients with predominantly dystonic or parkinsonian features typically worsen on neuroleptic therapies. Even the patient with disabling choreic features may not derive much functional benefit despite an appreciable reduction in chorea. Some patients seem dependent on their choreic movements during ambulation, and a lessening of chorea may have adverse consequences on gait and balance.

There has been no systematic appraisal of antidepressant and antipsychotic therapies in Huntington's disease. The tricyclics are the most widely used antidepressant drugs, but the attainment of therapeutic dosage is often limited by hypotension, hypertension, insomnia, somnolence and restlessness. Tricyclic antidepressants with minimal anticholinergic effects (e.g. desipramine) are usually preferred in situations where excessive sedation or exacerbation of chorea should be avoided. There has been no orderly evaluation of the use of monoamine oxidase inhibitors or electroconvulsive therapy in depressed patients with the disease. Antipsychotic drugs are used frequently for psychotic patients, but their worth has not been established. The dementia of Huntington's disease is not amenable to symptomatic therapy.

The inevitable and unremitting progression of the disease lends itself paradoxically to therapeutic strategies aimed at preventing or retarding clinical decline. Unlike the demyelinating diseases, there are no spontaneous remissions or exacerbations in Huntington's disease, which might complicate long-term evaluation. In contrast to other neurodegenerative disorders (e.g. Alzheimer disease), the hereditary nature of Huntington's disease affords a high degree of diagnostic precision. The emerging knowledge regarding pathogenesis provides an impetus for extending the experimental therapeutics beyond the scope of symptomatic intervention.

Kainic acid, a glutamate analogue, is toxic to local neurons when injected intrastriatally into experimental animals[7,27]. Kainate-lesioned animals show morphologic, chemical, pharmocologic and behavioral effects resembling Huntington's disease[8]. The integrity of the glutamate-containing corticostriatal pathway is a requisite for the development of kainate-induced neurotoxicity as demonstrated by lesioning and tissue culture studies[5,9,28,49]. Because the animal paradigm of kainate neurotoxicity develops acutely and is not based on genetic predisposition, it cannot be viewed as an exact model for Huntington's disease. On the other hand, the accumulated experience with kainic acid has generated the reasonable supposition that its pathogenesis is linked to a glutamate-dependent neurotoxic process[12,29,32]. This assertion has received recent support from Gray et al., who found that physiological concentrations of glutamate specifically induced a dose-dependent degeneration of fibroblasts[15, 16, 26]. These findings might logically be extended to the prophylactic treatment of patients using drugs which reduce the availability of glutamate in the striatum. Pharmacologic attenuation of glutamatergic neurotransmission may reasonably delay the process of progressive neuronal degeneration in Huntington's disease. A reliable early detection test would certainly be more appealing if therapeutic intervention halted or retarded the steady decline of the disease. Experimental studies are underway in an effort to test these strategies.

References

1 AVANZINI, G., GIROTTI, F., CARACENI, T. and SPREAFICO, R. Oculomotor disorders in Huntington's chorea. *Journal of Neurology, Neurosurgery and Psychiatry*, **42**, 581–589 (1979)

2 BARETTE, J. and MARSDEN, C. D. Attitudes of families to some aspects of Huntington's chorea. *Psychological Medicine*, **9**, 327–336 (1979)

3 BEHAN, P. O. and BONE, I. Hereditary chorea without dementia. *Journal of Neurology, Neurosurgery and Psychiatry*, **40**, 687–691 (1977)

4 BIRD, T. D., CEDERBAUM, S., VALPEY, R. W. and STAHL, W. L. Familial degeneration of the basal ganglia with acanthocytosis: a clinical, neuropathological, and neurochemical study. *Annals of Neurology*, **3**, 253–258 (1978)

5 BIZIERE, K. and COYLE, J. T. Effects of cortical ablation on the neurotoxicity and receptor binding of kainic acid in striatum. *Journal of Neuroscience Research*, **4**, 383–398 (1979)

6 BUXTON, M. Diagnostic problems in Huntington's chorea and tardive dyskinesia. *Comprehensive Psychiatry*, **17**, 325–333 (1976)

7 COYLE, J. T. and SCHWARCZ, R. Lesion of striatal neurons with kainic acid provides a model for Huntington's chorea. *Nature*, **263**, 244–246 (1976)

8 COYLE, J. T., McGEER, E. G., McGEER, P. L. and SCHWARCZ, R. Neostriatal injections: a model for Huntington's chorea. In *Kainic Acid as a Tool in Neurobiology*, edited by McGeer, E. G., Olney, J. W. and McGeer, P. L., 139–159. New York, Raven Press (1978)

9 COYLE, J. T., LONDON, E. D., BIZIERE, K. and ZACZEK, R. Kainic acid neurotoxicity: insights into the pathophysiology of Huntington's disease. *Advances in Neurology*, **23**, 593–608 (1979)

10 DAMASIO, H., ANTUNES, L. and DAMASIO, A. R. Familial nonprogressive involuntary movements of childhood. *Annals of Neurology*, **1**, 602–603 (1977)

11 DEWHURST, K., OLIVER, J. E. and KcKNIGHT, A. L. Social-psychiatric consequences of Huntington's disease. *British Journal of Psychiatry*, **116**, 255–258 (1970)

12 DIVAC, I. Possible pathogenesis of Huntington's chorea and a new approach to treatment. *Acta Neurologica Scandinavica*, **56**, 357–360 (1977)

13 FAHN, S. Treatment of choreic movements with perphenazine. *Advances in Neurology*, **1**, 755–763 (1973)

14 FISHER, M., SARGENT, J. and DRACHMAN, D. Familial inverted choreoathetosis. *Neurology*, **29**, 1627–1631 (1979)

15 GRAY, P. N. and MAY, P. C. Glutamate toxicity in Huntington's disease fibroblasts. *Society for Neuroscience Abstracts*, **10,** 405 (1980)
16 GRAY, P. N., MAY, P. C., MUNDY, L. and ELKINS, J. L-glutamate toxicity in Huntington's disease fibroblasts. *Biochemistry Biophysics Research Communication*, **95,** 707–714 (1980)
17 GUSELLA, J. F., KEYS, C., VARSANYI-BREINER, A., KOA, F., JONES, C., PUCK, T. T. and HOUSMAN, D. Isolation and localization of DNA segments from specific human chromosomes. *Proceedings of the National Academy of Sciences*, **77,** 2829–2833 (1980)
18 HANS, M. B. and KOEPPEN, A. H. Huntington's chorea. Its impact on the spouse. *Journal of Nervous and Mental Disease*, **168,** 209–214 (1980)
19 HARPER, P. S. Benign hereditary chorea: clinical and genetic aspects. *Clinical Genetics*, **13,** 85–95 (1978)
20 HARPER, P. S., TYLER, A., WALKER, D. A., NEWCOMBE, R. G. and DAVIES, K. Huntington's chorea: the basis for long-term prevention. *Lancet*, **ii,** 346–349 (1979)
21 KITO, S., ITOGA, E., HIROSHIGE, Y., MATSUMOTO, N. and MIWA, S. A pedigree of amyotrophic chorea with acanthocytosis. *Archives of Neurology*, **37,** 514–517 (1980)
22 KLAWANS, H. L., GOETZ, C. G. and PERLIK, S. Presymptomatic and early detection in Huntington's disease. *Annals of Neurology*, **8,** 343–347 (1980)
23 KORENYI, C. and WITTMAN, R. Prevalence of medical disorders other than Huntington's disease in offspring of symptomatic and at risk parents. *Disease of the Nervous System*, **35,** 17–19 (1974)
24 LANCE, J. W. Familial paroxysmal dystonic choreoathetosis and its differentiation from related syndromes. *Annals of Neurology*, **2,** 285–293 (1977)
25 MARTINDALE, B. and BOTTOMLEY, V. The management of families with Huntington's chorea: a case study to illustrate some recommendations. *Journal of Child Psychology and Psychiatry*, **21,** 343–351 (1980)
26 MAY, P. C. and GRAY, P. N. Altered glutamate/glutamine metabolism in Huntington's disease fibroblasts. *Journal of Cell Biology*, **87,** 75a (1980)
27 McGEER, E. G. and McGEER, P. L. Duplication of biochemical changes of Huntington's chorea by intrastriatal injections of glutamic and kainic acids. *Nature*, **263,** 517–519 (1976)
28 McGEER, E. G., McGEER, P. L. and SINGH, K. Kainate-induced degeneration of neostriatal neurons: dependency upon corticostriatal tract. *Brain Research*, **139,** 381–383 (1978)
29 McGEER, P. L. and McGEER, E. G. Use of the neurotoxic agents kainic acid and tetanus toxin in the extrapyramidal systems. *Advances in Cytopharmacology*, **3,** 437–446 (1979)
30 McKUSICK, V. A. The anatomy of the human genome. *American Journal of Medicine*, **69,** 267–276 (1980)
31 NEOPHYTIDES, A. N., DiCHIRO, G., BARRON, S. A. and CHASE, T. N. Computed axial tomography in Huntington's disease and persons 'at-risk' for Huntington's disease. *Advances in Neurology*, **23,** 189–191 (1979)
32 OLNEY, J. W. and DE GUBAREFF, T. Glutamate neurotoxicity and Huntington's chorea. *Nature*, **271,** 557–559 (1978)

33 PAULSON, G. W. Diagnosis of Huntington's disease. *Advances in Neurology*, **23**, 177–184 (1979)
34 PERICAK-VANCE, M. A., CONNEALLY, P. M., MERRITT, A. D., ROOS, R. P., VANCE, J. M., YU, P. L., NORTON, J. A. and ANTEL, J. P. Genetic linkage in Huntington's disease. *Advances in Neurology*, **23**, 59–72 (1979)
35 PROPERT, D. B. Presymptomatic detection of Huntington's disease. *Medical Journal of Australia*, **1**, 609–612 (1980)
36 RINGEL, S. P., GUTHRIE, M. and KLAWANS, H. L. Current treatment of Huntington's chorea. *Advances in Neurology*, **1**, 797–801 (1973)
37 ROSENBERG, R. N., NYHAN, W. L., COUTINHO, P. and BAY, C. Joseph's disease. *Advances in Neurology*, **21**, 33–57 (1978)
38 SHOULSON, I. Dementia in Huntington's disease and cognitive effects of muscimol therapy. In *Senile Dementia: A Biomedical Approach*, edited by K. Nandy, 251–258. Amsterdam, Elsevier (1978)
39 SHOULSON, I. Huntington's disease: overview of experimental therapeutics. *Advances in Neurology*, **23**, 751–758 (1979)
40 SHOULSON, I. Huntington's disease: function capacities in patients treated with neuroleptic and antidepressant drugs. *Neurology*, **31**, 1333–1335 (1981)
41 SHOULSON, I. and CHASE, T. N. Huntington's disease. *Annual Review of Medicine*, **26**, 419–426 (1975)
42 SHOULSON, I., CAINE, E., FAHN, S., KOBAYASHI, R., KOKMEN, E., SAX, D., WEINGARTNER, H. and WEXLER, N. S. Clinical care of the patient and family with Huntington's disease. In *Commission for the Control of Huntington's Disease and Its Consequences*, Vol. 11, 421–451. Department of Health, Education and Welfare (National Institute of Health) publication (1977)
43 SHOULSON, I. and FAHN, S. Huntington disease: clinical care and evaluation. *Neurology*, **29**, 1–3 (1979)
44 SHOULSON, I. and PLASSCHE, W. Huntington disease: the specificity of computed tomography measurements. *Neurology*, **30**, 382–383 (1980)
45 SHOULSON, I. and GOLDBLATT, D. Huntington disease (HD): effect of tetrabenazine and antipsychotic drugs on motoric features. *Neurology*, **31**, 79 (1981)
46 STERN, R. and ELDRIDGE, R. Attitudes of patients and their relatives to Huntington's disease. *Journal of Medical Genetics*, **12**, 217–223 (1975)
47 TAKAHATA, N., ITO, K., YOSHIMURA, Y., NISHIHORI, K. and SUZUKI, H. Familial chorea and myoclonus epilepsy. *Neurology*, **28**, 913–919 (1978)
48 WEXLER, N. Genetic 'Russian Roulette': the experience of being at risk for Huntington's disease. In *Genetic Counseling*, edited by S. Kessler, 199–220. New York, Academic Press (1979)
49 WHETSELL, W. O., ECOB-JOHNSTON, M. and NICKLAS, W. J. Studies of kainate-induced caudate lesions in organotypic tissue culture. *Advances in Neurology*, **23**, 645–654 (1979)
50 WHITTIER, J. R. Treatment of Huntington's disease. *Modern Treatment*, **5**, 332–350 (1968)

17.1
Surgical approaches to the dyskinesias: foreword

C. D. Marsden and Stanley Fahn

This section may seem unusual, for it consists of brief descriptions of the various neurosurgical approaches to the treatment of movement disorder, each written by an acknowledged expert in their particular craft. The editors did not ask for extensive technical description of the operative methods employed. Rather, they hope that each section would give some guidance to the practitioner on what the particular technique offers, which patients are suitable, what are the chances of success, and what are the unwanted consequences and risks of the operation in question. The editors will leave the reader to judge each approach, but in an afterword they describe their own use of these various techniques to manage the patients with movement disorders which they see.

17.2
Surgical approach to tremor
H. Narabayashi

INTRODUCTION

Treatment of tremor has been of great interest to neurosurgery, especially after the introduction of stereotaxic techniques for lesioning deep structures of the brain to improve involuntary movements. Most cases operated upon were those with parkinsonian tremor; but as a result of the rapid development of pharmacological treatment for this disease in the last 10 years, the number of patients suitable for surgery has decreased markedly. Levodopa and its modifications, such as the combination of levodopa and a peripheral decarboxylase inhibitor, proved sufficient to control tremor in most patients with Parkinson's disease. The addition of an anticholinergic drug also may be of benefit. However, there are still a number of parkinsonian patients who suffer from severe disabling unilateral or bilateral tremor which does not respond satisfactorily to medical treatment. Surgical treatment of such otherwise uncontrollable parkinsonian tremor must be considered.

Marked intention tremor or postural tremor due to various causes other than Parkinson's disease are not, in general, influenced or improved by medical therapy, with the exception of the effect of propranolol and other β-antagonists in some patients with benign essential tremor. For such patients with non-parkinsonian tremor, stereotaxic thalamotomy using a microelectrode approach is still today the only treatment which can eliminate this symptom almost totally usually without producing any side-effects.

ADVANCES IN SURGICAL TECHNIQUE

Radiological localization

Since the introduction of stereotaxic surgery for treating involuntary movements and other disorders, great effort always was made to improve the accuracy of target insertion. The first step in human stereoencephalotomy is neuroradiological measurement of the target structure with reference to a brain atlas giving three-dimensional co-ordinates. Many thalamic nuclei can be located by measuring exactly their relation in three dimensions to the anterior (CA) and posterior (CP) commissures, and to the connecting baseline, the CA–CP line.

Most patients, however, suffer from chronic degenerative diseases, stroke or trauma, so gross anatomical changes due to pathology almost always occur. In order to overcome individual variation in localizing the target, neurophysiological information has been investigated intensively.

Electrical stimulation

Firstly, observation and analysis of the effects of high-frequency stimulation of the target structure, such as an increase or decrease of tremor or of rigidity, and the change of sensation or of mental symptoms, have been used routinely since initiation of the stereotaxic technique around 1950.

Secondly, the technique of cortical potentials evoked by stimulation of different thalamic subnuclei at low frequency was started around 1964 by Yoshida et al.[15]. Detection by application of averaging techniques of negative–positive responses in the motor cortex may indicate insertion into the ventrolateral nucleus of the thalamus, which projects specifically to the motor area[15].

Thirdly, the microelectrode technique for detection and analysis of neuronal activity in each deep structure of the brain, especially the different thalamic nuclei, was introduced. Microelectrode methods, which are not widely used, will now be described.

Recording through a microelectrode

Recording of extracellular spike discharges through a microelectrode during a stereotaxic procedure was applied first by Albe-Fessard et al.[1] in 1963 and subsequently was used in many other centres[2, 5, 6]. The technique became available routinely in the author's surgical theatre in 1971, when remodelling of the theatre with full facility of electronics for this specific purpose was completed.

The size of the microelectrode is about 10 µm at the tip of the needle, which consists of a core electrode of bipolar, concentric electrodes, extending 0.5 mm from the sheath. The needle is introduced in an anterolateral–posteromedial direction through a small burr hole in the frontal area, about 3 cm lateral to the midline, by using a set of micromanipulators which advance the needle by millimetre to micrometre steps. Recording usually is unipolar. Scalp EEG at the frontal, pre- and postcentral, and occipital areas is recorded to monitor the patient's general cerebral activity[13].

When the needle tip reaches the ventral nuclei of the thalamus, the electrode is advanced in micrometre steps with the help of a remote control hydraulic micromanipulator (Narishige, Mo–8). As soon as stable spike discharges, especially burst discharges, are established after cessation of injury discharges, their characteristics are studied to separate them from background activity. The spike-discharges are displayed on a cathode-ray oscilloscope (Nihon Kohden VC–8), and are recorded on a running film and an FM magnetic tape.

RHYTHMIC BURSTS IN THE VENTRAL INTERMEDIATE NUCLEUS

In patients with tremor, either of parkinsonian, postural or intention type, the microelectrode is inserted to a tentative target calculated as 18–20 mm behind the anterior commissure and on the CA–CP baseline, when the distance between CA and CP is 24 mm. This coincides roughly with the ventral part of the ventral intermediate nucleus of the thalamus, the lateral distance of which is 14–17 mm from the midline, depending on the degree of enlargement of the third ventricle.

Figure 17.2.1 Unit recording of a ventral intermediate nucleus neuron in a man of 49 years with post-traumatic postural tremor. l.th. = Left thalamic ventral intermediate nucleus neuron; r.b. = right biceps brachii muscle; r.t. = right triceps brachii muscle; r.f. = right wrist flexor muscle; r.e. = right wrist extensor muscle; ▲ = quick passive stretch of extensor muscle. The right side muscles were recorded by surface EMG

The microelectrode passes through several structures, such as the frontal subcortical white matter, caudate nucleus, external lamella of the thalamus, and the dorsal thalamic nuclei, all of which are clearly identified by measuring the neural noise from each structure[4]. When the needle tip approaches an area several millimetres above the target, the ventral part of the ventral intermediate nucleus, rhythmic bursts of spike discharges often are encountered. Some of the rhythmic bursts are quite regular and are synchronous in phase and time-locked to tremor in a particular part of the contralateral extremities, neck or face (*Figure 17.2.1*); when tremor stops, such bursts disappear; when tremor starts, the rhythmic bursts reappear.

Neurons exhibiting bursts synchronous with tremor respond to passive stretching of certain muscles, or to movement of certain joints involved in that specific tremor; but they do not respond to tactile stimuli, suggesting that they are specifically receiving proprioceptive or kinaesthetic afferents from muscle or joint[10, 13]. These neurons seem to be arranged somatotopically within the ventral intermediate nucleus; leg neurons lie more laterally than arm or neck neurons, as do tactile neurons in the ventral posterior nucleus.

As previously reported[11], when the median or ulnar nerve is stimulated by subthreshold pulses, the neurons with rhythmic discharges synchronous to tremor at the wrist exhibit an evoked response with short latency of 11–12 ms, which gives a conduction velocity of about 70 m/s.

These observations suggest that the bursts of neuronal firing in the ventral intermediate nucleus synchronous with tremor are the result of projection of kinaesthetic afferents from muscles involved in tremor. The area of distribution of

Figure 17.2.2. Distribution of different type of bursts in thalamus superimposed on the schema of Bailey-Schaltenbrand's atlas (15 mm lateral from the midline). Asterisks indicate nonsynchronous bursts; hatching indicates a lesion in this area immediately abolishes tremor; crosses indicate the sensory nucleus. (From Narabayashi and Ohye[10], courtesy of the Publishers, *Physiological Tremor, Pathological Tremors and Clonus*)

296 *Surgical approach to tremor*

such tremor-locked bursts coincides with the confines of the nucleus as measured radiologically (*Figure 17.2.2*); such bursts cannot be detected in the ventrolateral or ventral posterior nuclei.

STIMULATION AND LESION IN THE VENTRAL INTERMEDIATE NUCLEUS

After recording and analysis of neuronal activities as described, high frequency stimulation (routinely with parameters of 2×10^{-5} nm (0.2 mA), 0.5 ms and 60 Hz) is applied in the chosen area through the same recording microelectrode, and suppression or enforcement of tremor of the corresponding body part is looked for. If accurate localization is established by recording and stimulation, a small surgical lesion is made by controlled hyperthermia (70°C for 30 s), which produces a lesion of about 3 mm in diameter around the coagulation electrode. Such a lesion abolishes tremor immediately and completely.

CLINICAL OBSERVATIONS

Since the small surgical lesion of about 3 mm diameter is made exactly in the neurons with tremor-synchronous bursts, it produces no unwanted effects such as slight paresis, speech disturbance, hypotonia of muscles or slight cerebellar signs[3, 12, 14]. The introduction of the microelectrode recording technique seems to be a

Figure 17.2.3. Frontal cut of the brain of women aged 69 years with parkinsonism, who died of cancer two years after a right ventral intermediate thalamotomy. (From Narabayashi and Ohye[11], courtesy of the Editor and Publishers, *Applied Neurophysiology*)

reliable method for defining the target area for tremor alleviation. *Figure 17.2.3* is a frontal cut of the brain of a woman of 69 years with parkinsonism. It shows the small coagulation-lesion in the base of the ventral intermediate nucleus, a lesion that was effective in abolishing tremor of the contralateral side of the body for two years after the operation until her death due to cancer[11].

As tremor disappears within a few seconds after placing the coagulation-lesion, normal skilled movement dramatically returns. *Figures 17.2.4a, b, c* and *d* are examples of handwriting before and after operation in cases with severe disabling tremor of various causes.

Figure 17.2.4 Pre- and postoperative handwriting in patients with (*a*) Parkinsonism under levodopa therapy; (*b*) Coarse postural tremor two years after cerebral haemorrhage; (*c*) Tremor-typed cerebral palsy, slightly athetoid; and (*d*) Idiopathic familial tremor, unchanged by propranolol

Immediate alleviation of tremor on the operating table was obtained in all 48 cases (except one) operated between October 1979 and December 1980. However, three cases showed recurrence of tremor within three weeks after operation. In these four cases, whose tremor did not improve or recurred, a second operation abolished their tremor permanently. At reoperation, the lesion was extended a little wider than in the first procedures, mostly in order to control tremor in the proximal arm.

There also were three additional cases in which tremor recurred slightly, but insufficient to interfere with the patient's activities. As seen from *Figure 17.2.5*, steady progress in the rate of sustained improvement has been established in the author's series of surgical cases, paralleling the application of the newer physiological devices over a 30-year history of stereotaxic surgery.

298 *Surgical approach to tremor*

Figure 17.2.5 Comparison of the effects of surgery throughout the period of investigation. (a) Pallidotomy, Mar. 52–Mar. 57, n = 120; (b) ventrolateral thalamotomy, Dec. 61–Feb. 63, n = 61; (c) ventrolateral and/or subventrolateral thalamotomy, Mar. 63–May 64, n = 51; (d) Subventrolateral and/or subventral intermediate thalamotomy, Jan. 70–May 71, n = 48 (e) Ventral intermediate thalamotomy, Oct. 79–Dec. 80, n = 48. (▨) Percentage improvement of rigidity examined by EMG within 2–3 weeks after operation. (□) Tremor. X-P indicates radiological control with air ventriculography. EMG = Observation of the EMG effects of thalamus stimulation on motor activity; EEG = thalamocortical evoked potential; Micro. = depth recording by microelectrode technique. (From Fukamachi et al.[3], courtesy of the Editor and Publishers, *Journal of Neurosurgery*)

In cases with postural tremor or intention tremor due to non-progressive causes, such as stroke, cerebral palsy or severe head injury, the beneficial effects of surgery have persisted for up to about 20 years. In parkinsonism, other signs of the disease such as akinesia and psychic symptoms still tend to progress after surgery, even though tremor and rigidity may not recur for up to 16 years after operation. The most disabling symptom, which incapacitates patients with disease lasting from more than 10 years, is the freezing phenomenon in gait, writing and speech, so-called paradoxical akinesia. Even levodopa treatment may have no influence on the phenomenon.

DISCUSSION

In the author's experience, a lesion of the ventral intermediate nucleus alleviates parkinsonian, postural or intention tremor equally well. Furthermore, tremor-locked rhythmic bursts in this nucleus, and the ability of stimulation in this area to suppress or modify tremor, are common observations in all three clinical types of tremulous movements. These facts may indicate that a common mechanism might be operating in this nucleus to generate or maintain tremor of three clinically different types. If this is true, what would be the key factor responsible for producing differences in these clinical types of tremor? As discussed in previous papers by the author[7, 8, 9], the critical difference may be in the grade of tone of muscles in the three conditions, but this was not be discussed in detail in this chapter[7].

References

1 ALBE-FESSARD, D., ARFEL, G. and GUIOT, G. Activités électriques caractéristiques de quelques structures cérébrales chez l'homme. *Annales de Chirurgie*, **17**, 1185–1214 (1963)

2 BERTRAND, G., JASPER, H. H., WONG, A. and MATHEWS, G. Microelectrode recording during stereotactic surgery. *Clinical Neurosurgery*, **16**, 328–355 (1969)

3 FUKAMACHI, A., OHYE, CH. and NARABAYASHI, H. Delineation of the thalamic nuclei with a microelectrode in stereotaxic surgery for parkinsonism and cerebral palsy. *Journal of Neurosurgery*, **39**, 214–225 (1973)

4 FUKAMACHI, A., OHYE, CH., SAITO, Y. and NARABAYASHI, H. Estimation of the neural noise within the human thalamus. *Acta Neurochirurgica*, Suppl. **24**, 121–136 (1977)

5 HARDY, J. Electrophysiological localization and identification. *Journal of Neurosurgery*, **24**, 410–414 (1966)

6 JASPER, H. H. and BERTRAND, G. Thalamic units involved in somatic sensation and voluntary and involuntary movements in man. In *The Thalamus*, edited by D. P. Purpura and M. D. Yahr, 365–390. New York, Columbia University Press (1966)

7 NARABAYASHI, H. Importance of muscle tone in production or modification of tremorous movements. In *Parkinson's Disease*, **2**, edited by J. Siegfried, 27–36. Bern, Hans Huber (1973)

8 NARABAYASHI, H. Involuntary movements and cerebellar pathology. In *Cerebro-Cerebellar Interactions*, edited by J. Massion and K. Sasaki, 231–248. Amsterdam, Elsevier (1979)

9 NARABAYASHI, H. A consideration of intention tremor. In *Integrative Control Function of the Brain*, **2**, edited by M. Ito, et al. 185–187. Tokyo, Kodan-sha (1979)

10 NARABAYASHI, H. and OHYE, C. Parkinsonian tremor and nucleus ventralis intermedius of the human thalamus. In *Physiological Tremor, Pathological Tremors and Clonus*, edited by J. E. Desmedt, *Progress in Clinical Neurophysiology*, **5**, 165–172. Basel, Karger (1978)

11 NARABAYASHI, H. and OHYE, CH. Importance of microstereoencephalotomy for tremor alleviation. *Applied Neurophysiology* **43**, 222–227 (1980)

12 OHYE, CH. and NARABAYASHI, H. Physiological study of presumed ventralis intermedius neurons in the human thalamus. *Journal of Neurosurgery*, **50**, 290–297 (1979)

13 OHYE, CH., SAITO, Y., FUKAMACHI, A. and NARABAYASHI, H. An analysis of the spontaneous rhythmic and non-rhythmic burst discharges in the human thalamus. *Journal of Neurological Sciences*, **22**, 245–259 (1974)

14 YASUI, N., NARABAYASHI, H., KONDO, T. and OHYE, C. Slight cerebellar signs in stereotactic thalamotomy and subthalamotomy for parkinsonism. *Applied Neurophysiology*, **39**, 315–320 (1976/77)

15 YOSHIDA, M., YANAGISAWA, N., SHIMAZU, H., GIVRE, A. and NARABAYASHI, H. Physiological identification of the thalamic nucleus. *Archives of Neurology*, **11**, 435–443 (1964)

17.3
Surgical approach to dystonia
Joseph M. Waltz

THALAMIC SURGERY

Dystonia is a symptom complex of abnormal muscle contraction, affecting a single muscle group in one patient, while presenting in another as a generalized neurological syndrome involving multiple muscle groups of the whole body. Dystonic postures caused by sustained involuntary muscle spasms have responded to thalamic surgery and every dystonic symptom potentially is reversible. However, there are many varieties of dystonia, and its response to lesions placed in the ventral tier of the lateral thalamus has been variable. In one patient, motor dysfunction may be relieved by a single lesion in the thalamus, yet in another the same symptoms are totally resistant to multiple lesions virtually destroying all of the thalamus, pulvinar and globus pallidus. Thalamotomy is not without risk and carries a definite mortality and morbidity. This becomes of great significance with bilateral thalamic surgery which causes a high incidence of pseudobulbar complications. However, in certain selected cases carefully placed sequential thalamic lesions may have to be utilized to reverse dystonic posturing and spasms[2,3]. The results and response of dystonia to a thalamic lesion support the theory that dystonia is a dysfunction of an abnormal sensory communication system. Interrupting and overriding these abnormal communications from the basal ganglia allows other intact portions of the central nervous system to be utilized and overcome the dystonia.

CERVICAL CORD STIMULATION

Introduction

The possibility of altering such sensory abnormalities via sensory input modulation prompted the author to apply minute electrical impulses to the surface of the spinal cord to improve motor function and reverse abnormal posturing. The use of spinal cord stimulation in the treatment of neurological disease was initiated by the 'gate theory' of pain as proposed by Melzack and Wall[4] in 1965. Its use in the treatment of pain appeared to be its only application until 1973, when improved motor function in patients with multiple sclerosis was observed[1]. This finding prompted the author initially in 1975 to investigate cord stimulation in the treatment of motor disorders, and now over 250 patients with cerebral palsy, dystonia, torticollis, post-stroke or post-traumatic spasticity, or epilepsy have been treated.

In the initial 100 patients, a preferred site for a positive response was observed[7]. The best results occurred with electrodes placed in the cervical area between C-2 and C-4. Conventional systems available at the time had two electrodes and allowed only single level stimulation. The author felt that an electrode permitting stimulation between C-2 and C-4 would improve the results and therefore designed a four-electrode system to allow such flexibility. His present stimulation system of four electrodes permits 18 different combinations, including single and double bipolar stimulation. Since 1978, this four-electrode system has been used exclusively and has yielded improve results compared with the older two-electrode system[8].

Technique

The electrodes are placed in the epidural space between C-2 and C-4. Initially, this required a cervical laminectomy[6]. During the past two years a percutaneous technique was developed with the four electrodes incorporated into a single fine

Figure 17.3.1 The multilevel 4-electrode catheter assembly with platinum electrodes 1.19 mm in diameter and spaced 1 cm apart from center to center

catheter (*Figure 17.3.1*), which is inserted through a 16 gauge epidural needle into the cervical epidural space under fluoroscopy (*Figure 17.3.2*), thus eliminating the need for a large cervical operation. The patients' response to stimulating specific electrode combinations is then studied; the analysis of the 18 possible electrode

Figure 17.3.2 Lateral cervical X-ray showing the 4-electrode system in place (arrow)

combination is crucial for therapeutic effectiveness. Once the best electrode combination is discovered, the system is permanently internalized with a subcutaneously-placed receiver. The external system consists of a radiofrequency transmitter and antenna. The antenna is placed over the receiver and, by transcutaneous induction, the radiofrequencies are converted into minute electrical impulses conveyed to the appropriate cervical electrodes. During the postoperative period, the patient is tested with frequencies ranging from 100 to 1400 Hz. There is great variability in the response to different frequencies; many respond to higher frequencies while others to a lower frequency. The earliest four-electrode system had four temporary percutaneous extensions for testing the various electrode combinations. Recently a computerized receiver has been developed which allows the complete system to be implanted initially with no percutaneous extensions. Therefore, all 18 combinations can be tried through the transmitter, eliminating the need for a second operation and allowing an indefinite period for the electrode analysis, which can be extremely beneficial in the dystonic patient.

Results

Torsion dystonia

During the past six years, spinal cord stimulation has been carried out in 55 patients with generalized torsion dystonia and in 26 patients with segmental axial dystonia. In the generalized torsion dystonia group, there were 35 males and 20 females, ranging in age from 8 to 64 years (mean 24.4 years). The duration of their illness ranged from 1.5 to 27 years (mean 10.6 years). Previous thalamic surgery had been carried out in 38 patients, 21 bilaterally and 17 unilaterally; 17 patients had no previous thalamic surgery. Twenty-five patients had implantation of the older two-electrode system and 30 patients had the four-electrode system inserted. Follow-up time ranged from 6 to 62 months. Earlier results[5], based almost exclusively on the two-electrode system, indicated that axial dystonia responded best, and that peripheral dystonia was less affected. However, results following use of the four-electrode system and more specific stimulation has led to the reversal this earlier conclusion. The author now feels that the peripheral and axial problems respond equally well. Since instituting the four-electrode system, he has seen not only improvement in peripheral dystonia, but also the improvement in the overall number of patients responding (*Table 17.3.1*). The number of patients with marked to moderate improvement rose from 52 to 70 percent, while those not improved fell from 48 to 17 percent.

Table 17.3.1 Results of spinal cord stimulation in dystonia: comparison of two-electrode (2E) and four-electrode (4E) systems

	Number		Marked improvement (%)		Moderate improvement (%)		Mild improvement (%)		No improvement (%)	
	2E	4E	2E	4E	2E	4E	2E	4E	2E	4E
Generalized torsion dystonia										
No previous thalamic surgery	4	14	–	4 (29)	–	4 (29)	–	3 (21)	4 (100)	3 (21)
Unilateral thalamic surgery	10	7	2 (20)	5 (71)	3 (30)	2 (29)	–	–	5 (50)	–
Bilateral thalamic surgery	11	9	3 (27)	3 (33)	5 (46)	3 (33)	–	1 (11)	3 (27)	2 (22)
Total	25	30	5 (20)	12 (40)	8 (32)	9 (30)	–	4 (13)	12 (48)	5 (17)
Segmental dystonia (Torticollis)	17	9	6 (35)	3 (33)	3 (18)	3 (33)	1 (6)	1 (11)	7 (41)	2 (22)

The effect of previous thalamic surgery on the results was most interesting. None of the four patients with no previous thalamic surgery implanted with the two-electrode system was improved, while 11 patients (79 percent) who had no thalamic surgery and implanted with the four-electrode system were helped, 58 percent being improved moderately to markedly. Reversal was noted in both the axial and the peripheral dystonic manifestations. In patients who had unilateral thalamotomy, all implanted with the four-electrode system improved, while only 50 percent with the two-electrode system improved. In patients who had bilateral thalamic surgery, 8 (73 percent) of the 11 implanted with the two-electrode system were improved while 7 (87 percent) of the 9 who had the four-electrode system improved. Often the most disabling symptoms from previous bilateral thalamic surgery were the residual pseudobulbar and pyramidal tract dysfunction. Patients with spinal cord stimulation have demonstrated improvement in dysarthric speech, chewing, swallowing and decrease in drooling. Walking was improved with decrease in spasticity and difficulties in balance, and residual dystonic symptoms of both an axial and peripheral type were improved.

Twenty-six patients with segmental axial dystonia (spasmodic torticollis) underwent spinal cord stimulation. These included 9 men and 17 women, with an age range of 30–61 years (mean 44.5 years). Duration of symptoms ranged from 8 months to 27 years (mean 5.3 years). Follow-up time ranged from 6 to 54 months. Marked to moderate improvement was noted in 15 patients (58 percent), mild improvement in 2 patients (8 percent), and no benefit in 9 patients (35 percent). Greater improvement was demonstrated in the four-electrode series (*Table 17.3.1*). Marked to moderate improvement was increased from 53 to 66 percent and unimproved cases fell from 41 to 22 percent. Patients who were noted as markedly improved showed no evidence of torticollis and had full range of motion of the head and neck. Moderately improved patients showed full motility but demonstrated some torticollis. Patients considered mildly improved had a decrease in torticollic posture, spasms and pain, but retained some element of torticollis and some limitation of motion.

Figure 17.3.3 (*a*) Focal torsion dystonia of 2 years duration in a 30-year-old man manifested by severe painful action spasms of the right hand, arm and shoulder. (*b*) Postoperatively the patient demonstrated improvement in deformity with relief of the dystonic posturing and pain

Dystonic patients with peripheral, axial and pseudobulbar abnormalities have responded to specific cervical cord stimulation with the four-electrode system. Dystonic posturing of the affected extremity has been improved or reversed, with restoration of hand function and dexterity (*Figure 17.3.3*). With reversal and improvement of the torsion deformity of the feet, walking is improved. The axial dystonic symptoms respond with straightening of the spine, reversal of scoliosis and

Figure 17.3.4(*a*) and (*b*) Axial dystonia in a 32-year-old man of 4 years duration, manifested by spastic dysphonia, postural-induced severe kyphosis and flexion deformity of the trunk and shoulders. (*c*) and (*d*) Postoperatively the patient demonstrated improvement in the axial deformity with improved walking and speech

306 Surgical approach to dystonia

Figure 17.3.5 Severe uncontrolled painful spasms had incapacitated this 31-year-old man for over 3 years. Preoperative photos show the patient's ability to temporarily overcome the constant spasms (*a*) by exerting pressure over his face and forehead (*b,c*). Postoperatively, (*d,e,f*) the patient demonstrates complete relief of torticollis. The patient now has complete range of motion of his neck and has been without painful cervical spasms for the past 3 years

lordosis, improved posture, and walking (*Figure 17.3.4*). Patients with torticollis are relieved of abnormal posturing of the neck and pain, and experience return of head and neck mobility (*Figure 17.3.5*). Patients with pseudobulbar problems noted improved balance and walking stability, lessening of drooling and improved swallowing and speech.

Complications

Complications have been infrequent in the series of over 250 patients. There have been no deaths and no serious morbidity. Broken electrodes have occurred in 9.7 percent of patients using the earlier system, but were easily repaired or replaced; this has not been a problem with the newer single catheter four-electrode system. Infections (4.9 percent) occurred with prolonged observation using the temporary percutaneous leads. however, with the computerized system this has not been a problem. Occasional electrode displacement (1.3 percent) in the vertical plane has been seen, but the electrode can easily be repositioned when necessary.

Discussion

Chronic epidural spinal stimulation is capable of altering and reversing many different neurological symptoms, including the torticollic neck, and dystonic trunk and extremity, spasticity, pseudobulbar dysfunction and intractable epilepsy[8]. Neuroaugmentation and modulation may result from direct electrical influence on nervous tissue, indirectly via some neurotransmitter substance, or perhaps both. The mechanism must be through some diffuse system accessible to the stimulating electrode, and most likely involves the ascending and/or descending reticular formation. The level at which these systems are stimulated, the polarity of the electrical field and the frequency of stimulation are critical in achieving a therapeutic result and these must be found for each patient with the four-electrode multilevel system. To improve the therapeutic response in dystonia, the clinical results must be correlated and analyzed with different stimulation parameters, including frequency, polarity, pulse width, impedance, site of stimulation and evoked potentials. The author is investigating the possible neurophysiological neurotransmitter mechanisms which may lead to further understanding the types of brain and spinal activity initiated or altered through spinal cord stimulation. This may further elucidate the mechanisms of stimulation in dystonia and perhaps the underlying abnormality of the disease.

References

1 COOK, A. W. and WEINSTEIN, P. Chronic dorsal column stimulation in multiple sclerosis: preliminary report. *New York Journal of Medicine*, **73**, 2868–2872 (1973)
2 COOPER, I. S. Twenty-year followup study of the neurosurgical treatment of dystonia musculorum deformans. *Advances in Neurology*, **14**, 423–452 (1976)
3 COOPER, I. S. Surgical approaches to treatment and physiological implications. In *The Basal Ganglia*, edited by M. D. Yahr, 369–383. New York, Raven Press (1976)
4 MELZACK, R. and WALL, R. D. Pain mechanisms: a new theory. *Science*, **150**, 971–979 (1965)
5 WALTZ, J. M. Spinal cord stimulation for palsies. *Patient Care*, **13**, 118–206 (1979)
6 WALTZ, J. M. and ANDREESEN, W. H. Multiple lead spinal cord stimulation: technique. *Applied Neurophysiology*, **44**, 30–36 (1981)
7 WALTZ, J. M. and PANI, K. C. Spinal cord stimulation in disorders of the motor system. *Proceedings of the Sixth International Symposium of External Control of Human Extremities*, 545–556 (1978)
8 WALTZ, J. M., REYNOLDS, L. O. and RIKLAN, M. Multi-lead spinal cord stimulation for control of motor disorders. *Applied Neurophysiology* (in press)

17.4
Surgical treatment of spasmodic torticollis

J. J. Maccabe

The cause of spasmodic torticollis is unknown. A focal manifestation of torsion dystonia, the disorder of muscular contraction which results in the abnormal movements and postures of the head and neck has no known pathological or pharmacological basis. The idea that it represents a functional manifestation of psychiatric illness no longer bears critical examination[21]. Movements resembling torticollis have been produced in the experimental animal, but the relevance of such models for the human condition is not easy to assess[10]. They are many and varied concepts of the origin and mechanism of the disorder.

There is little detailed information on the natural history of the condition. The usual patient is over 40 years. Jerking or turning movements of the head begin insidiously, and gradually increase in severity, leading ultimately to a more or less sustained deviation. Though the initial stages of the illness may suggest an inexorable deterioration several surveys indicate that for the majority of patients the condition soon becomes static[16, 25]. In a prolonged follow-up study of 41 patients, Meares[23] concluded that there might be three stages in the course of the illness. First, a period of slow progression, lasting some 5 years, during which there was a possibility of remission. Next a stationary period of perhaps 5 years, followed by a final stage during which some slight improvement might occur. Matthews et al.[22] came to a similar conclusion. For the majority of their 30 patients symptoms persisted largely unchanged over many years. Temporary complete remission is not unknown, especially in the early years of the illness, but relapse is also frequent. Substantial sustained improvement without treatment may occur – four examples are recorded by Matthews. Examination of patients after a number of years will reveal some with manifestations of dystonia elsewhere – usually in the shoulder, sometimes in the arm and trunk[6]. In about 10 per cent of patients there will be an associated postural tremor. The manifestations of torticollis vary widely from patient to patient. For those who are severely affected there can be no doubt as to the major disability which torticollis represents. The serious adverse social effect on the life and happiness of many patients is well documented. Pain in the neck, due to sustained muscular contraction or to associated degenerative joint disease may also be a problem. On the other hand, for those with milder symptoms, and for whom remission may be more likely, a full life and a normal working pattern are not impossible, as the findings of several series testify.

PERIPHERAL SURGERY

The participating head and neck muscles responsible for the varying posture of torticollis provide the most obvious and accessible target for surgical endeavour. Procedures designed to reduce or abolish their activity have a long history. In 1891 Keen[17] reported the division of the first three cervical nerves on one side by an extraspinal method. The first intraspinal operation was by Taylor (1915)[29].

How far it is possible or worthwhile to assess in detail by clinical examination and by electromyography those muscles primarily involved is a matter for conjecture. Myotomy of the selected muscle bellies is now rarely practised and despite a recent enthusiastic report on 60 patients so treated[3] is unlikely to be revived. Denervation has proved equally effective. However, denervation or ablation of only a limited group of muscles carries a high risk of failure or later recurrence of symptoms. Dandy[7] was emphatic that bilateral nerve section was essential for success. His recommendation of intradural section of the first three anterior cervical roots on both sides remains the basis of denervation procedures to the present day. Electromyography is used by some to help identify the affected muscles, and temporary nerve blocks may also be of assistance in assessing the individual problem[2,9].

The standard rhizotomy procedure consists of section of the cervical anterior roots 1–3 on both sides. An operating microscope is essential so that the fine arterioles accompanying the rootlets can be seen and preserved. The identification of the first cervical root may be difficult; failure to divide it may mean that the suboccipital muscles will continue to be active. McKenzie[20] pointed out an important contribution from the spinal accessory to the first cervical root, which also must be sought and divided. The same author advocated section of the fourth cervical root on the side showing greater posterior neck muscle contraction, but there is no evidence that this gives additional benefit. The spinal root of the accessory nerve may be divided at the level of the foramen magnum at the same operation. Bulbar tributaries of the vagus which travel with the accessory nerve may be at risk; their inadvertent damage has been held responsible for the postoperative difficulty with swallowing noted by some authors. As the trapezius muscle is infrequently involved in the involuntary movements, denervation of the sternomastoid muscle alone in the neck is to be preferred. Some advocate sternomastoid denervation as a first procedure, to allow easier assessment of other muscle activity.

There are many series of patients recording the beneficial effects of these denervation procedures. Hamby and Schiffer[11] stated that 79 per cent of their patients considered themselves much improved. Arseni and Meretsis[1] reported 74 per cent satisfactory results with 52 patients. Tasker[28] noted an immediate impressive amelioration of symptoms in 29 out of 47 patients, a further six having modest improvement. Scoville and Bettis[26] claimed eminently satisfactory results for most of their 23 patients. Fabinyi and Dutton[9] had 18 good results out of 20 patients.

Such figures need qualification. The operative procedure has complications for more than the occasional patient. Weakness of the neck muscles with a feeling of instability of the head is the most common. An occasional patient suffers a subluxation of the cervical spine, requiring fusion for its correction. Nearly one-third of the patients of Hamby and Schiffer[11] complained of difficulty with swallowing. The authors attributed this to the patient's inability to lift the head in the reflex act of swallowing. Ischaemic complications affecting the spinal cord or medulla, though extremely rare, can take the form of a temporary hemiparesis or hemianaesthesia, or there may be a permanent infarction[26]. An unusual variant with ultimately permanent weakness of both upper limbs was recorded by Sweet[27]. Such complications are the reason why some still advocate extradural root sections[2].

But the most serious complaint levelled against the procedure, by Meares[23], was that it often failed to abolish the distressing movements. Comparing operated and nonoperated groups, he concluded that those submitted to surgery fared worse, and that in some operation led to severe disability, something not seen in his unoperated group. In common with many other observers he was impressed by those untreated patients who continued to lead full lives.

STEREOTAXIC SURGERY

The neuronal mechanisms underlying the involuntary movements of the head and neck have been the subject of extensive experimental research. Direction-specific turning movements can be obtained by stimulation of many extrapyramidal structures in the mesodiencephalon. Contraversive turning movements have their main centre in the pallidum internum and its thalamic and other descending connexions[24]. Rotatory movements are obtained from the interstitial nucleus of Cajal and its connexions, notably those to the nucleus ventralis oralis internus of the thalamus[13]. Stimulation of the midline cerebellar nuclei and parts of the cerebellar peduncle will also produce a rotation of the head[18]. A state very similar to human torticollis was produced by Foltz et al.[10] in the monkey, with lesions involving parts of the medial reticular formation. These and other observations have provided the theoretical basis for a centrally directed stereotaxic surgical approach to treatment.

Cooper[4] was the first to report a series of 75 patients treated by a stereotaxic method. Observing that the nuchal hyperkinesis of Parkinson's disease and dystonia musculorum deformans could be modified or abolished by a thalamic lesion, and believing that torticollis was at least partly mediated by an abnormality of the motor-modulating sensory connections between the cerebellum and the motor cortex, he concluded that by interrupting these pathways at a thalamic level torticollis might be alleviated. The frequent association of tremor with torticollis and the knowledge that cerebellar tremor could be abolished by thalamic surgery seemed to support this theory. The immediate results of even unilateral thalamic surgery were often dramatic. Longer follow-up, however, very soon revealed the difficulty of achieving a permanent result. Bilateral lesions, though more effective, rarely abolished all abnormal movement. With an experience of 160 patients it had become clear that to achieve lasting relief of symptoms bilateral lesions of the ventrolateral thalamic nucleus combined with lesions of the ventroposteromedial and centrum medianum nuclei were essential[5]. Even then there was only a 60 per cent chance of improvement. For 40 per cent of the patients there was no satisfactory alleviation of symptoms. A major drawback was the development of dysphonic symptoms in nearly one-fifth of the patients.

The nucleus ventralis oralis internus (VOI) of the thalamus was selected as a target for torticollis surgery by Hassler and Riechert[14] because of its head and face representation. Their initially good results were of short duration. Study of head and neck movements suggested that there might be two different elements to be considered, each alleviated perhaps by a different neuronal circuit. Thus for pure turning movements of the head destruction of the pallidothalamic fibres might be appropriate, whereas with turning plus tilting or inclination of the head interruption of the interstitiothalamic fibres would be required in addition. These last could be most suitably interrupted in the posterior part of the nucleus VOI[12]. Reporting on 70 patients, Dieckmann[8] noted that with the above combination of lesions, in 47 per cent of patients torticollis was completely abolished, 29 per cent were said to have had a good result, whereas 9 per cent obtained no relief. The beneficial effects might not appear for several months after surgery. An important side-effect was a tendency to neglect the opposite extremities, a deficit appearing in some 16 per cent of patients.

The posterior part of the nucleus of VOI was also used by Bertrand et al.[2] who treated 14 patients – 10 with unilateral and 4 with bilateral surgery. With the patient awake and able to co-operate, microelectrode recording aided localization within the thalamic nuclei and stimulation was used to identify and protect structures surrounding the target area, in particular the corticospinal fibres. The moderate contralateral hypotonia that followed was rapidly compensated for by the patient. The only permanent complication was dysarthria in 1 of 4 patients undergoing bilateral thalamic surgery. These authors at that time regarded thalamic surgery as the procedure of choice in moderate to severe forms of torticollis, and felt it was effective in 70 per cent of cases. Since then, however, their view has changed (*see* Chapter 17.4).

A less optimistic view was taken by Laitenen and Vilkki[19]. While admitting that torticollis could be alleviated they found the effects were mostly short-lived; after a few months all the patients were dissatisfied. Detailed psychological assessment after surgery revealed unsuspected defects, especially with left-sided lesions, both receptive and expressive verbal efficiency being impaired. These authors were reluctant to recommend thalamotomy for torticollis.

CONCLUSIONS

It is not easy to assess the value of the present methods of surgical treatment, peripheral or central, available to the patient with torticollis. Though published reports relate to several hundred patients – the great majority treated by cervical rhizotomy – the criteria for recommending surgery are rarely stated. Some consider sternomastoid denervation appropriate for those whose symptoms are mild. Others operate only for 'real disability' – probably implying severe manifestations, perhaps with pain, where loss of employment threatens. Evidence of dystonia elsewhere makes many reluctant to offer surgical help. At what stage operation should be contemplated is equally unclear – though a few advocate early surgery to avoid the development of fibrotic and degenerative changes in the neck. A stable disability of at least 6 months' duration is required by Chen[3].

Results of surgical treatment are often quoted simply as 'excellent' or 'eminently satisfactory', terms which by themselves convey little. Who assesses the results, and when, are also important considerations. Hamby and Schiffer[11], adopting a more critical approach than most, admitted that with their 50 patients evaluation of results was difficult. They noted that some patients with what the authors regarded as excellent objective results remained unhappy with their status, while others, apparently more severely affected, were content. Only 72 per cent of their patients were glad that they had undergone surgery. Some residual head rotation was displayed by 53 per cent. Hernesniemi and Laitinen[15] in a follow-up of 56 patients treated by various methods observed that though the immediate effects of surgery were judged by them to be good or fair, at a later date most of their patients considered the results to be poor. Matthews et al.[22] found surgery to be either ineffective or palliative.

The natural history for the majority of patients is probably one of relatively unchanging disability over many years, most being able to continue at work. An effective treatment should abolish all involuntary movement, without risk of complication adding to the patients' burden. None of the present methods can achieve these aims. Whether the mildest symptoms should be treated at an early stage seems doubtful. Once manifestations are severe, cervical rhizotomy offers the best hope of long term palliation[28]. For a standard procedure, however, the results are not uniform. There is no way to predict what the result will be for each individual. When it fails it is usually because it is inadequate in controlling the movements.

The same uncertainty attaches to the stereotaxic method. Even among its practitioners, opinions are divided as to its suitability and indications. There can be no unqualified acceptance of this approach at present. Few neurologists refer torticollis patients for stereotaxic treatment nowadays, and few patients seek such a treatment, when the uncertainty of the outcome and the risk to speech of the bilateral lesions are explained.

References

1 ARSENI, C. and MARETSIS, M. The surgical treatment of spasmodic torticollis. *Neurochirurgia*, **14**, 177–180 (1971)

2 BERTRAND, C. Combined stereotactic and peripheral surgical approach for spasmodic torticollis. *Applied Neurophysiology*, **41**, 122–131 (1978)

3 CHEN, X. Selective resection and denervation of cervical muscles in the treatment of spasmodic torticollis: results in 60 cases. *Neurosurgery*, **8,** 681–688, (1981)
4 COOPER, I. S. Clinical and physiological publications of thalamic surgery. *Journal of Neurological Sciences*, **2,** 520–533 (1965)
5 COOPER, I. S. Neurosurgical treatment of the dyskinesias. *Clinical Neurosurgery*, **24,** 367–390 (1977)
6 COUCH, J. R. Dystonia and tremor in spasmodic torticollis. In *Dystonia*, edited by R. Eldridge and S. Fahn. *Advances in Neurology*, **14,** New York, Raven Press (1976)
7 DANDY, W. E. An operation for the treatment of spasmodic torticollis. *Archives of Surgery*, **20,** 1021–1032 (1930)
8 DIECKMANN, G. Stereotaxic treatment of extrapyramidal torticollis. *Neurochirurgie*, **22,** 568–571 (1976)
9 FABINYI, G. and DUTTON, J. The surgical treatment of spasmodic torticollis. *Australian and New Zealand Journal of Surgery*, **50,** 155–157 (1980)
10 FOLTZ, E. L., KNOPP, L. M. and WARD, A. A. Experimental spasmodic torticollis. *Journal of Neurosurgery*, **16,** 55–72 (1959)
11 HAMBY, W. B. and SCHIFFER, S. Spasmodic torticollis; results after cervical rhizotomy in 80 cases. *Clinical Neurosurgery*, **17,** 28–37 (1970)
12 HASSLER, R. and DIECKMANN, G. Stereotactic treatment of different kinds of spasmodic torticollis. *Confinia Neurologica*, **32,** 135–143 (1970)
13 HASSLER, R. and HESS, W. R. Experimentelli und Anatomische Befundi über die Drehbewegungen und ihre nervösin Apparate. *Archiv für Psychiatrie und Nervenkrankheiten*, **192,** 488–526 (1954)
14 HASSLER, R. and RIECHERT, T. Uber die Symptomatik und operative Behandberg der extrapyramidalin Bewegungsstörungen. *Medizinische Klinik*, **53,** 817–824 (1958)
15 HERNESNIEMI, J. and LAITENEN, L. Résultats tardifs de la chirurgie dans le torticolis spasmodique. *Neurochirurgie*, **23,** 123–131 (1977)
16 HERZ, E. and GLASER, G. H. Spasmodic torticollis II. *Archives of Neurology and Psychiatry*, **61,** 227–239 (1949)
17 KEEN, W. W. New operation for spasmodic wry neck, namely division or exsection of the nerves supplying the superior rotator muscles of the neck. *Annals of Surgery*, **13,** 44 (1891)
18 KOELLA, W. P. Motor effects from electrical stimulation of the basal cerebellum in the unrestrained cat. *Journal of Neurophysiology*, **18,** 558–573 (1955)
19 LAITENEN, L. V. and VILKKI, J. Observations on physiological and psychological function of the ventral oral internal nucleus of human thalamus. *Acta Neurologica Scandinavica*, **55,** 198–212 (1977)
20 McKENZIE, K. G. The surgical treatment of spasmodic torticollis. *Clinical Neurosurgery*, **2,** 37–43 (1955)
21 MARSDEN, C. D. Dystonia: the spectrum of the disease. In *Association for Research in Nervous and Mental Diseases*; *The Basal Ganglia, Research Publications*, **55,** edited by M. D. Yahr, 351–367. New York, Raven Press (1976)
22 MATTHEWS, W. B., BEASLEY, P., PARRY-JONES, W. and GARLAND, G. Spasmodic torticollis: a combined clinical study. *Journal of Neurology, Neurosurgery and Psychiatry*, **41,** 485–492 (1978)

23 MEARES, R. Natural history of spasmodic torticollis and effect of surgery. *Lancet*, **2,** 149–151 (1971)
24 MONTANELLI, R. P. and HASSLER, R. Motor effects elicited by stimulation of the pallido-thalamic system in the cat. In *Lectures on the Diencephalon*, edited by W. Bargmann and J. P. Schade, 56–66 Amsterdam, Elsevier (1964)
25 PATTERSON, R. M. and LITTLE, S. C. Spasmodic torticollis. *Journal of Nervous and Mental Disease*, **98,** 577–599 (1943)
26 SCOVILLE, W. B. and BETTIS, D. B. Motor tics of the head and neck: surgical approaches and their complications. *Acta Neurochirurgia*, **48,** 47–66 (1979)
27 SWEET, W. H. What should the neurosurgeon do when faced with a malpractice suit? *Clinical Neurosurgery*, **23,** 112–124 (1976)
28 TASKER, R. R. The treatment of spasmodic torticollis by peripheral denervation: the McKenzie operation. In *Current Controversies in Neurosurgery*, edited by T. P. Morley, 443–447. Philadelphia, W. B. Saunders (1976)
29 TAYLOR, A. S. Operations on the peripheral and cranial nerves. In *Operative Therapeusis*, **2,** edited by A. B. Johnson, New York, Appleton and Co. (1915)

17.5
Peripheral versus central surgical approach for the treatment of spasmodic torticollis

Claude M. Bertrand

Anterior cervical rhizotomy was the technique used in the author's department for the surgical treatment of distressing cases of torticollis even after 1954 when stereotaxic surgery was performed for many forms of involuntary movements, including generalized late-onset dystonias. The anterior roots of C1 down to and including the upper portion of C4 on the side of the most active posterior cervical group of muscles and the anterior roots of C1, C2 and C3 on the other side were sectioned; branches of the spinal accessory nerve were also interrupted in the neck whenever necessary. In 1960, following the report of Hassler and Hess[7], a lesion of VOI in the thalamus, as a rule bilaterally and in two stages, was done in a few patients. Satisfactory results were obtained in only 50 percent of the cases and rhizotomy was reverted to in spite of its shortcomings. Rhizotomy brings about an appreciable amount of relief in most cases[6]. However it produces an indiscriminate denervation both of the involved and uninvolved muscles, and denervation cannot be carried below C4 because of the roots of the phrenic nerve. It leaves an ungainly neck, and sometimes a significant portion of the symptoms persist. There may be subluxation or at least excessive lordosis of the cervical spine in the ensuring years, or recurrence of symptoms due to the multiple peripheral anastomoses of the roots which form the cervical plexus.

In 1968, after examining some patients who had had a thalamotomy a few years previously, the author was impressed by the almost total absence of symptoms in the successful cases. In the intervening period, while performing thalamotomies for more diffuse forms of late-onset dystonia, it was noted that the electromyographic discharges of involved muscles were increased by having the patient look to the side of the abnormal movements. This phenomenon was diminished or abolished by an effective lesion, presumably within VOI. Accordingly, thalamotomy was reintroduced for the treatment of spasmodic torticollis. Using this additional preoperative criterion, the percentage of favorable result was raised to 70 percent[6]. However, because VOI is situated in the thalamus in the same coronal plane as the corticobulbar fibers in the internal capsule, complications from involvement of these fibers may be as high as 10 percent in bilateral lesions, while they occur in 2 percent with a more posterior target for tremor or rigidity[3]. Unilateral thalamotomy and/or pallidotomy was then combined with peripheral denervation: the muscles which were still active were blocked with lidocaine (lignocaine) under EMG control and, later on, denervated peripherally. The results were excellent or good in 8 of 9 cases and there were no complications from these unilateral lesions. Four of these 9 patients were submitted to peripheral denervation in addition to stereotaxic procedures[1].

Because of the marked improvement noted during the peripheral nerve blocks, and the very satisfactory results obtained, it was decided to do lidocaine block of the involved muscles under EMG control and to proceed with peripheral denervation according to the results of the block and the EMG before considering stereotaxic surgery[2,4]. In fact, during the past 4 years stereotaxic surgery has been reserved for more generalized forms of dystonia or patients in whom spasmodic torticollis was accompanied by tremor.

The technique has been described elsewhere[1,2,4]. Briefly, the sternomastoid and the trapezius are blocked at the motor point. The posterior cervical group of muscles is blocked partially by injecting lidocaine at the level of C1 over the occipital bone, near the occipital foramen and close to the point of emergence of the posterior ramus of C2, C3 and sometimes C4, near the articular facettes, care being taken not to penetrate the deep venous vertebral plexuses.

Since denervation is performed selectively in order to spare the antagonists for retraining, it is essential to identify the involved muscles accurately. Although, in rotational torticollis, the sternocleidomastoid contralateral to the side to which the head turns and the ipsilateral posterior cervical group are the main offenders, other muscles such as the trapezius also may be involved. Likewise, in laterocollis, besides the ipsilateral posterior cervical group and the ipsilateral trapezius, the ipsilateral sternocleidomastoid among others, may contribute. In retrocollis, both posterior cervical groups are usually involved but a sternocleidomastoid muscle may also participate.

Surgical peripheral denervation is done under light anesthesia without curare in order to be able to use stimulation. In rotational torticollis only the branches of the spinal accessory nerve to the sternocleidomastoid muscle are sectioned and in laterocollis usually only those to the trapezius must be denervated. For these forms of torticollis, denervation of the posterior cervical group unilaterally is done with the patient lying on his side, again using light anesthesia. The incision has the form of an inverted L with the apex over the mastoid. The incision extends downwards, just posterior to the articular facettes, to the level of C6 or C7. C1 and C2 are first identified by stimulation. C1 is followed under the microscope up to its point of emergence over the posterior arch of the atlas, under the vertebral artery. Then, after stimulation, the posterior rami of C2, C3, C4, C5 and C6 are followed to their point of emergence and avulsed. Although sometimes ramicectomy is limited to C5, it may have to be carried down to C7. At the end of the procedure, stimulation over the articular facettes should not arouse any motor response from the posterior cervical group. In retrocollis, denervation has been carried down to the posterior ramus of C4 on one side and C5 on the other and in one instance, to C5 bilaterally with the patient being able to hold his head erect without difficulty.

Results have been reported on a group of 35 consecutive cases[2,4]. Of 30 patients with rotational or laterocollis or a combination thereof, 12 (40 percent) had an excellent result. In 16 (53 percent), the abnormal movements were so reduced that the patients were not concerned about them. Two (7 percent) were only slightly improved.

In retrocollis, since denervation must perforce be partial, the symptoms are not alleviated as completely. Of five patients, one had a very good result and two were markedly relieved. Two others, one of which had had a previous rhizotomy, were slightly improved.

The only permanent untoward effects of posterior cervical ramicectomy are anesthesia in the territory of C2, which three patients found to be disturbing, and localized atrophy in the posterior cervical region. There was transitory dysphagia in two cases. Since there is no laminectomy and only C1 and the posterior rami of the cervical branches are denervated, no major complications are anticipated. Besides its safety, since innervation of the uninvolved muscles is spared, rehabilitation is more rapid and complete. The patient can be up after 2 days and most of the normal movements of the neck are preserved. In 5 instances re-operation was required: twice to complete the denervation of C1, once to pursue denervation at C6 and C7 in one of the initial cases, and twice to denervate further the sternocleidomastoid muscle. Selective peripheral denervation requires an extensive study of the muscles involved. Avulsion of C1 with posterior ramicectomy down to C6 is a meticulous procedure. However, it is a benign operation which brings about total or sufficient relief in most cases. When an appreciable amount of rotation or inclination persists after satisfactory denervation, it is because other muscles are involved besides those normally contributing to the movement. Only in these circumstances is a more serious procedure such as a stereotacxic thalamotomy and /or pallidotomy now considered.

References

1 BERTRAND, C., MOLINA-NEGRO, P. and MARTINEZ, S. N. Combined stereotaxic and peripheral surgical approach for spasmodic torticollis. *Applied Neurophysiology*, **41,** 122–133 (1978)

2 BERTRAND, C., MOLINA-NEGRO, P. and MARTINEZ, S. N. Selective peripheral denervation for spasmodic torticollis. *Sixteenth Canadian Congress of Neurological Sciences*, (Calgary, June 25, 1981)

3 BERTRAND, C., MOLINA-NEGRO, P. and MARTINEZ, S. N. Stereotaxic targets for dystonias and dyskinesias: relationship to corticobulbar fibers and other adjoining structures; *Advances in Neurology*, **24,** edited by L. J. Poirier, T. L. Sourkes and P. J. Bédard, 395–399. New York, Raven Press (1979)

4 BERTRAND, C., MOLINA-NEGRO, P. and MARTINEZ, S. N. Technical aspects of selective peripheral denervation for spasmodic torticollis. (Presented at the 8th meeting of the World Society for Stereotaxic and Functional Neurosurgery jointly with the 5th meeting of the European Society for Stereotaxic and Functional Neurosurgery, Zurich, Switzerland, July 1981) *Applied Neurophysiology* (in press)

5 BERTRAND. C. The treatment of spasmodic torticollis with particular reference to thalamotomy. *Current Controversies in Neurosurgery*, edited by T. P. Morley, 455–459. Philadelphia, W. B. Saunders (1976)

6 HAMBY, W. B. and SCHIFFER, S. Spasmodic torticollis: results after cervical rhizotomy in 50 cases. *Journal of Neurosurgery*, **31,** 323–326 (1969)

7 HASSLER, R. and HESS, W. R. Experimentell und anatomische befunde über die Drehbewegungen und ihre nervosen Apparate. *Archiv für Psychiatrie und Nervenkrankheiten*, **192,** 488–526 (1954)

17.6
Surgical approach to blepharospasm: nerve thermolysis
Arthur F. Battista

In severe cases of blepharospasm which do not respond to medical treatment, surgical therapy may be considered. Various types of operations have been employed in the treatment of this condition. The ideal surgical procedures should relieve involuntary muscle spasms, with the production of minimal or no facial muscle paresis, and no or low morbidity. The facial nerve in its course from the stylomastoid foramen to the peripheral branches has been interrupted by injecting phenol or alcohol, or by sectioning the nerves surgically. In addition, to prevent nerve regeneration various surgical techniques have been applied[5, 8, 11, 12, 14]. The beneficial results from these operations in many patients have been temporary[9]. The injection of alcohol into branches of the facial nerve bilaterally in patients as reported by Henderson[6] in 1956 resulted in only very temporary relief of muscle spasms. Because of the associated complications, as well as only temporary benefit, he advocated a more direct surgical interruption of the branches of the facial nerve.

In 1967, Reynolds et al.[13] performed bilateral differential section of the facial nerve on 11 patients with blepharospasm. Although these patients had some change in facial expression, they reported that all were satisfied with the operation. In 1970 McCabe[10] reported on patients with blepharospasm who had undergone, in addition to resection of nerves to the orbicularis oculi, avulsion of the nerves in order to prevent nerve regeneration; 88 percent of the patients had marked improvement of their symptoms. In 1975, Bird and McDonald[3] reported on 7 cases with severe blepharospasm operated with the Reynolds technique of avulsing branches of the facial nerve. Two patients had partial recurrence of symptoms in the third year after operation (see also Chapter 17.7). Frueh et al. in 1976[7] reported the results of differential section of the VIIth nerve, using the Callahan technique in 100 patients with blepharospasm. They concluded that 50 percent of the patients operated with this technique obtained long-termed benefit[7].

Surgical transection and/or avulsion method of relieving blepharospasm may result in the following sequelae: drooping of the corner of the mouth, eyebrow drop, paralytic ectropion, and lagophthalmos[6, 9]. However these difficulties are usually easily corrected by simple procedures[4, 6, 13].

To minimize possible facial paresis and to diminish morbidity of facial nerve section and/or avulsion, the following surgical procedure for the treatment of blepharospasm was reported in 1977[1]. The patient is operated using local anesthesia and intravenous analgesia. Using a percutaneous approach, a needle probe* is passed and branches to the orbicularis oculi or other facial muscles are identified by electrical stimulation. When the appropriate neural elements are identified, a thermolytic lesion is produced to interrupt nerve conduction. With the patient conscious, voluntary facial movements can be evoked on request. This process is repeated until the spontaneous spasms are markedly decreased or abolished without producing significant muscle paresis. Eight to 35 unilateral lesions are usually required. The procedure may be lengthy, since it is performed bilaterally. For optimal benefit, exact identification of the neural elements involved in the involuntary spasms is required.

The assessment of improvement from medical or surgical therapy for blepharospasm is difficult, since there are many subjective variables. As reported in 1980[2], the symptoms and signs of 17 patients who had undergone bilaterally fractional thermolytic destruction of branches of the facial nerve for blepharospasm were graded pre- and postoperatively on a scale of 0 to 5. This study showed that 14 of the 17 patients, up to 1 September 1980, had 1–2 operations, ranging from 13 to 37 months (average 24 months) from their last operation; their improvement ranged from 50 to 90 percent with an average of 70 percent[2]. Overall evaluation of the 17 patients regardless of the number of operations indicated that a patient who had this operation for blepharospasm could expect an average of 69 percent improvement for an average of 20 months (*Table 17.6.1*).

Table 17.6.1 Results in 17 patients operated for blepharospasm one year after their first operation

Operations	Number of patients	Excellent	Results Good	Fair	None
1	6	3	2	1	–
2	8	4	1	3	–
3	2	–	2	–	–
4	1	–	–	–	1

The complications from this procedure have been minimal. All patients have facial swelling to varying degrees. This usually recedes in a few days and resolves in a week or so. In several cases there was minimal facial fullness for several weeks which completely cleared. In several early patients, eyelid closure was slightly slower on one side compared to the other which equalized in several weeks[2].

*Radio frequency generator Model RFG–5S, Radionics Burlington, Massachusetts 01803

Although the procedure of thermolytic fractional destruction of the branches of the facial nerve for the treatment of blepharospasm is not the optimal surgical therapy, it does have certain specific advantages: (1) because it is done under local anesthesia and intravenous analgesia, the risks of general anesthesia are avoided. This may be important in older patients. (2) With the patient alert and cooperative, constant monitoring of facial muscle minimizes the possibility of facial weakness. (3) Using electrical stimulation, it is possible to have exact control and affect the facial nerve from the stylomastoid region to the fine terminal branches. Because of the minimal scarring, the procedure can be performed in stages. The spasms of hemifacial spasm have been markedly decreased by this operation also[1].

References

1 BATTISTA, A. F. Hemifacial spasm and blepharospasm. *New York State Journal of Medicine*, **77**, 2234–2237 (1977)

2 BATTISTA, A. F. Blepharospasm: a surgical procedure for therapy. Presented at the *Eleventh Annual Scientific Symposium* (Chicago, Nov. 7–8th, 1980) American Society of Ophthalmic Plastic and Reconstructive Surgery

3 BIRD, A. C. and McDONALD, W. I. Essential blepharospasm. *Transactions of the Ophthalmological Society, UK*, **95**, 250–253 (1975)

4 COLES, W. H. Essential blepharospasm. *Southern Medical Journal*, **66**, 1407–1411 (1973)

5 DIAMANT, H., ENFORS, B. and WIBERG, A. Facial spasm with special reference to the chorda tympani function and operative treatment. *Laryngoscope*, **77**, 350–358 (1967)

6 DORTZBACH, R. K. Complications in surgery for blepharospasm. *American Journal of Ophthalmology*, **75**, 142–147 (1973)

7 FRUEH, B. R., CALLAHAN, A., DORTZBACH, R. K. WILKINS, R. B., BEALE, H. L., REITMAN, H. S. and WATSON, F. R. The effects of differential section of the VIIth nerve in patients with intractable blepharospasm. *Transactions of the American Academy of Ophthalmology and Otolaryngology*, **81**, 595–602 (1976)

8 GERMAN, W. J. Surgical treatment of spasmodic facial tic. *Surgery*, **11**, 192–194 (1942)

9 HENDERSON, J. W. Essential blepharospasm. *Transactions of the American Ophthalmological Society*, **54**, 453–520 (1956)

10 McCABE, B. F. Management of hyperfunction of the facial nerve. *Annals of Otolaryngology*, **79**, 252–258 (1970)

11 MIEHLKE, A. *Die Chirugie des Nervus Facialis*. Munich, Urban and Schwarzenberg (1960)

12 NOSIK, W. A. and WEIL, A. A. Selective partial neurectomy in hemifacial spasm and the electrophysiologic selection of patients. *Journal of Neurosurgery*, **13**, 596–602 (1956)

13 REYNOLDS, D. H., SMITH, J. W. and WALSH, T. J. Differential section of the facial nerve for blepharospasm. *Transactions of the American Academy of Ophthalmology and Otolaryngology*, **71**, 656–664 (1967)

14 SCOVILLE, W. B. Partial section of proximal seventh nerve trunk for facial spasm. *Surgery, Gynecology and Obstetrics*, **101**, 494–497 (1955)

17.7
The surgical management of essential blepharospasm

J. F. Talbot, Z. Gregor and A. C. Bird

Blepharospasm consists of involuntary sustained and forcible eyelid closure, which may occur spontaneously[13] (essential blepharospasm) or be precipitated by sensory stimuli (reflex blepharospasm)[7,14]. Essential blepharospasm may occur in the presence of signs of basal ganglia dysfunction or as an isolated abnormality[13,17].

OCULAR FEATURES

Henderson[13] comprehensively reviewed 135 patients from the Mayo Clinic and the authors' own experience differs little from his. The condition has an insidious onset at an average age of 52 years in men and 60 years in women. The age range is wide and the authors have seen a man with symptoms starting as early as 30 and a woman as late as 78 years; it occurs more commonly in women than in men. Initially the symptoms consist of brief and infrequent eye closure affecting one or both eyes, often triggered by bright light. At first they may be unnoticed by the patient, who is not disabled by them. With progression of the disease, however, it affects both eyes and lid closure becomes increasingly frequent and sustained, so that ultimately the patient becomes effectively blind. The degree of disability may vary from day to day and tends to be least marked during the first hours of the day. One patient was forced to complete all her housework and shopping by 10 o'clock in the morning because, after that time, she was invariably severely handicapped. Heightened emotion often causes prolonged lid closure, but increased attention or concentration may lessen the blepharospasm. This latter feature of the condition frequently causes difficulty when the patient is interviewed in a clinical environment as the lid closure may be dramatically improved under these circumstances, causing the clinician seriously to underestimate the severity of the patient's symptoms. It may be observed that the eyes close if the patient is ignored for a short period.

Patients are sometimes forced to employ techniques, which are occasionally bizarre, by which eye closure can be averted or the eyes can be induced to open.

Sometimes it is sufficient to prise the eyelids open manually, but merely touching the forehead or shaking the head may be enough to cause the lids to open. Most patients' lid closure was improved in darkness and one adopted the habit of covering her head with a black cloth to abort an attack of blepharospasm. Others find that enforced mental activity, such as arithmetic, may prevent the onset of lid closure. During an attack, a sudden surprise such as bumping into an object when the eyes are closed or being called by name may similarly terminate an attack. These devices gradually lose their effectiveness as the disease progresses, and eventually the patients' activities become increasingly restricted, until he loses his job and his social independence. In addition, many find their disorder a social barrier causing them to shun their friends and neighbours who are willing to help them. Lack of eye to eye contact may engender similar problems even within the home.

TREATMENT

Inability to identify the fundamental cause of essential blepharospasm and the failure of medical and psychiatric treatment, have led to a variety of surgical procedures by which the disease can be treated symptomatically. Henderson[13] has given a full account of surgical procedures which have been used during the last two centuries.

Operations designed to weaken the local effector muscle have a long history[13]. Attempts have been made to weaken the orbicularis by direct interference with the muscle, and Fox[9] described a patient with blepharospasm following encephalitis, who gained considerable relief after subtotal resection of the upper lid orbicularis muscle. However it appears that the symptoms were not completely abolished, and subsequent experience has shown that the residual movement in the eyelids renders this operation unsatisfactory[13, 21, 23]. Similarly, denervation of the orbicularis muscle by dividing the branches of the facial nerve as they enter the muscle from the lateral side, as described by Callahan[2], gives little relief of blepharospasm or is followed in a very short time by recurrence of eye closure[13, 21]. It is significant that Callahan[3] later recommended facial nerve section in the parotid gland as the operation of choice. Limited success has been reported after insertion of a frontalis sling using nonabsorbable material[19, 23], although this served to reduce the severity of the symptoms rather than to abolish them. This technique may have a place in the treatment of mild cases or of mild recurrences after other procedures[23], though other authors report poor results[21].

Facial denervation represents a more radical approach to this problem. This may be achieved by injection of alcohol into the facial nerve, and was the treatment most commonly used during the first half of this century. The injection was given at the point where the nerve emerged from the stylomastoid foramen[24], in the vicinity of its upper branches within the parotid gland[22], or to the branches as they entered the temporal side of the muscle[16]. The effect of the injection, although good, is short lived, less than half the patients experiencing relief for more than 3 months[13]. Repeated injections are less effective and one patient is reported to have received 19 injections without permanent cure of symptoms[13].

Surgical interruption of the facial nerve has become popular in recent years. Section of the nerve has been performed at the stylomastoid foramen, in the region of the parotid gland, and near the orbital margin. The most successful results have been achieved by dividing the upper branches of the nerve in the parotid gland, so that the orbicularis oculis was paralysed, but sparing the muscles of the lower face. The operation was described by Gurdjian and Williams[12] in America, and Frazier[10] introduced the technique of electrical stimulation of the nerves to identify the precise function of each nerve before it was divided. For the operation to achieve permanent and complete relief of blepharospasm, the whole of the orbicularis oculis should be denervated, together with all the other muscles in the face which overlie the orbicularis muscle and take part in the abnormal movements. Otherwise, orbicularis reinnervation from the overlying muscles can be expected with resumption of blepharospasm[25]. Previous experience supports this view. Callahan[3] made efforts to denervate the orbicularis muscle only, to preserve all the muscles of the lower face, and specifically to leave the innervation of the levator anguli oris. Of 26 patients operated on, only 8 had complete relief of symptoms. In a later review[8], he reported the results of surgery in 100 cases; 50 per cent had recurrence of blepharospasm in 3 years. Of 7 patients operated on by Dortzbach[5], three had rapid recurrence of symptoms although only one required further surgery. There appears, therefore, to be a direct relationship between the extent of the denervation and the completeness and duration of symptomatic relief.

Different surgical approaches to the facial nerve within the parotid gland have been recommended. Reynolds[20] identified the branches of the nerve at the anterior border of the parotid gland, which allows a greater degree of selectivity in the denervation. However, some branches may be small at this site and difficult to find and, for this reason, Dortzbach[5] identified the nerves as they entered the parotid and dissected forwards within the gland. It is evident that simple division of the nerve is inadequate since nerve regeneration occurs[4, 11, 18] and it is necessary to resect a length of nerve[10, 12, 13], or to tie back the proximal end of the nerve[3, 11]. Reynolds has recently popularized the technique of nerve avulsion in order to remove long filaments of nerve[20, 21].

Dvorak and Nemec[6] described an alternative surgical approach in which the facial area of the non-dominant motor cerebral cortex is undermined. Of 8 patients operated on, 5 have immediate relief of blepharospasm bilaterally without facial palsy, and in 4 the relief was long lasting. No further reports of this operation have appeared in the literature since the initial publication.

RESULTS OF TREATMENT

Bird and McDonald[1] reported the results of facial nerve avulsion in 7 patients. The cases described here include these and a further 15 patients that have had identical surgery in the ensuing interval. They have been followed up for 6 months or more and 18 have been seen for more than 18 months since surgery; 14 were women and 8 men.

The authors' own experience is limited to patients referred for advice concerning facial nerve surgery.

Essential blepharospasm appears to be remarkably resistant to medical therapy. The following, wide variety of drugs have been tried in an attempt to cure or at least reduce the disability:

Amantadine
Benzhexol (trihexyphenidyl)
Carbidopa
Clomipramine
Diazepam
Imipramine
Levodopa
Lorazepam
Orphenadrine
Tetrabenazine
Thiopropazate

Many of the authors' patients had received them without success. Eight had received no medical treatment. Tetrabenazine has been introduced more recently as a drug offering some hope to these individuals, but it rarely causes sufficient reduction in blepharospasm to give significant symptomatic relief, and is not now consistently used by this unit. It has the additional disadvantage of causing significant depression which may be severe, and tetrabenazine is usually used in conjunction with an antidepressant. Seven patients had received tetrabenzine alone or in combination.

Some patients reported psychiatric problems, particularly depression, but in only one did it predate the onset of blepharospasm. Seven had had psychiatric treatment, including electroconvulsive therapy. Psychotherapy has had no reported success, with one exception[15]. At best, medical treatment has caused minor improvement in symptoms, and in none has the condition been cured.

All patients underwent a neurological examination prior to surgery, and all were considered for a trial of medical therapy. The recommendation for surgery was based on an evaluation of the patient's social disability. It was important to obtain an objective assessment of this from the patient's spouse, as some patients were unaware as to whether or not they were visually directed in the home. Where there was doubt the patients were admitted for a period of observation. Essential activities such as driving may be critical for some patients' jobs, and such cases tended to come to surgery early. At the same stage of the disorder, surgery was not recommended for those with less visual demand. At the time of surgery most patients estimated that their eyes were closed for 60–90 per cent of the day.

The operation used was facial denervation with the technique described by Reynolds[20], with little modification. All temporal zygomatic and buccal branches were avulsed; the mandibular branch was identified and its function assessed by electrical stimulation. Any of its branches which caused contraction of the muscles of the upper face were also avulsed.

IMMEDIATE CONSEQUENCES OF SURGERY

All patients except one had complete immediate relief of blepharospasm. In this single instance, denervation was inadequate and required immediate reoperation, with subsequent symptomatic relief. Seventeen patients have remained free of blepharospasm or have had minimal return of symptoms, such as faintly discernible abnormal lid movements which do not interfere with life. Of the patients with otherwise successful results, two had persistent recurrent Bell's phenomenon sufficient to cause severe visual handicap. This abnormality ceased after 3 days in one, but has persisted in the other.

Complete denervation of the orbicularis muscle causes lagophthalmos but, as yet, only one patient has suffered significantly from corneal exposure. She was successfully managed with a soft contact lens in her affected eye. Lower lid ectropion occurred in 12 and required surgical correction in 5. Routine lid shortening techniques have been sufficient in all cases.

Orbicularis oris weakness caused 3 patients to dribble slightly for up to two weeks after surgery when drinking fluids, and 4 had some difficulty in eating or managing their dentures. In only one was this a long-standing problem after the convalescent period. This patient suffered from Parkinson's disease and was severely bradykinetic preoperatively; the reduction of his food intake after surgery increased the absorption of his medication, with consequent aggravation of his bradykinesia.

In 2 patients, parotid secretion into the tissues of the cheek was a transient postoperative problem, causing marked facial swelling. This was managed by repeated aspiration and in both cases the accumulation ceased after 3 weeks without the development of a fistula or dryness of the mouth.

An alteration in facial appearance was an inevitable consequence of denervation. The most notable changes were brow droop, due to loss of frontalis action, and weakness of the elevators of the corner of the mouth, giving rise to a flat, expressionless appearance. This frequently improved after several months, allowing limited facial mobility in some, but recovery of facial expression was never complete. Great care was always taken to explain this drawback of surgery to the patient, and only one has found his altered appearance a significant social handicap. The appearance of the face was symmetrical so that it was cosmetically acceptable after bilateral surgery, and was certainly preferable to the abnormal

Table 17.7.1 Postoperative complications of facial nerve avulsion in 22 patients

Ectropion	12	Brow droop	1
Epiphora	11	Ptosis	1
Difficulty eating	4	Lid swelling	1
Difficulty with dentures	3	Trichiasis	1
Dribbling	3	Corneal exposure	1
Blepharochalasis	2	Facial pain	1
Ectopic parotid secretion	2		

preoperative facial movements. Other complications and their management are listed in *Tables 17.7.1 and 17.7.2*. It should be emphasized that every patient except one was otherwise satisfied with their surgery.

Table 17.7.2 Secondary surgery required after facial nerve avulsion in 22 patients

Ectropion correction	5
Blepharoplasty	2
Brow elevation	1
Tarsorrhaphy	1
Ptosis correction	1
Face lift	1
Clot evuacation	1

All patients are routinely given an artifical tear preparation to be used through the day, and ointment at night. In addition, side-shields are fitted to their glasses if they have them; if not, spectacles are made for them.

RECURRENCE

Symptomatic recurrence is the inevitable risk of recovery of facial mucle function. Return of very little orbicularis power was sufficient to cause eye closure, presumably due to reflex inhibition of the levator palpebrae superioris. Nevertheless, only 4 patients have required a further operation for recurrence, and one has had a total of three procedures. The average time to reoperation in these cases was 14 months. It is notable that patients reported symptoms very soon after their recurrence and frequently demanded reoperation when their visual handicap was significantly less than that prior to their initial surgery.

Before further surgery was undertaken, innervation to the orbicularis from an unexpected source, either on the same or from the opposite side, was excluded. This was achieved by infiltration with local anaesthetic of the subcutaneous tissues over the ramus of the mandible on the affected side. In every case this caused the blepharospasm to cease, indicating the absence of abnormal innervation.

Reoperation was technically more difficult because of the scarring that ensues after surgery. Furthermore, the route of reinnervation is frequently tortuous and small nerves may be difficult to trace.

CONCLUSION

The most impressive features of these patients were the speed of social rehabilitation following surgery and the resolution of any affective disorder. Women unable to cope with their normal responsibilities within the home before surgery returned almost immediately to a full active life. Some had been housebound for more than two years. The two youngest male patients were at work of some kind within a few weeks, and most had returned to their normal employment within three months.

Symptoms may be alleviated temporarily in a few patients by less radical procedures. Nevertheless it is probably justified to attempt total and complete relief of eye closure by surgical means when the patient is severely visually handicapped, such that they are incapable of undertaking activities essential to their life. This is supported by the patients' sensitivity to recurrence. Permanent and total relief of eye closure can only be achieved with any consistency by radical upper facial denervation and it appears that bilateral upper facial weakness is not an unreasonable price to pay in patients who are severely affected by essential blepharospasm.

References

1 BIRD, A. C. and McDONALD, W. I. Essential blepharospasm. *Transactions of the Ophthalmological Society of the UK*, **95**, 250–253 (1975)

2 CALLAHAN, A. Blepharospasm with resection of part of orbicularis nerve supply. *Archives of Ophthalmology*, **70**, 508–511 (1963)

3 CALLAHAN, A. Intractable blepharospasm improvement by differential section of the facial nerve. In *Ophthalmic Plastic Update*, edited by J. Mustarde, L. Jones and A. Callahan, 107–111. Birmingham, Ala., Aesulapius Publishing Co, (1970)

3a COERS, C. and WOOLF, A. L. Pathological anatomy of the intramuscular motor innervation. In *Disorders of Voluntary Muscle*, edited by J. N. Walton, 238–260. London, Churchill Livingstone (1981)

4 COLEMAN, C. C. Surgical treatment of facial spasm. *Annals of Surgery*, **105**, 647–657 (1937)

5 DORTZBACH, R. K. Complications in surgery for blepharospasm. *American Journal of Ophthalmology*, **75**, 142–147 (1973)

6 DVORAK, M. and NEMEC, J. Beitrag zur Neurochirurgischen Therapie des hartnackigen Blepharospasmus. *Ophthalmologica (Basel)* **148**, 130–134 (1964)

7 FISHER, C. M. Reflex blepharospasm. *Neurology (Minneapolis)*, **13**, 77–78 (1963)

8 FRUEH, B. R., CALLAHAN, A., DORTZBACH, R. K., WILKINS, R. B. BEALE, H. L., REITMAN, H. S. and WATSON, F. R. The effects of differential section of the VIIth nerve on patients with intractable blepharospasm. *Transactions of the American Academy of Ophthalmology and Otolaryngology*, **81**, 595–602 (1976)

9 FOX, S. A. Relief of intractable blepharospasm. *American Journal of Ophthalmology*, **34**, 1351–1356 (1951)

10 FRAZIER, C. H. The surgical treatment of blepharospasm. *Annals of Surgery*, **93**, 1121–1125 (1931)

11 GERMAN, W. J. Surgical treatment of spasmodic facial tic. *Surgery*, **11**, 912–914 (1942)

12 GURDJIAN, E. S. and WILLIAMS, H. W. The surgical treatment of intractable cases of blepharospasm. *Journal of the American Medical Association*, (1928)

13 HENDERSON, J. W. Essential blepharospasm. *Transactions of the American Ophthalmological Society*, **54**, 453–520 (1956)
14 IRVINE, A. R., DAROFF, R. B., SANDERS, M. D. and HOYT, W. F. Familial reflex blepharospasm. *American Journal of Ophthalmology*, **65**, 889–890 (1968)
15 LANGWORTHY, O. R. Emotional issues related to certain cases of blepharospasm and facial tics. *Archives of Neurology*, **68**, 620–628 (1952)
16 VAN LINDT, M.A. Blepharospasme queri par injection d'alcool au rebord inferoexterne de l'orbite. *Annales d'Oculistique*, **158**, 463–464 (1921)
17 MARSDEN, C. D. The problem of adult-onset torsion and other isolated dyskinesias in adult life (including blepharospasm, oromandibular dystonia, dystonic writer's cramp, torticollis and axial dystonia). In *Dystonia*, edited by R. Eldridge and S. Fahn. *Advances in Neurology*, **13**, New York, Raven Press (1976)
18 DE MORSIER, G. and MONTANT, R. Le traitement du blepharospasme bilateral par la section des nerfs faciaux. *Revue d'Oto-neuro-ophalmologie*, **18**, 211–213 (1946)
19 PUTTERMAN, A. M. and URIST, M. Treatment of essential blepharospasm with frontalis sling. *Archives of Ophthalmology*, **88**, 278–281 (1973)
20 REYNOLDS, D. H. Differential section of the facial nerve for blepharospasm. In *Neuro-ophthalmology*, edited by J. L. Smith, St. Louis, Mo., C. V. Mosby (1968)
21 REYNOLDS, D. H., SMITH, J. L. S. and WALSH, T. J. Differential section of the facial nerve for blepharospasm. *Transactions of the Americam Academy of Ophthalmology and Otolaryngology*, **71**, 656–664 (1967)
22 SICARD, A. and BLOCH, M. Bi-spasme facial: Alcoolisation des branches de divisiondu nerf facial. *Revue Neurologique*, **20**, 119–121 (1910)
23 URIST, M. J. Bilateral blepharospasm. *Archives of Ophthalmology*, **58**, 520–529 (1957)
24 VALUDE, E. Le blepharospasme tracte par les injections profondes d'alcool au niveau de l'émergence du nerf facial. *Annales d'Oculistiques*, **134**, 436–439 (1905)

17.8
Surgical approach to hemifacial spasm: microvascular decompression
Peter J. Jannetta

Hemifacial spasm is a descriptive term of hyperactive, unilateral, abnormal facial movements presumably caused by an abnormality, usually vascular, at the point where the facial nerve leaves the brainstem before traversing the cerebellopontine angle[3-6]. The symptom complex usually starts in the orbicularis oculi muscle and gradually spreads down over the face, eventually causing platysma muscle involvement, recurrent sustained contractions which close the eye and pull the corner of the mouth over (the 'tonus phenomenon'), and mild but progressive weakness. It is more common in women than men, more common on the left than the right side of the face, and most commonly begins in middle age although the age distribution is the usual Gaussian curve. The patient population is described as follows:

229 patients: 150 females, 79 males
Involved side: 91 right, 137 left, 1 bilateral
Syndrome: 205 classical, 24 atypical
Median decade: 50–60 years of age
Median duration of symptoms: 5 years

No medication is useful in hemifacial spasm. Pulsatile compression by elongating arterial loops, most commonly the posterior inferior cerebellar artery (*Figure 17.8.1*), is most commonly found to be the cause. Tumors, aneurysms and arteriovenous malformations are rare causes of hemifacial spasm. Classical hemifacial spasm, described above, is caused by a blood vessel on the anterior caudal aspect of the facial nerve at the brainstem. 'Atypical' hemifacial spasm, which starts in the buccal muscles and progress rostrally up the face, is caused by a vessel on the rostral-posterior aspect of the nerve. This is harder to visualize and treat[5,6].

Before the application of the binocular dissecting microscope to cranial nerve hyperactive dysfunction problems, hemifacial spasm was said to be 'idiopathic' or 'cryptogenic', although Gardner[1,2] found arteries on the facial nerve in 9 of 16 patients, but he traumatized the nerve for treatment. Scoville[7] found a blood vessel on the facial nerve in one patient. Neither surgeon used the microscope, nor were they able to appreciate the root entry zone–vascular relationships. With the microscope, however, precise clinicopathological relationships have been found in a large series of patients (*Table 17.8.1*). Destructive procedures of various

Figure 17.8.1 Left facial nerve at brainstem through surgical binocular microscope (10 ×) in patient with hemifacial spasm. Exposure via retromastoid craniectomy with patient in lateral position. Self-retaining retractor blade gently holds cerebellum. PICA = posterior inferior cerebellar artery; VII, VIII and IX are cranial nerves

Table 17.8.1 Operative findings in hemifacial spasm, 229 patients (From Jannetta[6], courtesy of the Editor and Publishers, *Annals of Surgery*)

Arterial	Mixed	Venous	Tumor	Aneurysm	Arteriovenous malformation
210	10	4	3	1	1

magnitude have been used with temporary relief of hemifacial spasm, but usually relief has been associated with concurrent weakness and the symptoms tend to recur when facial muscle strength returns. Such therapy – partial section or crush of the facial nerve, alcohol injection or electrocoagulation techniques – was the best, and really the only treatment available for this condition which is economically, socially and psychologically disabling.

Definitive treatment of hemifacial spasm is now available in many centers. The operation, retromastoid craniectomy and microvascular decompression, may be performed safely and effectively by a microneurosurgeon with experience in the surgery of the cerebellopontine angle and preferably who has had the opportunity

Figure 17.8.2 Offending artery subsequently mobilized and held away with a small implant of shredded Teflon felt. VIII is the auditory nerve

Table 17.8.2 Operative results in hemifacial spasm, 229 patients (From Jannetta[6], courtesy of the Editor and Publishers, *Annals of Surgery*)

Operative Results	Number	Percent
No spasm after one operation	201	87.8
No spasm, second procedure necessary	12	5.2
Partially symptomatic (<25% of preoperative level)	11	4.8
Failure of therapy	5	2.2
Total	229	100.0

Table 17.8.3 Postoperative complications in hemifacial spasm, 229 patients

Cranial Nerve	Deficit	Number
Trigeminal	Hypalgesia	1
Facial	Postoperative weakness	9 (6 persist)
	Postoperative late onset weakness	7 (1 persists)
Acoustic	Hearing loss	18
	(deaf)	(8)
	(profound)	(8)
	(mild)	(2)

There complications occurred in 23 patients

to learn the important details of technique at a center where these cases are performed. In the operation, performed with the patient under general endotracheal anesthesia in the contralateral lateral decubitus position, a small (3–4 cm diameter) craniectomy is performed through a vertical retromastoid incision, the cerebellum is elevated minimally over the cranial nerves IX and X, the facial nerve root entry zone is identified, the offending blood vessel or vessels mobilized away from the nerve and held away with a small permanent implant of soft plastic felt (*Figure 17.8.2*). The results of operation in 229 patients followed from 2 to 15 years are collated in *Table 17.8.3*. There have been no operative deaths. The major risk is to hearing in the ipsilateral ear (*Table 17.8.4*). The incidence of ipsilateral deafness has dropped significantly as experience has grown, the operative technique has become more precise and gentle, and the implant materials have been improved.

References

1 GARDNER, W. J. Concerning the mechanism of trigeminal neuralgia and hemifacial spasm. *Journal of Neurosurgery*, **19**, 947–957 (1962)

2 GARDNER, W. J. and SAVA, G. A. Hemifacial spasm: a reversible patho-physiologic state. *Journal of Neurosurgery*, **19**, 240–247 (1962)

3 JANNETTA, P. J. Microsurgical exploration and decompression of the facial nerve in hemifacial spasm. *Current Topics in Surgical Research*, **2**, 217–220 (1970)

4 JANNETTA, P. J. HACKETT, E. R. and RUBY, J. R. Electromyographic and electron microscopic correlates in hemifacial spasm treated by microsurgical relief of neurovascular compression. *Surgical Forum*, **21**, 449–451 (1970)

5 JANNETTA, P. J. ABBASY, M., MAROON, J. C., RAMOS, F. M. and ALBIN, M. S. Etiology and definitive microsurgical treatment of hemifacial spasm: operative techniques and results in 47 patients. *Journal of Neurosurgery*, **47**, 321–328 (1977)

6 JANNETTA, P. J. Neurovascular compression in cranial nerve and systemic disease. *Annals of Surgery*, **192**, 518–525 (1980)

7 SCOVILLE, W. B. Hearing loss following exploration of cerebellopontine angle in treatment of hemifacial spasm. *Journal of Neurosurgery*, **31**, 47–49 (1969)

17.9
Cerebellar and deep brain stimulation in movement disorders

D. L. McLellan

Implantable electrodes suitable for chronic electrical stimulation of the human brain have been developed in the past fifteen years or so. This has encouraged attempts to reproduce the observations of experimental physiologists in patients suffering from neurological disease, notably spasticity, the torsion dystonias, severe tremor of various kinds and epilepsy.

CEREBELLAR STIMULATION: PHYSIOLOGICAL BACKGROUND

Only the principles relevant to human studies will be mentioned here. By the end of the last century, it was known that decerebrate rigidity in the cat could be lessened by the application of electrical stimulation to the surface of the cerebellum[21, 34]. Later, Dow and Moruzzi[14] described complex effects in animals depending upon the type of stimulation applied. Their results were found to depend critically upon the strength, rate and pattern of stimulation, the precise site at which it was applied, and the underlying state of the preparation at the time.

Following the first of the clinical studies described below, the interest of physiologists in cerebellar stimulation has been rekindled and some remarkable new observations have been made[1, 12, 19, 31, 37, 38]. Experiments in the cat and monkey have shown that surface stimulation activates mossy fibres and climbing fibres antidromically. This resulted in the monosynaptic activation of nuclear neurones via collaterals of the cerebellar afferent fibres. In addition, collateral branches of nuclear cells were demonstrated to project as mossy fibres to the cerebellar cortex. When these collaterals were fired antidromically by stimulation of the cerebellar surface, the main axons of the nuclear cells were activated directly. Although inhibitory Purkinje cells are nearer the cerebellar surface, neurons in the cerebellar nuclei are likely thus to be activated rather than inhibited by electrical stimulation of the surface, while other antidromic effects may alter activity in the olivary nucleus, locus coereleus, reticular formation and thalamus[3, 39].

These concepts have received circumstantial support from estimations of neurotransmitter turnover in the CSF of patients treated by chronic cerebellar stimulation. Noradrenaline turnover was increased but the turnover of γ-amino butyric acid, the transmitter used by Purkinje cells, was unexpectedly diminished[36, 44–46].

In monkeys rendered 'spastic' by bilateral ablation of the motor cortex[15], analysis of passive stretch responses has further shown that acute cerebellar stimulation does not simply reduce stretch response excitability. This particular spastic model was characterized by a marked tonic shortening reaction in biceps and triceps muscles with a strong triceps stretch response and a weak biceps stretch response. Cerebellar stimulation a little above the threshold necessary to activate the most superficial cortical elements had no effect. At higher strengths of stimulation, the shortening reactions in biceps and triceps were suppressed; concurrently the stretch response was diminished in triceps but increased in biceps, so that a complex 'dystonic' form of stretch response was converted to a more conventionally 'spastic' type. Higher levels or different frequencies of stimulation could reverse these effects. These changes took place concurrently with stimulation and reverted as soon as it stopped.

Such complex observations sound a clear warning to clinical investigators. Different patterns and strengths of stimulation can have critically different effects. Moreover, the methods used for clinical evaluation of the results of stimulation need to be sophisticated enough to detect complex, subtle and possibly contradictory changes in the patient's condition.

Figure 17.9.1 Diagram of 4- and 8-button electrodes on upper surface of cerebellum indicating the range of locations that have been reported most effective for spasticity. In an individual patient, symmetrical stimulation is used but the precise location of the electrodes on the superior surface does not appear to be critical in clinical studies, in contrast to observations made in experimental animals

CEREBELLAR SURFACE STIMULATION IN MAN: TECHNICAL ASPECTS

Chronic stimulation for human motor disorders was introduced by Cooper *et al.*[7] in 1973. Electrodes were implanted over the superior surface of the cerebellum (*Figure 17.9.1*) and activated from a passive radiofrequency receiver implanted under the skin of the chest wall. A transmitter carried by the patient controlled the amplitude and frequency of the pulses.

The electrode current must be measured at the time of implantation[24], but if there is any subsequenct alteration in electrode impedance or in the efficiency of radiofrequency coupling, the current will change during chronic use. Moreover, if tissue underneath the electrode becomes damaged, the effectiveness of stimulation is likely to alter even if the current remains constant.

CLINICAL STUDIES

Cooper and his colleagues have now published a number of reports, relating to 200 patients with cerebral palsy[6, 8], of whom 124 were analysed in detail[9]. When their stimulation was first switched on no immediate clinical change occurred but within a few hours in some cases, or a few days in most, patients reported a subjective sensation of muscular relaxation. The clinical changes could be delayed for over a month and appeared to accumulate for 6 months. The time course of these changes therefore differed considerably from the immediate physiological effects reported in animals.

The clinical gains described in these series were in subjective stiffness, articulation of speech, spastic postures especially those affecting the trunk and shoulders, athetoid movements and drooling. Improvement in spasticity by one or two out of five clinical grades was recorded in 73 per cent of patients; 61 per cent of patients reported similar improvements in athetosis. Voluntary control of the trunk and proximal segments of the limb improved more than manual or bimanual dexterity. 'Clinically useful improved vision' occurred in 15 per cent of patients, possibly due to improved extraocular muscle fixation. No changes could be detected in scoliosis, tendon reflexes, muscle strength or sphincter control. Other claims included 'increase in mental functioning' characterized by improved alertness, diminished anxiety, improved cognitive function and memory, and more cooperative behaviour[29].

An even larger group of 262 patients has recently been reported, though in less detail, by Davis *et al.*[13]. These studies too are uncontrolled. Davis' collaborators included a paediatrician with many years' experience of assessing patients with cerebral palsy. Different equipment was used and charge density levels were only a tenth of those employed by Cooper, but the pattern of clinical improvement was remarkably similar. The patients included a high proportion of children, some under 5 years old, making the results even harder to assess since children with cerebral palsy treated by conventional means tend to show gains in function if only as a result of maturation.

Table 17.9.1 The seven largest cerebellar stimulation studies showing the different patterns of stimulation that have been used

Reference	No. of patients	Location of electrode	No. of buttons	Orientation	Polarity	Rate (Hz)	Current (mA)	Pulse width (ms)	Charge density (µC/cm²)	On/off cycle for each button during stimulation	Hours of stimulation per 24 h
6, 9	200	A or A + P	8–32 mostly 16	Usually bipolar (coronal)	Constant or alternating	200	Not known ?3–12	0.5	Not known ?4–18	Usually 1 min	12–24
13	262	A	8	Bipolar (saggital) or monopolar	Constant or alternating	150–180	1.0	0.5	0.8	4–7 min	24
20	62	A or A + P	20–32	Bipolar (saggital) or monopolar (various)	Alternating	100	Not stated	0.25	13–16	Not stated	Not stated
27	17(10*)	A + P	8 or 32	Bipolar (saggital)	Alternating	20–30	1.67–13.33	0.5	0.25–10.25	1–20 min Usually 6–8	8–12
17	8*	A	8	Bipolar (saggital)	Alternating	175	Headache level: not known	0.5	?1.25–10.00	7 min	Not stated
42	17(8*)	A or A + P	10–32	6 bipolar (saggital) 2 monopolar (A to P)	Constant	100	Not known	0.25	Not known	Not stated	Not stated

*Controlled studies. A = Anterior; P = posterior

Similar uncontrolled observations have been made in a group of 62 patients by Larson et al.[20] and very marked improvements have been reported in a few cases suffering from severe extensor dystonia and impaired respiratory function[35]. Other case studies describe similar results[42].

Recent experience with chronic stimulation of the dentate nucleus itself, using an implanted wire electrode, has shown clinical effects in a single case that were similar to those reported after successful surface stimulation[33]. When the dentate nucleus was stimulated, this patient showed all the acute neurophysiological responses similar to those produced by stimulation of the cerebellar surface previously reported by Upton and Cooper[40].

In contrast to these optimistic accounts, double-blind studies in small numbers of patients have been unable to show convincing overall clinical change with stimulation, though one or two patients have stood out from the others as seeming to show an effect[17, 27, 43]. The clinical skills required to assess a patient with cerebral palsy are clearly far more highly developed in some clinicians than in others[43], a source of error to which insufficient attention has probably been paid. Unfortunately, two of these double-blind studies are unsatisfactory since the level of stimulation used was not measured (see Table 17.9.1). Penn's series[27] compared the results of a prospective open evaluation with a double-blind evaluation of the effect of discontinuing stimulation. The prospective results were in reasonable accord with the larger series, but very little useful clinical gain could be identified in the double-blind phase.

It is theoretically possible that permanent gains could be conferred by stimulation, so that no deterioration would take place when the current is turned off. However, unplanned equipment failures have occurred, correctly diagnosed by the patients who noted deterioration in their spasticity on the side of the body ipsilateral to the broken electrode. Since most patients feel no direct sensation when the electrodes are activated, this is convincing evidence of a genuine effect. But equipment failures have also been revealed by electrical testing in patients who have had no symptoms of deterioration.

In open studies of such innovative therapy it is impossible to disentangle placebo effects from the results of electrical stimulation itself. Evaluation of subtle changes in cerebral palsy can be extraordinarily difficult[28].

A second difficulty in comparing these reports is that different patterns of stimulation have been used in each study (*Table 17.9.1*). In one recent double-blind study the equipment was 'calibrated' by turning up the dial until headache developed[17]. This suggests that the implications of the physiological work in animals had not been fully digested.

UNWANTED EFFECTS OF STIMULATION

The unwanted effects of stimulation itself appear to be dose-related and infrequent. Headache may occur transiently at the onset of stimulation when the higher range of charge levels (above $5\,\mu C/cm^2$ per phase) are used, presumably because of activation of sensory endings in the tentorium. Only two patients have been reported to show transient abnormalities of motor control as a result of stimulation[20].

Biopsies taken at the time of implantation have suggested that the cerebellum is already abnormal in many of these patients before stimulation begins[41]. Tissue damage from electrical stimulation appears in experimental animals at charge densities of 30 μC/cm^2 per phase[5, 11, 18]. Autopsy studies in patients dying with stimulators *in situ* have shown that the electrodes tend to become coated in a fibrous sheath, especially when stimulation at the higher end of the clinical range has been used. The grooves in the cerebellar surface caused by the mass of the electrode and its lead wires are more likely than stimulation itself to lead histological damage, with the charge levels normally used[20, 30, 41].

The largest clinical series[9, 13] show a risk of approximately 0.5 per cent of death from postoperative haemorrhage. Hydrocephalus requiring shunting developed in 0.5 per cent, 3 per cent need re-exploration of the electrode site, 6–15 per cent require surgery for a broken electrode wire within 3 years, and 16 per cent experience accumulation of CSF (usually temporary) in the subcutaneous receiver pocket. Totally implantable units may need replacing every 2–5 years depending upon the level of stimulation used.

CLINICAL NEUROPHYSIOLOGICAL STUDIES OF CEREBELLAR STIMULATION IN MAN

Somatosensory evoked potentials are reduced by bursts of cerebellar stimulation lasting 1–20 min in most patients with cerebral palsy[2, 20, 40]. Suppression may be followed by rebound excitation, especially when high levels of stimulation are used. It is claimed that the level of stimulation that produces immediate effects is similar to that required for therapeutic effects and that physiological measurements can be relied upon for 'biocalibration'[20, 40]. Clinical benefit does not of course depend upon evoked potential amplitude and usually follows a very different time course; some patients show acute physiological changes and disappointing clinical responses while others with good results show no acute changes[23].

Acute changes in the amplitude of H and V responses have also been reported[40]. The compliance of the ankle joint may increase immediately after stimulation for 5 min with a further increase over chronic stimulation for 3 weeks; in other patients no such change could be detected[26]. Some patients show depression of F responses, reversal of the F response ratio in flexor and extensor muscles, or depression of H responses after 2–5 days of stimulation[16, 25]. These changes are consistent with the animal work and with the trend of clinical results but their relevance to the clinical benefits of chronic stimulation are still uncertain.

THE PRESENT ROLE OF CEREBELLAR STIMULATION FOR CEREBRAL PALSY

This form of therapy is potentially exciting but its introduction has been marred by a serious lack of properly controlled observations. This means that there is no objective body of data against which different investigators can test their own results. Despite treatment of hundreds of patients, the optimum charge levels, frequency levels, patterns of stimulation and electrode configuration have not been established. Since the results of stimulation are likely to depend rather critically upon these factors, it is important to identify them so that patients are not implanted with inappropiate equipment.

The present concensus of opinion among proponents of the technique is that stimulation of the superior or anterior surface of the cerebellum is more effective than stimulation of the posterior or inferior surface. Large electrodes may be more effective than small ones[32]. Bilateral stimulation is more effective than unilateral stimulation and monopolar cathodal stimulation using a distant anode is probably more effective than bipolar stimulation[9, 13]. The precise site of the electrodes in the coronal plane does not obviously alter the results (*see Figure 17.9.1*).

The patients most likely to respond have cerebral palsy, though some good responses have occurred in patients with cerebral infarction or head injury. They have a combination of moderate to severe spasticity and mild to moderate athetosis. Their intelligence and also some capacity for voluntary activation of the limbs should be preserved and they should be well motivated to capitalize on any gains achieved through stimulation. Those who seem likely to derive benefit from a small improvement in spasticity are most likely to achieve a useful functional gain. Small numbers of patients with dystonia, parkinsonian tremor, torticollis and ataxia have been treated, but the results are conflicting and no firm conclusions have yet emerged.

What is one to advise a patient who asks for this form of treatment? A conservative interpretation of the clinical results reported so far would be that fewer than half the patients implanted can expect significant functional improvement as a result of stimulation itself. Davis recently reported that only 84 of 178 patients fitted with a radiofrequency system (as opposed to a totally implantable system) were using it and benefitting from it. In those who do respond, improvements are usually slight or modest. Occasionally a patient is found who enjoys pronounced, even dramatic, improvement but as yet there is no means by which such good responders can be identified preoperatively. Such potential gains have to be balanced against the risks outlined above. The long term results of treatment are unknown and implantation should be attempted only by clinicians who have the technical resources to monitor and service the patient during years of follow-up[24].

CHRONIC ELECTRICAL STIMULATION OF OTHER TARGETS FOR THE TREATMENT OF MOVEMENT DISORDERS

The tremor of parkinsonism can be abolished by a stereotactically placed lesion in the ventrolateral nucleus of the contralateral thalamus. Electrical stimulation in the same site can inhibit the tremor temporarily and this is used by some neurosurgeons to help locate the target.

Another target deep to this region has recently been identified[4]. Its anatomical location is not certain; it may be in the ascending limb of the brachium conjunctivum, or in the internal capsule. Chronic contingent stimulation at this site in two severely ataxic patients with multiple sclerosis successfully abolished their severe intention tremor during a six-month period of follow-up. The effect of stimulation was established within 3 s and disappeared immediately stimulation ceased. This time course is totally different from the time course of the changes seen in spasticity with cerebellar stimulation. In order to minimize the dose of stimulation delivered to the brain, the radiofrequency transmitters were triggered by an EMG monitor over the patient's deltoid muscle. In this way the transmitter could be activated contingently whenever the limb was used.

Chronic stimulation of the nucleus ventralis posterolateralis (VPL) of the thalamus can suppress chronic pain caused by damage to sensory pathways in the region of the thalamus or by peripheral damage such as amputation of a limb. In both these disorders, involuntary movement sometimes occurs in the painful area. The involuntary movements associated with hyperpathia in brain damage resemble chorea or athetosis, while twitching movements or tremors may appear in the stump of an amputated limb – the so-called 'jumping stump'. Both these involuntary movement disorders have been reported to respond to chronic stimulation in VPL[22]. Stimulation there was reported also to have suppressed choreoathetosis in a patient with impaired sensation due to multiple sclerosis. No changes were seen in 12 other patients suffering from action tremor, parkinsonism or other types of dyskinesia not associated with sensory disturbance.

Similar therapeutic results have been obtained by chronic stimulation in the ventrolateral nucleus of the thalamus and internal capsule by Cooper et al.[10] Patients with a variety of conditions including spasticity due to spinal injury, idiopathic progressive ataxia, olivopontocerebellar degeneration, torsion dystonia and torticollis were reported improved. The suppression of intention tremor had a time-course very similar to the effects of subthalmic stimulation described above.

It is too soon to draw firm conclusions from these preliminary reports except to say that chronic electrical stimulation of discrete areas of the nervous system is now possible. This promises to be an exciting field of advancement in the treatment of movement disorders and of other forms of acquired neurological deficit.

References

1 BANTLI, H., BLOEDEL, J. R. and TOLBERT, D. Activation of neurones in the cerebellar nuclei and ascending reticular formation by stimulation of the cerebellar surface. *Journal of Neurosurgery*, **45**, 539–554 (1976)

2 BAROLAT-ROMANA, G. and DAVIS, R. Neurophysiological mechanisms in abnormal reflex activity in cerebral palsy and spinal spasticity. *Journal of Neurology Neurosurgery and Psychiatry*, **43**, 333–342 (1980)

3 BLOEDEL, J. R. and BANTLI, H. A spinal action of the dentate nucleus mediated by descending systems originating in the brain stem. *Brain Research*, **153**, 602–607 (1978)

4 BRICE, J. and McLELLAN, D. L. Suppression of intention tremor by contingent deep-brain stimulation. *Lancet*, **1**, 1221–1222 (1980)

5 BROWN, W. J., BABB, T. L., SOPER, H. V., LIEB, J. P., OTTINO, C. A. and CRANDALL, P. H. Tissue reactions to long-term electrical stimulation of the cerebellum in monkeys. *Journal of Neurosurgery*, **47**, 366–379 (1977)
6 COOPER, I. S., AMIN, I., UPTON, A. R. M., RIKLAN, M., WATKINS, E. S. and McLELLAN, D. L. Safety and efficacy of chronic stimulation. *Neurosurgery*, **1**, 203–205 (1977)
7 COOPER, I. S., CRIGHEL, E. and AMIN, I. Clinical and physiological effects of stimulation of the paleocerebellum in humans. *Journal of the American Geriatric Society*, **21**, 40–43 (1973)
8 COOPER, I. S., RIKLAN, M., AMIN, I., WALTZ, J. M. and CULLINAN, M. A. Chronic cerebellar stimulation in cerebral palsy. *Neurology (Minneapolis)*, **16**, 744–753 (1976)
9 COOPER, I. S., RIKLAN, M., TABADDOR, K., CULLINAN, T., AMIN, I. and WATKINS, E. S. A long-term follow-up of chronic cerebellar stimulation for cerebral palsy. In *Cerebellar Stimulation in Man*, edited by I. S. Cooper, 59–99. New York, Raven Press (1978)
10 COOPER, I. S., UPTON, A. R. M. and AMIN, A. Reversibility of chronic neurological deficits. Some effects of electrical stimulation of the thalamus and internal capsule in man. *Applied Neurophysiology* (in press)
11 DAUTH, G. W., DEFENDINI, R., GILMAN, S., TENNYSON, V. and KREMZNER, L. T. Long term surface stimulation of the cerebellum in the monkey. Light microscopic electrophysiologic and clinical observation. *Surgical Neurology*, **7**, 377–384 (1977)
12 DAUTH, G. W., DELL, S. and GILMAN, S. Alteration of Purkinje cell activity from transfolial stimulation of the cerebellum in the cat. *Neurology*, **28**, 265–660 (1978)
13 DAVIS, R., BAROLAT-ROMANA, G. and ENGLE, H. Chronic cerebellar stimulation for cerebral palsy – five year study. *Acta Neurochirurgia*, Suppl. 30, 317–332 (1980)
14 DOW, R. S. and MORUZZI, G. In *The Physiology and Pathology of the Cerebellum*, 103–358. Minneapolis, University of Minnesota Press (1958)
15 EBNER, T. J., VITEKM, J. L., SCHWARTZ, A. B. and BLOEDEL, J. R. Effects of cerebellar stimulation on abnormal proprioceptive reflexes in spastic primates. *Experimental Neurology*, **70**, 721–725 (1980)
16 FISHER, M. A. and PENN, R. D. Evidence for changes in segmental motoneurone pools by chronic cerebellar stimulation and its clinical significance. *Journal of Neurology Neurosurgery and Psychiatry*, **41**, 630–635 (1978)
17 GAHM, N. H., RUSSMAN, B. S., CERCIELLO, R. L., FIORENTINO, M. R. and McGRATHM, D. M. Chronic cerebellar stimulation for cerebral palsy: a double-blind study. *Neurology*, **31**, 87–90 (1981)
18 HAMBRECHT, F. T. Neural prostheses. *Annual Review of Biophysics and Bioengineering*, **8**, 239–67 (1979)
19 HEMMY, D. C., LARSON, S. J., SANCES, A. and MILLAR, E. A. The effect of cerebellar stimulation on focal seizure activity and spasticity in monkeys. *Journal of Neurosurgery*, **46**, 648–653 (1977)
20 LARSON, S. J., SANCES, A., HEMMY, D. C., MILLAR, E. A. and WALSH, P. R. Physiological and histological effects of cerebellar stimulation. *Applied Neurophysiology*, **40**, 160–174 (1977/8)

21 LÖWENTHAL, M. and HORSLEY, V. On the relations between the cerebellar and other centres (namely cerebral and spinal) with special reference to the action of antagonistic muscles. *Proceedings of the Royal Society of London*, **61**, 20–25 (1897)

22 MAZARS, G. MERIENNE, L. and CIOLOCA, C. Control of dyskinesias due to sensory deafferentiation by means of thalamic stimulation. *Acta Neurochirurgia*, Suppl. 30, 239–243 (1980)

23 McLELLAN, D. L., SELWYN, M. and COOPER, I. S. Time course of clinical and physiological effects of stimulation of the cerebellar surface in patients with spasticity. *Journal of Neurology, Neurosurgery and Psychiatry*, **41**, 150–160 (1978)

24 McLELLAN, D. L., WRIGHT, G. D. R. and RENOUF, F. Calibration of clinical cerebellar and deep brain stimulations systems. *Journal Neurology, Neurosurgery and Psychiatry*, **44**, 392–396 (1981)

25 PENN, R. D., ETZEL, M. L. Chronic cerebellar stimulation and developmental reflexes. *Journal of Neurosurgery*, **46**, 506–511 (1977)

26 PENN, R. D., GOTTLIEB, G. L. and AGARWAL, G. C. Cerebellar stimulation in man. Quantitative changes in spasticity. *Journal of Neurosurgery*, **48**, 779–786 (1978)

27 PENN, R. D., MYKLEBUST, B. M., GOTTLIEB, G. L., AGARWAL, G. C. and ETZEL, M. E. Chronic cerebellar stimulation for cerebral palsy: prospective and double-blind studies. *Journal of Neurosurgery*, **53**, 160–165 (1980)

28 RATUSNIK, D. L., WOLFE, V. I., PENN, R. D. and SCHEWITZ, M. S. Effects on speech of chronic cerebellar stimulation in cerebral palsy. *Journal of Neurosurgery*, **48**, 876–882 (1978)

29 RIKLAN, M., HALGIN, L., SHULMAN, M., CULLINAN, T. and COOPER, I. S. Behavioural alterations following acute, shorter term and longer term cerebellar stimulation in humans. In *Cerebellar stimulation in man*, edited by I. S. Cooper, 161–183. New York, Raven Press (1978)

30 ROBERTSON, L. T., DOW, R. S., COOPER, I. S. and LEVY, L. F. Morphological changes associated with chronic cerebellar stimulation in the human. *Journal of Neurosurgery*, **51**, 510–520 (1979)

31 ROBERTSON, L. T. and SMITH, W. L. Physiological and behavioural changes produced by cerebellar stimulation in the monkey. *Journal of Neurosurgery*, **53**, 533–540 (1980)

32 SANCES, A., LARSON, S. J., MYKLEBUST, J., SWIMTEK, T., MILLAR, E. A., CUSICK, J. F., HEMMY, P. C., JODAT, R. and ACKMANN, J. Evaluation of electrode configurations in cerebellar implants. *Applied Neurophysiology*, **40**, 141–159 (1977/78)

33 SCHVARCZ, J. R., SICA, R. E. and MORITA, E. Chronic self-stimulation of the dentate nucleus for the relief of spasticity. *Acta Neurochirurgica.*, Suppl. 30, 351–359 (1980)

34 SHERRINGTON, C. S. Decerebrate rigidity and the reflex coordination of movements. *Journal of Physiology (London)*, **22**, 319–332 (1898)

35 SUKOFF, M. H. and RAGATZ, R. E. Cerebellar stimulation for chronic extensor-flexor rigidity and opisthotonus secondary to hypoxia. *Journal of Neurosurgery*, **53**, 391–396 (1980)

36 TABADDOR, K., WOLFRON, L. I. and SHARPLESS, N. S. Ventricular fluid homovanillic acid and 5-hydroxy-indoleacetic acid concentrations in patients with movement disorders. *Neurology*, **28**, 1249–1253 (1978)

37 TOLBERT, D. L., BANTLI, H. and BLOEDEL, J. R. Anatomical and physiological evidence for a cerebellar nucleo-cortical projection in the cat. *Neuroscience*, **1**, 205–217 (1976)

38 TOLBERT, D. L., BANTLI, H. and BLOEDEL, J. R. The intracerebellar nucleocortical projection in the primate. *Experimental Brain Research*, **30**, 425–434 (1977)

39 TOLBERT, D. L., BANTLI, H. and BLODEL, J. R. Multiple branching of cerebellar efferent projections in cats. *Experimental Brain Research*, **31**, 305–316 (1978)

40 UPTON, A. R. M. and COOPER, I. S. Some neurophysiological effects of cerebellar stimulation in man. *Candian Journal of Neurological Sciences*, **3**, 237–254 (1976)

41 URICH, H., WATKINS, E. S., AMIN, I., COOPER, I. S. Neuropathological observations on cerebellar cortex lesions in patients with epilepsy and motor disorders. In *Cerebellar Stimulation in Man*, edited by I. S. Cooper, 145–159. New York, Raven Press (1978)

42 WINKELMÜLLER, W., SEIDEL, B. U. and DIETZ, H. Über die beeinflussung von bewegungs störungen beider infantilen cerebral parese durch chronische kleinhirn stimulation. *Neurochirurgia*, **20**, 179–185 (1977)

43 WHITTAKER, C. K. Cerebellar stimulation for cerebral palsy. *Journal of Neurosurgery*, **52**, 648–653 (1980)

44 WOOD, J. H., GLAESER, B. S., HARE, T. A., SODE, J., BROOKS, B. R. and VAN BUREN, J. M. Cerebrospinal fluid GABA reductions in seizure patients evoked by cerebellar surface stimulation. *Journal of Neurosurgery*, **47**, 582–589 (1977)

45 WOOD, J. H., LAKE, C. R., ZEIGLER, M. G., SODE, J., BROOKS, B. R. and VAN BUREN, J. M. Cerebrospinal fluid norepinephrine alterations during electrical stimulation of cerebellar and cerebral surfaces in epileptic patents. *Neurology*, **27**, 716–724 (1977)

46 WOOD, J. H., ZIEGLER, M. C., LAKE, C. R., SODE, J. BROOKS, B. R. and VAN BUREN, J. M. Elevations in cerebrospinal fluid norepinephrine during unilateral and bilateral cerebellar stimulation in man. *Neurology*, **1**, 260–264 (1977)

17.10
Surgical approaches to the dyskinesias: afterword

C. D. Marsden and Stanley Fahn

Although the editors rarely advise surgical treatment for their patients with Parkinson's disease today, an occasional patient is seen for whom the technique of stereotaxic thalamotomy as described by Narabayashi (Chapter 17.2) seems ideal. Such patients are young, have severe, disabling, preferably unilateral tremor interfering with their livelihood (for example, the teacher or the actress), and which has not responded to aggressive and prolonged medical therapy. The latter should include not only a levodopa preparation alone, but also combined with an anticholinergic drug. One of the editors (SF) is particularly fond of ethopropazine as being more effective against tremor than other anticholinergic preparations. It is worthwhile noting that some of the synthetic dopamine agonists have been reported to be more active against tremor than against other symptoms of Parkinson's disease. Further development of agents selectively effective against symptoms of the illness may be expected in the future. The editors would never advise more than a unilateral thalamotomy. Bilateral thalamotomies, even in the best of hands, carries about a 20 percent or even greater risk of *severe* speech impairment.

Similar considerations apply to their attitude to stereotaxic thalamotomy for other tremors. In a few patients, the preface 'benign' is a misnomer for their essential tremor. The tremor in such patients may be so severe as to prevent feeding, drinking, and self-care. In this situation, a careful, unilateral thalamotomy by a specialist stereotaxic surgeon active in this work may restore function of one hand and independence. Likewise, very rewarding results may be obtained in young patients with severe posttraumatic tremor or with poststroke tremor. The editors' experience with stereotaxic treatment of tremor in multiple sclerosis has not been favorable. Such patients usually have underlying severe cerebellar deficit, so that even if tremor is alleviated, function is not restored. Furthermore, exacerbations of their disease may be precipitated by surgery. Neither editor refers such patients for operation.

Stereotaxic surgery also has been used to treat torsion dystonia. In general, the results have not been so satisfactory. Bilateral lesions, with their risk to speech, are required for axial dystonia, such as spasmodic torticollis, and only a minority of these patients gain any useful benefit. The editors do not refer patients with spasmodic torticollis for stereotaxis and also are reluctant to refer patients with generalized dystonia. The latter frequently require multiple operations to produce very large lesions to gain any benefit, which increases the risks. Any benefit that does accrue is frequently only temporary; in a matter of months or years, progression of the disease or other unexplained factors lead to relapse, and the patients return to their previous level of disability.

Nevertheless, on occasions, a patient with generalized torsion dystonia may seem so severely incapacitated as to warrant the risks of surgery. However, the consequences of losing speech are so disastrous to such individuals that the editors resist recommending stereotaxis in this situation, particularly since the advent of the promising technique of cervical cord stimulation. It is too early to judge the overall place of this new method, but it carries little or no risk and appears to produce considerable benefit in some patients. Their approach, therefore, is first to explore pharmacotherapy to its limit (*see* Chapter 12); if unsuccessful, they next would recommend cervical cord stimulation; only if this approach also fails, would they consider stereotaxic thalamotomy, and only in patients who are willing fully to take the risk of speech impairment because of intolerable dystonia.

The editors have less reluctance in advising a unilateral stereotaxic thalamotomy for hemiplegic dystonia or focal dystonia affecting the opposite arm or leg. A unilateral lesion has little or no risk of causing a speech disturbance, and carries a less than 1 percent chance of producing hemiplegia in the hands of an experienced stereotaxic surgeon. Unlike axial dystonia, limb dystonia responds more reliably and more dramatically to thalamotomy, which can be recommended to the younger patient with severe disability that does not respond to drugs.

The problem of spasmodic torticollis requires further consideration. The mental anguish that this condition causes often prompts patients to seek a surgical cure. The editors have already stated their view that bilateral thalamotomy has no role in treatment of this condition today. They have no personal experience of the use of unilateral thalamotomy combined with peripheral denervation as described by Bertrand (Chapter 17.5). In general, limited peripheral denervation alone is not satisfactory unless extensive. This means section of all upper cervical motor roots and the accessory nerve at open laminectomy (as described by Maccabe in Chapter 17.4), which is not a minor undertaking. The patient is initially left with a floppy neck after such extensive surgery and, in the long term, there is a very real risk of the development of severe cervical spondylosis. Many such patients develop intractable pain, cervical radiculopathy and myelopathy. In any case, even such extensive denervation frequently does not abolish the torticollis, which is what the patient seeks. At present, the editors would try and dissuade any patient with spasmodic torticollis from this form of surgery, particularly now that the alternative, if still experimental, treatment with cervical cord stimulation is available.

Meige's syndrome, another focal dystonia, also deserves separate consideration. No surgical treatment will help muscle spasms of the mouth, jaw and tongue. However, if the spasms around the eyes occur so frequently, or are so prolonged, as to cause functional blindness, such blepharospasm may be abolished by selective destruction of the upper branches of the facial nerve. In Chapters 17.6 and 17.7 Battista and Bird describe different technical approaches to achieve this aim. The former uses thermolysis after needle exploration under local anesthesia, which may relieve blepharospasm without causing marked facial paresis, but may require multiple operations to cope with recurrence. The latter paralyzes orbicularis oculi and the upper half of the face at open operation under general anesthesia, and appears to have a lesser risk of recurrence.

The surgical approach to the treatment of hemifacial spasm outlined by Jannetta in Chapter 17.8 seems remarkably successful. However, such treatment does require posterior fossa exploration which is not without risks. These must be balanced against the disability caused by the condition, which is essentially cosmetic. Most of the editors' patients decline surgery for this condition.

Finally, in the editors' opinion, brain stimulation as a treatment of abnormal involuntary movements remains entirely experimental and not suitable for routine recommendation to any patient at present.

18.1
Dopamine receptors in movement disorders
Donald B. Calne

THE PROBLEM OF CLASSIFYING DOPAMINE RECEPTORS

Over the last few years the problem of characterizing dopamine receptors has occupied a large amount of space on the pages of journals of pharmacology and neurology. Much of the controversy has arisen as a consequence of different approaches to the study of dopamine receptors, which have been anatomical, biochemical and physiological.

In 1972, Kehr et al[13] stressed the importance of separating presynaptic dopamine receptors, located on the nerve endings or cell bodies of dopaminergic neurons, from postsynaptic receptors, situated on neurons which received synaptic input from dopaminergic cells. In the same year Kebabian et al.[12] reported a close association between a striatal dopamine receptor and an adenylate cyclase; it is important to emphasize that these workers did not claim that adenylate cyclase, the enzyme catalyzing the synthesis of cyclic adenosine monophosphate (AMP), was the recognition molecule (i.e. the receptor) for dopamine, but they did conceive of the cyclase being closely linked to the recognition site so that enhanced formation of cyclic AMP was an early consequence of dopamine occupying the receptor on the cell membrane.

The next important step was a separation of dopamine receptors, proposed by Cools and Van Rossum[4], based upon whether receptor occupation led to excitatory (D_e type) or inhibitory (D_i type) effects on the neuronal membrane.

The controversy rested here for several years, but was reopened following the development of a new series of dopamine agonists derived from ergot. The initial compounds to be studied, bromocriptine and lergotrile, were found to be extremely potent dopaminomimetic agents in such test systems as prolactin suppression and induction of rotation in animals with unilateral nigral lesions[5,6]. However, these compounds failed to stimulate the dopamine-sensitive adenylate cyclase in homogenates of rat striatum[11]; indeed they were shown to possess inhibitory properties in this test of dopaminergic activity. This paradox was resolved by the proposal that dopamine receptors be subdivided according to whether they did or did not stimulate an adenylate cyclase: those which induced formation of cyclic AMP were designated D-1 type (also referred to as DA-1 or β), while those which failed to excite a cyclase were termed D-2 type (also referred to as DA-2 or α)[10,21].

There followed an extensive flurry of publications in which the technique of ligand binding was applied to the task of characterizing the multiple categories of dopamine receptors. Initial reports endorsed the separation of D-1 and D-2 receptor types, and subsequent binding studies identified a third category, designated D-3[26] and more recently a fourth[20]. Later the specificity of the ligands, and the techniques employed for measuring binding, became the subject of heated debate. The wide range of observations, which were often in conflict, resulted in a refutation of all the inferences relating to multiple categories of dopamine receptor, and in the conclusion that since binding studies have failed, under critical scrutiny, to separate different types of dopamine receptor, all previous attempts to establish a subdivision must have been erroneous[14]. This position is clearly insecure from a logical viewpoint and represents an overreaction to the problem.

In this setting, it would seem reasonable to cast aside all evidence deriving from binding studies. Having done so, one is left with the irrefutable fact that there exist certain agonists, such as dopamine, which stimulate receptors of the types designated as D-1 and D-2, while there are others, such as bromocriptine and lergotrile, which stimulate only the D-2 category. We do not have satisfactory selective agonists for the D-1 type, and there is no complete agreement on the relative specificity of antagonists for D-1 and D-2 receptors. The acceptance of the classification of dopamine receptors into D-1 and D-2 types seems the most appropriate compromise between a totally nihilistic approach which ignores these facts and an unbridled enthusiasm which accepts uncritically every report in the extensive and perplexing literature. The D-1/D-2 classification also has the attraction of conformity with the precendent set by subdivisions of other receptor types, such as those for norepinephrine, where the β-receptor is linked to an adenylate cyclase.

In discussing the classification of dopamine receptors it should be stressed that all receptor mechanisms are complex, and that in general what is not known about the process of receptor activation far exceeds what is known. Receptor mechanisms have three tasks to perform: (1) they must selectively recognize minute concentrations of transmitter; (2) they must amplify the biochemical effect of interaction between the transmitter and the recognition molecule; (3) they must transduce the amplified signal into a form which has biological significance for the cell, such as an alteration in membrane polarization. In picking out one or two aspects of these processes which we can characterize, and employing these as criteria for classifying different types of receptor, we are only scratching the suface of knowledge, and the conclusions that are drawn must be regarded as our best guess at a particular time in the evolution of rapidly expanding perspectives. In spite of these reservations, the conceptual framework that is assembled from such an incomplete background can have important practical implications. For all receptor subgroups that have been identified, efforts have been made to treat human disease by developing compounds which can be used to manipulate one receptor type selectively. The

350 Dopamine receptors in movement disorders

examples of propranolol and cimetidine suffice to illustrate how this approach has yielded therapeutic results. No comparable success has yet been achieved in the case of dopamine receptors, but the problem is sufficiently new for the circumstances to be regarded as challenging.

DOPAMINE RECEPTORS AND MOTOR RESPONSES IN ANIMALS

The usual animal screening tests for motor responses to dopaminergic drugs include (1) stereotyped behavior, comprising repetitive sniffing, licking and gnawing; (2) turning in animals, with unilateral experimental lesions placed in the substantia nigra; (3) reversal of the akinetic state induced by reserpine and α-methyl-para-tyrosine; (4) decreased spontaneous electrical activity in single dopaminergic neurons of the substantia nigra. In addition to these tests, which are all performed on rats, there are primate models of movement disorders produced by lesions placed in the brainstem.

Current evidence indicates that both D-1 and D-2 receptors are located at several sites on the neuronal pathways between the substantia nigra and the brainstem[10] (*Figure 18.1.1*). Since the distribution of D-1 and D-2 receptors extends over

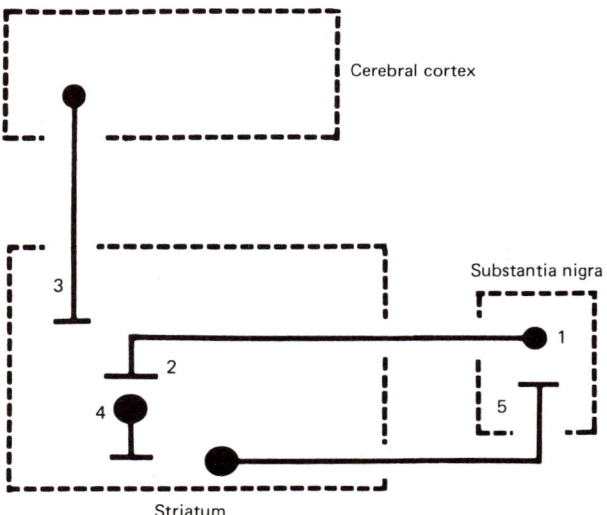

Figure 18.1.1 A schematic representation of the neurons in the nigrostriatal axis which contain dopamine receptors. The dopaminergic neurons contain autoreceptors which regulate either electrical firing of these cells in the substantia nigra (*site 1*) or tyrosine hydroxylase (*site 2*) on the terminals. Cortical neurons which project to the striatum possess binding sites for radiolabelled haloperidol which have been identified as dopamine receptors (*site 3*). Neurons intrinsic to the caudate contain the dopamine-sensitive adenylate cyclase (*site 4*). Finally, terminals of striatal neurons which project to the nigra also contain a dopamine-sensitive adenylate cyclase (*site 5*). The dopamine receptors at sites 1–3 have not been associated with adenylate cyclase activity; only the receptors at sites 4 and 5 regulate this enzyme. (From Kebabian and Calne[10], reprinted by permission from *Nature*, **277**, 93–96. Copyright © 1979 Macmillan Journals Limited)

macroscopically overlapping regions, it is difficult to explore the relative role of the two receptor types by lesioning experiments. An alternative approach is the use of drugs which act selectively on D-1 and D-2 receptors.

Selective D-1 agonists in animals

SK & F 38393 (tetra-hydro-dihydroxy-phenyl-benzazepine) appears to be a relatively selective agonist for D-1 receptors[19]. In the motor tests of dopaminergic function it produces rotation in rats with unilateral nigral lesions but fails to generate stereotyped behavior. It is only weakly effective in reversing the akinetic syndrome induced by reserpine and α-methyl-para-tyrosine. There is no information available on the effects of SK & F 38393 on the firing rate of nigral dopamine cells in the rat. In primates with experimental lesions, SK & F 38393 only ameliorates tremor at very high dosage, and it does not induce choreatic dyskinesia (Goldstein, personal communication). CF 25-397 resembles SK & F 38393 in causing rats with unilateral nigral lesions to turn, without generating stereotyped behavior[17]; however, it does not stimulate striatal adenylate cyclase so it cannot be classified as a D-1 agonist.

Selective D-2 agonists in animals

The most extensively studied D-2 agonists (bromocriptine, lergotrile and lisuride) all display inhibitory properties on D-1 receptors. Two new dopaminergic ergot derivatives, pergolide[15, 28] and CQ 32-084 (Aellig, personal communication), appear to stimulate both D-1 and D-2 receptors. A novel tricyclic ergot derivative, Ly 141865, is a relatively pure D-2 agonist[1], (Kebabian, personal communication).

From surveying the motor responses elicited with D-2 agonists, it becomes evident that taken as a group, these agents seem capable of eliciting all the reactions that have been listed as dopaminergic reactions, including induction of stereotyped behavior. There are some inconsistencies; for example, bromocriptine does not reverse the akinetic syndrome induced by reserpine plus α-methyl-para-tyrosine[9]. However, since the other D-2 ergot agonists are active in this test system, it seems more appropriate to interpret the findings in terms of an unexplained feature of bromocriptine, rather than a general manifestation of D-2 agonism.

D-1 antagonists

There are no specific D-1 antagonists.

D-2 antagonists

Three drugs are available as selective D-2 antagonists; these are sulpiride, molindone and metoclopramide. They block all the dopaminergic motor responses in which they have been tested.

Conclusions from animal studies

These findings indicate that there is quite extensive overlap between the motor responses elicited by D-1 and D-2 agonists. The most notable discriminant appears to be stereotypic behavior in rats, which is readily obtained with D-2, but not D-1, agonists.

DOPAMINE RECEPTORS AND MOTOR RESPONSES IN MAN

Observations on the involvement of dopamine in motor control in man derive from the study of Parkinson's disease and choreatic disorders. Over the last 25 years it has become established that dopamine agonists alleviate parkinsonism and induce chorea, while dopamine antagonists induce parkinsonism and alleviate chorea. In addition to these general statements, it must be admitted that there is a wide range of conflicting anecdotal evidence. Rare dystonic and athetoid patients have been reported to improve following the administration of levodopa[3, 18] and occasionally low doses of dopamine antagonists can help parkinsonian patients. More substantial reports claim that low doses of dopaminergic agents can alleviate chorea. This apparent paradox can be resolved by invoking selective stimulation of autoreceptors on nigrostrial neurons, activation of which leads to reduced release of dopamine onto postsynaptic cells in the striatum[7, 27].

In the following discussion, attention will be focused on the firmly based conclusion that in spite of a few poorly documented exceptions, deprivation of dopamine leads to parkinsonism and excess of dopamine causes chorea.

Selective D-1 agonists in man

There is no experience with selective D-1 agonists in man. It would be of considerable interest to know what, if any, action SK & F 38393 has in patients with extrapyramidal disease. It is of interest that CF 25–397 has no therapeutic activity in Parkinson's disease[23].

Selective D-2 agonists in man

Bromocriptine[25], lisuride[8], lergotrile[24], pergolide[16] and CQ 32-084 (Pakkenberg, personal communication) are all powerful therapeutic agents in Parkinson's disease[8, 16, 25]. The pharmacological profile of these ergot derivatives varies (*see also* Chapter 9), but they all share the property of D-2 agonism. Pergolide and CQ32-084 also stimulate D-1 receptors, but the other drugs are all D-1 antagonists.

The relationship between D-2 agonists and chorea is one of considerable interest. Levodopa, which is converted to dopamine and presumably stimulates both D-1 and D-2 receptors, induces choreic dyskinesia in the majority of parkinsonian patients. In contrast, selective D-2 agonists appear to be much less potent in producing chorea. The largest experience has been obtained with bromocriptine, and this drug only rarely generates choreic dyskinesia in patients who had not previously taken levodopa[22]. It is a curious and unexplained finding that bromocriptine quite frequently causes chorea in patients who had developed this adverse reaction during previous levodopa therapy, but even under these circumstances, the problem of disabling choreic dyskinesia is less common and less severe[2].

Selective D-1 antagonists in man

As already stated, there are no selective D-1 antagonists.

Selective D-2 antagonists in man

Sulpiride, molindone and metaclopramide are all relatively selective D-2 antagonists which induce or exacerbate parkinsonism. They have not been studied in choreic disease.

Conclusions from studies in man

The experience with drugs which act selectively on D-1 or D-2 receptors in man clearly indicates that in Parkinson's disease, a therapeutic response is elicited by stimulation of D-2 receptors. The evidence does not allow any firm conclusion on whether D-1 agonism might be beneficial or deleterious in parkinsonism.

The role of dopamine receptors in chorea is less precisely defined. The fact that choreic dyskinesia is a less severe and frequent problem when using selective D-2 agonists to treat parkinsonism perhaps may be construed as evidence for implicating D-1 agonists in the production of chorea.

GENERAL CONCLUSIONS

From a review of the function of dopaminergic mechanisms in motor control it is evident that some of the tools required for an adequate analysis, such as a D-1 receptor antagonist, are missing. Furthermore, elucidation of function in the basal ganglia is impeded by profound ignorance of the relevant neurophysiology. Nevertheless, the limited body of knowledge that is available is sufficient justification for a few somewhat tentative proposals. (1) Stereotyped behavior in rats appears to be a response mediated through selective stimulation of D-2 receptors. (2) Stereotyped activity seems to be the best animal motor response for testing anti-parkinsonian drugs. (3) While the therapeutic action of dopaminergic drugs in parkinsonism results from D-2 agonism, the possibility of an additional contribution from D-1 agonism cannot be completely excluded. (4) Chorea is more likely to be induced by activation of D-1 receptors; this statement carries the implication that selective D-1 antagonists might prove useful as therapeutic agents for choreatic disorders.

References

1 BACH, N. J., KORNFELD, E. C., JONES, N. D., CHANEY, M. O., DORMAN, D. E., PASCHAL, J. W., CLEMENS, J. A. and SMALSTIG, E. B. Bicyclic and tricyclic ergoline partial structures. Rigid 3-(2-aminoethyl)pyrroles and 3- and 4-(2-aminoethyl)pyrazoles as dopamine agonists. *Journal of Medicinal Chemistry*, **23,** 481–491 (1980)

2 CALNE, D. B., WILLIAMS, A. C., NEOPHYTIDES, A., PLOTKIN, C., NUTT, J. G. and TEYCHENNE, P. F. Long-term treatment of parkinsonism with bromocriptine. *Lancet*, **i,** 735–738 (1978)

3 COLEMAN, M. Preliminary remarks on the L-dopa therapy of dystonia. *Neurology*, **20,** 114 (1970)

4 COOLS, A. R. and VAN ROSSUM, J. M. Excitation-mediating and inhibition-mediating dopamine-receptors: a new concept towards a better understanding of electrophysiological, biochemical, pharmacological, functional and clinical data. *Psychopharmacologia (Berlin)*, **45,** 243–254 (1976)

5 CORRODI, H., FUXE, K., HOKFELT, T., LIDBRINK, P. and UNGERSTEDT, U. Effect of ergot drugs on central catecholamine neurons: evidence for a stimulation of central dopamine neurons. *Journal of Pharmacy and Pharmacology*, **25,** 409–412 (1973)

6 DEL POZO, E. and FLUCKIGER, E. Human prolactin. In *Proceedings of the International Symposium on Human Prolactin* (Brussels, June 12–14, 1973) 292–301. International Congress Series No. 308 (ISBN 90 219 0231 1) Amsterdam, Excerpta Medica (1973)

7 FRATTOLA, L., ALBIZZATIR, M. G. and TRABUCCHI, M. Bromocriptine and Huntington's chorea. *Archives of Neurology*, **35,** 60 (1978)

8 GOPINATHAN, G., TERAVAINEN, H., DAMBROSIA, J. M., WARD, C. D., SANES, J. N., STUART, W. K., EVARTS, E. V. and CALNE, D. B. Lisuride in parkinsonism. *Neurology* **31,** 371–376 (1981)

9 JOHNSON, A. M., LOEW, D. M. and BIOGURET, J. M. Stimulant properties of bromocriptine on central dopamine receptors in comparison to apomorphine, (+)-amphetamine and L-dopa. *British Journal of Pharmacology*, **56,** 59–68 (1976)

10 KEBABIAN, J. W. and CALNE, D. B. Multiple receptors for dopamine. *Nature*, **277,** 93–96 (1979)

11 KEBABIAN, J. W., CALNE, D. B. and KEBABIAN, P. R. Lergotrile mesylate: an in vivo dopamine agonist which blocks dopamine receptors in vitro. *Communications in Psychopharmacology*, **1,** 311–318 (1977)

12 KEBABIAN, J. W., PETZOLD, G. L. and GREENGARD, P. Dopamine-sensitive adenylate cyclase in caudate nucleus of rat brain and its similarity to the dopamine receptor. *Proceedings of the National Academy of Sciences of the United States of America*, **69,** 2145–2149 (1972)

13 KEHR, W., CARLSSON, A., LINDQVIST, M., MAGNUSSON, T. and ATACK, C. Evidence for a receptor-mediated feedback control of striatal tyrosine hydroxylase activity. *Journal of Pharmacy and Pharmacology*, **24,** 744 (1972)

14 LADURON, P. Dopamine receptor: from an in vivo concept towards a molecular characterization. *Trends in Pharmacological Sciences*, **1**, No. 2, 471–474 (1980)
15 LEMBERGER, L. and CRABTREE, R. E. Pharmacologic effects in man of a potent, long-acting dopamine receptor agonist. *Science*, **205**, 1151–1153 (1979)
16 LIEBERMAN, A. N., LEIBOWITZ, M., NEOPHYTIDES, A., KUPERSMITH, M., MEHL, S., KLEINBERG, D., SERBY, M. and GOLDSTEIN, M. Pergolide and lisuride for Parkinson's disease. *Lancet*, **2**, 1129–1130 (1979)
17 LOEW, D. M., VIGOURET, J. M. and JATON, A. L. *Dopaminergic Ergot Derivatives and Motor Functions*, edited by K. Fuxe and D. B. Calne, 129–140. Oxford, Pergamon Press (1979)
18 ROSENTHAL, R. K., McDOWELL, F. H. and COOPER, W. Levodopa therapy in athetoid cerebral palsy. *Neurology*, **22**, 1–11 (1972)
19 SETLER, P. E., SARAU, H. M., ZIRKLE, C. L. and SAUNDERS, H. L. The central effects of a novel dopamine agonist. *European Journal of Pharmacology*, **50**, 419–430 (1978)
20 SOHOLOFF, P., MARTRES, M. P. and SCHWARTZ, J. C. Three classes of dopamine receptor (D-1, D-3, D-4) identified by binding studies with ^{3}H-apomorphine and ^{3}H-domperidone. *Naunyn-Schmiedeberg's Archiv für Pharmacologie*, **315**, 89–102 (1980)
21 SPANO, P. F., GOVONI, S. and TRABUCCHI, M. Studies on the pharmacological properties of dopamine receptors in various areas of the central nervous system. *Advances in Biochemical Psychopharmacology*, **19**, 155–165 (1978)
22 STERN, G., LEES, A. and SHAW, K. *Dopaminergic Ergot Derivatives and Motor Functions*, edited by K. Fuxe and D. B. Calne, 337. Oxford, Pergamon Press (1979)
23 TEYCHENNE, P. F., PFEIFFER, R., BERN, S. M. and CALNE, D. B. Experience with a new ergoline (CF 25–397) in parkinsonism. *Neurology*, **27**, 1140–1143 (1977)
24 TEYCHENNE, P. F., PFEIFFER, R. G., BERN, S. M., McINTURFF, D. and CALNE, D. B. Comparison between lergotrile and bromocriptine in parkinsonism. *Annals of Neurology*, **3**, 319–324 (1978)
25 THORNER, M. O., FLUCKIGER, E. W. and CALNE, D. B. *Bromocriptine: A Clinical and Pharmacological Review*, 189. New York, Raven Press (1980)
26 TITELER, M., LIST, S. and SEEMAN, P. High affinity dopamine receptors (D_3) in rat brain. *Communications in Psychopharmacology*, **3**, 411–420 (1979)
27 TOLOSA, E. S. and SPARBER, S. B. Apomorphine in Huntington's chorea: clinical observations and theoretical considerations. *Life Sciences*, **15**, 1371–1380 (1975)
28 WONG, D. T. and REID, L. R. Activation of adenylate cyclase in rat striatum by an ergoline dopamine agonist, pergolide. *Communications in Psychopharmacology* (in press)

18.2
Interpretation of radioactive ligand binding to cerebral dopamine receptors
P. Jenner and C. D. Marsden

Ligand binding techniques utilize the capacity of highly labelled tritiated derivatives of selected drug molecules to interact with specific neuronal receptors in cerebral tissue preparations. The techniques are relatively easy to perform and require little expensive apparatus, so neuroscientists have turned to them to investigate a whole range of problems. As a result, clinicians have been inundated with a plethora of such data from animal experiments designed to illuminate neurological or psychiatric conditions, or from study of human autopsy brain material. However, although these techniques are easy to perform, they can be difficult to interpret. In this brief chapter we will examine the basic terminology of ligand binding experiments and some of the problems of interpretation that can arise, with particular reference to the dopamine systems of the brain (*see also* Yamamura *et al.*[37]).

BASIS OF LIGAND BINDING EXPERIMENTS

Before defining the terminology used in receptor binding studies it is necessary to explain briefly the principles of the experimental system used, *in vitro*, to obtain receptor binding data.

Ligand binding experiments start with the preparation of washed brain homogenates from the area containing the neuronal system of interest. The homogenates then are incubated to equilibrium with a range of concentrations of a radioactive ligand which attaches itself to the tissue. The ligand bound to the tissue preparation is separated from the free ligand using either vacuum filtration or rapid centrifugation. The radioactivity present in the resulting tissue residue is assessed by liquid scintillation counting. The ligands bind not only to specific receptors in the tissue, but also nonspecifically to other tissue components and even to glass or filter paper. Specific binding is measured by using a large concentration of an unlabelled compound acting on the same receptor to displace the ligand. Total binding (without the unlabelled compound) and non-specific binding (with the addition of the unlabelled compound) are measured in parallel. The difference between the two represents the specific binding.

TERMINOLOGY USED IN RECEPTOR BINDING EXPERIMENTS

The ligand: a highly tritiated (greater than 10 Ci/mmol) derivative of a molecule (usually but not always a drug) which has a high affinity for the receptor system under study.

The displacing agent: an unlabelled compound which will displace the radioactive ligand from its binding site.

The binding site: the site on tissue preparations occupied by the ligand. A binding site cannot be presumed to be identical with a receptor until certain criteria have been fulfilled (see later).

Total binding: binding of the ligand to the tissue in all forms irrespective of its pharmacological relevance (*Figure 18.2.1a*).

Non-specific binding: binding of the ligand to sites other than specific receptor sites (*Figure 18.2.1a*).

Specific binding: binding of the ligand to a limited population of sites which (1) can be saturated and (2) can be displaced by other agents known to interact with that receptor, preferably stereospecifically (*Figure 18.2.1a*).

Scatchard analysis: a linear transformation of the saturation curve for specific binding (*Figure 18.2.1b*).

B*max*: the maximum number of specific binding sites present in a tissue preparation assessed from an extrapolation of the Scatchard plot to intercept with its vertical axis (*Figure 18.2.1b*).

K_D: the dissociation constant, which provides an assessment of the affinity of the ligand for the receptor, is obtained from the slope of the Scatchard plot (*Figure 18.2.1b*).

Hill plot: a further linear transformation of specific binding data. A slope of unity signifies normal competitive binding to a single binding site. Slopes differing from unity indicate multiple binding sites or the existence of cooperativity. A slope less than one may signify the occurrence of negative cooperativity; slopes greater than one may signify positive cooperativity (*Figure 18.2.1c*).

Cooperativity: a change in the binding site that results either in an increase (positive cooperativity) or in a decrease (negative cooperativity) in the binding of ligand molecules subsequently interacting with the receptor.

Eadie-Hofstee plot: a further but more sensitive method of treating specific binding data to look for multiple sites or for cooperativity.

IC50 value: the concentration of displacing agent required to be added to cause a 50 per cent displacement of the ligand from its specific binding site.

K*i* *value*: the IC50 value corrected to account for the ligand concentration (C) employed to give the true binding affinity constant of the displacing drug

$$Ki = \frac{IC50}{1 + \frac{C}{K_D}}$$

Figure 18.2.1 Schematic diagrams to illustrate (*a*) saturation of specific binding (*b*) Scatchard analysis of specific binding data, (*c*) Hill plot analysis and (*d*) the definition of specific binding to show spirodecanone sites. T = total binding, NS = non-specific binding, SB = specific binding, F = free ligand concentration, FB = filter binding, SPD = spirodecanone site, SSB = stereoselective binding, SPI = spiperone, S = sulpiride, (+)−B = (+)−butaclamol (active) and (−)−B = (−)−butaclamol (inactive). (*a*) The linear increase in total and non-specific binding of ligand to tissue compared to the saturable specific component defined using an appropriate displacing agent. In (*b*) the saturable component has undergone linear transformation by Scatchard analysis to give the kinetic constants B_{max} and K_D. (*c*) Represents further analysis of specific binding data using a Hill plot to detect multiplicity of binding sites or co-operativity; (*d*) shows the difficulties inherent in the definition of specific binding using ^{3}H-spiperone as an example. Total binding consists of a number of components. Binding to filters is relatively small but note that spiperone itself cannot displace ^{3}H-spiperone from non-specific sites. In addition note that the component defined as specific binding using sulpiride is smaller than that obtained using spiperone. The difference represents the binding of ^{3}H-spiperone to a saturable non-physiological spirodecanone site, from which, it can only be displaced by close structural analogues. Lastly, note also the definition of stereoselective binding by the isomers of butaclamol as the difference between the displacement caused by the active and inactive enantiomers at a minimally effective concentration of the inactive isomer

DEFINITION OF SPECIFIC BINDING

Only specific binding gives an indication of the extent to which a ligand interacts with a receptor (*see also* Seeman[22]). Three major questions must be answered to define specific binding.

How much of the ligand attached to the tissue is linked to specific binding sites?

The total binding obtained is composed of a number of components:

(1) Binding to the filter paper, or even to glass or plastic tubes, used during separation of free from bound ligand.
(2) Non-specific and non-saturable binding, which cannot be displaced by incorporation of a high concentration of displacing agent.
(3) Non-specific but saturable binding, which can be displaced by close chemical analogues of the ligand but not by drugs of other chemical classes.
(4) Specific binding, which is the component displaced by pharmacologically related drugs of all chemical classes.
(5) Stereoselective binding, which is the difference between the binding of the ligand to the tissue in the presence of the pharmacologically active optical isomer of a drug compared to that obtained in the presence of the pharmacologically inactive form.

How much of the ligand specifically bound to the tissue is attached to one receptor?

Some ligands bind specifically to more than one receptor type; for example, ^{3}H-spiperone labels both dopamine and serotonin receptors in the frontal cortex[17]. The specific binding of the ligand to a single receptor type should be displaced by a single neurotransmitter substance, and by agonist and antagonist drugs acting only on the neuronal system.

To which neuronal receptor is the ligand binding specifically?

The identity of the neurotransmitter receptor to which a ligand specifically binds can be established by studies of the capacity of a range of agonist and antagonist drugs to displace it from those sites, and from their anatomical distribution. In such studies, the following criteria have to be met:

(1) There must be competition between the ligand and unlabelled drugs, although where the ligand binds irreversibly this does not apply.
(2) The number of binding sites must be limited.

(3) There should be good agreement between the displacing ability of drugs and their known pharmacological or clinical properties.
(4) Stereoselective displacement of specific binding must occur.
(5) The regional distribution of specific binding sites should correlate with that of the neurotransmitter or its marker substance.
(6) The subcellular distribution of specific binding sites should indicate association with synaptic membranes.

INTERPRETATION OF CHANGES IN SPECIFIC LIGAND BINDING

Using a single ligand concentration

Results obtained using a single ligand concentration should be viewed with scepticism. Such data will be very difficult to interpret because:

(1) an increase or a decrease in specific binding might be due to a change in either Bmax or K_D, depending on the ligand concentration employed;
(2) no change in specific binding at one ligand concentration does not necessarily mean that there is no change in either Bmax or K_D when a range of ligand concentrations is studied.

Scatchard analysis of specific binding obtained over a range of ligand concentrations

Changes in Bmax or K_D may not indicate real differences in receptor numbers or affinity:

(1) An increase in K_D, for example, may be attributed to the presence of competing drug in the tissue, particularly in autopsy material.
(2) A decrease in Bmax may be due to comparison with inappropriate control tissue, since numbers of receptors are known to decrease with age or agonal status.

Poor definition of specific binding

Unless specificity of binding of the ligand is properly defined, the data may be of little functional significance; for example:

(1) a single ligand may label two receptor sites;
(2) a ligand may label a non-specific but saturable binding site of no pharmacological significance, particularly if the unlabelled ligand itself or a close structural analogue is used to define specific binding.

The use of ^{3}H-spiperone to label dopamine receptors illustrates both these points. ^{3}H-Spiperone also labels serotonin receptors, and unlabelled spiperone displaces ^{3}H-spiperone from a physiologically irrelevant spirodecanone site[7] (*Figure 18.2.1d*).

Use of tissue pools

Pooling of tissue from different animals or subjects may be misleading since:

(1) variation between subjects may provide a false average result.
(2) each pool of tissue can only be regarded as a single observation, even though it may be derived from a large number of different individuals.

However, where saturation analysis cannot be achieved from Scatchard plots due to the small amount of tissue available, pooling of tissue is acceptable, although at least duplicate analysis of each tissue pool at each ligand concentration should be carried out.

CHARACTERIZATION OF CEREBRAL DOPAMINE RECEPTORS USING LIGAND BINDING ASSAYS

The previous chapter described the division of dopamine receptors into those linked to adenylate cyclase and those acting independently of this enzyme, as described originally by Kebabian and Calne[13]. Using this as a starting point, the present authors will describe how *in vitro* ligand binding assays have subsequently been used to advance the hypothesis of the existence of multiple dopamine receptors in brain, taking each of the current hypotheses in turn.

Adenylate cyclase linked and adenylate cyclase independent receptors

This hypothesis, as advanced by Kebabian and Calne[13], recognizes the existence of two classes of dopamine receptors:

(1) dopamine receptors linked to the enzyme adenylate cyclase–D-1;
(2) dopamine receptors acting independently of adenylate cyclase–D-2.

The differentiation of dopamine receptors dependent on their linkage to dopamine-sensitive adenylate cyclase is based on the fact that not all dopamine agonists will stimulate cyclic AMP formation, and not all dopamine antagonists will inhibit dopamine's capacity to stimulate adenylate cylase activity. Thus, some dopamine agonists, particularly ergot derivatives such as bromocriptine[19], not only do not stimulate basal adenylate cyclase activity in tissue preparations from dopamine-containing brain regions, but will inhibit the enhancement of cyclic AMP formation induced by dopamine. On the other hand, while thioxanthene and phenothiazine neuroleptics inhibit dopamine-induced adenylate cyclase activity, with a potency consistent with their known anti-dopamine activity and clinical potency, butyrophenone neuroleptics, such as haloperidol or spiperone, are much weaker antagonists than would be expected[21]. Indeed, substituted benzamide drugs, such as sulpiride and metoclopramide, are inactive in blocking adenylate cyclase activity[12], suggesting that they are selective D-2 antagonists.

The existence of adenylate cyclase linked and adenylate cyclase independent receptors is supported by differential labelling by different dopamine ligands. Thus, ^{3}H-haloperidol and ^{3}H-spiperone can be used to label D-2 receptors in concentrations which are 1000 times lower than those required to inhibit adenylate cyclase activity[9]. Newer ligands, such as ^{3}H-sulpiride[29, 36] and ^{3}H-domperidone[1, 20], can be used to label D-2 receptors even more selectively, for they are inactive in inhibiting adenylate cyclase activity. No selective ligands are available to identify only D-1 receptors, but ^{3}H-cis-flupenthixol and ^{3}H-piflutixol label both D-1 and D-2 receptors with equal affinity[8, 9, 10, 11]. Using the selective D-2 antagonist sulpiride in high concentration to mask D-2 receptors, it is possible to selectively examine D-1 receptors[6]. Indeed, the ability of neuroleptic drugs to inhibit adenylate cyclase activity correlates well with their ability to displace ^{3}H-cis-flupenthixol or ^{3}H-piflutixol from their specific binding site in rat striatal preparations[8, 9, 10, 11].

Adenylate cyclase linked and adenylate cyclase independent dopamine receptors also differ in their subcellular distribution[16] and in their anatomical locations within the striatal complex[24, 31]. Lesioning studies of the striatum have shown that both D-1 and D-2 receptors lie on striatal cell bodies, while D-2 receptors alone lie on the terminals of corticostriate glutamate fibres.

The main criticism of the division of dopamine receptors based on their linkage to adenylate cyclase is that there is no known functional correlate of drug action on D-1 receptors on *neurons in the central nervous system*, although there is a clear involvement of adenylate cyclase in *the synthesis and secretion of many hormones*. Both the behavioural effects in animals and the clinical actions of dopamine agonists and antagonists in man appear to correlate with their activity on D-2 receptors[15, 23]. Adenylate cyclase systems certainly are associated with many hormonal actions, but their role in neuronal function is not established. It may be that the dopamine linked adenylate cyclase system is concerned with long-term changes in neuronal receptor function, perhaps mediating the possible neuromodulator role of this amine.

Agonist and antagonist ligand binding sites

This hypothesis recognizes two dopamine receptors based on their relative affinity for agonist and antagonist compounds[4, 33]:

(1) Agonist binding sites show a high affinity for dopamine agonists but a low affinity for dopamine antagonists. The specific binding of ^{3}H-apomorphine to striatal preparations is displaced by nanomolar concentrations of apomorphine but only by micromolar concentrations of haloperidol.

(2) Antagonist binding sites show a high affinity for dopamine antagonists but a low affinity for dopamine agonists. The specific binding of ^{3}H-haloperidol to striatal preparations is displaced by nanomolar concentrations of haloperidol but only by micromolar amounts of apomorphine.

It was at first thought that agonist and antagonist binding sites represented interconvertible forms of the same dopamine receptor, but this concept has not been substantiated. Subsequently it has been proposed that they are in fact different binding sites, but whether the agonist and antagonist forms are functionally distinct dopamine receptors, or whether they represent different subunits of a single dopamine receptor[4], remains to be resolved.

D-1, D-2α and D-2β, and D-3 receptors

This classification recognizes three classes of dopamine receptors with one further subdivision[2]:

(1) *D-1 receptors* remain those dopamine receptors linked to adenylate cyclase.
  The other two classes of receptors are thought to be independent of adenylate cyclase.
(2) *D-2 receptors* are labelled with high affinity by both dopamine agonist and antagonist ligands but are subdivided according to the alteration of specific binding caused by guanine nucleotides:
  (a) *D-2α*. Interaction of dopamine-active compounds at this site is regulated by guanine nucleotides. The specific binding of ^{3}H-apomorphine to striatal preparations is reduced by the incorporation of guanine nucleotides *in vitro*, as is the ability of apomorphine to displace the specific binding of ^{3}H-haloperidol[5, 38].
  (b) *D-2β*. Interaction of dopamine-active compounds with this site is independent of the action of guanine nucleotides. The specific binding of ^{3}H-haloperidol is not affected by the incorporation of guanine nucleotides into the incubation medium, nor is the ability of haloperidol to displace ^{3}H-apomorphine.
(3) *D-3 receptors* are highly sensitive to the actions of dopamine agonists but are insensitive to dopamine antagonists[34, 35]. Thus, D-3 sites are only labelled by agonist ligands such as ^{3}H-dopamine or ^{3}H-apomorphine, and the specific binding of these ligands is displaced by apomorphine in the nanomolar range but by haloperidol only in micromolar concentrations. These sites are thought to lie mainly on the terminals of nigrostriatal dopaminergic fibres.

The mechanisms by which guanine nucleotides distinguish between D-2 receptor subtypes are unknown[3, 18]. Guanine nucleotides do act to facilitate the coupling of dopamine receptors to adenylate cyclase. However, it is not thought that they act in this manner in the *in vitro* systems used for ligand binding studies. Whether the differentiation of dopamine receptors based on the effect of guanine nucleotides has any physiological significance remains to be determined.

This division of dopamine receptors can be related to the D-1 and D-2 hypothesis of Kebabian and Calne[13], and also to the agonist–antagonist site hypothesis, for it is agonist ligands and drugs which are sensitive to the effects of guanine nucleotides, while antagonist ligands and antagonist compounds are not affected by such manipulation.

D-1, D-2, D-3 and D-4 receptors

This latest hypothesis recognizes four classes of dopamine receptors[22, 25, 26] (*Table 18.2.1*) which are distinguished as follows:

(1) D-1 receptors again are that population linked to adenylate cyclase. Both dopamine and haloperidol only have an effect on this receptor population in micromolar concentrations.

All the other forms of dopamine receptors are thought to be independent of adenylate cyclase:

(2) D-2 receptors are sensitive to low concentrations of both agonist and antagonist compounds. Both dopamine and haloperidol displace ligands from this site in nanomolar concentrations.
(3) D-3 receptors are sensitive to low concentrations of agonist compounds but insensitive to antagonist molecules. Dopamine displaces from D-3 sites in nanomolar concentrations while haloperidol only has an effect in micromolar concentrations.
(4) D-4 receptors are sensitive to low concentrations of antagonist compounds but insensitive to agonist molecules. Haloperidol displaces ligands from this site in nanomolar concentrations, but dopamine is only effective in the micromolar range.

Two versions of this hypothesis exist. The scheme described above is based on the work of Sokoloff *et al.*[25, 26]. In the version devised by Seeman[22] the definition of D-2 and D-4 receptors is reversed.

Table 18.2.1 The relative affinity of D-1, D-2, D-3 and D-4 dopamine ligand binding sites for dopamine and neuroleptics

Receptor site	Relative affinity (nM)			
	Sokoloff *et al.*[26]		Seeman[22]	
	Dopamine	*Haloperidol*	*Dopamine*	*Spiperone*
D-1	–	–	ca 3000	ca 2000
D-2 (D-4)	7	6	ca 15	ca 0.2
D-3	6	32	ca 3	ca 1500
D-4 (D-2)	1830	4	ca 5000	ca 0.3

The terminology proposed by Sokoloff *et al.*[26] is shown. It must be remembered that in the classification of Seeman[22], the D-2 receptors of Sokoloff *et al.* are called D-4 and *vice versa* (in parentheses).

These four different receptor sites also appear to be distinguished by different anatomical locations within the striatal complex[26]. D-1 receptors are, as before, thought to lie on striatal cell bodies, where D-2 receptors also are thought to exist. The majority of D-3 receptors lie on the terminals of the nigrostriatal dopamine fibres. D-4 receptors, on the other hand, mainly reside on the terminals of corticostriate glutamate fibres.

The neuroleptic-sensitive D-2 and D-4 receptors may mediate different dopamine-initiated behaviours[27]. Thus, neuroleptic agents such as sulpiride, which from the binding studies appears to have a greater affinity for D-4 than D-2 receptors, are more effective in preventing apomorphine-induced climbing behaviour than apomorphine-induced stereotypy.

Sodium-dependent and sodium-independent binding sites

This hypothesis recognizes two subcategories of adenylate cyclase independent binding sites:

(1) Sites to which the binding of the ligand or displacement of the ligand is critically dependent on the presence of sodium ions;
(2) Sites where binding or displacement is independent of sodium ions.

This division is based on two fundamental observations:

(1) The specific interaction of ^{3}H-sulpiride with its specific binding site shows an absolute requirement for the presence of sodium ions in the incubation buffer[30]. This effect is specific for sodium since it cannot be replaced by other ions in equimolar concentrations.
(2) The ability to displace the specific binding of ^{3}H-spiperone by sulpiride (and substituted benzamide drugs in general) is decreased by the omission of sodium ions from the incubation buffer[28]. The ability of other classes of neuroleptic drugs to displace the specific binding of ^{3}H-spiperone is unaffected by sodium.

The effect of sodium, which causes an alteration in the number of available ^{3}H-sulpiride binding sites rather than a change in receptor affinity[32], is not fully understood. It is possible that ^{3}H-sulpiride labels a different portion of the dopamine receptor complex to that identified by ^{3}H-spiperone, and that this represents an ionophore site concerned with the passage of ions across neuronal membranes.

CONCLUSIONS

The simplicity and power of ligand binding techniques to identify neurotransmitter receptors in the brain, and in many other tissues, has provided a new method of investigating central nervous system function. Their application to cerebral dopamine receptors has led to a number of conflicting divisions into separate categories.

No doubt future discoveries will clarify these issues, and will resolve present debate as to how many different classes of dopamine receptors exist and what their critical distinguishing features are. No doubt also that these techniques will be applied to many other neurotransmitter systems in the central nervous system to elucidate their functions.

References

1 BAUDRY, M., MATRES, M. P. and SCHWARTZ, J-C. ^{3}H-Domperidone: a selective ligand for dopamine receptors. *Naunyn-Schmiedeberg's Archiv für Pharmacologie*, **308**, 231–237 (1979)

2 CREESE, I. Dopamine receptors: subtypes, localization and regulation. Presented at Third World Congress of Biological Psychiatry (*Stockholm*) (1981)

3 CREESE, I. and SIBLEY, D. R. Radioligand binding studies: evidence for multiple dopamine receptors. *Communications in Psychopharmacology*, **3**, 385–395 (1979)

4 CREESE, I., BURT, D. R. and SNYDER, S. H. Dopamine receptor binding: differentiation of agonist and antagonist states with ^{3}H-dopamine and ^{3}H-haloperidol. *Life Sciences*, **17**, 993–1002 (1975)

5 CREESE, I., USDIN, T. and SNYDER, S. H. Guanine nucleotides distinguish between two dopamine receptors. *Nature*, **278**, 577–578 (1979)

6 FLEMINGER, S., JENNER, P. and MARSDEN, C. D. Differentiation of the binding of ^{3}H-piflutixol to D-1 and D-2 receptors using sulpiride. *British Journal of Pharmacology* (in press)

7 HOWLETT, D. R., MORRIS, H. and NAHORSKI, S. R. Anomalous properties of ^{3}H-spiperone binding sites in various areas of the rat limbic system. *Molecular Pharmacology*, **15**, 506–514 (1979)

8 HYTTEL, J. Effects of neuroleptics on ^{3}H-haloperidol and [^{3}H]*cis*(Z)flupenthixol binding and on adenylate cyclase activity in vitro. *Life Sciences*, **23**, 551–556 (1978)

9 HYTTEL, J. A comparison of the effect of neuroleptic drugs on the binding of ^{3}H-haloperidol and ^{3}H-*cis*(Z)flupenthixol and on adenylate cyclase activity in rat striatal tissue in vitro. *Progress in Neuro-Psychopharmacology*, **3**, 329–335 (1978)

10 HYTTEL, J. Further evidence that ^{3}H-*cis*(Z)flupenthixol binds to the adenylate cyclase-associated dopamine receptor (D-1) in rat corpus striatum. *Psychopharmacology*, **67**, 107–109 (1980)

11 HYTTEL, J. Similarities between the binding of [^{3}H]piflutixol and [^{3}H]flupenthixol to rat striatal dopamine receptors in vitro. *Life Sciences*, **28**, 563–569 (1981)

12 JENNER, P., ELLIOTT, P. N. C., CLOW, A., REAVILL, C. and MARSDEN, C. D. A comparison of in vitro dopamine receptor antagonism produced by substituted benzamide drugs. *Journal of Pharmacy and Pharmacology*, **30**, 46–48 (1978)

13 KEBABIAN, J. W. and CALNE, D. B. Multiple receptors for dopamine. *Nature*, **277**, 93–96 (1979)

14 LEYSEN, J. E. Unitary dopaminergic receptor composed of cooperatively linked agonist and antagonist sub-unit binding sites. *Communications in Psychopharmacology*, **3**, 397–410 (1979)

15 LEYSEN, J. E. Review on neuroleptic receptors: specificity and multiplicity of in vitro binding related to pharmacological activity. *Presented at Second International Meeting on Clinical Pharmacology in Psychiatry* (Tromso) (1980)

16 LEYSEN, J. and LADURON, P. Differential distribution of opiate and neuroleptic receptors and dopamine-sensitive adenylate cyclase in rat brain. *Life Sciences*, **20,** 281–288 (1977)

17 LEYSEN, J. E., NIEMEGEERS, C. J. E., TOLLENAERE, J. P. and LADURON, P. M. Serotonergic component of neuroleptic receptors. *Nature*, **272,** 168–171 (1978)

18 MARCHAIS, D. and BOCKAERT, J. Is there a connection between high affinity ^{3}H-spiperone binding sites and DA-sensitive adenylate cyclase in corpus striatum? *Biochemical Pharmacology*, **29,** 1331–1336 (1980)

19 MARKSTEIN, R., HERRLING, P. L., BURKI, H. R., ASPER, H. and RUCH, W. The effect of bromocriptine on rat striatal adenylate cyclase and rat brain monoamine metabolism. *Journal of Neurochemistry*, **31,** 1163–1172 (1978)

20 MARTRES, M.-P., BAUDRY, M. and SCHWARTZ, J.-C. Characterisation of ^{3}H-domperidone binding on striatal dopamine receptors. *Life Sciences*, **23,** 1781–1784 (1978)

21 SEEMAN, P. Anti-schizophrenic drugs: membrane receptor sites of action. *Biochemical Pharmacology*, **26,** 1741–1748 (1977)

22 SEEMAN, P. Brain dopamine receptors *Pharmacological Reviews*, **32,** 229–313 (1980)

23 SCHACHTER, M., BEDARD, P., DEBONO, A. G., JENNER, P., MARSDEN, C. D., PRICE, P., PARKES, J. D., KEENAN, J., SMITH, B., ROSENTHALER, J., HOROWSKI, R. and DOROW, R. The role of D-1 and D-2 receptors. *Nature*, **286,** 157–159 (1980)

24 SCHWARCZ, R., CREESE, I., COYLE, J. T. and SNYDER, S. H. Dopamine receptors localised on cerebral cortical afferents to rat corpus striatum. *Nature*, **271,** 766–768 (1978)

25 SOKOLOFF, P., MARTRES, M.-P. and SCHWARTZ, J.-C. ^{3}H-apomorphine labels both dopamine postsynaptic receptors and autoreceptors. *Nature*, **288,** 283–286 (1980)

26 SOKOLOFF, P., MATRES, M.-P. and SCHWARTZ, J.-P. Three classes of dopamine receptor (D-2, D-3, D-4) identified by binding studies with ^{3}H-apomorphine and ^{3}H-domperidone. *Naunyn-Schmiedeberg's Archiv für Pharmacologie*, **315,** 89–102 (1980)

27 SOKOLOFF, P., MARTRES, M.-P. and SCHWARTZ, J.-C. Multiple classes of dopaminergic receptors identified by radioligand and behavioural techniques. *Presented at Eighth International Congress of Pharmacology* (Tokyo) (1981)

28 STEFANINI, E., MARCHISIO, A. M., DEVOTO, P., VERNALEONE, F., COLLU, R. and SPANO, P. F. Sodium-dependent interaction of benzamides with dopamine receptors. *Brain Research*, **198,** 229–233 (1980)

29 THEODOROU, A., CROCKETT, M., JENNER, P. and MARSDEN, C. D. Specific binding of ^{3}H-sulpiride to rat striatal preparations. *Journal of Pharmacy and Pharmacology*, **31,** 424–426 (1979)

30 THEODOROU, A., HALL, M. D., JENNER, P. and MARSDEN, C. D. Cation regulation differentiates specific binding of ^{3}H-sulpiride and ^{3}H-spiperone to rat striatal preparations. *Journal of Pharmacy and Pharmacology*, **32,** 441–444 (1980)

31 THEODOROU, A., REAVILL, C., JENNER, P. and MARSDEN, C. D. Kainic acid lesions of striatum and decortication reduce specific [^{3}H]sulpiride binding in rats, so D-2

receptors exist post-synaptically on cortico-striate afferents and striatal neurons. *Journal of Pharmacy and Pharmacology*, **33,** 439–444 (1981)

32 THEODOROU, A., JENNER, P. and MARSDEN, C. D. Sodium ions alter the number of ^{3}H-sulpiride binding sites, not receptor affinity. *Life Sciences* (in press)

33 TITELER, M., WEINREICH, P., SINCLAIR, D. and SEEMAN, P. Multiple receptors for brain dopamine. *Proceedings of the National Academy of Sciences, USA*, **75,** 1153–1156 (1978)

34 TITELER, M., LIST, S. and SEEMAN, P. High affinity dopamine receptors (D3) in rat brain. *Communications in Psychopharmacology*, **3,** 411–420 (1979)

35 TITELER, M., TEDESCO, J. L. and SEEMAN, P. Selective labelling of presynaptic receptors by ^{3}Hdopamine, ^{3}Hapomorphine and [^{3}H]clonidine; labelling of postsynaptic sites by [^{3}H]neuroleptics. *Life Sciences*, **23,** 587–592 (1978)

36 WOODRUFF, G. N. and FREEDMAN, J. B. Binding of ^{3}H-sulpiride to purified rat striatal synaptic membranes. *Neuroscience*, **6,** 407–410 (1981)

37 YAMAMURA, H. I., ENNA, S. J. and KUHAR, M. J. *Neurotransmitter Receptor Binding*. New York, Raven Press (1978)

38 ZAHNISER, N. R. and MOLINOFF, P. B. Effect of guanine nucleotides on striatal dopamine receptors. *Nature*, **275,** 453–455 (1978)

Index

Acetyl choline, 41, 256
   in Parkinson's disease, 51
Action myoclonus, 215
Adenylate cyclase and dopamine receptors, 159, 349, 350, 362–366
Adult-onset focal dystonias, treatment, 195
Age and tardive dyskinesia, 251, 271
Ageing and Parkinson's disease, 9
Agoraphobia in Parkinson's disease, 6
Akinetic rigid syndrome, 2
Alcohol and control of tremor, 192, 193
Alzheimer's disease, 5, 287
   and dementia, 87–90
   Lewy bodies, 30–31, 37
   neurofibrillary tangles, 31–32, 37
Amantadine, 147, 329
   in Huntington's disease, 287
   and neuroleptics in rodents, 273
   in Parkinson's disease, 2, 4, 103, 105, 106
Amino acids, dietary, and levodopa, 105, 132
γ-Aminobutyric acid, *see* GABA
Amobarbital and control of tremor, 192
Amphetamine in rodents, 264–265, 271, 273
Animal models,
   Huntington's disease, 287
   Parkinson's disease, 148
   tardive dyskinesia, 263–267
Anomia in Parkinson's disease, 85
Anoxic encephalopathy, 5
β-Antagonists in tremor, 292
Anticholinergic drugs,
   in dystonia, 194
   in Huntington's disease, 287
   with levodopa, 147
   long duration responses, 103, 106

Anticholinergic drugs (*cont.*)
   and neuroleptic drugs, risks, 271
   in Parkinson's disease, 2, 4
   in tardive dyskinesia, 271
Antidepressant drugs in Huntington's disease, 287
Antipsychotic drugs,
   in dystonia, 194, 195
   in Huntington's disease, 286
   in tics, 193
Apomorphine, 48, 364, 366
   in Parkinson's disease, 151
   in rodents, 264–265, 267, 271–273
^{3}H-Apomorphine, 363, 364
Apomorphine derivatives, tolerance to, 105–106
Arteriosclerotic parkinsonism, 32, 82, 83
Asterixis, 197
Ataxia, cerebellar stimulation in, 340, 341
Atenolol and tremor control, 192
Athetosis, 251
Autonomic failure, *see* Progressive autonomic failure

Baclofen,
   in dystonia, 116, 195
   with levodopa, 147
Baltic myoclonus, 213–214
Barbiturates in myoclonus, 217
Beck depression index, 79, 80, 81
Benign essential tremor, 5
   β-antagonists, 292
   control, 192–193
Benserazide, 3, 147
   and levodopa, 150

Benzhexol, 329
  in Parkinson's disease, 105
Benzodiazepines,
  in dystonia, 194
  in Huntington's disease, 286
  in tics, 193
Biballism, 114, 119
Belpharospasm, 347
  clinical features, 326–327
  nerve thermolysis in, 319–321
  surgery in, 326–332
  treatment, 327–330
β-Blockers and control of tremor, 192
Brain neurotransmitters in Parkinson's disease, 45 (see also Neurotransmitters)
Brain pathology in myoclonus, 216 (see also Pathology)
Brain receptors, 1 (see also Receptors)
Brain surgery, 334 (see also Surgery)
Bromocriptine, 3, 48, 352, 353, 354, 362
  in autonomic failure, 186
  and dopamine receptors, 349, 350
  dyskinesias induced by, 116
  in Parkinson's disease, 1, 103, 105, 106, 109
    clinical studies, 152–154, 160
    compared with lergotrile, 155–156
    compared with lisuride, 158–159
    compared with pergolide, 157–158
  properties, 149, 150
Bucculinguo triad, 249, 250–251
  in animals, 264
Butyrophenones, 43, 46, 363
  in Huntington's disease, 286

Carbamazepine
  in dystonia, 194
  in myoclonus, 217, 219
Carbidopa, 3, 138, 167, 329
  and levodopa, 150
  in myoclonus, 217
Carbidopa–levodopa ratio, 147
Catecholamine receptors and ECT, 82
Catecholaminergic nerve cells, 35–37
Catechol-O-methyltransferase inhibitors
  and levodopa, 147
Cerebellar stimulation,
  background, 334–336
  in cerebral palsy and other disorders, 339–340
  clinical studies, 336–338
  neurophysiological studies, 339
  other targets, 340–341

Cerebellar stimulation (cont.)
  technical aspects, 336
  unwanted effects, 338–339
Cerebral dopamine receptors (see also Dopamine receptors)
  characterisation by ligand binding, 362–366
Cerebral palsy, 336–338, 339–341
Cervical cord stimulation, 347
  complications, 306
  technique, 301–302
  in torsion dystonia, 302–306
Cervical rhizotomy, 309–310, 315
CF 25–397, 352
  In Parkinson's disease, 353
  trials in man, 156
'Cheese effect' and monoamine oxidase inhibitors, 170–171
Children, myoclonus in, 209–210
Chlorpromazine,
  in guinea pigs, 264–265
  in rodents, 268–270, 271
Choline acetyltransferase, 184, 185
  and dementia, 88
  in Parkinson's disease, 50
Cholinergic nerve cells, 35–37
Cholinergic receptors in Parkinson's disease, 63–64, 68
Cholinesterase levels and dementia, 88
Chorea, 251
  and bromocriptine, 354
  distinction from myoclonus, 197
  dopamine receptors, role of, 354–355
  history, 198–199
  and Huntington's disease, 279, 281, 287
  induction by dopamine agonists and antagonists, 353–354
  in Parkinson's disease, 110, 111, 127
Cimetidine, 351
^{3}H-cis-Flupenthixol, 363
Clomipramine, 329
Clonazepam,
  in dystonia, 195
  and levodopa, 147
  in myoclonus, 216, 217
  in tics, 193
Clonidine, 193
Clorgyline and 'cheese effect', 170–171
Clozapine in rodents, 270–271
Cohort hypothesis of Parkinson's disease, 16–17
Community health services and Huntington's disease, 285
Compensated Parkinson's disease and dopamine, 49

Complicated end-of-dose effects in
    Parkinson's disease, 106–109, 132
Convulsive tremor, 202
Cooperativity, 358
Cortical myoclonus (*see also* Myoclonus)
    cortical reflex myoclonus, 225–229
    epilepsia partialis continua, 231
    spontaneous cortical myoclonus, 230–231
Coxsackie B meningoencephalitis, 17
CQ 32-084, 352, 353
Creutzfeld-Jakob disease, 18
    and myoclonus, 230
Crying spells in Parkinson's disease, 76
Cryptogenic myoclonic epilepsy, 210, 230
Cyclase-linked drugs in Parkinson's disease,
    159–160

D-1 Agonists, *see* Dopamine receptors
D-2 Agonists, *see* Dopamine receptors
D-2 Antagonists, *see* Dopamine receptors
Decompensated Parkinson's disease and
    dopamine, 49
Defective viruses and Parkinson's disease,
    19–20
Dementia, 4, 5
    of Huntington's disease, 287
    and Parkinson's disease, 75, 82–91
        characteristics, 84–85
        aetiology, 87
        levodopa, 90
        prevalence, 80, 82–84
        relationship to the disease, 86–87
Denervation,
    for blepharospasm, 327, 330–332
    in torticollis, 309–310, 316
Deprenyl,
    and levodopa, 147
    in Parkinson's disease, 2, 109
(−)Deprenyl,
    'cheese effect', 171
    formula, 169
    and levodopa, clinical trials, 167–168
    and monoamine oxidase, 166, 167
    in Parkinson's disease, 166–171
(+)Deprenyl, 168, 169
Depression in Parkinson's disease, 75–82,
    90–91
    characteristics, 79–81
    prevalence, 76–79
    treatment, 81–82
Desipramine,
    for depression in Parkinson's disease,
        81–82
    in Huntington's disease, 287

Diazepam, 116, 329
    in dystonia, 194
    and levodopa, 147
    in myoclonus, 217
Diet and response to levodopa, 137, 147
Dietary amino acids and levodopa effects,
    105, 132
Dietary protein and levodopa effects, 133
Diphenhydramine, 5
Disability,
    fluctuations in Parkinson's disease, 96, 123
    scales of, 277–278
DNA homology studies in Parkinson's
    disease, 18
Domperidone, 3
^{3}H-Domperidone, 363
Dopa decarboxylase, 45
Dopa decarboxylase inhibitors, 3
Dopamine,
    and dementia, 89
    and dopamine receptors, 365
    and fatigue, 126
    and freezing, 126
    function in the striatum, 41–43
    inhibition of degradation, 166
    levels,
        in the brain, 45
        in multiple system atrophy, 184
        and levodopa response, 102
        in Parkinson's disease, 45, 124–126
        in progressive autonomic failure, 185
    and levodopa efficacy, 102, 146–148
    metabolism, 43
    in Parkinson's disease, 43, 44, 32–33,
        128–134
    in tardive dyskinesia, 255–258
    treatment related fluctuations, 128–134
^{3}H-Dopamine, 364
Dopamine agonists, 351, 353–354, 364
    a comparison, 150
    in Parkinson's disease, 146–160, 353–355
        advantages, 148
        conclusions, 159–160
        ergolines, 152–159
        non-ergolines, 151–152
        rationale, 146–148
        selection, 148–151
Dopamine antagonists, 349, 364, 353–354
    in chorea, 353–355
    in Huntington's disease, 287
    side effects, 249
Dopamine deficiency and parkinsonian
    symptoms, 48–49
Dopamine depletion in treatment of
    Huntington's disease, 286

Dopamine β-hydroxylase in plasma, 184
Dopamine neurones, 42
  changes in Parkinson's disease,
    dopaminergic supersensitivity, 47
    presynaptic changes, 46–47
Dopamine receptors, 46, 48, 53, 360, 362
  adenylate cyclase, 362–363
  agonist and antagonist binding sites, 363–364
  blockers, 46
  blockage in Huntington's disease, 286
  cerebral, see Cerebral dopamine receptors
  classification, 59, 349–351, 362, 367
  D-1 agonists, 351, 353
  D-2 agonists, 352, 353–354
  D-2 antagonists, 352–354
  D-1, D-2α and D-2β and D-3 receptors, 364–365
  D-1, D-2, D-3, D-4 receptors, 365–366
  drugs affecting, 159
  and dyskinesias, 256, 263, 270
  and motor responses in animals, 351
  and neuroleptics binding, 265–266, 270–271
  non-striatal, 139
  and Parkinson's disease, 7, 59–62, 68
    clinical signs, 62
    neuroleptics, 61–62
    patient subgroups, 60
    response fluctuations, 132–133, 134–135, 139
    types, 148
    sodium dependent and independent binding sites, 366
Dopaminergic changes in Parkinson's disease, 46–48, 52–53
Dopaminergic drugs, screening tests, 351
Dopaminergic supersensitivity in animal models, 268
Dopamine synthesis,
  and end-of-dose deterioration, 105, 128
  and Parkinson's disease, 96
Dopamine synthesizing enzymes, 45, 46
DOPS and freezing in Parkinson's disease, 126
Drug holiday, 3–4, 53, 139, 147
  and tardive dyskinesias, 255
Drug-induced dyskinesia, 110–119, 134–141, 249–259, 263
  classification, 135–138, 138–141
  diphasic, 113–116, 134, 140
  early morning dystonia, 116–118, 135, 140–141
  myoclonus, 118, 135
  peak-dose, 110–113, 134, 137

Drug-induced dyskinesias (cont.)
  simultaneous dyskinesias and Parkinson's disease, 140
  Yo-yo-ing, 141
Drug-induced parkinsonism, 5, 9
Drug-induced response in Parkinson's disease,
  drug-resistant 'off' periods, 106, 131–132
  end-of-dose effects, 106–108, 129, 136
  long duration, 103–106, 128
  medium duration, 102, 128
  random oscillations, 109, 132–133
  resistant fluctuation, 109, 134
Drug failure in levodopa therapy, 5–7
Drug-resistant 'off' periods, 106, 132
Drugs in plasma, 103, 105, 129
Dyskinesias, (see also Drug-induced dyskinesias)
  and deprenyl, 167
  differentiation, 197–198
  in Parkinson's disease, 110–119, 134–141
    chorea, 110, 111, 127
    dystonia, 110, 111, 127
  tardive, see Tardive dyskinesias
  treatment by surgery, 291
Dyssynergia cerebellaris myoclonica, 203, 214
Dystonia, 251, 252, 308 (see also Torsion dystonia)
  cerebellar stimulation in, 338, 340, 341
  diagnosis and management, 193–195
  distinction from myoclonus, 197
  in Huntington's disease, 279
  in Parkinson's disease, 110, 112, 114, 116–118, 127
  surgery, 300–307, 338, 340, 341

Early morning dystonia, 116–118
EEG and myoclonus, 210–213, 215, 220–223, 226, 230–231, 233–237
Electric chorea, 196, 200
Electrical stimulation of the brain, 340–341 (see also Cerebellar stimulation)
Electrical stimulation in neurosurgery, 293
  cervical cord stimulation, 300–307
  microelectrodes, 293–294
Electroconvulsive therapy,
  in blepharospasm, 329
  in Huntington's disease, 287
  in Parkinson's disease, 82
Electromyogram in myoclonus, 220–223, 225, 230–231, 233–237
Electron microscopic study of Parkinson's disease, 33

Electrophysiology of myoclonus, 223–238
Emotion and Parkinson's disease symptoms, 99, 127
Encephalitis lethargica, 14
  cohort hypothesis, 16–17
  pathology, 14
  postencephalitic parkinson syndrome, 15, 16
Encephalopathy,
  anoxic, 5
  drug-induced, 252
  myoclonic, 206, 209
Enkephalin receptors, 65, 68
Environmental factors and Parkinson's disease, 13
Epilepsia partialis continua, 212, 224, 231, 232
Epilepsy,
  history, 198–204
  and myoclonus, 210–221, 224
Epileptic myoclonus, 204–206, 210–213, 230
  classification, 209, 224
  clinical features, 208–213
Ergoline derivatives and Parkinson's disease, 1
Ergoline dopamine agonists, 152–160
Ergot, 349, 362
Essential blepharospasm, surgery, 326–332
Essential myoclonus, 201–204, 206, 207–208, 217, 236
  classification, 224
Ethopropazine,
  in dystonia, 194, 195
  and tremor, 346
Extrapyramidal myoclonus, 220–224, 230
Eye movement in Huntington's disease, 280

Facial nerve, 319
  surgery, 327–328, 329–332
Facial paralysis after surgery, 319–320
Familial chorea, 281
Familial paroxysmal dystonic choreoathetosis, 281
Familial progressive myoclonic epilepsy, 212
Familial myoclonic epilepsy, 202–203, 213
Familial myoclonus, 281
Fatigue,
  in myasthenia, 102
  and Parkinson's disease symptoms, 99–102, 127
Fibrillary chorea, 201
Fludrocortisone, 186
Flying saucer syndrome, 211
Focal and segmental myoclonus, 217–220

Freezing,
  effect of surgery, 298
  in Parkinson's disease, 98, 126
Functional capacity in Huntington's disease, 277–278
Fusaric acid and levodopa, 147

GABA binding, 256, 270
GABA-containing nerve cells, 35–37, 41
GABA receptors in Parkinson's disease, 50–51, 64, 68
Gastric emptying and response to levodopa, 137
Gastrointestinal upset and levodopa, 138–139
Genetic counselling in Huntington's disease, 282
Genetic hypothesis of Parkinson's disease, 1, 9–13
  family studies, 10–12
  twin studies, 12–13
Gilles de la Tourette's syndrome, 191
  management of tics, 193
Glutamate-dependent neurotoxicity, 287
Glutamatergic neurotransmission, 288
Glutamic acid decarboxylase, 50, 184
Guanine nucleotides and dopamine receptors, 364

Habit spasm, 202 (see also Tics)
Hallucinations and drug treatment, 186, 192
Haloperidol, 60, 363
  and dopamine receptors, 365
  in dystonia, 194
  and levodopa, 147
  in rodents, 265–267, 270–272
  in tics, 193
^{3}H-Haloperidol, 363, 364
Headache and cerebellar stimulation, 338
Head injury, 5
Hemiballism, 114, 119, 251
Hemifacial spasm, surgery for, 321–325, 348
Hemiparkinsonism, 48
Hereditary ataxias, 281
Heredity and Parkinson's disease, 9–13
Herpes ophthalmicus, 17
Hiccough, 206
Histochemistry of Lewy bodies, 29 (see also Lewy bodies)
Homovanillic acid, 44–46
  in Parkinson's disease, 45
  in progressive autonomic failure, 165
Homovanillic acid: dopamine ratio, 46

Huntington's disease, 34, 191, 198–199, 250
   chronic care, 284–286
   early diagnosis, 279–281
   genetic counselling, 281–284
   HD gene, 279
   pharmacotherapy, 286–288
   treatment, 151
Hydrocephalus, 5
5-Hydroxyindoleacetic acid and myoclonus, 216
5-Hydroxytryptophan, 216, 217, 219
5-Hydroxytryptamine, see Serotonin
Hyperekplexia, 200
Hypertension and monoamine oxidase inhibitors, 170–171
Hyperthermia in surgery for tremor, 296
Hypnic jerks, 206, 208
Hypotension, postural, 177, 185–186
Hysteria and dystonia, 193

Idiopathic orthostatic hypotension, 2, 176, 184, 87
Imipramine, 81–82, 329
Immunohistochemistry in the study of Parkinson's disease, 29, 33–37
Impotence and progressive autonomic failure, 177
Incontinence in Parkinson's disease, 6
Indolamine receptors and ECT, 82
Indomethacin, 186
Infantile myoclonic encephalopathy, 209–210
Infantile spasms, 209, 230
Influenza and encephalitis, 14–15, 18
Insomnia in Parkinson's disease, 76
Intellectual defects in Parkinson's disease, 80, 84–85
Intention tremor, surgery, 298
Iproniazid and 'cheese effect', 170
Isocarboxazid and 'cheese effect', 170
Isoleucine and levodopa, 105
Isaacs' syndrome, 202

Japanese B encephalitis, 17
Joseph's disease, 281
Jumping Frenchman of Maine, 200, 207

Kainic acid in Huntington's disease, 287
Kinesis, paradoxic, 99
Kuru, 18

Lafora body disease and myoclonus, 213
Lagophthalmos, 320
Lance-Adams syndrome, 215–217
Lennox-Gastaut syndrome, 209–210
Lergotrile, 148, 149, 352, 353
   and dopamine receptors, 349, 350
   in Parkinson's disease,
      clinical studies, 154–155, 160
      compared with bromocriptine, 155–156
   properties, 150
Leucine and levodopa, 105
Levodopa, 329, 353
   in autonomic failure, 186
   and deprenyl, 167–168
   and dyskinesias, 110–119, 134
   in dystonia, 194
   in Huntington's disease, 287
   metabolism, 109
   and monoamine oxidase inhibitors, 166
   in myoclonus, 217
   in Parkinson's disease, 2
      dementia, 90
      depression, 81
      effect on dopamine and homovanillic acid, 52
      fatigue, 102
      and disability fluctuations, 96, 123
      freezing, 98
      lack of response, 177
      non-levodopa therapy, 160
      pharmacokinetic problems, 135–136, 138–139
      side-effects, 53
      plasma levels, 129, 131, 132, 133, 134
      and postencephalitic parkinsonism, 15
      response and meals, 137
      sensitivity and dopamine and homovanillic acid, 47
Levodopa: carbidopa,
   and haloperidol in rodents, 273
   ratio, 147
Levodopa therapy,
   accidental withdrawal effects, 3
   cholinergic receptors, 63–64
   cumulative 'on–off' chart technique, 106–108
   dopamine receptors, 61–62
   drug holiday, 3–4
   enkephalin receptors, 66–67
   psychiatric disturbances, 4
   primary drug failure, 5–6
   pyridoxine, 138
   responses,
      end-of-dose effects, 106–108, 132
      long duration response, 103, 128–129

Levodopa therapy (*cont.*)
  responses (*cont.*)
    medium duration response, 102, 128
    'off' periods, 106
    reasons for decline in efficacy, 146–148
    wearing off, 104–106, 129–131
  secondary drug failure, 6
  serotonin receptors, 65
  variations to combat fluctuations, 147–148
Lewy bodies, 25, 26–37, 174, 175, 181
  and Alzheimer's disease, 30
  anatomical distribution, 29–30
  composition and morphology, 26–29
  histochemistry, 29
  polymorphism, 29
  specificity for Parkinson's disease, 30, 87
Lidocaine, 316
Life expectancy in Parkinson's disease, 97
Ligand binding techniques, 350
  conclusions, 361
  definitions of binding, 360–361
  interpretation of changes, 361
  receptor classification and characterization, 362–367
  terminology, 358–359
Limbic forebrain dopamine, 44, 48–49
Lioresal, 116
Lipid storage disease and myoclonus, 213
Lisuride, 48, 149, 352, 353
  in dystonia, 116
  induced dyskinesias, 116
  in Parkinson's disease, 105, 109
    clinical studies, 158, 160
    compared with bromcriptine, 158–159
  properties, 150
Lithium and haloperidol in rodents, 272–273
Locus coerulus, 26, 27, 29
  ultrastructure, 33–35
Lorazepam, 329
Ly 141865, 352

Madopar, 3
Major depressive episodes in Parkinson's disease, 75–76
Manganese and dyskinesia, 268
Manganese parkinsonism, 44, 45
Meige's syndrome,
  surgery, 347–348
  treatment, 195
Memory defects in Parkinson's disease, 85
Mental syndromes in Parkinson's disease, 75, 76–82
Metabolites of levodopa, 137–138

3-Methyldopa, 137–138
  and levodopa, 147
α-Methyl-para-tyrosine, 351, 352
Methylphenidate in rodents, 265, 271
Methysergide, 118
  and levodopa, 147
Metoclopramide, 352, 354, 363
Metoprolol, 192
Microelectrodes in neurosurgery, 293
Microvascular decompression, 323–325
Molindone, 352
Monoamine oxidase inhibitors, 166, 168–171
  in Huntington's disease, 287
  and levodopa, 166
  in postural hypotension, 186
Monitoring levodopa therapy, 106–109, 130, 131, 133, 134
Muscarinic receptors, 63, 68
Muscle jerking, *see* Myoclonus
Muscle system atrophy, 2, 5, 7, 174, 181, 187
Myocardial infarction in Parkinson patients, 3
Myoclonic astatic epilepsy, 230
Myoclonus,
  classification, 204–207, 223–224
  definition, 196–197
  distinction from other dyskinesias, 197–198
  electrophysiological types, 224–233
  epileptic, 208–213, 224
  essential, 207–208, 224
  history, 198–204
  in Huntington's disease, 281
  in Parkinson's disease, 118, 139
  pathophysiology, 220
  symptomatic, 213
  in torticollis, 309

Neostriatum ultrastructure, 33–35
Nerve thermolysis, 319–321
Neurasthenia in Parkinson's disease, 100–102
Neurochemistry of progressive autonomic failure, 183–185
Neurofibrillary tangles, 29–30, 31–32, 37
  in Parkinson's disease, 31–32
Neurofilaments and Lewy bodies, 29 (*see also* Lewy bodies)
Neuroleptic drugs (*see also named drugs*)
  in animals, 268
  effect on dopamine receptors, 61, 63–64, 65, 363
  in Huntington's disease, 280, 286, 287

Neuroleptic drugs (*cont.*)
  indications for use, 258
  and tardive dyskinesias, 249–259, 263–274
Neuromelanin, 25
Neuronal loss and dementia, 88
Neuropathology, (*see also* Pathology)
  of Parkinson's disease, 25–26
  of tardive dyskinesia, 267–268
Neurophysiology of cerebellar stimulation, 339
Neurotoxins, 2, 287
Neurotransmitters, 360
  after cerebellar stimulation, 335
  in basal ganglia, 41–43
  desensitization, 132–133, 139
  in Parkinson's disease, 1
    changes, 41–52
    dysfunction, 50–53
    receptors, 124–126
  replacement therapy in Huntington's disease, 286–287
Nicotine and Parkinson's disease, 13
Nigrostriatal degeneration and tardive dyskinesia, 257
Nigrostriatal fibres, dopamine receptors, 366
Nigrostriatal neurones, 7
  neurotransmission, 286
Nocturnal myoclonus, 204, 208
Non-cyclase linked drugs, 159–160
Non-ergoline dopamine agonists, 151–152, 159–160
Noradrenaline,
  'cheese effect', 170, 171
  in Parkinson's disease, 50, 51–52, 125–126, 350
Normal pressure hydrocephalus, 5
Nortriptyline, 81–82
Nosology of myoclonus, *see* Myoclonus

Oestrogens in myoclonus, 217
Opiate receptors, 65, 66, 67, 68 (*see also* Enkephalin receptors)
  types, 67
Organic affective syndrome, 75, 81
Orofacial dyskinesia, *see* Tardive dyskinesia
Orphenadrine, 329

Palatal myoclonus, 217–219, 238
Pallidotomy for torticollis, 315–317
Paradoxical akinesia, effect of surgery, 298
Paradoxic kinesis in Parkinson's disease, 99, 126

Paralytic ectropion, 320
Paramyoclonus multiplex, 200, 201, 202, 207
Parkinson's disease (*see also named drugs*)
  animal modes, 148
  arteriosclerotic, 32
  brain neurotransmitter changes, (*see also* Dopamine, Neurotransmitters)
    in basal ganglion, 41–43
    clinical relevance, 52–53
    compensatory dopaminergic changes, 46
    dopamine symptomatology, 48–49
    dopamine metabolism, 43
    other neurotransmitter dysfunctions, 50
    striatal dopamine, 49
  brain neurotransmitter receptors (*see also* Dopamine, Receptors *and named receptors*)
    cholinergic, 63–64, 68
    dopamine, 59–62, 68, 353–354
    enkephalin, 65, 68
    GABA, 64–65, 68
    serotonin, 65, 68
  causes, 8
    cohort hypothesis, 16–17
    encephalitis lethargica, 14–20, 31–32
    environmental factors, 13–14, 31
    heredity, 9–13, 31
    seroepidemic surveys, 18–20
    viruses, 13, 18–20, 31
  dementia, 75, 82–91, (*see also* Dementia)
    and levodopa, 90
  depression, 75–82, 90–91
  differential diagnosis, 5
    from striatonigral degeneration, 174–175
  disability fluctuations, 96
    classification, 97
    dyskinesias, 110–119
    pathophysiology, 123
    treatment induced, 102
    variations, 98–102
  drug induced, 5, 9
  drug resistant 'off' periods, 106, 132
  and Huntington's disease, 279, 280, 286, 287 (*see also* Huntington's disease)
  levodopa, 2–7, 15 (*see also* Levodopa)
  life expectancy, 97
  manganese, 44–45
  non-classical, 32
  pathology,
    Alzheimer's disease, 30–31
    Lewy bodies, 25–27, 37
    neurofibrillary tangles, 31–32
    'new' pathology, 32–37
    other forms of Parkinson's disease, 32

Pathology (*cont.*)
  post-encephalic, 15–18, 30–34
  and progressive autonomic failure, 174, 177 (*see also* Progressive autonomic failure)
  sleep benefit, 99–100
  surgery, 294, 298, 346
  symptom pathophysiology, 124–125
  system degeneration, 174
  treatment, 103–106, 146–160
  tremor, 292
    cerebellar stimulation, 294, 340–341
Pathology (*see named diseases*)
Pathophysiology (*see named diseases*)
Perceptual motor impairment in Parkinson's disease, 84
Pergolide, 3, 352, 353
  discovery, 149
  in Parkinson's disease, 105, 109, 156–159, 160
    compared with bromocriptine, 157–158
  properties, 150
Perphenazine,
  in dystonia, 195
  in rats, 268
Peptidergic nerve cells, 35–37
Pharmacokinetics of levodopa, 135–136
  problems, 138–139
Pharmacological tolerance, 105–106
Phenelzine, 'cheese effect', 170
Phenothiazines, 43, 46, 363 (*see also* Neuroleptic drugs)
  in dystonia, 194
  in Huntington's disease, 286
Physiological myoclonus, 204, 206 (*see also* Myoclonus)
^{3}H-Piflutixol, 363
Pimozide, 194–195
  and levodopa, 147
  in tics, 193
Pindolol, 186
Piribidel in Parkinson's disease, 151–152
Platelet receptors, 180
Plasma, chemicals in,
  levodopa, 129–136, 148
  3-O-methyldopa, 138
Postencephalitic Parkinson's disease, 15, 16, 18, 146 (*see also* Parkinson's disease)
  chorea, 110
  dopamine, 44
Posthypoxic myoclonus, 215–217, 225–226, 228, 231, 233, 236 (*see also* Myoclonus)
Postural dizziness, 177, 185–186
Postural tremor, surgery, 298
Presynaptic dopamine, 7, 149

Primate model of dyskinesia, 264
Primidone, 192
Prochlorperazine in rodents 268–270
Progressive autonomic failure,
  classification, 176–177
  diagnosis, 177–178
  neurochemistry, 183–185
  pathology, 181–183
  physiological investigations, 178–179
  survival, 187
  treatment, 186–187
    postural hypotension, 185–186
Progressive familial myoclonus, 213
Progressive myoclonic encephalopathy, 206, 209, 228
Progressive supranuclear palsy, 5
Propranolol, 351
  in dyskinesia, 192
  in postural hypotension, 186
  in tremor, 292
N-propyl-noraporphine in Parkinson's disease, 151
N6-propyl-ergoline, *see* Pergolide
Prostatectomy, 6–7
Prostatic hypertrophy in Parkinson's disease, 6
Psychiatric disturbances and levodopa, 4
Psychotherapy in blepharospasm, 329
Purkinje cells, 213, 214, 334
Pyramidal myoclonus, 220–224, 230
Pyridoxine, 138

Radioactive ligands, *see* Ligand binding tests
Ramsay Hunt syndrome, 206, 214–215
Receptors, (*see also* Dopamine receptors, Neurotransmitters, Parkinson's disease)
  binding assays, *see* Ligand binding techniques
  in the brain, 1
  enkephalin, 65, 68
  indolamine, 82
  norepinephrine, 350
  opiate, 65–67, 68
  and Parkinson's disease 'off' periods, 105, 132
  platelet and lymphocyte, 180
Recombinant DNA analysis, 281
Reflex blepharospasm, 326
Reserpine, 43, 351, 352
  and dyskinesia, 255
  in Huntington's disease, 286
Resistant fluctuators, 109, 134
Response swings in Parkinson's disease, 97, 98–101, 102–119

Restless leg syndrome, 208
Rhizotomy, 302–310, 315
RO 84650 in levodopa resistant Parkinson's disease, 152
Rodent models, 148, 264–271

Saltatoric spasm, 196, 200
Schizophrenics, dyskinesia in, 250, 258
Screening tests for motor responses, 351
Segmental axial dystonia, 302–304
Segmental myoclonus, 203, 220–224, 238
Serological studies in Parkinson's disease, 18
  markers, 8
Serotonin,
  in myoclonus, 216
  in Parkinson's disease, 50–51, 65, 68, 125–126
Serotonin receptors, 65, 68, 360, 362
Sex hormones and tardive dyskinesias, 271
Shock in Parkinson's disease, 99
Shy-Drager syndrome, 2, 176
  definition, 176, 184
  and progressive autonomic failure, 177, 180, 183
  survival, 187
Sibling studies in Parkinson's disease, 11
SK & F 38393, 352, 353
Sleep and Parkinson's disease symptoms, 99, 100, 127
Smoking and Parkinson's disease, 13
Sodium ions and dopamine receptors, 366
Sotalol and tremor control, 192
Spasm, see Hemifacial spasm
Spasmodic torticollis 347 (see also Torticollis)
Spinal myoclonus, 219
Spinocerebellar degeneration and myoclonus, 213
Spiny nerve cells, 34–35
Spiperone, 60, 61, 65, 363
  and dopamine receptors, 365
^{3}H-Spiperone, 360, 362, 363
^{3}H-Spiperone binding, 366
Stereoencephalotomy, 293
Stereoselective binding and displacement, 360, 361
Stereotaxic surgery, 292–293, 310, 311, 315, 316
Stereotaxic thalamotomy, 292, 310, 311
Stress and Parkinson's disease symptoms, 99
Striatal cell bodies, dopamine receptors, 366
Striatal dopamine, 265
  deficiency and Parkinson's disease, 48–49, 53, 127
  and tardive dyskinesia, 255–258

Striatal neurones, chemical types, 41
Striatonigral degeneration, 2, 174
  differentiation from Parkinson's disease, 174–175
Subacute sclerosing panencephalitis, myoclonus in, 236
Subcortical myoclonus,
  reticular reflex myoclonus, 231–236
  spontaneous reticular myoclonus, 236
  others, 236–238
Substantia nigra,
  dopamine receptors, 351
  in Parkinson's disease,
    degeneration, 25, 27, 29, 31, 37
    loss of dopamine cell bodies, 43
  ultrastructure, 33–35
Suicide,
  and levodopa, 81
  in Parkinson's disease, 78, 79
'Suicide' enzyme inhibitors, 168
Sulpiride, 352, 354, 363, 366
^{3}H-Sulpiride, 363, 366
Surgery,
  for blepharospasm, 319–321, 326–332
  in cerebellar palsy, 336–338
  for dyskinesias, 291
  in dystonia, 300–307
  in hemifacial spasm, 322–325, 348
  in torticollis, 309–313, 315–317
Symptomatic myoclonus, 202–203, 205–206
  Baltic myoclonus, 213–214
  Electrophysiological classification, 224
  Ramsay Hunt syndrome, 214–215

Tardive dyskinesia,
  cause, 250
  classification, 252
  heavy metals, 268
  in Huntington's disease, 281, 287
  mechanism, 255–258
  primate models, 263–264
  risk factors, 254–255
  risk factors, animal models, 268–273
  rodent models, 263, 264–267, 268–271
  significance, 258–259
  subgroups, 253
Tay Sachs disease and myoclonus, 213
Tetrabenazine, 329
  and dyskinesia, 255
  in dystonia, 195
  in Huntington's disease, 286
Thalamic surgery, 300, 303, 315
Thalamotomy, 300, 315

Thalamotomy, stereotaxic, (see also
  Stereotaxic thalamotomy)
 in Parkinson's disease, 346
 in torticollis, 347
 in tremor, 346
Thermolysis, 319–321, 348
Thiopropazate, 329
Thioridazine, 5
 in rats, 264, 268–270
 and levodopa, 147
Thioxanthene neuroleptics, 363
 in Huntington's disease, 286
Tics, 251
 distinction from myoclonus, 197, 202
 and Huntington's disease, 279
 treatment and management, 193
Tomography (see also Computer
  tomography)
 in dyskinesias, 257
 in Huntington's disease, 281
 in myoclonus, 212
 in Parkinson's disease, 89
Torsion dystonia, 191, (see also Dystonia)
 stereotaxic surgery, 346–347
 treatment, 302–306, 308
Torticollis (see also Segmental axial
  dystonia)
 cerebellar stimulation, 340, 341
 pallidotomy, 315–317
 surgery, 308–313, 315–317
Tranylcypromine, 166
 'cheese effect', 170
Tremor, (see also Benign essential tremor),
 distinction from myoclonus, 198
 drug resistant, 292
 surgery, 292–296, 297, 346
Tricyclic antidepressants,
 in Huntington's disease, 287

Tricyctic antidepressants (cont.)
 and levodopa, 147
 in Parkinson's disease, 81–82
Trifluoperazine,
 in rats, 264, 266
 in rodents, 268–270
Trihexyphenidyl, 194
Tryptophan and levodopa, 147
Trivastal, see Piribidel
Twin studies in Parkinson's disease, 12–13
Tyramine, 186
Tyrosine hydroxylase, 184, 185
L-tyrosine hydroxylase, 45
Tyrosine-3-monooxygenase, 36

Valine and levodopa effect, 105
Valproate,
 and levodopa, 147
 in myoclonus, 217
Ventricular dilation, 88, 89
Viral antibodies in Parkinson's disease, 18
Viral encephalitis and Parkinson's disease,
  14–18
Viruses and Parkinson's disease, 1, 18–20
Visuospatial impairment in Parkinson's
  disease, 84, 85
Voluntary agencies, role in Huntington's
  disease, 285
Von Economo's encephalitis, 14 (see also
  Encephalitis lethargica)

Walking problems in Parkinson's disease,
  98, 99, 100
Western equine encephalitis, 17
Wilson's disease, 250, 281

Movement Disorders 2

Butterworths International Medical Reviews

Neurology 6

Published titles

1 **Clinical Neurophysiology**
  Erik Stålberg and Robert R. Young

2 **Movement Disorders**
  C. David Marsden and Stanley Fahn

3 **Cerebral Vascular Disease**
  Michael J. G. Harrison and Mark L. Dyken

4 **Peripheral Nerve Disorders**
  Arthur K. Asbury and R. W. Gilliatt

5 **The Epilepsies**
  Roger J. Porter and Paolo L. Morselli

6 **Multiple Sclerosis**
  W. I. McDonald and Donald H. Silberberg

Movement Disorders 2

Edited by

C. David Marsden, FRS, DSc, MSc, MB BS, MRCPsych, FRCP
Professor of Neurology, University Department of Neurology, Kings College Hospital Medical School and Institute of Psychiatry; and Consultant Neurologist, King's College Hospital and Bethlem Royal and Maudsley Hospitals, London, UK

and

Stanley Fahn, MD
N. Houston Merritt Professor of Neurology, Columbia University College of Physicians and Surgeons, Neurological Institute, New York, New York, USA

Butterworths
London   Boston   Durban   Singapore   Sydney   Toronto   Wellington

All rights reserved. No part of this publication may be reproduced or transmitted in any form or by any means, including photocopying and recording, without the written permission of the copyright holder, application for which should be addressed to the Publishers. Such written permission must also be obtained before any part of this publication is stored in a retrieval system of any nature.

This book is sold subject to the Standard Conditions of Sale of Net Books and may not be re-sold in the UK below the net price given by the Publishers in their current price list.

First published, 1987

© **Butterworth & Co. (Publishers) Ltd, 1987**

British Library Cataloguing in Publication Data

Movement disorders 2.—(Butterworths international medical reviews. Neurology, ISSN 0260-0137; 7)
1. Movements disorders
I. Marsden, C. David   II. Fahn, Stanley
616.7′4   RC385

ISBN 0-407-02299-6

Photoset by Butterworths Litho Preparation Department
Printed and bound in England by Robert Hartnoll Ltd, Bodmin, Cornwall

Foreword

For almost a quarter of a century (1951–1975), subjects of topical interest were written about in the periodic volumes of our predecessor, *Modern Trends in Neurology*. Although both that series and its highly regarded editor, Dr Denis Williams, are now retired, the legacy continues in the present Butterworths series in Neurology. As was the case with *Modern Trends*, the current volumes are intended for use by physicians who grapple with the problems of neurological disorder on a daily basis, be they neurologists, neurologists in training, or those in related fields such as neurosurgery, internal medicine, psychiatry, and rehabilitation medicine.

Our purpose is to produce annually a monograph on a topic in clinical neurology in which progress through research has brought about new concepts of patient management. The subject of each monograph is selected by the Series Editors using two criteria: first, that there has been significant advance in knowledge in that area and, second, that such advances have been incorporated into new ways of managing patients with the disorders in question.

This has been the guiding spirit behind each volume, and we expect it to continue. In effect we emphasize research, both in the clinic and in the experimental laboratory, but principally to the extent that it changes our collective attitudes and practices in caring for those who are neurologically afflicted.

C. D. Marsden
A. K. Asbury
Series Editors

Contributors

Yves Agid, MD, PhD
Professor, Laboratoire de Médicine Expérimentale, INSERM U289; and Clinique de Neurologie et Neuropsychologie, CHU Pitié-Salpêtrière, Paris, France

Xandra O. Breakefield, PhD
Director, Department of Molecular Neurogenetics, E. K. Shriver Center, Waltham, Massachusetts; and Associate Professor, Neuroscience Program (Neurology), Harvard Medical School, Boston, Massachusetts, USA

Susan Bressman, MD
Assistant Professor of Clinical Neurology, Dystonia Clinical Research Center and Neurological Institute, Columbia University College of Physicians and Surgeons, New York, USA

Richard G. Brown, BA, MPhil
Research Psychologist, MRC Movement Disorder Research Group, University Department of Neurology and Parkinson's Disease Society Research Centre, Institute of Psychiatry, London, UK

Donald B. Calne, DM, FRCP, FRCPC
Professor of Medicine, Division of Neurology, University of British Columbia, Vancouver, British Columbia, Canada

Roger C. Duvoisin, MD
Professor and Chairman, Department of Neurology, University of Medicine and Dentistry of New Jersey, Robert Wood Johnson Medical School, New Brunswick, New Jersey, USA

Stanley Fahn, MD
H. Houston Merritt Professor of Neurology, Columbia University College of Physicians and Surgeons, Neurological Institute, New York, New York, USA

Leslie J. Findley, MB, ChB, MRCP, DCH
Consultant Neurologist, Regional Centre for Neurology and Neurosurgery, Oldchurch Hospital, Romford, Essex and Queen Elizabeth Military Hospital, Woolwich, London; and Research Neurologist, MRC Neuro-Otology Unit, National Hospital, Queen Square, London, UK

Denis R. Giblin, MD
Associate Professor, Department of Neurology, Albert Einstein College of Medicine, New York, USA

A. E. Harding, MD, MRCP
Senior Lecturer in Neurology, Institute of Neurology, Queen Square and the Royal Postgraduate Medical School, London, UK

Joseph Jankovic, MD
Associate Professor, Department of Neurology, Baylor College of Medicine, Texas Medical Center, Houston, Texas, USA

France Javoy-Agid, PhD
Mâtre de Recherche, Laboratoire de Médecine Expérimentale, INSERM U289, CHU Pitié-Salpêtrière, Paris, France

K. Jellinger, MD
Professor of Neurology and Neuropathology Ludwig-Boltzmann Institute of Clinical Neurobiology, Lainz-Hospital, Vienna, Austria

J. William Langston, MD
Director, Parkinson's Research and Clinical Programs, The Institute for Medical Research and The Santa Clara Valley Medical Center, San Jose, California, USA

Robert G. Lee, MD, FRCP(C)
Professor and Head, Department of Clinical Neurosciences, University of Calgary, Calgary, Alberta, Canada

A. J. Lees, MD, MRCP
Consultant Neurologist, The National Hospitals for Nervous Diseases, Queen Square, London, UK

C. David Marsden, FRS, DSc, MSc, MB BS, MRCPsych, FRCP
Professor of Neurology, University Department of Neurology, King's College Hospital Medical School and Institute of Psychiatry, London, UK

W. R. Wayne Martin, MD, FRCP(C)
Division of Neurology, Department of Medicine, University of British Columbia, Health Sciences Centre Hospital, Vancouver, British Columbia, Canada

Jose A. Obeso, MD
Consultant Neurologist and Head of Movement Disorders Unit, Department of Neurology, Clinica Universitaria, University of Navarra, Pamplona, Spain

Mary M. Robertson, MD, DPM, MRCPsych
Senior Registrar, The Maudsley Hospital, London, UK

John C. Rothwell, PhD
Royal Society Research Fellow, University Department of Neurology, Institute of Psychiatry and King's College Hospital Medical School, London, UK

Merle Ruberg, PhD
Chargée de Recherche Laboratoire de Médecine Expérimentale, INSERM U289, CHU Pitié-Salpêtrière, Paris, France

I. Herbert Scheinberg, MD
Professor of Medicine and Head, Division of Genetic Medicine, Albert Einstein College of Medicine, New York, USA

Bruce S. Schoenberg, MD, DPH, FACP
Chief, Neuroepidemiology Branch, Intramural Research Program, National Institute of Neurological and Communicative Disorders of Stroke, National Institutes of Health, Bethesda, Maryland; and Clinical Professor, Department of Neurology, Georgetown University School of Medicine, Washington DC, USA

Gerald Stern, MD, FRCP
Consultant Neurologist, Faculty of Clinical Sciences, University College, London, UK

Irmin Sternlieb, MD
Professor of Medicine and Associate Director, Liver Research Center, Albert Einstein College of Medicine, New York, USA

Michael R. Trimble, MD, FRCP, FRCPsych
Consultant Physician to the Department of Psychological Medicine, National Hospitals for Nervous Diseases, Queen Square, London; and Senior Lecturer in Behavioural Neurology, Institute of Neurology, Queen Square, London, UK

G. Frederick Wooten, MD
Mary Anderson Harrison Professor of Neurology, Department of Neurology, University of Virginia Medical Center, Charlottesville, Virginia, USA

Contents

Part I Introduction 1

1 General introduction 3
   S. Fahn and C. D. Marsden

2 Imaging techniques and movement disorders 4
   W. R. W. Martin and D. B. Calne
   Colour plates opposite p. 6

3 Epidemiology of movement disorders 17
   B. S. Schoenberg

4 Molecular genetics of movement disorders 33
   X. O. Breakefield and S. Bressman

Part II Parkinson's disease and other akinetic–rigid syndromes 63

5 Problems in Parkinson's disease and other akinetic–rigid syndromes 65
   C. D. Marsden and S. Fahn

6 MPTP: The promise of a new neurotoxin 73
   J. W. Langston

7 Prognosis in Parkinson's disease 91
   G. Stern

8 Neuropsychology and cognitive function in Parkinson's disease: an overview 99
   R. G. Brown and C. D. Marsden

9 The pathology of parkinsonism 124
   K. Jellinger

10 Biochemistry of neurotransmitters in Parkinson's disease   166
    Y. Agid, F. Javoy-Agid and M. Ruberg

11 Pharmacokinetics of levodopa   231
    G. F. Wooten

12 The olivopontocerebellar atrophies   249
    R. C. Duvoisin

    Commentary: Olivopontocerebellar atrophy is not a useful concept   269
    A. E. Harding

13 The Steele–Richardson–Olszewski syndrome (progressive supranuclear palsy)   272
    A. J. Lees

14 Wilson's disease   288
    I. Sternlieb, D. R. Giblin and I. H. Scheinberg

Part III   Dyskinesias   303

15 Problems in the dyskinesias   305
    C. D. Marsden and S. Fahn

16 The anatomical and physiological basis of torsion dystonia   313
    J. C. Rothwell and J. A. Obeso

17 Classification and investigation of dystonia   332
    S. Fahn, C. D. Marsden and D. B. Calne

18 The treatment of dystonia   359
    S. Fahn and C. D. Marsden

19 The neurology of tics   383
    J. Jankovic

20 The psychopathology of tics   406
    M. R. Trimble and M. M. Robertson

21 The pathophysiology of essential tremor   423
    R. G. Lee

22 The pharmacology of essential tremor   438
    L. J. Findley

    Index   459

Part I
Introduction

1
General introduction
S. Fahn and C. D. Marsden

The first volume on Movement Disorders in this series was published in 1982. As we stated then: 'This book is not a textbook on movement disorders and does not encompass all that has been written on the subject in recent years'. We selected topics that appeared to have 'reached a stage that warrants definitive discussion'. So much has happened since then that we believe a second volume is required to review advances that have occurred in the last five years, and to deal with new topics that were not considered previously.

As before, we selected a number of areas for discussion, and invited as authors those with particular expertise on these subjects to present their personal viewpoints. Our editing of all chapters makes us share equally with the authors any responsibility for errors, omissions or misinterpretations.

This volume is introduced by three general chapters on disciplines which have and will contribute greatly to the understanding of movement disorders. Donald Calne and Wayne Martin review imaging techniques in Chapter 2, Bruce Schoenberg surveys epidemiology in Chapter 3, and Xandra Breakefield and Susan Bressman look at molecular genetics in Chapter 4. As before, the remainder of the book is divided into two halves. The first deals with aspects of parkinsonism, the second with various dyskinesias. Each of these halves is prefaced by an introductory chapter in which we discuss our reasons for including the subjects dealt with by the invited authors, and we also give brief reviews of other items which may be of practical interest to the reader. We hope that this book will be of value to neurologists-in-training, and those in research or in practice. We trust that its clinical content will again help in the practical management of patients with movement disorders, while its more scientific sections may aid in understanding of the background to the field.

We wish to thank the publishers for preparing this volume, the authors for sharing our enthusiasm for the need for this second volume and for their timely cooperation, and our wives for their patience and understanding.

2
Imaging techniques and movement disorders
W. R. W. Martin and D. B. Calne

Imaging of the central nervous system is one of the most impressive developments to have taken place in medicine in the last decade. Although the ultimate implications of the newer techniques, magnetic resonance imaging (MRI) and positron emission tomography (PET), are not yet discernible, enough has been achieved in the field of CNS imaging to claim that it represents a step in the evolution of neurology comparable to the developments in electrophysiology 40 years ago and neuropharmacology 20 years ago. X-ray computed tomography (CT) has already revolutionized the practice of neurology. While MRI and PET scanning may not prove to have the same impact on diagnosis, they should play a major role in helping to elucidate the anatomical and functional substrates of many neurological diseases including movement disorders.

In this chapter, initially there is a brief discussion concerning the techniques of CT, MRI and PET. Then the individual categories of movement disorders are reviewed where MRI and PET have proved useful, and speculation is made on what these techniques may have to offer in the future.

METHODS

Computed tomography

X-ray computed tomography has been widely applied to the practice of clinical neurology over the last ten years, and the results are well known. The development and implementation of the technique resulted in the award of the Nobel Prize for Medicine to Drs Godfrey N. Hounsfield and Allan M. Cormack in 1979. The principles are well described in their Nobel lectures (Cormack, 1980; Hounsfield, 1980). The initial equipment has been refined so that high quality pictures can now be obtained and reconstructed in about 20 s/slice; the resolution is approximately 0.5 mm and reasonable distinction between grey and white matter can usually be achieved. The technique measures the attenuation of X-ray beams which are directed through the brain from many angles. From these measurements an image of the brain corresponding primarily to electron density is reconstructed. The main limitations of the technique are the predeliction for artefacts in tissues adjacent to bone, and relative difficulty in discriminating minor differences in tissue density.

Magnetic resonance imaging

This imaging technology has developed rapidly over the last few years. MRI is superior to CT in the depiction of structural detail, especially with regard to differentiation of grey from white matter. It does not involve ionizing radiation, and it permits direct multiplanar imaging independent of patient positioning. The latter capability provides for higher resolution coronal and sagittal imaging. The technique is based on the magnetic properties of hydrogen nuclei, i.e. protons, and their response to externally applied magnetic fields, and the excitation of those nuclei within such a field by a radiofrequency pulse. When the radiofrequency pulse is terminated, the protons lose energy in the form of a radiofrequency signal, the intensity and temporal decay pattern of which is related to the chemical milieu of the protons. The recorded signal is dependent upon the imaging parameters as well as tissue properties such as mobile proton density and relaxation times T_1 and T_2. Further details regarding the theory and methodology of MRI have been well summarized in recent reviews (Norman and Brant-Zawadzki, 1985; Oldendorf, 1985). Although some examples of the application of MRI to the study of movement disorders are included in this chapter, the technique is in its infancy and has not yet achieved widespread use.

Positron emission tomography

This is an imaging technique whereby the concentration of positron-emitting radionuclides may be measured in the living human brain. By combining this technique with the use of appropriately labelled compounds and tracer kinetic models, it is possible to quantify regionally selective biochemical and physiological processes in health and disease. The application of PET to the study of movement disorders has involved two general types of measurements: that of cerebral metabolism and blood flow and, more recently, the measurement of both presynaptic and postsynaptic function in dopaminergic pathways.

The distribution of regional cerebral blood flow (rCBF), regional cerebral oxygen metabolism ($rCMRO_2$) and regional glucose metabolism (rCMRG) is related to neuronal and synaptic functional activity. The major energy expenditure in the brain is for the ion transport mechanisms responsible for pumping sodium and potassium across neuronal membranes in order to maintain the electrochemical gradients necessary for the generation of action potentials (Mata *et al.*, 1980). Because aerobic glucose metabolism is responsible for most of the necessary energy production, the mapping of $rCMRO_2$ or rCMRG provides a functional image of brain metabolic activity.

The most commonly used approach that has been employed for the measurement of rCMRG is based on the 2-[^{14}C]deoxyglucose tissue autoradiographic method (Sokoloff *et al.*, 1977). This depends upon the unique biochemical properties of 2-[^{14}C]deoxyglucose. The bidirectional transport of 2-[^{14}C]deoxyglucose across the blood–brain barrier and its hexokinase-catalysed phosphorylation is similar to that of glucose. However, unlike glucose, the phosphorylated product cannot be metabolized further and is dephosphorylated by glucose-6-phosphatase only very slowly. 2-[^{14}C]Deoxyglucose-6-phosphate is thus trapped within the tissue and its accumulation is directly related to the rate of 2-[^{14}C]deoxyglucose phosphorylation by hexokinase. Sokoloff *et al.* (1977) derived an operational equation expressing glucose utilization per unit mass of tissue in terms of measurable variables. This method has been used extensively in animals for the measurement of rCMRG in both physiological and pathological situations (Sokoloff, 1981).

The original implementation of this method required the direct measurement of tissue radioactivity following 2-[^{14}C]deoxyglucose administration and therefore the method could not be applied to rCMRG studies in man. It became possible to make similar measurements non-invasively, however, with the development of PET. Reivich et al. (1979) demonstrated the use of this model for the measurement of rCMRG in man with PET and the tracer [^{18}F]fluoro-2-deoxyglucose (FDG) which behaves in a similar fashion to 2-[^{14}C]deoxyglucose. The glucose-6-phosphatase catalysing dephosphorylation of FDG was thought to become significant and thus introduce an error at the later scanning times employed with PET measurements, so the original Sokoloff model was expanded (Phelps et al., 1979). This modified version has become the standard model employed for PET measurements of rCMRG in man. A normal FDG image is illustrated in *Plate 1* (opposite p. 6).

Cerebral oxygen extraction is measured with inhaled ^{15}O-labelled oxygen. A steady-state approach employing continuous tracer inhalation has been widely used (Jones, Chesler and Ter-Pogossian, 1976; Subramanyam et al., 1978; Frackowiak et al., 1980). Laboratories using this method also employ a steady-state approach for the measurement of rCBF with inhaled C^{15}O$_2$. More recently an approach has been described and validated (Mintun et al., 1984a) which combines the data obtained from the PET measurement of the cerebral distribution of radioactivity following a bolus administration of H$_2$^{15}O with regional data from a single breath inhalation of ^{15}O$_2$. Laboratories using this method typically employ the autoradiographic method for rCBF measurement with H$_2$^{15}O administered as a bolus (Raichle et al., 1983). With either technique rCMRO$_2$ is calculated from the extraction, rCBF and arterial oxygen content.

The *in vivo* labelling of presynaptic dopaminergic nerve endings has been made possible by the development of 6-[^{18}F]fluoro-L-dopa (6-FD) which behaves as an analogue of L-dopa (Garnett, Firnau and Nahmias, 1983). Fluorodopa is a substrate for aromatic L-amino acid decarboxylase (Firnau et al., 1975) and is thought to be decarboxylated to fluorodopamine within terminals of nigrostriatal neurones to result in accumulation of radioactivity in the striatum. This accumulation of activity has been well demonstrated in both baboon (Garnett et al., 1983) and man (Garnett, Firnau and Nahmias, 1983). One unanswered question is whether the fluorodopamine formed remains trapped within intraneuronal vesicles or is further metabolized to fluorinated analogues of homovanillic acid and dihydroxyphenylacetic acid. A normal 6-FD study is illustrated in *Plate 2* (opposite p. 6).

At present, the interpretation of 6-FD studies is semiquantitative and does not provide precise values for the kinetics of dopa metabolism. Radioactive imaging techniques, whether tissue autoradiography in animals or '*in vivo* autoradiography' in man with PET, are able to quantify the distribution of the radioactive label only. The compounds to which the label is attached cannot be determined from these studies alone. When 6-FD is administered several labelled metabolites are potentially present in the brain analogous to the situation seen with [^{3}H]dopa in animal studies (Horne, Cheng and Wooten, 1984). These include 3-*O*-methyl-6-FD formed by catechol *O*-methyl transferase as well as those listed previously. Ultimately, one would like to apply tracer kinetic modelling techniques to make quantitative measurements of meaningful biochemical indices. Initial attempts at

Plate 1 Normal male subject scanned with the fluorodeoxyglucose techniques. The two coronal sections are oriented perpendicular to the transverse sections at the levels marked by the horizontal lines. Figures on the colour scale refer to CMRG in mg/100 g per min.

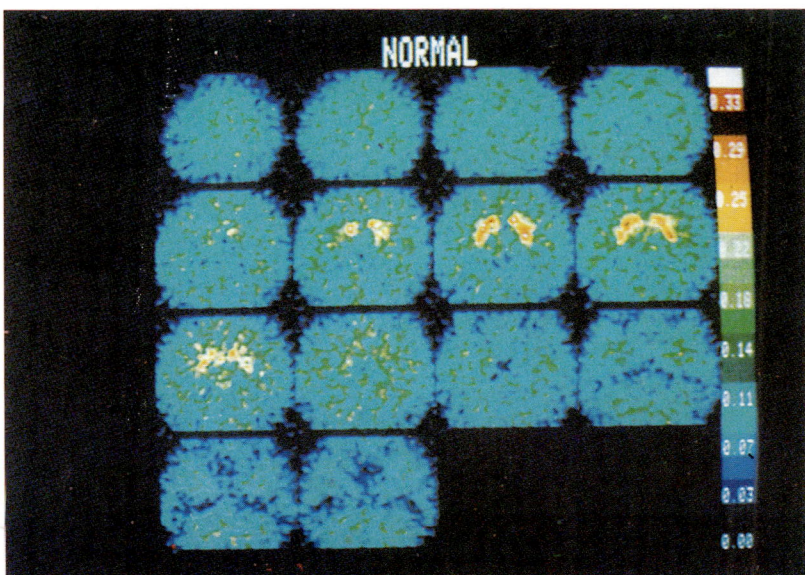

Plate 2 Normal male subject scanned with 6-fluorodopa. Images are spaced at 7 mm intervals with the highest image placed in the upper left corner; axial resolution is about 14 mm. Figures on the colour scale refer to radioactivity in arbitrary units. Note the high uptake of radioactivity in the striatum.

(a)

(b)

Plate 3 Images from a male subject with asymmetric Parkinson's disease (PD), affecting the right side of the body more than the left. The patient's right side is on the right side of the image. Figures on the colour scale refer to radioactivity in arbitrary units. (*a*) Axial sections; (*b*) axial sections with the planes of coronal sections (*Plates 3c* and *d*) marked.

(c)

(d)

Plate 3(c) Coronal sections in a normal subject, with planes as marked in *Plate 3b*. Section 1 is the most anterior. Intersection spacing is 8 mm. (d) Coronal sections in the same PD patient, with planes as marked in *Plate 3b*

Plate 4 Images from comparable levels in a normal subject and a patient with Huntingdon's disease. The colour scale is calibrated in CMRG in mg/100 g per min.

Plate 5

Plate 6

Plate 5 Axial 6-fluorodopa image from a patient with hemidystonia secondary to infarction of the putamen. The colour scale is calibrated in arbitrary units of radioactivity.

Plate 6 PET images of $CMRO_2$ from a patient with paroxysmal hemidystonia. Note the decreased $CMRO_2$ in basal ganglia opposite the affected limbs. (From Perlmutter and Raichle (1984) by courtesy of the Publishers of *Annals of Neurology*.)

developing such techniques have been reported (Garnett *et al.*, 1980; Martin *et al.*, 1985), but much work remains to be done.

The study of radiopharmaceuticals which are believed to bind to receptor sites has been useful for *in vitro* and *in vivo* studies of receptor function (Snyder, 1984). The neuroleptic ligand 3-*N*-methylspiperone binds preferentially to D-2 dopamine and S-2 serotonin receptors. Initial results using ^{11}C-labelled 3-*N*-methylspiperone with PET in man demonstrate maximal activity in the basal ganglia and are considered to reflect D-2 receptor binding (Wagner *et al.*, 1983). These studies (*Figure 2.1*) show a lesser degree of uptake in cerebral cortex where accumulation is thought to reflect S-2 receptor binding (Wong *et al.*, 1984). Numerous other positron emitting dopamine-receptor ligands labelled with positron-emitting isotopes have been synthesized (Arnett *et al.*, 1984; Maziere *et al.*, 1984; Arnett *et al.*, 1985a,b; Baron *et al.*, 1985).

The use of tracer kinetic modelling techniques in conjunction with these radiolabelled ligands may permit *in vivo* quantitative analysis of dopamine

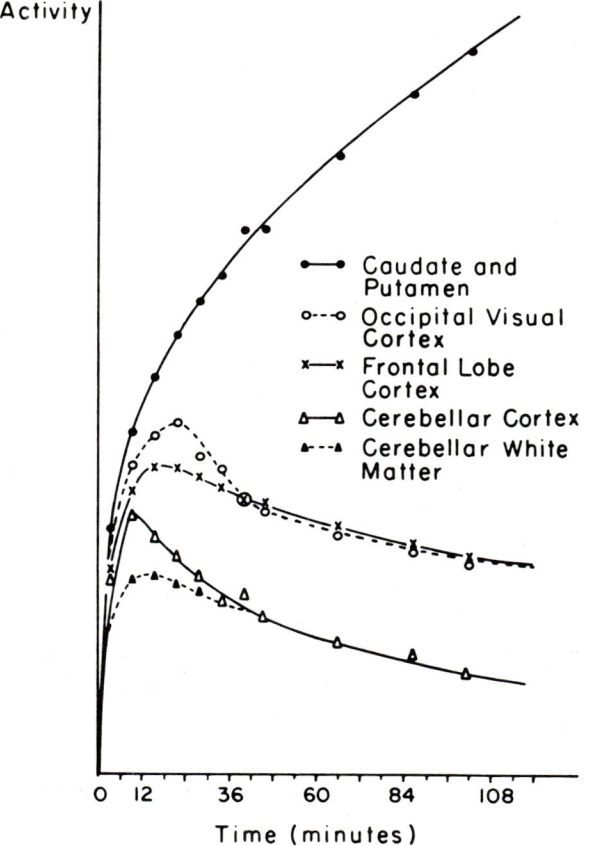

Figure 2.1 Time–activity curve following an intravenous injection of 3-N-[^{11}C]methylspiperone. [From Inoue *et al.* (1985) by courtesy of the Publishers of *Journal of Computer Assisted Tomography*.]

receptors. One such approach is that reported by Mintun et al. (1984a). Their model makes use of sequential PET scans following tracer administration to characterize the dynamic interplay between the ligand and its binding site. These data are combined with PET measurements of other local physiological variables such as blood flow and blood volume to determine the 'binding potential' of the tissue. In this model, binding potential is equivalent to the product of the binding affinity and the number of binding sites. The application of this model to the measurement of [^{18}F]spiperone binding in baboons has been studied (Mintun et al., 1984a); the same techniques may be applied to man. An alternative approach has been reported by Wong et al. (1984).

IMAGING NORMAL SUBJECTS

CT and MRI scans on normal subjects provide information on the morphology of the brain and spinal cord. These images provide in vivo representations almost comparable to macroscopic examination postmortem. Structures less than 1 cm in diameter can easily be delineated provided their properties are reasonably different from the surrounding tissue. The age-related changes found in autopsy material have confirmed the CT and MRI findings, indicating that the major alterations with advancing years are increased sulcal width and ventricular diameter.

Imaging of functional anatomy in terms of glucose utilization has been performed by PET systems in normal subjects at rest (Mazziotta et al., 1981; Duara et al., 1983) and during varying degrees of sensory deprivation and activation (Phelps and Kuhl 1981; Phelps et al., 1981; Mazziotta et al., 1982a,b). Studies performed during visual (Phelps and Kuhl, 1981; Phelps et al., 1981) and auditory (Mazziotta et al., 1982a) stimulation have confirmed that this technique provides significant information regarding brain function as opposed to brain structure. The importance of the type and rate of repetitive stimuli has been addressed in rCBF studies during visual activation (Fox and Raichle, 1984, 1985).

Most studies concerned with cerebral activation have dealt with the brain's response to sensory stimulation. Few studies have been directed at the cerebral control of voluntary movement. Roland et al. (1982) reported increased rCBF in the supplementary motor area bilaterally during performance of a task involving complex repetitive finger movement on one side. They noted, in addition, bilateral basal ganglia changes. Mazziotta, Phelps and Wapenski (1985) observed increased rCMRG in contralateral motor cortex, but not basal ganglia, in subjects performing a similar task. In contrast, contralateral basal ganglia activation in subjects asked to sign their name repeatedly was reported (Mazziotta, Phelps and Wapenski, 1985). These studies suggest that the cerebral control of previously learned tasks differs significantly from control of newly learned tasks. Much further work is required to shed additional light on the physiology of movement in health and disease.

PARKINSON'S DISEASE

CT/MRI

The findings in Parkinson's disease are essentially normal. An early claim (Bydder et al., 1982) that the substantia nigra could be visualized and appeared to be atrophied has not been confirmed.

PET

Measurements of cerebral metabolism and blood flow in patients with predominantly unilateral Parkinson's disease have been reported by several investigators. Asymmetric basal ganglia metabolism with increased $CMRO_2$ (Raichle, Perlmutter and Fox, 1984; Wolfson et al., 1985) and CBF (Wolfson et al., 1985) has been found contralateral to the most severely affected limbs. Preliminary CMRG studies showed similar changes in basal ganglia glucose utilization in some, but not all, patients (Martin et al., 1984a). These findings are consistent with animal studies in which unilateral substantia nigra lesions led to increased ipsilateral pallidal CMRG (Wooten and Collins, 1981). Perlmutter and Raichle have used a stereotactic method for anatomical localization (Fox, Perlmutter and Raichle, 1985) which permits more precise evaluation of specific neuronal groups, and have reported that right and left pallidal blood flows were significantly less tightly coupled in hemiparkinsonian patients than in controls (Perlmutter and Raichle, 1985). In their patients, pallidal blood flow was not necessarily increased contralateral to the patients' symptoms. These studies suggest that abnormalities in pallidal function are present in Parkinson's disease, but that the situation is more complex than would be expected from Wooten and Collins' data (Wooten and Collins, 1981). As Perlmutter and Raichle (1985) suggest, different clinical symptoms may reflect different functional abnormalities of specific basal ganglia nuclei. Confirmation of this possibility must await further studies.

Abnormalities of cortical function have been reported in the frontal lobe contralateral to affected limbs in asymmetrically affected patients. Wolfson et al. (1985) noted a decrease in both $CMRO_2$ and CBF in contralateral frontal cortex. Perlmutter and Raichle (1985), with their stereotactic method, localized the reduction in frontal CBF to 'mesocortex' receiving dopaminergic input from the ventral tegmental area.

Patients with bilateral parkinsonian symptoms have also been studied. Wolfson et al. (1985) reported a widespread decrease in CBF unaccompanied by changes in $CMRO_2$ and suggested the presence of vasoconstriction due to loss of dopaminergic innervation of blood vessels. Studies of rCMRG with FDG have shown either no consistent difference when compared to normal subjects (Rougemont et al., 1983), or a moderate generalized reduction (Kuhl, Metter and Reige, 1984).

The effect of L-dopa on CBF and $CMRO_2$ has been studied. A diffuse increase was found in CBF unaccompanied by changes in $CMRO_2$ in both normal subjects and patients with Parkinson's disease, suggesting a direct vasodilatation of cerebral blood vessels (Leenders et al., 1985). This is consistent with dopamine-induced dilatation demonstrated in the feline cerebral vasculature (Edvinsson et al., 1978) and increased CBF in man after administration of dopamine agonists (Gnell et al., 1982; Bes et al., 1983). In contrast, Perlmutter and Raichle (1985) found no effect from L-dopa on global CBF, possibly because a smaller dose of L-dopa was used.

Studies of 6-FD uptake in non-demented patients with asymmetric Parkinson's disease have recently been reported. Patients with purely unilateral symptoms were found to have normal caudate radioactivity but impaired putamen activity (Nahmias et al., 1985). Patients with somewhat more advanced disease (bilateral involvement, but with significant clinical asymmetry) as a group had symmetric, mildly decreased caudate isotope accumulation, and more severely decreased putamen activity (*Plate 3,* opposite p. 6) (Martin et al., 1986). In both of these reports putamenal activity was asymmetric with the most marked depression being contralateral to the most severely affected limbs. These results are consistent with neurochemical studies which have reported more severe dopamine depletion in the putamen than in the caudate in patients with Parkinson's disease (Hornykiewicz, 1981). Results from our studies are illustrated in *Figure 2.2*.

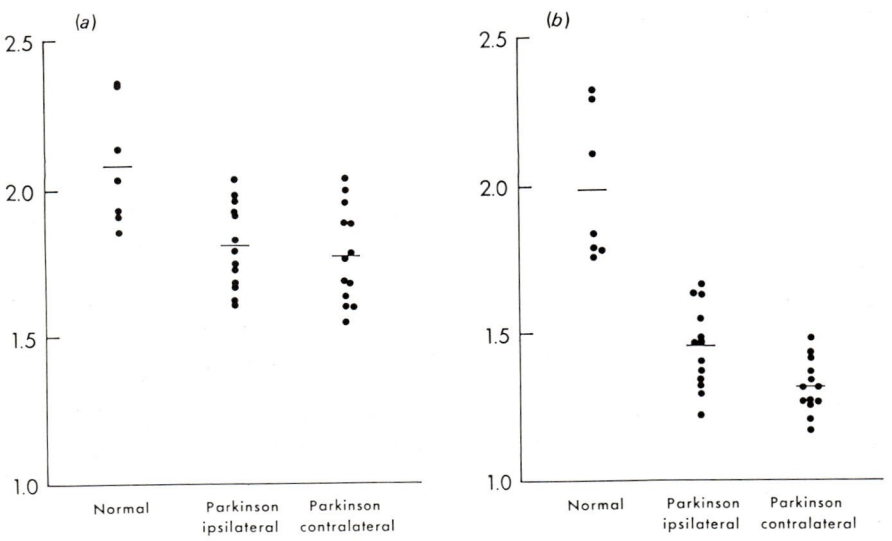

Figure 2.2 Striatum/cerebellum activity ratios from normal subjects ($n = 7$) and patients with asymmetric Parkinson's disease ($n = 13$). Values ipsilateral and contralateral to the most severely affected limbs are indicated for the Parkinson's disease patient. (*a*) Caudate; (*b*) putamen.

Loss of dopamine receptors has been inferred in progressive supranuclear palsy. The D-2 antagonist bromospiperone was employed with PET to study seven patients and the results were thought to suggest a 60% loss of striatal receptor sites, although a mathematical model of ligand–receptor binding interactions was not utilized (Baron *et al.*, 1985).

HUNTINGTON'S DISEASE

CT/MRI

In Huntington's disease cerebral atrophy occurs with prominent loss of cerebral cortex and basal ganglia. In a study of 12 patients, CT measurements have been correlated with clinical deficits (Stober, Wussow and Schimrigk, 1984). From this and related work an index has been derived which seems to be a satisfactory measure of caudate tissue loss. This is the distance between the caudate nuclei, referred to as the bicaudate diameter. One study of Huntington's disease gave a mean value of 21.8 mm ± 3.4(s.d.) (Stober, Wussow and Schimrigk, 1984) and another reported 22.5 mm ± 5.2(s.d.) (Oepen and Ostertag, 1981). These results compare with 12.5 ± 0.6 mm and 14.9 ± 2.92 mm in normal subjects. Attempts to derive ratios between the bicaudate diameter and other brain or skull measurements failed to increase the discriminative capacity of the bicaudate diameter (Stober, Wussow and Schimrigk, 1984). Morphometric examinations of pathological materials confirm that, in Huntington's disease, atrophy is most marked in the head of the caudate nucleus and the anterior putamen (Lange et al., 1976).

PET

The pioneer studies of cerebral metabolism in Huntington's disease were performed at UCLA by Kuhl et al. (1982). They reported a characteristic rCMRG decrease in the striatum. Although many of their patients had CT evidence of ventricular dilatation and caudate atrophy, it was postulated that the local hypometabolism appears early, preceding bulk tissue loss. More recently, Martin and coworkers have studied a series of patients with early Huntington's disease and minimal or no caudate atrophy on CT (*Plate 4,* opposite p. 6) (Martin et al., 1984b). These patients had definite caudate hypometabolism, supporting the conclusions that the rCMRG changes reflect true alterations in neuronal function rather then artefactual changes related to the partial volume effect. Glucose utilization typically remains normal throughout the rest of the brain (Kuhl et al., 1982; Martin et al., 1984b).

Do the changes in caudate metabolism precede the development of clinical symptoms? Kuhl, Metter and Reige (1984), in their initial study, reported the presence of caudate hypometabolism in 6 of 15 asymptomatic subjects at risk for Huntington's disease. Over the subsequent 2-year period, 3 of these subjects developed signs of Huntington's disease (Kuhl et al., 1985), suggesting that the presence of caudate hypometabolism in at-risk subjects may be predictive for the development of symptomatic Huntington's disease.

Decreases in striatal rCMRG have also been reported in benign hereditary chorea (Suchowersky et al., 1983); these changes therefore are not specific for Huntington's disease, but must be interpreted in conjunction with the clinical findings.

DYSTONIA

Idiopathic and genetically determined dystonia

There is no convincing evidence that any structural changes can be detected by CT or MRI in idiopathic or genetically determined dystonia. This is hardly surprising since there are no macroscopic or microscopic morphological alterations evident. In contrast, PET studies do provide evidence of metabolic abnormalities in the basal ganglia. Stoessl et al. (1986) studied 16 patients with idiopathic torticollis using FDG and a correlative analysis of regional activity. They found a bilateral

12 Imaging techniques and movement disorders

breakdown in the normal relationships between the thalamus and the basal ganglia, and postulated that uncoupling might relate to dysfunction in thalamostriate or pallidothalamic projections. In collaboration with Dr M. Meunter we have encountered decreased isotope uptake in the striatum in 6-FD studies of a patient with bilateral diurnal dystonia.

Secondary dystonia

A large series of CT, and more recently MRI, reports have implicated lesions of the basal ganglia in dystonia secondary to various focal lesions of the brain. Abnormalities have been reported in the putamen, pallidum and caudate, but the most consistent thread running through these various findings is pathology involving the putamen. It is clear that several factors are important in the genesis of dystonia as a result of cerebral lesions. It seems that the clinical outcome can be modulated by both macro-anatomical and micro-anatomical factors. Thus the effect of a putamenal lesion will be influenced by concomitant pathology involving the pallidum, the caudate, and the internal capsule. For example, a lesion that affects capsular corticospinal pathways may preclude the expression of any movement disorder. Correspondingly, the relative involvement of the various neuronal components of the putamen will have a profound impact on the pattern of motor dysfunction. A lesion primarily affecting the nigrostriatal dopaminergic pathway will be expressed as parkinsonism, whereas loss of output from the putamen can cause dystonia. Some of these differences are most readily evident from PET scanning. We have observed decreased accumulation of radioactivity in the affected putamen after administering 6-FD to a patient with hemidystonia secondary to a putamenal infarct (*see Figure 2.3* and *Plate 5*, opposite p. 6). In

Figure 2.3 Axial and coronal MRI (inversion recovery) images from a patient with hemidystonia secondary to infarction of the putamen.

Parkinson's disease there is similarly decreased putamenal isotope accumulation after 6-FD, but the putamen is intact on CT and MRI. In a patient with post-traumatic paroxysmal hemidystonia, Perlmutter and Raichle (1984) have reported decreased $CMRO_2$ in the basal ganglia contralateral to the hemidystonia (*Plate 6*, opposite p. 6).

Many types of focal pathology can cause dystonia by inducing appropriate putamenal pathology. In adults atheromatous disease is a common cause (Burton *et al.*, 1984), but tumours can also elicit dystonia (Narbona *et al.*, 1984). In children, Leigh's disease is a relatively common underlying pathology, but there are many others, including the uraemic haemolytic syndrome, ceroid lipofuscinosis, and metachromatic leucodystrophy. Metal deposition in the basal ganglia can lead to dystonia in children or adults, as in Wilson's disease, Hallervorden–Spatz disease, manganese intoxication and some cases of Fahr's syndrome.

Subcortical abnormalities have been reported in Wilson's disease with MRI (Lawler *et al.*, 1983; Littrup and Gemarski, 1985; Starosta-Rubinstein *et al.*, 1985) and CT (Williams, John and Walshe, 1981). Dystonia was found to correlate with lesions of the putamen, caudate, and nigra (Starosta-Rubinstein *et al.*, 1985). Studies of rCMRG in Wilson's disease showed a decrease in all areas of the brain examined (Hawkins *et al.*, 1983). This decrease was present in patients with and without neurological symptoms, but was more severe in the former.

In two patients with a clinical diagnosis of Hallervorden–Spatz disease, MRI demonstrated marked loss of brain substance, predominantly involving the brainstem and cerebellum (Littrup and Gebarski, 1985). In addition, areas of decreased signal intensity were evident in the lentiform nuclei and perilentiform white matter. It was thought that the lentiform abnormality was related either to disordered myelination or to abnormal iron storage.

BALLISM

Focal lesions of the subthalamic nucleus have been associated with ballism, because of long-established clinicopathological correlations. The advent of CT and MRI has allowed *in vivo* observations, from which it is evident that lesions in the thalamus can also induce ballism (Johnson and Fahn, 1977).

CONCLUSIONS

The advent of CT and MRI scanning has already established a new era in the elucidation of correlations between morphological lesions and disorders of movement. The development of PET scanning promises an extension of this advance into the realms of biochemical pathology; the technique has particular potential for the elucidation of fundamental disturbances in movement disorders in which macroscopic and microscopic examination of the structure of the brain have failed to reveal any abnormality.

References

ARNETT, C. D., FOWLER, J. S., WOLF, A. P., LOGAN, J. and MacGREGOR, R. R. (1984) Mapping brain neuroleptic receptors in the live baboon. *Biological Psychiatry*, **19**, 1365–1375

ARNETT, C. D., FOWLER, J. S., WOLF, A. P., SHIUE, C-Y. and McPHERSON, D. W. (1985a) [^{18}F]-N-Methylspiroperidol: The radioligand of choice for PET studies of the dopamine receptor in human brain. *Life Sciences,* **36,** 1359–1366

ARNETT, C. D., SHIUE, C-Y., WOLF, A. P., FOWLER, J. S., LOGAN, J. and WATANABE, M. (1985b) Comparison of three ^{18}F-labeled butyrophenone neuroleptic drugs in the baboon using positron emission tomography. *Journal of Neurochemistry,* **44,** 835–844

BARON, J. C., COMAR, D., ZARIFIAN, E., AGID, Y., CROUZEL, C., LOO, H. *et al.* (1985) Dopaminergic receptor sites in human brain: positron emission tomography. *Neurology,* **35,** 16–24

BARON, J. C., MAZIERE, B., LOC'H, C., SGOUROPOULOS, P., BONNET, A. M. and AGID, Y. (1985) Progressive supranuclear palsy: loss of striatal dopamine receptors demonstrated *in vivo* by positron tomography. *Lancet,* **i,** 1163–1164

BES, A., GUELL, A., FABRE, N., ARNE-BES, M. C. and GERAUD, G. (1983) Effects of dopaminergic agonists (piribedil and bromocriptine) on cerebral blood flow in parkinsonism. *Journal of Cerebral Blood Flow and Metabolism,* **3** (Suppl. 1), S490–S491

BURTON, K., FARRELL, K., LI, D. and CALNE, D. B. (1984) Lesions of the putamen and dystonia: CT and magnetic resonance imaging. *Neurology,* **34,** 962–965

BYDDER, G. M., STEINER, R. E., YOUNG, I. R., HALL, A. S., THOMAS, D. J., MARSHALL, J. *et al.* (1982) Clinical NMR imaging of the brain: 140 cases. *American Journal of Radiology,* **139,** 215–236

CORMACK, A. M. (1980) Early two-dimensional reconstruction (CT scanning) and recent topics stemming from it. *Journal of Computer Assisted Tomography,* **4,** 658–664

DUARA, R., MARGOLIN, R. A., ROBERTSON-TCHABO, E. A., LONDON, E. D., SCHWARTZ, M., RENFREW, J. W. *et al.* (1983) Cerebral glucose utilization, as measured with positron emission tomography in 21 resting healthy men between the ages of 21 and 83 years. *Brain,* **106,** 761–775

EDVINSSON, L., HARDEBO, J. E., McCULLOCH, J. and OWMAN, C. (1978) Vasomotor response of cerebral blood vessels to dopamine and dopaminergic agonists. *Advances in Neurology,* **20,** 85–96

FIRNAU, G., GARNETT, E. S., SOURKES, T. L. and MISSALA, K. (1975) [^{18}F]FluoroDopa: a unique gamma emitting substrate for dopa decarboxylase. *Experientia,* **31,** 1254–1255

FOX, P. T., PERLMUTTER, J. S. and RAICHLE, M. E. (1985) A stereotactic method of anatomical localization for positron emission tomography. *Journal of Computer Assisted Tomography,* **9,** 141–153

FOX, P. T. and RAICHLE, M. E. (1984) Stimulus rate dependence of regional cerebral blood flow in human striate cortex, demonstrated by positron emission tomography. *Journal of Neurophysiology,* **51,** 1109–1120

FOX, P. T. and RAICHLE, M. E. (1985) Stimulus rate determines regional brain blood flow in striate cortex. *Annals of Neurology,* **17,** 303–305

FRACKOWIAK, R. S. J., LENZI, G-L., JONES, T. and HEATHER, J. D. (1980) Quantitative measurement of regional cerebral blood flow and oxygen metabolism in man using ^{15}O and positron emission tomography: theory, procedure, and normal values. *Journal of Computer Assisted Tomography,* **4,** 727–736

GARNETT, E. S., FIRNAU, G. and NAHMIAS, C. (1983) Dopamine visualized in the basal ganglia of living man. *Nature,* **305,** 137–138

GARNETT, S., FIRNAU, G., NAHMIAS, C. and CHIRAKAL, R. (1983) Striatal dopamine metabolism in living monkeys examined by positron emission tomography. *Brain Research,* **280,** 169–171

GARNETT, E. S., FIRNAU, G. NAHMIAS, C., SOOD, S. and BELBECK, L. (1980) Blood–brain barrier transport and cerebral utilization of dopa in living monkeys. *American Journal of Physiology,* **238,** 318–327

GUELL, A., GERAUD, G., JAUZAC, P., VICTOR, G. and ARNE-BES, M. C. (1982) Effects of a dopaminergic agaonist (piribedil) on cerebral blood flow in man. *Journal of Cerebral Blood Flow and Metabolism,* **2,** 255–257

HAWKINS, R. A., PHELPS, M. E., MAZZIOTTA, J. C. and KUHL, D. E. (1983) A study of Wilson's disease with F-18 FDG and positron tomography. *Journal of Cerebral Blood Flow and Metabolism,* **3** (Suppl. 1), 498–499

HORNE, M. K., CHENG, C. H. and WOOTEN, G. F. (1984) The cerebral metabolism of L-dihydroxyphenylalanine. *Pharmacology,* **28,** 12–26

HORNYKIEWICZ, O. (1981) Brain neurotransmitter changes in Parkinson's disease. In *Movement Disorders,* Eds. C. D. Marsden and S. Fahn, pp. 41–58. London: Butterworth Scientific

HOUNSFIELD, G. N. (1980) Computed medical imaging. *Journal of Computer Assisted Tomography,* **4,** 665–674

INOUE, Y., WAGNER, H. N. JR, WONG, D. F., LINKS, J. M., FROST, J. J., DANNALS, R. F. *et al.* (1985) Atlas of dopamine receptor images (PET) of the human brain. *Journal of Computer Assisted Tomography,* **9,** 129–140

JOHNSON, W. G. and FAHN, S. (1977) Treatment of vascular hemiballism and hemichorea. *Neurology,* **27,** 634–636

JONES, T., CHESLER, D. A. and TER-POGOSSIAN, M. M. (1976) The continuous inhalation of oxygen-15 for assessing regional oxygen extraction in the brain of man. *British Journal of Radiology*, **49**, 339–343

KUHL, D. E., MARKHAM, C. H., METTER, E. J., RIEGE, W. H., PHELPS, M. E. and MAZZIOTTA, J. C. (1985) Local cerebral glucose utilization in symptomatic and presymptomatic Huntington's disease. In *Brain Imaging and Brain Function*. Ed. L. Sokoloff, pp. 199–209. New York: Raven Press

KUHL, D. E., METTER, E. J. and REIGE, W. H. (1984) Patterns of local cerebral glucose utilization determined in Parkinson's disease by the [^{18}F]fluorodeoxyglucose method. *Annals of Neurology*, **15**, 419–424

KUHL, D. E., PHELPS, M. E., MARKHAM, C. H., METTER, E. J., RIEGE, W. H. and WINTER, J. (1982) Cerebral metabolism and atrophy in Huntington's disease determined by ^{18}FDG and computed tomographic scan. *Annals of Neurology*, **12**, 425–434

LANGE, H., THORNER, G., HOPF, A. and SCHRODER, K. F. (1976) Morphometric studies of the neuropathological changes in choreatic diseases. *Journal of Neurological Sciences*, **28**, 401–425

LAWLER, G. A., PENNOCK, J. M., STEINER, R. E., JENKINS, W. J., SHERLOCK, S. and YOUNG, I. R. (1983) Nuclear magnetic resonance (NMR) imaging in Wilson's disease. *Journal of Computer Assisted Tomography*, **7**, 1–8

LEENDERS, K. L., WOLFSON, L., GIBBS, J. M., WISE, R. J. S., CAUSON, R., JONES, T. and LEGG, N. J. (1985) The effects of L-dopa on regional cerebral blood flow and oxygen metabolism in patients with Parkinson's disease. *Brain*, **108**, 171–191

LITTRUP, P. J. and GEBARSKI, S. S. (1985) MR imaging of Hallervorden–Spatz disease. *Journal of Computer Assisted Tomography*, **9**, 491–493

MARTIN, W. R. W., BECKMAN, J. H., CALNE, D. B., ADAM, M. J., HARROP, R., ROGERS, J. G. et al. (1984a) Cerebral glucose metabolism in Parkinson's disease. *Canadian Journal of Neurological Sciences*, **11**, 169–173

MARTIN, W. R. W., BOYES, B. E., LEENDERS, K. L. and PATLAK, C. S. (1985) A method for the quantitative analysis of 6-fluorodopa uptake data from positron emission tomography. *Journal of Cerebral Blood Flow and Metabolism*, **5** (Suppl. 1), 5593–5594

MARTIN, W. R. W., HAYDEN, M. R., SUCHOWERSKY, O., BECKMAN, J., ADAM, M., AMMANN, W. et al. (1984b) Striatal metabolism in Huntington's disease and in benign hereditary chorea. *Annals of Neurology*, **16**, 126

MARTIN, W. R. W., STOESSL, J., ADAM, M. J., AMMANN, W., BERGSTROM, M., HARROP, R. et al. (1986) Positron emission tomography in Parkinson's disease: glucose and dopa metabolism. In *Advances in Neurology, Parkinson's Disease* (in press)

MATA, M., FINK, D. J., GAINER, H., SMITH, C. B., DAVIDSEN, L., SAVAKI, H. et al. (1980) Activity-dependent energy metabolism in rat posterior pituitary primarily reflects sodium pump activity. *Journal of Neurochemistry*, **34**, 213–215

MAZIERE, B., LOC'H, C., HANTRAYE, P., GUILLON, R., DUQUESNOY, N., SOUSSALINE, F. et al. (1984) ^{76}Br-Bromospiroperidol: a new tool for quantitative *in vivo* imaging of neuroleptic receptors. *Life Sciences*, **35**, 1349–1356

MAZZIOTTA, J. C., PHELPS, M. E., CARSON, R. E. and KUHL, D. E. (1982a) Tomographic mapping of human cerebral metabolism: auditory stimulation. *Neurology*, **32**, 921–937

MAZZIOTTA, J. C., PHELPS, M. E., CARSON, R. E. and KUHL, D. E. (1982b) Tomographic mapping of human cerebral metabolism: sensory deprivation. *Annals of Neurology*, **12**, 435–444

MAZZIOTTA, J. C., PHELPS, M. E., MILLER, J. and KUHL, D. E. (1981) Tomographic mapping of human cerebral metabolism: normal unstimulated state. *Neurology*, **31**, 503–516

MAZZIOTTA, J. C., PHELPS, M. E. and WAPENSKI, J. (1985) Human cerebral motor system metabolic responses in health and disease. *Journal of Cerebral Blood Flow and Metabolism*, **5** (Suppl.), 5213–5214

MINTUN, M. A., RAICHLE, M. E., KILBOURNE, M. R., WOOTEN, G. F. and WELCH, M. J. (1984a) A quantitative model for the *in vivo* assessment of drug binding sites with positron emission tomography. *Annals of Neurology*, **15**, 217–227

MINTUN, M. A., RAICHLE, M. E., MARTIN, W. R. W. and HERSCOVITCH, P. (1984b) Brain oxygen utilization measured with 0–15 radiotracers and positron emission tomography. *Journal of Nuclear Medicine*, **25**, 177–187

NAHMIAS, C., GARNETT, E. S., FIRNAU, G. and LANG, A. (1985) Striatal dopamine distribution in Parkinsonian patients during life. *Journal of the Neurological Sciences*, **69**, 223–230

NARBONA, J., OBESO, J. A., TUNON, T., MARTINEZ-LAGE, J. M. and MARSDEN, C. D. (1984) Hemi-dystonia secondary to localized basal ganglia tumour. *Journal of Neurology, Neurosurgery and Psychiatry*, **47**, 704–709

NORMAN, D. and BRANT-ZAWADZKI, M. (1985) Magnetic resonance imaging of the central nervous system. In *Brain Imaging and Brain Function*. Ed. L. Sokoloff, pp. 259–269. New York: Raven Press

OEPEN, G. and OSTERTAG, C. (1981) Diagnostic value of CT in patients with Huntington's chorea and their offspring. *Journal of Neurology*, **225**, 189–196

OLDENDORF, W. H. (1985) Principles of imaging structure by NMR. In *Brain Imaging and Brain Function*. Ed. L. Sokoloff, pp. 245–257. New York: Raven Press

PERLMUTTER, J. S. and RAICHLE, M. E. (1984) Pure hemidystonia with basal ganglion abnormalities on positron emission tomography. *Annals of Neurology,* **15,** 228–233

PERLMUTTER, J. S. and RAICHLE, M. E. (1985) Regional blood flow in hemiparkinsonism. *Neurology,* **35,** 1127–1134

PHELPS, M. E., HUANG, S. C., HOFFMAN, E. J., SELIN, D., SOKOLOFF, L. and KUHL, D. E. (1979) Tomographic measurement of local cerebral glucose metabolic rate in humans with (F-18)2-fluoro-2-deoxy-D-glucose: validation of method. *Annals of Neurology,* **6,** 371–388

PHELPS, M. E. and KUHL, D. E. (1981) Metabolic mapping of the brain's response to visual stimulation: studies in humans. *Science,* **211,** 1445–1448

PHELPS, M. E., MAZZIOTTA, J. C., KUHL, D. E., NUWER, M., PACKWOOD, J., METTER, J. and ENGEL, J. JR (1981) Tomographic mapping of human cerebral metabolism: visual stimulation and deprivation. *Neurology,* **31,** 517–529

RAICHLE, M. E., MARTIN, W. R. W., HERSCOVITCH, P., MINTUN, M. A. and MARKHAM, J. (1983) Brain–blood flow measures with intravenous $H_2{}^{15}O$. II. Implementation and validation. *Journal of Nuclear Medicine,* **24,** 790–798

RAICHLE, M. E., PERLMUTTER, J. S. and FOX, P. T. (1984) Parkinson's disease: metabolic and pharmacological approaches with positron emission tomography. *Annals of Neurology* (Suppl.), **15,** 131–132

REIVICH, M., KUHL, D., WOLF, A., GREENBERG, J., PHELPS, M., IDO, T. *et al.* (1979) The [^{18}F]fluorodeoxyglucose method for the measurement of local cerebral glucose utilization in man. *Circulation Research,* **44,** 127–137

ROLAND, P. E., MEYER, E., SHIBASAKI, T., YAMAMOTO, Y. L. and THOMPSON, C. J. (1982) Regional cerebral blood flow changes in cortex and basal ganglia during voluntary movements in normal human volunteers. *Journal of Neurophysiology,* **48,** 467–480

ROUGEMONT, D., BARON, J. C., COLLARD, P., BUSTANY, P., COMAR, D. and AGID, Y. (1983) Local cerebral metabolic rate of glucose (1CMRG1c) in treated and untreated patients with Parkinson's disease. *Journal of Cerebral Blood Flow and Metabolism,* **3** (Suppl. 1), 504–505

SNYDER, S. H. (1984) Drug and neurotransmitter receptors in the brain. *Science,* **224,** 22–31

SOKOLOFF, L. (1981) Localization of functional activity in the central nervous system by measurement of glucose utilization with radioactive deoxyglucose. *Journal of Cerebral Blood Flow and Metabolism,* **1,** 7–36

SOKOLOFF, L., REIVICH, M., KENNEDY, C., DES ROSIERS, M. H., PATLAK, C. S., PETTIGREW, K. D. *et al.* (1977) The [^{14}C]deoxyglocose method for the measurement of local cerebral glucose utilization: theory, procedure, and normal values in the conscious and anesthetized albino rat. *Journal of Neurochemistry,* **28,** 897–916

STAROSTA-RUBINSTEIN, S., YOUNG, A. B., KLUIN, K., HILL, G. M., AISEN, A. M., GABRIELSEN, T. and BREWER, G. J. (1985) Quantitative clinical assessment of 25 Wilson's patients: correlation with structural changes on MRI. *Neurology* (Suppl. 1), **35,** 175

STOBER, T., WUSSOW, W. and SCHIMRIGK, K. (1984) Bicaudate diameter – the most specific and simple CT parameter in the diagnosis of Huntington's disease. *Neuroradiology,* **26,** 25–28

STOESSL, A. J., MARTIN, W. R. W., CLARK, C., ADAM, M. J., AMMAN, W., BECKMAN, J. H. *et al.* (1986) PET studies of cerebral glucose metabolism idiopathic torticollis. *Neurology,* **36,** (in press)

SUBRAMANYAM, R., ALPERT, N. M., HOOP, B. JR, BROWNELL, G. L. and TRAVERS, J. M. (1978) A model for regional cerebral oxygen distribution during continuous inhalation of $^{15}O_2$, $C^{15}O$ and $C^{15}O_2$. *Journal of Nuclear Medicine,* **19,** 48–53

SUCHOWERSKY, O., HAYDEN, M., MARTIN, W. R. W., LI, D. K., BERGSTROM, M., HARROP, R. *et al.* (1984) Benign hereditary chorea: clinical, radiological and PET findings. *Canadian Journal of Neurological Science,* **11,** 329

WAGNER, H. N. JR, BURNS, H. D., DANNALS, R. F., WONG, D. F., LANGSTROM, B., DUELFER, T. *et al.* (1983) Imaging dopamine receptors in the human brain by positron tomography. *Science,* **221,** 1264–1266

WILLIAMS, F., JOHN, B. and WALSHE, J. M. (1981) Wilson's disease. An analysis of the cranial computerized tomographic appearances found in 60 patients and the changes in response to treatment with chelating agents. *Brain,* **104,** 735–752

WOLFSON, L. I., LEENDERS, K. L., BROWN, L. L. and JONES, T. (1985) Alterations of regional cerebral blood flow and oxygen metabolism in Parkinson's disease. *Neurology,* **35,** 1399–1405

WONG, D. F., WAGNER, H. N. JR, DANNALS, R. F., LINKS, J. M., FROST, J. J., RAVERT, H. T. *et al.* (1984) Effects of age on dopamine and serotonin receptors measured by positron tomography in the living human brain. *Science,* **226,** 1393–1396

WOOTEN, G. F. and COLLINS, R. C. (1981) Metabolic effects of unilateral lesions of the substantia nigra. *Journal of Neurosciences,* **1,** 285–291

3
Epidemiology of movement disorders
Bruce S. Schoenberg

GENERAL CONSIDERATIONS

Neuro-epidemiology may be defined as the study of the distribution and dynamics of neurological diseases in human populations and the factors that affect those characteristics (Schoenberg, 1978). Whereas the clinician is concerned with disease in the individual patient, the neuro-epidemiologist is concerned with the occurrence of neurological disease in the entire community. Studies of the distribution of disease involve identifying the particular segments of the population affected. For example, does the disease occur more often in men or in a particular age group? Investigations of the dynamics of disease address the question of whether the disease is changing over time. Is it increasing or decreasing? Are the clinical manifestations changing?

The patterns of disease in the community, as derived from descriptive epidemiological studies, provide important information for formulating aetiological hypotheses. Thus, if the incidence of a given disease has remained stable over several decades, a cause must be searched for which has been present in the environment of the community for a considerable period of time.

The two most important considerations for the neuro-epidemiologist in the design of studies are the representativeness of the population selected for investigation and the accuracy of the diagnoses in that population.

On the basis of their experience, clinicians review patients' signs and symptoms, establish a diagnosis and a prognosis, and institute appropriate forms of therapy. But how representative is the physician's personal experience? This is a critical concern for the epidemiologist. Certain physicians practising in the community may specialize in Parkinson's disease or other movement disorders, whereas other clinicians in the same community may rarely treat patients with these problems. Because of a lack of financial resources and limited access to neurological expertise, some individuals with the disease of interest may never seek medical care or may never be correctly diagnosed. The situation is analogous to blind-folded men examining different parts of an elephant, with each coming to an entirely different conclusion as to the characteristics of the beast. To avoid this problem, the neuro-epidemiologist attempts to identify all cases of a particular neurological disease in a well-defined population. In drawing conclusions from investigating disease occurrence in a population, the characteristics of that population must be known. Very different conclusions can be arrived at by examining residents of a retirement community, as contrasted with inhabitants of a military base. One must therefore be certain that the community which has been studied is *representative* of the larger population to which the results are to be generalized.

Of equal importance is the problem of diagnostic accuracy. The results of the most sophisticated analysis are no better than the quality of the original data. This problem was recognized earlier in this century by the British statistician, Sir Josiah Stamp (1929), who wrote:

> The government are very keen on amassing statistics – they collect them, add them, raise them to the *n*th power, take the cube root and prepare wonderful diagrams. But what you must never forget is that every one of those figures comes in the first instance from the . . . village watchman, who puts down what he damn pleases.

For neuro-epidemiological studies, the clinician represents the village watchman. The greater the accuracy and completeness of the physician's data, the greater the validity of the epidemiological information concerning the spectrum of disease in the community under investigation. If residents of a community have little or no access to physicians with neurological expertise, then it may be necessary to have a neurologist review all suspected cases. In comparing the results of several different studies, it is important to consider the criteria for making a diagnosis. Some investigations simply accept the diagnosis made by a physician. Other surveys set up strict criteria, i.e. to make a diagnosis of parkinsonism the patient must exhibit a resting tremor, rigidity, and bradykinesia. It is also important to note the criteria employed to distinguish secondary parkinsonism from idiopathic Parkinson's disease.

The magnitude of the disease burden in the community is usually expressed in terms of the population at risk. To say how many people had or died of a particular disease has little meaning unless it is also stated how many people were at risk of having or dying from that specific disease. To adjust for this, the epidemiologist usually expresses disease magnitude as a rate or ratio, in which the frequency of disease (numerator) is related to the population at risk of having disease (denominator). The magnitude of the disease burden in the population is usually defined in terms of certain epidemiological indices, such as mortality, incidence, and prevalence. These are briefly defined in *Table 3.1*.

Epidemiological studies of Parkinson's disease pose some special problems. The parkinsonian syndrome can result from: tumours or other focal lesions of the basal ganglia; as a sequela to von Economo's type A encephalitis; from exposure to certain toxins, such as manganese or carbon monoxide; following the use of pharmacological agents such as phenothiazines. It may be difficult in evaluating all cases in a community to distinguish between secondary parkinsonism and idiopathic Parkinson's disease. Studies of the incidence of Parkinson's disease require an accurate determination of disease onset. This may be extremely difficult in a situation in which the signs and symptoms develop insidiously. Parkinson's disease occurs primarily among the elderly. Careful evaluation may be required to distinguish the characteristic features of Parkinson's disease from other signs observed in the elderly patient, e.g. essential tremor or a general slowing and hesitancy of movement due to the pain and stiffness of arthritis. This problem is compounded by the fact that adequate data are not generally available concerning

Table 3.1 Common epidemiological indices

Mortality measures the frequency of deaths within a specific population and is calculated for a given time interval and given place. It is often expressed as a death rate: deaths from a given disease per 100 000 persons at risk of dying of the disease per year

Prevalence measures the frequency of all current cases of disease within a specific population and is calculated for a given time and given place. It is usually expressed as a prevalence ratio: the number of persons with a given disease at a specified time per 100 000 persons capable of having the disease at the same specified time*

Incidence measures the rapidity with which a disease occurs or the frequency of addition of new cases of a disease within a specific population. It is calculated for a given time interval and given place, and is often expressed as an incidence rate: the number of new cases of a given disease during a specified period (usually 1 year) per 100 000 persons at risk of having the disease for the first time per year

---
*Prevalence and incidence are related to each other as follows: prevalence approximately equals incidence multiplied by the average duration of the disease.
Reproduced with permission from Schoenberg, 1981.

the functional neurological status of older individuals without diseases of the nervous system. The concept of what defines 'normal' must be carefully reconsidered. Patients in this age group are often afflicted by multiple disorders, and sorting out the specific cause of disability may be a formidable task. Finally, we must consider the patient's accessibility to and desire to utilize expert neurological care. The elderly patient or his family may feel that tremor and a slowness of movement and difficulty in walking are part of the ageing process and may not seek medical care. Hence, a correct diagnosis is never established.

Of the various movement disorders, Parkinson's disease has been the most extensively studied, both because of its frequency and its effect as a major cause of morbidity. The majority of this report will therefore focus on the results of epidemiological investigations relating specifically to Parkinson's disease.

PARKINSON'S DISEASE

Mortality data

Mortality tabulations have a number of advantages. Many countries have routine systems for collecting such information in a centralized registry. Furthermore, such procedures have been in effect for many years. Thus, with mortality data, readily available information exists for many countries, covering large populations over many years. Unfortunately, when dealing with Parkinson's disease, mortality data do not adequately reflect the frequency of the disorder. Although the disease may be listed on the death certificate, some other condition is often specified as the single, underlying cause of death. In fact, tabulating the number of times Parkinson's disease appears anywhere on US death certificates and comparing it to the number of times it is listed as the underlying cause of death, the former figure is nearly four times greater than the latter (Chandra, Bharucha and Schoenberg, 1984). Another difficulty is the accuracy of the diagnoses appearing on the death certificate. This document may not even be filled out by a physician. Even if a doctor has this responsibility, problems can arise. For example, a physician not previously involved in the care of a patient may be called on to pronounce that person dead. Lacking adequate medical records, he may get this information from relatives and use these unconfirmed data in filling out the certificate. Despite these deficiencies, interesting patterns emerge when analysing data from the USA (Chandra, Bharucha and Schoenberg, 1984). The mortality rates are negligible for people under the age of 45. When considering only the underlying cause of death, the rates increase steadily with advancing age, reaching a peak at the ages of 75 through to 84, and then declining among the oldest age group. If the tabulations are based on all listings of Parkinson's disease on US death certificates, the mortality rates continue to increase with advancing age. Another interesting observation is that Parkinson's disease death rates for the USA and for England and Wales have remained relatively stable over time (Duvoisin and Schweitzer, 1966; Kurtzke and Kurland, 1984).

Incidence data

Morbidity information is much more difficult to obtain, since such data require special surveys. Incidence rates from several such investigations are summarized in *Table 3.2*. Since incidence rates for Parkinson's disease vary greatly with age, it is important to use age-specific or age-adjusted figures in any comparison. Incidence rates derived from surveys with good case ascertainment provide figures near 20 new cases per 100000 per year. After the age of 30–40, the incidence rates increase with age to reach a maximum at about 75, with a decline in the rate of new cases after that (*Figure 3.1*). It may be that very elderly people who first develop signs of parkinsonism do not seek expert medical care for their condition, and hence are not correctly diagnosed. A further problem with calculating incidence data is that an

Table 3.2 Incidence rates for Parkinson's disease from selected studies

Population	Time period	New cases per 100000 per year	
		Observed	Age-adjusted to 1960 US population
Rochester, Minnesota			
Kurland et al., 1969	1955–66	19.3	17.9*
Rajput et al., 1984a	1967–79	19.7†	18.6†
Carlisle, England			
Brewis et al., 1966	1955–61	12.1	9.4*
Iceland			
Gudmundsson, 1967	1954–63	16.0	18.2*
Gippsland, Victoria, Australia			
Jenkins, 1966	1959–64	7.0	7.7*
South-west Finland			
Martilla and Rinne, 1976	1968–70	14.8	11.6*

*Data from Kessler, 1978.
†Includes drug-induced parkinsonism.

Figure 3.1 Average annual age-specific incidence rates for parkinsonism from three population-based studies. (●) Rochester, Minnesota; (■) Iceland; (▲) Carlisle, England. (Reproduced in modified form with permission from Kurtzke and Kurland, 1984).

accurate determination of disease onset is required. This may be extremely difficult with a condition such as Parkinson's disease. The actual shape of the age-specific incidence curve is of more than academic interest, since it has important aetiological implications. If the incidence rates rise to a maximum at a specific age and then decline it could mean that the number of susceptible individuals at that age is beginning to decrease or that susceptible individuals are exposed to a putative aetiological agent for a limited number of years.

Of particular interest are incidence rates based on studies of a stable population in the United States (Rochester, Minnesota) covering a 35-year period (Kurland *et al.*, 1973; Rajput *et al.*, 1984a). From 1945 through to 1979 the rates varied within the narrow range of 16–21 new cases per 100 000 per year, with no general trend showing either a consistent increase or decrease over time. Furthermore, wherever morbidity surveys of Parkinson's disease have been carried out, Rochester, Minnesota has one of the highest reported incidence rates (probably reflecting an excellent level of case ascertainment). These data imply that whatever causes Parkinson's disease must have been present in the non-industrialized environment of Rochester at a fairly steady level over a period of some 35 years.

Prevalence data

There have been several studies providing estimates of the prevalence of parkinsonism in general or Parkinson's disease in particular. Selected findings are summarized in *Table 3.3*. Because of the change in prevalence ratios with age, it is

Table 3.3 Prevalence ratios of Parkinson's disease from selected studies

Population	Date	Cases per 100000	
		Observed	Age-adjusted to 1960 US population
Goteborg, Sweden Broman, 1963	Jan. 1, 1960	67.5	69.5*
Carlisle, England Brewis et al., 1966	Jan. 1, 1961	112.5	90.2*
Iceland Gudmundsson, 1967	Dec. 31, 1963	162.6	179.8*
Rochester, Minnesota Kurland et al., 1969	Jan. 1, 1965	156.9	165.5*
Gippsland, Victoria Jenkins, 1966	Jan. 1, 1965	84.3	95.4*
South-west Finland Martilla and Rinne, 1976	Dec. 31, 1971	120.1	93.5*
Baltimore, Maryland Kessler, 1972			
Whites	1967–69	125.0	124.5
Blacks	1967–69	21.4	30.4
Copiah County, Mississippi Schoenberg et al., 1985			
Whites	Jan. 1, 1978	159.2	93.1†
Blacks	Jan. 1, 1978	102.9	90.4†
Yonago, Japan Harada, Nishikawa and Takahashi, 1983	Apr. 1, 1980	80.6	73.3†
Six cities, People's Republic of China Li et al., 1985	Jan. 1, 1983	44	57

*Data from Kessler, 1978.
†Calculated from data given in the corresponding published report.

important that any comparisons utilize age-specific or age-adjusted figures. The different surveys reported in *Table 3.3* employed different methods of case identification. In rather unique circumstances, such as exist for residents of Rochester, Minnesota, it is possible to obtain accurate statistics by applying defined diagnostic criteria to information available in medical records. By means of a records-linkage system, data concerning all medical contacts, i.e. outpatient records, inpatient records, house calls, emergency room visits etc., are kept together in a single computerized file. Furthermore, the population has easy access to expertise in neurological diagnosis, and this access is not generally limited because of a lack of financial resources. Finally, the medical records contain sufficient details concerning the findings of the medical history, the physical examination, and the results of laboratory tests to allow retrospective review of the diagnosis. Only in such special instances is it possible to rely on medical records to obtain most or all of the cases within a community. *Figure 3.2* outlines the various steps involved in the identification of cases. One can use medical records as the sole method of case ascertainment only if: (*a*) those with signs or symptoms have sufficient motivation and resources to seek medical care; (*b*) neurological expertise is readily available to members of the community; (*c*) uniform diagnostic criteria are utilized to establish the diagnosis; (*d*) sufficient detail is available in the medical record to allow for retrospective review. If the diagnosis is uncertain in some

Figure 3.2 Factors to be considered in choosing the optimal procedure for the identification of cases in morbidity surveys of Parkinson's disease.

instances, it may be necessary for the neurologist to re-examine these selected cases. In situations in which these criteria are not fulfilled, it is necessary to use door-to-door survey techniques to identify all cases of Parkinson's disease within the community. Such survey methods were employed in investigations carried out in rural, biracial Copiah County, Mississippi, USA (Schoenberg, Anderson and Haerer, 1985) and in urban areas of the People's Republic of China (Li *et al.*, 1985).

Based on earlier studies carried out in Baltimore on cases coming to medical attention, it appeared that Parkinson's disease is much more prevalent among Whites as compared to Blacks (*Table 3.3*) (Kessler, 1972, 1978). However, because of a concern that Whites and Blacks might not have availed themselves of medical services to the same extent, this reported racial difference in prevalence was tested in a door-to-door survey of all residents of a biracial county in the southern part of the USA. In contrast to the Baltimore findings, the results of the door-to-door survey in Mississippi revealed virtually no differences in the age-adjusted prevalence ratios of Parkinson's disease among Blacks and Whites residing in Copiah County (*Table 3.3*). Of particular interest is that 32% of the cases among Whites and 58% of the cases among Blacks were newly diagnosed at the time of the survey (Schoenberg, Anderson and Haerer, 1985). These cases would have been missed in an investigation relying on medical records or previously established physician diagnoses. A similar procedure was carried out among a sample population of 63 195 in six urban centres of the People's Republic of China, yielding much lower prevalence ratios (*Table 3.3*) (Li *et al.*, 1985). The same techniques are now being employed in Nigeria, India, and various South American countries (Schoenberg, 1982, 1983). Preliminary data from the door-to-door survey in Nigeria indicate a much lower prevalence ratio of Parkinson's disease among rural

West African Blacks (Osuntokun *et al.*, 1986) as compared to Blacks in rural Mississippi (Schoenberg, Anderson and Haerer, 1985). Osuntokun and his colleagues believe the differences in prevalence figures are too large to be explained by possible differences in survival between Blacks with Parkinson's disease in Africa and in the USA. The finding is consistent with the hypothesis that an environmental agent(s) may be responsible for the observed differences.

Unlike the data for incidence, the age-specific prevalence ratios for Parkinson's disease generally show consistently increasing figures with increasing age (*Figure 3.3*). These increasing prevalence ratios have important implications for the future.

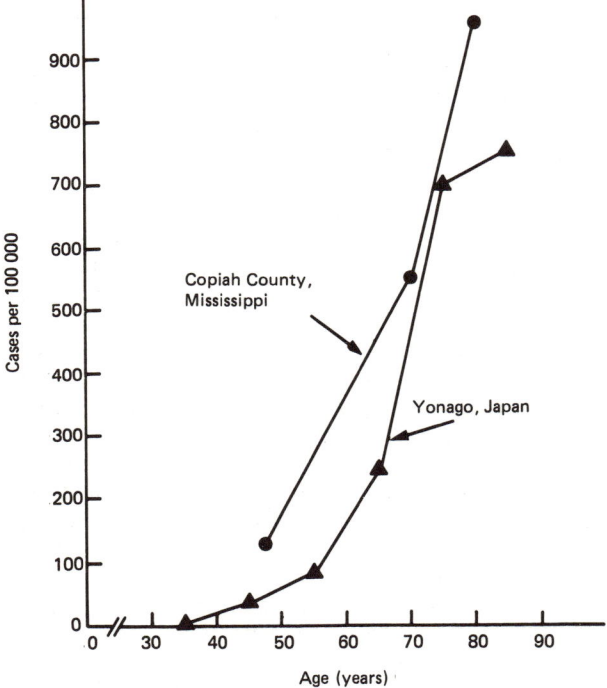

Figure 3.3 Age-specific prevalence ratios of Parkinson's disease from two population-based studies.

Based on projections from the US Bureau of the Census, the age group 65 and over is expected to increase in size over the next 15 years, moving from 25 million in 1980 to an estimated 32 million in the year 2000. The proportion of the aged in the total population is also expected to rise, from 11.2% in 1980 to 12.2% in the year 2000, to 15.5% in the year 2020 (Siegel, 1980). Finally, current tabulations indicate that the recent reduction in the mortality rate for the extremely aged (persons 85 years and older) is larger than that exhibited by other adult age groups (Rosenwaike, Yaffe and Sagi, 1980). Thus, the segment of the population at greatest risk of Parkinson's disease is anticipated to increase in size, resulting in many more expected cases. With improvements in survival as a result of more effective therapeutic measures (Sweet and McDowell, 1975), these projections will increase even further.

As standardized methods and diagnostic criteria are implemented throughout the world, we shall obtain more accurate information on the actual international distribution of Parkinson's disease. These data could provide valuable aetiological clues.

Analytical studies: risk factors

On the basis of descriptive studies of the distribution of Parkinson's disease, it is possible to formulate hypotheses concerning the causation of disease. For example, the stable incidence rates demonstrated for the population of Rochester, Minnesota, suggest that whatever causes Parkinson's disease must have been present in this non-industrialized community for a considerable period of time. Such hypotheses can be formally tested using the techniques of analytical epidemiology, which is primarily aimed at identifying factors that are associated with either a high or a low risk of disease. The study of the occurrence of natural experiments is the domain of this area of epidemiology. During the course of our lives, different individuals are exposed to a variety of different factors or conditions, some of which may play an important role in the occurrence of disease. There are two general approaches to this type of study: case-control and prospective.

With a case-control investigation, one begins with a group of individuals who have the disease of interest (cases) and a group of individuals without the disease (controls). One then explores the present characteristics (in a cross-sectional study) or the history (in a retrospective study) of these two groups for the presence or absence of factors thought to be related to the occurrence of the disease. Obviously, one looks for factors that are distributed differentially among the cases as compared to the controls. In order to evaluate a possible association between a particular disease and a particular attribute, it is always necessary to have a control group against which to compare this association.

With the prospective approach, we begin with a group or cohort exposed to a particular factor(s) and a group not exposed to the specific factor(s). The two groups are observed over time to see how many in each group develop the disease under investigation. The frequency of disease in the cohort exposed to the factor is compared to the frequency in the unexposed cohort.

Since case-control studies provide information relatively quickly and at much lower cost than the prospective approach, most analytical investigations of Parkinson's disease have used the case-control design. In analysing the results of analytical epidemiological studies, we must always consider whether the results are artefactual, i.e. due to differences between the groups other than the factor(s) being studied, and whether the findings are statistically significant, i.e. the possibility that the findings occurred simply on the basis of chance. It is also important to remember that an association should *not* be equated with the cause of the disease. A particular characteristic may be only indirectly related to a biologically significant factor. However, there are a number of features of epidemiological associations which suggest causal inferences. For example, one must consider whether the disease appears to follow exposure to a given agent after an appropriate period of time consistent with current knowledge concerning the latency of the agent's known effects. One must also consider the strength of the association and whether exposure to the given agent appears to lead to the specific neurological disease of interest. If the link between a given factor and a specific disease is consistent with available knowledge of pathogenesis, i.e. there is a plausible biological explanation as to how the factor can cause the disease, a possible aetiological role of the factor is more likely. Finally, one must examine the results of multiple studies to verify the consistency of a reported association. These principles have been applied in several analytical investigations of Parkinson's disease.

Results from prospective studies of the relationship between smoking and mortality from various chronic diseases yielded some unexpected findings: mortality from Parkinson's disease was *inversely* associated with smoking (Hammond, 1966; Kahn, 1966). This finding has since been confirmed in a series of case-control investigations (Nefzger, Quadfasel and Kark, 1968; Kessler and Diamond, 1971; Martilla and Rinne, 1980; Baumann et al., 1980; Haack et al., 1981; Ward et al., 1983; Bharucha et al., 1986). Only one case-control study to date has failed to demonstrate this inverse association (Rajput, 1984). This last investigation was based on smoking histories available in medical records. Unfortunately, such information is not uniformly recorded in general patient histories available for residents of Rochester, Minnesota, where the investigation was conducted. Although some have suggested that some product in cigarette smoke may provide a protective effect against Parkinson's disease (Kessler, 1978), this is not consistent with descriptive epidemiological patterns. Although smoking habits in the USA have been changing dramatically over the last 40–50 years, available data on the incidence of Parkinson's disease indicate stable rates over time (Kurland et al., 1973; Rajput et al., 1984a).

Another interesting observation involves the pre-morbid personality of those with Parkinson's disease (Todes and Lees, 1985). This question has only recently been addressed in case-control studies because of the difficulties in reliably measuring the pre-morbid personality. A case-control study of twin pairs discordant for Parkinson's disease indicated that the affected twin tended to be more 'introverted' and 'self-controlled' (Ward et al., 1983; Eldridge and Rocca, 1986).

Although several studies have suggested the importance of genetic factors in the pathogenesis of Parkinson's disease, the low concordance rates among monozygotic twins implies that heredity plays a minor role (Duvoisin et al., 1981; Ward et al., 1983; Eldridge and Rocca, 1986). Attention has therefore been focused on possible environmental factors. A variety of such factors have been investigated with regard to a possible association with Parkinson's disease. These included other medical conditions (especially infections of the nervous system), a previous history of head injury, vaccinations, exposures to specific drugs or anaesthetic agents, birth order, birth weight, alcohol consumption, coffee consumption etc. There have been no consistent and reproducible findings between studies, however (Eldridge and Rocca, 1986).

The discovery that 1-methyl-4-phenyl-1,2,3,6-tetrahydropyridine (MPTP) can produce a disorder which simulates the clinical features of Parkinson's disease (Burns et al., 1985) has led to renewed interest in the possible role of neurotoxins in the pathogenesis of Parkinson's disease (Calne and Langston, 1983; Snyder, 1984). Based on the findings of a recent study of the frequency of Parkinson's disease in an area near Montreal, Quebec, Canada, Barbeau and his colleagues found an association between disease frequency and pesticide use (Lewin, 1985). In a study of patients with Parkinson's disease with onset before age 41 in Saskatchewan, Canada, Rajput et al. (1984c) found such cases occurred in rural areas more often than expected and that they used underground (well) water. They hypothesized that some agent in the water may be responsible for Parkinson's disease. The findings of these two Canadian studies await confirmation. The stability of the incidence rates in Rochester, Minnesota, would argue against a major aetiological role for a newly introduced toxin, however (Eldridge, Rocca and Ince, 1986). Case-control studies have investigated exposure to potential neurotoxins, but have failed to demonstrate any significant associations (Eldridge and Rocca, 1986). Similarly, although manganese intoxication is a recognized cause of parkinsonism, it has not been implicated as a major cause in analytical investigations (Kurtzke and Kurland, 1984; Eldridge and Rocca, 1986).

Based on the increasing age of cases seen at a given medical institution, Poskanzer and Schwab (1963) hypothesized that the majority of cases were the result of a prior epidemic of encephalitis lethargica. This led them to predict a decline in the incidence of new cases. Stable incidence rates from Rochester, Minnesota, contradict this theory, however (Kurtzke and Kurland, 1984; Rajput et al., 1984a). Furthermore, the proportion of incident cases classifiable as 'postencephalitic' has been declining among the Rochester, Minnesota, population (Rajput et al., 1984a).

Further analytical investigations are being conducted in an attempt to discover as yet unrecognized factors associated with an increased risk of Parkinson's disease. Findings of such studies will hopefully provide much needed information for the development of prevention strategies for this major public health problem.

EPIDEMIOLOGY OF OTHER MOVEMENT DISORDERS

Parkinsonism–dementia of Guam

Parkinsonism–dementia is observed predominantly among the Chamorro people of Guam in the western Pacific and has been reported to account for 7% of all adult deaths in that population (Kurtzke and Kurland, 1984). This is the same group in which amyotrophic lateral sclerosis occurs in very high frequency. Some patients show evidence of both disorders, leading some to speculate that the two conditions may represent different manifestations of the same underlying disease. Careful studies on Guam over many years indicate that this phenomenon cannot be explained simply on the basis of a genetic factor, and several searches for environmental causes have been undertaken (Kurtzke and Kurland, 1984).

Essential tremor

There have been five published investigations reporting the descriptive epidemiology of essential tremor among well-defined populations in four countries: Papua-New Guinea (Hornabrook and Nagurney, 1976), Sweden (Larsson and Sjogren, 1960), Finland (Rautakorpi, 1978), the biracial population of Copiah

County, Mississippi (USA) (Haerer, Anderson and Schoenberg, 1982) and the population of Rochester, Minnesota (USA) (Rajput et al., 1984b). The Scandinavian investigations found essential tremor to be more common among men than among women, while the Papua-New Guinea and Copiah County studies reported the reverse. With the exception of the last report (which did not provide age-specific prevalence figures), all of the investigations found that for broad age groups the prevalence ratio of essential tremor increases with age, for both men and women. Although the age-specific pattern of prevalence ratios is similar in all studies for which such data are available, the actual magnitude of the prevalence figures differs considerably. If we restrict our comparisons to cases over the age of 39 years and age adjust the reported data, we obtain the figures shown in *Table 3.4*. These disparate figures cannot be readily explained and may be the result of different definitions of essential tremor and variations in study procedures. Furthermore, it is possible that some of the geographical areas were selected for study because they were suspected of having unusually high frequencies of essential tremor.

Table 3.4 Prevalence ratios (ages 40+ years) of essential tremor from selected studies

Population	Date	Cases per 100 000	
		Observed	Age-adjusted*
Xa-Sjo, Sweden Larsson and Sjogren, 1960	1950	3725.4	3975.0
Kamano, Auyana, Gadsup, Tairora, and Agarabe populations, Papua-New Guinea Hornabrook and Nagurney, 1976	1970–72	1635.1	1976.8
Sakyla and Koylio, Finland Rautakorpi, 1978	Jan. 1, 1973 (ages 40–64) Jan. 1, 1974 (ages 65+)	5565.1	5565.1
Copiah County, Mississippi Haerer, Anderson and Schoenberg, 1982	Jan. 1, 1978	414.6	381.0

*Age-adjusted to Finnish population by indirect method.

Based on a review of medical records for residents of Rochester, Minnesota, for 1935–79, Rajput et al. (1984b) were able to provide age- and sex-specific incidence rates. The overall incidence rate is 15.6 per 100 000 per year and is virtually the same for either sex. The incidence rates rise with age. The investigators reported no increased risk for subsequent Parkinson's disease or hypertension among the incident cases of essential tremor, nor was there any difference between expected and observed survival of identified cases. Rajput et al. (1984b) also measured the prevalence for this population as of January 1, 1979 (305.6 per 100 000; age adjusted to the 1970 US White population). Unfortunately, the information provided in the report concerning the community of Rochester does not permit comparison with the age-adjusted data given in *Table 3.4*.

Torsion dystonia

There have as yet been no formal community-based surveys of torsion dystonia (Kurtzke and Kurland, 1984). Although Larsson and Sjogren (1966) reported clinical and genetic information on 121 cases from a rural area of northern Sweden, reliable prevalence figures cannot be derived from these data. Based on his review of available reports, Eldridge estimated the prevalence ratios of torsion dystonia for various segments of the US population as follows: 3/1 000 000 for the total US; 25/1 000 000 for the US Jewish population; 0.3/1 000 000 for the US Black population (Eldridge, 1970). These estimates are not derived from actual population surveys, however.

Huntington's disease

Mortality data for Huntington's disease have been extensively analysed (Krutzke and Kurland, 1984). Death rates for US Whites are approximately 1.6/1 000 000 per year. Corresponding rates for non-Whites in the US are only one-third this figure. Rates reported from Japan are also considerably lower than figures for US Whites. Available morbidity data are consistent with the patterns derived from the mortality tabulations. The cluster of Huntington's disease in the Lake Maricaibo region of Venezuela (estimated prevalence ratio of 7/1000; Kurtzke and Kurland, 1984) has been of enormous importance in the recent advances in the molecular genetics of Huntington's disease.

Wilson's disease

The only available morbidity data for Wilson's disease are provided in a study of the Icelandic population (Gudmundsson, 1969). The prevalence ratio was 1.6/100 000 and the incidence rate was 0.2 per 100 000 per year.

CONCLUSIONS

In the last thirty years there have been several studies reporting morbidity rates for Parkinson's disease. Prevalence ratios from these investigations document that this disorder is a major cause of morbidity among the elderly. Data from one population (Rochester, Minnesota, USA) indicate virtually no change in the incidence rates over a period of 35 years. Whatever is the primary cause of Parkinson's disease has been present in the non-industrialized community of Rochester for many years. In general, reported prevalence figures have been higher among Caucasians when compared to Black or Oriental populations. Studies show an increasing prevalence ratio with age, and many reveal a higher risk for men. However, these investigations usually relied on records of health care providers (mainly hospitals and medical practitioners) in the identification of cases. Excluded from the resulting morbidity data are individuals who failed to seek medical attention for their symptoms or individuals who were improperly diagnosed. Among the various investigations, the differences in study methods, levels of case ascertainment, and definitions of Parkinson's disease could account for the variation in the reported morbidity estimates. To minimize these problems a standard methodology using a door-to-door survey technique and uniform diagnostic criteria was developed. This study design was implemented in surveys conducted in a biracial population (Blacks and Whites) in the USA and in urban populations of the People's Republic of China. In contrast to earlier investigations, the US study revealed no substantial differences in age-adjusted prevalence ratios by race. The prevalence ratios derived from the sample population of 63 195 in urban areas of China are lower than the US figures based on the same methods of case identification. As this standardized methodology is implemented in other parts of the world, more accurate information will be obtained on the actual international distribution of Parkinson's disease. Analytical studies of factors related to an increased risk of Parkinson's disease have revealed an inverse association with cigarette smoking, i.e. smokers have a lower risk. Available epidemiological evidence does not support a direct protective effect of smoking, however. Further such investigations are required to discover as yet unknown factors which heighten the risk of this major health problem.

ACKNOWLEDGEMENT

The author wishes to thank Ian C. Schoenberg for help in preparing this manuscript.

References

BAUMANN, R. J., JAMESON, H. D., McKEAN, H. E. et al. (1980) Cigarette smoking and Parkinson's disease. I. A comparison of cases with matched neighbors. *Neurology*, **30**, 839–843

BHARUCHA, N. E., STOKES, L., SCHOENBERG, B. S. et al. (1986) A case-control study of twin pairs discordant for Parkinson's disease: A search for environmental risk factors. *Neurology*, **36**, 284–288

BREWIS, M., POSKANZER, D. C., ROLLAND, C. et al. (1966) Neurological disease in an English city. *Acta Neurologica Scandinavica*, Suppl. 24, **42**

BURNS, R. S., LEWITT, P. A., PAKKENBERG, H. et al. (1985) The clinical syndrome of striatal dopamine deficiency: MPTP-induced parkinsonism. *New England Journal of Medicine*, **312**, 1418–1421

BROMAN, T. (1963) Parkinson's syndrome, prevalence and incidence in Goteborg. *Acta Neurologica Scandinavica*, Suppl. 4, **39**, 95–101

CALNE, D. B. and LANGSTON, J. W. (1983) Hypothesis: Aetiology of Parkinson's disease. *Lancet*, **ii**, 1457–1459

CHANDRA, V., BHARUCHA, N. E. and SCHOENBERG, B. S. (1984) Mortality data for the U.S. for deaths due to and related to twenty neurologic diseases. *Neuroepidemiology*, **3**, 149–168

DUVOISIN, R. C., ELDRIDGE, R., WILLIAMS, A. et al. (1981) Twin study of Parkinson disease. *Neurology*, **31**, 77–80

DUVOISIN, R. C. and SCHWEITZER, M. D. (1966) Paralysis agitans mortality in England and Wales, 1855–1962. *British Journal of Preventive Medicine*, **20**, 27–33

ELDRIDGE, R. (1970) The torsion dystonias: Literature review and genetic and clinical studies. *Neurology*, **20**, Issue 11, part 2, 1–78

ELDRIDGE, R. and ROCCA, W. A. (1986) Parkinson disease: Etiologic considerations. In *The Genetic Basis of Common Disease*. Ed. by R. A. King, J. I. Rotter and A. G. Motulsky. New York: McGraw-Hill (in press)

ELDRIDGE, R., ROCCA, W. A. and INCE, S. E. (1986) Parkinson's disease: Evidence against a toxic etiology and for an alternative theory. In *MPTP: A Neurotoxin Producing A Parkinsonian Syndrome*. Ed. by S. P. Markey, N. Castagnoli, M. Trevor and I. J. Kopin. New York: Academic Press (in press)

GUDMUNDSSON, K. R. (1967) A clinical survey of parkinsonism in Iceland. *Acta Neurologica Scandinavica*, Suppl. 33, **43**, 9–61

GUDMUNDSSON, K. R. (1969) The prevalence and occurrence of some rare neurological diseases in Iceland. *Acta Neurologica Scandinavica*, **45**, 114–118

HAACK, D. G., BAUMANN, R. J., McKEAN, H. E. et al. (1981) Nicotine exposure and Parkinson's disease. *American Journal of Epidemiology*, **114**, 191–200

HAERER, A. F., ANDERSON, D. W. and SCHOENBERG, B. S. (1982) Prevalence of essential tremor. *Archives of Neurology*, **39**, 750–751

HAMMOND, E. C. (1966) Smoking in relation to the death rates of one million men and women. In *Epidemiological Study of Cancer and Other Chronic Diseases*, pp. 127–204. National Cancer Institute Monograph 19. Washington, DC: US Government Printing Office

HARADA, H., NISHIKAWA, S. and TAKAHASHI, K. (1983) Epidemiology of Parkinson's disease in a Japanese city. *Archives of Neurology*, **40**, 151–154

HORNABROOK, R. W. and NAGURNEY, J. T. (1976) Essential tremor in Papua New Guinea. *Brain*, **99**, 659–672

JENKINS, A. C. (1966) Epidemiology of parkinsonism in Victoria. *Medical Journal of Australia*, **2**, 496–502

KAHN, H. A. (1966) The Dorn study of smoking and mortality among US veterans; report on eight and one-half years of observation. In *Epidemiologic Approaches to the Study of Cancer and Other Chronic Diseases*, pp. 1–125. National Cancer Institute Monograph 19. Washington, DC: US Government Printing Office

KESSLER, I. I. (1972) Epidemiologic studies of Parkinson's disease. III. A community-based survey. *American Journal of Epidemiology*, **96**, 242–254

KESSLER, I. I. (1978) Parkinson's disease in epidemiologic perspective. In *Advances in Neurology*, Vol. 19. *Neurological Epidemiology: Principles and Clinical Applications*. Ed. by B. S. Schoenberg. pp. 355–384. New York: Raven Press

KESSLER, I. I. and DIAMOND, E. L. (1971) Epidemiologic studies of Parkinson's disease. I. Smoking and Parkinson's disease: A survey and explanatory hypothesis. *American Journal of Epidemiology*, **94**, 16–25

KURLAND, L. T., HAUSER, W. A., OKAZAKI, H. et al. (1969) Epidemiologic studies of parkinsonism with special reference to the cohort hypothesis. In *Proceedings of the Third Symposium on Parkinsonism*. Ed. by F. J. Gillingham and J. M. Donaldson. pp. 12–16. Edinburgh: E. and S. Livingstone

KURLAND, T. L., KURTZKE, J. F., GOLDBERG, I. D. et al. (1973) Parkinsonism. In *Epidemiology of Neurologic and Sense Organ Disorders*. Ed. by L. T. Kurland, J. F. Kurtzke and I. D. Goldberg. pp. 41–63. Cambridge, Massachusetts: Harvard University Press

KURTZKE, J. F. and KURLAND, L. T. (1984) The epidemiology of neurologic disease. In *Clinical Neurology*, Vol. 4, Chap. 66. Ed. by A. B. Baker and L. H. Baker. pp. 55–60. Philadelphia: Harper and Row

LARSSON, T. and SJOGREN, T. (1960) Essential tremor: A clinical and genetic population study. *Acta Neurologica Scandinavica*, Suppl. 14, **36**, 1–176

LARSSON, T. and SJOGREN, T. (1966) Dystonia musculorum deformans: A genetic and clinical population study of 121 cases. *Acta Neurologica Scandinavica*, Suppl. 17, **42**, 3–233

LEWIN, R. (1985) Parkinson's disease: An environmental cause? *Science*, **229**, 257–258

LI, S. C., SCHOENBERG, B. S., WANG, C. C. et al. (1985) A prevalence survey of Parkinson's disease and other movement disorders in the People's Republic of China. *Archives of Neurology*, **42**, 655–657

MARTILLA, R. J. and RINNE, U. K. (1976) Epidemiology of Parkinson's disease in Finland. *Acta Neurologica Scandinavica*, **53**, 81–102

MARTILLA, R. J. and RINNE, U. K. (1980) Smoking and Parkinson's disease. *Acta Neurologica Scandinavica*, **62**, 322–325

NEFZGER, M. D., QUADFASEL, F. A. and KARK, V. C. (1968) A retrospective study of smoking in Parkinson's disease. *American Journal of Epidemiology*, **88**, 149–158

OSUNTOKUN, B. O., ADEUJA, A. O. G., SCHOENBERG, B. S. et al. (1986) Neurological disorders in Nigerian Africans: A community-based study. Submitted for publication

POSKANZER, D. C. and SCHWAB, R. S. (1963) Cohort analysis of Parkinson's disease: evidence for a single etiology related to sub-clinical infection about 1920. *Journal of Chronic Diseases*, **16**, 961–973

RAJPUT, A. H. (1984) Epidemiology of Parkinson's disease. *Canadian Journal of Neurological Sciences*, Suppl. 1, **11**, 156–160

RAJPUT, A. H., OFFORD, K. P., BEARD, C. M. et al. (1984a) Epidemiology of parkinsonism: Incidence, classification, and mortality. *Annals of Neurology*, **16**, 278–282

RAJPUT, A. H., OFFORD, K. P., BEARD, C. M. et al. (1984b) Essential tremor in Rochester, Minnesota: a 45-year study. *Journal of Neurology, Neurosurgery and Psychiatry*, **47**, 466–470

RAJPUT, A. H., STERN, W., CHRIST, A. et al. (1984c) Abstract – Etiology of Parkinson's disease: environmental factors. *Neurology*, Suppl. 1, **34**, 207

RAUTAKORPI, I. (1978) *Essential Tremor: An Epidemiological, Clinical, and Genetic Study.* Research Report No. 12. Turku, Finland, Department of Neurology, University of Turku

ROSENWAIKE, I., YAFFE, N. and SAGI, P. (1980) The recent decline in mortality of the extreme aged: An analysis of statistical data. *American Journal of Public Health*, **70**, 1074–1080

SCHOENBERG, B. S. (1978) Principles of neurological epidemiology. In *Advances in Neurology*, Vol. 19. *Neurological Epidemiology: Principles and Clinical Applications.* Ed. by B. S. Schoenberg. pp. 11–54. New York: Raven Press

SCHOENBERG, B. S. (1981) Neurologic disease in the elderly: Epidemiologic considerations. *Seminars in Neurology*, **1**, 5–12

SCHOENBERG, B. S. (1982) Clinical neuroepidemiology in developing countries: Neurology with few neurologists. *Neuroepidemiology*, **1**, 137–142

SCHOENBERG, B. S. (1983) Neuroepidemiologic generalizations: High tax on importing data, low tax on importing principles. *Neuroepidemiology*, **2**, 117–120

SCHOENBERG, B. S., ANDERSON, D. W. and HAERER, A. F. (1985) Prevalence of Parkinson's disease in the biracial population of Copiah County, Mississippi. *Neurology*, **35**, 841–845

SIEGEL, J. S. (1980) Recent and prospective demographic trends for the elderly population and some implications for health care. In *Second Conference on the Epidemiology of Aging.* Ed. by S. G. Haynes and M. Feinleib. pp. 289–315. Washington, DC: US Government Printing Office

SNYDER, S. H. (1984) Clues to aetiology of Parkinson's disease from a toxin. *Nature*, **311**, 514–515

STAMP, J. (1929) *Some Economic Factors in Modern Life.* pp. 258–259. London: P. S. King and Son Ltd

SWEET, R. D. and McDOWELL, F. H. (1975) Five years' treatment of Parkinson's disease with levodopa: Therapeutic results and survival of 100 patients. *Annals of Internal Medicine*, **83**, 456–463

TODES, C. J. and LEES, A. J. (1985) The pre-morbid personality of patients with Parkinson's disease. *Journal of Neurology, Neurosurgery and Psychiatry*, **48**, 97–100

WARD, C. D., DUVOISIN, R. C., INCE, S. E. *et al.* (1983) Parkinson's disease in 65 pairs of twins and in a set of quadruplets. *Neurology*, **33**, 815–825

4
Molecular genetics of movement disorders
Xandra O. Breakefield and Susan Bressman

INTRODUCTION

Recent attention to the genetics of neurological diseases stems from advances in molecular genetics that allow inheritance itself to be used as a tracking scheme for identifying defective genes causing these diseases. Effective use of these genetic schemes requires accurate clinical diagnosis, careful choice of families for study and clear understanding of the genetic principles involved. Many of the movement disorders are well suited for this type of analysis, as they follow patterns of inheritance indicating defects in single genes, large families with multiple affected members are available, and the symptoms are readily discernible. The goal of genetic studies is ultimately to determine the defective molecule that underlies the aetiology of a disease. In fact, these studies form only the first step in the logical pursuit of this goal. In most cases genetic analysis will elucidate only where the gene is in the genome and serve to label the defective gene in affected families. This information, itself, can be used in genetic counselling for determining carriers of the defective gene and affected fetuses *in utero*. To proceed from locational to causative information will require the collaborative efforts of neurochemists, neurophysiologists and neurologists, as well as molecular geneticists.

This chapter will focus on clinical considerations important for molecular genetic studies, and on the genetic methodology itself. Examples will be given of genetic research carried out for several neurological diseases associated with abnormal involuntary movements originating in the basal ganglia. Several excellent books are available which review symptoms, disease classification and patterns of inheritance of neurological diseases – *see* Adams and Lyon (1982), Baraitser (1982) and Ionasescu and Zellweger (1983). For discussion of general genetic principles *see* Stanbury *et al.* (1983) and Rosenberg, Hansen and Breakefield (1985).

CLINICAL AND GENETIC CONSIDERATIONS
Clinical considerations

The most critical clinical aspects for molecular genetic analyses of human diseases involve diagnosis and disease classification. Simply stated, the genetic schemes are designed to find a single defective gene responsible for a particular disease, and they will not work well if more than one defective gene, or if environmental factors, can produce the 'same' disease state. For this reason it is best to focus attention on the largest affected family available, as all affected members will very likely have the same aetiology. It is difficult to rule out environmental factors, but if the pattern of inheritance is clearcut, e.g. autosomal recessive, autosomal dominant or X-linked, there is a strong suggestion that a single defective gene is responsible. This interpretation must be modulated by considerations of how frequently the same symptoms can be produced by drugs, trauma and other environmental factors, and by possible problems in interpreting the pattern of inheritance.

Diagnosis even within a family must be rigorous, as one unaffected individual misclassified as affected can rule out the possibility of finding the responsible gene. Also, affected members may deny the disease and require non-intrusive testing to elicit symptoms. To this end, all family members should receive a careful neurological examination and provide a medical history. Videotapes should be made of all affected and possibly affected members to allow confirmation of their clinical status by other neurologists. Symptoms should be evaluated individually and rated in severity. There is always the possibility that some of the symptoms may be caused by environmental factors or another genetic problem in the family, or may not always be expressed in a given genetic disease, so it could be important to differentiate different subsets of symptoms for analysis. Information regarding age of onset should also be obtained to evaluate which asymptomatic individuals are still at risk of developing the disease. Although it may be difficult to obtain this information, since it depends on knowledge of the disease and memory of family members, estimates of the range and mean age at onset are helpful for linkage analysis.

Genetic considerations

Some simple principles of genetics underlie the clinical considerations discussed above. First of all, the same disease state can be caused by different mutations at the same gene locus or at different gene loci. This is referred to as 'genetic heterogeneity'. The latter can present a serious problem for linkage analysis and is the primary reason for focusing on single families where possible. Information can be compiled across families with confidence only if the disease is rare, restricted to a particular ethnic population and/or diagnostically distinctive. Second, even within a family where all cases of the disease are caused by the same gene defect, the disease may manifest itself with different subsets of symptoms and different degrees of severity, termed 'variable expressivity'. In dominantly inherited diseases, defective genes may not be expressed at all in some individuals carrying them, or may cause only minor neurological problems (formes frustes). This is termed 'incomplete gene penetrance' and probably reflects the interaction of other modifying genes or environmental influences on phenotypic expression of the defective gene.

The mode of inheritance of a disease state can be difficult to interpret for a number of reasons: human pedigrees tend to be small; rare recessive conditions appear infrequently and may be difficult to distinguish from environmental causes; incomplete gene penetrance in dominantly inherited diseases may make them difficult to distinguish from recessive diseases with a relatively high frequency of carriers; some diseases have a high rate of new mutations; and many diseases interfere with reproductive fitness. In general, the following guidelines are useful in examining pedigrees. For autosomal dominant disorders, successive generations should be affected with about half the children of an affected parent having the disease and with males and females being equally affected. New mutations may produce the disease state in a single generation, and hence there is an increase in the frequency of these diseases with advanced paternal age. Dominant diseases tend to be characterized by onset in childhood or adult life, variable expressivity and incomplete penetrance. For autosomal recessive disorders, the disease should appear in the offspring of two unaffected carriers of the same defective gene at a frequency of 25%, with males and females being equally affected. The rarer the disease gene in the population, the more likely that the disease will result from consanguineous marriages. These diseases usually present from birth or in early childhood, and tend to have more uniform clinical features. For X-linked disorders, most of which are 'recessive', the pattern of inheritance is more obvious with many more males than females being affected and no father-to-son transmission. Female carriers have a 50% chance of producing affected male offspring. Fortunately, it is possible to consider several different modes of inheritance within a family in linkage analysis if the pattern is not obvious.

The terms 'dominant' and 'recessive' can cause confusion as they can vary for the same disease state depending on the level of expression being considered. Clinically, dominant refers to a condition where one copy of a defective gene produces the disease state, and recessive when two copies of the same defective gene or one copy without a normal counterpart are needed to cause the condition. At the cellular or biochemical level, however, if the product of the defective gene can be detected, the phenotypic state is referred to as co-dominant. At the DNA level, since all defective genes can ultimately be distinguished from their normal counterparts, they are all co-dominant.

CHROMOSOMAL LOCATION OF DEFECTIVE GENES

Clues to chromosomal location

Establishing the location of a defective gene in the human genome is important in providing genetic counselling, as well as serving as a first step in the identification of the nature and function of the gene. If the disease follows an X-linked pattern of inheritance, the search for the defective gene is limited to that chromosome which represents about 8% of the coding information of the total genome. Since the X-chromosome is almost completely saturated with marker DNA sequences (*see below*), the search for the defective gene is simplified. For autosomal conditions the search must cover the rest of the genome and any information that can limit or focus the search is useful. Such information might be the chromosomal map position of a mutation causing a similar condition in other mammals, as chromosomal regions have been redistributed in blocks during the evolution of species, and thus a particular region, in for instance the mouse, corresponds to a comparable region in humans (Roderick *et al.*, 1984). Another source of information can be chromosomal rearrangements that result in an imbalance in genetic information. Chromosomal imbalances associated with monosomy or trisomy of discrete chromosomal regions, which cause neurological abnormalities, can implicate these regions. Usually, if the imbalances are large enough to be

36   Molecular genetics of movement disorders

visible microscopically, they result in a plethora of developmental anomalies. Examples of these rearrangements include translocations involving the short (p) arm of the X-chromosome which have resulted in gene deletions causing Duchenne's muscular dystrophy (Monaco et al., 1985); discrete deletions in a specific region of chromosome 13q causing hereditary retinoblastoma (Sparkes et al., 1980); and translocations involving chromosome 21q which define the subregion of this chromosome that, when present in three copies, is responsible for mental retardation in Down's syndrome (Hagemeijer and Smit, 1977; Kitsiou-Tzeli et al., 1984).

Linkage analysis

The main breakthrough provided by molecular genetics has been in expanding the capacity of linkage analysis to search the whole genome, so that a defective gene cannot elude detection (Botstein et al., 1980; Davies, 1981; White et al., 1985). Linkage analysis is based on the observation that the closer two genes are to each other in the linear sequence of a chromosome, the more likely they are to stay together through meiosis and be transmitted in the same gamete. During meiosis there are an average of three recombinational events between each set of homologous chromosomes serving to redistribute genes between them. If the homologous copies (alleles) of a gene can be distinguished from each other, one can assess how frequently each of them is transmitted with specific alleles at other gene loci. In the case of an inherited disease, one looks for the frequency with which a particular disease state (caused by a defective allele at one gene locus) co-inherits with alleles at other loci, thereby determining whether the genes are close to each other in the genome.

Linkage analysis has traditionally been carried out by distinguishing alleles for genes coding for proteins on the basis of variations in DNA sequence that affect

Undigested DNA Sequences	Type of change	Length of fragments hybridizing to probe (kb)
		3, 4
	single b.p. substitution	3, 6
	deletion	3, 3
	insertion	3, 5
	inversion	3, 2

Figure 4.1 Hypothetical changes in DNA sequence that could cause variations in restriction-fragment lengths. (From Rosenberg, Hansen and Breakefield (1985) with permission of the Publishers.)

Chromosomal location of defective genes 37

(a)

(b)

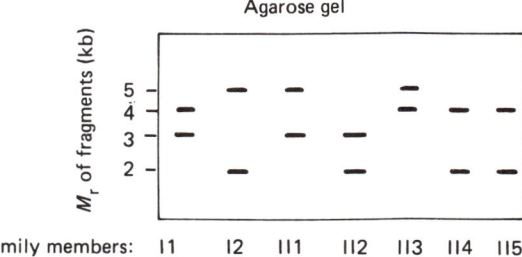

(c)

Figure 4.2 Family with autosomal recessive disease: theoretical diagram of the inheritance of mutant alleles that cause a disease and the use of RFLPs near these alleles to identify their presence in family members. (*a*) Shaded symbols, affected carriers; half-shaded, unaffected carriers; clear, unaffected non-carriers. Chromosomes A, B, C, and D, homologous copies of the same autosome. (●) Centromere; (□) normal allele; (■) mutant allele. (*b*) Theoretical positions of specific restriction endonuclease cleavage sites (↓) in the DNA around responsible gene (□■) from different chromosomes and sizes of DNA fragments generated by cleavage and hybridization to a cloned DNA probe (□). (*c*) DNA isolated from family members, digested with restriction endonuclease and resolved by agarose gel electrophoresis. The position of fragments containing the responsible gene is determined by hybridization to a radioactively labelled DNA probe, followed by autoradiography. The allelic contributions from each parent can be distinguished on the basis of the fragment size that hybridizes to the probe. If, as in this ideal example, the DNA probe hybridizes to DNA sequences within or very near to the gene of interest, there is essentially no chance of recombination between them, and a specific fragment will identify the mutant allele. (From Rosenberg, Hansen and Breakefield (1985) with permission of the Publishers.)

biochemical or immunological properties of the protein. The limitation in the use of protein polymorphisms is that analyses require a number of different immunological and electrophoretic techniques, only a relatively small number of genes can be examined, and the frequency of polymorphisms among alleles is relatively low.

Molecular genetics has expanded the number of 'gene loci' that can be used by being able to recognize the many DNA sequences represented once or several times in the haploid genome by hybridization to cloned probes of genomic or cDNA. Human probes are usually most useful as they hybridize most efficiently with human genomic sequences, but probes from other species, which have a high degree of homology to corresponding human sequences, can also be used. The number of different alleles that can be distinguished at a given loci is also increased by DNA technology. Alleles are distinguished by discrete variations in DNA sequence that alter cutting sites for restriction endonucleases (*Figure 4.1*). Such variations can be visualized by cutting genomic DNA with restriction endonucleases and hybridizing fragments to a given DNA probe (*Figures 4.2* and *4.3*).

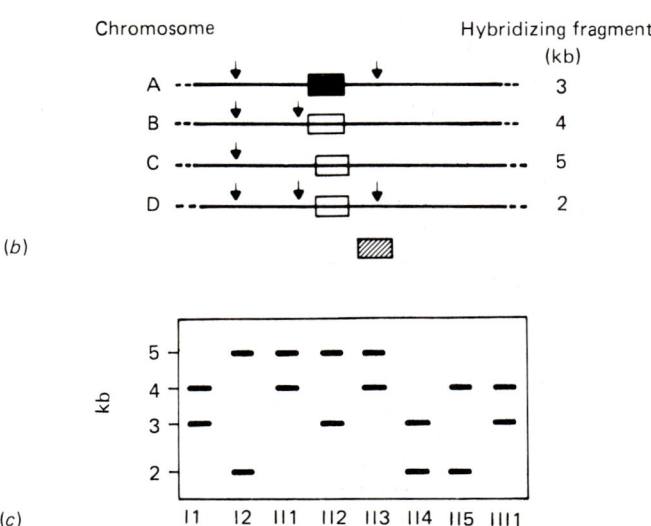

Figure 4.3 Family with autosomal dominant disease. See caption to *Figure 4.2* for symbols. (From Rosenberg, Hansen and Breakefield (1985) with permission of the Publishers.)

When such variations occur relatively frequently among alleles in the human population, they are referred to as polymorphisms. Hence, the term 'restriction fragment length polymorphism' (RFLP) refers to the way alleles are distinguished using DNA probes.

The frequency of variations in unique DNA sequence among alleles is relatively low – about one nucleotide variation per 100 nucleotides (Neel, 1984). These variations are more common in non-coding, as compared to coding, regions of the genome, as the latter have been more highly conserved during evolution. The more frequently an RFLP appears for a particular gene in the human population, the more useful it is in studying families in general. By screening for RFLPs using the 100-or-so restriction endonucleases in common usage, it is usually possible to mark alleles for any given gene within a family. Although it is not necessary to know the chromosomal location of the sequences used in linkage analysis, this information eventually becomes critical in helping to establish how many 'genes' the DNA probe detects in the human genome and, if more than one, whether they are located on different chromosomes, or how close they are on the same chromosome. Theoretical examples of RFLPs and tight linkage between marker DNA sequences and diseases causing recessively and dominantly inherited diseases, are illustrated in *Figures 4.2* and *4.3*, respectively. Current information on marker genes for inherited neurological diseases is presented in *Table 4.1*.

Table 4.1 Neurological diseases for which linked markers have been identified

Chromosome*	Disease
1	Charcot–Marie-Tooth disease
3	G_{M1} gangliosidosis
	Morquio's disease
4	Huntington's disease
5	Sandhoff's disease
6	Spinocerebellar ataxia
11	Acute porphyria
	Wilm's tumour with mental retardation
13	Retinoblastoma, Wilson's disease
15	Prader–Willi syndrome
	Tay–Sachs disease
17	Pompe's disease
18	Amyloid polyneuropathy
19	Myotonic dystrophy
22	Metachromatic leucodystrophy
	Hurler–Scheie syndrome
X	Muscular dystrophy
	Adrenoleucodystrophy
	Lesch–Nyhan syndrome
	Fragile X-syndrome
	Retinitis pigmentosa
	Hunt's disease
	Menkes' kinky hair disease
	Charcot–Marie-Tooth neuropathy 2
	Albinism – deafness
	Cerebellar ataxia
	Pelizaeus–Merzbacher disease

* Rowland, 1983; Rosenberg *et al.*, 1985.

Figure 4.4 Repeated DNA sequences used to generate restriction fragment length polymorphisms: theoretical diagram. (*a*) Varying numbers of repeated units (R1–RN) of two different sets ('1' and '2') of homologous chromosomes from two individuals. Arrows indicate restriction endonuclease cutting sites. (*b*) Autoroadiogram showing size of genomic fragments hybridizing to a probe for the repeated unit after cutting genomic DNA from individuals 1 and 2 with this restriction endonuclease. (*See also Figure 4.2c.*) (Modified from Jeffreys, Wilson and Lay Thein (1985).)

In the initial paper describing the use of RFLPs in linkage analysis (Botstein et al., 1980), it was estimated that about 165 probes for unique sequence DNA spaced at intervals of 20 centimorgans (cM; 20% recombination per meiotic event) would be sufficient to detect any disease gene within a recombination distance of 10 cM (10% recombination). In practice, a much larger number of probes is needed at the present time since: (a) it will take a number of years more before probes detecting useful polymorphisms are available at appropriate distances in the genome; (b) the original estimate assumed a single linear stretch of total genomic DNA, whereas the DNA is actually distributed among 22 autosomes and X- and Y-chromosomes; (c) within a particular family it may be hard to obtain statistically significant linkage information out to 10 cM on either side of a given probe.

Two general strategies can be employed at the present time in linkage analysis of a particular disease state. First, a set of probes can be used that hybridize to sequences distributed at known linkage intervals along a particular chromosome. One can then assess linkage of the disease locus to several other loci simultaneously by multipoint analysis which expands the extent of chromosomal material that can be examined (Lathrop et al., 1984). Sets of probes are being developed for different chromosome regions and are now available, for example for 11p (Kittur et al., 1985), 21q (Watkins et al., 1985) and the X-chromosome (Monaco et al., 1985). Second, highly polymorphic regions of DNA can be used which increase the chance of carrying out informative linkage analysis in any family. These regions can occur through the presence of multiple polymorphic restriction endonuclease sites within them, e.g. for the β-globin gene (Orkin and Kazazian, 1984). Alternatively, they may result from the presence of variable numbers of short, tandemly repeated sequences in the genome (Jeffreys, Wilson and Lay Thein, 1985). By using a DNA probe homologous to the repeated unit and cutting genomic DNA with a restriction endonuclease that does not have a site within this unit, it is possible to distinguish many RFLPs at a given locus (*Figure 4.4*). Further, the same repeated unit may be present at a number of different places in the genome, so a number of chromosomal regions may be assessed at the same time. There is so much variation among individuals in the length of fragments hybridizing to these repeated units that the relative positions of fragments can be used to uniquely 'fingerprint' individuals.

Families

The type of family appropriate for linkage analysis varies, depending on the disease being studied and the chromosomal location of the gene causing the disease. For autosomally inherited diseases it is easiest to analyse a single, large family with multiple affected members where there is clear evidence of a dominant mode of transmission, phenocopies of the disease are rare, onset of the disease is relatively early in life and reproductive fitness is not affected (*Table 4.2*). A theoretical estimate can be made of how large such a family must be to confirm or exclude linkage to marker sequences within 10 cM of the disease gene based on the number of 'informative gametes' in the family (Kidd and Ott, 1984; Breakefield et al., 1986). Informative gametes in a dominant family are defined as those produced by an affected parent who is heterozygous for the marker sequence where both alleles can be distinguished, e.g. *a/b*, and where the other parent is unaffected and homozygous for either of those alleles or heterozygous for different alleles at the marker locus, e.g. *a/a, b/b, c/c* or *c/d*. Such a family would require 15–20 offspring

Table 4.2 Factors making a disease amenable to linkage analysis

Single gene defect
Mendelian inheritance
  (X-linked or autosomal dominant easier
  than autosomal recessive)
Large pedigrees available
Early age of onset
Defect does not interfere with reproductive fitness
Complete gene penetrance
Diagnosis clearcut
No phenocopies

of affected individuals, implying that the family would probably have to consist of 50–200 members depending on its structure.

If the pattern of inheritance is recessive (and not X-linked), the number of informative gametes per family size will be smaller as the status of individuals with respect to the disease gene is only known for individuals with the disease or those producing affected offspring. X-linked recessive disease genes are easier to track as all male carriers of the defective gene will be affected. However, unless a female has produced more than one affected son, or her sister or mother has also produced one, it will not be clear whether she is a gene carrier or whether the mutation arose *de novo* in her germline. In some cases of recessive and X-linked disease, it may be necessary to pool information from more than one family manifesting similar clinical syndromes, in order to obtain a sufficient number of informative gametes. Since the same syndrome can be caused by mutations at different loci, it may be important to carry out linkage analysis on subsets of the families, which will require more families. If linkage to a marker sequence is found in all or a subset of families, it will indicate that in these cases the syndrome is caused by the same defective gene.

Lod scores

Linkage data is usually evaluated by the lod score method using the FORTRAN computer program LIPED (Ott, 1976; Hodge *et al.*, 1979). Basically, the likelihood is determined that alleles at two different gene loci are distributed to the offspring in the pattern observed within a given pedigree if they are linked at different distances (from 0 to 50 cM), as compared to if they are not linked (>50 cM). A very large ratio of these two expectations favours linkage. The lod score is the logarithm of the probability of obtaining the pedigree at a given recombination distance (<50 cM) divided by the probability at 50 cM (50% recombination or random assortment). The logarithmic value is used so that information can be summed among families as appropriate. As a general practice, lod scores of >+3 are considered highly indicative of linkage (equivalent to 1000 times the chance that the two genes are linked at a given distance compared to their being unlinked) and those of <−2 (1/100th the chance) are taken to rule out linkage. It should be noted that it is easier to exclude regions closer to the marker sequence as compared to those further away (*see* Sutton, 1975, for further discussion of lod scores).

In linkage analysis it is important to include correction factors for variable age-of-onset, reduced gene penetrance, and frequency of phenocopies so that unaffected family members can be weighted as to their likelihood of carrying the defective gene. The frequency of the defective gene in the population should also be set at a realistic level based on the prevalence of the disease in the ethnic group of the family being studied.

NATURE OF DEFECTIVE GENES

Correlation with neurochemical data

Of the 50 000–100 000 or so genes thought to be expressed in the nervous system (Chaudhari and Hahn, 1983), biochemical and/or immunological information is available on only several hundred of the gene products. A large number of gene products have been compared in patients with inherited neurological diseases and normals using tissues, such as skin fibroblasts, blood cells, serum, CSF and nerve or brain biopsies, as well as autopsy specimens of nervous tissue. These studies are limited by which proteins are expressed in these accessible tissues, as well as by how much of the protein is available. An understanding of the aetiology of a number of inherited neurological diseases has come about through such studies, e.g. the Lesch–Nyhan syndrome, phenylketonuria and a number of lysosomal storage disorders.

The number of gene products that can be examined, albeit indirectly, has been expanded by the availability of cloned DNA probes corresponding to these genes (Rosenberg, Hansen and Breakefield, 1985). By linkage analysis using DNA polymorphisms targeted to gene loci, it is possible to determine whether or not these genes are defective in an inherited neurological disease. If there are some clues as to what gene(s) may be defective, and if cloned probes for those genes are available, this type of analysis has several advantages. First, much smaller families can be used, since one is looking at only a very small region of the genome (a 10-kb sequence, the approximate size of a gene, occupies a linkage distance of roughly 0.01 cM), and asking whether a restriction endonuclease site polymorphism and the defective sequence occur within that region. There is essentially no chance of recombination over this genetic distance within a generation, so even families with two affected members can be informative. Second, no matter where the mutational defect occurs in the gene – including intron, exon or flanking sequences – its presence will be apparent through linkage to the DNA polymorphism, although in most cases the defect will not be responsible for that polymorphism. A few cases have been described, however, in which the defect does produce a change in a restriction endonuclease site, e.g. for the defect in sickle-cell β-globin (Orkin and Kazazian, 1984), a pre-albumin variant associated with amyloid polyneuropathy (Sasaki et al., 1984), and a defective hypoxanthine phosphoribosyl transferase (HPRT) causing gout (Wilson, Young and Kelly, 1983). Targeted mapping can be more efficient in establishing a gene defect than nucleotide sequencing, as there is a substantial amount of nucleotide variation among normal alleles of a gene, especially in non-coding regions, and defects in non-coding as well as coding sequences can disrupt gene function.

Excluding a gene by targeted mapping is relatively easy. If two affected children in the same family carrying a recessively inherited disease have different alleles for the test gene, that gene is not responsible. It is more difficult to prove that a defective gene and test gene are one and the same in small families, as it has to be established that no recombination has occurred between them in a number of meiotic events. It is even more difficult to rule out that the defect is not in another tightly linked gene. Still, given that the test gene was selected originally as having a possible role in the disease process, it is likely that a linked gene would be a member of the same gene family clustered together in the genome. This type of targeted linkage analysis has been used to exclude the gene for β-nerve growth factor in families with peripheral neurofibromatosis (Darby et al., 1985) and familial dysautonomia (Breakefield et al., 1984), as well as the pro-opiomelanocortin gene in a family with the autosomal dominant form of torsion dystonia (Breakefield et al., 1986).

Molecular strategies to identify defective genes

In many cases, linkage analysis will be useful in finding a marker DNA sequence that is near a defective gene in the genome. The marker sequence may be from 1 to 10 cM (very approximately 10^3–10^4 kb) away from the defective gene. The next steps include obtaining accurate map distances and finding marker sequences as close to the gene as possible and preferably on both sides of it. Gaining this information depends on the number of informative gametes available in the pedigree(s). For instance, to obtain accurate linkage distances of 0.1 cM (~100 kb) one would have to evaluate over 1000 informative gametes and find one recombinational event. Two other approaches can be taken for limiting the region of DNA sequence containing the defective gene. One approach is to identify deletion mutations that cause the disease state and determine which DNA probes map to these deletions; this has been pursued for Duchenne's muscular dystrophy (Monaco et al., 1985). Another is to use DNA probes for linked marker sequences to screen genomic libraries and thus obtain clones that share some overlapping sequences with the marker sequence, but which may extend closer to the defective gene (chromosome walking; Gusella et al., 1984).

Several strategies have been discussed to move on from linkage information to identifying the defective gene. It may be realistic in a very large family, such as the Venezuelan Huntington's disease pedigrees (see below), to find markers within 0.1 cM of the defective gene. It should be noted, however, that there are hot spots of recombination in the human genome (Chakravarti et al., 1984) so that this linkage distance could represent <10 to >1000 kb of nucleotide sequence. It is not reasonable to sequence >10 kb of DNA and, even if one did, it might be difficult recognizing genes within it. In order to find genes within a large fragment of DNA, vectors can be used which distinguish open reading frames (nucleotide sequences that lack a termination codon and can code for a stretch of amino acids: potential exons), and cDNAs from normal individuals can be hybridized to them. (For further discussion of strategies for identifying defective genes see Roses et al., 1983; Gusella et al., 1984.) As yet, no one has moved from linkage information to identification of a defective gene locus, so although there are a number of theoretical ways by which this could be achieved, the most effective has yet to be established. The excitement of this approach lies in the fact that it is logically and technically possible to go from genetic information on the inheritance of the disease state to characterization of the defective gene. Further, it appears likely that these genes will code for, as yet unknown, proteins important in the development and integrity of the nervous system.

DYSTONIA

Dystonia refers to both a type of involuntary movement that is twisting, repetitive and continuous, and a group of neurological disorders in which dystonic contractions are a principal feature (*see* Chapter 17). Dystonia, as a group or class of disorders, has been subcategorized according to aetiology as idiopathic (primary) and symptomatic (secondary) dystonia. The symptomatic dystonias include cases secondary to metabolic abnormalities such as Wilson's disease, G_{M1} and G_{M2} gangliosidoses, as yet poorly understood inherited disorders, such as Hallervorden–Spatz syndrome, and a multitude of environmental causes, i.e. hypoxia, trauma, infection, stroke and exposure to neuroleptics. Pathology, when present in these secondary causes, frequently involves lesions of the basal ganglia.

Often secondary dystonia can be distinguished from primary dystonia on the basis of history and examination of the patient. Unlike primary dystonia, in which the only or major neurological abnormality is dystonic contractions, the secondary dystonias often manifest other neurological signs such as spasticity, ataxia, ocular dysmobility or cognitive impairment. However, it should be mentioned that tremor, stuttering and myoclonus are considered, by some, to represent aspects of the clinical spectrum that may be seen in primary dystonia. The course a patient follows (in primary dystonia usually one of insidious onset and slow progression of symptoms) and the results of laboratory studies (normal in primary dystonia) may also help to distinguish primary and secondary dystonias. Details on clinical classification and investigation of dystonia are presented in Chapter 17.

Clinical heterogeneity

Even, however, with careful evaluation, the diagnosis of primary dystonia does not denote a homogenous disorder, clinically or genetically. This heterogeneity is a major consideration in any strategy to understanding how genes contribute to and act in this disorder.

Clinical heterogeneity (Fahn, 1982; 1984) has been observed on various levels involving a variety of clinical features, such as age-of-onset, distribution of dystonia, presence of fluctuations in symptoms and concurrence of other involuntary movements, such as myoclonus or tremor. For example, childhood and adolescent onset primary dystonia (often referred to as dystonia musculorum deformans) is more likely to involve the legs, to progress to other body regions, and to lead to significant disability, particularly with walking (Marsden and Harrison, 1974; Marsden, Harrison and Bundey, 1976). On the other hand, adult-onset dystonia more frequently begins with craniocervical or upper limb dystonia and tends to remain focal or segmental. In one study by Bundey, Harrison and Marsden (1975), most patients with onset of dystonia before 20 years (a clinically homogenous group described above) were thought to have a genetic disorder that was either autosomal recessive (based on sib or first cousin involvement) or due to new dominant mutation (based on increased paternal age). On the other hand, patients with adult onset were a clinically heterogeneous group with a variety of focal and segmental dystonias and most were thought to be non-genetic due to absence of dystonia in first degree relatives. This issue of mode of inheritance, which is controversial, is discussed partially in Chapter 17 and will be discussed again below.

Other unusual clinical variants based on the temporal characteristics of the movements, rather than on age-of-onset or distribution, have been described. These include dystonia with marked diurnal fluctuations (or Segawa variant) (Segawa et al., 1976) and paroxysmal dystonia (Lance, 1977). The former describes a group of patients with childhood-onset dystonia that is virtually absent early in the day and after sleep, and which becomes prominent in the afternoons and evenings. Several of these patients had affected sibs and cousins and there is dramatic benefit from levodopa therapy. Paroxysmal dystonia, on the other hand, refers to discrete bouts of dystonia lasting minutes to hours, often induced by alcohol, caffeine, prolonged exercise and intense emotion. Paroxysmal kinesiogenic choreoathetosis is another disorder of intermittent involuntary movements that may be dystonic. These movements last less than five minutes and occur upon sudden movement and with startle. Both autosomal dominant inheritance and sporadic cases (Lance, 1977; Fahn and Bressman, 1983) of these paroxysmal disorders have been reported. Another more controversial clinical variant of dystonia is so-called 'myoclonic dystonia' (Obeso et al., 1983; Quinn and Marsden, 1984; Kurlan et al., 1985). These patients have both dystonia and more rapid shock-like or myoclonic movements that are considered by some to represent a phenomenon distinct from dystonia. Again, both sporadic cases and autosomal dominant inheritance have been reported. These variants are discussed in Chapter 17.

Genetic heterogeneity

The issue of clinical heterogeneity is inseparable from that of the probable genetic heterogeneity of this disorder. Discrete genotypes based on clinical variants, such as myoclonic and paroxysmal dystonia and dystonia with diurnal variation, have been proposed. One unique clinical and genetic subclass of dystonia that has been described in the Philippines has an X-linked recessive mode of inheritance (Lee et al., 1976). These patients are unusual clinically in that dystonia begins in adult life and subsequently generalizes.

Although there is considerable information about inheritance in primary torsion dystonia, much is unknown or controversial. According to several previous studies, 30–50% of patients have family histories of dystonia. At the Dystonia Clinical Research Center of Columbia–Presbyterian Medical Center, 20% (117/575) of all patients with primary dystonia (regardless of age at onset or distribution) have a family history of dystonia. The significance of these percentages regarding pattern of inheritance is unclear. Furthermore, the issue of whether focal dystonias are milder phenotypes of the same genetic lesions causing generalized dystonia has not been addressed in a controlled study. Nevertheless, it is clear that dystonia can occur in some families with an apparent autosomal dominant mode of inheritance.

Beginning with one of the earliest descriptions of dystonia by Schwalbe (1908), numerous families with apparent dominant inheritance have been described. In 1967, Zeman and Dyken firmly consolidated the notion of dystonia as an inherited disorder and concluded that all familial cases were autosomal dominant. They stressed the need to examine family members and described the occurrence of diminished expression or formes frustes in family members. This included dystonia that involved only one body region (such as graphospasm or torticollis), dystonia with action (but not at rest) and non-progressive dystonia. They calculated a penetrance of 0.52 and gene frequency of 1:200 000 in the general population and 1:38 000 for American Jews. However, it is not at all clear that dystonia in reported large dominant families results from the same genetic defect. For example, in one American family of Johnson, Schwartz and Barbeau (1962), average age of onset was 10, whereas in a large Swedish family age of onset was 30 (Larsson and Sjorgren, 1966). This clinical difference suggests either different mutations at the same or different loci, or the influence of other genes and environmental factors on the manifestation of the same mutation.

After the study by Zeman and Dyken (1967) the pattern of inheritance of dystonia was reassessed by Eldridge (1970) and a conflicting conclusion drawn. Eldridge also found a particularly high frequency of dystonia among Jews, specifically Ashkenazim. He noted that these patients had earlier age of onset, greater initial limb involvement and more rapid progression of dystonia as compared to non-Jews. Parent and child were rarely both affected and there was close agreement between the number of observed and expected sibs affected for a recessive mode of inheritance. He concluded that there were at least two modes of inheritance: autosomal recessive among Ashkenazim and autosomal dominant among non-Jews.

Subsequent reports have cast doubt on the notion that clinical distinctions can be made between cases of presumed recessive and dominant inheritance. Rather, the key determinant of clinical course is age of onset, earlier onset being associated with leg involvement and more severe disease (Bundey, Harrison and Marsden, 1975; Burke et al., 1985). Most recently the notion of recessive inheritance among Jews has been challenged altogether by Zilber et al. (1984) studying the population in Israel. They, too, found a marked increase in the frequency of primary dystonia among European (Ashkenazi) Jews (1:23 000 compared to 1:117 000 among Afro-Asian Jews). However, they did not find that a recessive model fitted their data unless a much higher frequency of the disease gene was postulated. Further, consanguinity was too infrequent, the observed number of affected parents, offspring, aunts, uncles and cousins was too high and the observed number of affected sibs from presumed heterozygous parents was lower than would be expected for recessive inheritance. An autosomal dominant pattern with a penetrance of 51% was considered the best explanation (*Figure 4.5*).

Figure 4.5 Inheritance of dystonia in Israeli families. Solid symbols, affected with dystonia; shaded symbols, possible forme fruste. T = tremor, ST = stutter, BL = blepharospasm; (*) assigned carrier when either parent is a possible carrier. (From Zilber et al. (1984) with permission of the Authors and Publishers.)

The mode of inheritance in the Jewish population, then, remains to be clarified. There may be dominant inheritance with low penetrance or recessive inheritance, with 'pseudo-dominance' occurring when an affected parent marries a normal carrier of the same defective gene. It is also possible that more than one autosomal mutation causes dystonia in the Jewish population and that these different mutations follow different modes of inheritance.

One way to begin sorting out the genetics of dystonia is to select large families amenable to extensive linkage analysis, to locate the chromosomal position of the defective gene in each of those families, and to establish whether the same gene is involved in these and other smaller families. By using a single family, the odds are increased that all affected individuals will have the same genetic cause. Even within a family, however, there may be difficulty in interpreting the status of some individuals. For example, some people who have dystonic posturing at an early age may not manifest any symptoms in later life; some individuals may begin to have clearly defined dystonia only in their adult life, whereas most individuals in the family have onset in their teens; and some apparently unaffected individuals with an affected parent may produce affected children. It is particularly critical in linkage analysis that an unaffected individual is not misclassified as affected. Also one must assign a probability score to an unaffected individual as to whether they are carrying the defective gene, taking into account the chance that they will express the disease at their present age if they carry the defective gene. Assigning this probability requires reasonable estimates of gene penetrance, average and range of age-of-onset, and gene frequency in the ethnic population under study.

Linkage analysis using DNA polymorphisms has been undertaken in one large family manifesting an apparently autosomal dominant form of dystonia (Breakefield *et al.*, 1986). Four strategies are being used. First, where possible, cloned DNA probes for genes coding for proteins thought to be defective in this disease have been used in targeted mapping. Thus, the genes for propiomelanocortin and glutamic acid decarboxylase have been excluded as causing dystonia in this family. Second, chromosomal abnormalities associated with dystonic symptoms are considered as possible clues to the location of dystonia genes. For example, an individual with mental retardation and dystonic symptoms carrying a translocation between chromosomes 18p and 21q and being monosomic for portions of these chromosomes, may implicate them in harbouring the responsible gene. Third, a systematic search using sets of linked probes for given chromosomes has been used, in order to 'scan' larger regions of the chromosomes by multipoint analysis. Fourth, highly polymorphic random probes are being used as they provide maximal information in linkage analysis. So far no linked marker has yet been identified in this family in over 100 tested. Since the probes available for this analysis are essentially unlimited, however, it should only be a matter of time before a linked marker is found.

HUNTINGTON'S DISEASE

Prevalence and age of onset

The disease has appeared in a large number of ethnic populations. In the US and the United Kingdom, prevalence rates have ranged from 5 to 9 per 100 000 (Conneally, 1984). Prevalences among South African Blacks (Hayden and

Beighton, 1982) and Japanese (Kishimoto, Nakamura and Sotokawa, 1957) are thought to be lower and the highest rates have been reported in regions where affected individuals have resided for many generations (i.e. Lake Maracaibo region, Venezuela). Average age of onset reported is between 35 and 42 years (Martin, 1984) with a range of 4 (Byers, Gilles and Fung, 1973) to over 75 (Myers et al., 1985a) years. In one study, 6% of patients exhibited symptoms before the age of 21 and 28% after 50 (Martin, 1984).

Variability in age of onset is greater among, than within, families (Newcombe, Walker and Harper, 1981), although intrafamilial variability can be considerable. This familial similarity suggests that either common environmental or genetic mechanisms can modify age of onset. Twin studies (Sudarsky, Myers and Walsh, 1983) have shown very high concordance in age of onset and clinical features of homozygous twins even when raised apart. This supports the hypothesis that age of onset is substantially determined by genetic factors.

It has also been noted that juvenile cases present more frequently with a variant of Huntington's disease known as the Westphal or rigid form (Martin, 1984). In this form, akinesia and rigidity, rather than chorea, are present. In addition, juvenile onset Huntington's disease is characterized by marked behavioural and cognitive changes and seizures. Furthermore, unlike adult-onset Huntington's disease, which generally runs a 15-year course, juvenile onset is rapidly progressive with a fatal outcome in less than 10 years (Bruyn, 1968). On the other hand, the late-onset form (first symptoms at age 50 or older) appears to be associated with slower progress and less severe cognitive impairment; postmortem findings reveal less severe neuronal atrophy (Myers et al., 1985a).

One of the most interesting aspects of the age of onset issue is the effect of the sex of the affected parent. Specifically, paternal transmission is associated with early onset (Conneally, 1984), while cases with late onset are more frequently inherited from an affected mother (Myers, 1985b). This has led to various hypotheses about maternally transmitted protective factors that modify onset. These include production of a neuronal growth factor that crosses the placenta and partially protects the basal ganglia from later degenerative changes and amelioration of the effects of the Huntington gene, through genes in the maternally derived mitochondria.

Pathology and clinical features

Pathologically, Huntington's disease is characterized by severe loss of neurones in the caudate and putamen. Neuronal loss is also found in the globus pallidus and cerebral cortex (Martin, 1984). Recent studies of Golgi impregnations of neostriatum suggest that dendrites of medium-sized spiny neurones may be selectively involved (Graveland, Williams and Figliam, 1985). PET scanning indicates that metabolism in the basal ganglia may decrease some years before onset of symptoms and precedes bulk tissue loss as demonstrated by CT scan (Kuhl et al., 1985). The biochemical defect underlying neuronal cell death is unknown. Examinations of postmortem brain tissue have found altered levels of a number of neurotransmitters, enzymes and receptor binding sites. *Table 4.3* summarizes some of the neurotransmitter changes that have been noted.

Clinically, Huntington's disease is characterized by chorea and neurobehavioural changes that include both psychiatric symptoms and intellectual deficits. Usually,

Table 4.3 Neurotransmitter changes in Huntington's disease

Neurotransmitters that are decreased:
   Gamma-aminobutyric acid and glutamic acid decarboxylase
   Acetylcholine (and choline acetyltransferase)
   Substance P
   Enkephalins
   Cholecystokinin

Neurotransmitters that are unchanged:
   Dopamine
   Serotonin
   Vasoactive intestinal polypeptide
   Noradrenaline

Neurotransmitters that are increased:
   Dopamine*
   Thyrotropin-releasing hormone
   Somatostatin
   Neurotensin

* Reported to be increased in some studies but not in others

onset of symptoms is insidious and may consist of behavioural changes, involuntary movements or both. The most diagnostic feature of the disorder is chorea – an abrupt, rapid, random movement that is not patterned and tends to flow from one muscle to another. These movements may involve limb, axial and cranial musculature. Also there is motor impersistence that produces the inability to sustain a contraction such as tongue protrusion. The gait becomes noticeably abnormal and develops a stuttering, lurching or dance-like quality. Gait analysis has shown reduced stride length, fewer steps per minute, and varied swing phase speed in each walking cycle (Koller and Trimble, 1985). The speech often becomes jerky, and impaired control of swallowing becomes evident (Leopold and Kagel, 1985).

Mental symptoms include disorders of affect, a schizophrenia-like syndrome and personality disorders (Caine and Shoulson, 1983). Family members often describe early symptoms of withdrawal, apathy, silence or emotional lability. Psychological testing often shows the patient to be less apathetic than disorganized with an inability to initiate, plan and sequentially arrange. Furthermore, there appears to be an overall deficiency of arousal (Caine and Fisher, 1985). Memory is affected and defects in all aspects of new learning, retention and retrieval occur. On the other hand, language function is generally well preserved. Other neurological abnormalities which may be seen include impaired ocular fixation, saccades and smooth pursuit (Leigh and Folstein, 1983), hypotonia and hyperactive reflexes (Martin, 1984).

Molecular genetics

Molecular genetic studies of Huntington's disease have been at the forefront in demonstrating the power of linkage analysis using DNA polymorphisms. Linkage analysis using DNA polymorphisms was undertaken by Gusella and coworkers

Huntington's disease 51

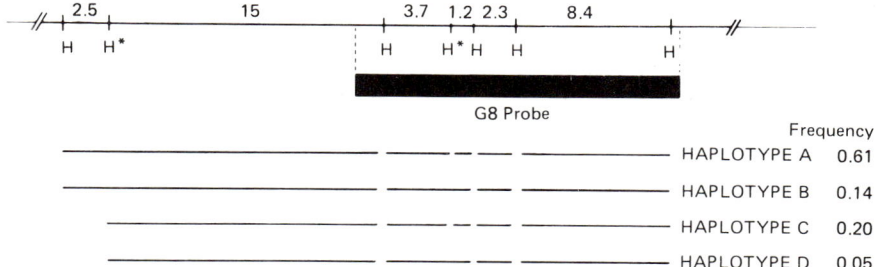

Figure 4.6 G8 locus showing restriction site polymorphisms on chromosome 4. Top line, genomic sequence hybridizing to the G8 cloned sequence (solid bar) of chromosome 4. Numbers on top of line, site of restriction fragments in kb. H under line, position of sites for restriction endonuclease Hind III (* = variable sites). Four haplotype lines (A, B, C, and D) indicate size of fragments generated. The frequency of each haplotype in the human population is indicated on the right. (From Gusella (1984) with permission of the Author and Publishers.)

(1983) using the very large Venezuelan pedigree. A random genomic probe, G8, was found to serve as a linked marker for the Huntington gene. Several restriction endonuclease site polymorphisms can be used to distinguish alleles at the G8 locus (*Figure 4.6*). Within this pedigree, a particular allele (C) was found to co-inherit with the Huntington gene 96% of the time (*Figure 4.7*), which is not to say that this allele is always associated with the Huntington gene. The genomic sequence corresponding to G8 is located 4 cM proximal to the Huntington gene on the short arm (p) of chromosome 4. The availability of this probe has allowed elucidation of two issues. First, using the Venezuelan pedigree where two affected individuals

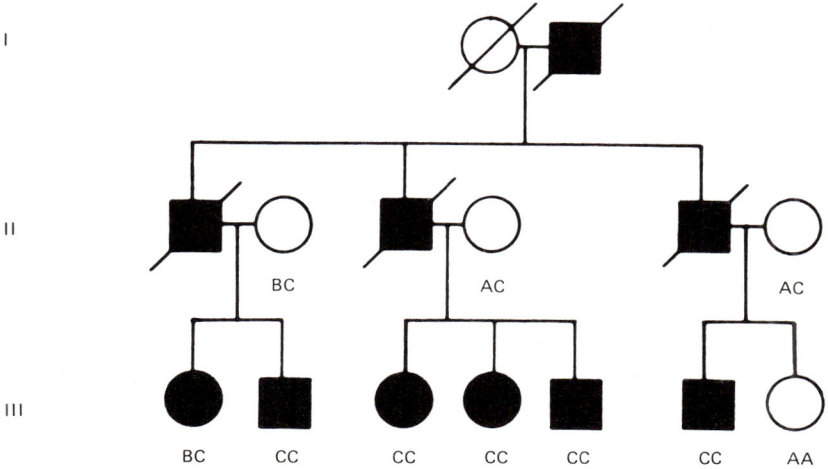

Figure 4.7 Venezuelan pedigree showing inheritance of Huntington gene and G8 marker alleles. Solid symbols, affected with Huntington's disease. A, B and C refer to haplotypes for G8 shown in *Figure 4.6*. Huntington gene co-segregates with haplotype C in this small portion of the Venuzuelan pedigree. (From Gusella (1984) with permission of the Author and Publishers.)

have produced affected offspring, it appears that individuals inheriting two copies of the Huntington gene have a similar clinical course to those inheriting only one copy (Wexler et al., 1985). Second, in at least three other families from America and Europe, the same gene appears to be causing Huntington's disease, although it is not clear yet whether the same mutation in that gene is responsible.

In order to use the linked marker in genetic counselling and identification of the mutant gene, it would be very useful to find markers closer to the gene and preferably on both sides of it. One approach towards this end taken by Gusella et al. (1985) has been to use genomic DNA from cells of patients with the Wolf–Hirschhorn syndrome, which is caused by the loss of the terminal portion of chromosome 4p, in order to identify genomic clones which map to this region. These genomic clones have been prepared from a rodent–human hybrid cell line containing only human chromosome 4 in a background of rodent chromosomes. Rodent and human DNA clones can be distinguished by hybridization to repetitive DNA sequences unique to each (Gusella et al., 1980). Although a number of clones have been isolated corresponding to sequences near the terminal of 4p, none is as yet any closer to the Huntington gene, apparently due to the fact that this gene is very near the terminus.

The inability to localize the Huntington gene more accurately has hindered attempts to identify it. Proposed strategies for identifying this gene include: (*a*) walking or leaping closer to it using G8 to recognize genomic clones containing adjacent DNA sequences; (*b*) cloning sequences in the Huntington gene region and looking for open reading frames corresponding to genes; (*c*) preparing cDNA libraries from basal ganglia and determining whether any of these cDNAs are encoded in this region (Gusella, 1984). Similar strategies are currently being employed to use linked markers to assist in identification of defective genes responsible for Duchenne's muscular dystrophy and retinoblastoma. In these cases, small deletions or translocations have been described which cause the disease state and help to define the position of the responsible genes (Sparkes et al., 1980; Worton et al., 1984; Monaco et al., 1985).

LESCH–NYHAN SYNDROME

Clinical aspects

Although not considered a movement disorder as such, individuals with the Lesch–Nyhan syndrome frequently have choreoathetotic and dystonic movements (Watts et al., 1982).

The syndrome is associated in most cases with virtually complete deficiency of the enzyme hypoxanthine guanine phosphoribosyltransferase (HPRT) (Wilson, Young and Kelly, 1983). This enzyme deficiency may be caused by abnormalities in catalytic function or by diminished intracellular concentration of the enzyme. Most patients with Lesch–Nyhan syndrome have diminished or absent enzyme concentrations, although a point mutation producing normal concentrations of a catalytically incompetent variant may also produce the syndrome. On the other hand, cases of 'partial HPRT deficiency' which result in hyperuraemia and gout are not associated with neurological illness. In both cases different mutations at the HPRT locus can produce a range of symptoms.

Clinical symptoms of the Lesch–Nyhan syndrome usually become apparent at between 3 and 5 months of age with a delay in motor development. By 8–12 months involuntary movements appear. These include athetoid limb movements and axial dystonia, particularly opisthotonic spasms. Soon after, long tract signs including scissoring of gait develop. Dysarthria is invariably present and patients cannot walk. Mental retardation is often present and may be mild. In almost all cases physical growth and development is retarded. Uric acid production is excessive and may lead to nephrolithiasis and obstructive uropathy. Treatment with allopurinol will prevent urate nephropathy, but has no effect on neurological function.

The most striking clinical feature of this syndrome is compulsive self-destructive behaviour (Christie, Bay and Kaufman, 1982). Onset ranges from infancy to mid-teens. Usually patients bite fingers, lips, and buccal mucosa, often leading to loss of tissue. They may also bang their head or limbs and may exhibit aggressiveness towards others. The degree of self-mutilation varies and may not be evident unless the patient is stressed. Patients are very aware of their behaviour but have great difficulty with control and are managed with physical restraints.

The abnormal movements are presumably mediated through changes in neuronal function in the basal ganglia. No neuropathological abnormalities have been described in the brains of these patients, but significant reductions in several parameters of dopamine metabolism and in choline acetyltransferase activity have been noted in the basal ganglia (Lloyd et al., 1981). These neurochemical changes have been attributed to a decrease in arborization of dopamine neurones, since no comparable changes are seen in the substantia nigra containing the cell bodies of these neurones. Similarly, in an experimental animal model of this syndrome, rats treated neonatally with 6-hydroxydopamine show decreased arborization of dopamine neurones in the basal ganglia and supersensitivity of D-1 dopamine receptors, as well as self-mutilatory behaviour on treatment with L-dopa (Breese et al., 1985).

It is not clear why a lack of HPRT activity, and hence a deficiency in the purine salvage pathway, would disrupt dopaminergic function in the basal ganglia. This area of the brain, however, normally has the highest level of HPRT activity in the body (Stout et al., 1985) and presumably depends on this pathway for some specific function(s). Possibly, neurotransmission through purines is disrupted and this secondarily affects other neurones in this region. The Lesch–Nyhan syndrome is an example of how, even when the gene locus and the defective product are known, it can still be difficult to understand the nature of the neurological defect.

Genetics

The Lesch–Nyhan syndrome follows a typical X-linked recessive mode of inheritance with males being primarily affected (for review see Wilson, Young and Kelley, 1983). Carrier females can be detected by the presence of about 50% normal levels of HPRT activity in lymphocytes, and either normal or absent HPRT activity in the clonal progeny of hair follicles (due to random X-inactivation). Since affected males do not reproduce, about one-third of the affected males represent new mutations occurring in the germline of the mother (Francke et al., 1976). Thus, although the same gene locus is defective in all patients, many different mutational events account for these defects. Biochemical analysis of HPRT deficiency states, where the mutant protein can be analysed, have identified four different amino acid

54   *Molecular genetics of movement disorders*

substitutions leading to loss of enzyme activity that can be accounted for by single base-pair substitutions in the HPRT gene (Wilson, Young and Kelley, 1983).

The availability of cloned DNA sequences for HPRT have allowed a more detailed analysis of mutational changes in the HPRT locus (Jolly *et al.*, 1982; Yang *et al.*, 1984). More is known now about alterations in DNA sequence causing this disease than for any other inherited neurological condition. There is a single active HPRT locus located on the q arm of the X-chromosome between bands 26 and 27 (*Figure 4.8*). This gene is about 40 kb in length, contains nine exons (*Figure 4.9*) and codes for a 1.6-kb poly(A)$^+$ mRNA. Southern blot analysis of genomic DNA from lymphocytes of 28 unrelated Lesch–Nyhan patients revealed that five of them (18%) contained substantial DNA rearrangements that result in altered or missing sequences in the HPRT gene (*Figure 4.9*). None of the deletion mutations produced detectable mRNA for HPRT by Northern blotting using mRNA from patients' lymphocytes and neither did at least one of the non-rearrangement mutations. In addition to rearrangements, we can anticipate that defective expression of the HPRT gene will be associated with discrete changes in flanking,

Figure 4.8 Gene map of part of human X-chromosome. Selected loci on the long arm of the X-chromosome are indicated. The bands identified by the Giesma method are numbered on the left side of the chromosome; G6PD is glucose-6-phosphate dehydrogenase. (From Stout and Caskey (1986) with permission of the Authors and Publishers.)

Figure 4.9 HPRT gene. Diagram at top indicates HPRT gene with numbered boxes for exons and double lines between for introns. Point mutations causing alterations in amino acid (a.a.) sequence are indicated (*see* Wilson, Young and Kelley, 1983). Extent of deletion, insertion and duplication mutations described in humans are shown below. (From Stout and Caskey (1986) with permission of the Authors and Publishers.)

exon (coding) and intron regions of the gene as observed for the β-globin gene (Orkin and Kazazian, 1984).

Changes in DNA sequences associated with HPRT deficiency can also be used to track the mutant gene in families. One of the rearrangements represents an apparent partial duplication of genetic material and can be identified by the appearance of a unique hybridizing fragment on Southern blots (Yang *et al.*, 1984). Analysis of DNA from members of the affected family revealed that the mutation took place in the germline of the maternal grandmother or grandfather (*Figure 4.10*). Another base-pair substitution in the HPRT gene causing gout is correlated with loss of a specific restriction endonuclease site and a change in the size of hybridizing fragments (Wilson, Young and Kelley, 1983). In addition, a restriction endonuclease site polymorphism near the HPRT gene has been described that can be used to follow the inheritance of alleles in a number of families (Nussbaum *et al.*, 1983).

There are no natural animal models available for the Lesch–Nyhan syndrome, but several strategies have been proposed for generating them. These include generation of mosaic mice containing both normal cells and cells derived from embryonic carcinoma cells selected for HPRT deficiency in culture (Dewey *et al.*, 1977). If such mice contained HPRT-deficient (HPRT$^-$) germ cells, they could be used to foster an HPRT-deficient mouse colony. Another approach would be to insert an HPRT gene in the reverse orientation with respect to a promoter for RNA transcription into the genome of fertilized mouse eggs by microinjection. This

Figure 4.10 Inheritance of defective HPRT gene in family of patient GM 1662. (*a*) Southern blot of DNA from family shown in (*b*) digested with restriction endonuclease Bgl II. XY, normal male. Arrow, 4.1-kb Bgl II band associated with the gene alteration in GM 1662. (*b*) Solid symbol, individual with Lesch–Nyhan syndrome (GM 1662, *see Figure 4.9*); symbol with dot, carrier females. (From Yang *et al.* (1984) with permission of the Authors and Publishers. Copyright © 1984 Mamillan Journals Limited.)

inserted gene would produce an 'antisense' RNA which could hybridize to the normal mRNA for HPRT and block its processing and/or translation (Izant and Weintraub, 1984). Thus the resulting mice would be functionally HPRT deficient. A decrease of >98% activity would be necessary, however, to produce a biochemical situation comparable to the Lesch–Nyhan syndrome and it is not clear that this would be possible.

One interesting aspect of the HPRT deficiency state is the possibility of reversion to normal activity through introduction of a functional HPRT gene into the genome (gene therapy). Expression of HPRT activity in HPRT$^-$ cells has been achieved through retroviral-mediated integration into cultured cells and bone marrow cells (Miller *et al.*, 1983; Willis *et al.*, 1983; Williams *et al.*, 1984). In the latter case, introduction of these cells back into the bone marrow of mice, previously irradiated to kill off their own bone marrow cells, has resulted in continued expression of the foreign HPRT activity in blood cells *in vivo*. This indicates that haemopoietic stem cells have been transformed and are able to give rise continuously to progeny cells expressing this new phenotype. In other studies, foreign HPRT gene has been injected into fertilized mouse eggs and given rise to mice that express activity in most or all tissues of their body, with particularly high expression in the brain (Stout *et al.*, 1985). The issue of how to confer HPRT activity into brain cells of Lesch–Nyhan patients remains unsolved, however. It might be possible to introduce the gene by a replication-defective retroviral vector into discrete areas of the brain, such as the basal ganglia, but the level of expression would not be regulated. Further, it is not clear whether delivery of HPRT activity to this area of the brain would alleviate neurological symptoms. It does appear that it is possible to have metabolic cooperation between HPRT$^+$ and HPRT$^-$ cells within a limited tissue domain, so not all cells in an area would have to be transfected (Gruber *et al.*, 1985). Overall the Lesch–Nyhan syndrome illustrates the many ways molecular genetic techniques can be used to explore an inherited neurological disease once the gene defect is known.

OTHER DISEASES

There are a number of reports in the literature of families manifesting apparently inherited movement disorders. Depending on the size of the family and mode of inheritance some of these may be amenable to linkage analysis. Two are selected for discussion here: Gilles de la Tourette syndrome and Parkinson's disease.

Gilles de la Tourette syndrome

Gilles de la Tourette syndrome has followed an interesting history, being first thought to be a psychiatric condition and then recognized to be an inherited neurological disease. Interpretation of the genetics of the disease was confounded by the multiple manifestations the defective gene can have and the apparently frequent occurrence of phenocopies (Comings *et al.*, 1984). One important aspect of elucidating the genetics has been a nationally standardized criterion for diagnosis (DSM-III as recommended by the American Psychiatric Association). It was noted early that more males were affected than females (approximately 4:1) and that other members of the family might have chronic multiple tics rather than the Gilles de la Tourette syndrome (TS) as such. There are examples of sex-modified penetrance of gene expression and variable expressivity, respectively. Careful family and twin studies revealed that multiple tics were another manifestation of the TS gene (Pauls et al., 1981; Price et al., 1985). Another interesting aspect of this variable expression is that 60–80% of affected individuals with TS also have obsessive–compulsive illness (Nee et al., 1980). Recent data suggest obsessive–compulsive symptoms also occur in the relatives of TS gene patients and that this latter manifestation of the disease is more frequently seen in females (D. L. Pauls, unpublished data). Several recent studies support the inheritance of the TS gene in an autosomal dominant mode with about 50% gene penetrance (Comings et al., 1984; Devor, 1984). A large pedigree, 528 members with 52 affected, has been described which is appropriate for linkage analysis (Kurlan et al., 1986). Although the mode of inheritance in all families is not resolved, this disease demonstrates how careful clinical and genetic investigations can bring clarity in cases where neither the disease entity nor the mode of inheritance are obvious.

Parkinson's disease

Parkinsonism is again a set of symptoms as well as a disease entity. This condition demonstrates the problem of trying to establish whether a genetic defect occurs, when most, but not all, the cases are probably produced environmentally. Parkinsonian symptoms are noted in depression, olivopontocerebellar atrophy and Joseph's disease, each of which could be an inherited syndrome in its own right (Barbeau, Roy and Boyer, 1984). Symptoms seen in combination with amyotrophic lateral sclerosis and dementia have been reported both in Guam, where the condition seems to reflect an environmental imbalance of heavy metal ions at an early age (Gajdusek, 1985), and in Germany, where it appears to be a familial syndrome (Schmitt, Emser and Heimes, 1984).

Most cases of Parkinson's disease do not appear to be familial. With the high incidence of the disease (1% of individuals over 60 years of age), however, affected individuals frequently have affected relatives. Recent findings indicate that parkinsonism can be produced in humans by a chemical, 1-methyl-4-phenyl-1,2,3,6-tetrahydropyridine (Javitch et al., 1985), and support the idea that exogenous or endogenous toxins can cause the degeneration of dopaminergic neurones in the substantia nigra. The finding that monozygotic twins show no concordance for Parkinson's disease probably reflects the fact that most cases are sporadic, and does not exclude some families having an inherited form of the disease (Ward et al., 1984).

There appears to be a subset of Parkinson's patients where inheritance does have a role. Barbeau and coworkers (1974) have described two familial forms of Parkinson's disease. One is referred to as essential tremor related parkinsonism. Transmission of essential tremor follows a dominant pattern in families, with parkinsonism symptoms occurring apparently randomly, but with a five-fold greater incidence in these families than in the general population. A recent study of the prevalence of Parkinson's disease in a population with essential tremor found it to be 24-fold higher than in the normal population, again suggesting an association between these symptoms (Geraghty, Jankovic and Zetusky, 1985). Although families with dominantly inherited essential tremor without parkinsonism have been described, it is possible that inherited essential tremor is genetically heterogeneous and that Parkinson's disease is associated with only one form. Barbeau, Roy and Boyer (1984) also described a few families with an akinetic–rigid form of Parkinson's disease that appears to follow an autosomal recessive mode of inheritance. It becomes important in diseases such as this, which appear to have more than one cause, to select families for molecular genetic study very carefully.

References

ADAMS, R. D. and LYON, G. (1982) *Neurology of Hereditary Metabolic Diseases of Children*. New York: McGraw-Hill
BARAITSER, M. (1982) *The Genetics of Neurological Disorders*. Oxford: Oxford University Press
BARBEAU, A., ROY, M. and BOYER, L. (1984) Genetic studies in Parkinson's disease. *Advances in Neurology*, **40**, 333–339
BOTSTEIN, D., WHITE, R. L., SKOLNICK, M. and DAVIS, R. W. (1980) Construction of a genetic linkage map in man using restriction fragment length polymorphisms. *American Journal of Human Genetics*, **32**, 314–331
BREAKEFIELD, X. O., BRESSMAN, S. B., KRAMER, P. L., OZELIUS, L., MOSKOWITZ, C., TANZI, R. *et al.* (1986) Linkage analysis in a family with dominantly-inherited torsion dystonia: Exclusion of the pro-opiomelanocortin and glutamic acid decarboxylase genes, and other chromosomal regions using DNA polymorphisms. *Journal of Neurogenetics*, 159–175
BREAKEFIELD, X. O., ORLOFF, G., CASTIGLIONE, C., COUSSENS, L., AXELROD, F. B. and ULLRICH, A. (1984) The gene for beta-nerve growth factor is not defective in familial dysautonomia. *Proceedings of the National Academy of Sciences of the USA*, **81**, 4213–4216
BREESE, G. R., NAPIER, T. C. and MUELLER, R. A. (1985) Dopamine agonist-induced locomotor activity in rats treated with 6-hydroxydopamine at differing ages: functional supersensitivity of D-1 dopamine receptors in neonatally lesioned rats. *Journal of Pharmacology and Experimental Therapeutics*, **234**, 447–455
BUNDEY, S., HARRISON, M. J. G. and MARSDEN, C. D. (1975) A genetic study of torsion dystonia. *Journal of Medical Genetics*, **12**, 12–19
BURKE, R. E., FAHN, S., BRIN, M. F. *et al.* (1985) The clinical course of autosomal dominant torsion dystonia. *Neurology*, **35**, 273
BRUYN, G. W. (1968) Huntington's chorea: historical, clinical and laboratory synopsis. In *Handbook in Clinical Neurology*, Eds. P. J. Vinken and G. W. Bruyn, Vol. 6, pp. 278–298. Amsterdam: Elsevier
BYERS, R. K., GILLES, F. H. and FUNG, C. (1973) Huntington disease in children. *Neurology*, **23**, 561–569
CAINE, E. D. and FISHER, J. M. (1985) Dementia in Huntington's disease. In *Handbook of Clinical Neurology*, Eds. P. Vinken, G. W. Bruyn, H. K. Klawans and J. A. M. Frederics, Vol. 2 (46), *Neurobehavioural Disorders*. Amsterdam: Elsevier
CAINE, E. D. and SHOULSON, I. (1983) Psychiatric syndromes in Huntington's disease. *American Journal of Psychology*, **140**, 728–733
CHAKRAVATI, A., BUETOW, K. H., ANTONARKIS, S. E., WABER, P. G., BOEHM, C. D. and KAZAZIAN, H. H. (1984) Nonuniform recombination within the human beta-globin gene cluster. *American Journal of Human Genetics*, **36**, 1239–1258
CHAUDHARI, N. and HAHN, W. E. (1983) Genetic expression in developing brain. *Science*, **220**, 924–928
CHRISTIE, R., BAY, C. and KAUFMAN, I. A. (1982) Lesch–Nyhan disease: clinical experience with nineteen patients. *Developmental Medicine and Child Neurology*, **24**, 293–306
COMINGS, D. E., COMINGS, B. G., DEVOR, E. J. and CLONINGER, C. R. (1984) Detection of major gene for Gilles de la Tourette syndrome. *American Journal of Human Genetics*, **36**, 586–600
CONNEALLY, P. M. (1984) Huntington disease: genetics and epidemiology. *American Journal of Human Genetics*, **36**, 506–526
DARBY, J. K., FEDER, J., SELBY, M., RICCARDI, V., FERRELL, R., SIAO, D. *et al.* (1985) A discordant sibship analysis between beta-NGF and neurofibromatosis. *American Journal of Human Genetics*, **37**, 52–57
DAVIES, K. E. (1981) The application of DNA recombinant technology to the analysis of the human genome and genetic disease. *Human Genetics*, **58**, 351–357
DEVOR, E. J. (1984) Complex segregation analysis of Gilles de la Tourette syndrome: further evidence for a major locus mode of transmission. *American Journal of Human Genetics*, **36**, 704–709
DEWEY, M. J., MARTIN, D. W. JR, MARTIN, G. R. and MINTZ, B. (1977) Mosaic mice with teratocarcinoma-derived mutant cells deficient in hypoxanthine phosphoribosyltransferase. *Proceedings of the National Academy of Sciences of the USA*, **74**, 5564–5568

ELDRIDGE, R. (1970) The torsion dystonias: Literature review and genetic and clinical studies. *Neurology*, **20** (Part 2), 1–78
FAHN, S. (1982) Torsion dystonia: clinical spectrum and treatment. *Seminars in Neurology*, **2**, 316–323
FAHN, S. (1984) The varied clinical expressions of dystonia. *Neurological Clinics*, **2**, 541–554
FAHN, S. and BRESSMAN, S. (1983) Sporadic paroxysmal dystonic choreathetosis. *Neurology*, **33**, 131
FRANCKE, U., FELSENSTEIN, J., GARTLER, S. M., MIGEON, B. R., DANCIS, J., SEEGMILLER, J. E. *et al.* (1976) The occurrence of new mutants in the X-linked recessive Lesch-Nyhan disease. *American Journal of Human Genetics*, **28**, 123–137
GAJDUSEK, D. C. (1985) Hypothesis: Interference with axonal transport of neurofilament as a common pathogenetic mechanism in certain diseases of the central nervous system. *New England Journal of Medicine*, **312**, 714–719
GERAGHTY, J. J., JANKOVIC, J. and ZETUSKY, W. J. (1985) Association between essential tremor and Parkinson's disease. *Annals of Neurology*, **17**, 329–333
GRAVELAND, G. A., WILLIAMS, R. S. and FIGLIAM, D. (1985) Evidence for degenerative and regenerative changes in neostriatal spiny neurons in Huntington's disease. *Science*, **227** (4688), 770–773
GRUBER, H. E., KOENKER, R., LUCHTMAN, L. A., WILLIS, R. C. and SEEGMILLER, J. E. (1985) Glial cells metabolically cooperate: A potential requirement for gene replacement therapy. *Proceedings of the National Academy of Sciences of the USA*, **82**, 6662–6666
GUSELLA, J. (1984) Genetic linkage of the Huntington's disease gene to a DNA marker. *Le Journal Canadien des Sciences Neurologiques*, **11**, 421–425
GUSELLA, J., KEYS, C., VARSANYI-BREINER, A., KAO, F. T., JONES, C., PUCK, T. and HOUSMAN, D. (1980) Isolation and localization of DNA segments from specific human chromosomes. *Proceedings of the National Academy of Sciences of the USA*, **77**, 2829–2833
GUSELLA, J. F., TANZI, R. E., ANDERSON, M. A., HOBBS, W., GIBBONS, K., RASCHTCHIAN, R. *et al.* (1984) DNA markers for nervous system diseases. *Science*, **225**, 1320–1326
GUSELLA, J. F., TANZI, R. E., BADER, P. I., PHELAN, M. C., STEVENSON, R. and HAYDEN, M. R. *et al.* (1985) Deletion of Huntington's disease-linked G8 (D4S10) locus in Wolf–Hirschhorn syndrome. *Nature*, **318**, 75–78
GUSELLA, J. F., WEXLER, N. S., CONNEALLY, P. M., NAYLOR, S. L., ANDERSON, M. A., TANZI, R. E. *et al.* (1983) A polymorphic DNA marker genetically linked to Huntington's disease. *Nature*, **306**, 234–238
HAGEMEIJER, A. and SMIT, E. M. E. (1977) Partial trisomy 21: Further evidence that trisomy of band 21q22 is essential for Down's phenotype. *Human Genetics*, **38**, 15–23
HAYDEN, M. R. and BEIGHTON, P. H. (1982) Genetic aspects of Huntington's chorea: results of a national survey. *American Journal of Human Genetics*, **11**, 135–141
HODGE, S. E., MORTON, L. A., TIDEMAN, S., KIDD, K. K. and SPENCE, M. A. (1979) Age-of-onset correction available for linkage analysis (LIPED). *American Journal of Human Genetics*, **31**, 761–762
IONASESCU, V. and ZELLWEGER, H. (1983) *Genetics in Neurology*. New York: Raven Press
IZANT, J. G. and WEINTRAUB, H. (1984) Inhibition of thymidine kinase gene expression by anti-sense RNA: A molecular approach to genetic analysis. *Cell*, **36**, 1007–1015
JAVITCH, J. A., D'AMATO, R. J., STRITTMATTER, S. M. and SNYDER, S. H. (1985) Parkinsonism-inducing neurotoxin, N-methyl-4-phenyl-1,2,3,6-tetrahydropyridine: Uptake of the metabolite N-methyl-4-phenylpyridine by dopamine neurons explains selective toxicity. *Proceedings of the National Academy of Sciences of the USA*, **82**, 2173–2177
JEFFREYS, A. J., WILSON, V. and LAY THEIN, S. (1985) Hypervariable 'minisatellite' regions in human DNA. *Nature*, **314**, 67–73
JOHNSON, W., SCHWARTZ, G. and BARBEAU, A. (1962) Studies on dystonia musculorum deformans. *Archives of Neurology*, **7**, 301–313
JOLLY, D. J., ESTY, A. C., BERNARD, H. U. and FRIEDMANN, T. (1982) Isolation of a genomic clone partially encoding human hypoxanthine phosphoribosyltransferase. *Proceedings of the National Academy of Sciences of the USA*, **79**, 5038–5041
KIDD, K. K. and OTT, J. (1984) Power and sample size in linkage studies. *Cytogenetics and Cell Genetics*, **37**, 510–511
KISHIMOTO, K., NAKAMURA, M. and SOTOKAWA, Y. (1957) Population genetics study of Huntington's chorea in Japan. *Annual Report of the Research Institute of Environment Medicine*, **9**, 195–211
KITSIOU-TZELI, S., HALLETT, J. J., ATKINS, L., LATT, S. A. and HOLMES, L. B. (1984) Brief clinical report: Familial t(4;21)(q24;q22) leading to unbalanced offspring with partial duplication of 4q and of 21q without manifestations of the Down syndrome. *American Journal of Medical Genetics*, **18**, 725–729
KITTUR, S. D., HOPPENER, J. W. M., ANTONARAKIS, S. E., DANIELS, J. D. J., MEYERS, D. A. and MAESTRI, N. E. *et al.* (1985) Linkage map of the short arm of human chromosome 11: Location of the genes for catalase, calcitonin, and insulin-like growth factor II. *Proceedings of the National Academy of Sciences of the USA*, **82**, 5064–5067

KOLLER, W. J. and TRIMBLE, J. (1985) The gait abnormality of Huntington's disease. *Neurology,* **35,** 1450–1454
KUHL, D. E., MARKHAM, C. H., RIEGE, E. J., PHELPS, M. E. and MAZZIOTTA, J. C. (1985) Local cerebral glucose utilization in symptomatic and presymptomatic Huntington's disease. *Research Publication, Association for Research in Nervous and Mental Disorders,* **63,** 199–209
KURLAN, R., BEHR, J., MEDRED, L., SHOULSON, I., PAULS, D., KIDD, J. *et al.* (1986) Familial Tourette syndrome: Report of a large pedigree and potential for linkage analysis. *Neurology,* in press
KURLAN, R., BEHR, J., MILLER, C. and SHOULSON, I. (1985b) Inherited myoclonic dystonia. *Annals of Neurology,* **18,** 164
LANCE, J. W. (1977) Familial paroxysmal dystonic choreoathetosis and its differentiation from related syndromes. *Annals of Neurology,* **2,** 285–293
LARSSON, T. and SJORGREN, T. S. (1966) Dystonia musculoram deformans: A genetic and clinical population study of 121 cases. *Acta Neurologica Scandinavica,* **42,** 1–235
LATHROP, G. M., LALOUEL, J. M., JULIER, C. and OTT, J. (1984) Strategies for multilocus linkage analysis in humans. *Proceedings of the National Academy of Sciences of the USA,* **81,** 3443–3446
LEE, L. V., PASCASIO, F. M., FUENTES, F. D. and VITERBO, G. H. (1976) Torsion dystonia in Panay, Philippines. *Advances in Neurology,* **14,** 137–151
LEIGH, R. J., FOLSTEIN, S. E. *et al.* (1983) Abnormal ocular motor control in Huntington's disease. *Neurology,* **33,** 1268–1275
LEOPOLD, N. A. and KAGEL, M. C. (1985) Dysphagia in Huntington's disease. *Archives of Neurology,* **42,** 57–60
LLOYD, K. G., HORNYKIEWICZ, O., DAVIDSON, L., SHANNAK, K., FARLEY, I., GOLDSTEIN, M. *et al.* (1981) Biochemical evidence of dysfunction of brain neurotransmitters in the Lesch–Nyhan syndrome. *New England Journal of Medicine,* **305,** 1106–1111
MARSDEN, C. D., HARRISON, M. J. G. and BUNDEY, S. (1976) Natural history of idiopathic torsion dystonia. *Advances in Neurology,* **14,** 177–187
MARSDEN, C. D. and HARRISON, M. J. G. (1974) Idiopathic torsion dystonia. *Brain,* **97,** 793–810
MARTIN, J. B. (1984) Huntington's disease: new approaches to an old problem. The Robert Wartenberg lecture. *Neurology,* **34,** 1059–1072
MILLER, A. D., JOLLY, D. J., FRIEDMAN, T. and VERMA, I. M. (1983) A transmissible retrovirus expressing human hypoxanthine phosphoribosyltransferase (HPRT): Gene transfer into cells obtained from humans deficient in HPRT. *Proceedings of the National Academy of Sciences of the USA,* **80,** 4709–4713
MONACO, A. P., BERTELSON, C. J., MIDDLESWORTH, W., COLLETTI, C. A., ALDRIDGE, J., FISCHBECK, K. H. *et al.* (1985) Detection of deletions spanning the Duchenne muscular dystrophy locus using a tightly linked DNA segment. *Nature,* **316,** 842–845
MYERS, R. H., SAX, D. S., SCHOENFIELD, M., BIRD, E. D. *et al.* (1985a) Late onset of Huntington's disease. *Journal of Neurology, Neurosurgery and Psychiatry,* **48,** 530–534
MYERS, R. H., CUPPLES, L. A., SCHOENFIELD, M. *et al.* (1985b) Maternal factors in onset of Huntington's disease. *American Journal of Human Genetics,* **37,** 511–523
NEE, L. E., CAINE, E. D., POLINSKY, R. J., ELDRIDGE, R. and EBERT, M. H. (1980) Gilles de la Tourette syndrome: Clinical and family study of 50 cases. *Advances in Neurology,* **7,** 41–49
NEEL, J. V. (1984) A revised estimate of the amount of genetic variation in human proteins: implications for the distribution of DNA polymorphisms. *American Journal of Human Genetics,* **36,** 1135–1148
NEWCOMBE, R. G., WALKER, D. A. and HARPER, P. S. (1981) Factors influencing age at onset and duration of survival in Huntington's chorea. *Annals of Human Genetics,* **45,** 387–396
NUSSBAUM, R., BRENNAND, J., CHINAULT, C., FUSCOE, J., KONECKI, D., MELTON, D. *et al.* (1983) Molecular analysis of the hypoxanthine phosphoribosyltransferase locus. In *Recombinant DNA Applications to Human Disease,* Eds. C. T. Caskey and R. L. White, pp. 81–89. Cold Spring Harbor: Cold Spring Harbor Press
OBESO, J. A., ROTHWELL, J. C., LANG, A. E. *et al.* (1983) Myoclonic dystonia. *Neurology,* **33,** 825–830
ORKIN, S. H. and KAZAZIAN, H. H. (1984) The mutation and polymorphism of the human beta-globin gene and its surrounding DNA. *Annual Review of Genetics,* **18,** 131–171
OTT, J. (1976) A computer program for linkage analysis of general human pedigrees. *American Journal of Human Genetics,* **28,** 528–529
PAULS, D. L., COHEN, D. J., HEIMBUCH, R., PHIL, M., DETLOR, J. and KIDD, K. K. (1981) Familial pattern and transmission of Gilles de la Tourette syndrome and multiple tics. *Archives of General Psychiatry,* **38,** 1091–1093
PRICE, R. A., KIDD, K. K., COHEN, D. J., PAULS, D. L. and LECKMAN, J. F. (1985) A twin study of Tourette syndrome. *Archives of General Psychiatry,* **42,** 815–820

QUINN, N. P. and MARSDEN, C. D. (1984) Dominantly inherited myoclonic dystonia with dramatic response to alcohol. *Neurology,* **34** (Suppl. 1), 236

RODERICK, T. H., LALLEY, P. A., DAVISSON, M. T., O'BRIEN, J. J., WOMACK, J. E., CREAN-GOLDBERG, N. *et al.* (1984) Report of the committee on comparative mapping. *Cytogenetics and Cell Genetics,* **37**, 312–339

ROSENBERG, M. B., HANSEN, C. and BREAKEFIELD, X. O. (1985) Molecular genetic approaches to neurologic and psychiatric diseases. *Progress in Neurobiology,* **24**, 95–140

ROSES, A. D., PERICAK-VANCE, M. A., YAMAOKA, L. H., STUBBLEFIELD, E., STAJICH, J., VANCE, J. M. *et al.* (1983) Recombinant DNA strategies in genetic neurological diseases. *Muscle and Nerve,* **6**, 339–355

ROWLAND, L. P. (1983) Molecular genetics, pseudogenetics and clinical neurology. *Neurology,* **33**, 1179–1195

SASAKI, H., SAKAKI, Y., MATSUO, H., GOTO, I., KUROIWA, Y., SAHASHI, I. *et al.* (1984) Diagnosis of familial amyloidotic polyneuropathy by recombinant DNA techniques. *Biochemical and Biophysical Research Communications,* **125**, 636–642

SCHMITT, H. P., EMSER, W. and HEIMES, C. (1984) Familial occurence of amyotrophic lateral sclerosis, parkinsonism, and dementia. *Annals of Neurology,* **16**, 642–648

SCHWALBE, W. (1908) *Eine eigentumliche tonische krampfform mit hysterischen Symptomen.* Berlin: G. Schade

SEGAWA, M., HOSAKA, A., MIYAGAWA, F. *et al.* (1976) Hereditary progressive dystonia with marked diurnal fluctuation. *Advances in Neurology,* **14**, 215–233

SPARKES, R. S., SPARKES, M. C., WILSON, M. G., TOURNER, J. W., BENEDICT, W., MURPHEE, A. L. *et al.* (1980) Regional assignment of genes for human esterase D and retinoblastoma to chromosome band 13 q14. *Science,* **208**, 1042–1044

STANBURY, J. B., WYNGAARDEN, J. B., FREDRICKSON, D. S., GOLDSTEIN, J. L. and BROWN, M. S. (1983) *The Metabolic Basis of Inherited Disease,* Chaps. 1, 2. New York: McGraw-Hill

STOUT, J. T. and CASKEY, C. T. (1986) HPRT gene structure, expression and mutation. *Annual Review of Genetics,* 127–148

STOUT, J. T., CHEN, H. Y., BRENNAND, J., CASKEY, C. T. and BRINSTER, R. L. (1985) Expression of human HPRT in the central nervous system of transgenic mice. *Nature,* **317**, 250–252

SUDARSKY, L., MYERS, R. H. and WALSH, T. M. (1983) Huntington's disease in monozygotic twins reared apart. *Journal of Medical Genetics,* **20**, 408–411

SUTTON, H. E. (1975) *An Introduction to Human Genetics.* New York: Holt, Rinehart and Winston

WARD, D. D., DUVOISIN, R. C., INCE, S. W., NUTT, J. D., ELDRIDGE, R., CALNE, D. B. *et al.* (1984) Parkinson's disease in twins. *Advances in Neurology,* **40**, 341

WATKINS, P. C., TANZI, R. E., GIBBONS, K. P., TRICOLI, J. V., LANDIS, G., EDDY, R. *et al.* (1985) Isolation of polymorphic DNA segments from human chromosome 21. *Nucleic Acid Research,* **13**, 6075–6088

WATTS, R. W. E., SPELLACY, E., GIBBS, D. A., ALLSOP, J., McKERAN, R. O. and SLAVIN, G. E. (1982) Clinical, post-mortem, biochemical and therapeutic observations on the Lesch–Nyhan syndrome with particular reference to the neurological manifestations. *Quarterly Journal of Medicine,* **201**, 43–78

WEXLER, N. S., YOUNG, A., TANZI, R., STAROSTA, S., GOMEZ, F., TRAVERS, H. *et al.* (1985) Huntington's disease heterozygotes detected. *American Journal of Human Genetics,* **37**, a82

WHITE, R., LEPPERT, M., BISHOP, D. T., BARKER, D., BERKOWITZ, J., BROWN, C. *et al.* (1985) Construction of linkage maps with DNA markers for human chromosomes. *Nature,* **313**, 101–105

WILLIAMS, D. A., LEMISCHKA, I. R., NATHAN, D. G. and MULLIGAN, R. C. (1984) Introduction of new genetic material into pluripotent haematopoietic stem cells of the mouse. *Nature,* **310**, 476–480

WILLIS, R. C., JOLLY, D. J., MILLER, A. D., PLENT, M. M., ESTY, A. C., ANDERSON, P. J. *et al.* (1983) Partial phenotypic correction of human Lesch–Nyhan (hypoxanthine-guanine phosphoribosyltransferase-deficient) lymphoblasts with a transmissible retroviral vector. *Journal of Biological Chemistry,* **259**, 7842–7849

WILSON, J. M., YOUNG, A. B. and KELLEY, W. N. (1983) Hypoxanthine-guanine phosphoribosyltransferase deficiency. *New England Journal of Medicine,* **309**, 900–910

WORTON, R. G., DUFF, C., SYLVESTER, J. E., SCHMICKEL, R. D. and WILLARD, H. F. (1984) Duchenne muscular dystrophy involving translocation of the dmd gene next to ribosomal RNA genes. *Science,* **224**, 1447–1448

YANG, T. P., PATEL, P. I., CHINAULT, A. C., STOUT, J. T., JACKSON, J. G., HILDEBRAND, B. M. *et al.* (1984) Molecular evidence for new mutation at the HPRT locus in Lesch–Nyhan patients. *Nature,* **310**, 412–413

ZEMAN, W. and DYKEN, P. (1967) Dystonia musculorum deformans; clinical, genetic and pathoanatomical studies. *Psychiatria Neurologia Neurochirurgia,* 77–121

ZILBER, N., KORCZYN, A. D., KAHANA, E., FRIED, K. and ALTER, M. (1984) Inheritance of idiopathic torsion dystonia among Jews. *Journal of Medical Genetics,* **21**, 13–20

Part II
Parkinson's disease and other akinetic–rigid syndromes

5
Problems in Parkinson's disease and other akinetic–rigid syndromes
C. D. Marsden and Stanley Fahn

INTRODUCTION

In the previous volume *Movement Disorders* in 1982, Roger Duvoisin discussed what was known about the cause of Parkinson's disease. Much has happened since then. In particular, the full report on Parkinson's disease in twins has been published (Ward *et al.*, 1983), suggesting that inheritance does not play a major part and the first environmental toxin known to produce pure parkinsonism, 1-methyl-4-phenyl-1,2,3,6-tetrahydropyridine or MPTP, has been identified (Langston *et al.*, 1983). This latter discovery has generated enormous excitement in the clinical and research community, for it may have provided a new clue to the cause of Parkinson's disease. Accordingly, we invited Bill Langston to review, at first hand, the MPTP story in Chapter 6. The discovery that MPTP-induced destruction of the substantia nigra can be prevented in the experimental animal by inhibition of monoamine oxidase B, and by inhibition of dopamine re-uptake, has focused attention on the possibility of treatments designed to slow or prevent progression of Parkinson's disease. Clinical evaluation of such preventive therapy will depend upon knowledge of the natural history of Parkinson's disease. So Gerald Stern reviews what is known of the prognosis of this illness in Chapter 7.

In the previous volume, Richard Mayeux discussed depression and dementia in Parkinson's disease. Both are important practical and theoretical problems. However, since then, considerable attention has been given to the frequency, nature and significance of more subtle cognitive changes in parkinsonian patients who are not demented or depressed. These aspects of selective cognitive deficits are reviewed by Richard Brown in Chapter 8.

The morphological and biochemical pathology of Parkinson's disease were discussed by Lysia Forno, Oleh Hornykiewicz and Urpo Rinne in the previous volume. New data have appeared since then and current concepts of the neuropathology of Parkinson's disease are reviewed by Kurt Jellinger in Chapter 9, and of the neurochemistry by Yves Agid and colleagues in Chapter 10.

In 1982, it was recognized that the appearance of fluctuations of response to chronic levodopa therapy was one of the major long-term problems in treating Parkinson's disease. This was reflected in the previous volume by chapters on the clinical features and pathophysiology of such fluctuations by the editors, along with

David Parkes and Niall Quinn. At that time there was debate as to whether these fluctuations were due to long-term receptor changes or to alterations in the pharmacokinetic handling of levodopa. Since then it has been shown that continuous intravenous infusions of levodopa (Hardie, Lees and Stern, 1984; Quinn, Parkes and Marsden, 1984), or other dopamine agonists such as lisuride, can produce a stable response to levodopa in many patients who have developed the 'on–off' problem. This has focused attention on the pharmacokinetics of levodopa, discussed here by Fred Wooten in Chapter 11.

Patients with an akinetic–rigid parkinsonian syndrome who do not respond to levodopa are increasingly realized to have illnesses other than Parkinson's disease. In the last volume Roger Bannister and David Oppenheimer discussed the complex inter-relationships between the clinical syndromes of progressive autonomic failure, parkinsonism and ataxia, and their pathological counterparts of central autonomic, striatonigral and olivopontocerebellar degeneration – the multiple-system atrophies. Since then, the discovery of a partial deficiency of glutamate dehydrogenase in some patients with olivopontocerebellar degeneration has focused attention on this entity, which is reviewed by Roger Duvoisin in Chapter 12. Because of difficulties in the clinical diagnosis of this condition, we invited another expert, Anita Harding, to comment on Duvoisin's chapter. Steele–Richardson–Olszewski disease (progressive supranuclear palsy) is another common cause of parkinsonism not generally responsive to levodopa. Andrew Lees reviews this condition in Chapter 13.

Finally, in this section, the crucial importance of Wilson's disease, one of the few movement disorders that can be prevented by attacking its root cause, is recognized by inviting Irmin Sternlieb and Herb Scheinberg to review their extensive experience of this illness in Chapter 14.

As before, many other practical problems that face the practitioner in the management of a patient with Parkinson's disease are not discussed, because it remains difficult to provide a definitive statement on these matters. To cover these gaps, and to give some guidance on present views, the editors state their own approach to coping with some of these problems.

WHEN AND HOW SHOULD TREATMENT BE STARTED?

Whether to start levodopa (or bromocriptine) as soon as the diagnosis of Parkinson's disease is made, or whether to delay such treatment until disability, social or occupational, warrants it remains controversial. No new prospective studies of early versus late levodopa therapy have been published to resolve this dilemma. The original claim by Markham and Diamond (1981) that the response to levodopa is determined by the duration of the disease rather than the duration of therapy, with the implication that delaying levodopa treatment results in loss of its efficiency, has been disputed (Fahn and Bressman, 1984). The editors still advise their patients to delay levodopa until disability requires it. Until that point is reached we employ a simpler treatment with an anticholinergic and/or amantadine. However, we have become more hesitant in employing anticholinergics, in view of the emerging evidence for the role of cholinergic mechanisms in the cognitive problems and dementia of Parkinson's disease, and the possible role of anticholinergic drugs in aggravating such problems (*see* Chapter 10). Particularly in the elderly, who are very susceptible to the toxic effects of anticholinergic drugs, levodopa is begun early rather than late. However, the general principle of tailoring therapy to each individual patient's needs remains paramount. The young executive trying to preserve his employment despite Parkinson's disease may require early levodopa therapy; likewise the active elderly patient with a limited life-expectancy. However, the recently retired individual who can manage all his/her social and occupational affairs on simpler treatment (or on no treatment at all) may be advised to delay. No simple rule governs this decision; each patient's requirements require individual judgement.

One of the major reasons for caution in the introduction of levodopa therapy has been the realization that many individuals develop problems after some years of treatment. Fluctuations in response and unpleasant dyskinesias appear with increasing frequency as time goes by. One hope of avoiding these problems has been the possibility of introducing a directly acting dopamine agonist, such as bromocriptine, as the first line of treatment when disability requires it. A number of studies have been published in recent years to support this view. Long-term bromocriptine treatment may cause fewer problems of dyskinesias and fluctuations than levodopa therapy. The matter has been complicated by a debate on whether low doses (less than 20 mg/day) or higher doses of bromocriptine should be employed. Teychenne has championed the view that low doses of bromocriptine are adequate for new patients, providing patience is maintained to await the response (Teychenne *et al.*, 1982). Others, including ourselves, generally have found that higher doses of bromocriptine are required for most patients when the drug is used by itself. This debate is not as polarized as some of the literature would suggest. A recent unpublished double-blind study of low dose (up to 25 mg/day introduced over six months) versus high dose (up to 100 mg/day introduced over six months) bromocriptine treatment of a total of 134 *de novo* patients by the UK Bromocriptine Trial Group drew the following conclusions: fewer patients will achieve significant improvement on lower doses, but many do although they take longer to do so; the incidence of severe side-effects requiring withdrawal from bromocriptine surprisingly is no different in slow and fast regimes, although more in the fast group experience minor side-effects. (Minor and some major side-effects may be prevented by the co-administration of domperidone, which is routine practice in the UK.) The overall conclusion is the the dose of bromocriptine required varies from patient to patient, as does the rate of increment. It seems that more severely affected individuals may require larger doses, whilst those mildly affected can manage on low doses.

This still leaves the question as to whether bromocriptine or levodopa is the drug of choice for *de novo* patients. Our own experience, and that of others (Lees and Stern, 1981; Rinne, 1985), suggests that only a minority of such individuals can be managed on bromocriptine alone. In the UK Bromocriptine Trial, only 50% of patients had achieved adequate benefit within six months, and the studies of Rinne (1985) suggest that after three years of treatment with bromocriptine alone, less than a third of patients maintain an adequate therapeutic response.

With this in mind, the editors and others have adopted a different therapeutic strategy. The aim is to use levodopa as the main and first drug (when disability warrants it), but to keep the dose of levodopa to a minimum. New patients are started on Sinemet (levodopa/carbidopa) [or Madopar (levodopa/benserazide) where it is available], but the dose is kept to no more than about four levodopa/carbidopa 25/100 tablets per day. If the therapeutic response is inadequate, bromocriptine is added in low dosage and then gradually increased until an adequate response is achieved. Rinne (1985) has provided evidence that this strategy may reduce dyskinesias and fluctuations compared to treatment with levodopa alone. Combined treatment with levodopa and bromocriptine seems to represent the best current method of using these drugs so as to obtain optimum benefit with the least risk of problems during long-term therapy.

NEW DOPAMINE AGONISTS

What of the other newer directly acting dopamine agonists? Much effort has gone into clinical studies of a variety of such new agonists, but the results generally have been disappointing. Some have been withdrawn because of toxicity – lergotrile caused liver disturbance, mersulergine and ciladopa because they caused tumours in rodents. Lisuride, although effective as an antiparkinsonian agent, is too short acting for routine oral use. (Lisuride may find a place for chronic continuous subcutaneous infusions – *see below*.) Pergolide remains, but, although effective, it has shown no obvious advantages over bromocriptine, and has not yet been licensed for general use. The overall impression of these various dopamine agonists has been that, although they differ in their pharmacological specificity for different dopamine receptors, their antiparkinsonian actions and side-effects broadly have been the same. Patients who fail to respond to levodopa and/or bromocriptine have rarely responded to any of the other dopamine agonists. Those who have run into severe problems of resistant fluctuations in response to levodopa generally have not responded better to the newer dopamine agonists than they have to bromocriptine. So far, the new dopamine agonists have not improved greatly on existing therapy, although some patients will respond better to one agonist compared to another. Many other compounds of this category are being prepared for clinical trial, and may prove valuable in the future.

MANAGEMENT OF FLUCTUATIONS AND DYSKINESIAS

These remain major problems. Unfortunately, there is no reliable way of reducing dyskinesias without worsening the parkinsonism. Reduction of levodopa dosage often provokes an unacceptable return of loss of mobility, and although many other drugs have been added to levodopa to try to decrease dyskinesias selectively, none has proved generally effective. Particularly distressing are 'off-period' or diphasic dystonias, which often are painful. Some success in relieving such dystonia has been obtained with the addition of baclofen or pergolide.

Severe fluctuations also remain difficult to manage. The first sign of this complication, namely the appearance of the 'wearing-off' phenomenon or 'end-of-dose deterioration', can initially be controlled by closer spacing of individual levodopa doses, or the addition of bromocriptine (or deprenyl where it is available – *see below*). However, many patients subsequently escape from control and begin to experience increasingly severe and unpredictable variations in mobility (and dyskinesias). As discussed above, the newer dopamine agonists generally have not solved this problem. For this reason a number of workers have turned to constant infusions of dopamine agonists to try and maintain a stable response.

The principle is similar to the use of constant subcutaneous infusions of insulin to stabilize the brittle diabetic. Constant intravenous infusions of levodopa can dramatically smooth out fluctuations in brittle parkinsonism. Unfortunately, levodopa is unstable, not very soluble, and acidic, and so is not an ideal candidate for such an approach. Lisuride, on the other hand, is highly potent and water soluble at a neutral pH. Constant subcutaneous infusions of lisuride have proved effective in restoring reliable mobility in initial trials (Obeso et al., 1983). Development of this strategy, perhaps using lisuride or other similar dopamine agonists, is awaited with interest.

Other methods of delivery of levodopa, to try to maintain more constant plasma levels, are also under trial. Longer-acting preparations of both levodopa/carbidopa and levodopa/benzerazide are being investigated.

The role of drug holidays in patients with Parkinson's disease has become clearer since it was discussed in the last volume. In general, most neurologists, including ourselves, have not found drug holidays to be of value in restoring a stable response to levodopa in those with uncontrollable fluctuations. Any initial benefit soon disappears, and there is a price to pay. The severe deterioration that occurs when such patients are withdrawn from levodopa for any length of time is psychologically disastrous, and sometimes physically dangerous; deep vein thrombosis, aspiration pneumonia and other problems can occur. Accordingly, we do not see this as a practical means of coping with the severely fluctuating response to long-term levodopa therapy.

However, shorter periods of drug withdrawal can be useful in those with toxic effects of levodopa, particularly psychiatric problems. 'Weekend withdrawal', stopping the drug for one or two days over the weekend, may reduce toxic psychosis over the next week, and sometimes can be a useful strategy.

Finally, much media publicity has been given to attempts to restore function in Parkinson's disease by transplantation. Research work in rodents clearly has shown that transplants of fetal substantia nigra into the denervated striatum can survive, grow, secrete dopamine, and restore some functional deficits. Whether this is true in primates is not yet known. A few speculative attempts at a similar strategy have been made in Scandinavia. The patient's adrenal medulla, which also secretes dopamine, has been transplanted into the striatum of a few patients with Parkinson's disease, but without success. Clearly, this is an area where much more basic scientific research is required before further human experiments can be undertaken, and one in which ethical issues will have to be resolved.

TREATMENT OF THE CAUSE OF PARKINSON'S DISEASE

One of the major outcomes of the MPTP story has been the discovery of how this agent is specifically toxic to the nigrostriatal dopamine system (see Chapter 6). MPTP itself is not the toxic agent, but requires conversion to the 1-methyl-4-phenylpyridinium ion MPP^+. This involves the enzyme monoamine oxidase B, and probably occurs in glia. Monoamine oxidase B inhibitors, such as deprenyl, prevent MPTP toxicity in rodents and primates.

These observations have led to the suggestion that patients with Parkinson's disease should be treated with deprenyl from the moment of diagnosis, to try and prevent progression of the disease. The assumption is that Parkinson's disease is caused by something like MPTP, either present in the environment or generated by faulty metabolism in the brain.

Deprenyl was introduced into the treatment of Parkinson's disease in Europe in the mid-1970s (see Chapter 10 by Merton Sandler and Gerald Stern in the previous volume *Movement Disorders*). The initial rationale was that brain dopamine in man is catabolized by monoamine oxidase B, so that inhibition of this enzyme might prolong the duration of action of levodopa, thus improving fluctuations in response. Certainly this turned out to be the case; some patients with the 'wearing-off' effect are undoubtedly improved by the addition of deprenyl. The drug has been used for this purpose routinely in Europe for many years now.

However, the MPTP story has thrown an entirely new light on the potential value of deprenyl, as a drug that might slow or halt progression of the disease. Indeed, from his considerable experience of the use of deprenyl, Birkmayer (Birkmayer and Riederer, 1984) has published data to suggest that this might be the case. In his material, life expectancy in those treated with deprenyl and levodopa is claimed to be longer than in those treated with levodopa alone. Not everyone would accept his claim, and certainly general experience has shown that deprenyl does not stop progression, but it might slow it. Obviously what is now required, urgently, is the appropriate randomized 'blind' study to prove or disprove this hypothesis. But it will take at least five years to obtain the answer, and the question is what to do now.

The matter is not simple. Whilst deprenyl does prevent experimental MPTP toxicity, it may not prevent that of MPP^+. Another facet of the story is that the toxicity of MPP^+ may depend upon uptake into dopaminergic neurones by the dopamine re-uptake system. MPP^+ toxicity may be prevented by dopamine re-uptake blockers. By chance, one such agent, benztropine, has been in use in Parkinson's disease as an anticholinergic for about a quarter of a century. There is no suggestion that benztropine has halted or slowed the progression of Parkinson's disease, but it may not have been employed clinically in doses adequate to block dopamine re-uptake (and by inference to prevent MPP^+-type toxicity).

This issue is not settled and requires further research. Meanwhile, because deprenyl appears a safe non-toxic drug, there seems little to be lost in using it in newly diagnosed patients with Parkinson's disease.

OTHER AKINETIC–RIGID SYNDROMES

Failure of a patient with an akinetic–rigid syndrome to respond to levodopa at all is a strong clue that the cause is not Parkinson's disease, but some other pathological condition. The commonest alternatives are multiple-system atrophy, progressive supranuclear palsy, and cerebrovascular disease. Other rarer conditions include normal pressure hydrocephalus, pugilistic or traumatic parkinsonism, and some newly recognized conditions such as corticostrionigrodentate degeneration. Failure to respond to levodopa should thus prompt full investigation to discover an alternative diagnosis to Parkinson's disease. However, often this is difficult to establish in the early stages of the illness.

For example, postural hypotension in a patient with parkinsonism may be due to Lewy body disease or multiple-system atrophy. Only time will tell whether more profound autonomic failure will develop to indicate the latter. The eye movement disorder of progressive supranuclear palsy may not be apparent to begin with and may take many years to evolve. Indeed, there now are pathological reports of this condition in patients not noted to have the characteristic eye movement disturbance in life. It is also difficult to judge what degree of gaze palsy warrants a diagnosis of progressive supranuclear palsy. Patients with levodopa-responsive Parkinson's disease, due to Lewy body degeneration, may exhibit defects of voluntary and pursuit horizontal and up-gaze. A diagnosis of progressive supranuclear palsy cannot be made in the absence of a significant defect of down-gaze. Even then there are difficulties, for a typical clinical syndrome of a progressive supranuclear palsy, including down-gaze, in an akinetic-rigid patient may not indicate the pathology of Steele–Richardson–Olszewski disease; a similar clinical picture can be seen in multiple-system atrophy and a few other rare system degenerations.

Recently, new data on the pathological biochemistry of Steele–Richardson–Olszewski disease have been obtained (Kish et al., 1985; Ruberg et al., 1985). Dopamine concentrations in striatum and substantia nigra were profoundly reduced, as in Parkinson's disease. However, in contrast to Parkinson's disease, dopamine levels in nucleus accumbens and most areas of cerebral cortex were unaffected, and levels of noradrenaline and serotonin generally were not altered. This raises the interesting question as to the origin of the cognitive changes so characteristic of progressive supranuclear palsy. The two studies reported different findings with regard to cortical acetylcholine content; one group (Ruberg et al., 1985) found modest reductions in choline acetyltransferase activity in cerebral cortex and greater losses in substantia innominata; the other (Kish et al., 1985) reported values within the normal range. The reason for the profound decrease in glucose utilization in frontal cortex of patients with progressive supranuclear palsy (D'Antona et al., 1985) remains unexplained.

Treatment with levodopa or other dopamine agonist drugs in this illness generally is ineffective. Some improvement in mobility may be seen in the occasional patient, for a limited period of time, but usually such treatment has little or no effect. This may be explained by the finding of a considerable reduction in the number of dopamine receptors in the striatum, measured using the potent D-2 antagonist [^{3}H]spiperone (Ruberg et al., 1985). A similar loss of striatal dopamine receptors has been shown in life by PET scanning using the tracer [^{76}Br]bromospiperone (Baron et al., 1985). Unfortunately, the treatment of Steele–Richardson–Olszewski's disease remains unsatisfactory.

The treatment of the neurological symptoms and progressive autonomic failure in multiple system atrophy also is difficult. Parkinsonian symptoms sometimes may respond to levodopa, at least temporarily, although postural hypotension may be aggravated. Other dopamine agonists, such as bromocriptine, lisuride and pergolide also occasionally give benefit, but again worsening postural syncope or adverse psychiatric effects may limit their use. The management of symptomatic postural hypotension likewise is difficult. A simple measure to increase the patient's blood volume by head-up tilt at night may be effective initially. Head-up body tilt at night is thought to operate by reducing renal arterial pressure, thus promoting renin release leading to angiotensin II formation and aldosterone stimulation. If nocturnal head-up tilt is insufficient, fludrocortisone is usually added. A variety of pressor drugs have been tried, but with inconsistent results and often with unacceptable recumbent hypertension. Indomethacin has been reported to be of some benefit, thought to be due to its actions in increasing vasoconstrictor sensitivity to endogenous noradrenaline and angiotension II, as well as to its effects as a prostaglandin inhibitor.

References

BARON, J., MAZIERE, B., LOC'H, C., SGOUROPOULOS, P., BONNET, A. M. and AGID, Y. (1985) Progressive supranuclear palsy: loss of striatal dopamine receptors demonstrated in vivo by positron tomography. Lancet, i

BIRKMAYER, W. and RIEDERER, P. (1984) Deprenyl prolongs the therapeutic efficacy of combined L-DOPA in Parkinson's disease. In Advances in Neurology. Eds. R. G. Hassler and J. F. Christ, Vol. 40, pp. 475–481. New York: Raven Press

D'ANTONA, R., BARON, J. C., SAMSON, Y., SERDARU, M., VIADER, F., AGID, Y. and CAMBIER, J. (1985) Subcortical dementia: frontal cortex hypometabolism detected by positron tomography in patients with progressive supranuclear palsy. *Brain,* **108,** 785–799

FAHN, S. and BRESSMAN, S. B. (1984) Should levodopa therapy for parkinsonism be started early or late? Evidence against early treatment. *Canadian Journal of Neurological Science,* **11,** 200–206

HARDIE, R. J., LEES, A. J. and STERN, G. M. (1984) On–off fluctuations in Parkinson's disease: A clinical and neuropharmacological study. *Brain,* **107,** 487–506

KISH, S. J., CHANGE, L. J., MIRCHANDANI, L., SHANNAK, K. and HORNYKIEWICZ, O. (1985) Progressive supranuclear palsy: relationship between extrapyramidal disturbances, dementia and brain neurotransmitter markers. *Annals of Neurology,* **18,** 530–536

LANGSTON, J. W., BALLARD, P., TETRUD, J. W. and IRWIN, I. (1983) Chronic parkinsonism in humans due to a product of meperidine–analog synthesis. *Science,* **219,** 979–980

LEES, A. J. and STERN, G. M. (1981) Sustained bromocriptine therapy in previously untreated patients with Parkinson's disease. *Journal of Neurology, Neurosurgery and Psychiatry,* **44,** 1020–1023

MARKHAM, C. H. and DIAMOND, S. G. (1981) Evidence to support early levodopa therapy in Parkinson's disease. *Neurology,* **31,** 125–131

OBESO, J. A., MARTINEZ-LAGE, J. M., LUQUIN, M. R. and BOLIO, N. (1983) Intravenous lisuride infusion for Parkinson's disease. *Annals of Neurology,* **14,** 252

QUINN, N., PARKES, J. D. and MARSDEN, C. D. (1984) Control of on/off phenomenon by intravenous infusion of levodopa. *Neurology (Cleveland),* **34,** 1131–1136

RINNE, U. K. (1985) Early combination of bromocriptine and levodopa in the treatment of Parkinson's disease. In *Approaches to the Use of Bromocriptine in Parkinson's Disease.* Eds. S. Fahn, C. D. Marsden, P. Jenner and P. Teychenne, pp. 7–14. New York: Raven Press

RINNE, U. K. (1985) Combined bromocriptine–levodopa therapy early in Parkinson's disease. *Neurology,* **35,** 1196–1198

RUBERG, M., JAVOY-AGID, F., HIRSCH, E., SCATTON, B., LHEUREUX, R., HAUW, J. J. et al. (1985) Dopaminergic and cholinergic lesions in progressive supranuclear palsy. *Annals of Neurology,* **18,** 523–529

TEYCHENNE, P. F., BERGSRUD, D., RACY, A., ELTON, R. L. and VERN, B. (1982) Bromocriptine: low-dose therapy in Parkinson's disease. *Neurology,* **32,** 577–583

WARD, C. D., DUVOISIN, R. C., INCE, S. E., NUTT, J. D., ELDRIDGE, R. and CALNE, D. B. (1983) Parkinson's disease in 65 pairs of twins and a set of quadruplets. *Neurology (Cleveland),* **33,** 815–824

6
MPTP: The promise of a new neurotoxin
J. William Langston

It has been known for over 60 years that idiopathic Parkinson's disease is characterized pathologically by death of neurones in the zona compacta of the substantia nigra (Tretiakoff, 1919). While this is not the only pathological feature of the disease (Forno, 1982), it is the most prominent, and damage to this structure has been repeatedly incriminated as the major, if not sole, cause for the classical clinical findings seen in the disease (Hornykiewicz, 1966; Fahn, 1982). In spite of a great deal of interest and research, no one knows why these cells die in Parkinson's disease, or precisely what the mechanism underlying their death is. The potential importance of answering these questions may, at least in part, explain the great surge of interest in the newly described neurotoxin 1-methyl-4-phenyl-1,2,3,6-tetrahydropyridine (MPTP) (Lewin, 1984a). This compound appears to be selectively toxic to the cells of the zona compacta of the substantia nigra (Burns *et al.*, 1983; Langston *et al.*, 1984a) and is capable of inducing virtually all the signs and symptoms of Parkinson's disease in humans (Ballard, Tetrud and Langston, 1985).

In this chapter the author will review some of the scientific dividends which have resulted from the recognition of the biological effects of MPTP, and look at the future promise this newly described neurotoxin may hold. The discovery of MPTP has already led to the development of an animal model for Parkinson's disease, to increasing interest in possible environmental causes for the disease, and even to hints of a strategy for the prevention of the disease (Langston, 1985a).

HISTORICAL REVIEW

For a compound which had never appeared in the title of an article before 1983, MPTP has an interesting though somewhat chequered history. Soon after it was synthesized in 1947 by Ziering and coworkers (1947), the compound underwent testing as a possible therapeutic agent (Langston, Langston and Irwin, 1984). But primates, after receiving MPTP, became rigid and unable to move and eventually died. Six humans were given the compound, but two died during or shortly after the study, and MPTP was apparently abandoned as a possible therapeutic agent

(Langston, Langston and Irwin, 1984). In what seems in retrospect an astonishing irony, the compound was being tested as a possible anti-parkinsonian agent. Although this was a less than promising therapeutic debut, in retrospect it was the first clue that a powerful experimental neurotoxin was at hand.

Only after another compound, 1-methyl-4-propionoxypiperidine (MPPP) began finding its way into the laboratories of clandestine chemists interested in synthesizing narcotics for illicit use, were the biological effects of the compound clearly recognized (Langston *et al.*, 1983). MPPP, which is a reverse ester of meperidine and a potent narcotic, apparently achieved popularity because it is relatively easy to synthesize, and until very recently was uncontrolled, and hence possession was not illegal. Unfortunately, the synthesis of MPPP typically results in varying amounts of MPTP as a byproduct. This problem was to have disastrous consequences for a number of young drug abusers, but was of little if any concern at the time since the toxic effects of MPTP had yet to be identified.

The first instance of parkinsonism in an individual using the Ziering formula, of which we have a detailed account, occurred in 1976 (Davis *et al.*, 1979). The story is that of a young college student who successfully synthesized and abused MPPP as a heroin substitute for approximately six months. However, on one occasion he rushed the synthesis and made a 'sloppy batch' after which he became severely parkinsonian. He died two years later, at which time pathological examination of his brain revealed cell loss limited to the substantia nigra. In fact, the lesions in the nigra were indistinguishable from those seen in moderately advanced Parkinson's disease (Lysia Forno, 1982, personal communication). Although it was not clear at the time which compound had been the offending agent, the case was eventually published in 1979 under the title of 'Chronic parkinsonism secondary to intravenous injection of meperidine analogues' (Davis *et al.*, 1979). In 1980 a young drug abuser in Vancouver, Canada, attempted to synthesize MPPP using a different formula (Schmidle and Mansfield, 1956). Of particular interest was the fact that he used the compound intranasally rather than intravenously, yet its effects were equally devastating (Wright *et al.*, 1984), as this young man became rigid and unable to move. He was eventually hospitalized on a psychiatric unit, where he remained for one year until his underlying parkinsonian condition was recognized and treated. However, once again the offending agent was not identified with certainty. This young man died two years later in a drowning accident, but unfortunately the time delay in obtaining the brain prevented a complete neuropathological examination.

In the summer of 1982 in northern California, MPPP was again produced for illicit use (personal communication, 1982, James Heagy), but this time it was destined for mass distribution. It was widely sold in northern California as heroin, synthetic heroin, Mexican brown heroin ('organic heroin'), and even China White (supposedly high-grade heroin from south-east Asia). Predictably, it was not long before contaminated batches containing MPTP (one contained almost pure MPTP) began appearing on the streets, the consequences of which were dramatic. Young drug abusers began arriving in various emergency rooms at hospitals in northern California with what appeared to be advanced Parkinson's disease. After tracking down samples of the 'heroin' and searching out additional cases, it was eventually possible to identify MPTP as the probable offending agent (Langston *et al.*, 1983; Lewin, 1984b; Langston, 1985b). Based on the clinical findings, response to therapy, and spinal fluid examinations in these patients, as well as pathological data from the previously reported student (Davis *et al.*, 1979) (which we concluded was likely to have been a case of MPTP intoxication as well), it was suggested that this compound was selectively toxic to the substantia nigra (Langston et al., 1983), something which has since been proven to be the case.

INSIGHTS FROM THE CLINICAL SYNDROME

Assessing MPTP neurotoxicity from a purely clinical standpoint, the most striking aspect is the complete and unalloyed parkinsonism which it produces (Ballard, Tetrud and Langston, 1985). While there are other agents which cause clinical parkinsonism, such as manganese, carbon disulphide, and carbon monoxide, none of these consistently produce such a pure and complete parkinsonian state (Ballard, Tetrud and Langston, 1985). Not only do patients with MPTP-induced parkinsonism manifest all of the typical features seen in Parkinson's disease (*Table 6.1*), but subtle features of the disease such as seborrhoea and certain tests of cognitive function typically seen in non-demented patients with Parkinson's disease (such as difficulties with visual spatial tasks) are seen as well (Ballard, Tetrud and Langston, 1985; Stern and Langston, 1985). These observations are of particular interest because they have direct bearing on the anatomical site of the origin of the signs and symptoms in Parkinson's disease.

Because the pathological lesions in Parkinson's disease extend well beyond the substantia nigra (Forno, 1982), it has been difficult to discern which symptoms are due to loss of cells in the nigra as opposed to other affected areas in brain. This issue has remained a matter of some debate, although the suggestion that most if not all of the motor symptoms are in fact due to the lesions of the substantia nigra was first put forth by Hornykiewicz in 1966, and has since been championed by others (Fahn, 1982). While these arguments have stood the test of time, direct proof has, by and large, been lacking. Because all the evidence to date suggests that patients with MPTP-induced parkinsonism have lesions limited to the substantia nigra (Ballard, Tetrud and Langston, 1985), and they exhibit virtually all of the clinical features of this disease, these patients provided powerful support for the argument that most if not all of the motor symptoms and signs in Parkinson's disease can be produced by lesions of the substantia nigra. This is particularly interesting in regard to signs such as tremor, which has been thought to require additional damage to the cerebellofugal system (Poirier et al., 1975), and freezing, a clinical phenomenon often thought to reflect involvement of the mesiolimbic system (Price, Farley and Hornykiewicz, 1978). This is not to say that lesions in other areas of the brain may not produce some of the phenomenology of Parkinson's disease, or that these phenomena may not be augmented by involvement of other systems, but rather that they are not required for the production of the wide array of signs and symptoms seen with the idiopathic disease.

On the other hand, dementia which clearly occurs in some patients with Parkinson's disease, was not seen in patients with MPTP-induced parkinsonism, suggesting that a loss of dopaminergic nigrostriatal neurones does not cause major cognitive deficits. Certainly these findings are compatible with the recent suggestions that dementia, particularly memory loss, may be secondary to involvement of cholinergic systems in the CNS (Whitehouse et al., 1983). Finally, depression has been a prominent feature in four of our original seven patients. Interestingly, this has been observed in all three females, and only one of the four

Table 6.1 Signs of Parkinson's disease in MPTP patients

Features of idiopathic Parkinson's disease	Severity in untreated MPTP patients						
	1	2	3	4	5	6	7
Bradykinesia	+++	+++	+++	+++	+++	+	++
Rigidity	+++	++	+++	++	+++	+	++
Resting tremor	O	++	O	O	++	+++	+++
Flexion posture	++	++	+++	++	++	++	++
Loss of postural reflexes	++	+	+++	++	+++	+	++
Loss of associated movements	+++	++	+++	++	+++	++	++
Shuffling, petit pas gait	++	++	+++	++	+++	+	++
En bloc turning	++	++	+++	++	+++	+	++
Difficulty initiating movement	++	++	+++	++	+++	+	++
Cogwheeling	++	++	+	+	+++	+++	+++
Loss of finger dexterity	++	++	+++	++	+++	++	++
Micrographia	++	++	+++	++	+++	+	+
Masked facies	+++	++	+++	++	+++	++	++
Reduced blink rate	+++	+++	+++	++	+++	++	++
Widened palpebral fissure	+++	+++	+++	++	+++	++	+
Limitation of upward gaze	++	+	++	++	O	O	O
Glabellar sign	+++	++	+++	++	+++	++	+
Hypophonia	+++	++	+++	++	+++	++	+
Drooling	++	++	+++	++	+++	++	+
Difficulty swallowing	++	++	+++	+	+++	++	O
Freezing	*	*	*	*	*	O	*
Kinesia paradoxica	*	*	*	*	*	O	O
Seborrhea	+	+++	+	+	+++	++	O
Diaphoresis	O	O	O	O	O	++	O
Hoehn and Yahr score	V	V	V	IV	V	IV	IV

O = absent.
+ = mild.
++ = moderate.
+++ = severe.
* = present, but not rated.
Reproduced from Ballard, Tetrud and Langston (1985).

males. At present we have no good explanation for this apparent disparity between males and females.

Our experience with MPTP-induced parkinsonism and its treatment may also be relevant to current controversies surrounding the timing of initiation of L-dopa therapy (Langston and Ballard, 1984). The concern is that L-dopa therapy itself may be responsible for some or all of the complications of therapy which typically occur over time, including end-of-dose deterioration (or 'wearing off'), peak-dose dyskinesias, on–off phenomenon, and psychiatric complications, particularly hallucinations. The alternative explanation is that some or all of these side-effects of therapy are related to severity of disease, which increases with time. When issues such as this remain unresolved, it is often not only a statement as to their complexity, but often an indication that both factors may be at work to some degree. In any case, the issue has proved a particularly knotty one, and answers may vary depending on which complication is under discussion.

Observations in our patients are most compelling in regard to the wearing-off effect, which refers to the gradual loss of the long duration, smooth response to L-dopa which may be seen early in the course of treatment. In two of our original seven cases, a short duration response (1–2 hours) with rapid wearing-off was apparent literally as soon as a therapeutic response was evident. Since all of these patients started out with advanced disease, and duration of therapy could not have been a factor, these observations suggest in a fairly convincing way that severity of disease may be a major determinant in regard to the appearance of this therapeutic problem. Peak-dose dyskinesias were seen within 3–5 weeks of initiation of therapy in these same two patients, and have now occurred in all but one of these patients. This unusually early and high rate of occurrence would again suggest that severity of disease may, to at least some degree, predispose to 'dopa dyskinesias'. Interestingly, primates given single but very high doses of L-dopa may exhibit dyskinesias (Mones, 1972), suggesting that flooding even the normal nervous system with enough L-dopa can produce dyskinesias. It may be that the very high doses of medication required from the very beginning in these patients, perhaps combined with relative intactness of the rest of their nervous system (and possibly young age), may have a bearing on the early onset of this particular side-effect of therapy. Finally, five of these seven patients began experiencing 'on–off' fluctuations within a year of onset of therapy, again an unusually early and high incidence rate. Somewhat unexpectedly, psychiatric complications have become dose limiting in four of our patients after three years of therapy, something which is of interest in view of their young age. In this group, at least, it can be said that dementia (and particularly senile dementia of the Alzheimer type) does not appear to be a factor predisposing to L-dopa-induced hallucinations. One possibility is that the prior history of drug abuse has in some way predisposed these relatively young people to this disabling complication of L-dopa therapy, but for the moment this remains a point of speculation.

In summary, clinical observations in this unique group of patients have already provided some interesting new insights into the clinical phenomenology of Parkinson's disease. It may be hoped that we shall learn much more from this group of patients as they are followed over time.

AN ANIMAL MODEL FOR PARKINSON'S DISEASE

Given the faithful reproduction of parkinsonian signs and symptoms observed in the humans, it was not difficult to surmise that this compound would be highly effective in producing a good animal model for Parkinson's disease, the absence of which has been one of the factors retarding basic research into the disease. While there have been many animal models developed for the study of Parkinson's disease, most if not all have been subject to certain limitations or criticisms. On the other hand, MPTP has proved dramatically effective in reproducing classical parkinsonism in primates (Burns et al., 1983; Jenner et al., 1984; Langston et al., 1984a), and has provided what appears to be a highly useful model for the testing of new forms of therapy, and studying the pathophysiology of the motor deficits in the disease (Tatton et al., 1984; Doudet et al., 1985). These animals may also provide models for complications of therapy as well. For example, we have repeatedly encountered dyskinesias in animals undergoing L-dopa therapy. Hence, this animal model may offer the first opportunity to answer directly some of the questions regarding the pathophysiology and anatomy of this phenomenon. This model should be particularly attractive as these 'dopa dyskinesias' are so clearly analogous to those observed in humans with MPTP-induced parkinsonism and the latter are indistinguishable from those seen in patients with the idiopathic disease (Langston and Ballard, 1984).

As exciting as this new primate model of Parkinson's disease may be, it has been a matter of both disappointment and frustration that rodents are much more resistant to the effects of MPTP (Boyce *et al.*, 1984; Chiueh *et al.*, 1984). While the compound has been effective in producing dopamine depletion in virtually every animal reported in the literature to date (Langston, 1985c), from new world monkeys to the medicinal leech (Charles Lente, 1985, personal communication), clearcut evidence of cell loss in the substantia nigra has proved to be more difficult to achieve, although this has been reported in mouse (Heikkila, Hess and Duvoisin, 1984), guinea-pig (but only after direct injection into the nigra) (Paul Carvey, 1985, personal communication), cat (Schneider, Yuwiler and Markham, 1985) and the beagle (Burns, 1985). However, none of these animals has demonstrated a persistent behavioural syndrome typical of well-developed Parkinson's disease (with the possible exception of the cat). Particularly interesting in this regard is the beagle, where in spite of a marked depletion of nigral neurones and a greater than 95% dopamine depletion in the striatum, near-complete recovery of clinical symptomatology after three months is observed. It may be that with evolution primates have become much more dependent on the nigrostriatal system and, therefore, more vulnerable to its destruction. Perhaps this has made the substantia nigra more vulnerable to damage from intrinsic or extrinsic factors as well, which could explain why the disease is limited to primates, i.e. humans. On the other hand, perhaps other animals do get Parkinson's disease but do not express it clinically.

HOW GOOD A MODEL IS MPTP-INDUCED PARKINSONISM?

The answer to this question depends on the use for which the model is intended. But perhaps the first point to make is that MPTP-induced parkinsonism is *not* Parkinson's disease. If it were, it would no longer be a model. However, as a clinical or behavioural model for the disease, MPTP-induced parkinsonism would appear to be ideal (tragically, we are in the unique position of being able to judge precisely how analogous the model is to the human condition). Further, from a standpoint of response to therapy and even complications of therapy, the parallel continues unabated (Langston and Ballard, 1984). So what are the differences? There are several.

First, as noted earlier, the pathological changes in MPTP-induced parkinsonism are much more selective than those seen in idiopathic Parkinson's disease. In the latter, other structures such as the locus ceruleus, dorsal motor nucleus of the vagus, and the dopaminergic ventral tegmental area are affected (Forno, 1982). Based on these observations, one would expect the neurochemical changes to be more restricted in MPTP-induced parkinsonism than in Parkinson's disease, something which appears to be the case, at least in the more chronic stages of toxicity (Burns et al., 1983). The second difference is also to be found at the neuropathological level, and has to do with Lewy bodies. These eosinophilic concentric inclusion bodies are considered a hallmark of idiopathic Parkinson's disease (although they are by no means unique to this entity), but they have yet to be convincingly demonstrated in MPTP-induced parkinsonism. Do these differences mean that MPTP or related compounds have nothing to do with the idiopathic disease? In the author's opinion such a conclusion would be quite premature. There are several possibilities which might bring these two syndromes even closer together.

First, it may be that the model used in primates, which employs a relatively acute, high-dose exposure, is insufficient to reproduce these additional pathological features of Parkinson's disease. Lewy bodies may require months, or even years, to develop. Further, chronic low-grade exposure to MPTP or similar toxins might much more closely mimic low-grade exposure to an environmental toxin; the latter possibility could be much closer to what happens in the idiopathic disease if it is indeed due to an environmental agent. It is an axiom in neurotoxicology that the chronic effects of a compound may be far different pathologically than those typically seen after acute exposure (Spencer and Schaumburg, 1984). Another possibility is that MPTP-like compounds exist that produce more extensive pathological damage, which might in turn more closely mirror the distribution of lesions in the idiopathic disease. We are already aware of at least one other compound which appears to be more toxic than MPTP itself based on its ability to provoke dopamine depletion in the mouse striatum (Wilkening et al., 1986). It will be of great interest to see if these compounds produce more extensive lesions in the primate CNS. On the other hand, it may be that subtle species differences may prove to be relevant. There are now preliminary reports of damage to other areas of the brain in certain primate species, including the hypothalamus (Gibb et al., 1986). Some of these changes would again bring us closer to the idiopathic disease. Moving from higher primates to the human might represent just such another change. Finally, ageing could represent another such variable, and will be discussed later in this chapter. In any event, the situation is unique, and benefits should accrue either way. The selectivity of MPTP makes the compound an extremely useful experimental neurotoxin; on the other hand, the ability to produce more widespread changes would make the move even closer to Parkinson's disease.

ENVIRONMENTAL NEUROTOXINS AND PARKINSON'S DISEASE

While the possibility that an environmental toxin might play a role in Parkinson's disease has been entertained for many years, there can be little doubt that the discovery of a relatively simple molecule which is highly toxic to the substantia nigra has served as an invigorating tonic for this particular hypothesis. Further, kindling interest in the possibility of an environmental cause for Parkinson's disease has been the accumulation of data from twin studies suggesting that the disease is not hereditary in nature (Ward et al., 1983). The author's own interest in MPTP as a potential environmental toxin was heightened rather abruptly when, shortly after his original report on MPTP-induced parkinsonism appeared in 1983 (Langston et al., 1983), a letter was received from a pharmaceutical chemist who had developed Parkinson's disease at age 38 while working with MPTP. He was using the compound as a chemical intermediate while synthesizing various analgesics

(Langston and Ballard, 1983). The only possible routes of exposure were via cutaneous contact or vapour inhalation. While it might be argued that this may have simply been a coincidence, several additional cases of parkinsonism have now been identified in chemists who were working with the compound for legitimate purposes, and a higher incidence of parkinsonian findings on physical examination has been reported in industrial workers exposed to MPTP when compared to a matched group of unexposed individuals examined in a blind fashion (Barbeau, Roy and Langston, 1985). Finally, as noted earlier, the two drug abusers in Vancouver were using the compound via the nasal route (Wright *et al.*, 1984). Hence the evidence is relatively strong that parenteral exposure is not required for MPTP to exert its parkinsonian effects.

Could MPTP or a similar substance in the environment be a cause of Parkinson's disease? At the moment there is no evidence that this substance or a similar one exists in either the man-made or natural environment, but then to the best of the author's knowledge it has never been searched for either. The only hint that such a compound might be present in the environment also comes from California, and that is the entity of yellow star thistle toxicity, also known as pallidonigral degeneration (Young, Brown and Klinger, 1970): it occurs in horses when they eat large amounts of this wild growing plant, which is found primarily in the Sacramento Valley. The syndrome has been of interest not only to veterinarians but to neurologists as well, because of its similarity to Parkinson's disease. Affected animals become rigid, have difficulty eating or swallowing, and drooling may be prominent. Damage in the nervous system is severe, but exquisitely localized to the substantia nigra and the globus pallidus. In the latter respect it differs from MPTP neurotoxicity, but it does suggest there are other toxins in the environment which may cause selective damage to the basal ganglia structures. It is currently being investigated whether or not an MPTP-like compound may be involved in this syndrome.

Donald Calne and the author have recently proposed an environmental hypothesis for Parkinson's disease which is testable (Calne and Langston, 1983). This suggests that the disease may result from an environmental insult to the substantia nigra at some time in early to mid-adult life. Since an 80% loss of striatal dopamine (and presumably an equivalent number of cells in the substantia nigra) is required for symptoms to develop (Reiderer and St Wuketich, 1976), most if not all of affected individuals would most likely remain asymptomatic. It has been shown that there is an approximately 5–8% cell loss in the substantia nigra per decade of life. Hence, an individual with a 50–60% cell loss due to an environmental insult at age 30 might well reach the critical 80% loss of striatal dopamine in his/her 60s or 70s, thereby explaining the age-related aspects of the disease. Alternatively, it could be that the increased dopamine turnover, which would occur as a compensatory mechanism after a partial cell loss in the nigra, would in turn result in an increased generation of toxic byproducts (such as free radicals or peroxides) (Barbeau, 1984). This in turn could cause additional damage to nigral neurones (Cohen, 1983). Thus, one could easily envision the development of a classic vicious cycle, with ever-increasing nigral cell death and dopamine turnover. In this system the degeneration of other neuronal systems would have to be a secondary phenomenon, something which might well occur within other catecholaminergic systems, although involvement of cholinergic systems in the CNS of patients with Parkinson's disease would be more difficult to explain in this scheme (unless there was initial damage to this system as well).

In any case we now have available the unique opportunity to study this hypothesis clinically. We are now aware of over 400 individuals in northern California who are likely to have been exposed to meperidine analogues, and many if not most of these were likely to have been exposed to MPTP (Ruttenbur et al., 1986). Hence we have a population of patients with a high probability of pre-existent nigral damage induced by an environmental event (in this case, intravenous exposure to MPTP) who as yet do not have clinically diagnosable parkinsonism. To the best of the author's knowledge this represents the first opportunity to prospectively follow a group of 'pre-parkinsonian' patients to see whether or not with time their disease will become clinically manifest. For this reason it is believed that long-term follow-up of this patient cohort is crucial.

Will MPTP-induced parkinsonism prove to be a progressive condition? We now have several tantalizing bits of evidence that it may be, but the case is by no means proven. We recently carried out a preliminary study of 40 subjects, all of whom had a high degree of probability of MPTP exposure (Langston, 1986). All of these patients were asymptomatic after recovering from the acute phase of MPTP toxicity (Langston, 1985d). Two years after initial exposure to MPTP, 20 of these individuals had begun to experience symptoms very suggestive of early Parkinson's disease. Because the study depends on historical data, and hence is not objective, we are reluctant to draw any firm conclusions from this data as yet. However, we have encountered an intriguing patient who has developed progressive micrographia as documented by measures of figure height from her extensive record-keeping efforts as a book-keeper (Langston, 1986). These show that the height of her handwriting began gradually diminishing beginning about six months after her exposure to MPTP in the summer of 1982, a phenomenon which has continued through to the present. She also has minimal parkinsonian features on examination. Whether or not the observations in this patient represent the first objective evidence that MPTP exposure can result in a progressive neurodegenerative process remains to be seen as this is just a single case. If long-term follow-up of these patients does eventually provide definite evidence of progressive disease, it would represent important evidence that time-limited insult *can* produce a progressive neurodegenerative process which may have a delayed onset. This principle would have implications, not only for Parkinson's disease, but for other neurodegenerative diseases as well.

A final observation in this regard relates to experience with drug holidays in three of the author's original seven patients. Using videotape analysis, there is clear evidence of progression in two of the three (Langston, 1986). However, one could argue that drug therapy may have contributed to this functional decline (presumably through chronic receptor bombardment and desensitization), as both had been on high doses of dopamine precursor and agonist agents. The third patient lost all voluntary movement except for lateral eye movements after three days of medication withdrawal, a condition fairly close to that seen at the time of his original admission. However, since there was so little left to lose, progression might have been difficult to detect in this patient. In the author's opinion, issues such as effects of prior therapy make it all the more important to study untreated individuals exposed to MPTP.

In looking to the future it seems likely that there will be increasing interest in potential environmental factors which might contribute to Parkinson's disease. Unfortunately the disease is not a reportable one and, therefore, most epidemiological studies to date have been hampered. The only study which is not subject to this problem is that from Rochester, Minnesota (Nobrega, Glattre and Kurland, 1967). The evidence from this study suggests that the incidence of the disease is not changing, something which has been interpreted as an argument against an environmental cause of Parkinson's disease. However, these data span only a few decades (1935–1966), and the only safe conclusion is that, in Rochester between these years, the incidence is relatively stable. Over the next few years it is likely that increasingly sophisticated epidemiological data on Parkinson's disease will be generated, and more than a few studies designed to identify specific factors in the environment are likely to appear. In fact, one such study, the results of which are very provocative, has already emerged from Canada. Barbeau and colleagues (Lewin, 1985; Barbeau et al., 1986), struck by the similarity between a metabolite of MPTP and the herbicide paraquat, carried out a detailed study of the prevalence of Parkinson's disease in a Quebec province (where it is routinely reported by virtue of the billing requirements in the health care system). These investigators found that the highest incidence of the disease was in the so-called 'bread basket' of the province, where most of the agricultural industry is located. Further, there was a remarkably high degree of correlation between the use of pesticides and the occurrence rate of Parkinson's disease (Spearman's rank coefficient 0.967). It is perhaps too early to begin drawing definite conclusions regarding the aetiology of Parkinson's disease from such data, but the point I would like to make here is that there are likely to be many more such studies, and for the neuroepidemiologist these should be lively times.

THE MECHANISM OF ACTION OF MPTP

Although recognition of the biological effects of MPTP has attracted a great deal of attention, it is at the basic science level that the activity has been the most intense (Lewin, 1984a). At the heart of this excitement are basically four questions which investigators are intent on answering. These are: (*a*) What is the mechanism of action of MPTP in causing cell death in the substantia nigra? (*b*) Why is the compound selectively toxic to the substantia nigra? (*c*) Why are primates so much more sensitive to the effects of MPTP than lower species, particularly the rodent? (*d*) Will the answers to one or more of the first three questions shed light on the factors underlying the death of nigral neurones and their selective vulnerability in Parkinson's disease? While one could argue that answers to the first three questions are of primarily academic interest, the last, if answered in the affirmative, could have major implications for the study of the aetiopathogenesis of Parkinson's disease.

The evolution of understanding of the mechanism of action of MPTP has been fast paced and fascinating (Lewin, 1985). The first discovery was the identification of a major metabolite of MPTP, 1-methyl-4-phenylpyridinium ion, or MPP^+ (Chiba, Trevor and Castagnoli, 1984; Langston et al., 1984b; Markey et al., 1984). This product of biotransformation represents approximately 80% of the CNS metabolites (Markey et al., 1984; Irwin, I. and Langston, J. W., 1984, unpublished observations), but this conversion also occurs throughout the rest of the body, with the exception of the eye (Langston et al., 1984b). Hence the production of MPP^+ *per se* cannot be invoked to explain the anatomical selectivity of the compound. If MPP^+ is indeed the neurotoxic culprit, it will be necessary to either invoke a quantitative explanation or identify a unique property of nigral neurones which would make them selectively vulnerable to its effects.

It is now known that the biotransformation of MPTP to MPP$^+$ is mediated by monoamine oxidase (Chiba, Trevor and Castagnoli, 1984; Gessner et al., 1984; Heikkila, Hess and Duvoisin, 1985; Singer, Salach and Crabtree, 1985). This finding was somewhat of a surprise as quaternary amines are not generally thought to be good substrates for monoamine oxidase, an enzyme which is more typically involved in the process of deamination (Singer, Salach and Crabtree, 1985). This discovery was first reported in an *in vitro* rat brain mitochondrial preparation by Chiba and colleagues (1984). Independently, Mytilineou and Cohen (1984) found that pargyline (a non-specific monoamine oxidase inhibitor) blocked the toxic effects of MPTP on dopaminergic cells in tissue culture from the rat mesencephalon, suggesting that monoamine oxidase was involved in mediating the toxic effects of MPTP. It was quickly shown that inhibition of monoamine oxidase blocks the dopamine depleting effects of MPTP in the mouse striatum (Heikkila et al., 1984; Markey et al., 1984), and evidence of nigral cell death and clinical parkinsonism in the primate (Cohen et al., 1984; Langston et al., 1984c). This was coincident with near complete inhibition of the transformation of MPTP to MPP$^+$ (Langston et al., 1984c; Markey et al., 1984). These findings have led to interest in the use of monoamine oxidase inhibitors in Parkinson's disease, as we shall see later (Lewin, 1984a).

It has now been shown that MPTP is metabolized by both the A and B forms of the enzyme but that the rate is much higher with the B form (approximately 14 times faster) (Singer, Salach and Crabtree, 1985). Hence, the B form is probably far more important biologically, a fact which may explain why selective monoamine oxidase B inhibitors are effective in preventing neurotoxicity (Cohen et al., 1984), and monoamine oxidase A inhibitors are not (Heikkila et al., 1984). Interestingly, MPTP and its metabolites are also inhibitors of both monoamine oxidase A and B forms, although they have a much higher affinity for the A form. This probably explains the finding that MPTP is primarily a monoamine oxidase A inhibitor *in vivo* (Fuller and Hemrick-Luecke, 1985b). While it may act initially as a competitive inhibitor of the A and B forms of the enzyme, with time this inhibition becomes irreversible, resulting in non-competitive inhibition (Singer, Salach and Crabtree, 1985).

Because MPP$^+$ is a charged compound, it was first thought that it was generated within nigral neurones, where it would then become trapped (Langston et al., 1984b; Markey et al., 1984). A number of investigators, including the author's own group, thought that it was likely that MPTP gained entrance into dopaminergic neurones via the dopamine uptake system because of its structural similarity to dopamine. Hence, when it was reported by Javitch and colleagues that MPP$^+$ (Javitch et al., 1985), but not MPTP, was taken up by the dopamine uptake system, it was again somewhat of a surprise. These investigators suggested that the biotransformation was taking place outside the nigrostriatal neurones, perhaps in glia (*Figure 6.1*). Consistent with this hypothesis is the fact that dopamine uptake blockers do indeed prevent the dopamine depleting effects of MPTP on the mouse striatum (Ricaurte et al., 1986), and the increasing evidence that monoamine oxidase A, not the B form, is the primary form of the enzyme located within nigral neurones – while the B form is located primarily within glia and serotonergic neurones (Westlund et al., 1986).

The fact that MPP$^+$ may be generated before ever reaching nigral neurones poses serious problems for one of the more attractive hypotheses regarding the mechanism of neurotoxicity of MPTP. It has frequently been speculated that during the biotransformation of MPTP either the intermediate dihydropyridine (known as 1-methyl-4-phenyl-2,3-dyhydropyridine or MPDP$^+$) (Chiba *et al.*, 1985), is neurotoxic, or that the liberation of free radicals or peroxides generated in the process actually causes cell damage. However, if this biotransformation is occurring elsewhere it is unlikely to be damaging to nigral neurones (rather it should be killing glia or perhaps serotonergic neurones).

Figure 6.1 Scheme showing the current concepts regarding the sequence of events after systemic administration of MPTP. It is still not entirely clear at what point the actual toxic event occurs, and it is very likely that this conceptualization will be modified repeatedly over the next few years as knowledge of the mechanism of action of MPTP continues to unfold.

How far does all of this take us in terms of answering some of the questions posed at the beginning of this section? The fact that MPP$^+$ is taken up by the dopamine uptake system may begin to explain why only dopaminergic cells in the brain are affected, but does not explain why only one of these, the nigrostriatal system, is singled out. Although there have been occasional reports of damage to other dopaminergic-containing areas of the brain such as the hypothalamus (Gibb *et al.*, 1985), most have not seen these changes, and at the very least we can say with certainty that the dopaminergic cells of the substantia nigra appear to be by far the most sensitive to this compound.

While other factors have been invoked to explain the selectivity of MPTP, such as neuromelanin and dopamine, neither of these are unique to the substantia nigra. Further, the fact that the cat (Schneider, Yuwiler and Markham, 1985) and young beagles (Burns, 1986) appear to have clearcut damage from MPTP, neither of which have neuromelanin, militates against neuromelanin as a factor. Recently, experimental evidence has begun to accumulate against a role for dopamine in the neurotoxic effects of MPTP as well, with the finding that dopamine depletion at the time of exposure to MPTP does not ameliorate long-term dopamine depleting effects in the striatum of the mouse (Fuller and Hemrick-Leucke, 1985a; Ricaurte, G. A., Langston, J. W. and Irwin, I., 1985, unpublished observations).

The reason for the species variability remains unexplained, but we have recently suggested (Langston et al., 1986) that a contributing factor may be that in rodents MPP^+ is rapidly cleared (how this occurs is not yet understood) before much of this metabolite can be taken up by nigral neurones (presuming that MPP^+ is generated outside of nigrostriatal neurones). It has been shown that the half-life of MPP^+ in rodent brain is only several hours (Markey et al., 1984; Langston et al., 1986). On the other hand, MPP^+ remains in the primate brain for a lengthy period of time (Markey et al., 1984; Langston et al., 1986). Hence it may be that in the primate the compound remains trapped in a compartment outside nigrostriatal neurones (it is not yet clear whether this represents glia, serotonergic neurones, or some other CNS compartment) from which it is then gradually released. This slow release might then result in the gradual poisoning of nigral neurones, which because of continuing low-grade exposure could eventually accumulate enough MPP^+ to cause cell death. We have shown that nigral neurones in fact accumulate MPP^+ for up to three days after exposure to MPTP (Irwin and Langston, 1985), an observation which is certainly compatible with this hypothesis. This sequence of events could also explain a puzzling feature of MPTP neurotoxicity, and that is the gradual and even delayed onset of toxicity observed in a number of our patients (Ballard, Tetrud and Langston, 1985; Langston, 1985d).

Precisely how MPP^+ kills nigral neurones once inside cells is still a mystery (if it is indeed the actual toxic agent), although interference with mitochondrial oxidation (Heikkila et al., 1985) or cellular redox reactions (Johannessen et al., 1985) have been suggested. However, there are other metabolites of MPTP in the CNS (Langston et al., 1986), and it is still conceivable that one or more of these might be the responsible agent.

Before leaving the experimental work, the latest development which relates to ageing will be touched on. Parkinson's disease is one of the two major neurodegenerative diseases of ageing, Alzheimer's being the other. Hence, if there is a relationship between a neurotoxin and an age-related disease, the effects of that toxin should be age dependent. Evidence is rapidly evolving that such may be the case with MPTP, at least in the rodent. It has recently been found that while MPTP does little if any damage to cell bodies in the young mature mouse using the Fink–Heimer silver staining technique for neuronal degeneration, it does affect cell bodies in the aged mouse, strongly suggesting an age-dependent effect for neurotoxicity (Ricaurte et al., 1985). Jarvis and Wagner (1985) have shown that the dopamine-depleting effects of MPTP increase with age in the rat and a similar effect in the mouse has been noted (1985, unpublished observation). Further, it has been reported that mazindol binding in the striatum (presumably a marker of dopamine nerve terminals) decreases to a greater extent after exposure to MPTP in older mice than in young mature mice (Sershon et al., 1985). Perhaps the most exciting possibility is that in the aged animal the neuropathological features of MPTP might more closely resemble those of idiopathic Parkinson's disease. This possibility is being actively studied at the present time. It is believed that these findings may have important implications for the study of diseases of ageing, such as Parkinson's disease, and possibly even for the ageing process itself.

THERAPEUTIC IMPLICATIONS

Although one might not have expected new ideas to emerge regarding the treatment of Parkinson's disease at such an early date after the discovery of MPTP, research on this compound has already had potential implications in this regard. The fact that monoamine oxidase inhibition completely prevents MPTP-induced experimental parkinsonism has raised the interesting possibility that this class of compounds might retard the process of progressive nigral cell death in Parkinson's disease itself. However, sceptics would be right in pointing that there is as yet no proven relationship between the idiopathic disease and MPTP. In this light, the findings of Birkmayer and colleagues (1984) are most relevant, as these investigators have reported in a retrospective study that patients receiving deprenyl, a selective monoamine oxidase B inhibitor, appear to progress more slowly than those who do not. Hence, there may be empirical evidence that cell death can be retarded in the idiopathic disease with monoamine oxidase inhibitor therapy. It is worth noting that there is also a theoretical rationale for using monoamine oxidase inhibitor therapy in Parkinson's disease. This relates to the suggestion that the nigral cell death seen in Parkinson's disease results from the high rate of oxidation of dopamine, a process which would be blocked by monoamine oxidase inhibition (Cohen, 1983). It is believed that these three very separate lines of evidence constitute enough of a case to initiate a prospective trial with deprenyl to see if indeed the course of the disease can be altered. Another approach is to try antioxidant therapy beginning early in the course of the disease, a strategy which is currently being attempted by Fahn and colleagues (1985, personal communication).

In a project which at first might appear unrelated, the author and his colleagues have recently begun studying individuals exposed to MPTP, who do not have clinically diagnosable parkinsonism, using positron emission tomography (PET) techniques. Preliminary findings have shown for the first time that a preclinical striatal dopamine deficiency can be demonstrated in the human (Calne *et al.*, 1985). The implications could be most important for a variety of reasons. For example, it allows a hypothetical strategy to be presented for the prevention of clinical parkinsonism. If PET scan techniques are eventually refined to the stage that they can be used as a screening technique, then it might be possible to screen all individuals at risk for Parkinson's disease, i.e. those over 50 to 60 years of age. Those who have preclinical parkinsonism based on a certain degree of striatal dopamine depletion could then be placed on one or more forms of therapy designed to retard further cell loss if any of the previously discussed clinical trials are successful. Although this is only a research strategy and may well carry on into the twenty-first century, it is of interest that these concepts can even be discussed, particularly as they are based on a story which began with the discovery of a bad batch of synthetic heroin.

EPILOGUE

In a day and age when the lines between basic research and the practice of clinical medicine seem to be more clearly demarcated than ever, the discovery of the biological effects of MPTP, which occurred at the bedside, should be heartening to the clinician. In a way, it seems to be saying that no matter how technologically advanced we become, there will always be an opportunity for clinicians to contribute to basic discoveries in medicine, and that clinical medicine will always continue to make significant contributions to the progress of basic research, just as the discoveries in the basic science laboratory so often affect the general practice of medicine. Given the refractoriness of basic laboratory animals, i.e. rodents, to MPTP, one must wonder when, if ever, its effects would have been discovered had it not been for simple clinical observation combined with a basic knowledge of human disease.

Addendum

As hinted at in this chapter, age may be a highly relevant factor in regard to the MPTP model of Parkinson's disease. The author's group have recently completed a preliminary study of six squirrel monkeys, all of which were five years or older in age (Forno *et al.*, 1986). Using repeated injections of MPTP, they were able to produce unequivocal evidence of locus ceruleus degeneration in five of six animals, a lesion which brings the MPTP model more into line with the neuropathological features seen in Parkinson's disease. Perhaps of even more interest, in the three oldest animals (age range 15–20 years – probably the equivalent of 60 years or older in the human), eosinophilic intraneuronal inclusion bodies were seen in a number of areas in the central nervous system, including the substantia nigra. Whether or not these represent a 'Lewy body equivalent' in the squirrel monkey, or are perhaps the precursors of true Lewy bodies, remains to be proven. However, many of these structures demonstrated the peripheral halo typical of Lewy bodies. Further, they have been seen only in known predilection sites for Lewy bodies in humans. These findings appear to take us a step closer to Parkinson's disease and, in the opinion of the author, should further fuel the search for MPTP-like substances in the envinronment.

References

BALLARD, P. A., TETRUD, J. W. and LANGSTON, J. W. (1985) Permanent human parkinsonism due to 1-methyl-4-phenyl-1,2,3,6-tetrahydropyridine (MPTP): 7 cases. *Neurology*, **35**, 949–956

BARBEAU, A. (1984) Etiology of Parkinson's disease: A research strategy. *Canadian Journal of Neurosciences*, **11**, 24–28

BARBEAU, A., ROY, M. and LANGSTON, J. W. (1985) Neurological consequence of industrial exposure to 1-methyl-4-phenyl-1,2,3,6-tetrahydropyridine. *Lancet*, **i**, 747

BARBEAU, A., ROY, M., CLOUTIER, T., PLASSE, L. and PARIS, S. (1986) Environmental and genetic factors in the etiology of Parkinson's disease. In *Advances in Neurology*. Ed. M. D. Yahr. New York: Raven Press (in press)

BIRKMAYER, W., KNOLL, J., RIEDERER, P. and YOUDIM, M. B. H. (1983) Deprenyl leads to prolongation of L-Dopa efficacy in Parkinson's disease. *Modern Problems of Pharmacopsychiatry*, **19**, 170

BOYCE, S., KELLY, E., REAVILL, C., JENNER, P. and MARSDEN, C. D. (1984) Repeated administration of N-methyl-4-phenyl-1,2,5,6-tetrahydropyridine to rats is not toxic to striatal dopamine neurons. *Biochemical Pharmacology*, **33**, 1747–1752

BURNS, R. S., CHIUEH, C. C., MARKEY, S. P., EBERT, M. H., JACOBOWITZ, D. M. and KOPIN, I. J. (1983) A primate model of parkinsonism: Selective destruction of dopaminergic neurons in the pars compacta of the substantia nigra by N-methyl-4-phenyl-1,2,3,6-tetrahydropyridine. *Proceedings of the National Academy of Sciences*, **80**, 4546–4550

BURNS, R. S., CHUIUEH, C. C., PARIS, J., MARKEY, S. P. and KOPIN, I. J. (1986) In *Recent Developments in Parkinson's Disease*. Eds. S. Fahn, C. D. Marsden, P. Jenner and P. Teychenne. pp. 127–136. New York: Raven Press
CALNE, D. B. and LANGSTON, J. W. (1983) On the etiology of Parkinson's disease. *Lancet*, ii, 1457–1459
CALNE, D. B., LANGSTON, J. W., MARTIN, W. R., STOESSEL, A. J., RUTH, T. J., ADAM, M. J., PATE, B. D. and SCHULZER, M. (1985) Observations relating to the cause of Parkinson's disease: PET scans after MPTP. *Nature*, 317, 246–248
CHIBA, K., TREVOR, A. and CASTAGNOLI, JR, N. (1984) Active uptake of MPP$^+$, a metabolite of MPTP, by brain synaptosomes. *Biochemical and Biophysical Research Communications*, 120, 574–578
CHIBA, K., PETERSON, L. A., CASTAGNOLI, K. P., TREVOR, A. J. and CASTAGNOLI, JR, N. (1985) Studies on the molecular mechanism of bioactivation of the selective nigrostriatal toxin 1-methyl-4-phenyl-1,2,3,6-tetrahydropyridine (MPTP). *Drug Metabolism and Disposition*, 13, 342–347
SCHIUEH, C. C., MARKEY, S. P., BURNS, R. S., JOHANNESSEN, J. N., JACOBOWITZ, D. M. and KOPIN, I. J. (1983) N-Methyl-4-phenyl-1,2,3,6-tetrahydropyridine, a parkinsonian syndrome causing agent in man and monkey, produces different effects in guinea pig and rat. *Pharmacologist*, 25, 131
CHIUEH, C. C., MARKEY, S. P., BURNS, R. S., JOHANNESSEN, J. N., JACOBOWITZ, D. M. and KOPIN, I. J. (1984) Selective neurotoxic effects of 1-methyl-4-phenyl-1,2,3,6-tetrahydropyridine (MPTP) in subhuman primates and man: A new animal model of Parkinson's disease. *Psychopharmacological Bulletin*, 20, 548–553
COHEN, G. (1983) The pathobiology of Parkinson's disease: Biochemical aspects of dopamine neuron senescence. *Journal of Neural Transmission*, 19 (Suppl.), 89–103
COHEN, G., PASIK, P., COHEN, B., LEIST, A., MYTILINEOU, C. and YAHR, M. D. (1984) Pargyline and deprenyl prevent the neurotoxicity of 1-methyl-4-phenyl-1,2,3,6-tetrahydropyridine (MPTP) in monkeys. *European Journal of Pharmacology*, 106, 209–210
DAVIS, G. C., WILLIAMS, A. C., MARKEY, S. P., EBERT, M. H., CAINE, E. D., REICHERT, C. M. and KOPIN, I. J. (1979) Chronic parkinsonism secondary to intravenous injection of meperidine analogues. *Psychiatry Research*, 1, 249–254
DOUDET, D., GROSS, C., LEBRUN-GRANDIE, P. and BIOULAC, B. (1985) MPTP primate model of Parkinson's disease: A mechanographic and electromyographic study. *Brain Research*, 335, 194–199
FAHN, S. (1982) Fluctuations of disability in Parkinson's disease: Pathophysiology. In *Movement Disorders*. Eds. C. D. Marsden and S. Fahn, pp. 123–145. London: Butterworth Scientific
FORNO, L. S. (1982) Pathology of Parkinson's disease. In *Movement Disorders*. Eds. C. D. Marsden and S. Fahn, pp. 25–40. London: Butterworth Scientific
FORNO, L. C., LANGSTON, J. W., DELANNEY, L. E., IRWIN, I. and RICAURTE, G. R. (1986) Loius ceruleus lesions and eosinophilic inclusions in MPTP-treated monkeys. *Annals of Neurology*, (in press)
FULLER, R. W. and HEMRICK-LEUCKE, S. K. (1985a) Effects of amfonelic acid, alpha-methyltyrosine, Ro 4-1284 and haloperidol pretreatment of the depletion of striatal dopamine by 1-methyl-4-phenyl-1,2,3,6-tetrahydropyridine in mice. *Research Communications in Chemical Pathology and Pharmacology*, 48, 17–25
FULLER, R. and HEMRICK-LEUECKE, S. K. (1985b) Inhibition of types A and B monoamine oxidase by 1-methyl-4-phenyl-1,2,3,6-tetrahydropyridine. *Journal of Pharmacology and Experimental Therapeutics*, 232, 696–701
GESSNER, W., BROSSI, A., SHEN, R., FRITZ, R. R. and ABELL, C. W. (1984) Conversion of 1-methyl-4-phenyl-1,2,3,6-tetrahydropyridine (MPTP) and its 5-methyl analog into pyridinium salts. *Helvetica Chimica Acta*, 67, 2037–2042
GIBB, W. R. G., LEES, A. J., WELLS, F. R., BARNARD, R. O., JENNER, P. and MARSDEN, C. D. (1986) The neuropathology of parkinsonism in the marmoset induced by N-methyl-4-phenyl-1,2,5,6-tetrahydropyridine. In *Advances in Neurology* Ed. M. D. Yahr. New York, Raven Press (in press)
HEIKKILA, R. E., HESS, A. and DUVOISIN, R. C. (1984) Dopaminergic neurotoxicity of 1-methyl-4-phenyl-1,2,5,6-tetrahydropyridine in mice. *Science*, 224, 1451–1453
HEIKKILA, R. E., MANZINO, L., CABBAT, F. S. and DUVOISIN, R. C. (1984) Protection against the dopaminergic neurotoxicity of 1-methyl-4-phenyl-1,2,5,6-tetrahydropyridine by monoamine oxidase inhibitors. *Nature*, 311, 467–469
HEIKKILA, R. E., HESS, A. and DUVOISIN, R. C. (1985) Dopaminergic neurotoxicity of 1-methyl-4-phenyl-1,2,5,6-tetrahydropyridine (MPTP) in the mouse: Relationships between monoamine oxidase, MPTP metabolism and neurotoxicity. *Life Sciences*, 36, 231–236
HEIKKILA, R. E., NICKLAS, W. J., HESS, A. and DUVOISIN, R. C. (1985) 1-Methyl-4-phenyl-1,2,5,6-tetrahydropyridine (MPTP) induced dopaminergic neurotoxicity, monoamine oxidase and parkinsonism. In *Advances in Neurology*. Ed. M. D. Yahr. New York, Raven Press (in press)
HORNYKIEWICZ, O. (1966) Dopamine (3-hydroxytyramine) and brain function. *Pharmacological Reviews*, 18, 925–962

IRWIN, I. and LANGSTON, J. W. (1985) Selective accumulation of MPP$^+$ in the substantia nigra: A key to neurotoxicity? *Life Sciences*, **36**, 207–212

JARVIS, M. F. and WAGNER, G. C. (1985) Age-dependent effects of 1-methyl-4-phenyl-1,2,3,6-tetrahydropyridine (MPTP). *Neuropharmacology*, **24**, 581–583

JAVITCH, J. A., D'AMATO, R. M., STRITTMATTER, S. M. and SNYDER, S. H. (1985) Parkinsonism-inducing neurotoxin, *N*-methyl-4-phenyl-1,2,3,6-tetrahydropyridine: Uptake of the metabolite *N*-methyl-4-phenylpyridine by dopamine neurons explains selective toxicity. *Proceedings of the National Academy of Sciences of the United States of America*, **82**, 2173–2177

JENNER, P., RUPNIAK, N. M. J., ROSE, S., KELLEY, E., KILPATRICK, G., LEES, A. and MARSDEN, C. D. (1984) 1-Methyl-4-phenyl-1,2,3,6-tetrahydropyridine-induced parkinsonism in the common marmoset. *Neuroscience Letters*, **50**, 85–90

JOHANNESSEN, J. N., CHIUEH, C. C., BURNS, R. S. and MARKEY, S. P. (1985) Differences in the metabolism of MPTP in the rodent and primate parallel differences in sensitivity to its neurotoxic effects. *Life Sciences*, **36**, 219–224

LANGSTON, J. W. (1985a) Parkinson's disease and MPTP: Implications for future research and treatment. In *Future Trends in the Treatment of Parkinson's Disease and Epilepsy*. Ed. F. Kerry. pp. 9–12. London, Franklin Scientific Publishers

LANGSTON, J. W. (1985b) The case of the tainted heroin. *The Sciences*, **25**, 34–40

LANGSTON, J. W. (1985c) MPTP and Parkinson's disease. *Trends in Neuroscience*, **80**, 79–83

LANGSTON, J. W. (1985d) MPTP neurotoxicity: An overview and characterization of phases of toxicity. *Life Sciences*, **36**, 201–206

LANGSTON, J. W. (1986) MPTP-induced parkinsonism: How good a model is it? In *Recent Developments in Parkinson's Disease*. Eds. S. Fahn, C. D. Marsden, P. Jenner and P. Teychenne, pp. 119–126. New York, Raven Press

LANGSTON, J. W. and BALLARD, P. A. (1983) Parkinson's disease in a chemist working with 1-methyl-4-phenyl-1,2,5,6-tetrahydropyridine (MPTP). *New England Journal of Medicine*, **309**, 310

LANGSTON, J. W. and BALLARD, P. A. (1984) Parkinsonism induced by 1-methyl-4-phenyl-1,2,3,6-tetrahydropyridine: Implications for treatment and the pathophysiology of Parkinson's disease. *Canadian Journal of Neurosciences*, **11**, 160–165

LANGSTON, J. W., BALLARD, P., TETRUD, J. W. and IRWIN, I. (1983) Chronic parkinsonism in humans due to a product of meperidine-analog synthesis. *Science*, **219**, 979–980

LANGSTON, J. W., FORNO, L. S., REBERT, C. S. and IRWIN, I. (1984a) 1-Methyl-4-phenyl-1,2,5,6-tetrahydropyridine causes selective damage to the zona compacta of the substantia nigra in the squirrel monkey. *Brain Research*, **292**, 390–394

LANGSTON, J. W., IRWIN, I., LANGSTON, E. B. and FORNO, L. S. (1984b) 1-Methyl-4-phenylpyridinium ion (MPP$^+$): Identification of a metabolite of MPTP, a toxin selective to the substantia nigra. *Neuroscience Letters*, **48**, 87–92

LANGSTON, J. W., IRWIN, I., LANGSTON, E. B., DELANEY, L. E. and RICAURTE, G. A. (1986) MPTP-induced parkinsonism in humans: A review of the syndrome and observations relating to the phenomenon of tardive toxicity. In *MPTP: A neurotoxin producing a Parkinsonian Syndrome*. Eds S. P. Markey, N. Castagnoli, Jr, A. J. Trevor and I. J. Kopin. New York, Academic Press (in press)

LANGSTON, J. W., IRWIN, I., LANGSTON, E. B. and FORNO, L. S. (1984c) Pargyline prevents MPTP-induced parkinsonism in primates. *Science*, **225**, 1480–1482

LANGSTON, J. W., LANGSTON, E. B. and IRWIN, I. (1984) MPTP-induced parkinsonism in human and non-human primates – Clinical and experimental aspects. *Acta Neurologica Scandinavica*, **70** (Suppl. 100), 49–54

LEWIN, R. (1984a) Brain enzyme is the target of drug toxin. *Science*, **225**, 1460–1462

LEWIN, R. (1984b) Trail of ironies to Parkinson's disease. *Science*, **224**, 1083–1085

LEWIN, R. (1985) Parkinson's disease: An environmental cause? *Science*, **229**, 257–258

MARKEY, S. P., JOHANNESSEN, J. N., CHIUEH, C. C., BURNS, R. S. and HERKENHAM, M. A. (1984) Intraneuronal generation of a pyridinium metabolite may cause drug-induced parkinsonism. *Nature*, **311**, 464–467

MONES, R. J. (1972) Levodopa-induced dyskinesia in the normal rhesus monkey. *Mount Sinai Journal of Medicine*, **39**, 197–201

MYTILINEOU, C. and COHEN, G. (1984) 1-Methyl-4-phenyl-1,2,3,6-tetrahydropyridine destroys dopamine neurons in explants of rat brain mesencephalon. *Science*, **225**, 529–531

NOBREGA, F. T., GLATTRE, E. and KURLAND, L. T. (1967) Comments on the epidemiology of parkinsonism including prevalence and incidence statistics for Rochester, Minnesota, 1935–1966. *Excerpta Medica International Congress Series #175*, 474–485

POIRIER, L. J., PECHADRE, J. C., LAROCHELLE, L., DANKOVA, J. and BOUCHER, R. (1975) Stereotaxic lesions and movement disorders in monkeys. In *Primate Models of Neurological Disorders*. Eds B. S. Meldrum and C. D. Marsden. *Advances in Neurology*, Vol. 10, pp. 5–22. New York: Raven Press

PRICE, K. S., FARLEY, I. J. and HORNYKIEWICZ, O. (1978) Neurochemistry of Parkinson's disease: Relation between striatal and limbic dopamine. In *Dopamine Advances in Biochemical Psychopharmacology.* Eds P. J. Roberts, G. N. Woodruff and L. L. Iversen, Vol. 19, pp. 293–300. New York: Raven Press

REIDERER, P. and WUKETICH, S. (1976) Time course of nigrostriatal degeneration in Parkinson's disease. *Journal of Neural Transmissions,* **39,** 277–301

RICAURTE, G. A., LANGSTON, J. W., DELANNEY, L. E., IRWIN, I. and BROOKS, J. D. (1985) Dopamine uptake blockers protect against the dopamine depleting effects of MPTP in the mouse striatum. *Neuroscience Letters,* **59,** 259–264

RICAURTE, G. A., LANGSTON, J. W., IRWIN, I., DELANNEY, L. E. and FORNO, L. S. (1985) The neurotoxic effect of MPTP on the dopaminergic cells of the substantia nigra in mice is age-related. *Society for Neuroscience,* Abstract, **11,** 631

RUTTENBUR, A. J., GARBE, P. L., KALTER, H. D., CASTRO, K. G., TETRUD, J. W., PORTER, P., IRWIN, I. and LANGSTON, J. W. (1986) Meperidine analogue exposure in California narcotics abusers: Initial epidemiologic findings. In *MPTP: A Neurotoxin producing a Parkinsonian Syndrome.* Eds S. P. Markey, N. Castagnoli Jr, A. J. Trevor and I. J. Kopin. New York, Academic Press (in press)

SCHMIDLE, C. J. and MANSFIELD, R. C. (1956) The aminomethylation of olefins. IV. The formation of 1-alkyl-4-aryl-1,2,3,6-tetrahydropyridines. *Journal of American Chemistry,* **78,** 425–428

SCHNEIDER, J. S., YUWILER, A. and MARKHAM, C. H. (1986) Behavioral, biochemical and pathological changes of an MPTP model of Parkinson's disease in the cat. *Experimental Neurology,* **91,** 293–307

SERSHEN, H., MASON, M. F., HASHIM, A. and LAJTHE, A. (1985) Effect of N-methyl-4-phenyl-1,2,3,6-tetrahydropyridine (MPTP) on age-related changes in dopamine turnover and transporter function in the mouse striatum. *European Journal of Pharmacology,* **113,** 135–136

SINGER, T. P., SALACH, J. I. and CRABTREE, D. (1985) Reversible inhibition and mechanism-based irreversible inactivation of monoamine oxidases by 1-methyl-4-phenyl-1,2,3,6-tetrahydropyridine (MPTP). *Biochemical and Biophysical Research Communications,* **127,** 707–712

SPENCER, P. S. and SCHAUMBURG, H. H. (1984) An expanded classification of neurotoxic responses based on cellular targets of chemical agents. *Acta Neurologica Scandinavica,* **70** (Suppl. 100), 9–19

STERN, Y. and LANGSTON, J. W. (1985) Intellectual changes in patients with MPTP-induced parkinsonism. *Neurology,* **35,** 1506–1509

TATTON, W. G., EASTMAN, M. J., BEDINGHAM, W., VERRIER, M. C. and BRUCE, I. C. (1984) Defective utilization of sensory input as the basis for bradykinesia, rigidity and decreased movement repertoire in Parkinson's disease: A hypothesis. *The Canadian Journal of Neurological Sciences,* **11,** 136–143

TRETIAKOFF, C. (1919) Contribution a l'étude de l'anatomie pathologique du locus niger de soemmering avec quelques deductions relatives à la pathogenic de troubles du tonus musculaire et de la maladie de Parkinson. *Thèse de Paris*

WARD, C. D., DUVOISIN, R. C., INCE, S. E., NUTT, J. D., ELDRIDGE, R. and CALNE, D. B. (1983) Parkinson's disease in 65 pairs of twins and in a set of quadruplets. *Neurology,* **33,** 815–824

WESTLUND, K. N., DENNEY, R. M., KOCHERSPERGER, L. M., ROSE, R. M. and ABELL, C. W. (1985) Distinct monoamine oxidase A and B populations in primate brain. *Science,* **230,** 181–183

WHITEHOUSE, P., HEDREEN, J. C., WHITE, C., DELONG, M. and PRICE, D. L. (1983) Basal forebrain neurons in the dementia of Parkinson's disease. *Annals of Neurology,* **13,** 243–248

WILKENING, D., VERNIER, V. G., ARTHAUD, L. E., TREACY, G., KENNEY, J. P., CLARK, R., SMITH, D. H. and SMITH, C. (1986) A Parkinson-like neurologic deficit in primates is caused by a novel 4-substituted piperidine. *Brain Research,* in press

WRIGHT, J. M., WALL, R. A., PERRY, T. L. and PATY, D. W. (1984) Chronic parkinsonism secondary to the intranasal administration of a product of meperidine-analogue synthesis. *New England Journal of Medicine,* **310,** 325

YOUNG, S., BROWN, W. W. and KLINGER, B. (1970) Nigropallidal encephalomalacia in horses caused by ingestion of weeds of the genus centaurea. *Journal of the American Veterinary Medical Association,* **157,** 1602–1605

ZIERING, A., BERGER, L., HEINEMAN, S. D. and LEE, J. (1947) Piperidine derivatives. Part III. 4-Ayrlpiperidines. *Journal of Organic Chemistry,* **12,** 894–903

7
Prognosis in Parkinson's disease
Gerald Stern

While an overall picture of the natural history of Parkinson's disease during the levodopa era can be obtained from the literature, it is now difficult and perhaps impossible to determine how this compares with the untreated disorder prior to 1960. Accurate statistics of the kind that would satisfy a clinical epidemiologist were not available and it seems legitimate to assume that there will never be a controlled clinical trial of the true impact of levodopa on the currently prevailing malady, whatever developments there may be in our knowledge of the causes and treatments of the illness. Thus, it is unlikely that we shall ever know whether the constellation of motor deficits that we now call 'Parkinson's disease' was identical in aetiology, clinical and epidemiological features to that observed in the nineteenth century. Nevertheless, making due allowance for historical constraints and inaccuracies and the inherent problems of patient selection, by reading through the accounts of astute clinicians writing in the nineteenth and the first half of the twentieth century, some sort of image emerges, albeit fragmentary and incomplete, of the illness before effective treatments appeared. In this chapter a few of the major studies will be briefly and sequentially reviewed before considering contemporary data.

PRE-LEVODOPA ERA

In 1817 James Parkinson, with characteristic succinctness and clarity, posed the problem: 'from the little knowledge of its nature, acknowledged by the physician who attended; and from the mode of its termination; excited an eager wish to acquire some further knowledge of its nature and cause.' His shrewd observations on only six patients made him aware of the significance of presenting tremor and of the importance – not pursued again until Schwab (1960) and Hoehn and Yahr (1967) in the 1960s – of the potential prognostic importance of categories and staging. 'It seldom happens that the agitation extends beyond the arms within the first two years; which period therefore, if we were disposed to divide disease into stages, might be said to comprise the first stage.'

Aware of timespan of deterioration and its attendant problems in the assessment of treatments, Parkinson wrote: 'that in this disease there is one circumstance that demands particular attention; the long period to which it may extend. One of its peculiar symptoms, Scelotyrb festinans, may not occur until the disease has existed ten or twelve years or more . . .'. In his pithy summary of the salient characteristics he wrote: 'the disease . . . is of a nature highly afflictive . . . an evil, from the domination of which he had no prospect of escape . . . is of long duration . . . requires a continuance of observation of the same case or at least a correct history of its symptoms even for several years . . . a tedious and most distressing malady.' Acknowledging the contribution of one of his predecessors, 'the celebrated Cullen', James Parkinson referred to 'his accustomed accuracy', but surely this compliment applies equally to himself.

The great clinicians who were the founders of modern clinical neurology working in the latter part of the nineteenth into the first two decades of this century, began to collate distinctive features of the illness. Thus, Charcot (1880) affirmed that Parkinson's disease was the fifth most common disease treated at Sâlpetrière, ranking next to locomotor ataxia and affecting those over 40 or 50 years of age; Buzzard (1882), in a clinical lecture on the shaking palsy, confirmed Charcot's observations concerning age of onset and emphasized that the illness 'has a slow march and little or no tendency to curtail longevity. Hence there are always about a certain number of persons afflicted with paralysis agitans who have arrived at a ripe old age.' However, he was aware of the variations: 'it is sometimes acute in its progress and, I think, is more often the case when the patient is comparatively young.' In questioning the possible cause of the illness in a patient aged 38, Buzzard (1882) was clearly affected by Victorian puritanism in drawing attention to the history of excessive sexual intercourse immediately preceding the commencement of symptoms. During this era, despite the prevalence of the malady, there is no detailed record of the characteristics of the illness even though it is clear that on occasions such an approach could be diligently and profitably pursued. For example, in the same volume of *Brain* that contains Buzzard's clinical observations there is a most impressive and detailed statistical analysis concerning rheumatic chorea by Angela Money: 'Dr Gower suggested to me that in the records of University College Hospital there would be a number of cases of Chorea Sancti Viti which had up to the present never been worked up.' There follows a meticulous account of 236 patients, including month of birth, duration of chorea, clinical details and intervals between relapses which would have satisfied the most demanding of clinical epidemiologists save for the problems of sampling. Characteristically, Gower was probably the first in his manual of diseases of the nervous system (1888) to address himself with comparable attention to paralysis agitans. In his personal experience of 80 patients he noted that 'the malady usually commences after forty years of age. Nearly half the cases begin between fifty and sixty and about one-fifth in each of the two decades, 40–50 and 60–70, but on account of the lessened number of persons living, it is probably twice as frequent in the latter as in the former decade. It occasionally begins between thirty and forty, very rarely under thirty.' He was aware of others where the disease had begun still earlier, as at 21, quoted by Buzzard, at 19 by Duchenne and at 17 by Berger. He thought that presentation over the age of 65 was rare and that it was 'essentially a disease of degenerative period of life not of extreme senility . . . I have found the exact age of commencement to be the same in each sex, fifty-two years.'

'The disease has been thought to be more frequent in the labouring classes but the influence of station in life and also of occupation has been certainly exaggerated by some writers. Exciting causes cannot be traced in more than one-third of the cases and vary much in character. The most frequent are emotion, physical injury and acute disease. Prolonged anxiety and severe emotional shock often precede the onset. A woman was much shocked at a neighbour being killed in a railway accident; she went to the funeral carrying a heavy child on her left arm; the arm felt very tired afterwards, and the feeling of fatigue persisted and gradually changed to one of stiffness, which proved to be the local commencement of paralysis agitans.' In addition to other shrewdly observed clinical features he was clearly aware of one of the few inaccuracies in James Parkinson's essay. 'The intellect may be unaffected throughout, except by the irritability which usually accompanies the physical restlessness. Often there is mental depression; it may be difficult to say whether this is more than the natural result of the physical ailment. Pronounced mental symptoms are occasionally present, however, in the later stages of the disease, commonly limited to mental weakness and loss of memory, but sometimes accompanied by a tendency to delusions.' With respect to the course of the illness and its duration and cause of death, he remarks that 'the disease is always chronic and usually progressive in its course . . . the shortest time in which I have known all four limbs to be affected in a case beginning locally was nine months . . . very rarely the tremor lessens as the disease advances and rigidity fixes the limbs . . . The variations and extension are thus so great as to make it difficult to tell the course of a commencing case. Paralysis agitans does not directly cause death and the advanced age of most of its subjects renders its duration and its influence in shortening life difficult to determine . . . The longest case which has come under my own observation had existed for ten years but the disease has been known to last for thirty years. Death sometimes occurs from exhaustion, bed sores etc. in the later stage; more frequently from intercurrent affections especially of the respiratory organs facilitated by the progressive muscular weakness, which involves the thoracic muscles as well as others. The tremor has been observed to cease before death.'

Purves Stewart (1898), when a senior house officer to The National Hospital for the Paralysed and Epileptic, Queen Square, remarked that since Parkinson wrote his classical description 'so little has been added to its symptomatology since and the disease now appears at first sight to be, clinically at least, so thoroughly worked out that to many it may seem a superfluous task to traverse once more a subject so well worn.' However, in his personal examination of 28 patients whose age of onset of symptoms ranged from 22 to 73 years, he was able to provide further intriguing observations. With respect to the significance of the history of fright or emotional disturbance he described: 'another patient was at a menagerie when a lion escaped from its cage and caused considerable alarm among the spectators. On the next day the patient's illness is said to have commenced, his first symptom being stiffness of the left leg.' Another patient was threatened as a blackleg by his fellow workers on the railway which was on strike and ever afterwards he found his right hand stiff and his handwriting unusually slow. Purves Stewart was able to draw attention to a new feature of the illness which he had recognized in five of his 28 patients, namely dystonic posturing of the feet usually provoked by exercise but occasionally relieved by walking and which could be the first symptom of the malady well before generalized features could be recognized. A salutary example of the importance of scrutinizing past literature because, at one stage, foot dystonia was thought to be a unique complication of levodopa therapy.

By the early years of the twentieth century clinicians were able to muster relatively large personal series of patients. Thus, Hart (1904) reviewed 219 patients who had attended a large neurological department between 1888 and 1904; Bing (1915) described similar experiences from Basel. He remarked that 'although many authors assert that the poorer classes of the population are more frequently attacked . . . in our region there is no evidence of a less predisposition to it in the higher classes of society. The prognosis of the disease is not unfavourable as to life, but very unfavourable as to recovery; remissions occur but unfortunately they are not usually of long duration. Death follows either in marasmus or from internal diseases among which cerebral haemorrhage is relatively frequent.' Other clinical studies continued to emerge about this period, such as an analysis of 146 patients by Patrick and Levy (1922). When Russell Brain (1933) published the first edition of his textbook of the diseases of the nervous system, in a chapter related to neurological diseases and life insurance with particular reference to the hazards of developing Parkinson's disease after encephalitis, he drew attention to an author of a standard textbook on such risks who advised that it 'may be accepted as standard six to twelve months after complete recovery' – this, dryly observed Brain, 'is somewhat misleading'. He thought that those who had recovered from encephalitis lethargica should be regarded as uninsurable for at least ten years after an acute attack. 'After this period if he appears to be in normal health he may be accepted for a double endowment plan or with a heavy lieu.' He emphasized that the disease is always progressive, although cases differ considerably in rates of progress and that symptoms may be confined to one limb for months or years. 'The average duration of the disease is about ten years and death occurs usually from complications such as pneumonia or bed sores. Occasionally there is a transient stage of lethargy passing into coma.' Dimsdale (1946), at the suggestion of Russell Brain, examined the clinical features of 320 patients collected from records in an attempt to assess change in aetiology and modifications of the syndrome during the twentieth century. She felt it important to make due allowance for the epidemic of encephalitis, arteriosclerotic parkinsonism, syphilitic mesencephalitis and the syndrome described by Jakob (1921). By dividing her material into three groups, those presenting between 1900 and 1919, 1920 and 1930 and 1931 and 1942, it was possible to make appropriate clinical analyses with respect to pattern and aetiology. Those occurring in the first period were cases of paralysis agitans developing in the second half of life, presenting with tremor and only rarely affected with abnormal mental states, excessive salivation and who had normal oculomotor function. The second group with greater ocular anomalies, mainly weakness of convergence, tended to develop severe incapacities within short periods of time and were associated with common mental symptoms and disorders of sleep. In the third group there was an equal mixture of idiopathic disease (paralysis agitans) and those presumably related to the encephalitis. She accepted Jakob's view that post-encephalitic disease was due to sublethal damage to the ganglion cells by a virus resulting in degeneration at deferred intervals.

Markovich and Schwab (1952), when attempting to identify those factors which determined prognosis and progression in Parkinson's disease, suggested that those with easy going rather placid personalities showed the slowest progression and those with driving competitive personalities, as well as vulnerable personalities, deteriorated rapidly. Schwab (1960) came back to the same problem when he challenged the prevailing view of 'the gloomy picture of the inevitable invalidism after seven or eight years with demise' and suggested that this was not an accurate description of the true state of the disease. He maintained that slow inevitable progression, such that seven or eight years from onset patients are completely dependent on others for everyday activities and that release from this hopeless state by death from intercurrent infection and malnutrition followed, was not necessarily true for all parkinsonian patients. He presented evidence of patients whose disease altered only slowly and some whose signs and symptoms did not progress in any measurable way from year to year: 'some patients after as many as twenty-five years since onset of the disease are still independent and even at work.' In support of the very wide range of clinical possibilities, he was among the pioneers who proposed a simple but workable effective staging system (his involved five grades) and was able to demonstrate 40 patients who had survived for 25–29 years since the onset of symptoms and that one-half remained independent. He found no correlation with prognosis or progression in relation to age of onset or duration of disease, but was still impressed that there might be some link between rates of progression and individual adaptiveness and strength of personality. He thought that early evidence of akinesia was a poor prognostic sign usually associated with rapid progression and also that when the disease becomes bilateral within the first year this too carries a less favourable prognosis. He emphasized that long persistence of unilateral parkinsonism is generally a good prognostic sign, associated with slow progress; early involvement of memory and loss of intellectual faculties, marked changes in personality, and loss of drive also indicated a poor outcome.

This generally more favourable assessment has to be compared with a Scandinavian study which indicated that 50% of patients were completely disabled or incapable of full employment four years after the onset of the disease (Mjones, 1949). Kurland (1958) found an excess mortality of only 1.4 in 44 patients followed between 1940 and 1954, and Pollock and Hornabrook (1966) reported that 25% of their patients were alive and still active as long as 18 years after their first symptom. So diverse were the prognostic extremes of optimism and pessimism that a dispassionate observer might well wonder whether the several clinicians were describing the same disease.

Duvoisin *et al.* (1963) analysed six of the larger patient review papers published between 1885 and 1962 and showed that the mean age of onset throughout this span varied little, from 52.7 to 56.8 years, and thought it unlikely that the illness would become less frequent as the epidemic of encephalitis became more remote.

Hoehn and Yahr (1967) published the best known and the most influential statement concerning the onset, progression and mortality of the disease and introduced a staging system which has stood the test of time. They considered 866 patients attending one hospital between 1949 and 1964 and, although fully conscious of the inherent problems of sampling such as omissions, death from other causes, those who were lost to follow-up and other distortions, they were able to present the most accurate picture of the disease in the immediate pre-levodopa era. The mean age of onset was 55.3 years and they felt able to conclude that youth at onset of disease was not necessarily a favourable prognostic sign. They drew attention to the difficulty in obtaining accurate mortality statistics – only 15% of their patients had such death certificates, which were frequently inaccurate and incomplete as to the actual cause of death. Approximately a quarter who had the disease for less than five years were already severely disabled or dead; of those with a disease duration of five to nine years, two-thirds were dead and of those with an illness span of 10–14 years, 80% were dead. Regardless of age of onset the observed mortality was three times that of the general population of the same age, sex and colour. They found no evidence that the currently available methods of

BRAIN, W. R. (1933) Diseases of the nervous system in relation to life insurance. *Diseases of the Nervous System*, pp. 807–815. London: Oxford University Press
BUZZARD, R. (1882) A clinical lecture on the shaking palsy. *Brain*, **4**, 473
CALNE, D. B., SPIERS, A. S. D., STERN, G. M. and LAURENCE, D. R. (1969) L-Dopa in post-encephalitic parkinsonism. *Lancet*, **i**, 744
CASTAIGNE, P., RONDOT, P., RIBADEAU-DUMAS, J. L. and CARDON, P. (1975) Long-term treatment of Parkinson's disease with L-dopa alone and in combination with a decarboxylase inhibitor. In *Advances in Parkinsonism*, Eds. W. Birkmayer and O. Hornykiewicz. *New England Journal of Medicine*, **276**, 374
CHARCOT, J. M. (1880) *Lecons sur les maladies du systeme nerveux faites a la Salpetriere*, 4th edn. Collected and published by Bournville, Paris. Delahaye and Lecrosier, p. 186
COTZIAS, G. C. (1971) Levodopa in the treatment of Parkinsonism. *Journal of the American Medical Association*, **218**, 1903
CURTIS, L., LEES, A. J., STERN, G. M. and MARMOT, M. G. (1984) Effect of L-dopa on course of Parkinson's disease. *Lancet*, **ii**, 211–212
DIMSDALE, H. (1946) Changes in the Parkinsonian syndrome in the twentieth century. *Quarterly Journal of Medicine*, **59**, 155–170
DUVOISIN, R. C., YAHR, M. D., SCHWEITZER, M. D. and MERRITT, H. H. (1963) Parkinsonism before and since the epidemic of encephalitis lethargica. *Archives of Neurology*, **9**, 232–241
GOWERS, W. R. (1888) *Diseases of the Nervous System*, Vol. 2. London: J. & A. Churchill
HART, T. S. (1904) Paralysis agitans: some clinical observations based on the study of 219 cases seen in the clinic of Professor M. Allen Starr. *Journal of Nervous and Mental Disease*, **31**, 177–188
HEIKKILA, R. E., MANZINO, L., CABBAT, F. C. and DUVOISIN, R. C. (1984) Protection against the dopaminergic toxicity of 1-methyl-4-phenyl-1,2,5,6-tetrahydropyridine by monoamine oxidase inhibitors. *Nature*, **311**, 467–469
HOEHN, M. D. and YAHR, M. M. (1967) Parkinsonism: onset, progression and mortality. *Neurology*, **17**, 427–442
HUNTER, K. R., SHAW, K. M., LAURENCE, D. R. and STERN, G. M. (1973) Sustained levodopa therapy in Parkinsonism. *Lancet*, **ii**, 929
JAKOB, A. (1921) Uber eigenertige erkrankungen des zentralnerven-systems mit bemerkenswarten anatomischen befunden. Spastische pseudosklerose-encephalomyelopathie mit disseminierten degenerationsherden. *Zeitschrift für das gesamte Neurologie und Psychiatrie*, **64**, 146
KURLAND, L. T. (1958) Epidemiology, incidence, geographic distribution, genetic considerations (of Parkinsonism). In *Pathogenesis and Treatment of Parkinsonism*, Ed. W. S. Fields. Springfield, Illinois: C. C. Thomas & Co.
MARKHAM, C. H., TRECIOKAS, L. J. and DIAMOND, S. G. (1974) Parkinson's disease and levodopa: a five year follow-up and review. *Western Journal of Medicine*, **121**, 188
MARKOVICH, S. and SCHWAB, R. S. (1952) Prognosis and progression in Parkinson's disease in patients under medical treatment. *Archivio internazionale di Studi neurologici*, **2**, 1–9
MARSDEN, C. D. and PARKES, J. D. (1977) Success and problems in long-term levodopa therapy in Parkinson's disease. *Lancet*, **i**, 345–349
MARTILLA, R. J., RINNE, U. K., SIIRTOLA, T. and SONNINEN, V. (1977) Mortality of patients with Parkinson's disease treated with levodopa. *Journal of Neurology*, **216**, 147
MJONES, H. (1949) Paralysis agitans: a clinical and genetical study. *Acta Psychiatrica Scandinavica*, Supplementum, **54**, 1
PARKINSON, J. (1817) *An Essay on the Shaking Palsy*. London: Sherwood, Neely & Jones
PATRICK, H. T. and LEVY, D. M. (1922) Parkinson's disease – a clinical study of one hundred and forty-six cases. *Archives of Neurology and Psychiatry*, **7**, 711
POLLOCK, M. and HORNABROOK, R. W. (1966) The prevalence, natural history and dementia of Parkinson's disease. *Brain*, **89**, 429
SCHWAB, R. S. (1960) Progression and prognosis in Parkinson's disease. *Journal of Nervous and Mental Disease*, **130**, 556–566
SHAW, K. M., LEES, A. J. and STERN, G. M. (1980) The impact of treatment with levodopa on Parkinson's disease. *Quarterly Journal of Medicine*, **49**, 283–293
STEWART, P. (1898) Paralysis agitans: with an account of a new symptom. *Lancet*, 1258–1260
SWEET, R. D. and McDOWELL, F. H. (1975) Five years treatment of Parkinson's disease with levodopa – therapeutic results and survival of 100 patients. *Archives of Internal Medicine*, **83**, 456–463
YAHR, M. D. (1975) Evaluation of long-term therapy in Parkinson's disease: mortality and therapeutic efficacy. In *Advances in Parkinsonism*. Eds. W. Birkmayer and O. Hornykiewicz, p. 435. Basel: Roche Scientific Presse
ZUMSTEIN, H. and SIEGFRIED, J. (1976) Mortality among Parkinsonian patients treated with L-dopa combined with a decarboxylase inhibitor. *European Neurology*, **14**, 321

expectancy appeared to be normal. However, when the same group of patients was reviewed (Curtis *et al.,* 1984) after 12 years of sustained therapy, the ratio of observed to expected deaths had risen to 2.59. Thus, although levodopa probably improved life expectancy during the first six years of therapy, this protective effect subsequently declined. While it is posible to show that there are potentially significant differences between the several long-term reviews – selection of patients, differences in age and sex distributions and proportions of mildly and severely affected patients as well as the possibility that some of the diagnoses may have been incorrect – few would dispute the general conclusions of the effects of levodopa on the course of Parkinson's disease in the second half of the twentieth century.

We are currently passing through a phase of intense neuropharmacological excitement and exploration. Trials abound describing the effects of a wide variety of drugs – dopaminergic agonists alone or in combination with levodopa, selective monoamine oxidase inhibitors – and whatever the effect such drugs may have in ameliorating symptoms, signs, incapacities and complications of the disease, it is premature to conclude whether any of these stratagems will fundamentally alter the prognosis or the mortality of Parkinson's disease.

At the time of writing – such is the cadence of events that current research and hypotheses speedily become disregarded history – there is considerable interest in the speculation that the addition of L-deprenyl, a selective monoamine type-B inhibitor, to conventional levodopa therapy results in increased life expectancy for patients with Parkinson's disease. This proposal (Birkmayer *et al.,* 1985) stems from an open, uncontrolled, retrospective analysis of 941 patients in which it is presumed that there were no significant demographic differences between two groups studied over a period of nine years. Like any study of this kind it is not beyond criticism – for example, the daily levodopa dosage for the group treated only with this drug was 524 mg while that in the group that also took L-deprenyl, which has levodopa-sparing effects, was 627 mg – but it could be argued that the adjunct prevents or retards degeneration of dopaminergic neurones in the striatum. Since there is evidence (Heikkila *et al.,* 1984) that L-deprenyl may selectively prevent degeneration of such neurones induced in animals by the drug 1-methyl-4-phenyl-1,2,3,6-tetrahydropyridine (MPTP), the notion is not all that romantic. Confirmation of this claim of improved life expectancy by controlled randomized patients in sufficient numbers to allow such differences to become evident will be lengthy and arduous, but the possibility remains that in a decade when a further attempt is made to record the history and prognosis of Parkinson's disease, more favourable conclusions might be drawn.

References

BARBEAU, A. (1969) L-Dopa therapy in Parkinson's disease: a critical review of nine years experience. *Canadian Medical Association Journal,* **101,** 39

BARBEAU, A. (1976) Six years of high-level levodopa therapy in severely akinetic Parkinsonian patients. *Archives of Neurology,* **33,** 333

BING, R. (1915) Paralysis agitans. In *A Textbook of Nervous Diseases for Students and Practising Physicians.* Translated by C. L. Allen. pp. 86–90. London: Heinemann

BIRKMAYER, W. and HORNYKIEWICZ, O. (1962) Der L-dioxyphenylalanin-effect beim Parkinson syndrome des menschen. *Archiv für Psychiatrie und Nerven Krankheiten,* **203,** 560–571

BIRKMAYER, W., KNOLL, J., RIEDERER, P., YOUDIM, M. B. H., HARS, V. and MARTON, J. (1985) Increased life expectancy resulting from addition of L-deprenyl to Madopar treatment in Parkinson's disease: a longterm study. *Journal of Neural Transmission,* **64,** 113–127

BRAIN, W. R. (1933) Diseases of the nervous system in relation to life insurance. *Diseases of the Nervous System*, pp. 807–815. London: Oxford University Press
BUZZARD, R. (1882) A clinical lecture on the shaking palsy. *Brain*, **4**, 473
CALNE, D. B., SPIERS, A. S. D., STERN, G. M. and LAURENCE, D. R. (1969) L-Dopa in post-encephalitic parkinsonism. *Lancet*, **i**, 744
CASTAIGNE, P., RONDOT, P., RIBADEAU-DUMAS, J. L. and CARDON, P. (1975) Long-term treatment of Parkinson's disease with L-dopa alone and in combination with a decarboxylase inhibitor. In *Advances in Parkinsonism*, Eds. W. Birkmayer and O. Hornykiewicz. *New England Journal of Medicine*, **276**, 374
CHARCOT, J. M. (1880) *Lecons sur les maladies du systeme nerveux faites a la Salpetriere*, 4th edn. Collected and published by Bournville, Paris. Delahaye and Lecrosier, p. 186
COTZIAS, G. C. (1971) Levodopa in the treatment of Parkinsonism. *Journal of the American Medical Association*, **218**, 1903
CURTIS, L., LEES, A. J., STERN, G. M. and MARMOT, M. G. (1984) Effect of L-dopa on course of Parkinson's disease. *Lancet*, **ii**, 211–212
DIMSDALE, H. (1946) Changes in the Parkinsonian syndrome in the twentieth century. *Quarterly Journal of Medicine*, **59**, 155–170
DUVOISIN, R. C., YAHR, M. D., SCHWEITZER, M. D. and MERRITT, H. H. (1963) Parkinsonism before and since the epidemic of encephalitis lethargica. *Archives of Neurology*, **9**, 232–241
GOWERS, W. R. (1888) *Diseases of the Nervous System*, Vol. 2. London: J. & A. Churchill
HART, T. S. (1904) Paralysis agitans: some clinical observations based on the study of 219 cases seen in the clinic of Professor M. Allen Starr. *Journal of Nervous and Mental Disease*, **31**, 177–188
HEIKKILA, R. E., MANZINO, L., CABBAT, F. C. and DUVOISIN, R. C. (1984) Protection against the dopaminergic toxicity of 1-methyl-4-phenyl-1,2,5,6-tetrahydropyridine by monoamine oxidase inhibitors. *Nature*, **311**, 467–469
HOEHN, M. D. and YAHR, M. M. (1967) Parkinsonism: onset, progression and mortality. *Neurology*, **17**, 427–442
HUNTER, K. R., SHAW, K. M., LAURENCE, D. R. and STERN, G. M. (1973) Sustained levodopa therapy in Parkinsonism. *Lancet*, **ii**, 929
JAKOB, A. (1921) Uber eigenertige erkrankungen des zentralnerven-systems mit bemerkenswarten anatomischen befunden. Spastische pseudosklerose-encephalomyelopathie mit disseminierten degenerationsherden. *Zeitschrift für das gesamte Neurologie und Psychiatrie*, **64**, 146
KURLAND, L. T. (1958) Epidemiology, incidence, geographic distribution, genetic considerations (of Parkinsonism). In *Pathogenesis and Treatment of Parkinsonism*, Ed. W. S. Fields. Springfield, Illinois: C. C. Thomas & Co.
MARKHAM, C. H., TRECIOKAS, L. J. and DIAMOND, S. G. (1974) Parkinson's disease and levodopa: a five year follow-up and review. *Western Journal of Medicine*, **121**, 188
MARKOVICH, S. and SCHWAB, R. S. (1952) Prognosis and progression in Parkinson's disease in patients under medical treatment. *Archivio internazionale di Studi neurologici*, **2**, 1–9
MARSDEN, C. D. and PARKES, J. D. (1977) Success and problems in long-term levodopa therapy in Parkinson's disease. *Lancet*, **i**, 345–349
MARTILLA, R. J., RINNE, U. K., SIIRTOLA, T. and SONNINEN, V. (1977) Mortality of patients with Parkinson's disease treated with levodopa. *Journal of Neurology*, **216**, 147
MJONES, H. (1949) Paralysis agitans: a clinical and genetical study. *Acta Psychiatrica Scandinavica*, Supplementum, **54**, 1
PARKINSON, J. (1817) *An Essay on the Shaking Palsy*. London: Sherwood, Neely & Jones
PATRICK, H. T. and LEVY, D. M. (1922) Parkinson's disease – a clinical study of one hundred and forty-six cases. *Archives of Neurology and Psychiatry*, **7**, 711
POLLOCK, M. and HORNABROOK, R. W. (1966) The prevalence, natural history and dementia of Parkinson's disease. *Brain*, **89**, 429
SCHWAB, R. S. (1960) Progression and prognosis in Parkinson's disease. *Journal of Nervous and Mental Disease*, **130**, 556–566
SHAW, K. M., LEES, A. J. and STERN, G. M. (1980) The impact of treatment with levodopa on Parkinson's disease. *Quarterly Journal of Medicine*, **49**, 283–293
STEWART, P. (1898) Paralysis agitans: with an account of a new symptom. *Lancet*, 1258–1260
SWEET, R. D. and MCDOWELL, F. H. (1975) Five years treatment of Parkinson's disease with levodopa – therapeutic results and survival of 100 patients. *Archives of Internal Medicine*, **83**, 456–463
YAHR, M. D. (1975) Evaluation of long-term therapy in Parkinson's disease: mortality and therapeutic efficacy. In *Advances in Parkinsonism*. Eds. W. Birkmayer and O. Hornykiewicz, p. 435. Basel: Roche Scientific Presse
ZUMSTEIN, H. and SIEGFRIED, J. (1976) Mortality among Parkinsonian patients treated with L-dopa combined with a decarboxylase inhibitor. *European Neurology*, **14**, 321

8
Neuropsychology and cognitive function in Parkinson's disease: an overview
R. G. Brown and C. D. Marsden

Why study cognitive function in Parkinson's disease? The question is not a trivial one, as the aims behind the many studies are varied, and an understanding of those aims may help put the research into perspective.

Neuropsychological research may be divided into two broad fields, clinical and experimental. Considerable overlap may occur between the two areas, but important differences exist in their aims and methods. The contributions of these two branches of neuropsychology to our knowledge of cognitive changes in Parkinson's disease will be considered separately.

ISSUES IN CLINICAL NEUROPSYCHOLOGICAL RESEARCH

Clinical neuropsychological research is concerned with providing information which may be of value in the diagnosis and management of individual patients with brain disorders. The questions addressed by clinical research reflect those asked most commonly in clinical practice with individual patients. With respect to research into Parkinson's disease, three key issues are:

(1) Is there evidence of cognitive impairment in Parkinson's disease?
(2) Is there an increased risk of dementia in Parkinson's disease?
(3) What are the effects of treatment on cognitive function in Parkinson's disease?

These three questions are integrally related in clinical practice. If cognitive impairment is found in a patient, it is important to determine its nature and possible cause. Mild cognitive impairment may be a relatively benign manifestation of normal ageing, or it may be the early stages of a progressive dementia. Alternatively, the changes may be related to the treatment which the patient is receiving. Modification of that treatment may lead to an improvement in the patient's cognitive status.

Is there evidence of cognitive impairment in Parkinson's disease?

Studies which have addressed this question can be divided into those which assessed a wide range of cognitive functions and those which focused upon a single area. The latter class of studies will be considered in detail later in this chapter.

patients (Anthony et al., 1982; Dick et al., 1984). Such a criterion seems unsuitable for providing accurate estimates of the prevalence of dementia in Parkinson's disease. Indeed some authors have doubted the usefulness of the whole exercise. Pirozzolo et al. (1982) analysed the data from a neuropsychological battery and found a near normal distribution of test scores in the patient group. There was no evidence of bimodality to suggest the presence of a specific demented subgroup. Any diagnostic criterion based upon test performance would have been arbitrary and subject to the same errors of misclassification as mental state examination scores.

Despite these criticisms, it can be stated with certainty that some patients with Parkinson's disease will dement during the course of their illness. Less certain is the increased risk of this happening above that found in the general population. Unknown is the relationship between the unequivocal dementia found in some patients, and the mild cognitive changes shown by the group as a whole. The most crucial issue, and one which has yet to be addressed fully by the literature, is whether early evidence of mild cognitive impairment is predictive of later dementia. This issue will only be answered when the necessary longitudinal study is conducted.

However, while the prevalence of dementia is debatable, some clinically significant cognitive loss clearly is present in a proportion of patients. The nature of this dementia is uncertain, with the main issue being its relationship to the cognitive changes of Alzheimer's disease. While a few studies have compared Alzheimer patients with patients with Parkinson's disease (Gainotti et al., 1980; Bentin, Silverberg and Gordon, 1981; Mayeux et al., 1983), none have compared two groups of patients matched for severity of dementia. Instead, comparisons between the two groups have been restricted to clinical impressions. Benson (1984) has proposed that the dementia of Parkinson's disease is an example of a subcortical dementia with features distinct from the cortical dementia of Alzheimer's disease. However, the cortical–subcortical distinction seems to be an inappropriate one to use with Parkinson's disease. Rather, as Albert (1978) suggests, the dementia of Parkinson's disease might best be considered as one of the 'fronto-subcortical' system. An understanding of the precise nature of the dementia, and of the functional significance of its underlying mechanisms, will have important clinical and theoretical implications.

One factor which complicates all studies of dementia in Parkinson's disease, particularly longitudinal studies, is the progressive nature of the illness and the constant changes in treatment which that necessitates. Cognitive changes seen late in the illness may be qualitatively, as well as quantitatively, different from those seen earlier. A clear understanding of the effects of treatment, both in the short term and in the long term, is crucial if the changes in cognitive function are to be understood.

What are the effects of treatment on cognitive function in Parkinson's disease?

In the 1950s and 1960s, a large proportion of the neuropsychological research on Parkinson's disease focused upon the effects of stereotaxic surgery for the symptomatic relief of tremor (McFie, 1960; Riklan et al., 1960; Levita and Riklan, 1967; Almgren et al., 1969; Asso et al., 1969; Perret and Siegfried, 1969;

8
Neuropsychology and cognitive function in Parkinson's disease: an overview
R. G. Brown and C. D. Marsden

Why study cognitive function in Parkinson's disease? The question is not a trivial one, as the aims behind the many studies are varied, and an understanding of those aims may help put the research into perspective.

Neuropsychological research may be divided into two broad fields, clinical and experimental. Considerable overlap may occur between the two areas, but important differences exist in their aims and methods. The contributions of these two branches of neuropsychology to our knowledge of cognitive changes in Parkinson's disease will be considered separately.

ISSUES IN CLINICAL NEUROPSYCHOLOGICAL RESEARCH

Clinical neuropsychological research is concerned with providing information which may be of value in the diagnosis and management of individual patients with brain disorders. The questions addressed by clinical research reflect those asked most commonly in clinical practice with individual patients. With respect to research into Parkinson's disease, three key issues are:

(1) Is there evidence of cognitive impairment in Parkinson's disease?
(2) Is there an increased risk of dementia in Parkinson's disease?
(3) What are the effects of treatment on cognitive function in Parkinson's disease?

These three questions are integrally related in clinical practice. If cognitive impairment is found in a patient, it is important to determine its nature and possible cause. Mild cognitive impairment may be a relatively benign manifestation of normal ageing, or it may be the early stages of a progressive dementia. Alternatively, the changes may be related to the treatment which the patient is receiving. Modification of that treatment may lead to an improvement in the patient's cognitive status.

Is there evidence of cognitive impairment in Parkinson's disease?

Studies which have addressed this question can be divided into those which assessed a wide range of cognitive functions and those which focused upon a single area. The latter class of studies will be considered in detail later in this chapter.

The approach of administering a wide ranging battery of tests is applicable to clinical practice with the individual patient or to a group study. The aim in both cases is to provide a comprehensive picture of the cognitive function of the individual/group. As such, the purpose of the investigation is largely descriptive.

The particular battery of tests used has varied from study to study. The most popular measure, either in isolation or in conjunction with other tests, has been the Wechsler Adult Intelligence Scale (WAIS) (Wechsler, 1955) or its predecessor the Wechsler–Bellvue Intelligence Test (Wechsler, 1944). Results from these tests have been reported in many studies (Riklan et al., 1960; Riklan, Levita and Cooper, 1966; Perret and Siegfried, 1969; Asso, 1969; Christensen et al., 1970; Meier and Martin, 1970; Beardsley, and Puletti, 1971; Reitan and Boll, 1971; Loranger et al., 1972, 1973; Riklan, Whelihan and Cullinan, 1976; Matthews and York-Haaland, 1979; Portin and Rinne, 1980; Fischer and Findley, 1981; Lees and Smith, 1983; Portin, Raininko and Rinne, 1984; Weingartner et al., 1984). To summarize the results, mean verbal IQ has ranged from 97 (Riklan, Whelihan and Cullinan, 1976) to 113 (Riklan, Levita and Cooper, 1966) with a mean IQ across studies of 105. Mean performance IQ has ranged from 90 (Meier and Martin, 1970) to 105 (Riklan, Levita and Cooper, 1966; Reitan and Boll, 1971; Matthews and York-Haaland, 1979) with a mean of 98. In other words, the mean IQ of patients with Parkinson's disease lies well within the normal range. However, it is likely that these results are not representative of the whole parkinsonian population. Patients with severe intellectual loss will have been excluded from many of these studies, particularly those concerned with evaluating the effects of treatment, either levodopa or thalamotomy, both of which may be contraindicated in demented patients. Furthermore, patients with severe motor disability may have been unable or unwilling to participate. These biases, whether explicit or not, are probably present in the majority of studies on cognitive function in Parkinson's disease.

One consistent finding from these studies is a mean performance IQ lower than the corresponding verbal IQ. For example, Loranger et al. (1972) found a discrepancy of more than 20 IQ points in almost 60% of the Parkinson's disease group, compared to only 2% of a normal, age-matched control group. Large discrepancies between verbal and performance IQ are often indications of lateralized brain disorder, or more specifically, of impairment of spatial skills compared to verbal. Such a conclusion is difficult to make in the case of Parkinson's disease, as many of the performance subtests have a motor speed component which in itself would compromise the patients with Parkinson's disease.

As mentioned, several studies have administered the WAIS as part of a more extensive battery of neuropsychological assessment measures. The most comprehensive assessments have been those carried out by Reitan and Boll (1971), Pirozzolo et al. (1982) and Portin and Rinne (1980). The batteries in these studies included measures of language ability, motor skills, memory, perceptual function, visuospatial function, praxis, problem solving and conceptual ability. Results revealed deficits on a wide range of tests covering most aspects of cognitive function. This apparent global impairment is supported by the study of Villardita et al. (1982), which employed a less comprehensive battery of tests. One study which stands out is that of Talland (1962), which, almost uniquely, failed to show a widespread cognitive impairment in the patient group.

Two trends have so far emerged. First, that the mean IQ of patients with Parkinson's disease tends to be within the normal range. Second, that (as a group) they appear to show evidence of impairment on a wide range of tests of cognitive function. How can this apparent contradiction be resolved? First, it suggests that global measures such as IQ may be inappropriate for describing cognitive changes in Parkinson's disease. Mean IQs may be within the normal range, yet still represent a small but significant decline from premorbid levels. Second, a distinction must be drawn between statistically significant differences between groups, and clinically significant impairment. The studies mentioned have demonstrated the former but not the latter. In none of the studies was the mean performance of the patients within the pathological range for any of the tests, except for measures of motor speed. It may be concluded that patients with Parkinson's disease show a mild impairment, relative to normals, in their performance on a wide range of tests of cognitive function, but that this impairment may only be evident in a group study.

Is there evidence of dementia in Parkinson's disease?

The question of clinically significant cognitive impairment raises the issue of dementia in Parkinson's disease. Some patients with Parkinson's disease will also have dementia, if only because of the normal prevalence of the condition within the general population. The question of both practical and theoretical importance is whether dementia is present to an increased degree in the population of patients with Parkinson's disease. From the studies considered so far, it is clear that dementia is not an inevitable feature of the disease. However, group means do not indicate the range and distribution of performance, and it is possible that the results conceal an increased prevalence of dementia.

Problems start to arise at this point. In order to classify a patient as demented or non-demented, or to describe degrees of impairment, it is necessary to have a set of criteria for describing what is meant by dementia. The notion of 'clinical significance', mentioned above, is encompassed within the primary criterion of DSM-III (American Psychiatric Association, 1980) for the diagnosis of dementia, namely that the individual must have a 'loss of intellectual abilities of sufficient severity to interfere with social or occupational functioning'. Unfortunately, this criterion, while essential, is especially difficult to assess in Parkinson's disease. The presence of progressive, incapacitating motor impairment itself interferes with these aspects of life. The majority of studies which have looked at dementia in Parkinson's disease have failed to address themselves to this problem, resorting instead to more operational criteria such as cut-off scores on mental status examinations. The problems involved with this approach, and with the study of dementia in Parkinson's disease in general, have been discussed in detail elsewhere (Brown and Marsden, 1984). In the same paper, the authors evaluated the studies which have given estimates for the prevalence of dementia in Parkinson's disease, and suggested that a figure of 15–20% may be more realistic than the 33% often quoted in the literature. Likely reasons for the overestimation are: over-inclusive criteria for the diagnosis of dementia, failure to discriminate between dementia, confusional states, depression or even normal ageing, and the inclusion of patients without idiopathic Parkinson's disease, particularly those with arteriosclerotic changes. The cut-off scores employed on the mental state examinations are arbitrary, and depend upon the sensitivity and selectivity levels which the investigator chooses. Commonly, cut-offs which classify correctly the majority of demented patients also classify incorrectly a significant number of non-demented patients (Anthony et al., 1982; Dick et al., 1984). Such a criterion seems unsuitable for providing accurate estimates of the prevalence of dementia in Parkinson's disease. Indeed some authors have doubted the usefulness of the whole exercise. Pirozzolo et al. (1982) analysed the data from a neuropsychological battery and found a near normal distribution of test scores in the patient group. There was no evidence of bimodality to suggest the presence of a specific demented subgroup. Any diagnostic criterion based upon test performance would have been arbitrary and subject to the same errors of misclassification as mental state examination scores.

Despite these criticisms, it can be stated with certainty that some patients with Parkinson's disease will dement during the course of their illness. Less certain is the increased risk of this happening above that found in the general population. Unknown is the relationship between the unequivocal dementia found in some patients, and the mild cognitive changes shown by the group as a whole. The most crucial issue, and one which has yet to be addressed fully by the literature, is whether early evidence of mild cognitive impairment is predictive of later dementia. This issue will only be answered when the necessary longitudinal study is conducted.

However, while the prevalence of dementia is debatable, some clinically significant cognitive loss clearly is present in a proportion of patients. The nature of this dementia is uncertain, with the main issue being its relationship to the cognitive changes of Alzheimer's disease. While a few studies have compared Alzheimer patients with patients with Parkinson's disease (Gainotti et al., 1980; Bentin, Silverberg and Gordon, 1981; Mayeux et al., 1983), none have compared two groups of patients matched for severity of dementia. Instead, comparisons between the two groups have been restricted to clinical impressions. Benson (1984) has proposed that the dementia of Parkinson's disease is an example of a subcortical dementia with features distinct from the cortical dementia of Alzheimer's disease. However, the cortical–subcortical distinction seems to be an inappropriate one to use with Parkinson's disease. Rather, as Albert (1978) suggests, the dementia of Parkinson's disease might best be considered as one of the 'fronto-subcortical' system. An understanding of the precise nature of the dementia, and of the functional significance of its underlying mechanisms, will have important clinical and theoretical implications.

One factor which complicates all studies of dementia in Parkinson's disease, particularly longitudinal studies, is the progressive nature of the illness and the constant changes in treatment which that necessitates. Cognitive changes seen late in the illness may be qualitatively, as well as quantitatively, different from those seen earlier. A clear understanding of the effects of treatment, both in the short term and in the long term, is crucial if the changes in cognitive function are to be understood.

What are the effects of treatment on cognitive function in Parkinson's disease?

In the 1950s and 1960s, a large proportion of the neuropsychological research on Parkinson's disease focused upon the effects of stereotaxic surgery for the symptomatic relief of tremor (McFie, 1960; Riklan et al., 1960; Levita and Riklan, 1967; Almgren et al., 1969; Asso et al., 1969; Perret and Siegfried, 1969;

Christensen *et al.*, 1970). A consistent, although not universal, finding from these studies was that surgery led to an immediate post-operative deficit after which there was a partial, but never complete, recovery of function. Of some theoretical interest was the suggestion of laterality effects, with impairment of language function being more common following left thalamic lesions, and visuospatial deficits after right-sided lesions (McFie, 1960; Riklan *et al.*, 1960; Almgren *et al.*, 1969).

The first widely effective treatment of Parkinson's disease came with the advent of levodopa. With it came a string of studies, aimed at evaluating the impact of the drug upon the cognitive status of the patients (Beardsley and Puletti, 1971; Loranger *et al.*, 1972, 1973; Riklan, 1972; Riklan *et al.*, 1973; Bowen *et al.*, 1975, 1976; Hamel and Riklan, 1975; Riklan, Whelihan and Cullinan, 1976; Halgin, Riklan and Misiak, 1977; Morel-Maroger, 1977; Portin and Rinne, 1980; Fischer and Findley, 1981; Portin, Raininko and Rinne, 1984). Given the dramatic improvement in motor function, it was hoped that similar improvements would be seen in cognitive function. Short-term studies seemed to confirm this hypothesis, but with follow-up over a period of years, patients were found to return to pre-levodopa levels and below. Furthermore, some patients were found to experience acute reactions to the drug involving depression, delusions, hallucinations and confusional states (Parkes, 1981).

Adverse reactions are not confined to levodopa. Particularly important when considering cognitive function are the effects of the anticholinergics, which still play an important role in the treatment of Parkinson's disease. These drugs may induce confusional states in the elderly and already impaired patient (Parkes, 1981; De Smet *et al.*, 1982), and, even in non-demented patients they may lead to disturbances in memory function (Koller, 1984).

These results imply that consideration of current treatment (and prior treatment in the case of thalamotomy) is of considerable importance in evaluating studies of cognitive function in Parkinson's disease.

Before finishing this section on clinical issues, one further area deserves mention. This is the area of treatment. As has been discussed, mild cognitive changes may be the norm in Parkinson's disease, and in some cases these will be noticeable to the patient. This is particularly true if concentration, memory and the taking in of new information are affected, and the patient is still relatively active. Some patients may even consider these problems to be their primary handicap. There is no evidence to suggest that cognitive changes in Parkinson's disease are functionally different from those resulting from other central nervous system damage. Consequently, patients should benefit from the same behavioural strategies developed to remedy cognitive deficits for other clinical groups (Wilson and Moffat, 1984). It is hoped that this area will receive increasing attention from clinical neuropsychologists in the future.

ISSUES IN EXPERIMENTAL NEUROPSYCHOLOGICAL RESEARCH

It might be argued that many of the clinical studies described in the previous section were 'experimental' in that they used standardized procedures and comparison groups. However, a better description for such studies might be 'controlled'. By 'experimental' is meant the design of studies to test specific hypotheses about cognitive function. These hypotheses relate most frequently to the relationship between the cognitive status of the patients and theories and models of brain function.

Parkinson's disease provides one of the best (albeit imperfect) models of the effects of disruption of normal striatal and dopaminergic function in man (Marsden, 1982). It is argued that the profound depletion of dopamine in the striatum in Parkinson's disease must cause abnormal function of this major input zone of the striopallidal complex. As a result, the internal machinery of the striatum should generate abnormal striatal output to pallidum and substantia nigra pars reticulata, so that the final output from these latter regions to the thalamus would be disrupted. Cognitive abnormalities in Parkinson's disease thus might give clues as to the function of the striopallidal complex in normal cognitive function.

There are obvious caveats to this simple argument. The pathology of Parkinson's disease is not confined to striatal dopamine depletion. Cortical dopamine and noradrenaline are compromised, and the cholinergic projection from substantia innominata to cerebral cortex is involved. Furthermore, the depletion of striatal dopamine in Parkinson's disease is not uniform. The 'motor striatum' or putamen is always affected more severely than the caudate. Although caudate dopamine is reduced considerably, compensatory mechanisms to preserve function (e.g. postsynaptic receptor supersensitivity and increased activity in remaining intact presynaptic dopamine neurones) may be sufficient to prevent caudate dysfunction, at least initially in Parkinson's disease. However, nature has provided few other opportunities to study isolated abnormal striopallidal function. The devastation of the intrinsic striatal neuronal population in Huntington's disease is complicated by associated cortical atrophy (although the exact significance and extent of this pathology is not clear). Isolated bilateral lesions of the globus pallidus and substantia nigra motor complex are rare, e.g. Hallervorden–Spatz disease. So, accepting the limitations, Parkinson's disease is worthy of study.

Clinical neuropsychologists interested in this area have been joined by psychologists from two other fields: animal experimental neuropsychologists who study the behavioural and cognitive effects of controlled brain lesions and neurochemical manipulations (Divac and Oberg, 1979), and human cognitive psychologists who study the function of the intact human brain. In both of these disciplines, models and theories of the structural and functional organization of the brain abound. However, the strength and validity of those theories need to be tested in other conditions. For this reason cognitive and animal experimental psychologists have turned their attention to Parkinson's disease, bringing with them their theories and methods.

The questions addressed by such experimental research are too numerous to list. However, the following will give a flavour of the research:

(1) What is the functional role of the striatum in cognition?
(2) What is the relationship between striatal function and that of other areas such as the frontal cortex?
(3) What pathways are involved in the processing of different types of information in the brain?
(4) What is the functional role of dopamine systems in the regulation of behaviour?
(5) What is the nature of the cognitive changes found in Parkinson's disease, and what is their relationship to the deficits found in Alzheimer's disease?

These points will not be discussed individually. Instead, research on three main areas of cognitive function will be reviewed: (i) visuospatial function, (ii) memory function, and (iii) conceptual ability and regulation of behaviour. While not providing an exhaustive review of the experimental study of cognitive function in

Parkinson's disease, research in these three areas covers the majority of the published literature, and reflects the attention of researchers in the field. Within the context of reviewing these areas, and in the final discussion, most of the above issues will be considered.

Visuospatial function

The presence of a deficit in visuospatial function in Parkinson's disease, together with the idea of a high prevalence of dementia, form the two most pervasive themes to be found in the literature. In both cases, adequate definition of terms is an essential prerequisite if confusion is to be avoided. Boller *et al.* (1984) offer an operational definition of visuospatial function that involves:

(a) The appreciation of the relative positions of stimulus objects in space.
(b) The integration of those objects into a coherent spatial framework.
(c) The performing of mental operations involving those spatial concepts.

Possible evidence for a visuospatial deficit in Parkinson's disease may be found, at the most basic level, in the consistent finding that patients have lower performance IQs than verbal IQs. The high spatial loading on many of the tests in the performance scale suggests a spatial deficit as a plausible explanation for the results. However, a more parsimonious explanation can be found in the fact, as mentioned earlier, that the same tests also have a large motor-speed component. This leaves open the possibility that the results simply confirm that patients with Parkinson's disease are slow in their movements. Despite this possibility, some authors assert that the verbal-performance difference reflects a true spatial deficit (Meier and Martin, 1970; Loranger *et al.*, 1972). Unfortunately, the WAIS in the standard administration does not allow the spatial and speed components to be dissociated functionally, and so the issue has remained unresolved.

This raises a general problem, namely the nature of many of the standard clinical neuropsychological tests used in both clinical and experimental research. These tests were designed, or adopted, mainly for their usefulness in answering clinical questions relating to diagnosis: either the presence/absence of organic damage or the localization of that damage. The tests were seldom intended for use in isolation, but rather in the context of a comprehensive neuropsychological assessment. It is a characteristic of virtually all neuropsychological tests that, while aimed at a specific aspect of cognitive function, test failure may be due to a wide range of factors. Patients with Parkinson's disease are likely to have impaired performance on cognitive tests for many reasons other than specific cognitive impairment (*see Table 8.1*). In a clinical assessment, qualitative features of the patient's performance give

Table 8.1 Factors other than cognitive changes likely to influence the performance of patients with Parkinson's disease on tests of cognitive function

---
(1) Natural age-related decline
(2) Impaired motor speed and manual dexterity
(3) Mental and physical fatiguability
(4) Psychiatric disturbance, particularly depression
(5) Distraction by pain and dyskinesia
(6) Sedation, confusion, hallucinations and other drug side-effects
---

important clues as to the contribution of some of these factors. Steps may then be taken to adapt or devise tests to assess these ideas directly, such as relaxing time constraints if it is believed that the patient is failing because of impaired motor speed (Shapiro, 1973). Typically, qualitative information and flexibility in test administration are absent from experimental situations. Instead, the various factors contributing to test performance must be anticipated, and the experiment designed to exclude those components, or to measure each one separately so that its contribution to test performance may be evaluated. Unfortunately, such experiments tend to be the exception. Studies derived from the clinical background make the frequent error of placing too much faith in the power of individual tests to measure, unambiguously, specific cognitive functions. At the end of an experiment, often all that may be said is that the patient performed poorly on a particular task. Poor performance is not, in itself, evidence of a deficit in the assumed underlying function. This can only be proposed after the exclusion of alternative explanations for the performance deficit.

With that cautionary note, how strong is the evidence for a visuospatial impairment in Parkinson's disease?

Judging the orientation of a line in space, either with the body upright or tilted, satisfies the criteria for a spatial test. Patients with Parkinson's disease are impaired in performing this simple task (Proctor *et al.*, 1964). Danta and Hilton (1975) performed a similar study, but without the condition of body tilt, and found impaired performance in 29% of patients with Parkinson's disease. The experiments were carried out in the absence of external visual cues so that the task could only be performed by matching the line orientation to a vertical, judged from the individual's own body orientation. Errors in such a task might not be due to failure to appreciate the spatial orientation of the external stimulus, but to misinterpretation of one's own position in space. Some have claimed proprioceptive deficits in Parkinson's disease (Dinnerstein *et al.*, 1964). It is also possible that the subject's external and internal spatial appreciation might be unimpaired but that errors are made in matching the two components of the task, namely the perceived orientation of the line and the perceived orientation of the body. Indeed, visual matching deficits have been shown in Parkinson's disease in a number of studies (Portin and Rinne, 1980; Bentin, Silverberg and Gordon, 1981; Mortimer *et al.*, 1982; Pirozzolo *et al.*, 1982). Matching, while involved in some spatial tasks, is not in itself a spatial function. This component of the task needs to be separated out before a spatial deficit can be assumed. To try to avoid such difficulties, and to explore further the nature of the cognitive deficit in Parkinson's disease, other tasks have been utilized.

Bowen, Hoehn and Yahr (1972) found patients with Parkinson's disease to be impaired in performing a route-finding task (Semmes *et al.*, 1963). Nine discs were laid out on the floor in a 3 × 3 square. The same array was shown on paper which traced a path between the points. Holding this map, the subjects had to walk the path on the floor, but without turning the map as they did so. In a second study (Bowen *et al.*, 1976), patients were impaired on a body-schema task (Weinstein *et al.*, 1964). Subjects were shown a dorsal and ventral representation of a human figure on which parts of the body were numbered. Each subject had to point, in order, to the parts of their own body that corresponded to the numbered parts on the figure. Patients committed disproportionately more errors on the two tasks, in the conditions where their own perspective was the reverse of that represented on the map or the figure, thus obliging the subject to 'reverse' mentally his own body orientation. This is a spatial skill. However, it was a feature of both tasks that the subjects had repeatedly to switch from 'normal' to 'reverse' orientation and back again. As later evidence will indicate, this ability seems to be impaired in Parkinson's disease (Bowen et al., 1975; Lees and Smith, 1983; Canavan et al., 1984; Cools et al., 1984). This offers a plausible non-spatial explanation for the deficits in both experiments, an explanation favoured by the authors of the studies.

Mortimer et al. (1982) analysed the relative contributions of visual discrimination and visual memory to the visuospatial deficit in Parkinson's disease. In contrast to earlier studies, they found no evidence of impairment in matching line orientation or angle. However, introducing a delay of ten seconds between the model being shown, and the target line/angle, led to a disproportionate decrement in the patient's performance. The authors concluded that this is evidence for an impairment in spatial memory. However, this deficit is not restricted to spatial tasks. De Lancey Horne (1971) found a similar deficit in a delayed matching task, where a visual but not spatial match was required. It is parsimonious to assume that the common deficit in both experiments is at the level of visual memory, and is not specific to any spatial component.

In contrast to the studies reviewed so far, a number of studies have failed to find evidence of spatial impairment in Parkinson's disease. Boller et al. (1984) assessed spatial memory, perception, organization and mental manipulation. While patients were impaired on some of the tests of perceptual matching and on tasks with significant motor components, they were unimpaired on tests of visual recognition memory, perception of spatial location and the manipulation of spatial concepts.

Brown and Marsden (1985) assessed right–left discrimination and the ability to manipulate mental representations of spatial information. Subjects were presented with an arrow pointing up, down, left or right, and a target square to one side (*see Figure 8.1*). Subjects had to orient themselves to the arrow, and judge whether the target lay to the right or to the left. Mean reaction time and error rates for the four orientations are shown in *Figure 8.2*. Also shown are the mean simple reaction time for the two groups. No difference was found between the groups for total errors, nor any interaction between groups for the errors in the four orientations. For the reaction time data, patients were slower than the controls for all conditions, including the non-spatial, simple reaction time task. However, there was no difference in mean reaction times between the groups for the different conditions. This implies that increasing the spatial complexity of the task, while keeping the motor demands constant, did not lead to any increased difficulty for the patient group.

Finally, Della Sala et al. (1985) used a spatial task with two levels of complexity. In the first condition, subjects were shown a tilted line which, if continued, would intercept a horizontal baseline. The subject's task was to mentally extrapolate the first line and judge the point of interception with the baseline. In the second condition, the first line was pointed away from the baseline, and would only intercept after 'rebounding' from an upper line parallel to the baseline. Once again, the subject had to judge the point of interception, but this time after 'rebound'. Overall, no difference was found between the accuracy of the patient and control groups on the two tasks, and no interaction was found between group and task difficulty. It is of interest to mention at this point a study by Stern et al. (1983). In that study, subjects were also asked to extrapolate a line between two points, or to fill in portions missing from a saw-tooth pattern. In contrast to the Della Salla study, the patients were impaired on the tasks, particularly the more complex ones.

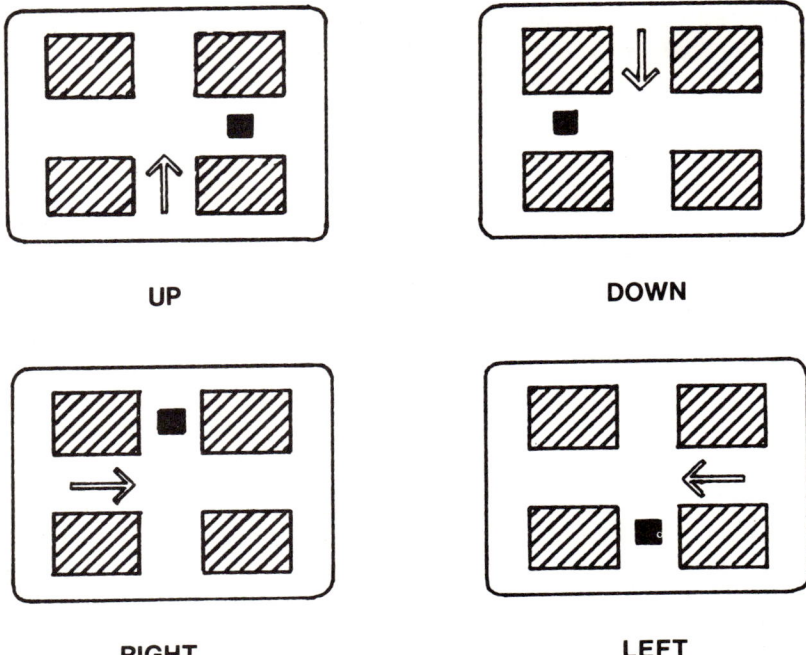

Figure 8.1 Examples of the stimulus configurations, showing the four possible arrow orientations (up, down, right and left)

Figure 8.2 Mean total reaction time for a simple reaction time task, and for the four arrow orientations of the spatial task. (Open bars = Parkinson's disease group; solid bars = control group)

Both studies involved similar visuospatial skills, yet only in the latter study was the subject required to use those skills for the control of movement. It is conceivable that deficits may only be found in visuospatial tests under such circumstances. The issue then becomes whether one is still talking about visuospatial skills or the utilization of those skills for the control of movement.

The results of these recent experiments, paired with the ambiguity of many of the earlier studies, offers little support for the hypothesis that Parkinson's disease is associated with a global deficit in spatial function. It is possible that consistent spatial deficits will be found in future studies, using different tasks and patient groups. If such deficits are found, then their nature and the conditions under which they are found will allow a finer, more useful definition of the putative 'spatial' impairment. However, at present, there appears to be no convincing proof of any specific deficit in visuospatial function in Parkinson's disease.

Memory

Patients with Parkinson's disease frequently complain of problems with their memory. Some unpublished data from our own laboratory (Gotham, personal communication) lends empirical support to this clinical observation. Ninety-three patients with Parkinson's disease (mean age: 65.2 years; mean duration of illness: 8.5 years) and 83 healthy controls (mean age: 69.4 years), completed a subjective memory questionnaire (Bennett-Levy and Powell, 1980). Subjects were asked to rate their memory for a range of everyday tasks, such as remembering people's names, birthdays and shopping lists. The subjects also rated the frequency with which they experienced common types of memory failure. Results confirmed that patients with Parkinson's disease, in their own opinion, have poorer memories than healthy controls, despite the fact that the patient group was significantly younger. Warburton (1967) assessed patients' autobiographical memory, and she too found a significant impairment in the Parkinson's disease group. However, research typically has ignored such real-life aspects of memory, relying instead upon traditional, laboratory-based tests. An enormous variety of procedures exist for assessing memory, derived from a long tradition of research in the clinical, animal and cognitive fields. Recently, a more integrated approach has started to bring together the diverse methods and theories (Baddeley, 1982).

Memory function is extremely sensitive to any factor which interferes with the efficiency of the central nervous system. Memory impairment is often the most prominent cognitive effect of centrally active drugs, of brain damage, and of normal ageing. While a considerable amount of research has focused on memory function in Parkinson's disease, the problem is to distinguish between memory deficits due to the organic changes of the disease and deficits due to normal ageing, drug side-effects or depression. Also, heterogeneity within the parkinsonian population means that results may vary depending on the nature of the sample. Unfortunately, most of the published research does not allow any firm conclusions to be drawn about the nature and cause of the apparent memory impairment in Parkinson's disease. Rather than reviewing individual studies, the general trends in the literature will be summarized. Attention will then be focused on a number of more recent experimental studies.

In clinical practice and in research, distinctions are often drawn between the modality of memory being assessed (verbal or visual), the manner in which it is tested (recall or recognition), and whether testing occurs immediately or after a delay. This simple scheme will be used here.

Immediate verbal memory is assessed commonly in clinical practice by use of the digit span (the number of digits which a subject can repeat back accurately after a single presentation). Despite its high face validity, the test is of doubtful utility as a measure of memory impairment. Commonly, patients with even gross memory impairment resulting from organic amnesia will have normal digit spans (Zangwill, 1946; Drachman and Arbit, 1966). Indeed, digit span may be better thought of as reflecting attention and alertness rather than memory (Cummings and Benson, 1983). Accordingly, most studies have failed to find any difference between parkinsonian patients and controls on this test (Asso, 1969; Asso et al., 1969; Horn, 1974; Hamel and Riklan, 1975; Riklan et al., 1976; Portin and Rinne, 1980; Lees and Smith, 1983) with only three exceptions (Reitan and Boll, 1971; Halgin, Riklan and Misiak, 1977; Pirozzolo et al., 1982).

This is in itself of interest, for it suggests that, at the simplest level, alertness is not impaired in Parkinson's disease. However, little research has been directed at the area of attention and alertness in Parkinson's disease. Part of the problem is that many of the clinical tests of attention are assessed by motor speed, for example in letter cancellation. However, the use of appropriate control conditions allows valid measures of attention to be made. Talland and Schwab (1964) and De Lancey Horne (1973) both used this technique. The results reveal that the patients are slow compared to the controls under all levels of task complexity, with no disproportionate increase in time with increasing task difficulty. Similarly, patients made more errors, but, again, the proportion of errors in the simple and complex conditions were similar to those shown by the controls. The results of such studies are difficult to interpret. Studies are needed which utilize the methods available from experimental psychology on sustained and directed attention, tasks in which the motor components are minimal or controlled experimentally.

All valid cognitive testing depends upon adequate alertness, attention and vigilance. The importance of this fact is reflected clinically in the need to judge patients' attentional state in making the differential diagnosis between dementia and confusional state. While the patients seen in experimental studies are typically neither confused nor demented, the tasks used are much more sensitive than many of those used in clinical situations. The extent to which attentional disturbance in Parkinson's disease influences performance on tests of memory or, indeed, on any cognitive test, is unknown at present. The effect, if any, needs to be evaluated.

In contrast to tests which assess the span of immediate memory, there are other tests which involve presenting the subject with more information than they can remember, and assessing what percentage they can recall/recognize and/or how long it takes them to learn the new material. The material may be a list of words or nonsense syllables, or a short story. When immediate recall for such material is assessed, groups of patients with Parkinson's disease frequently show a deficit compared to the mean performance of age-matched controls (Bowen et al., 1976; Halgin, Riklan and Misiak, 1977; Pirozzolo et al., 1982; Tweedy, Langer and McDowell, 1982; Weingartner et al., 1984). The one exception is the study of Talland (1962). Another common paradigm is paired associate learning, in which the subject must learn the associations between pairs of words read out in a list, usually over several trials. With this method too, immediate recall is impaired (Bowen et al., 1976; Riklan et al., 1976; Halgin et al., 1977; Pirozzolo et al., 1982; Portin and Rinne, 1982).

With delayed recall the subject's memory for the same information is assessed after a period which may vary from minutes to hours. Given that patients show deficits in the immediate recall of verbal material, it is not surprising that they also show deficits in recall after a delay (Talland, 1962; Halgin, Riklan and Misiak, 1977; Portin and Rinne, 1980; Pirozzolo et al., 1982; Weingartner et al., 1984). A single exception is found in one of the conditions of Talland's (1962) experiment, when the patients were required to learn and remember a list of non-meaningful syllables. The other experiments all used meaningful material. The possible significance of this difference will be discussed later.

In contrast to the large number of studies which have tested memory using recall, only a few have used a recognition paradigm. In such paradigms the information to be remembered is presented together with information new to the individual. The subject's task is to indicate the material which was presented previously. Garron et al. (1972) found no impairment on a recognition version of the digit span, while Asso et al. (1969) found no impairment on a recognition form of a visual–verbal paired associate task. Negative results were also reported by Lees and Smith (1983), Weingartner et al. (1984) and Flowers, Pearce and Pearce (1984). In the latter case, no deficit was found, even after a delay. Only one study (Tweedy, Langer and McDowell, 1982) has shown a significant impairment for the recognition of verbal material.

Visual memory in Parkinson's disease has received less attention than verbal memory, possibly due to difficulties in assessing recall where the subject is required to draw the response. Interpretation of the patient's response is complicated by the motor impairment. Nevertheless, some results have been reported. Asso et al. (1969) failed to find any deficit in immediate recall on a visual–visual paired associate task, although Weingartner et al. (1984), using a similar task, found a deficit when recall was assessed after a five-minute delay. However, deficits in immediate recall of visual material have been shown by Riklan et al. (1976), Bowen et al. (1976), Halgin, Riklan and Misiak (1977), Pirozzolo et al. (1982) and Portin and Rinne (1982). For recognition memory, motor impairment is not a problem as reproduction of the test material is not required. This makes the paradigm an attractive one for assessing visual memory in Parkinson's disease. Despite this it has been used only on a handful of occasions. Asso et al. (1969), Lees and Smith (1983) and Flowers, Pearce and Pearce (1984), have assessed visual memory using a recognition paradigm, and none were able to demonstrate any deficit for the patient's performance. The study of Flowers, Pearce and Pearce (1984) was particularly thorough in that it used a wide variety of materials ranging from words and meaningful pictures to non-meaningful groups of letters and abstract designs. In addition, two methods of assessing recognition were used, with both immediate and delayed testing. Whatever the material, and whichever method was used, both immediately and after delay, patients failed to show any consistent deficit compared to normal controls.

To summarize these results, patients with Parkinson's disease show impaired performance in the free recall of both visual and verbal material, both immediately and after a delay. In contrast, the majority of studies have shown normal recognition memory for verbal and visual material. Intact recognition memory implies that the information is being registered and stored accurately. The problem seems to be in the access to that information in the free recall task.

Some recent studies have sought to investigate the nature of this memory deficit in more detail.

In the review above, it was noted that Talland (1962) found normal recall of verbal material, both immediately and after a delay. This study was unique in that it used non-meaningful verbal material as stimuli. These were pronounceable but meaningless consonant–syllable–consonant triagrams such as TUZ. When a stimulus has a meaning (as in all of the other studies of recall of verbal material), the subject has access to previously stored representations of words and their meanings to aid in the encoding, storage and retrieval of the new information. It is possible that patients with Parkinson's disease are impaired in their ability to utilize this store of semantic information. Some support for this hypothesis can be found in patients' own reports of difficulty in word finding in spontaneous speech. This 'tip-of-the-tongue' phenomenon has been confirmed empirically. Matison *et al.* (1982) presented subjects with pictures to name. Patients with Parkinson's disease were able to name less items, but were often able to give the correct answer when given a phonetic or semantic cue. This implies that they knew the words but were unable to access them without help. In the same study, two types of verbal fluency were assessed: the first for words beginning with the letter 'f', 'a' or 's', and second, words in the semantic category 'animals'. The patient's performance was impaired only on the second condition. This suggests that while access to phonologically coded information was intact, access to semantically coded information was impaired.

These experiments offer some support for the hypothesis that the memory impairment in Parkinson's disease is linked in some way to the nature of the system of verbal semantic information. However, while the hypothesis may have value in explaining the deficits in verbal memory, it is unable to account for the impairments in visual memory, unless the visual material is verbally encodable. Either a separate memory deficit must be assumed, or another hypothesis proposed which can explain both types of result.

Weingartner *et al.* (1984) tested the theory of Hasher and Zacks (1979) which proposes that the crucial component is not the semantic content of the material, but the effort required to perform the task. To test this hypothesis, a variety of tasks were administered which were assumed to vary along a continuum 'effort demanding'–'automatic'. Some tasks assessed both modes. For example, subjects were given a set of 32 stimulus pairs. Some were word–word pairs, some picture–picture pairs, and some word–picture pairs. After a five minute delay subjects were asked to recall as many of the items as they could in a free recall test (effort-demanding). Following this, a list of the words or names of the pictures were read to the subject, who was asked to state whether the item had been shown as a word or as a picture (automatic task). Patients were impaired at the effort-demanding (recall) component, but unimpaired on the automatic task. Overall, results revealed that subjects were impaired only on the effort-demanding tasks, and that the degree of impairment was proportional to the amount of effort assumed to be required.

An additional study by the same group, this time on normal subjects, is worth mentioning. Newman *et al.* (1984) evaluated the effects of levodopa on normal subjects' ability to perform 'automatic' and effort-demanding learning tasks. Access to semantic information and automatic processes was unaffected but the drug reliably facilitated subject performance on the effortful memory processing.

The 'effort' theory offers an interesting alternative hypothesis to explain the memory deficits observed in Parkinson's disease. However, sample sizes in the above studies were small and it is too early to generalize from a single result. The strength (and possible weakness) of the theory comes in its applicability to areas of cognition other than memory. If 'cognitive effort' is viewed as a superordinate dimension, then whatever the task, be it visuospatial, conceptual or memory, the more effort required, the worse the patients should perform. However, the hypothesis will have little theoretical value unless a way can be found of defining, *a priori*, the precise 'effort demand' of each task. If this cannot be done, then there is the danger of defining as 'effortful' those tasks on which patients do badly.

The 'effort' theory shares many of the strengths and weaknesses of attention theories. In fact, Hasher and Zacks (1979) view the 'automatic'–'effortful' continuum as an elaboration of earlier attentional theories. As discussed earlier, attention and alertness are essential prerequisities for performing any cognitive task. However, similar problems arise in defining, *a priori*, the attentional demand of a task.

Another theory which may be useful in explaining the memory, and other deficits in Parkinson's disease, is that of 'working memory' (Baddeley and Hitch, 1974). This theory extends and elaborates the model of primary memory (or short-term memory) developed by Atkinson and Shiffrin (1968). Working memory is seen as comprising three subsystems. A modality-independent 'central executive', and two modality-specific, short-term memory storage systems: an 'articulatory loop' for holding limited amounts of phonological information (e.g. numbers being used in a mental calculation) and an equivalent system of visual material, called the 'visuospatial sketch pad'. Working memory, and in particular the central executive, is seen as playing a crucial role in cognition, both in the processing of incoming information, and in the access and utilization of stored information.

The model has proved useful in explaining the deficits observed in a number of amnesic disorders (Shallice and Warrington, 1970; Vallar and Baddeley, 1984) and has been proposed as a useful model for understanding the deficits found in normal ageing (Rabbitt, 1981; Welford, 1981) and dementia (Morris, 1984). As yet, the model has not been applied to Parkinson's disease.

It is clear that an important development will be the testing of such models in studies which compare directly the nature of the memory deficits in different disorders and in normal ageing. Such studies may provide clues to the functional nature of different pathological changes in cognitive function. They may also help explain why only some patients with Parkinson's disease (all of whom suffer striatal dopamine depletion) suffer significant memory loss. The possible role of the striatum in memory function is still uncertain, although the models just reviewed suggest that the concept of viewing memory as a separate system may be misleading, and that concepts such as attention, effort, or the processes of the central executive may provide more useful and plausible roles for the striatum in memory function.

Conceptual ability and the regulation of behaviour

In everyday life, an organism is surrounded by more stimuli than it can deal with. Much of that information is irrelevant to ongoing behaviour. It is necessary to extract the essential information and ignore the irrelevant. Once the organism has focused on the relevant information, it must maintain attention on those attributes to guide ongoing behaviour. However, changes in the organism or its environment may mean that the salience of a stimulus suddenly changes. It is essential that the organism monitors continuously the relationship between the environment and its behaviour. When necessary it must have the flexibility to shift attention from one stimulus to another and, at the same time, ignore the previously relevant stimulus.

The most popular neuropsychological test used to assess these complex functions is the Wisconsin Card Sorting Test (WCST) (Berg, 1948). The test consists of cards, each of which may be distinguished by three attributes (colour, number and shape). The subject must determine the relevant attribute, and use it as the basis for sorting the cards. When signalled by the examiner, the subject must switch attention to a different attribute and use that to categorize and sort the cards. This switching is repeated a number of times. Measures include the total number of successful sorts or categorizations by the subject, the total number of errors, and the total number of perseverative errors, which may be a 'sort' according to the previously correct, but now incorrect category (Milner, 1963), or a 'sort' according to a category which had been identified as incorrect on the immediately preceding trial (Nelson, 1976).

The WCST has been given to patients with Parkinson's disease on several occasions. Bowen et al. (1975) found that the patients sorted less categories and made more errors, but did make more perseverative errors by Milner's criteria. Flowers (1982) also found impaired performance, although its characteristics were not described. Lees and Smith (1983) and Canavan et al. (1984) both found a decrease in the number of categories in their patient groups, and an increase in the number of perseverative errors. However, in the former study the increase in perseverative errors was significant only when defined according to Milner's criteria.

The Halstead categories test (Halstead, 1947) is presumed to assess similar functions to the WCST. Impaired performance in Parkinson's disease has been found by Reitan and Boll (1971) and Matthews and York-Haaland (1979), although, in the latter study, only in patients with a duration of illness greater than six years. Canavan et al. (1984) also found an increased impairment on the WCST in patients with a longer duration of illness, although significant impairment was found also in some of the recently diagnosed groups. However, the patients in the Lees and Smith study had a mean disease duration of less than three years, suggesting that duration of illness is not necessarily a crucial factor in the appearance of these deficits.

Flowers and Robertson (1984) used a simple categorization task. In one condition, the stimuli consisted of three figures. Two were the same shape but different sizes, and two were the same size but different shapes. Depending on whether the crucial attribute was shape or size, one of the three figures could be classified 'odd-man-out'. As in the WCST, the subject had to find the correct attribute, and then in this case identify the odd-man-out. Subjects were told correct/incorrect. After ten sorts by the first rule, the subject was told to use the other rule. After ten more sorts he was told to use the first rule again. This alternation was repeated for eight groups of sorts. All subjects could identify the two rules. For the control subjects errors increased after the first switch, but performance improved with repeated alternations. In contrast, the patient's performance was characterized by a persistent tendency, after the first switch, to lapse into the incorrect category. The problem seemed to be one of maintaining attention on the (temporarily) relevant attribute and suppressing the (temporarily) irrelevant one. This deficit did not seem to be in switching *per se*.

However, a study by Cools et al. (1984) suggests that the ability to 'switch' is impaired in Parkinson's disease under some circumstances. A variety of motor and non-motor tasks were administered, which had the common feature of being divided into two phases. In a verbal fluency task, the first phase was generating animal names and the second phase, the names of professions. In another task, cards bearing the names of animals were sorted according to the dimension 'bird–mammal'. Subjects had to learn the rule by trial-and-error. After seven consecutive sorts the rule was changed to 'domestic–wild'. The measure was the number of trials to discover the new rule. A block sorting task was administered in an analogous fashion, with colour and size being the two attributes for the subject to discover. Finally, there was a motor task involving two different finger-tap sequences. In all cases, the crucial measure was the patient's performance on the second, 'switch' phase. Performance in the first phase of each task was used to control for different overall levels in performance between groups. For all tasks, patients performed proportionately worse in the 'switch' phase than in the initial baseline phase.

The results from these experiments suggest that patients with Parkinson's disease are impaired in the regulation of behaviour, in terms of maintaining and shifting response 'sets'. The term 'set' is used frequently in psychology to describe a state of behaviour in which, through repetition of an event, an organism becomes better able to process information relevant to that class of events. It is thus a process of focused and sustained attention on an aspect of the internal or external environment, with an accompanying facilitation of central nervous system activity involved in processing the stimulus or generating a response.

It is pertinent at this point to introduce the idea of 'cues'. A cue may be defined as a piece of information which guides the processing of subsequent information. One such cue may be the instruction to attend to shape or colour in WCST. If this is not the first category, then the cue may be called a 'shift cue'. Other shift cues may be feedback from the outcome of a response, or an internal decision to change. Another class of cues are those which allow the organism to maintain or 'hold' the set. Once again, these cues may be an instruction or aspect of the stimulus configuration, or an internal 'self-reminder' of what is relevant and what is irrelevant currently.

The evidence described above suggests that patients with Parkinson's disease may have difficulty in utilizing both 'shift' cues and 'hold' cues. However, there is an accumulation of evidence that a crucial aspect of the cues may be whether they are provided by an external source, or are internal to the organism. This distinction may be important for understanding the deficits of Parkinson's disease and those following frontal lobe lesions and of normal ageing.

In the visuospatial study of Brown and Marsden (1985) described previously, subjects had to alternate between different spatial orientations. Examination of the data revealed that the patients acquired a 'set' in that they became faster with repetition of the same arrow orientation, but were not handicapped when called upon to switch from making left–right decisions from the normal orientation, to decisions with the arrow inverted through 180 degrees. In this task, the arrow serves as either a shift cue or a hold cue for each individual trial. Thus, for each trial, there was an external cue telling the subject what was required. This is in contrast to tests such as the WCST or the 'odd-man-out' test in which there is nothing in the stimulus itself to tell the subject what is the relevant attribute, and set maintenance must be achieved by a mixture of internal cues or reminders and feedbacks. The question of internal versus external cues is raised by the issue of motor control in Parkinson's disease. It is a common clinical observation that a patient who is unable to walk spontaneously (through internal control) may be able to walk up stairs or if lines are drawn on the floor (external cues). Further evidence about the importance of the specific nature of cues is provided by some recent animal research (Passingham, 1985). Monkeys with lesions to prefrontal cortex were unable to learn to associate a particular colour with a particular action to obtain a food reward if the colour (cue) was spatially separated from the response handle. The same animals, however, could learn a similar task where the cue was contiguous with the handle. Similar deficits have been demonstrated when the cue occurs before rather than at the same time as the response is required (Goldman et al., 1971). Finally, there is a suggestion that the ability to utilize different types of cues may be affected by normal ageing. In the original version of the WCST (Berg, 1948), the cue to shift categories was feedback from the experimenter to the subject that the last response was wrong. Under such conditions, normal elderly subjects were found to have difficulty progressing beyond the first category and to perseverate. In an alternative version of the test (Nelson, 1976) subjects are told specifically when to shift to a new category. Canavan et al. (1984), applying this method, found normal elderly subjects to be essentially unimpaired on the task. Thus, with age, the ability to modify behaviour from information resultant on one's own actions may be compromised more than the ability to modify behaviour on external command.

It would seem from this gradual accumulation of evidence that the specific nature of the cues used to control motor and cognitive behaviour is an encouraging area for future research in Parkinson's disease.

The above discussion has been concerned with the control of behaviour. It has not been concerned with the more 'cognitive' component of conceptual ability. In the context of the tests used to assess it, this may be defined as the ability to identify alternative ways of analysing and classifying a stimulus configuration. Whether the ability to identify concepts is affected in Parkinson's disease is not clear. A decrease in the number of categories or concepts achieved in the tasks described above may be an artefact of increased errors due to set maintenance or shifting difficulty. The issue of conceptual ability separate from the regulation of behaviour has yet to be assessed.

DISCUSSION

What general conclusions can be drawn from the research considered so far? At present we would suggest:

(1) On average, groups of patients with Parkinson's disease perform less well than age-matched controls on a wide range of tests of cognitive function.
(2) A proportion of patients with Parkinson's disease will exhibit dementia, perhaps 15–20% in comparison to 5–10% of the general population of the same age.
(3) Such dementia will inevitably contribute to the impaired cognitive performance in studies with unselected clinical populations. However, even if care is taken to exclude those with dementia, it is clear that some patients with Parkinson's disease still exhibit cognitive deficits.
(4) The precise nature of these cognitive changes is still far from clear. Whether they consist of a collection of isolated deficits, in areas such as in 'memory' and 'visuospatial function', or whether a deficit in some superordinate process can be seen as responsible has yet to be determined.

Our models of memory and visuospatial function have been derived largely from neuropsychological studies on cortical dysfunction. Such is the tradition of neuropsychology, with subcortical structures being a relatively recent interest. If visuospatial function is linked traditionally with the parietal cortex, and memory function with the temporal cortex, then the cognitive functions discussed in the last section on conceptual ability and 'set' are most closely linked with the frontal cortex (Stuss and Benson, 1984). However, it is likely, with more detailed experimental analysis, that the memory impairment (and putative visuospatial impairment) seen in Parkinson's disease will be shown to differ qualitatively from that found with cortical damage. However, the parallels between the deficits resulting from lesions to the basal ganglia or the prefrontal cortex may be more than just an artefact of oversimplistic models and methods of assessment.

Anatomically, the frontal cortex is intimately linked with the basal ganglia. De Long, Georgopoulos and Crutcher (1983) describe two parallel loops connecting the two regions (see Figure 8.3). The first, the 'motor loop', runs from motor cortex to putamen, then separately to the substantia nigra and globus pallidus and thence

Figure 8.3 Schematic depiction of the suggested segregation of pathways from the 'association' (complex loop) and sensorimotor areas (motor loop) through the basal ganglia and thalamus. GP = globus pallidus; SN_{pr} = substantia nigra pars reticulata. (Reproduced with permission from De Long, Georgopoulos and Crutcher (1983))

to premotor cortex via the ventrolateral nuclei of the thalamus. The second 'complex loop' runs from prefrontal cortex to the caudate, and then in parallel but separate from the motor loop, via the globus pallidus and substantia nigra to the thalamus, this time via the ventrodorsal nuclei, and thence back to the prefrontal cortex. In addition, a third loop connects the basal ganglia and limbic system. This runs from the ventral tegmental area and limbic cortex to the ventral striatum (accumbens), then to the ventral pallidum and thence to the limbic cortex via the mediodorsal nucleus of the thalamus.

It is with the 'complex loop' that recent theorizing on the cognitive role of the striatum has been focused. The fibres from cortex to caudate are topographically mapped (Goldman and Nauta, 1977). Animal lesion experiments have revealed that the same behavioural effects can be produced by either a lesion to the prefrontal cortex, or to the area of the caudate onto which it projects (Rosvold and Szwarcbart, 1964; Divac, 1971; Oberg and Divac, 1975). This functional homogeneity suggests that the two areas may be best thought of as a functional system. Indeed, as described above, the link is in the form of a loop, with the output from the caudate being directed eventually back to the prefrontal cortex. The nature of the innervation from substantia nigra to cortex is also dopaminergic (Berger et al., 1976; Bjorklund, Divac and Lindvall, 1978). Dopamine levels in this mesocortical system are known to be affected in Parkinson's disease (Javoy Agid et al., 1981), which lends further weight to the hypothesis that a crucial impairment in Parkinson's disease may lie in the functional status of the 'complex' frontostriatal system. The functional significance of this dopaminergic loss has yet to be evaluated. Further research is needed to investigate how much of the widespread cognitive change seen in Parkinson's disease can be explained in terms of disturbance in this functional system. However, in addition to the research reviewed above, further parallels can already be found between the neuropsychological impairments of patients with Parkinson's disease and those with damage to frontal cortex.

The studies of Bowen et al. (Bowen, Hoehn and Yahr, 1972; Bowen et al., 1976) have already been mentioned, in which patients' performance on two tasks of left–right orientation seemed to be characterized by difficulty in switching from one orientation to another. The deficit in setting visual and postural vertical (Proctor et al., 1964; Danta and Hilton, 1975) is also shown by patients with frontal cortical lesions (Teuber and Mishkin, 1954). A large number of other behavioural deficits, described in studies on patients with Parkinson's disease, have also been known to be associated with lesions to the prefrontal cortex. These include: delayed matching-to-sample (De Lancey Horne, 1971), increased sensitivity to proactive interference in short-term memory tasks (Tweedy, Langer and McDowell, 1982), increased spontaneous Necker Cube alternations and decreased ability to 'freeze' the cube (Talland, 1962), impaired performance in carrying out simultaneous motor acts (Talland and Schwab, 1964; De Lancey Horne, 1973), anomia (Matison et al., 1982), impaired prism adaptation (Canavan et al., 1984), impaired performance on conditional learning tasks (Canavan et al., 1984), impaired ability to reproduce a sequence of gestures (Morel-Maroger, 1977) and difficulty in responding to a gesture with a predetermined different gesture (Morel-Maroger, 1977; Flowers, 1982). One of the few omissions to this list is the lack of a consistent deficit on verbal fluency tasks. Lees and Smith (1983) also failed to find a deficit on the cognitive estimates test (Shallice, 1982) although there are doubts about the test's reliability as an indicator of frontal lobe damage (Shallice, 1982).

CONCLUSION

Is there any final conclusion which may be drawn from consideration of the diverse body of data considered in this chapter? If there is any conclusion, it is that we are only slowly approaching the stage where we are asking the right questions to guide research. First, it is not logical to think of the striatum as being either cognitive or motor. It may be both, and the functions may be separate as suggested by the anatomical evidence, or parallel as implied by some of the behavioural work. Second, whatever the function of the basal ganglia in cognition, it is probably misleading to use models derived from studies of cortical lesions. Instead it is likely that more superordinate functions are involved with diverse effects on behaviour, both motor and cognitive. It is hoped in this way, through the study of Parkinson's disease and related diseases, that a more integrated understanding may be achieved of the complex functioning of the brain.

References

ALBERT, M. L. (1978) Subcortical dementia. In *Alzheimer's Disease: Senile Dementia and Related Disorders. Aging*, Vol. 7. Ed. by R. Katzman, R. D. Terry and K. L. Bick, pp. 173–180. New York: Raven Press

ALMGREN, P.-E., ANDERSSON, A. L. and KULLBERG, G. (1969) Differences in verbally expressed cognition following left and right ventrolateral thalamotomy. *Scandinavian Journal of Psychology*, **10**, 243–249

AMERICAN PSYCHIATRIC ASSOCIATION (1980) *Diagnostic and Statistical Manual of Mental Disorders*, 3rd edn. Washington DC: American Psychiatric Association

ANTHONY, J. C., LE RESCHE, L., NIAZ, U., VONKORFF, M. R. and FOLSTEIN, M. F. (1982) Limits of the 'mini mental state' as a screening test for dementia and delerium among hospital patients. *Psychological Medicine*, **12**, 397–408

ASSO, D. (1969) WAIS scores in a group of parkinson patients. *British Journal of Psychiatry*, **115**, 555–556

ASSO, D., CROWN, S., RUSSELL, J. A. and LOGUE, V. (1969) Psychological aspects of the stereotactic treatment of parkinsonism. *British Journal of Psychiatry*, **115**, 541–553

ATKINSON, R. C. and SHIFFRIN, R. M. (1968) Human memory: a proposed system and its control processes. In *The Psychology of Learning and Motivation*, Vol. 2. Ed. by K. W. Spence and J. T. Spence. New York: Academic Press

BADDELEY, A. D. (1982) Implications of neurpsychological evidence for theories of normal memory. *Philosophical Transactions of the Royal Society of London, Series B*, **298**, 59–72

BADDELEY, A. D. and HITCH, G. J. (1974) Working memory. In *The Psychology of Learning and Motivation*, Vol. 8. Ed. by G. A. Bower. New York: Academic Press

BEARDSLEY, J. V. and PULETTI, F. (1971) Personality (MMPI) and cognitive (WAIS) changes after levodopa treatment. Occurrence in patients with Parkinson's disease. *Archives of Neurology*, **25**, 145–150

BENNETT-LEVY, J. and POWELL, G. E. (1980) The subjective memory questionnaire (SMQ). An investigation into the self-reporting of 'real-life' memory skills. *British Journal of Social and Clinical Psychology*, **19**, 177–188

BENSON, D. F. (1984) Parkinsonian dementia: cortical or subcortical? In *Parkinson-specific Motor and Mental Disorders. Role of the Pallidum: Pathophysiological, Biochemical and Therapeutic Aspects. Advances in Neurology*, Vol. 40. Ed. by R. G. Hassler and J. F. Christ, pp. 235–240. New York: Raven Press

BENTIN, S., SILVERBERG, R. and GORDON, H. W. (1981) Asymmetrical cognitive deterioration in demented and parkinson patients. *Cortex*, **17**, 533–544

BERG, E. A. (1948) A simple objective technique for measuring flexibility in thinking. *Journal of General Psychology*, **39**, 15–22

BERGER, B., THIERRY, A. M., TASSIN, J. P. and MOYNE, M. A. (1976) Dopaminergic innervation of the rat prefrontal cortex: a fluorescence histochemical study. *Brain Research*, **106**, 133–145

BJORKLUND, A., DIVAC, I. and LINDVALL, D. (1978) Regional distribution of catecholamines in monkey cerebral cortex, evidence for a dopaminergic innervation of the primate prefrontal cortex. *Neuroscience Letters*, **7**, 115–119

BOLLER, F., PASSAFIUME, D., KEEFE, N. C., ROGERS, K. and KIM, Y. (1984) Visuospatial impairment in Parkinson's disease. *Archives of Neurology*, **41**, 485–490

BOWEN, F. P., BURNS, M. M., BRADY, E. M. and YAHR, M. D. (1976) A note on alterations of personal orientation in parkinsonism. *Neuropsychologia*, **14**, 425–429

BOWEN, F. P., BURNS, M. M. and YAHR, M. D. (1976) Alterations in memory processes subsequent to short- and long-term treatment with L-dopa. In *Advances in Parkinsonism*. Ed. by W. Birkmeyer and O. Hornykiewicz, pp. 488–491. Geneva, Roche

BOWEN, F. P., HOEHN, M. M. and YAHR, M. D. (1972) Parkinsonism: alterations in spatial orientation as determined by a route walking test. *Neuropsychologia*, **10**, 355–361

BOWEN, F. P., KAMIENNY, R. S., BURNS, M. M. and YAHR, M. D. (1975) Parkinsonism: effects of levodopa on concept formation. *Neurology*, **25**, 701–704

BROWN, R. G. and MARSDEN, C. D. (1984) How common is dementia in Parkinson's disease? *Lancet*, **ii**, 1262–1265

BROWN, R. G. and MARSDEN, C. D. (1985) Visuospatial function in Parkinson's disease. Paper presented at the European Neuroscience Association meeting on Clinical Neuropsychology, Zurich, Switzerland, 1985

CANAVAN, A. G. M., PASSINGHAM, R. E., MARSDEN, C. D., POLKEY, C. E., QUINN, N. and WYKE, M. (1984) Cognitive deficits in patients with Parkinson's disease. Poster presented at the European Training Programme Winter School on New Developments in the Investigation of the Human Brain, Zuoz, Switzerland

CHRISTENSEN, A. L., JUUL-JENSEN, P., MALMROS, R. and HARMSEN, A. (1970) Psychological evaluation of intelligence and personality in parkinsonism before and after stereotaxic surgery. *Acta Neurologica Scandinavica*, **46**, 527–537

COOLS, A. R., VAN DEN BERCKEN, J. H. L., HORSTINK, M. W. I., VAN SPAENDONCK, K. P. M. and BERGER, H. J. C. (1984) Cognitive and motor shifting aptitude disorder in Parkinson's disease. *Journal of Neurology, Neurosurgery and Psychiatry*, **47**, 443–453

CUMMINGS, J. L. and BENSON, D. F. (1983) *Dementia: a Clinical Approach*. Boston: Butterworths

DANTA, G. and HILTON, R. C. (1975) Judgement of the visual vertical and horizontal in patients with parkinsonism. *Neurology*, **25**, 43–47

DE LANCEY HORNE, D. J. (1971) Performance on delayed response tasks by patients with parkinsonism. *Journal of Neurology, Neurosurgery and Psychiatry*, **34**, 192–194

DE LANCEY HORNE, D. J. (1973) Sensorimotor control in parkinsonism. *Journal of Neurology, Neurosurgery and Psychiatry*, **36**, 742–746

DELLA SALA, S., DI LORENZO, G., GIORDANA, A. and SPINNLER, H. (1985) 'Directional forecast': a specific visuo-spatial impairment of parkinsonians? Paper presented at the joint meeting of the Polish and Italian Societies of Neurology, Rome, Italy

DE LONG, M. R., GEORGOPOULOS, A. P. and CRUTCHER, M. D. (1983) Cortico-basal ganglia relations and coding of motor performance. *Experimental Brain Research*, Supplement 7, 30–40

DE SMET, Y., RUBERG, M., SERDARU, M., DUBOIS, B., LHERMITTE, F. and AGID, Y. (1982) Confusion, dementia and anticholinergics in Parkinson's disease. *Journal of Neurology, Neurosurgery and Psychiatry*, **45**, 1161–1164

DICK, J. P. R., GUILOFF, R. J., STEWART, A., BLACKSTOCK, J., BIELAWSKA, C., PAUL, A. E. and MARSDEN, C. D. (1984) Mini-mental state examination in neurological patients. *Journal of Neurology, Neurosurgery and Psychiatry*, **47**, 496–499

DINNERSTEIN, A. J., LOWENTHAL, M., BLAKE, G. and MALLIN, R. E. (1964) Tactile delay in parkinsonism. *Journal of Nervous and Mental Disorders*, **139**, 521–524

DIVAC, I. (1971) Frontal lobe system and spatial reversal in the rat. *Neuropsychologia*, **9**, 175–183

DIVAC, I. and OBERG, R. G. E. (Eds) (1979) *The Neostriatum*. Oxford: Pergamon

DRACHMAN, D. A. and ARBIT, J. (1966) Memory and the hippocampal complex. *Archives of Neurology*, **15**, 52–61

FISCHER, K. and FINDLEY, L. (1981) Intellectual changes in optimally treated patients with Parkinson's disease. In *Research Progress in Parkinson's Disease*. Ed. by F. C. Rose and R. Capildeo. pp. 43–52. London: Pitman Medical Press

FLOWERS, K. A. (1982) Frontal lobe signs as a component of parkinsonism. *Behavioural and Brain Research*, **5**, 100

FLOWERS, K. A., PEARCE, I. and PEARCE, J. M. S. (1984) Recognition memory in Parkinson's disease. *Journal of Neurology, Neurosurgery and Psychiatry*, **47**, 1174–1181

FLOWERS, K. A. and ROBERTSON, C. (1985) The effects of Parkinson's disease on the ability to maintain a mental set. *Journal of Neurology, Neurosurgery and Psychiatry*, **48**, 517–529

GAINOTTI, G., CALTAGIRONE, C., MASULLO, C. and MICELL, G. (1980) Patterns of neuropsychological impairment in various diagnostic groups of dementia. In *Aging of the Brain and Dementia. Aging*, Vol. 13. Ed. by L. Amaducci, A. N. Davison and P. Antuono. pp. 245–250. New York: Raven Press

GARRON, D. C., KLAWANS, H. L. and NARIN, F. (1972) Intellectual functioning in persons with idiopathic parkinsonism. *Journal of Nervous and Mental Diseases*, **154**, 445–452

GOLDMAN, P. S. and NAUTA, W. J. H. (1977) An intricately patterned prefronto-caudate projection in the rhesus monkey. *Journal of Comparative Neurology*, **171**, 369–386

GOLDMAN, P. S., ROSVOLD, H. E., VEST, B. and GALLCIN, T. W. (1971) Analysis of the delayed-automation deficit produced by dorsolateral prefrontal lesions in the rhesus monkey. *Journal of Comparative Physiology and Psychology*, **73**, 212–220

HALGIN, R., RIKLAN, M. and MISIAK, H. (1977) Levodopa, parkinsonism and recent memory. *Journal of Nervous and Mental Diseases*, **164**, 268–272

HALSTEAD, W. C. (1947) *Brain and Intelligence: a Quantitative Study of the Frontal Lobes*. Chicago: University of Chicago Press

HAMEL, A. R. and RIKLAN, M. (1975) Cognitive and perceptual effects of long-range L-dopa therapy in parkinsonism. *Journal of Clinical Psychology*, **31**, 321–323

HASHER, L. and ZACKS, R. T. (1979) Automatic and effortful processes in memory. *Journal of Experimental Psychology*, **108**, 356–388

HORN, S. (1974) Some psychological factors in parkinsonism. *Journal of Neurology, Neurosurgery and Psychiatry*, **37**, 27–31

JAVOY-AGID, F., TAQUET, H., PLOSKA, A., CHERIF-ZAHAR, C., RUBERG, M. and AGID, Y. (1981) Distribution of catecholamines in the ventral mesencephalon of human brain, with special reference to Parkinson's disease. *Journal of Neurochemistry*, **36**, 2101–2105

KOLLER, W. C. (1984) Disturbance of recent memory function in parkinsonian patients on anticholinergic therapy. *Cortex*, **20**, 307–311

LEES, A. R. and SMITH, E. (1983) Cognitive deficits in the early stages of Parkinson's disease. *Brain*, **106**, 257–270

LEVITA, E. and RIKLAN, M. (1967) Patterns of psychological function before, after unilateral, and after bilateral thalamic surgery. *Perceptual and Motor Skills*, **24**, 619–626

LORANGER, A. W., GOODELL, H., McDOWELL, F. H., LEE, J. E. and SWEET, R. D. (1972) Intellectual impairment in Parkinson's syndrome. *Brain*, **95**, 405–412

LORANGER, A. W., GOODELL, H., McDOWELL, F. H., LEE, J. E. and SWEET, R. D. (1973) Parkinsonism, L-dopa and intelligence. *American Journal of Psychiatry*, **130**, 1386–1389

McFIE, J. (1960) Psychological effects of stereotaxic operations for the relief of parkinsonian symptoms. *Journal of Mental Science*, **106**, 1512–1517

MARSDEN, C. D. (1982) The mysterious motor function of the basal ganglia: the Robert Wartenberg lecture. *Neurology*, **32**, 514–539

MATISON, R., MAYEUX, R., ROSEN, J. and FAHN, S. (1982) 'Tip-of-the-tongue' phenomenon in Parkinson's disease. *Neurology*, **32**, 567–570

MATTHEWS, C. G. and YORK-HAALAND, K. Y. (1979) The effect of symptom duration on cognitive and motor performance in parkinsonism. *Neurology*, **29**, 951–956

MAYEUX, R., STERN, Y., ROSEN, J. and BENSON, D. F. (1983) Is 'subcortical dementia' a recognizable clinical entity? *Annals of Neurology*, **14**, 278–283

MEIER, M. J. and MARTIN, W. E. (1970) Intellectual changes associated with levodopa therapy. *Journal of the American Medical Association*, **213**, 465–466

MILNER, B. (1963) Effects of different brain lesions on card sorting: the role of the frontal lobes. *Archives of Neurology*, **9**, 90–100

MOREL-MAROGER, A. (1977) Effects of levodopa on 'frontal' signs in parkinsonism. *British Medical Journal*, **2**, 1543–1544

MORRIS, R. G. (1984) Dementia and the function of the articulatory loop system. *Cognitive Neuropsychology*, **1**, 143–157

MORTIMER, J. A., CHRISTENSEN, M. A., KUSKOWSKI, P., EISENBERG, P. and WEBSTER, D. D. (1982) The visuospatial disorder of Parkinson's disease. Paper presented at the meeting of the International Neuropsychological Society. Deauville, France

NELSON, H. E. (1976) A modified card sorting test sensitive to frontal lobe defects. *Cortex*, **12**, 313–324

NEWMAN, R. P., WEINGARTNER, H., SMALLBERG, S. A. and CALNE, D. B. (1984) Effortful and automatic memory: effects of dopamine. *Neurology*, **34**, 805–807

OBERG, R. G. E. and DIVAC, I. (1975) Dissociative effects of selective lesions in the caudate nucleus of cats and rats. *Acta Neurobiologica Experimentia*, **35**, 675–689

PARKES, J. D. (1981) Adverse effects of antiparkinsonian drugs. *Drugs*, **21**, 341–352

PASSINGHAM, R. E. (1985) Cortical mechanisms and cues for action. *Philosophical Transactions of the Royal Society of London, Series B*, **308**, 101–111

PERRET, E. and SIEGFRIED, J. (1969) Memory and learning performance of parkinsonian patients before and after thalamotomy. In *Proceedings from the Third Symposium on Parkinson's Disease*. Ed. by F. J. Gillingham and I. M. L. Donaldson. pp. 164–168. Edinburgh: Livingstone

PIROZZOLO, F. J., HANSCH, E. C., MORTIMER, J. A., WEBSTER, D. D. and KUSKOWSKI, M. A. (1982) Dementia in Parkinson's disease: a neuropsychological analysis. *Brain and Cognition*, **1**, 71–83

PORTIN, R., RAININKO, R. and RINNE, U. K. (1984) Neuropsychological disturbance and central atrophy determined by computerized tomography in parkinsonian patients with long-term levodopa treatment. In *Parkinson-specific Motor and Mental Disorders. Role of the Pallidum: Pathophysiological, Biochemical and Therapeutic Aspects. Advances in Neurology*, Vol. 40. Ed. by R. G. Hassler and J. F. Christ. pp. 219–229. New York: Raven Press

PORTIN, R. and RINNE, U. K. (1980) Neuropsychological responses of parkinsonian patients to long-term levodopa therapy. In *Parkinson's Disease: Current Progress, Problems and Management*. Ed. by M. Klinger and G. Stamm. pp. 271–304. Amsterdam: Elsevier/North Holland

PROCTOR, F., RIKLAN, M., COOPER, I. S. and TEUBER, H.-L. (1964) Judgement of visual and postural vertical by parkinsonian patients. *Neurology (Minneapolis)*, **14**, 287–293

RABBITT, P. (1981) Cognitive psychology needs models for changes in performance with old age. In *Attention and Performance IX*. Ed. by J. B. Long and A. D. Baddeley. Hillsdale, NJ: Lawrence Erlbaum Associates

REITAN, R. M. and BOLL, T. J. (1971) Intellectual and cognitive functions in Parkinson's disease. *Journal of Consulting and Clinical Psychology*, **37**, 364–369

RIKLAN, M. (1972) Levodopa and behaviour. *Neurology* (Supplement), **22**, 43–54

RIKLAN, M., DILLER, L., WEINER, H. and COOPER, I. S. (1960) Psychological studies on effects of chemosurgery of the basal ganglia in parkinsonism. I. Intellectual functioning. *Archives of General Psychiatry*, **2**, 22–32

RIKLAN, M., HALGIN, R., MASKIN, M. and WEISSMAN, D. (1973) Psychological studies of longer range L-dopa therapy in parkinsonism. *Journal of Nervous and Mental Disorders*, **157**, 452–464

RIKLAN, M., LEVITA, E. and COOPER, I. S. (1966) Psychological effects of bilateral subcortical surgery for Parkinson's disease. *Journal of Nervous and Mental Diseases*, **141**, 403–409

RIKLAN, M., WHELIHAN, W. and CULLINAN, T. (1976) Levodopa and psychometric test performance in parkinsonism – 5 years later. *Neurology*, **26**, 173–179

ROSVOLD, H. E. and SZWARCBART, M. K. (1964) Neural structures involved in delayed response performance. In *The Frontal Granular Cortex and Behaviour*. Ed. by J. M. Warren and K. Akbert, pp. 1–15. New York: McGraw-Hill

SEMMES, J., WEINSTEIN, S., GHENT, L. and TEUBER, H.-L. (1963) Correlates of impaired orientation in personal and extrapersonal space. *Brain*, **86**, 747–772

SHALLICE, T. (1982) Specific impairments in planning. *Philosophical Transactions of the Royal Society of London, Series B*, **298**, 199–209

SHALLICE, T. and EVANS, M. E. (1978) The involvement of the frontal lobes in cognitive estimation. *Cortex*, **14**, 294–303

SHALLICE, T. and WARRINGTON, E. (1970) Independent function of verbal memory stores, a neuropsychological study. *Quarterly Journal of Experimental Psychology*, **22**, 261–273

SHAPIRO, M. B. (1973) Intensive assessment of the single case: and inductive–deductive approach. In *The Psychological Assessment of Physical and Mental Handicap*. Ed. by P. E. Mittler, pp. 645–666. London: Methuen

STERN, Y., MAYEUX, R., ROSEN, J. and ILSON, J. (1983) Perceptual motor dysfunction in Parkinson's disease: A deficit in sequential and predictive voluntary movement. *Journal of Neurology, Neurosurgery and Psychiatry*, **46**, 145–151

STUSS, D. T. and BENSON, D. F. (1984) Neuropsychological studies of the frontal lobes. *Psychological Bulletin*, **95**, 3–28

TALLAND, G. A. (1962) Cognitive function in Parkinson's disease. *Journal of Nervous and Mental Disorders*, **135**, 196–205

TALLAND, G. A. and SCHWAB, R. S. (1964) Performance with multiple sets in Parkinson's disease. *Neuropsychologia*, **2**, 45–53

TEUBER, H.-L. and MISHKIN, M. (1954) Judgement of the visual and postural vertical after brain injury. *Journal of Psychology*, **38**, 161–175

TWEEDY, J. R., LANGER, K. G. and McDOWELL, F. H. (1982) The effects of semantic relations on the memory deficit associated with Parkinson's disease. *Journal of Clinical Neuropsychology*, **4**, 235–247

VALLAR, G. and BADDELEY, A. D. (1984) Fractionation of working memory: neuropsychological evidence for a phonological short-term store. *Journal of Verbal Learning and Verbal Behaviour*, **23**, 151–162

VILLARDITA, C., SMIRNI, P., LE PIRA, F., ZAPPALA, G. and NICOLETTI, F. (1982) Mental deterioration, visuoperceptive disabilities and constructional apraxia in Parkinson's disease. *Acta Neurologica Scandinavica*, **66**, 112–120

WARBURTON, J. W. (1967) Memory disturbance and the Parkinson syndrome. *British Journal of Medical Psychology*, **40**, 169–171

WECHSLER, D. (1944) *The Measurement of Adult Intelligence*, 3rd edn. Baltimore: Williams and Wilkins
WECHSLER, D. (1955) *The Wechsler Adult Intelligence Scale (Manual)*. New York, Psychological Corporation
WEINGARTNER, H., BURNS, S., DIEBEL, R. and LE WITT, P. A. (1984) Cognitive impairment in Parkinson's disease: distinguishing between effort-demanding and automatic cognitive processes. *Psychiatry Research*, **11,** 223-235
WEINSTEIN, S. (1964) Deficits concomitant with aphasia or lesions of either cerebral hemisphere. *Cortex*, **1,** 151-159
WELFORD, A. T. (1980) Memory and age: a perspective view. In *New Directions in Memory and Aging*. Ed. by J. L. Poon, L. S. Fozad, D. Cermak, D. Arenberg and L. W. Thompson. pp. 1-14. Hillsdale, NJ: Lawrence Erlbaum
WILSON, B. A. and MOFFAT, N. (EDS) (1984) *Clinical Management of Memory Problems*. London: Croon Helm
ZANGWILL, O. L. (1946) Some qualitative observations on verbal memory in cases of cerebral lesions. *British Journal of Psychology*, **37,** 8-19

9
The pathology of parkinsonism
K. Jellinger

Parkinsonism occurs in a variety of disorders of the central nervous system (CNS) affecting basically the pigmented neuronal systems of the brainstem, often as part of a more widespread process. The predominant damage to the dopaminergic nigrostriatal pathway due to lesions in the zona compacta of substantia nigra, known since Tretiakoff (1919) as the major site of pathological changes in Parkinson's disease, is frequently associated with:

(a) Non-specific degenerative or age-related changes in other parts of the brain.
(b) Variable non-specific neuronal changes including Lewy bodies (Lewy, 1913) and various types of neurofibrillary degeneration.
(c) A variety of other and/or coincidental lesions elsewhere in the CNS.

Since Foix and Nicolesco (1925) reported on the major pathological findings in Parkinson's disease, many morbid anatomy studies of this disorder have been published (Hassler, 1938; Klaue, 1940; Greenfield and Bosanquet, 1953; Hallervorden, 1957; Forno, 1966, 1982; Richardson, 1965; Earle, 1968; Forno and Alvord, 1971; Lewis, 1971; Escourolle, Recondo and Gray, 1971; Alvord et al., 1974; Jellinger, 1974, 1986; Pearce, 1979; Jacob, 1978, 1983; Blackwood, 1981). The present overview will outline:

(a) The morbid anatomy of the different entities of parkinsonism.
(b) The major morphological basis of neurotransmitter changes in parkinsonism.
(c) Some anatomical correlates of dementia in Parkinson's disease.

MAJOR TYPES OF PARKINSONISM

In a large autopsy series including personal material of over 500 cases, degenerative forms of parkinsonism account for 75–90%, including idiopathic parkinsonism, or Parkinson's disease ranging from 60 to 75% and other multisystem degenerations (about 15%). About 5–8% are associated with cerebrovascular disease, while the incidence of post-encephalitic parkinsonism is decreasing (13% before 1970, and 3% in a recent series) (Jellinger, 1986). Confirmed cases of parkinsonism due to trauma, tumours, intoxications and drugs are rare, some of the latter presenting morphological changes characteristic of Parkinson's disease (Rajput *et al.*, 1982). A small number of cases remain unclassified. A survey of the different entities of parkinsonism, their average incidence and the major type and distribution of brain lesions is given in *Table 9.1*.

Parkinson's disease

Parkinson's disease (idiopathic parkinsonism), encompassing 66–85% of all pathologically confirmed parkinsonism cases, is characterized by variable unilateral, or more often symmetrical, focal loss of melanin-containing neurones mainly involving the central and caudal parts of the zona compacta of substantia nigra associated with slight to moderate gliosis, and neuronal loss in the locus ceruleus and dorsal vagal nucleus with variable involvement of the nucleus basalis of Meynert and other subcortical nuclei. In 82–100% of cases, Lewy bodies are seen in many aminergic and other subcortical nuclei, spinal cord, sympathetic ganglia and, occasionally, in cerebral cortex (*Table 9.2*). These intracytoplasmic inclusions are composed of proteins, free fatty acids, sphingomyelin, and polysaccharides (Hartog-Jager, 1969). Electron probe microanalysis has demonstrated a high sulphur content, indicating products of degenerated proteins (Kimula

Figure 9.1 Lewy body in substantia nigra (inset). Ultrastructure of 'brainstem type' with both granular and filamentous materials, densely packed in a central core. N = nucleus. × 5120

Table 9.1 Classification, incidence and histopathology of different types of parkinsonism

Disease entity	Incidence (%)		Age of onset (years)	Duration (years)	Neurological findings				
	Literature* (mean)	Jellinger, 1985 (520 cases)			Substantia nigra	LB (%)	NFT (%)	Brainstem	Extranigral lesions / Other CNS regions
Parkinson's disease (idiopathic parkinsonism)	44–94 (76)	67.4	50–69	9–12	Focal damage neurone + melanin loss, gliosis	99	10	Neurone loss, gliosis: L.cer. dorsal vagus n., n.basalis, n.dorsalis raphe	Non-specific or age-related
Other degenerative parkinsonism	0–30 (6)	15.0							
'Senile' parkinsonism	?	6.0	~80	2–3	Mild neurone + melanin loss	40	40	Neurone loss l.cer. NFT + SP brainstem	Severe senile lesions–SDAT
Diffuse Lewy body disease	?	0.5	38–75	4–13	Focal neurone + melanin loss + gliosis	100	80	Widespread LB + neurone loss	Widespread LB and frequent NFT + SP
Striatonigral degeneration	?	3.0	45–60	2–7	Focal neurone loss + gliosis	90	0	Multiple system degenerations, no NFT	Atrophy + hyperpigmentation putamen, OPCA
Multisystem atrophies	?	2.3	40–50	Many	Focal or diffuse neurone loss	Frequent	Rare	Olivopontocerebellar, spinocerebellar degeneration	Motor neurone disease Joseph disease
Progressive supranuclear palsy	?	1.8	20–60	4–20	Diffuse neurone loss + gliosis	0	100	Systemic neurone loss + gliosis + straight NFT	Little or no cortical lesions

Condition	Age range	%	Age	N	Gross lesions	%	%	Microscopic lesions	Other features
Parkinson–dementia complex	? (Guam, Europe)	0.6	40–50	4	Neuronal loss + gliosis	0	90	Neurone loss + gliosis + NFT tegmentum + n. basalis Meynert	NFT hippocampus, thalamus, pallidum
Post-encephalitic parkinsonism	4–35 (13)	4.8	30–40	25	Severe diffuse neurone loss + depigmentation gliosis	0	95	Neurone loss + NFT upper brainstem	NFT hippocampus, hypothalamus No senile plaques
Vascular parkinsonism	0–15 (2)	7.5	70–80	3–4	Vascular lesions Lacunar state	10	6	Vascular lesions Lacunar state basal ganglia	Multi-infarct encephalopathy
Post-traumatic parkinsonism	0–1 (0.2)	0.6	Any	Many	Traumatic or vascular focal necroses	0	0	Primary or secondary traumatic lesions in brainstem and/or basal ganglia	
Dementia pugilistica	?	0	40–60	Many	Neurone loss + NFT	0	100	Multiple NFT brainstem	Multiple NFT No senile plaques
Toxic and CO, CS, MPTP, drugs, manganese	?	0.9	Any	Many	Diffuse or focal damage, gliosis	0	0	Damage gl.pallidum Non-specific lesions	Non-specific Caudate nucleus (neuroleptic-induced parkinsonism)
Symptomatic parkinsonism	?	2.7	Any	Many	Local damage	Rare	0	Various lesions: tumours, multiple sclerosis, Alzheimer's disease, Hallervorden–Spatz disease, neurolipidoses, SSPE, Creutzfeldt–Jakob disease etc.	
Unclassified	0–19 (2.6)	1.9	Any	Many	Focal damage	Occasional	?	Various non-specific lesions	

* Hassler (1938); Klaue (1940); Beheim-Schwarzbach (1952); Greenfield and Bosanquet (1953); Hallervorden (1957); Forno (1966); Richardson (1965); Stadlan, Duvoisin and Fahr, (1966); Earle (1968); Escourolle, Recondo and Gray (1971); Yahr et al. (1971); Forno and Alvord (1971); Alvord et al., (1974); Jacob (1978, 1983).

LB = Lewy bodies; NFT = neurofibrillary tangles; OPCA = olivopontocerebellar atrophy; SDAT = senile dementia of Alzheimer type; SP = senile plaques; SSPE = subacute sclerosing panencephalitis; ST = straight filament tangles.

Table 9.2 Distribution of Lewy bodies in Parkinson's disease

Affected region	Frequent	Rare
Cerebral cortex		X
Substantia innominata	XX	
Hypothalamus, lateral, posterior	X	
Subthalamic nucleus		X
Peri-aqueductal gray		X
Substantia nigra	XX	
Nucleus parabrachialis pigmentosus	XX	
Nucleus paranigralis	XX	
Nucleus of Westphal–Edinger	X	
Nucleus of Darkschewitsch		X
Supratrochlear nucleus		X
Nucleus tegmenti pedunculopontinus	X	
Central pontine gray		X
Locus ceruleus	XX	
Nucleus subceruleus	X	
Nucleus pontis centralis oralis	X	
Central superior nucleus of raphe		X
Processus griseum pontis supralemnisc.	X	
Dorsal motor nucleus of vagus	XX	
Nucleus of Roller		X
Nucleus gigantocellularis		X
Nucleus paragigantocellularis lateralis		X
Nucleus medullae oblongongatae centralis		X
Spinal cord, intermediolateral column		X
Spinal cord, anterior horn		X
Autonomic ganglia	XX	

See Hartog-Jager and Bethlem (1960); Ishii (1966); Ohama and Ikuta (1976); Hunter (1985); Jellinger (1986).

et al., 1983). Ultrastructurally two types have been distinguished. The 'brainstem type' of Lewy bodies (*Figure 9.1*) consists of granular and filamentous materials densely packed in a central core surrounded by radially arranged fragmentary filaments of 7–8 nm (Duffy and Tennyson, 1965; Forno, 1969; Roy and Wolman, 1969). The 'cortex type' (*Figure 9.2*) is rather homogeneous without a marked dense central core and random arrangement of the filaments in the outer zone (Ikeda *et al.,* 1978; Kosaka, 1978; Kosaka *et al.*, 1984). Lewy bodies are similar to other hyaline cytoplasmic inclusions (Roy and Wolman, 1969) and to intracytoplasmic acidophilic granules in nigral neurones composed of aggregates of parallel beaded or twisted 9.5-nm filaments (Schochet, Wyatt and McDormick, 1970). They show positive immunoreaction with human neurofilament protein antibodies (Forno, Sternberger and Eng, 1983; Goldman *et al.*, 1983; Nakazato *et al.*, 1984), but not with human brain microtubule antibodies acting with both Alzheimer neurofibrillary tangles and straight filament tangles (Yen, Horoupian and Terry, 1983). Despite their different ultrastructure (Tellez-Nagel and Wisniewski, 1973; Wisniewski and Wen, 1985), these tangles are made up of proteins and polypeptides which apparently share some antigenic determinants among each

Figure 9.2 Lewy bodies in cerebral cortex (inset, H.E. × 680). Ultrastructure of 'cortical type' showing no marked density of filamentous materials. × 20 250

other and the neurofilaments, suggesting some common disorganization of neurofibrillary protein metabolism (Wisniewski and Merz, 1985). Monoclonal antibodies against Lewy bodies were raised in parkinsonian brains (Hirsch, 1985), but their metabolic background is unknown. Lewy bodies frequently affect aminergic neurones (Ohama and Ikuta, 1976), and in the cerebral cortex show a distribution partly corresponding to that of dopaminergic axon terminals (Yoshimura, 1983). However, they appear not to represent a degeneration product specific for aminergic neuronal systems. They occur in about 5% of normal controls over age 65, in 10–23% of all cases of Alzheimer's disease–senile dementia of Alzheimer type (Beheim-Schwarzbach, 1952; Forno, 1969; Jellinger, 1986) and in other CNS disorders (ataxia-telangiectasia, Hallervorden–Spatz disease, chronic panencephalitis etc.). They are not pathognomonic for Parkinson's disease, but are considered probably to be more characteristic for this disease than the Alzheimer's neurofibrillary tangles for Alzheimer's disease–senile dementia of Alzheimer type (Forno, 1982). Alzheimer's neurofibrillary tangles in the brainstem, being a major finding in post-encephalitic parkinsonism and frequently occurring in Alzheimer's disease–senile dementia of Alzheimer type, are rarely seen in typical Parkinson's disease, but may occur in Parkinson's disease cases of advanced age or combined with Alzheimer's disease–senile dementia of Alzheimer type (*Table 9.3*). In addition to degenerative changes in other cortical and subcortical systems, the Parkinson's disease brain may show various age-related and/or vascular changes in other brain areas (Escourolle, Recondo and Gray, 1971; Richardson, 1965; Forno and Alvord, 1971; Jacob, 1978; Boller *et al.*, 1979; Hakim and Mathieson, 1979; Pearce, 1979). However, the incidence of coincidental cerebrovascular lesions in Parkinson's disease is about the same as in age-matched controls (*Table 9.3*).

Other degenerative types of parkinsonism

About 15% of the autopsy cases of parkinsonism are associated with multisystem degenerations, ageing disorders or other degenerative lesions exceeding the characteristic pattern of Parkinson's disease.

'Senile parkinsonism'

A small group of demented patients clinically presenting moderate parkinsonism signs (tremor, akinesia and gait disorders) with onset around the age of 80 years, short duration (average two years), and severe mental side-effects to otherwise ineffective levodopa treatment, is morphologically featured by severe cortical Alzheimer's lesions associated with mild damage to substantia nigra and locus ceruleus, and occurrence of both Lewy bodies and Alzheimer's neurofibrillary tangles in the brainstem and other subcortical areas in about 40% (*Table 9.3*). This group, accounting for almost 6% of our autopsy series of parkinsonism, shows the anatomical features of both senile dementia of Alzheimer type and of mild Parkinson's disease and, therefore, has been tentatively referred to as 'senile' parkinsonism (Jellinger, Grisold and Vollmer, 1983; Jellinger and Riederer, 1984). Whether it represents a distinct subset of Parkinson's disease population with less advanced nigral damage in old age, or a variant of senile dementia of Alzheimer type with mild, but clinically relevant, degenerative lesions of the pigmented brainstem nuclei, remains to be elucidated. It should be emphasized, however, that mild to moderate damage to substantia nigra is seen in 50–75% of the cases of Alzheimer's disease and senile dementia of Alzheimer type, where the loss of nigral neurones ranges from 8.4 to 23.8% (Mann, Yates and Hawkes, 1983) to 47% (Tabaton *et al.*, 1985), and is associated with Lewy bodies in the substantia nigra in 14–25% and in the locus ceruleus in 24–44%, respectively (*Table 9.3*). Based on morphology findings a distinction between Parkinson's disease with severe Alzheimer's pathology and of Alzheimer's disease–senile dementia of Alzheimer type with considerable involvement of the pigmented brainstem nuclei, appears impossible, and true coincidence of combination of both disorders may occur.

Diffuse Lewy body disease

Diffuse Lewy body disease is a rare disorder, clinically presenting as Parkinson's disease with or without dementia (Okazaki, Lipkin and Aronson, 1961; Forno,

Table 9.3 Brainstem lesions in parkinsonism, senile and presenile dementia, and controls

Lesion	Parkinson's disease (N = 270) (%)	Senile parkinsonism (N = 32) (%)	Vascular parkinsonism (N = 32) (%)	Postenceph. parkinsonism (N = 18) (%)	SDAT (N = 216) (%)	Alzheimer's disease (N = 92) (%)	Controls (N = 261) (%)
S. nigra							
Neuronal 3+	92.6	0	30.0	100.0	0	7.6	0
loss 2+	7.4	6.2	36.7	0	1.9	6.5	23.8
1+	0	93.4	33.3	0	72.2	44.6	13.4
Lewy bodies	99.3	40.6	9.3	0	25.4	14.1	4.7
Neurof. deg.	7.4	40.6	9.3	94.4	26.4	32.6	1.8
L. ceruleus							
Neurone loss	100.0	69.4	15.6	100.0	40.8	23.7	12.4
Lewy bodies	98.5	15.6	6.3	5.9	44.5	23.7	12.4
Neurof. deg.	5.8	31.2	9.3	94.4	55.0	55.0	1.8
Dors. X. nucl.							
Neurone loss	87.3	31.2	0	11.8	NE	NE	2.8
Lewy bodies	82.2	3.1	0	11.8	NE	NE	2.8
Axon. dystrophy							
Retic. nigra	78.6	87.5	70.0	87.5	62.5	52.5	27.3
Pontine SP	1.0	40.6	16.3	0	24.5	30.4	0.8
Tegmentum NFT	16.5	40.6	6.3	98.0	60.6	65.0	1.9
Lacunar state	30.0	37.5	100.0	50.0	31.0	5.6	20.4
Old infarcts	4.8	15.6	86.3	5.9	5.3	3.3	2.9
Amyloid angiopathy	2.7	12.5	0	0	66.7	67.5	0.5
Lewy bodies cortex	7.8	6.2	0	0	1.8	0.5	0

SP = senile plaques; NFT = neurofibrillary tangles; NE = not examined; SDAT = senile dementia of Alzheimer type.

Barbour and Norville, 1978; Ikeda *et al.*, 1978; Kosaka and Mehraein, 1979; Monmy *et al.*, 1979; Yoshimura, 1983), Shy–Drager syndrome (Kono, Matubara and Imagaki, 1976; Yoshimura, 1983), or as progressive dementia with or without parkinsonism (Clark and Lehman, 1983; Kosaka *et al.*, 1984). It is morphologically characterized by widespread distribution of Lewy bodies with frequent involvement of the cerebral cortex and variable degenerative changes in the brainstem, often accompanied by severe Alzheimer's lesions. The disorder has been separated into three types (Kosaka *et al.*, 1984): type A or 'diffuse type' with widespread occurrence of Lewy bodies in the brainstem, basal ganglia, and cerebral cortex, often accompanied by severe Alzheimer's lesions suggesting a combination of Lewy bodies disease with Alzheimer's disease; type B or 'transitional' type, with numerous Lewy bodies in brainstem and diencephalon, but less frequent in basal ganglia and cerebral cortex; type C or 'brainstem type' with many Lewy bodies in the brainstem, but few or none in the cerebral cortex, apparently identical with idiopathic Parkinson's disease. While types B and C clinically present as Parkinson's disease, the diffuse type A is particularly featured by progressive dementia with little parkinsonian symptoms. Lewy body disease has been considered as a clinicopathological entity (Kosaka *et al.*, 1984), but there are transitions between Parkinson's disease with cortical Lewy bodies (Ikeda *et al.*, 1978; Yoshimura, 1983) and the diffuse type, considered as a special presenile form of the disease. Accordingly, it remains unknown whether this disorder represents one end of a spectrum including idiopathic and atypical Parkinson's disease, presenile dementia or a combination of these disorders, or a single entity with various subtypes. Choline-acetyltransferase activity in the neocortex has been found to be extremely reduced (Clark and Lehman, 1983) which might correlate with most severe degeneration of the cholinergic nucleus basalis of Meynert (Jellinger, 1985).

Multisystem degenerations

Multisystem degenerations include a variety of disorders often associated with parkinsonism and involvement of pigmented brainstem nuclei that have been described under several headings. In striatonigral degeneration (Adams, Bogaert and Van der Ecken, 1964), focal damage to substantia nigra and locus ceruleus with or without Lewy bodies is associated with severe atrophy of the hyperpigmented putamen due to deposition of haematin pigment, neuromelanin and lipofuscin in astroglia (Koeppen, Barron and Cox, 1971; Borit, Rubinstein and Urich, 1975), moderate damage to the caudatum and multiple brainstem lesions (Jellinger and Danielczyk, 1968; Kan, 1978; Takei and Mirra, 1973). It can be associated with olivopontocerebellar atrophy (Adams, Bogaert and Van der Ecken, 1964; Johnson *et al.*, 1966) which also shows frequent damage to the substantia nigra and other brainstem systems in both hereditary and sporadic cases clinically presenting with or without parkinsonism (Jellinger and Tarnowsky-Dziduszko, 1971; Berciano, 1982). Orthostatic hypotension or Shy–Drager syndrome is featured by degenerative changes of several neuronal systems, one subtype associated with widespread occurrence of Lewy bodies, the other with multiple system atrophy of the olivopontocerebellar atrophy and striatonigral degeneration type, intermediolateral column cell loss being the only damage common to all cases (Johnson *et al.*, 1966; Schochet, Wyatt and McCormick, 1970;

Vanderhaeghen, Olivier and Sternon, 1970; Roessmann, Van der Nourt and McFarland, 1971; Oppenheimer, 1983). Hereditary multisystem degenerations include Joseph- or Machado–Joseph disease, an autosomal dominant ataxic multisystem disorder (Nakano, Dawson and Spence, 1972; Rosenberg, 1984) with variable combinations of primary nigral or nigrosubthalamopallidal atrophy with degeneration of cerebellofugal (dentatorubral) and cerebellopetal systems (Woods and Schaumberg, 1972; Romanul *et al.*, 1977; Sachdev, Forno and Kane, 1982; Rosenberg, 1984), and related hereditary combined spinocerebellar and extrapyramidal degenerations (Kaiya, 1974; Mizutani *et al.*, 1983), some associated with taurine deficiency (Perry *et al.*, 1975; Purdy *et al.*, 1979).

Parkinson–dementia complex

Parkinson–dementia complex, a combination of parkinsonism with dementia and frequent amyotrophic lateral sclerosis, occurring endemically with familial aggregation on Guam, is characterized by diffuse cortical atrophy with abundant Alzheimer's neurofibrillary tangles and Hirano bodies associated with multisystem neuronal loss and gliosis, rare Lewy bodies in the locus ceruleus, but absence of senile plaques (Hirano, Malamud and Kurland, 1961; Brody, Hirano and Scott, 1971). Similar syndromes have been observed in Japan (Shiraki and Yase, 1975; Kaiya and Mehraein, 1975), West Guinea (Chen *et al.*, 1982), USA (Mata *et al.*, 1983), and West Germany (Schmitt, Emser and Heimes, 1984). Concurrence of Parkinson's disease with motor neurone disease and/or dementia, whether occurring familially or sporadically (Greenfield and Matthews, 1954; Brait, Fahn and Schwarz, 1973; Forno, Barbour and Norville, 1978; Hudson, 1981) or Pick's disease has been reported infrequently (Neumayer, 1971), although considerable damage to substantia nigra and locus ceruleus is often seen in both conditions (Escourolle, Recondo and Gray, 1971; Jellinger, 1968, 1974).

Progressive supranuclear palsy

Progressive supranuclear palsy, a progressive sporadic Parkinson-like disorder with ophthalmoplegia, axial dystonia, rigid akinesia, pseudobulbar palsy and dementia (Steele, Richardson and Olszewski, 1964; Kristensen, 1985), shows widespread neurofibrillary filament tangles and multisystem neuronal loss and gliosis, with no or little involvement of the hippocampus and neocortex. The distribution of lesions and the ultrastructure of the neurofibrillary filament tangles made of 15-nm straight filaments (*Figure 9.3*) are different from those in post-encephalitic parkinsonism and in Guam–parkinsonism–dementia complex (Tellez-Nagel and Wisniewski, 1973; Powell, London and Lampert, 1974; Ishino, Ikeda and Otsuki, 1975; Bugiani *et al.*, 1979; Jellinger, Riederer and Tomonaga, 1980), but concurrence of straight neurofilament tangles with paired helical filaments in the same patient or even in the same diseased nerve cell (Ghatak, Nochlin and Hadfield, 1980; Takauchi, Mizumara and Miyashi, 1983; Tomonaga, 1977, 1979; Yagishita *et al.*, 1979), and of 10-nm filaments with Alzheimer's neurofibrillary tangles have been observed in this disorder (Probst, 1977).

Figure 9.3 Progressive supranuclear palsy. Neurofibrillary tangles in substantia nigra (inset: (*a*) cresyl violet and (*b*) Bodian × 1200). Ultrastructure showing parallel and interlacing bundles of straight tubules, × 28 800. Inset: detail of straight filaments with well-defined borders and superimposed electron-dense granular cytoplasmic material. × 96 000

Post-encephalitic parkinsonism

Post-encephalitic parkinsonism as a residual deficit of encephalitis lethargica and other viral infections of the CNS (Duvoisin and Yahr, 1965; Miyasaki and Fujita, 1977; Rail, Scholtz andSwash, 1981) shows extensive bilateral diffuse degeneration and gliosis of the substantia nigra (*Figure 9.4a*) and locus ceruleus in the absence of Lewy bodies, with damage to other parts of the upper brainstem, and widespread occurrence of neurofibrillary filament tangles in the brainstem particularly in substantia nigra, locus ceruleus, and mesencephalic tegmentum, in the hypothalamus and hippocampus, with no or little involvement of the neocortex (Hassler, 1938; Klaue, 1940; Greenfield and Bosanquet, 1953; Torvik and Meen, 1966; Ishii, 1966; Ishii and Nakamura, 1981; Rail, Scholtz and Swash, 1981). Their ultrastructure is that of paired helical filaments (*Figure 9.4b*) as seen in Alzheimer's disease–senile dementia of Alzheimer type and Guam–parkinsonism–dementia complex (Wisniewski, Terry and Hirano, 1970; Hirano, 1971), and only occasionally of straight neurofilament tangles in locus ceruleus neurones, but coexistence of both types of tangles in a single neurone of the locus ceruleus has been observed (Ishii and Nakamura, 1981). The pathogenesis of post-encephalitic parkinsonism is unknown, but the distribution of neuronal loss and of neurofibrillary filament tangles in the most severely affected sites and the demonstration of antibodies to influenza B by immunofluorescence technique (Gamboa *et al.*, 1974) suggests some relation with a viral agent.

Vascular or 'arteriosclerotic' parkinsonism

Vascular or 'arteriosclerotic' parkinsonism is widely recognized as pathologically unproved (Schwab and England, 1968; Lewis, 1971). Although vascular lesions (lacunar state, small infarcts) may occur in typical Parkinson's disease brains (Alvord *et al.*, 1974; Earle, 1968; Escourolle, Recondo and Gray, 1971; Jacob, 1983), their incidence is about the same as in age-matched controls (Jellinger, 1986). In autopsy series of parkinsonism, 1.8–7% have been classified as being of vascular origin (Earle, 1968; Bernheimer *et al.*, 1973; Tohgi, 1977; Jellinger, 1974), while in a personal series of over 500 Parkinson's disease brains, 7.4% revealed multi-infarct atrophy, hypertensive or Binswanger-type encephalopathy, with lacunar or small infarctions in the basal ganglia and/or brainstem, with no or only mild degenerative nigral changes. The presence of Lewy bodies in 9.3% of these cases was twice as high as in aged controls, suggesting a combination of Parkinson's disease with cerebrovascular disorders, thus reducing the incidence of acceptable vascular parkinsonism to about 6%.

Post-traumatic parkinsonism

Post-traumatic parkinsonism has been observed in rare cases of destruction of the substantia nigra by bullet injury (Morsier, 1960), direct traumatic impact or herniation contusion of the upper brainstem (Lindenberg, 1964; Huhn and Jakob, 1971), or secondary damage to the midbrain and basal ganglia resulting from vascular compression in transtentorial herniation and raised intracranial pressure (Lindenberg, 1964; Jellinger, 1966). Concurrence of post-traumatic brain damage with idiopathic Parkinson's disease may occur. Dementia pugilistica or boxer's

Figure 9.4 Post-encephalitic parkinsonism. (*a*) Diffuse neuronal loss and gliosis of substantia nigra. H.E. × 20. (*b*) Ultrastructure of neurofibrillary tangle consisting of twisted tubules. × 85 000

dementia shows diffuse cortical atrophy, severe neuronal loss from locus ceruleus and substantia nigra with numerous neurofibrillary filament tangles, but no senile plaques, spread widely throughout the CNS (Corsellis, Bruton and Freeman-Browne, 1973).

Toxic parkinsonism

In toxic parkinsonism due to carbon monoxide, carbon disulphide and cyanide intoxication or postnarcotic encephalopathies, the anoxic damage to the globus pallidus and/or substantia nigra is well documented (Peiffer, 1963; Lapresle and Fardeau, 1967; Jellinger, 1968; Uitti et al., 1985), although postmortem studies of cases with post-CO parkinsonism are rare (Brzezicki, 1930; Yakovlew, 1944; Escourolle, Recondo and Gray, 1971). Manganese encephalopathy shows widespread neuronal loss and gliosis, most prominent in the globus pallidus, and minor damage to substantia nigra with occasional Lewy bodies (Bernheimer et al., 1973; Stadler, 1936; Parnitzke and Peiffer, 1956). The pathology of neuroleptic and other drug-induced parkinsonism is poorly understood, since the minor changes seen in the substantia nigra and midbrain (Christensen, Möller and Faurbye, 1970) are considered as age-related findings (Jellinger, 1977), while the demonstration of neuronal loss with Lewy bodies in substantia nigra and locus ceruleus with reduced homovanillic acid levels in the striatum (Rajput et al., 1982) may indicate the presence of subclinical Parkinson's disease in some of these cases.

In MPTP (1-methyl-4-phenyl-1,2,3,6-tetrahydroxypyridine)-induced parkinsonism, neuropathology findings performed in one human case (Davis et al., 1979) and in experimental monkeys and beagles (Langston et al., 1984; Chiueh et al., 1985) have shown similar results: the brain of a male aged 23 years who developed parkinsonism following the self-administration of the drug and died 18 months later, showed destruction of the zona compacta of substantia nigra with neuromelanin pigment within microglial cells, and a considerable astrocytic response with focal glial scarring. The changes were present throughout the zona compacta of the substantia nigra, but were more severe in the caudal portion. No unequivocal Lewy bodies were identified except for one single questionable eosinophilic inclusions; the locus ceruleus and motor vagus nucleus were intact (Davis et al., 1979; Langston et al., 1983). The lesions in experimental animals were also restricted to the zona compacta of the substantia nigra, showing severe neuronal loss, astrocytosis, and free melanin pigment. The lesions were seen throughout the zona compacta of the substantia nigra, maximal or with focal accentuation in the medial third of the caudal substantia nigra (Langston et al., 1983) or in the medial and lateral portion (Chiueh et al., 1985). No unequivocal Lewy bodies were identified, and there was no damage to any other CNS regions, the reticular zone of substantia nigra, locus ceruleus, paranigral nucleus, ventral tegmental area and motor vagus nucleus being spared. Only in one severely affected monkey were axonal spheroids seen in the substantia nigra reticulata and medial pallidum (Parisi and Burns, 1985). Electron microscopy showed loss of granular endoplasmic reticulum and substance of Nissl in the few remaining nigral neurones, many macrophages, and large numbers of intact small unmyelinated axons. Dendrites were surrounded by normal-appearing axon terminals with synaptic complexes (Langston et al., 1984). Immunocytochemical studies of TH-containing neurones showed significant loss of dopaminergic cell bodies in the A-9 region with sparing of the interpeduncular A-10 area containing the cell bodies of the dopaminergic mesolimbic system (Chiueh et al., 1985). Despite greater than 80% decrease in A-9 nigral cell bodies, the dopamine content of striatum decreased only by 50%, indicating some sprouting of the surviving nigral neurones which was observed histochemically, by TH-immunochemistry, and biochemically (Chiueh et al., 1985). Although the lesions in MPTP-induced parkinsonism are similar to those of idiopathic Parkinson's disease, they are more selective than in this disorder, are not associated with the occurrence of Lewy bodies, and obviously spare other neuronal systems most frequently affected in Parkinson's disease.

Symptomatic parkinsonism

Symptomatic parkinsonism is seen in a large variety of disorders (Fahn, 1977; Jellinger, 1986), e.g. brainstem tuberculoma (Blocq and Marinesco, 1894), gliomas and lymphomas of the brainstem (Gherardi et al., 1985) or solid tumours causing damage to the substantia nigra and its dopaminergic projections via brainstem compression (Garcia de Yebenes et al., 1982), syringomyelia of brainstem (Hardy and Stevenson, 1957), viral encephalitis with acute destruction of substantia nigra (Bojinov, 1971), subacute sclerosing panencephalitis (Mossakowski and Mathieson, 1961) or calcification of the basal ganglia (Klawans, Lupton and Simon, 1976). It may also occur in neurolipidoses with protein-containing cytoplasmic inclusions in substantia nigra neurones (Seitelberger et al., 1967), Creutzfeldt–Jakob disease (Roos, Gajdusek and Gibbs, 1973), Alzheimer's disease with frequent damage to the substantia nigra and locus ceruleus (Sjögren, Sjögren and Lindgren, 1952; Sugimara, Yamasaki and Ando, 1977; Pearce, 1979; Rosenblum and Ghatak, 1979; Jakob, 1983), or late-onset Hallervorden–Spatz disease (Jellinger and Neumayer, 1972; Jankovic et al., 1985).

MORPHOLOGICAL BASIS FOR PATHOBIOCHEMISTRY

Consistent degeneration of the dopaminergic nigrostriatal neuronal system in Parkinson's disease is variably associated with widespread damage to other transmitter systems that may, at least in part, explain the many pathobiochemical data in this disorder. The pathological basis of the major neurotransmitter changes in Parkinson's disease is now well established, although the morphological background for many other biochemical changes and their causative mechanism is unclear.

Dopaminergic systems

Degeneration affects the nigrostriatal, mesocorticolimbic and hypothalamic dopaminergic systems arising from the pigmented neurones of the substantia nigra and the ventral tegmental area. Damage to the dopaminergic nigral neurones has been confirmed by quantitative studies in various types of parkinsonism (*Table 9.4*). In Parkinson's disease, the substantia nigra shows a decrease of fresh volume by 25% with loss of pigmented neurones ranging from 50 to 85%, with considerable reduction to nucleolar and perikaryal volumes and loss of melanin up to 88% of controls. A similar loss of pigmented neurones occurs in olivopontocerebellar

Table 9.4 Quantitative changes in the substantia nigra in parkinsonism

Author	Disease group	N	Age, mean	Fresh volume (% control)	Neuronal loss (% control)	Nucleolar volume (% control)	Volume perikarya (% control)	Melanin content (% control)
Pakkenberg and Brody (1965)	PD	10	68	–	59† (total) 66‡ (pigm.) 39† (unpigm.)	–	–	–
Tolppanen (1971)	PD	10	62	–	50–70	–	–	–
Javoy-Agid et al. (1984a)	PD	2	?	–	77.3	–	–	–
Mann and Yates (1983a)	PD	8	68	–	80‡	15*	–	15†
	PD (untreated)	4	63	–	76.3‡	11.4	–	17.4†
	PD (treated)	4	73	–	85.4‡	11.9	–	12.7*
Bogerts, Häntsch and Herzer (1983)	PD	5	72	28† (l) 24 (m)	66‡ (l) 63† (m)	60* (l) 17 (m)	39* (l) 24 (m)	–
	PEP	6	54	70‡ (l) 62‡ (m)	94‡ (l) 95‡ (m)	39* (l) 24 (m)	52‡ (l) 36* (m)	–
Takeda et al. (1982)	PDC	?	?	–	80‡ (total) 96‡ (pigm.) 42* (unpigm.)	–	–	–
	OPCA	?	?	–	61.8‡ (total) 83.3‡ (pigm.) 23 (unpigm.)	–	–	–

PD = Parkinson's disease; PEP = post-encephalitic parkinsonism; PDC = Parkinson–dementia complex; OPCA = olivopontocerebellar atrophy; * = $P<0.05$; † = $P<0.01$; ‡ = $P<0.001$; – = not examined; l = lateral; m = medial; pigm. = pigmented; unpigm. = unpigmented.

atrophy, while in post-encephalitic parkinsonism up to 96% of such neurones are lost. The degree of neuronal loss in substantia nigra correlates with the decrease of dopamine and homovanillic acid in striatum and ventral tegmentum (Bernheimer *et al.*, 1973), and with loss of activity of tyrosine hydroxylase (TH), the rate-limiting enzyme of catecholamine synthesis in these regions (McGeer and McGeer, 1976; Nagatsu *et al.*, 1981; Birkmayer and Riederer, 1983; Gaspar and Gray, 1984).

Immunocytochemistry shows a substantial loss of TH-immunoreactive neurones in the substantia nigra, nucleus paranigralis and ventral tegmentum (Pearson, 1983; Nakashima, Kumanishi and Ikuta, 1983; Javoy-Agid *et al.*, 1984), and a marked diminution of TH-immunoreactive processes (axons and dendrites) in the

Figure 9.5 Schematic distribution of tyrosine-hydroxylase immunoreactive neurones (left) and fibres or terminal (right) in midbrain of normal human (upper) and Parkinson's disease brain (lower)

nigrostriatal pathway and ventral tegmental area (*Figure 9.5*). While Lewy bodies in catecholaminergic neurones positively stain with TH antisera, suggesting that TH enzyme may play a role in the production of Lewy bodies (Nakashima and Ikuta, 1984b), positive TH-immunoreactivity of neurones in substantia nigra and locus ceruleus affected by neurofibrillary filament tangles in Parkinson's disease, progressive supranuclear palsy, parkinsonism–dementia complex and Alzheimer's disease indicate that these neurones still contain TH enzyme protein and that formation of Alzheimer's neurofibrillary tangles, except in final states when the neurone is entirely replaced by them, develops independently from TH protein synthesis (Nakashima and Ikuta, 1984b). Most of the remaining melanin-laden neurones of the substantia nigra show negative immunoreaction with TH indicating loss of TH enzyme activity. TH-immunoreactivity is related to the quantity of this rate-limiting enzyme of catecholamine synthesis in the tissue (Benno *et al.*, 1982), and therefore is an excellent marker for catecholaminergic pathways in the human postmortem CNS (Pearson *et al.*, 1983; Nakashima, Kumanishi and Ikuta, 1983; Dietl, 1985). These data indicate disappearance of catecholaminergic neurones and severe damage to the dopaminergic pathways with disappearance of dopaminergic terminals in the striatum. It is generally concluded that loss of nigral neurones and dopamine deprivation in the striatum need to reach a critical level before parkinsonism symptoms become apparent; the limit lies at a 70–80% depletion (Bernheimer *et al.*, 1973; Hornykiewicz, 1982; Birkmayer and Riederer, 1983), and correlates well with the morphometric findings in various types of parkinsonism and the greater loss of the substantia nigra in advanced states of Parkinson's disease (Mann, Yates and Marcyniuk, 1983).

Although deprivation of the normal input may cause degeneration of most dopaminergic terminals in the striatum (Mann and Yates, 1983a), there is little change in striatal morphology. It does not show any considerable reduction of its fresh volume and wet weight, nor definite loss of striatal neurones (*Table 9.5*). Ultrastructural studies have not revealed any definite abnormalities in the synaptic organization of the striatum in Parkinson's disease (Forno and Norville, 1981). The immunoelectrophoretic demonstration of normal concentration of synaptic marker antigens related to rat brain D_2 and D_3 protein in putamen extracts of Parkinson's disease (Jørgensen *et al.*, 1982) also suggests absence of major neuronal degeneration. The globus pallidus, in contrast to previously suggested severe neuronal loss (Martin, 1965), according to recent morphometric studies, shows only 30% neuronal loss in the external segment without changes in the cell density in both Parkinson's disease and post-encephalitic parkinsonism (*Table 9.5*). Demonstration of loss of TH-immunoreactivity in the striatum following experimentally induced damage to the substantia nigra suggesting striatal denervation (Pearson, 1983; Arluison, Dietl and Thibault, 1984), is extremely difficult in human postmortem brain to show for methodological reasons (Javoy-Agid *et al.*, 1984a; Dietl, 1985). In addition, there is considerable reduction of TH-immunoreactive neurones and fibres in the mesolimbic system and hypothalamus (Javoy-Agid *et al.*, 1984a; Gaspar and Gray, 1984), and also in some areas of the human spinal cord that shows similar distribution but considerably reduced density of TH-immunoreactive neurones, fibres and varicosities compared to controls, with predominant loss of thin TH-immunoreactive fibres (*Figure 9.6*). Together with reduced TH activity in the adrenal medulla (Riederer *et al.*, 1977), these data may indicate a *generalized* damage to the dopaminergic system in Parkinson's disease.

Table 9.5 Quantitative changes in the striopallidum in Parkinsonism

Author	Disease	N	Mean age (years)	Volume/weight (% control)			Cell count (% control)			Cell density (% control)
				Caudate	Putamen	Pallidum	Caudate	Putamen	Pallid. ext.	Pallid. ext.
Pakkenberg (1963)	PD	?	?	–	–	–	–	–	100	–
Sabuncu (1969)	PD	8	62	–	–	–	–	–	100	–
Dom, Baro and Brucher (1973)	PD	?	?	–	–	–	–	100	–	–
Bøttcher (1975)	PD	9	75	–	–	–	–	100	100	–
Wuketich et al. (1980)	PD	11	76	96.2(W)	96(W)	99(W)	–	–	–	–
Bugiani et al. (1980)	PD	14	63	–	–	–	50(l)	65(s)	–	–
Lange and Bogerts (1982)	PD	5	72	93(V)	100(V)	100(V)	89(s)	100	85	–
	PEP	6	54	85(V)	100(V)	93(V)	90(s)	93(l)	71	–
Arendt et al. (1983)	PD	14	59	–	–	–	–	–	92	105
	PEP	7	59	–	–	–	–	–	100	98

PD = Parkinson's disease; PEP = post-encephalitis parkinsonism; V = volume; s = small cells; W = weight (fresh); l = large cells.

Morphological basis for pathobiochemistry   143

Figure 9.6 Schematic distribution of catecholamine (tyrosine-hydroxylase immunoreactive) neurones and fibres in normal and Parkinson's disease spinal cord

Noradrenergic system

The locus ceruleus is the main source of widespread noradrenergic innervation of most CNS regions, with the dorsal vagal nucleus and the supra-optic and paraventricular nuclei of the hypothalamus forming its major projection fields (Mann, Yates and Hawkes, 1983). In Parkinson's disease, progressive supranuclear palsy, Parkinson–dementia complex and olivopontocerebellar atrophy there is a loss of pigmented neurones ranging from 50 to 80%. This is similar to the reduction found in both Alzheimer's disease–senile dementia of Alzheimer type and

Table 9.6 Quantitative changes in locus ceruleus in parkinsonism and senile dementia

Author	Disease	N	Mean age (years)	Cell loss (% age-matched controls)	Nucleolar volume (% age-matched controls)	Melanin content (% age-matched controls)
Mann, Yates and Hawkes (1983)	PD	6	65.4	78.5*	101	–
Mann and Yates (1983b)	PD	8	68.2	78.8*	100	24.6*
	PD untreated	4	63.0	72.2*	104.8	24.0*
	PD treated	4	73.2	85.3*	97.3	20.0*
Mann, Yates and Hawkes (1983)	PSP	4	56.0	50.7*	–	–
Takeda (1982)	PDC	?	?	49.6*	–	–
	OPCA	?	?	63.9*	–	–
Mann, Yates and Hawkes (1983)	SDAT	19	84.7	54.5*	82.3*	–
Mann, Yates and Marcyniuk (1984)	AD+SDAT	22	74.5	70.3*	68.5*	–
Mann, Yates and Hawkes (1983)	DP	4	55.0	65.8*	74.4*	–
Vijayashankar-Brody (1979)	SDAT	24	75–87	40.0*	–	–
Tomlinson, Irving and Blessed (1981)	SDAT	15	81.0	52–56*	–	–
Bondareff, Mountjoy and Roth (1982)	SDAT	20	78±7	80.0*	–	–

PD = Parkinson's disease; PDC = Parkinson–dementia complex; PSP = progressive supranuclear palsy; SDAT = senile dementia of the Alzheimer type; OPCA = olivopontocerebellar atrophy; DP = dementia pugilistica; * = $P<0.001$.

dementia pugilistica (*Table 9.6*), but less than in senile controls where it amounts to about 40% (Mann, Yates and Hawkes, 1983). Synaptic morphology of the locus ceruleus in both Parkinson's disease and Alzheimer's disease shows little change except for an accumulation of large dense core vesicles in axon terminals and nerve cell processes. This may be due to accumulation of biogenic amines, particularly noradrenaline, in the affected terminals deprived of their postsynaptic components due to degeneration of nerve cells and their dendrites (Forno and Norville, 1981). Despite involved protein synthesis capacity of the remaining locus ceruleus cells in normal aged individuals and in Parkinson's disease and progressive supranuclear palsy, the reduction of neurones, nucleolar volume and cytoplasmic RNA within cells of the dorsal vagal nucleus, paraventricular and supra-optic nuclei indicate that this cell loss leads to marked decrease of the function within the noradrenergic projection nuclei of the locus ceruleus (*Table 9.7*), causing gross depletion of brain noradrenaline levels (Birkmayer and Riederer, 1983; Javoy-Agid *et al.*, 1984a). In our autopsy series of Parkinson's disease, dorsal vagal nucleus showed neuronal loss in 87.3% and Lewy bodies in 82% as compared to 31% in senile parkinsonism, 12% in post-encephalitic parkinsonism and only 2.8% in aged controls (*Table 9.3*). Lewy bodies and neurofibrillary filament tangles are widely scattered throughout the hypothalamus (Ohama and Ikuta, 1976; Mann and Yates, 1983a).

Serotoninergic system

Damage to the dorsal raphe nucleus, giving rise to the ascending serotoninergic pathways (Ungerstedt, 1971), has been reported in both Parkinson's disease and post-encephalitic parkinsonism (Lewis, 1971; Escourolle, Recondo and Gray, 1971), with reduction of the RNA content and nucleolar volume by 9–19% (*Table 9.7*). These data did not seem to reflect the decrease of serotonin in many brain areas in Parkinson's disease (Birkmayer and Riederer, 1983; Javoy-Agid *et al.*, 1984a). Some dorsal raphe nucleus neurones contain Lewy bodies, while Alzheimer's neurofibrillary tangles in Parkinson's disease are rare, in contrast to Alzheimer's disease–senile dementia of Alzheimer type, where the dorsal raphe nucleus has the highest Alzheimer's neurofibrillary tangles incidence of the brainstem (Ishii, 1966; Jellinger Riederer and Tomonaga, 1980; Yamada and Mehraein, 1977). Recent studies, however, documented severe loss of large dorsal raphe nucleus neurones in both Alzheimer's disease–senile dementia of Alzheimer type and Guam–parkinsonism– dementia complex, ranging in average from 36.8 to 80% with reduction of the nucleolar volumes by 33.7 ± 9% (Yamamoto and Hirano, 1985a; Tabaton *et al.*, 1985), and affection of 2.25–91% of the neurones by Alzheimer's neurofibrillary tangles (Curcio and Kemper, 1984). In Parkinson's disease we observed an average loss of large dorsal raphe nucleus neurones of 57.8% compared to 36.8–55.8% in Alzheimer's disease and 41.8% in senile dementia of Alzheimer type, with similar reduction in neuronal density (*Figure 9.7*). Of the dorsal raphe nucleus neurones 4.5% contained Lewy bodies, and 6.5% Alzheimer's neurofibrillary tangles (*Table 9.7*) which indicates a considerable functional damage to the serotoninergic system in both Parkinson's disease and Alzheimer's disease–senile dementia of Alzheimer type.

Figure 9.7 Total number (*a*) and mean density/mm^2 (*b*) of large neurones in human nucleus dorsalis raphe in Parkinson's disease, Alzheimer's disease and senile dementia of the Alzheimer type (SDAT). --- mean; — s.e.m.

Cholinergic systems

The nucleus basalis of Meynert in the substantia innominata, known to be the main source of the widespread cholinergic innervation of the neocortex and hippocampus (Mesulam *et al.*, 1983; Hedren *et al.*, 1984), was one of the nuclei in which Lewy bodies were first observed in Parkinson's disease (Lewy, 1913; Foix and Nicolesco, 1925), and neuronal loss has long been known to occur in this condition (Hassler, 1938; Buttlar-Brentano, 1955). Morphometric studies show neuronal loss in the nucleus basalis of Meynert ranging from 32 to 87% with a mean of 50–60% in Parkinson's disease (Arendt *et al.*, 1983; Whitehouse *et al.*, 1983; Gaspar and Gray, 1984; Tagliavini *et al.*, 1984a; Jellinger, 1986) as compared to 44% in progressive supranuclear palsy (Tagliavini *et al.*, 1984a), over 60% in

Table 9.7 Quantitative changes in other subcortical nuclei in Parkinson's disease

Nucleus	Nerve cell number (% controls)	Nucleolar volume (% controls)	RNA content	Lewy bodies (% neurones)	Neurofibr. tangles (% neurones)	No. of cases	Mean age (years)	Author
Supra-optic nucleus	100	72.6†	76.4†	–	–	8	68.2	Mann and Yates (1983a)
Paraventricular nucleus	100	68.8†	71.3†	–	–			
Nucleus basalis of Meynert	–	78.1†	75.8†	–	–			
Westphal–Edinger nucleus	46*	–	–	3.0	3.0	2	76.5	Hunter (1985)
Dorsal raphe nucleus	100	91.3	83.7†	–	–	8	68.2	Mann and Yates (1983a)
	57.8†	–	–	4.5	6.7	28	78.5	Jellinger (1986)
Dorsal motor vagus nucleus	102	83.4‡	87.2‡	–	–	8	68.2	Mann, Yates and Hawkes (1983)

* = $P<0.001$; † = $P<0.01$; ‡ = $P<0.05$.

olivopontocerebellar atrophy (Tagliavini and Pilleri, 1985) and 93% in Guam–parkinsonism–dementia complex (Nakano and Hirano, 1983) and in 'diffuse Lewy body disease' (Jellinger, 1986), with a similar reduction of the maximum and mean neuronal densities from 35 to 85% in various types of parkinsonism (*Figure 9.8*).

Figure 9.8 Total number (*a*) and mean density (*b*) of large cholinergic neurones in the nucleus basalis of Meynert in demented and non-demented Parkinson's disease (PD), Alzheimer's disease (AD), senile dementia of the Alzheimer type (SDAT) and controls

Only post-encephalitic parkinsonism shows no or very little damage to the nucleus basalis of Meynert (Arendt *et al.*, 1983; Whitehouse *et al.*, 1983; Jellinger, 1986). Neuronal loss affects predominantly the large cholinergic neurones in the middle and posterior part of the nucleus basalis of Meynert and loss of the anterior part with comparative preservation of the nucleus of Broca's diagonal bundle (McGeer, McGeer and Suzuki, 1984; Rogers, Brogan and Mirra, 1985). The severity of neuronal loss is much higher in demented Parkinson's disease cases (60–77%), where it is similar to that in Alzheimer's disease ranging from 57 to 90% (Whitehouse *et al.*, 1983; Rogers, Brogan and Mirra, 1985; Jellinger, 1986), than in non-demented Parkinson's disease cases (34–49%), where it approaches the values seen in senile dementia of Alzheimer type ranging from 33 to 59% (*Figure 9.8*), while the normal aged population show a 30–50% reduction of the magnocellular population of the nucleus basalis of Meynert (Mann, Yates and Hawkes, 1983; McGeer, McGeer and Suzuki, 1984). The remaining nucleus basalis of Meynert neurones show a considerable decrease in protein synthesis capacity, with reduction of nucleolar volume and RNA content in Parkinson's disease of 22–24% as compared to 30–33% in Alzheimer's disease (*Table 9.7*). The incidence of Lewy bodies in the nucleus basalis of Meynert ranges from 84 to 96.5% and that of Alzheimer's neurofibrillary tangles from 29 to 65% (Gaspar and Gray, 1984; Jellinger, 1986). Senile plaques, usually seen in nucleus basalis of Meynert in Alzheimer's disease–senile dementia of Alzheimer type (Rudelli, Ambler and Wisniewski, 1984), have almost never been observed in Parkinson's disease (Gaspar and Gray, 1984; Nakano and Hirano, 1984; Jellinger, 1986). The degeneration of the cholinergic innominatocortical pathway associated with reduction of the activity of postsynaptic cholinergic markers, choline-acetyltransferase and acetylcholinesterase (AChE) in the nucleus basalis of Meynert and neocortex in Parkinson's disease (Candy et al., 1983; Perry et al., 1983b; Gaspar and Gray, 1984) and in Alzheimer's disease–senile dementia of Alzheimer type (Coyle, Price and De Long, 1983; Davies, 1983; Perry et al., 1983a; Wilcock and Esiri, 1982; Rossor et al., 1984) have been implicated in the disturbances of cognitive functions in these disorders.

The Westphal–Edinger nucleus is a visceral subdivision of the oculomotor complex, giving rise to cholinergic parasympathetic preganglionic fibres to the ciliary ganglion regulating pupilloconstriction. Recently, this nucleus has been shown to suffer from 54% neuronal loss in Parkinson's disease; 2–3% of the neurones in this nucleus and in the nucleus of Darkschewitsch are affected by Lewy bodies and Alzheimer's neurofibrillary tangles (Hunter, 1985). The frequent involvement of the neurones in these nuclei by Alzheimer's neurofibrillary tangles in Alzheimer's disease–senile dementia of Alzheimer type (Ishii, 1966; Hunter, 1985), confirmed by personal studies, may explain some of the neuro-ophthalmological dysfunctions in both Parkinson's disease and senile dementia of Alzheimer type.

Peptidergic systems

In Parkinson's disease several peptidergic systems are affected, as indicated biochemically by the reduction of substance P, met-enkephalin, and cholecystokinin-8 in the substantia nigra pars compacta and external pallidum, while somatostatin is affected in cortical areas (Javoy-Agid et al., 1984b; Dubois et al., 1985). However, in contrast to the severe reduction of immunoreactivity for substance P and met-enkephalin in Huntington's chorea, the pallidum and substantia nigra in Parkinson's disease and post-encephalitic parkinsonism show intense immunoreactivity for these substances (Grafe, Forno and Eng, 1983; Zech and Bogerts, 1985), or even increased immunoreactivity for substance P (Constantinides, Bouras and Richard, 1983). Somatostatin, however, in contrast to normal immunoreactivity in Huntington's chorea, shows considerable reduction or even absence of immunoreactivity in the basal ganglia in both Parkinson's disease and Alzheimer's disease (Ferrante et al., 1985; Forno, Gardiner and Eng, 1985). Hence, degeneration of peptidergic neuronal systems appears to be limited to comparatively small populations in the Parkinson's disease brain (Javoy-Agid et al., 1984b).

MORPHOLOGICAL BASIS OF DEMENTIA

Intellectual impairment, estimated to occur in 30–93% of Parkinson's disease patients (Lieberman et al., 1979; Mayeux and Stern, 1983; Ball, 1984), has been related to cerebral atrophy, to senile and other extranigral brain lesions (Alvord *et al.*, 1974; Boller *et al.*, 1979; Hakim and Mathieson, 1979; Jacob, 1983; Yoshimura, 1983), and to involvement of the mesolimbic cortical dopaminergic, noradrenergic, cholinergic, and somatostatin systems (Mann and Yates, 1983b; Perry *et al.*, 1983b; Whitehouse *et al.*, 1983; Gaspar and Gray, 1984; Hornykiewicz and Kish, 1984; Javoy-Agid *et al.*, 1984b; Dubois *et al.*, 1985). CT studies have shown a more severe cerebral atrophy in demented Parkinson's disease patients than in non-demented ones and age-matched controls (Schneider *et al.*, 1979; Jellinger, Grisold and Volmer, 1983; Steiner *et al.*, 1985), only cortical atrophy being related to both age and duration of Parkinson's disease (Sroka *et al.*, 1981). Postmortem demonstration of severe brain atrophy, with significantly reduced average brain weight (Hakim and Mathiesons, 1979), more pronounced cortical degeneration (Alvord *et al.*, 1974), and a six- to ten-fold increase of Alzheimer's lesions than in age-matched controls (Boller *et al.*, 1979), suggested an increased incidence of Alzheimer's disease in patients with Parkinson's disease and some links between the (as yet unknown) disturbance underlying Parkinson's and Alzheimer diseases (Hakim and Mathieson, 1979; Boller, 1985). In demented aged people without Parkinson's disease, a significant correlation was found between the presence and severity of dementia and the number of Alzheimer's neurofibrillary tangles, and to a lesser extent with senile plaques in the cortex (Wilcock and Esiri, 1982). However, no differences in the mean numbers of senile plaques and Alzheimer's neurofibrillary tangles (Mann, Yates and Marcyniuk, 1984) and the 'adjusted tangle index' were found between demented and non-demented Parkinson's disease cases (Ball, 1984), while Perry *et al.* (1983b) saw pathological evidence of coexistent Alzheimer's disease in only one of seven demented cases of Parkinson's disease.

According to recent autopsy studies, the average fresh brain weight (after opening of the ventricles) of controls (without neuropsychiatric disorders) was within the range of comparable samples (Dekaban, 1978; Ho *et al.*, 1980), and was *not* significantly higher than in Parkinson's disease, the latter showing an average reduction of 1.5%; senile parkinsonism, post-encephalitic parkinsonism, senile dementia of Alzheimer type and Alzheimer's disease showed a significant reduction of brain weight between 4 and 9.4% (*Figure 9.9*). Independent evaluation of brain weights for males and females showed similar results; only male Alzheimer's disease and senile dementia of Alzheimer type were below the 95% confidence range of brain weight for white humans (Jellinger, 1986). Regression analysis showed that in Parkinson's disease, but not in Alzheimer's disease, the loss of brain weight was related to both the age and duration of illness, although reduction in brain weight was accelerated after the onset of Parkinson's disease. This was more pronounced in Parkinson's disease cases with onset after the age of 60 years (Jellinger, 1986), which confirms previous time-course CT studies in Parkinson's disease (Schneider *et al.*, 1979).

Semiquantitative evaluation of the histological changes, using a four-degree scale of intensity, showed that neuronal loss and higher amount/severe density of senile plaques and Alzheimer's neurofibrillary tangles in both frontal cortex and hippocampus were higher in Parkinson's disease than in age-matched controls. However, in contrast to other authors (Hakim and Mathieson, 1979; Boller *et al.*, 1979), these differences were not significant (Jellinger, Grisold and Vollmer, 1983; Mann, Yates and Hawkes, 1983; Jellinger and Riederer, 1984). In the third layer of the isocortex of Parkinson's disease brains, an increased number of small to medium-sized pyramidal cells with lipofuscin-filled extensions of their proximal

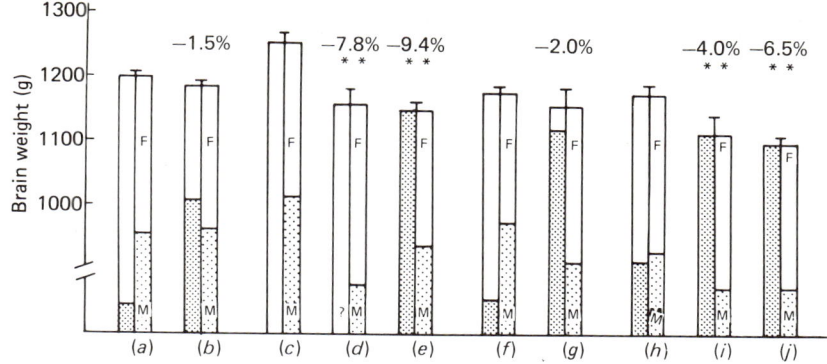

Figure 9.9 Comparison of fresh brain weights in different types of parkinsonism, Alzheimer's disease, senile dementia of the Alzheimer type and age-matched controls. ☐ percentage dementia; I s.e.m.; **$P<0.005$ (student's t test); M = male; F = female. (*a*) Controls ($N = 262$) 73.2 ± 0.6 years; (*b*) Parkinson's disease ($N = 255$) 73.4 ± 0.9 years; (*c*) controls ($N = 85$) 64.8 ± 0.8 years; (*d*) post-encephalitic parkinsonism ($N = 90$) 63.6 ± 1.9 years; (*e*) Alzheimer's disease ($N = 90$) 65.6 ± 0.5 years; (*f*) controls ($N = 180$) 76.3 ± 1.1 years; (*g*) vascular parkinsonism ($N = 32$) 77.2 ± 1.2 years; (*h*) controls ($N = 180$) 80.6 ± 0.5 years; (*i*) senile parkinsonism ($N = 32$) 82.9 ± 1.1 years; (*j*) senile dementia of the Alzheimer type ($N = 206$) 80.7 ± 0.4 years

axons has been reported (Stockhausen and Braak, 1984), but the significance of these age-related cortical changes is unknown. Significant reduction of large cortical neurones, as seen in senile dementia of Alzheimer type (Terry, 1983), associated with reduction of cortical somatostatin neurones (Joynt and McNeill, 1984), could be suggested from reduced cortical somatostatin content (Javoy-Agid *et al.*, 1984b), but has not been quantitatively documented in Parkinson's disease. Association of lesions characteristic of both Parkinson's disease and Alzheimer's disease was seen in 16.9% of all our Parkinson's disease patients dying under age 70 years, while 32.4% of the older cases showed additional signs of senile dementia of Alzheimer type (*Figure 9.10*). This does not confirm the previously suggested significantly increased incidence of Alzheimer's disease in Parkinson's disease populations (Alvord *et al.*, 1974; Boller *et al.*, 1979; Hakim and Mathieson, 1979). However, Parkinson's disease patients with severe dementia show a significantly older age at death, much lower brain weight and significantly increased Alzheimer's lesions in frontal cortex and hippocampus. Although severely demented Parkinson's disease cases usually have later onset with shorter duration of the illness (Boller *et al.*, 1979; Lieberman *et al.*, 1979; DeSmedt *et al.*, 1982), no difference in the duration of illness was found between demented and non-demented Parkinson's disease patients, except for 'senile' parkinsonism which showed the shortest clinical course and most severe Alzheimer's lesions (*Figure 9.10*). The severity of cortical Alzheimer's lesions, expressed as a total Alzheimer score using four degrees of intensity for both senile plaques and Alzheimer's neurofibrillary tangles in frontal cortex and hippocampus, in Parkinson's disease patients with no or only mild dementia similar to aged controls, was correlated with age, but no such age relation was seen in severely demented Parkinson's disease cases associated with Alzheimer's disease or senile dementia of Alzheimer type

152 Pathology of parkinsonism

Figure 9.10 Comparison of age, duration of illness, brain weight and cortical Alzheimer's scores in Parkinson's disease patients with and without senile dementia. A = senile plaques and neurofibrillary tangles (4 degrees each) frontal/hippocampus (max. score = 16). B = combination with Alzheimer's disease: $N = 13$ (16.9% of all Parkinson's disease cases dying under age 70 years – $N = 77$); combination with senile dementia of the Alzheimer type: $N = 56$ (32.4% of all Parkinson's disease cases dying over age 70 years $-N = 173$). *$P < 0.005$; **$P < 0.001$. ▨ Frontal cortex; ☐ hippocampus

(*Figure 9.11*). In both normal ageing and in the majority of Parkinson's disease cases, the presence and severity of dementia shows a good correlation with the intensity of cortical Alzheimer's lesions, particularly Alzheimer's neurofibrillary tangles in frontal cortex and hippocampus (Gaspar and Gray, 1984; Jellinger, 1986). However, a number of Parkinson's disease patients with severe dementia have no significant Alzheimer's pathology, suggesting other causes of their intellectual impairment (Gaspar and Gray, 1984; Heilig *et al.*, 1985). Recent studies emphasize the association of dementia with dysfunctions of the cholinergic magnocellular forebrain system (Coyle, Price and De Long, 1983; Whitehouse *et al.*, 1983; Price *et al.*, 1983; Hedren *et al.*, 1984), showing a 30–50% loss of large nucleus basalis of Meynert neurones in normal aged humans, of 35–59% in senile dementia of Alzheimer type and of 62–90% in Alzheimer's disease with a reduction of protein synthesis capacity of the remaining neurones by 40% (Mann, Yates and Marcyniuk, 1984; McGeer, McGeer and Suzuki, 1984; Rogers, Brogan and Mirra, 1985). In Parkinson's disease, the decrease in cell numbers and density in the nucleus basalis of Meynert averages from 46 to 77%, with significantly less reduction of 34–49% in non-demented than in demented cases, where it averages from 60 to 77%, similar to Alzheimer's disease (Arendt *et al.*, 1983; Whitehouse *et al.*, 1983; Gaspar and Gray, 1984; Jellinger, 1986). Almost total depletion of the magnocellular portion of nucleus basalis of Meynert has been observed in Guam–parkinsonism–dementia complex (Nakano and Hirano, 1983) and in 'diffuse Lewy body disease' (Jellinger, 1986). Comparative studies show that in non-demented Parkinson's disease patients, neuronal loss from nucleus basalis of Meynert ranges from 15 to 62% and is accompanied by no or only mild cortical Alzheimer's lesions; in severely demented patients nucleus basalis of Meynert neuronal loss ranging from 64 to 90% is often but inconsistently associated with

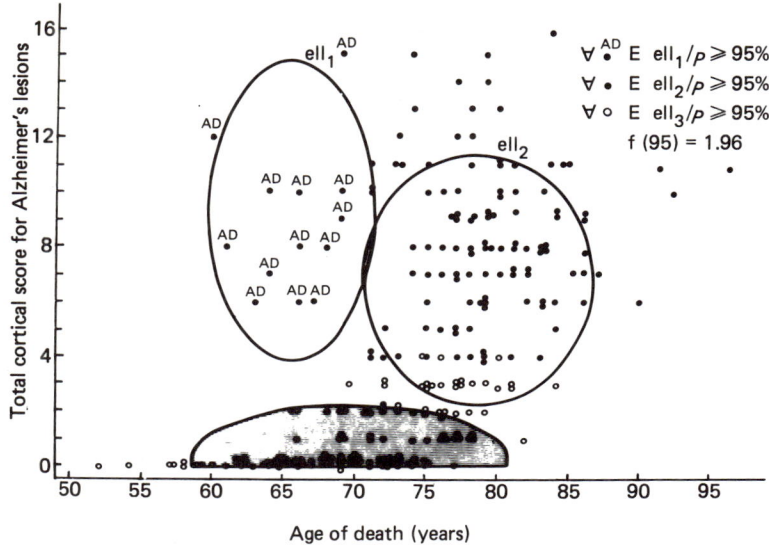

Figure 9.11 Relation of cortical Alzheimer's score (senile plaques and neurofibrillary tangles in frontal cortex and hippocampus) to age in 218 cases of Parkinson's disease using cluster analysis. ○ = non-demented ($N = 141$); ● = demented ($N = 107$); AD● = demented/Parkinson's + Alzheimer's disease ($N = 13$)

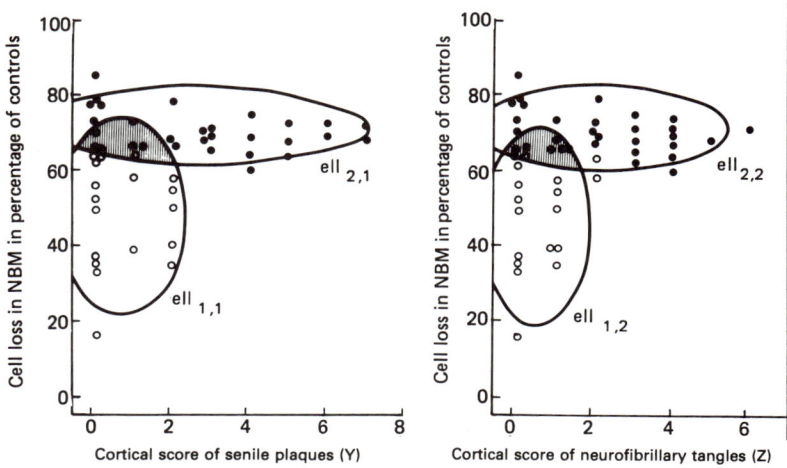

Figure 9.12 Relation between neuronal loss in nucleus basalis of Meynert (NBM) and Alzheimer's lesions in frontal cortex and hippocampus (4 degrees of intensity) in 50 autopsy cases of Parkinson's disease. ○ = Non-demented; ● = demented; $ell_{1,1}$, $ell_{1,2}$ = 95% of non-demented; $ell_{2,1}$, $ell_{2,2}$ = 95% of demented. Regression analysis: $ell_{2,1} : ell_{1,1} = P < 0.001$; $ell_{2,2}$ $ell_{1,2} = P < 0.001$; $r(ZX)$ $P < 0.05$, $r(ZY)$ = not significant, $r(YX)$ $P < 0.05$, $r(XYZ)$ $P < 0.01$, where X = percentage loss of nucleus basalis of Meynert, Y = senile plaques score, Z = cortical neurofibrillary tangle score

severe cortical Alzheimer's lesions (*Figure 9.12*). These data and the biochemical demonstration of greater reduction of choline acetyltransferase levels in both nucleus basalis of Meynert and neocortex in demented compared with non-demented Parkinson's disease patients (Perry *et al.*, 1983b; Gaspar and Gray, 1984; Javoy-Agid *et al.*, 1984a), and similar findings in senile dementia of Alzheimer type (McGeer, McGeer and Suzuki, 1984) suggest that:

(*a*) Dementias associated with reduced neocortical choline-acetyltransferase activity, such as Alzheimer's disease–senile dementia of Alzheimer type and Parkinson's disease with dementia, are related to dysfunction or selective degeneration of nucleus basalis of Meynert neurones.

(*b*) The cholinergic deficit related to selective loss of nucleus basalis of Meynert neurones and decreased protein synthesis capacity of the remaining ones must reach a critical level before dementia becomes apparent. The threshold lies around 60–70% neuronal depletion and reduction of neocortical choline-acetyltransferase activity. This suggests considerable functional compensatory capacities for the cholinergic forebrain system as has been demonstrated for the dopaminergic nigrostriatal system in producing Parkinson's disease symptoms (Hornykiewicz, 1982; Birkmayer and Riederer, 1983). Since no strict correlation was found between the neuronal loss from nucleus basalis of Meynert and the decreased choline-acetyltransferase activities in both nucleus basalis of Meynert and neocortex in both Parkinson's disease (Perry *et al.*, 1983b; Gaspar and Gray, 1984; Dubois *et al.*, 1985) and Alzheimer's disease (McGeer, McGeer and Suzuki, 1984), the mechanism of selective dysfunction of the cholinergic forebrain system remains unclear. Recent studies in Alzheimer's disease suggest reduction of choline-acetyltransferase synthesis with or without disruption of choline-acetyltransferase transport (Younkin *et al.*, 1985).

In contrast to Alzheimer's disease, where neuronal loss from the nucleus basalis of Meynert is related to neuritic plaques in the cortex (Arendt *et al.*, 1985), Parkinson's disease brains, in general, show no relationship between the intensity of nucleus basalis of Meynert cell loss and of cortical Alzheimer changes. The latter may be totally absent in Parkinson's disease brains despite severe selective damage to the nucleus basalis of Meynert (Candy *et al.*, 1983; Gaspar and Gray, 1984; Nakano and Hirano, 1984; Jellinger, 1986). A similar dissociation between nucleus basalis of Meynert neuronal loss and cortical senile plaques has been observed in Guam–parkinsonism–dementia complex (Nakano and Hirano, 1983) and in dementia pugilistica (Uhl *et al.*, 1982), both disorders being characterized by abundance of Alzheimer's neurofibrillary tangles in the absence of senile plaques. The failure to demonstrate a consistent relationship between neuronal loss in nucleus basalis of Meynert and cortical senile plaques, and the fact that senile plaques are observed in many brain areas, including the nucleus basalis of Meynert (Rudelli, Ambler and Wisniewski, 1984; Saper, German and White, 1985), do *not* support the dying-back degeneration hypothesis of cholinergic terminals as the initiator of senile plaque formation (Struble *et al.*, 1982; Price *et al.*, 1983). These data and the immunohistochemical demonstration of noradrenergic and multiple peptidergic markers in senile plaques rather suggest that pathology in both Alzheimer's disease and Parkinson's disease involves *multiple* transmitter-specific systems (Struble *et al.*, 1985; Jellinger, 1986). The relationship of selective degeneration in both the dopaminergic and the cholinergic forebrain systems in Parkinson's disease are unknown, although the demonstration of TH-immunoreactive fibres and terminals in the nucleus basalis of Meynert (Jellinger, 1986), and the biochemical demonstration of dopamine and homovanillic acid in the basal forebrain (Riederer *et al.*, unpublished data), suggest some dopaminergic innervation of these structures.

CONCLUDING REMARKS

The pathology in the majority of cases of parkinsonism, and in particular of Parkinson's disease and multisystem disorders, demonstrates many degenerative changes. In addition to the predominantly affected dopaminergic nigrostriatal system, a variety of other subcortical and cortical systems are involved, causing a multitransmitter dysfunction due to neuronal loss, reduction of synthesis capacity of the remaining neurones, and disorders of specific transport mechanisms. The causative mechanisms underlying the morphological degenerative changes in the affected neuronal systems are unknown. It remains unclear whether degenerative changes and neuronal loss in transmitter-specific systems represent a 'down-regulation' of transmitter production as the primary sequelae of neuronal dysfunction, or are caused by trans-synaptic interaction with other systems, or are due to other mechanisms. Degenerative types of Parkinson's disease, representing the vast majority of parkinsonian disorders, have been separated by Alvord *et al.* (1974) into two major groups: a 'Lewy body disease' which is relatively stereotyped and shows a good correlation of the degree of parkinsonism symptoms with that of neuronal loss from substantia nigra, and an 'Alzheimer tangle disease', possibly a variant of senile dementia of Alzheimer type, in which the degree of cortical degeneration correlates with dementia. More recent data allow a subdivision into several clinicopathological groups:

(*a*) 'Typical' Parkinson's disease without dementia, pathologically featured by predominant degenerative changes with Lewy bodies in the pigmented brainstem nuclei without higher degrees of brain atrophy, or of extranigral and cortical Alzheimer's lesions as compared to age-matched controls. Although duration of illness is not predictive of either the mental status or the severity of Alzheimer's lesions, reduction of brain weight is related to both age and duration of illness, the age dependency of both brain weight and Alzheimer's pathology being more pronounced. The latter appears to be superimposed on the basic degenerative disease process causing Parkinson's disease.
(*b*) Demented cases of Parkinson's disease show a significantly higher degree of brain atrophy and cortical Alzheimer's lesions than non-demented Parkinson's disease and age-matched control populations which, at least in part, appears due to their more advanced age at death. Severe dementia in Parkinson's disease can be related with the following pathology lesions:
  (i) Combination of typical Parkinson's disease changes with Alzheimer's brain pathology, suggesting an association of Parkinson's disease with Alzheimer's disease or senile dementia of Alzheimer type. In our material, its incidence was 14.6 and 32.5%, respectively, and was much less frequent than in other series ranging from 33 to 62.5% (Boller *et al.*, 1979; Hakim and Mathieson, 1979).

(ii) Demented Parkinson's disease cases without Alzheimer's pathology showing degeneration or dysfunction of the cholinergic forebrain or other transmitter-specific systems.
(iii) Rare Parkinson's disease cases featured by abundance of Lewy bodies with or without substantial Alzheimer's lesions – 'diffuse Lewy body disease'.
(iv) Aged demented Parkinson's disease patients with severe cortical Alzheimer's pathology and little degenerative damage to the substantia nigra and other pigmented brainstem nuclei, referred to as 'senile' parkinsonism. This may present either a distinct subset of the aged Parkinson's disease population with superimposed senile dementia of Alzheimer type, or a variant of senile dementia of Alzheimer type with nigral damage surpassing the age-related levels.
(v) Parkinsonism in other ageing and degenerative processes associated with damage to the nigrostriatal system, e.g. in multisystem degenerations, or associated with or superimposed by multifocal cerebrovascular disease.

The morphological changes related to motor dysfunction in Parkinson's disease mainly include degeneration of the TH-immunoreactive dopaminergic nigrostriatal and mesolimbic systems and are associated, particularly in advanced stages of the disease, with degenerative changes in the noradrenergic locus coeruleus and dorsal vagus nucleus, serotoninergic dorsal raphe system and some cholinergic parts of the oculomotor system. The pathological changes related to intellectual deterioration in Parkinson's disease include:

(a) Neuronal loss and Alzheimer's pathology in neocortex and hippocampus which, as in other aged people, show good correlation with the degree of dementia. The concept of dysfunction of cortical somatostatin transmission as a possible basis of 'cortical' dementia needs further morphological documentation.
(b) Dysfunction of the cholinergic forebrain system related to selective degeneration of the nucleus basalis of Meynert with disorders of synthesis and/or transport of specific enzymes.
(c) Dysfunction of other transmitter systems due to degeneration and neuronal dysfunction in their projecting nuclei, e.g. of the ascending noradrenergic system due to damage to the locus ceruleus, the mesolimbic dopaminergic system due to damage to the ventral tegmentum (Uhl, Hedren and Price, 1985), and the serotoninergic system related to damage to the dorsal raphe nucleus etc.
(d) Combination of degeneration of subcortical systems with cortical and/or subcortical Alzheimer's pathology. It should be emphasized that degeneration of the subcortical neuronal systems related to the 'subcortical' type of dementia (Cummings and Benson, 1984) is not necessarily associated with cortical Alzheimer's pathology.

The variable topography of morphological lesions in the Parkinson's disease brain does not indicate dysfunction of a single transmitter-specific system, but rather a multitransmitter dysfunction of variable extent and severity which is related to motor and mental impairment in this disorder. Further studies are needed to elucidate the basic mechanisms of the degenerative pathobiology of Parkinson's disease and their relations to ageing processes in the brain.

References

ADAMS, R. D., BOGAERT, L. VAN and VAN DER EECKEN, H. (1964) Striato-nigral degeneration. *Journal of Neuropathology and Experimental Neurology*, **23**, 584–608

ALVORD, E. D., FORNO, L., KUSSKE, J. A., KAUFMANN, R. J., RHODES, J. S. and GOETOWSKI, C. R. (1974) The pathology of parkinsonism. A comparison of degeneration in cerebral cortex and brainstem. *Advances in Neurology*, **5**, 175–193

ARENDT, T., BIGL, V., ARENDT, A. and TENNSTEDT, A. (1983) Loss of neurons in the nucleus basalis of Meynert in Alzheimer's disease, paralysis agitans and Korsakoff's disease. *Acta Neuropathologica*, **61**, 101–108

ARENDT, A., BIGL, V. and TENNSTEDT, A. (1985) Neuronal loss in different parts of the nucleus basalis is related to neuritic plaque formation in cortical areas in Alzheimer's disease. *Neurosciences*, **14**, 1–14

ARLUISON, M., DIETL, M. and THIBAULT, J. (1984) Ultrastructural morphology of dopaminergic nerve terminals and synapses in the striatum of the rat using tyrosine hydroxylase immunocytochemistry. A topographical study. *Brain Research Bulletin*, **13**, 269–285

BALL, M. J. (1984) The morphological basis of dementia in Parkinson's disease. *Canadian Journal of Neurological Sciences*, **11**, 180–184

BEHEIM-SCHWARBACH, D. (1952) Über Zelleibverännderungen im Nucleus coeruleus bei Parkinsonsymptomen. *Journal of Nervous and Mental Diseases*, **116**, 619–632

BENNO, R. H., TUCKER, L. W., JOH, T. H. and REIS, D. J. (1982) Quantitative immunocytochemistry of tyrosine hydroxylase in rat brain. *Brain Research*, **246**, 225–236

BERCIANO, J. (1982) Olivopontocerebellar atrophy. A review of 117 cases. *Journal of the Neurological Sciences*, **53**, 253–272

BERNHEIMER, H., BIRKMAYER, W., HORNYKIEWICZ, O., JELLINGER, K. and SEITELBERGER, F. (1973) Brain dopamine and the syndromes of Parkinson and Huntington. *Journal of the Neurological Sciences*, **20**, 415–455

BIRKMAYER, W. and RIEDERER, P. (1983) *Parkinson's Disease*. New York: Springer Verlag

BLACKWOOD, W. (1981) Morbid anatomy. In *Research Progress in Parkinson's Disease*. Eds. F. C. Rose and R. Capildeo, pp. 25–31. London: Pitman

BLOCQ, P. and MARINESCA, G. (1894) Sur un cas de tremblement parkinsonian hémiplégique symptomatique d'une tumeur du pédoncule cérébral. *Revue neurologique*, **2**, 265

BOGERTS, B., HÄNTSCH, J. and HERZER, M. (1983) A morphometric study of the dopamin-containing cell groups in the mesencephalon of normals, Parkinson patients, and schizophrenics. *Biological Psychiatry*, **18**, 951–969

BOJINOV, S. (1971) Encephalitis with acute parkinsonian syndrome and bilateral inflammatory necrosis of the substantia nigra. *Journal of the Neurological Sciences*, **12**, 383–415

BOLLER, F. (1985) Parkinson's disease and Alzheimer's disease – Are they associated? In *Senile Dementia of the Alzheimer Type*. Eds J. T. Hutton and A. D. Kenny. *Neurology and Neurobiology*, Vol. 18, pp. 119–130. New York: Alan Liss

BOLLER, F., MIZUTANI, T., ROESSMANN, U. and GAMBETTI, P. (1979) Parkinson's disease, dementia and Alzheimer disease: Clinicopathological correlations. *Annals of Neurology*, **7**, 329–335

BONDAREFF, N., MOUNTJOY, C. Q. and ROTH, M. (1982) Loss of neurons of origin of the adrenergic projections to the cerebral cortex (nucleus locus coeruleus) in senile dementia. *Neurology*, **32**, 165–168

BORIT, A., RUBINSTEIN, L. J. and URICH, H. (1975) The striatonigral degeneration – Putaminal pigments and nosology. *Brain*, **98**, 101–112

BØTTCHER, J. (1975) Morphology of the basal ganglia in Parkinson's disease. *Acta Neurologica Scandinavica*, **52**, Suppl. 62

BRAIT, K., FAHN, S. and SCHWARZ, G. A. (1973) Sporadic and familial parkinsonism and motor neuron disease. *Neurology (Minneapolis)*, **23**, 990–1002

BRZEZICKI, E. (1930) Der Parkinsonismus symptomaticus. V. Zur Frage des Parkinsonismus bei Kohlenoxydvergiftung. *Arbeiten aus dem Neurologischen Institut der Wiener Universität*, **32**, 148–208

BRODY, J. A., HIRANO, A. and SCOTT, R. M. (1971) Recent neuropathologic observations in amyotrophic lateral sclerosis and parkinsonism dementia in Guam. *Neurology (Minneapolis)*, **21**, 528–536

BUGIANI, L., MANCARDI, G. L., BRUSA, A. and EDERLI, E. (1979) The fine structure of subcortical neurofibrillary tangles in progressive supranuclear palsy. *Acta Neuropathologica*, **45**, 147–152

BUGIANI, O., PERDELLI, F., SALVARINI, S., LEONARDI, A. and MANCARDI, G. L. (1980) Loss of striatal neurons in Parkinson's disease: a cytometric study. *European Neurology*, **19**, 339–344

BUTTLAR-BRENTANO, K. VON (1955) Das Parkinsonsyndrom im Lichte der lebensgeschichtlichen Veränderungen des Nucleus basalis. *Journal für Hirnforschung*, **2**, 55–76

CANDY, J. M., PERRY, R. H., PERRY, E. K., IRVING, D., BLESSED, G., FAIRBAIRN, A. F. and TOMLINSON, B. E. (1983) Pathological changes in the nucleus of Meynert in Alzheimer's and Parkinson's disease. *Journal of Neurological Sciences*, **54**, 277–289

CHEN, K.-M., MAKIFUCHI, T., GARRUTO, R. M. and GAJDUSEK, D. C. (1982) Parkinson-dementia in a Filipino migrant: A clinicopathologic case report. *Neurology*, **32**, 1221–1226

CHIUEH, C. C., BURNS, R. S., MARKEY, S. P., JACOKOBOWITZ, D. M. and KOPIN, I. J. (1985) Primate model of parkinsonism: Selective lesion of nigrostriatal neurons by 1-methyl-4-phenyl-1,2,3,6-tetrahydropyridine produces an extrapyramidal syndrome in rhesus monkeys. *Life Sciences*, **36**, 213–218

CHRISTENSEN, E., MÖLLER, J. E. and FAURBYE, A. (1970) Neuropathological investigation of 28 brains from patients with dyskinesias. *Acta Psychiatrica Scandinavica*, **46**, 14–23

CLARK, A. W. and LEHMANN, J. (1983) Dementia with widespread Lewy bodies: Studies of the neocortical cholinergic system. *Abstract of the Canadian Association of Neuropathologists, 23rd Annual Meeting*, Sept. 29–30

CONSTANTINIDIS, J., BOURAS, C. and RICHARD, J. (1983) Putative neurotransmitters in human neuropathology; a review of topography and clinical implications. *Clinical Neuropathology*, **2**, 47–54

CORSELLIS, J. A. N., BRUTON, C. J. and FREEMAN-BROWNE, D. (1973) The aftermath of boxing. *Psychological Medicine*, **3**, 270–303

CUMMINGS, J. L. and BENSON, D. F. (1984) Subcortical dementia. Review of an emerging concept. *Archives of Neurology*, **41**, 874–879

CURCIO, C. A. and KEMPER, T. (1984) Nucleus raphe dorsalis in dementia of the Alzheimer type: Neurofibrillary changes and neuronal packing density. *Journal of Neuropathology and Experimental Neurology*, **43**, 359–368

COYLE, J. T., PRICE, D. and DE LONG, M. R. (1983) Alzheimer's disease: a disorder of cortical cholinergic innervation. *Science*, **219**, 1184–1190

DAVIES, P. (1983) Neurotransmitters and neuropeptides in Alzheimer's disease. In *Biological Aspects of Alzheimer's Disease*. Ed. R. Katzman. Banbury Report 15, pp. 255–261. Cold Spring Harbor Lab.

DAVIS, G. C., WILLIAMS, A. C., MARKEY, S. P., EBERT, M. H., CAINE, E. D., REICHERT, C. M. and KOPIN, I. J. (1979) Chronic parkinsonism secondary to intravenous injection of meperidine analogues. *Psychiatric Research*, **1**, 249–254

DEKABAN, A. S. (1978): Changes in brain weights during the span of human life. *Annals of Neurology*, **4**, 345–356

DeSMET, Y., RUBERG, M., SERDARU, M., DUBOIS, B. et al. (1982) Confusion, dementia and anticholinergic in Parkinson's disease. *Journal of Neurology, Neurosurgery and Psychiatry*, **45**, 1161–1164

DIETL, M. (1985) Etude immunocytochimique de la cholecystokinine et la tyrosine hydroxylase dans la moelle épinière chez le rat et chez l'homme. *Thèse*, Paris

DOM, R., BARO, F. and BRUCHER, J. M. (1973) Cytometric study of the putamen in different types of Huntington's chorea. *Advances in Neurology*, **1**, 369–385

DUBOIS, B., HAUW, J. J., RUBERG, M., SERDARU, M., JAVOY-AGID, F. and AGID, Y. (1985) Dementia and Parkinson's disease: Biochemical and clinico-pathological correlations. *Revue Neurologique*, **141**, 184–193

DUFFY, P. and TENNYSON, V. M. (1965) Phase and electron microscopic observations of Lewy bodies and melanin granules in the substantia nigra and locus coeruleus in Parkinson's disease. *Journal of Neuropathology and Experimental Neurology*, **24**, 398–414

DUVOISIN, R. C. and YAHR, M. D. (1965) Encephalitis and parkinsonism. *Archives of Neurology*, **12**, 227–239

EARLE, K. M. (1968) Studies on Parkinson's disease including X-ray fluorescent spectroscopy of formalin fixed brain tissue. *Journal of Neuropathology and Experimental Neurology*, **27**, 1–14

ESCOUROLLE, R., RECONDO, J. DE and GRAY, F. (1971) Etude anatomo-pathologique des syndromes parkinsonism. In *Monoamines et Noyaux Gris Centraux*. Eds. J. Ajuriaguerry and G. Gauthier, pp. 173–229. Geneva: Georg-Masson

FAHN, S. (1977) Secondary parkinsonism. In *Scientific Approaches to Clinical Neurology*. Eds. E. S. Goldensohn and S. H. Appel, pp. 1159–1189. Philadelphia: Lee and Febiger

FERRANTE, R. J., KOWALL, W. W., MARINT, J. B. and RICHARDSON, E. P. JR (1985) Characteristics of a selectively spared subset of neurons in Huntington's chorea (Abst.). *Journal of Neuropathology and Experimental Neurology*, **44**, 325

FOIX, C. and NICOLESCO, J. (1925) *Les Noyaux Gris Centraux et la Région Mésencéphalo-sous-optique*. Paris: Masson

FORNO, L. S. (1966) Pathology of parkinsonism. *Journal of Neurosurgery*, **24**, Suppl. II, 266–271

FORNO, L. S. (1969) Concentric hyaline intraneuronal inclusions of Lewy type in the brains of elderly persons (50 incidental cases): Relationship to parkinsonism. *Journal of the American Geriatric Society*, **17**, 557–575

FORNO, L. S. (1982) Pathology of Parkinson's disease. In *Movement Disorders*. Eds. D. Marsden, and S. Fahn, pp. 25–30. London: Butterworth Scientific
FORNO, L. S. and ALVORD, E. C. JR (1971) The pathology of Parkinsonism. In *Recent Advances in Parkinson's Disease*. Eds. F. H. M. McDowell and C. H. Markham, pp. 120–130. Philadelphia: F. A. Davis
FORNO, L. S., BARBOUR, P. J. and NORVILLE, R. L. (1978) Presenile dementia with Lewy bodies and neurofibrillary tangles. *Archives of Neurology*, **35**, 816–822
FORNO, L. S., GARDINER, R. E.. and ENG, L. F. (1985) Somatostatin-like immunoreactivity in the human basal ganglia (Abst.). *Journal of Neuropathology and Experimental Neurology*, **44**, 326
FORNO, L. S. and NORVILLE, R. L. (1981) Synaptic morphology in the human locus coeruleus. *Acta Neuropathologica*, **53**, 7–14
FORNO, L. S., STERNBERGER, N. R. and ENG, L. F. (1983) Immunocytochemical staining of neurofibrillary tangles and of the periphery of Lewy bodies with a monoclonal antibody to neurofilaments (Abst.). *Journal of Neuropathology and Experimental Neurology*, **42**, 342
GAMBOA, E. T., WOLF, A., YAHR, M. D. et al. (1974) Influenza virus antigen in post-encephalitic parkinsonism brain. Detection by immunofluorescence. *Archives of Neurology*, **31**, 228–232
GARCIA DE YEBENES, J., GERVAS, J. J., INGLESIAS, J., MENAJ et al. (1982) Biochemical finding in a case of parkinsonism secondary to brain tumor. *Annals of Neurology*, **11**, 313–316
GASPAR, P. and GRAY, F. (1984) Dementia in idiopathic Parkinson's disease. A neuropathological study of 32 cases. *Acta Neuropathologica*, **64**, 43–52
GHATAK, N. R., NOCHLIN, D. and HADFIELD, M. G. (1980) Neurofibrillary pathology in progressive supranuclear palsy. *Acta Neuropathologica*, **52**, 73–76
GHERARDI, R., ROUADES, B., FLEURY, J., PROBST, C. et al. (1985) Parkinsonian syndrome and central nervous system lymphoma involving the substantia nigra. *Acta Neuropathologica*, **65**, 338–343
GOLDMAN, J. E., YEN, S.-H., CHIU, F.-C. and PERESS, N. S. (1983) Lewy bodies of Parkinson's disease contain neurofilament antigens. *Science*, **221**, 1082–1084
GRAFE, M. R., FORNO, L. S. and ENG, L. F. (1983) Substance P and met-enkephalin immunoreactivity in Parkinson's, Huntington's and Alzheimer's disease (Abst.). *Journal of Neuropathology and Experimental Neurology*, **42**, 345
GREENFIELD, J. G. and BOSANQUET, F. D. (1953) The brain-stem lesions in parkinsonism. *Journal of Neurology, Neurosurgery and Psychiatry*, **16**, 213–226
GREENFIELD, J. G. and MATTHEWS, W. B. (1954) Postencephalitic parkinsonism with amyotrophy. *Journal of Neurology, Neurosurgery and Psychiatry*, **17**, 50–60
HAKIM, A. M. and MATHIESON, G. (1979) Dementia in Parkinson disease: A neuropathologic study. *Neurology*, **29**, 1209–1214
HALLERVORDEN, J. (1957) Paralysis agitans. In *Handbuch der speziellen pathologischen Anatomie und Histologie*. Ed. W. Scholz, Vol. XIII/1A, pp. 900–924. Berlin: Springer Verlag
HARDY, R. C. and STEVENSON, L. D. (1957) Syringomesencephalia. Report of a case with signs of Parkinson's disease having a syrinx of the substantia nigra. *Journal of Neuropathology and Experimental Neurology*, **16**, 356
HARTOG-JAGER, W. A. (1969) Sphingomyelin in Lewy inclusion bodies in Parkinson's disease. *Archives of Neurology*, **21**, 615–619
HARTOG-JAGER, W. A. and BETHLEM, J. (1960) The distribution of Lewy-bodies in the central and autonomic nervous systems in idiopathy paralysis agitans. *Journal of Neurology, Neurosurgery and Psychiatry*, **23**, 283–290
HASSLER, R. (1938) Zur Pathologie der Paralyse agitans und des postenzephalitischen Parkinsonism. *Journal für Psychologie und Neurologie*, **48**, 387–476
HEDREN, J. C., STRUBLE, R. G., WHITEHOUSE, P. J. and PRICE, D. L. (1984) Topography of the magnocellular basal forebrain system in human brain. *Journal of Neuropathology and Experimental Neurology*, **43**, 1–21
HEILIG, C. W., KNOPMAN, D. S., MASTRI, A. R. and FREY, W. (1985) Dementia without Alzheimer pathology. *Neurology*, **35**, 762–765
HIRANO, A. (1971) Electron Microscopy in Neuropathology. In *Progress in Neuropathology*. Ed. H. M. Zimmrman, Vol. I, pp. 1–61. New York: Grune and Stratton
HIRANO, A., MALAMUD, N. and KURLAND, L. T. (1961) Parkinsonism–dementia complex, an endemic disease on the island of Guam. II – Pathological features. *Brain*, **84**, 662–679
HIRSCH, E., RUBERG, M., DARDENNE, M., PORTIER, M. M., JAVOY-AGID, F., BACH, J. F. and AGID, Y. (1985) Monoclonal antibodies raised against Lewy bodies in brains from subjects with Parkinson's disease. *Brain Research*, **345**, 374–378
HO, K. C., ROESSMANN, U., STRAUMFJORD, J. V. and MONROE, G. (1980) Analysis of brain weight. *Archives of Pathology and Laboratory Medicine*, **104**, 635–639

HORNYKIEWICZ, O. (1982) Brain neurotransmitter changes in Parkinson's disease. In *Movement Disorders*. Eds. C. D. Marsden and S. Fahn, pp. 41–58. London: Butterworths
HORNYKIEWICZ, O. and KISH, S. J. (1984) Neurochemical basis of dementia in Parkinson's disease. *Canadian Journal of Neurological Sciences*, **11**, 185–190
HUDSON, A. J. (1981) Amyotrophic lateral sclerosis and its association with dementia, parkinsonism, and other neurological disorders. A review. *Brain*, **104**, 217–247
HUHN, B. and JAKOB, H. (1971) Traumatische Hirnstammläsionen mit vieljähriger Überlebensdauer. Beitrag zur Pathologie der Substantia nigra und der oralen Brückenhaube. *Nervenarzt*, **41**, 326–334
HUNTER, S. (1985) The rostral mesencephalon in Parkinson's and Alzheimer's disease. *Acta Neuropathologica* (in press)
IKEDA, K., IKEDA, S., YOSHIMURA, T., KATO, H. and NAMBA, M. (1978) Idiopathic parkinsonism with Lewy-type inclusions in cerebral cortex. A case report. *Acta Neuropathologica*, **41**, 165–168
ISHII, T. (1966) Distribution of Alzheimer's neurofibrillary tangles in the brainstem and hypothalamus in senile dementia. *Acta Neuropathologica*, **6**, 181–187
ISHII, T. and NAKAMURA, Y. (1981) Distribution and ultrastructure of Alzheimer's neurofibrillary tangles in postencephalitic parkinsonism of Economo type. *Acta Neuropathologica*, **55**, 59–62
JACOB, H. (1978) Neuropathologie des Parkinson-Syndroms und die Demenz des Gehirns. In *Langzeitbehandlung des Parkinsonsyndroms*. Ed. P. A. Fischer, pp. 5–25. Stuttgart: Schattauer
JACOB, H. (1983) Klinische Neuropathologie des Parkinsonismus. In *Pathophysiologie, Klinik und Therapie des Parkinsonismus*. Eds. H. Gänshirt, P. Berlit and G. Haack, pp. 5–18. Basle: ed.Roche
JANKOVIC, J., KIRKPATRICK, J. B., BLOMQUIST, K. A., LANGLAIS, P. J. and BIRD, E. D. (1985) Late-onset Hallervorden–Spatz disease presenting as familial parkinsonism. *Neurology*, **35**, 227–234
JAVOY-AGID, F., RUBERG, M., TAQUER, H., BOBOBZA, B. and AGID, Y. (1984) Biochemical neuropathology of Parkinson's disease. *Advances in Neurology*, **40**, 189–197
JAVOY-AGID, F., TAQUET, H., CESSELIN, F., EPELBAUM, J., GROUSELLE, D., MAUBORGNE, A., STUDLER, J. M. and AGID, Y. (1984) Neuropeptides in Parkinson's disease. In *Catecholamines: Neuropharmacology and Central Nervous System – Therapeutic Aspects*. Ed. E. Usdin, pp. 35–42. New York: A. R. Liss
JELLINGER, K. (1966) Läsionen des extrapyramidalen Systems bei akuten und protrahierten Komazuständen. *Wiener Zeitschrift für Nervenheilkunde*, **23**, 40–73
JELLINGER, K. (1968) Degenerations and exogenous lesions of the globus pallidus, caudate and lenticular nucleus. In *Handbook of Clinical Neurology*. Eds. P. Vinken and G. W. Bruyn, Vol. 6, pp. 632–693. Amsterdam: North Holland
JELLINGER, K. (1974) Pathomorphologie des Parkinson-Syndroms. *Aktuelle Neurologie*, **1**, 83–98
JELLINGER, K. (1977) Neuropathologic findings after neuroleptic long-term therapy. In *Neurotoxicology*. Eds. H. Shiraki and N. Grcevic, pp. 25–42. New York: Raven Press
JELLINGER, K. (1986) Pathology of parkinsonism. In *Recent Developments in Parkinsonism*. Eds. S. Fahn, C. D. Marsden and R. Duvoisin, pp. 33–66. New York: Raven Press
JELLINGER, K. and DANIELOZYK, W. (1968) Striato-nigrale degeneration. *Acta Neuropathologica*, **10**, 242–257
JELLINGER, K., GRISOLD, W. and VOLLMER, R. (1983) Hirnatrophie bei Morbus Parkinson und (prä)seniler Demenz. In *Fortschritte der klinischen Neurologie*. Eds. G. Schnaberth and K. Pateisky, pp. 151–164. Stuttgart: G. Thieme
JELLINGER, K. and NEUMAYER, E. (1972) Unusual late-onset type of Hallervorden–Spatz disease: clinico-pathological study of a case presenting as parkinsonism. *Zeitschrift für die gesamte Neurologie*, **203**, 105–118
JELLINGER, K. and RIEDERER, P. (1984) Dementia in Parkinson's disease and (pre)senile dementia of Alzheimer type: Morphological aspects and changes in the intracerebral MAO activity. *Advances in Neurology*, **40**, 199–210
JELLINGER, K., RIEDERER, P. and TOMONAGA, M. (1980) Progressive supranuclear palsy: Clinico-pathological and biochemical studies. *Journal of Neural Transmission*, **16**, 111–128
JELLINGER, K. and TARNOWSKY-DZIDUSZKO, E. (1971) Die ZNS-Veränderungen bei den olivo-ponto-zerebellaren Atrophien. *Zeitschrift für Neurologie*, **199**, 192–214
JØRGENSEN, O. S., REYNOLDS, G. P., RIEDERER, P. and JELLINGER, K. (1982) Parkinson's disease putamen: Normal concentration of synaptic membrane marker antigens. *Journal of Neural Transmissions*, **54**, 171–179
JOHNSON, R. H., LEE, G. DE J., OPPENHEIMER, D. R. and SPALDING, J. M. K. (1966) Autonomic failure with orthostatic hypotension due to intermediolateral column degeneration. *Quarterly Journal of Medicine*, **35**, 276–292
JOYNT, R. J. and McNEILL, T. H. (1984) Neuropeptides in aging and dementia. *Peptides*, **5** (Suppl. 1), 269–274
KAIYA, H. (1974) Spino-olivo-ponto-cerebello-nigral atrophy with Lewy bodies and binucleated nerve cells. A case report. *Acta Neuropathologica*, **30**, 263–269

KAIYA, H. and MEHRAEIN, P. (1974) Zur Klinik und pathologischen Anatomié des Muskelatrophie – Parkinsonismus–Demenz–Syndroms. *Archiv für Psychiatrie und Nervenkrankheiten*, **219**, 13–27
KAN, A. (1978) Striatonigral degeneration. *Pathology*, **10**, 54–57
KIMULA, Y., UTSUYAMA, M., YOSHIMURA, M. and TOMONAGA, M. (1983) Element analysis of Lewy and adrenal bodies in Parkinson's diseae by electron probe microanalysis. *Acta Neuropathologica*, **59**, 233–236
KLAUE, R. (1940) Parkinsonsche Krankheit (Paralysis agitans) und postenzephalitischer Parkinsonismus. Versuch einer klinisch-anatomischen Differentialdiagnose. *Archiv für Psychiatrie und Nervenkrankheiten*, **111**, 251–321
KLAWANS, H. L., LUPTON, M. and SIMON, L. (1976) Calcification of the basal ganglia as a cause of levodopa resistant parkinsonism. *Neurology*, **26**, 221–225
KOEPPEN, A. H., BARRON, K. D. and COX, G. L. (1971) Striato-nigral degeneration. *Acta Neuropathologica*, **19**, 10–19
KONO, C., MATUBARA, M. and INAGAKI, T. (1976) Idiopathic orthostatic hypotension with numerous Lewy bodies in the sympathetic ganglia. *Neurological Medicine*, **4**, 568–570
KOSAKA, K. (1978) Lewy bodies in cerebral cortex. Report of three cases. *Acta Neuropathologica*, **42**, 127–134
KOSAKA, K. and MEHRAEIN, P. (1979) Dementia–Parkinsonism syndrome with numerous Lewy bodies and senile plaques in cerebral cortex. *Archiv für Psychiatrie und Nervenkrankheiten*, **226**, 241–250
KOSAKA, K., YOSHIMURA, M., IKEDA, K. and BUDKA, H. (1984) Diffuse type of Lewy body disease. *Clinical Neuropathology*, **3**, 185–192
KRISTENSEN, M. O. (1985) Progressive supranuclear palsy – 20 years later. *Acta Neurologica Scandinavica*, **71**, 177–189
LANGE, H. N. and BOGERTS, B. (1982) Postencephalitic and idiopathic parkinsonism. Quantitative change of tel-, di-, mesencephalon and basal ganglia (Abst.). *Neurosciences*, Suppl. 17, 127
LANGSTON, J. W., BALLARD, P., TETRUD, J. W. and IRWIN, I. (1983) Chronic parkinsonism in humans due to a product of meperidine-analog synthesis. *Science*, **219**, 979–980
LANGSTON, J. W., FORNO, L. S., REBERT, C. S. and IRWIN, J. (1984) Selective nigral toxicity after systemic administration of 1-methyl-4-phenyl-1,2,5,6-tetrahydropyridine (MPTP) in the squirrel monkey. *Brain Research*, **292**, 390–394
LAPRESLE, J. and FARDEAU, M. (1967) The central nervous system and carbon monoxide poisoning. II. Anatomical study of brain lesions following intoxication with carbon monoxide (22 cases). *Progress in Brain Research*, **24**, 31–74
LEWIS, P. D. (1971) Parkinsonism – neuropathology. *British Medical Journal*, **3**, 690–697
LEWY, F. H. (1913) Zur pathologischen Anatomie der Paralysis agitans. *Deutsche Zeitschrift für Nervenheilkunde*, **50**, 50–55
LIEBERMAN, A. M., DZIATOLOWSKI, M., KUPERSMITH, M., SERBY, M., GOODGOLD, A., KORBIN, J. and GOLDSTEIN, M. A. (1979) Dementia in Parkinson's disease. *Annals of Neurology*, **6**, 355–359
LINDENBERG, R. (1964) Die Schädigungsmechanismen der Substantia nigra bei Hirntraumen und das Problem des posttraumatischen Parkinsonismus. *Deutsche Zeitschrift für Nervenheilkinde*, **185**, 637–663
McGEER, P. L. and McGEER, E. G. (1976) Enzymes associated with metabolism of catecholamines, acetylcholine and GABA in human controls and patients with Parkinson's disease and Huntington's chorea. *Journal of Neurochemistry*, **26**, 65–76
McGEER, P. L., McGEER, E. G. and SUZUKI, J. (1984) Aging, Alzheimer's disease, and the cholinergic system of the basal forebrain. *Neurology*, **34**, 741–745
MANN, D. M. A. and YATES, P. O. (1983a) Pathological basis for neurotransmitter changes in Parkinson's disease. *Neuropathology and Applied Neurobiology*, **9**, 3–19
MANN, D. M. A. and YATES, P. O. (1983b) Possible role of neuromelanin in the pathogenesis of Parkinson's disease. *Mechanism of Ageing and Development*, **21**, 193–203
MANN, D. M. A., YATES, P. O. and HAWKES, J. (1983) The pathology of the human locus coeruleus. *Clinical Neuropathology*, **2**, 1–7
MANN, D. M. A., YATES, P. O. and MARCYNIUK, B. (1984) Changes in nerve cells of the nucleus basalis of Meynert in Alzheimer's disease and their relationship to aging and to the accumulation of lipofuscin pigment. *Mechanism of Ageing and Development*, **25**, 189–204
MARTIN, J. P. (1965) The globus pallidus in post-encephalitic parkinsonism. *Journal of the Neurological Sciences*, **2**, 344–365
MATA, M., DOROVINI-ZIS, K., WILSON, M. and YOUNG, A. B. (1983) A new form of familial Parkinson-dementia syndrome: Clinical and pathologic findings. *Neurology*, **33**, 1439–1443
MAYEUX, R. and STERN, Y. (1983) Intellectual dysfunction and dementia in Parkinson disease. In *The Dementias*. Eds. R. Mayeux and W. G. Rosen. New York: Raven Press

MESULAM, M. M., MUFSON, E. J., LEVEY, A. L. et al. (1983) Cholinergic innervation of cortex by the basal forebrain. *Journal of Comparative Neurology*, **214**, 170–197

MIZUTANI, T., ODA, M., ABE, H., FUKUDA, S., OIKAWA, H. and KOSAKA, K. (1983) Hereditary multisystemic degeneration with unusual combination of cerebellipetal, dentato-rubral, and nigro-subthalamo-pallidal degeneration. *Clinical Neuropathology*, **2**, 147–153

MIYASAKI, K. and FUJITA, T. (1977) Parkinsonism following encephalitis of unknown etiology. *Journal of Neuropathology and Experimental Neurology*, **34**, 1–8

MONMY, Y., TAKAMATU, K., OGASAWARA, S. and ITO, T. (1979) An autopsy case of atypical presenile dementia with numerous Lewy bodies. *Advances in Neurological Sciences*, **23**, 398–599

MORSIER, G. DE (1960) Parkinsonism consecutif à une lesion traumatique du noyau rouge et du locus niger. *Psychiatrica et Neurologia (Basel)*, **139**, 60–84

MOSSAKOWSKI, M. J. and MATHIESON, G. (1961) A parkinsonian syndrome in the course of subacute encephalitis. *Neurology (Minneapolis)*, **11**, 461–469

NAGATSU, T., OKA, K., YAMAMOTO, T., MATSUI, H. et al. (1981) Catecholaminergic enzymes in Parkinson's disease and related extrapyramidal diseases. In *Transmitter, Biochemistry of Human Tissue*. Eds. P. Riederer and E. Usdin, pp. 291–302. London: Macmillan

NAKANO, K. K., DAWSON, D. M. and SPENCE, A. (1972) Machado disease: a hereditary ataxia in Portuguese immigrants to Massachusetts. *Neurology (Minneapolis)*, **22**, 49–55

NAKANO, I. and HIRANO, A. (1983) Neuron loss in the nucleus basalis of Meynert in Parkinson-dementiaa complex of Guam. *Annals of Neurology*, **13**, 87–91

NAKANO, I. and HIRANO, A. (1984) Parkinson's disease: Neuron loss in the nucleus basalis without concomitant Alzheimer's disease. *Annals of Neurology*, **15**, 415–418

NAKASHIMA, S. and IKUTA, F. (1984a) Catecholamine neurons with Alzheimer's neurofibrillary changes and alteration of tyrosine hydroxylase: Immunohistochemical investigation of tyrosine hydroxylase. *Acta Neuropathologica*, **64**, 273–280

NAKASHIMA, S. and IKUTA, F. (1984b) Tyrosin hydroxylase proteins in Lewy bodies of parkinsonism and senile brain. *Journal of Neurological Sciences*, **66**, 91–96

NAKASHIMA, S., KUMANISHI, T. and IKUTA, F. (1983) Immunohistochemistry on tyrosine hydroxylase in the substantia nigra of human autopsied cases. *Brain and Nerve*, **35**, 1023–1029

NAKAZATO, Y., SASAKI, A., HIRATO, J. and ISHIDA, Y. (1984) Immunohistochemical localization of neurofilament protein in neuronal degenerations. *Acta Neuropathologica*, **64**, 30–36

NEUMAYER, E. (1971) Kombination von Morbus Parkinson mit anderen zentralnervösen Krankheiten. *Zeitschrift für die gesamte Neurologie*, **199**, 306–318

OHAMA, E. and IKUTA, F. (1976) Parkinson's disease. Distribution of Lewy bodies and monoamine neuron system. *Acta Neuropathologica*, **34**, 311–319

OKAZAKI, H., LIPKIN, L. E. and ARONSON, S. M. (1961) Diffuse intracytoplasmic ganglionic inclusions (Lewy type) associated with progressive dementia and quadriparesis in flexion. *Journal of Neuropathology and Experimental Neurology*, **20**, 237–244

OPPENHEIMER, D. R. (1983) Multiple system atrophy and the Shy–Drager syndrome. In *Spinocerebellar Degenerations*. Ed. I. Sobue, pp. 165–169. Tokyo: Tokyo University Press

PAKKENBERG, H. (1963) Globus pallidus in parkinsonism. *Acta Neurologica Scandinavica*, **39**, 139–144

PAKKENBERG, H. and BRODY, H. (1965) The number of nerve cells in the substantia nigra in paralysis agitans. *Acta Neuropathologica*, **5**, 320–324

PARISI, J. E. and BURNS, R. S. (1985) MPTP-induced parkinsonism in man and experimental animals (Abst.) *Journal of Neuropathology and Experimental Neurology*, **44**, 325

PARNITZKE, K. H. and PEIFFER, J. (1956) Zur Klinik und pathologischen Anatomie der chronischen Braunsteinvergiftung. *Archiv für Psychiatrie und Nervenkrankheit*, **192**, 405–427

PEARCE, G. W. (1979) The neuropathology of parkinsonism. In *Recent Advances in Neuropathology*. Eds. W. T. Smith and J. B. Canavagh, Vol. I, pp. 299–320. London: Churchill-Livingstone

PEARSON, J. (1983) Neurotransmitter immunocytochemistry in the study of human development, anatomy and pathology. *Progress in Neuropathology*, **5**, 41–97

PEARSON, J., GOLDSTEIN, M., MARKEY, K. and BRANDEIS, L. (1983) Human brain stem catecholamine neuronal anatomy as indicated by immunocytochemistry with antibodies to tyrosine hydroxylase. *Neuroscience*, **8**, 3–32

PEIFFER, J. (1963) Symmetrische Pallidum- und Nigranekrosen nach unbemerkt gebliebenem Zwischenfall bei Barbituratnarkose. *Deutsche Zeitschrift für Nervenheilkunde*, **184**, 586–606

PERRY, R. H., CANDY, H., PERRY, E. K., IRVING, D., BLESSED, G. et al. (1983a) Extensive loss of choline acetyltransferase activity is not reflected by neuronal loss in the nucleus basalis of Meynert in Alzheimer's disease. *Neuroscience Letters*, **33**, 311–315

PERRY, R. H., TOMLINSON, B. E., CANDY, J. M., BLESSED, G. et al. (1983b) Cortical cholinergic deficit in mentally impaired Parkinsonian patients. *Lancet*, **ii**, 789–790

PERRY, T. L., BRATTY, P. J. A., HANSEN, S. et al. (1975) Hereditary mental depression and parkinsonism with taurine deficiency. *Archives of Neurology,* **32,** 108–113

POWELL, H. C., LONDON, G. W. and LAMPERT, P. W. (1974) Neurofibrillary tangles in progressive supranuclear palsy. Electron microscopic observations. *Journal of Neuropathology and Experimental Neurology,* **33,** 98–106

PRICE, D. L., WHITEHOUSE, P. J., STRUBLE, R. G. et al. (1983) Basal forebrain cholinergic neurons and neuritic plaques in primate brain. In *Biological Aspects of Alzheimer's Disease.* Ed. R. Katzman. Banbury Report 15, pp. 65–77. Cold Spring Harbor Lab.

PROBST, A. (1977) Dégenérescence neurofibrillaire sous-corticale sénile avec presence de tubule contournés et de filaments droits. *Revue Neurologique,* **133,** 417–428

PURDY, A., HAHN, A., BARNETT, H. J. M., BRATTY, P. et al. (1979) Familial fatal Parkinsonism with alveolar hypoventilation and mental depression. *Annals of Neurology,* **6,** 523–531

RAIL, D., SCHOLTZ, C. and SWASH, M. (1981) Post-encephalitic parkinsonism: current experience. *Journal of Neurology, Neurosurgery and Psychiatry,* **44,** 670–676

RAJPUT, A. H., ROZDILSKY, B., HORNYKIEWICZ, O., SHANNAK, K. et al. (1982) Reversible drug-induced Parkinsonism. Clinicopathologic study of two cases. *Archives of Neurology,* **39,** 644–646

RICHARDSON, E. P. JR (1965) Remarks on the pathology of Parkinson's disease. In *Parkinson's Disease: Trends in Research and Treatment.* Eds. A. Barbeau, L. J. Doshay and E. A. Spiegel, pp. 63–68. New York: Grune and Stratton

RIEDERER, P., BIRKMAYER, W., SEEMANN, D. and WUKETICH, S. (1977) Brain noradrenalin and 3-methoxy-4-hydroxy-phenylglycol in Parkinson's syndrome. *Journal of Neural Transmission,* **41,** 241–251

ROESSMANN, U., VAN DER NOURT, S. and McFARLAND, D. E. (1971) Idiopathic orthostatic hypotension. *Archives of Neurology,* **24,** 503–510

ROGERS, J. D., BROGAN, D. and MIRRA, S. S. (1985) The nucleus basalis of Meynert in neurological disease: A quantitative morphological study. *Annals of Neurology,* **17,** 163–170

ROMANUL, F. C. A., FOWLER, H. L., RADVANY, J., FELDMAN, R. G. and FEINGOLD, M. (1977) Azores disease of the nervous system. *New England Journal of Medicine,* **296,** 1505–1508

ROOS, R., GAJDUSEK, D. C. and GIBBS, C. J. JR (1973) The clinical characteristics of transmissible Creutzfeldt–Jakob disease. *Brain,* **96,** 1–30

ROSENBERG, N. (1984) Joseph disease, an autosomal motor system degeneration. *Advances in Neurology,* **41,** 179–194

ROSENBLUM, W. I. and GHATAK, N. R. (1979) Lewy bodies in the presence of Alzheimer's disease. *Archives of Neurology,* **36,** 170–171

ROSSOR, M. N., SVEDSEN, C., HUNT, S. P., MOUNTJOY, C. Q., ROTH, M. and IVERSEN, L. I. (1984) The substantia innominata in Alzheimer's disease; An histochemical and biochemical study of cholinergic marker enzymes. *Neuroscience Letters,* **28,** 217–222

ROY, S. and WOLMAN, L. (1969) Ultrastructural observations in parkinsonism. *Journal of Pathology,* **99,** 39–44

RUDELLI, R. D., AMBLER, M. W. and WISNIEWSKI, H. M. (1984) Morphology and distribution of Alzheimer neuritic (senile) and amyloid plaques in striatum and diencephalon. *Acta Neuropathologica,* **64,** 273–281

SABANCU, N. (1969) Quantitative Untersuchungen am Pallidum beim Parkinsonsyndrom. *Deutsche Zeitschrift für Nervenheilkunde,* **196,** 40–48

SACHDEV, H. S., FORNO, L. S. and KANE, C. A. (1982) Joseph disease a multisystem degenerative disorder of the nervous system. *Neurology,* **32,** 192–195

SAPER, C. B., GERMAN, D. C. and WHITE, C. L. III (1985) Neuronal pathology in the nucleus basalis and associated cell groups in senile dementia of the Alzheimer's type: Possible role in cell loss. *Neurology,* **35,** 1089–1095

SCHMITT, H. P., EMSER, W. and HEIMES, C. (1984) Familial occurrence of amyotrophic lateral sclerosis, parkinsonism and dementia. *Annals of Neurology,* **16,** 642–648

SCHNEIDER, E., BECKER, H., FISCHER, P. A. et al. (1979) The course of brain atrophy in Parkinson's disease. *Archiv für Psychiatrie und Nervenkrankheit,* **227,** 89–95

SCHOCHET, S. S., WYATT, R. and McCORMICK, W. F. (1970) Intracytoplasmic acidophilic granules in the substantia nigra. *Archives of Neurology,* **22,** 550–555

SCHWAB, R. and ENGLAND, A. D. (1968) Parkinson syndromes due to various specific causes. In *Handbook of Clinical Neurology.* Eds. P. Vinken and G. W. Bruyn, Vol. 6, pp. 227–247. Amsterdam: North Holland

SEITELBERGER, F., JACOB, H., PEIFFER, J. and COLMANT, J. (1967) The myoclonic variant of cerebral lipidosis. In *Inborn Disorders of Spingolipid Metabolism.* Eds. St. M. Aronson and B. W. Volk, pp. 43–47. New York: Macmillan-Pergamon

SHIRAKI, H. and YASE, Y. (1975) Amyotrophic lateral sclerosis in Japan. In *Handbook of Clinical Neurology*. Eds. P. Vinken and G. W. Bruyn, Vol. 22, pp. 353–419. Amsterdam: Elsevier
SJÖGREN, T., SJÖGREN, H. and LINDGREN, A. G. H. (1952) Morbus Alzheimer and Morbus Pick. A genetic, clinical and pathoanatomical study. *Acta Psychiatrica Scandinavica Supplementum*, **81**, 1–152
SROKA, H., ELIZAN, T. S., YAHR, M. O. et al. (1981) Organic mental syndrome and confusional states in Parkinson's disease. *Archives of Neurology*, **38**, 339–342
STADLAN, E. M., DUVOISIN, R. and YAHR, M. D. (1966) The pathology of parkinsonism. *Proceedings of the 5th International Congress of Neuropathologists*. ICS 100, pp. 569–471. Amsterdam: Excerpta Medica
STADLER, H. (1936) Zur Histopathologie des Gehirns bei Manganvergiftung. *Zeitschrift für die gesamte Neurologie*, **154**, 62–76
STEELE, J. C., RICHARDSON, J. C. and OLSZEWSKI, J. (1964) Progressive supranuclear palsy. *Archives of Neurology*, **10**, 333–359
STEINER, I., GOMORI, J. M. and MELAMED, E. (1985) Features of brain atrophy in Parkinson's disease. A CT scan study. *Neuroradiology*, **27**, 158–160
STOCKHAUSEN, P. and BRAAK, H. (1984) Morphological changes of the isocortex in Morbus Parkinson. *Clinical Neuropathology*, **3**, 206–209
STRUBLE, R. G., CORK, L. C., WHITEHOUSE, P. J. et al. (1982) Cholinergic innervation in neuritic plaques. *Science*, **216**, 413–415
STRUBLE, R. G., POWERS, R. E., CASANOVA, M. F., KITT, C. A., O'CONNOR, D. T. and PRICE, D. L. (1985) Multiple transmitter-specific markers in senile plaque in Alzheimer's disease (Abstr). *Journal of Neuropathology and Experimental Neurology*, **44**, 325
SUGIMURA, K., YAMASAKI, Y. and ANDO, K. (1977) Parkinson's disease accompanied by dementia. A case of concurrent Parkinson's and Alzheimer's diseases. *Rinsho Shin*, **12**, 513–519
TABATON, M., SCHENONE, A., ROMAGNOLI, P. and MANCARDI, G. L. (1985) A quantitative and ultrastructural study of substantia nigra and nucleus centralis superior in Alzheimer's disease. *Acta Neuropathologica*, **68**, 218–223
TAGLIAVINI, F. and PILLERI, G. (1983) Basal nucleus of Meynert. A neuropathological study in Alzheimer's disease, simple senile dementia, Pick's disease and Huntington's chorea. *Journal of Neurological Sciences*, **62**, 243–260
TAGLIAVINI, F. and PILLERI, G. (1985) Neuronal loss in the nucleus basalis of Meynert in a patient with olivopontocerebellar atrophy. *Acta Neuropathologica*, **66**, 127–133
TAGLIAVINI, F., PILLERI, G., BOURAS, C. and CONSTANDINIDIS, J. (1984a) The nucleus basalis of Meynert in idiopathic Parkinson's disease. *Acta Neurologica Scandinavica*, **69**, 20–28
TAGLIAVINI, F., PILLERI, G., BOURAS, C. and CONSTANTINIDIS, J. (1984b) The basal nucleus of Meynert in patients with progressive supranuclear palsy. *Neuroscience Letters*, **44**, 37–42
TAKAUCHI, S., MIZUMARA, T. and MIYOSHI, K. (1983) Unusual paired helical filaments in progressive supranuclear palsy. *Acta Neuropathologica*, **59**, 225–228
TAKEDA, S., OHAMA, E., IZUMO, S. et al. (1982) Substantia nigra and locus coeruleus in Parkinson-dementia complex of Guam and OPCA. In *Abstract of the IXth International Congress of Neuropathologists*. Eds. F. Seitelberger, H. Lassmann and K. Jellinger, p. 115. Vienna, Wiener Medizinische Akademie
TAKEI, Y. and MIRRA, S. S. (1973) Striatonigral degeneration, a form of multisystem atrophy with clinical parkinsonism. In *Progress in Neuropathology*, Ed. H. M. Zimmerman, Vol. 2, pp. 217–251. New York: Grune and Stratton
TELLEZ-NAGEL, I. and WISNIEWSKI, H. M. (1973) Ultrastructure of neurofibrillary tangles in Steele–Richardson–Olszewski syndrome. *Archives of Neurology*, **29**, 324–327
TERRY, R. D. (1983) Cortical morphometry in Alzheimer disease. In *Biological Aspects of Alzheimer's Disease*. Ed. R. Katzman, Banbury Report 15, pp. 95–103. Cold Spring Harbor Lab.
TOHGI, H. (1977) Arteriosclerotic parkinsonism: a reassessment. *Eleventh World Congress of Neurologists, International Congress series 427*, p. 200. Amsterdam: Excerpta Medica
TOLPPANEN, L. (1971) Quantitativ-mikroskopische Untersuchungen an der Substantia nigra des Menschen. Fälle ohne Bewegungsstörungen in Vergleich mit Fällen von Parkinson-Syndrom. Dissertation, Universität Göttingen
TOMLINSON, B. E., IRVING, D. and BLESSED, G. (1981) Cell loss in the locus coeruleus in senile dementia of the Alzheimer type. *Journal of Neurological Sciences*, **49**, 419–428
TOMONAGA, M. (1977) Ultrastructure of neurofibrillary tangles in progressive supranuclear palsy. *Acta Neuropathologica*, **37**, 177–181
TOMONAGA, M. (1979) Neurofibrillary tangles and Lewy bodies in the locus coeruleus neurons of the aged brain. *Acta Neuropathologica*, **53**, 165–168
TORVIK, A. and MEEN, C. (1966) Distribution of the brain stem lesions in postencephalitic parkinsonism. *Acta Neurologica Scandinavica*, **42**, 414–425

TRETIAKOFF, C. (1919) Contribution à l'étude d l'anatomia pathologique du locus niger. *Thèse*, Université de Paris
UHL, G. R., HEDREEN, J. C. and PRICE, D. L. (1985) Parkinson's disease: Loss of neurons from the ventral tegmental area contralateral to therapeutical surgical lesions. *Neurology*, **35**, 1215–1218
UHL, G. R., McKINNEY, M., HEDREEN, J. C., WHITE, C. L., COYLE, J. T., WHITEHOUSE, P. J. and PRICE, D. L. (1982) Dementia pugilistica: loss of basal forebrain cholinergic neurons and cortical cholinergic markers. *Annals of Neurology*, **12**, 99
UITTI, R. J., RAJPUT, A. H., ASHENHURST, E. M. and ROZDILSKY, B. (1985) Cyanide-induced parkinsonism: A clinicopathologic study. *Neurology (Minneapolis)*, **35**, 921–925
UNGERSTEDT, U. (1971) Sterotaxic mapping of the monoamine pathways in the rat brain. *Acta Physiologica Scandinavica*, **64** (Suppl. 247), 37–118
VANDERHAEGHEN, J. J., OLIVIER, P. and STERNON, J. (1970) Pathological findings in idiopathic hypotension, its relationship with Parkinson's disease. *Archives of Neurology and Psychiatry*, **22**, 207–214
VIJAYASHANKAR, N. and BRODY, H. (1979) A quantitative study of the pigmented neurons in the nucleus locu-coeruleus and subcoeruleus in man as related to aging. *Journal of Neuropathology and Experimental Neurology*, **38**, 490–497
WHITEHOUSE, P. J., HENDREEN, J. C., WHITE, C. L. and PRICE, D. L. (1983) Basal forebrain neurons in the dementia of Parkinson's disease. *Annals of Neurology*, **13**, 243–248
WHITEHOUSE, P. J., PRICE, D. L., STRUBLE, R. G., CLARK, A. W. et al. (1982) Alzheimer's disease and senile dementia: Loss of neurons in the basal forebrain. *Science*, **215**, 1227–1229
WILCOCK, G. K. and ESIRI, M. M. (1982) Plaques and dementia: A quantitative study. *Journal of the Neurological Sciences*, **56**, 343–356
WISNIEWSKI, H. M. and MERZ, G. S. (1985) Neuropathology of the aging brain and dementia of Alzheimer type. In *Aging 2000; Our Health Care Destiny*. Eds. C. H. Haitz and T. Samorajski, Vol. 1 Biomedical Issue, pp. 231–243. Berlin: Springer
WISNIEWSKI, H. M., TERRY, R. D. and HIRANO, A. (1970) Neurofibrillary pathology. *Journal of Neuropathology and Experimental Neurology*, **29**, 163–176
WISNIEWSKI, H. M. and WEN, G. Y. (1985) Substructures of paired helical filaments from Alzheimer neurofibrillary tangles. *Acta Neuropathologica*, **66**, 173–176
WOODS, B. T. and SCHAUMBURG, H. H. (1972) Nigro-spinal-dental degeneration with nuclear ophthalmoplegia. *Journal of the Neurological Sciences*, **17**, 149–166
WUKETICH, S., RIEDERER, P., JELLINGER, K. and AMBROZI, L. (1980) Quantitative dissection of human brain areas. *Journal of Neural Transmission*, Suppl. 16, 53–67
YAGISHITA, S., ITOH, Y., AMANO, N., NAKANO, T. and SAITOH, A. (1979) Ultrastructure of neurofibrillary tangles in progressive supranuclear palsy. *Acta Neuropathologica*, **48**, 27–30
YAHR, M. D., WOLF, A., ANTUNES, J.-L., MIYOSHI, K. and DUFFY, P. (1972) Autopsy findings in parkinsonism following treatment with levodopa. *Neurology*, Suppl. 56–71
YAKOVLEW, P. I. (1944) Anatomo-clinical report of a case of carbon monoxide poisoning with survival for forty-nine years. Correlation of evolution of extrapyramidal symptoms and structural organization of motor pathways of the forebrain. *Archives of Neurology and Psychiatry*, **51**, 494
YAMADA, M. and MEHRAEIN, P. (1977) Verteilungsmuster der senilen Veränderungen in den Hirnstammkernen. *Folia Psychiatrica Neurologica Japanica*, **31**, 219–224
YAMAMOTO, T. and HIRANO, A. (1985a) Nucleus raphe dorsalis in Alzheimer's disease. Neurofibrillary tangles and loss of neurons. *Annals of Neurology*, **17**, 573–577
YAMAMOTO, T. and HIRANO, A. (1985b) Nucleus raphe dorsalis in Parkinson's dementia complex of Guam. *Acta Neuropathologica*, **67**, 296–299
YEN, S. H., HOROUPIAN, D. S. and TERRY, R. D. (1983) Immunocytochemical comparison of neurofibrillary tangles in senile dementia of Alzheimer type, progressive supranuclear palsy, and postencephalitic parkinsonism. *Annals of Neurology*, **13**, 172–175
YOSHIMURA, M. (1983) Cortical changes in the Parkinsonian brain: A contribution to the delineation of "diffuse Lewy body disease". *Journal of Neurology*, **229**, 17–32
ZECH, M. and BOGERTS, B. (1985) Methionine, enkephalin and substance P in the basal ganglia of schizophrenics; a quantitative immunohistochemical comparison with Huntington and Parkinson patients. *Acta Neuropathologica*, **68**, 32–38

10
Biochemistry of neurotransmitters in Parkinson's disease

Yves Agid, France Javoy-Agid and Merle Ruberg

In 1817, James Parkinson published the seminal description of the disease to which his name is given. In 1912, Lewy described a neuropathological anomaly, thereafter known as the 'Lewy body', necessary for a confirmed diagnosis of Parkinson's disease. In 1919, Tretiakoff demonstrated that cell loss is localized in the substantia nigra. Thus emerged the anatomoclinical concept of Parkinson's disease, distinguishing idiopathic Parkinson's disease from other parkinsonian syndromes, some of which are reversible, such as neuroleptic-induced parkinsonism, and some not. Certain syndromes are rare: post-encephalitic parkinsonism (following the Von Economo encephalitis epidemic), toxic syndromes induced by carbon monoxide, manganese or MPTP (1-methyl-4-phenyl-1,2,3,6-tetrahydropyridine) and trauma-induced syndromes, as observed in professional boxers. More frequent are the degenerative parkinsonian syndromes, the most common of which is Parkinson's disease itself, an entity that must be distinguished from progressive supranuclear palsy (characterized histologically by the diffuse presence of neurofibrillary tangles), olivopontocerebellar atrophy and multiple-system atrophies (including striatonigral degeneration, Shy–Drager syndrome) and many others (*see* Escourolle, De Recondo and Gray, 1970).

In the 1960s, the biochemistry underlying Parkinson's disease began to be analysed. Carlsson showed that reserpine administered to rats caused catatonia, associated with decreased brain dopamine concentrations, that could be reversed by restoring normal dopamine concentrations with the dopamine precursor levodopa (Carlsson, Lindquist, Magnusson, 1957; Carlsson *et al.*, 1958). In 1960, Ehringer and Hornykiewicz showed that dopamine concentrations were decreased in the striatum of parkinsonian subjects. This discovery, in addition to showing that it is possible to perform biochemical assays in postmortem human brain, led to the administration of *dl*-dopa (then levodopa) to patients with improvement in their symptoms (Barbeau, 1961; Birkmayer and Hornykiewicz, 1961). This was the beginning of a vast movement towards research on neurotransmitters in the central nervous system, and the specialization of a growing number of research centres in the biochemical exploration of the human brain. Twenty-five years later, the time has come to evaluate the advances made. Within the limits of the possible, a critical attitude has been adopted in the hope of sifting out the essential observations and some hypotheses are advanced as to the physiopathology of parkinsonian symptoms and their implications for treatment. Although this review aims for completeness, it is not exhaustive; neglected authors and informed readers are begged to excuse us in advance.

DEGENERATION OF DOPAMINERGIC NEURONES

The dopamine-containing neurones in human brain, observed in fetal material (Nobin and Bjorklund, 1973), are organized into ascending (principally nigrostriatal, mesocorticolimbic and hypothalamic) and descending (to the spinal cord) neuronal systems which are similar to those that have been identified in studies on rat brain (Lindvall and Bjorklund, 1978). Destruction of the nigrostriatal neurones, and the consequent decrease in striatal dopamine (Ehringer and Hornyckiewicz, 1960), is the most distinctive biochemical characteristic of Parkinson's disease and parkinsonian-like degenerative syndromes, such as post-encephalitic parkinsonism and progressive supranuclear palsy (Hornykiewicz, 1966, 1972, 1975, 1979a, 1982b; Rinne, Sonninen and Laaksonen, 1979; Birkmayer and Riederer, 1980; Javoy-Agid et al., 1984b, 1986). This very important observation has given rise to a cascade of questions.

Is striatal dopamine deficiency specific to parkinsonian syndromes? Can it be regarded, along with the motor symptoms, as an unequivocal hallmark of Parkinson's disease? Are the nigrostriatal dopamine neurones damaged selectively or are the other dopamine systems also affected? Is cell loss restricted to central dopaminergic neurones, or are peripheral systems affected as well? Does the physiological state of the surviving dopaminergic neurones change in response to the decrease in striatal dopamine release? What neurochemical mechanisms underlie the beneficial effects of levodopa and subsequent side-effects often seen in patients? Do the various clinical signs of Parkinson's disease result uniquely from loss of dopaminergic neurones? How much cell loss can be tolerated before symptoms appear?

Biochemical abnormalities affecting the dopamine-containing neurones

Nigrostriatal system

The diagnosis of Parkinson's disease is classically confirmed by neuropathological evidence of cell loss in the substantia nigra. The observation of a dramatic decrease in striatal and nigral dopamine concentrations indicate that these cells correspond to the nigrostriatal dopaminergic neurones (*Figure 10.1*). Loss of these neurones follows an identifiable topographic pattern. The decrease in dopamine concentrations is greater in the rostral striatum (Fahn, Libsch and Cutler, 1971; Kish et al., 1986). The putamen is more severely affected than the caudate nucleus (Ehringer and Hornykiewicz, 1960; Bernheimer et al., 1973; Nyberg et al., 1983), perhaps because cell loss in the substantia nigra is more severe in those caudal and internal portions of the structure which projects preferentially to the putamen. In the substantia nigra, the dopamine deficit is more pronounced in the pars reticulata (which contains the dendrites of the nigrostriatal neurones) than in the pars compacta (which contains the cell bodies) (Ehringer and Hornykiewicz, 1960; Javoy-Agid et al., 1981). In addition to this dopamine deficiency, a number of other biochemical observations converge in support of the hypothesis that the

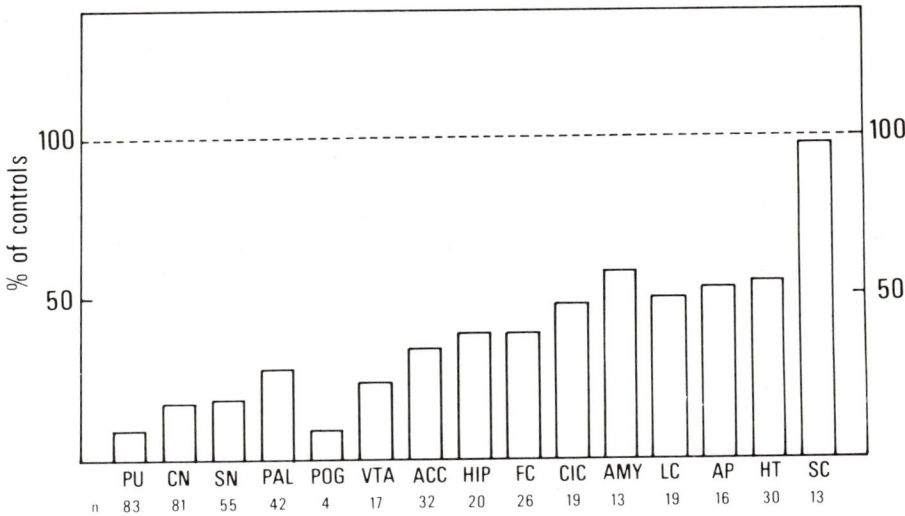

Figure 10.1 Brain dopamine content in Parkinson's disease. Data expressed as percentage of controls are the mean of data obtained from the literature: Erhinger and Hornykiewicz, 1960; Hornykiewicz, 1963; Fahn, Libsch and Cutler, 1971; Bernheimer *et al.,* 1973; Rinne *et al.,* 1973, 1977; Lloyd, Davidson and Hornykiewicz, 1975; Price, Farley and Hornykiewicz, 1978; Javoy-Agid *et al.,* 1981, 1984a; Ploska *et al.,* 1982; Scatton *et al.,* 1982, 1983, 1986; Bokobsa *et al.,* 1984; Cash *et al.,* 1986. n = number of brains. The dopamine content is statistically different from controls in all areas except spinal cord.
ACC, nucleus accumbens; AMY, amygdala; AP, area postrema; Cer, cerebellum; CIC, cingular cortex (Brodmann area 24); CN, caudate nucleus; EC, entorhinal cortex; FC, frontal cortex (Brodmann area 9); HIP, hippocampus; HT, hypothalamus; LC, locus ceruleus; PAL, pallidum; POG, parolfactory gyrus (Brodmann area 25); PU, putamen; RN, raphe nuclei; SC, spinal cord; SI, substantia innominata; SN, substantia nigra; SNC, substantia nigra, pars compacta; SNR, substantia nigra, pars reticulata; ST, subthalamic nucleus; VL, thalamus ventrolateral nucleus; VTA, ventral tegmental area of the mesencephalon

dopaminergic projections from the substantia nigra to the striatum degenerate in Parkinson's disease. (*a*) The activities of tyrosine hydroxylase and DOPA decarboxylase, enzymes involved in dopamine synthesis, are decreased in the substantia nigra and striatum (*Table 10.1*); (*b*) specific markers of aminergic nerve endings, such as the binding of [^{3}H]tetrabenazine (a ligand with high affinity for monoaminergic synaptic vesicles) (Scherman, D., Raisman, R., Agid, Y., personal communication) and [^{3}H]cocaine (which binds to the dopamine transport complex in the striatum) (Schoemaker *et al.,* 1985) decrease in the striatum of parkinsonians.

The metabolites of dopamine, dihydroxyphenylacetic acid (DOPAC) and homovanillic acid (HVA) also decrease in the substantia nigra and the striatum (Bernheimer *et al.,* 1973; Lloyd Davidson and Hornykiewicz, 1975; Rinne, Sonninen and Laaksonen, 1979; Bokobza *et al.,* 1984). This might be reflected in the reduced levels of HVA found in urine (Barbeau, Murphy and Sourkes, 1961; Weil-Malherbe and Van Buren, 1969) and CSF (Olson and Roos, 1968; Gottfries,

Gottfries and Roos, 1969) of patients. Interestingly, dopamine metabolities are less reduced than the amine itself. This may, in part, be explained by postmortem diffusion of dopamine from its storage sites and subsequent degradation by enzymes. Indeed, monoamine oxidase A and B (the former more specific for serotonin, the latter representing 35% of brain monoamine oxidase activity, more specific for dopamine) and catechol-O-methyltransferase (COMT), are not affected by the disease (they are primarily located outside the dopamine neurones) (*Table 10.1*). The difference between the dopamine deficiency and that of its metabolites may not be exclusively due to non-specific transformation postmortem (Sloviter and Connor, 1977), but may also result from an increased activity of the surviving neurones (*see below*).

Table 10.1 Enzyme activities in brains from parkinsonian patients

Enzyme* activity		Putamen	Caudate nucleus	Pallidum	Substantia nigra	Ventral tegmental area	References
Tyrosine hydroxylase		18 (75)	29 (78)	41 (59)	28 (67)	43 (7)	a,b,c,d,e,f
DOPA-decarboxylase		25 (66)	45 (66)	69 (66)	31 (41)		a,d,f
Monoamine oxidase	Total	108 (10)	101 (10)	138 (5)	81 (5)		a
	A	95 (7)	140 (7)		94 (7)		g
	B	107 (18)	125 (7)		133 (15)		a,h
Catechol-O-methyl transferase		82 (9)	70 (9)		82 (5)		a

* Values are expressed as a percentage of respective controls.
Numbers in parentheses represent the number of patients.
Data obtained from: (a), Lloyd *et al.*, 1975; (b), McGeer and McGeer, 1976; (c), Riederer *et al.*, 1977; (d), Rinne *et al.*, 1979; (e), Javoy-Agid and Agid, 1980; (f), Nagatsu *et al.*, 1982; (g), Jellinger and Riederer, 1984; (h), Yong and Perry, 1986.

Low striatal dopamine content, strikingly correlated with cell loss in the substantia nigra (Bernheimer *et al.*, 1973) (*Figure 10.2*), is a common feature of parkinsonian syndromes with different aetiologies: idiopathic Parkinson's disease, progressive supranuclear palsy (Bokobza *et al.*, 1984; Kish *et al.*, 1985; Ruberg *et al.*, 1985), striatonigral degeneration (Sharpe *et al.*, 1973) and post-encephalitic or manganese-induced parkinsonism (Bernheimer *et al.*, 1973). In post-encephalitic parkinsonism and progressive supranuclear palsy, however, unlike the idiopathic forms, the dopamine deficiency is particularly severe and affects the caudate nucleus and putamen to the same extent (Bernheimer *et al.*, 1973; Ruberg *et al.*, 1985). This biochemical observation is compatible with the histopathological evidence for a severe and uniform neuronal loss in the substantia nigra in these diseases (Greenfield and Bosanquet, 1953; Hassler, 1953; Escourolle, De Recondo and Gray, 1970).

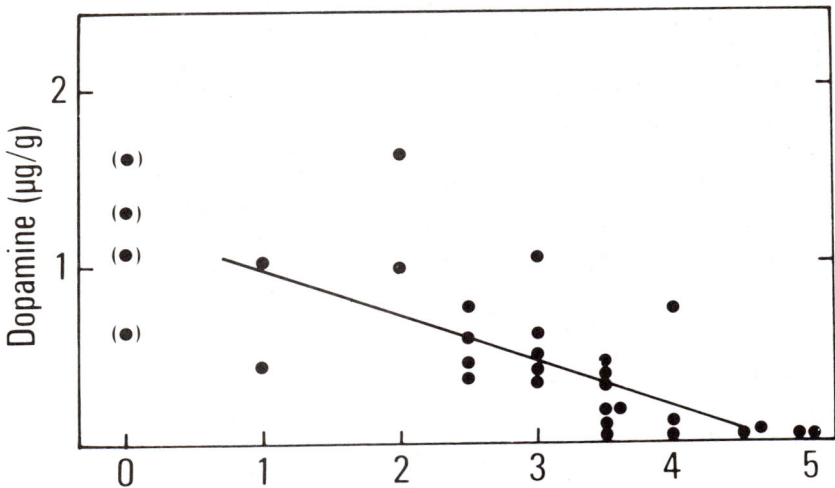

Figure 10.2 Correlation between dopamine concentrations in the caudate nucleus and the degree of cell loss in the substantia nigra. Correlation coefficient, $r = -0.67$, $P<0.001$. Values in parentheses have not been included in the calculation of the regression line. (Data redrawn from Bernheimer *et al.*, 1973)

Mesocorticolimbic system

The mesolimbic and mesocortical dopaminergic systems seem to exist in human brain as well as in animals (Lindvall and Bjorklund, 1978): (*a*) in the mesencephalon, high levels of dopamine in the ventral tegmental area (Javoy-Agid *et al.*, 1981) indicate the presence of dopaminergic perikarya, which have been visualized by histofluorescence in human fetuses (Nobin and Bjorklund, 1973) and by immunohistochemical staining of tyrosine hydroxylase in adult brain (Gaspar *et al.*, 1983); (*b*) in cortical and limbic regions substantial amounts of dopamine can be detected (Price, Farley and Hornykiewicz, 1978; Scatton *et al.*, 1983), indicating that the structures are innervated by dopaminergic neurones, although it cannot be ruled out that the dopamine may in part by located in noradrenergic fibres and/or in blood vessels. Dopaminergic fibres have been vizualized, however, by histofluorescence (Berger *et al.*, 1980). Dopaminergic innervation of the cortical areas is sparse compared to that of the striatum, in the order of 1/500 (Scatton *et al.*, 1983).

There is evidence that the mesocorticolimbic dopamine neurones degenerate in Parkinson's disease. Dopamine, DOPAC and HVA levels are subnormal (40–60%) in limbic (nucleus accumbens, parolfactory gyrus, cingulate and entorhinal cortex, hippocampus, olfactory tubercles) and neocortical (frontal, temporal, occipital) areas, indicating that dopamine afferents are damaged (Price, Farley and Hornykiewicz, 1978; Scatton *et al.*, 1983). Furthermore, morphological and biochemical changes are detected in the ventral tegmental area (VTA) suggesting loss of dopamine-containing cell bodies: (*a*) cell counts on serial sections of the nucleus paranigralis (the ventral part of the VTA) from two control and two

Figure 10.3 Human nucleus paranigralis (the ventral region of the ventral tegmental area) in cryostat sections obtained from a control brain (bottom figure). The tyrosine hydroxylase content of the neurones is shown using a specific antibody revealed with the indirect fluorescence method. The loss in tyrosine hydroxylase-containing neurones in the parkinsonian case is evidenced in the top figure. (Figure kindly provided by Drs B. Berger and P. Gaspar, Laboratoire Charles Foix, Hôpital de la Salpêtrière, Paris, France)

parkinsonian brains provide evidence of neuronal loss (Javoy-Agid *et al.*, 1984b; Uhl, Hedreen and Price, 1985); (*b*) the density of neurones containing tyrosine hydroxylase-like immunoreactivity is reduced (Javoy-Agid *et al.*, 1984b) (*Figure 10.3*); (*c*) the activity of tyrosine hydroxylase (Javoy-Agid, Ploska and Agid, 1982) and dopamine concentrations (Javoy-Agid *et al.*, 1981) are decreased.

Hypothalamic systems

Dopamine concentrations decrease by 60% in the hypothalamus (disregarding intrastructural variations) of patients with Parkinson's disease compared to controls) (*Figure 10.1*) indicating that the dopaminergic innervation of the hypothalamus is damaged.

(*a*) Dopaminergic systems seem to be selectively altered since the levels of other neuromediators (adrenaline, serotonin), enzymes (choline acetyltransferase, glutamic acid decarboxylase) and neuropeptides (β-endorphin, γ-lipotropin, somatostatin, methionine- and leucine-enkephalin, cholecystokinin-8) are not affected (Javoy-Agid et al., 1984a; Conte-Devolx et al., 1985; Pique et al., 1985).

(b) Discrete biochemical deficiencies restricted to specific hypothalamic nuclei, undetectable in studies on the whole structure, cannot be excluded however. Intrinsic dopaminergic neurones (Hökfelt et al., 1978) may be damaged, as suggested by the presence of Lewy bodies in the hypothalamus (Langston and Forno, 1978), but the decrease may also be due to degeneration of nigrohypothalamic afferents, since neuropathological data suggest that the melanin-containing neurones in the hypothalamus are intact (Matzuk and Saper, 1985).

Other dopaminergic systems
See Figure 10.1

BRAINSTEM

The concentrations of dopamine are subnormal in a number of other brain areas innervated by dopaminergic neurones of the mesencephalon, i.e. the internal and external parts of the pallidum and the subthalamic nucleus, which are basal ganglia nuclei connected to the striatum and involved in motor control. Dopamine levels also decrease in brainstem nuclei such as the locus ceruleus and the area postrema. The dopamine deficiency in the locus ceruleus suggests that the putative mesoceruleal dopaminergic system degenerates. Decreased dopaminergic transmission in the locus ceruleus may alter the activity of the main ascending noradrenergic pathway which originates in this structure. Similarly, the dopamine deficit in the area postrema, the chemoreceptor trigger area implicated in emesis, may be of physiological importance.

SPINAL CORD

According to studies in animals, dopamine neurones in the periventricular grey matter of the caudal thalamus and posterior and dorsal hypothalamus, project to the spinal cord (Skagerberg and Lindvall, 1985). Biochemical evidence suggests that the human spinal cord also receives dopaminergic afferents although these are only a small fraction of catecholamine input to the structure. Spinal dopamine levels, less than one-tenth of the concentration of noradrenaline, are comparable to those found in the cerebral cortex (Scatton et al., 1984). Yet, the high HVA/dopamine ratio (an indirect estimation of dopamine turnover) compared to that of the striatum, indicates that despite their low density the spinal cord dopaminergic neurones may have an important functional role.

In parkinsonian patients, dopamine and HVA concentrations in the ventral and dorsal horns of the lumbar spinal cord are not significantly different from those of controls (Scatton et al., 1986), suggesting that the descending dopaminergic system is spared in this disease. At present, these would seem to be the only dopaminergic neurones that are spared. The data must be considered with caution, however, until other segments of the spinal cord are examined.

Conclusions

The main biochemical feature of Parkinson's disease is the decrease in brain dopamine concentrations due to degeneration of central dopaminergic neurones (*Figure 10.4*).

Figure 10.4 Schematic representation of the central dopaminergic systems in Parkinson's disease. Broken lines: the nigrostriatal, the mesocorticolimbic and the hypothalamic systems degenerate in Parkinson's disease. For abbreviations *see Figure 10.1*

(1) The neuronal systems do not all degenerate to the same degree. *The nigrostriatal pathway is more severely affected than the mesocortical or the mesolimbic systems.* Within the striatum, dopaminergic denervation is not uniform: the anterior part of the striatum, and particularly of the putamen, is preferentially affected. Given the role of the putamen in the control of motor function, this might explain why motor disability is, in most cases, the first and then predominant symptom of the disease.

(2) *Not all dopaminergic systems degenerate.* The observation that the descending dopaminergic projection to the lumbar spinal cord seems to be spared suggests that the disease does not strike selectively dopamine-containing neurones only because they are dopaminergic, although it cannot be excluded that the survival of some dopaminergic neurones is related to a particular local resistance to the pathogenic process. The assumption that Parkinson's disease is not associated with a generalized dopamine abnormality (as suggested by Barbeau, 1969) must be confirmed by pursuing the investigation of all (central and peripheral) dopaminergic systems.

(3) The average degree of striatal dopamine deficit in Parkinson's disease is a general estimation in groups of subjects. Striatal dopamine levels differ from one patient to another, however. Differences in the degree of dopamine deficiency in individual patients might explain, at least partly, *the variability in the clinical pictures from one patient to another.*

(4) *A massive lesion of the nigrostriatal dopaminergic neurones is the characteristic abnormality of Parkinson's disease.* The resulting 'striatal dopamine deficiency' (Hornykiewicz, 1972) is essentially, if not exclusively, the cause of the major parkinsonian symptoms. This is suggested by the drug-induced degeneration of the nigrostriatal dopamine neurones in patients intoxicated with MPTP (*N*-methyl-4-phenyl-1,2,3,4, 6-tetrahydropyridine) which results in an unequivocal parkinsonian syndrome (Langston *et al.*, 1983; Langston, 1985a) (*see below*).

(5) *It is generally thought that the first parkinsonian signs appear only when at least 70–80% of the nigrostriatal dopaminergic system is damaged.* This hypothesis is based on two observations: (*a*) in a case of hemi-parkinsonism, a dopamine deficit of more than 80% has been reported in the contralateral striatum, whereas in the homolateral striatum (contralateral to the side with no clinical signs), the dopamine deficit was less than 75% of normal (Barolin, Bernheimer and Hornykiewicz, 1964); (*b*) from an investigation performed in 39 patients, a dopamine deficiency in the caudate nucleus of about 70% seems to be necessary before parkinsonian symptoms become apparent; the dopamine deficit then increases in relation to the evolution of the disease, but not in a linear manner (Riederer and Wuketich, 1976). It can therefore be assumed that central dopamine denervation is progressive and begins long before the consequences become clinically evident (*see below*).

(6) *The biochemical abnormality is not necessarily restricted to the dopamine deficiency.* It cannot be ruled out that the dopamine deficiency is the exclusive characteristic of some forms of parkinsonism, especially in young patients, at the onset of the disease. In most cases, however, other neurotransmitter-containing systems are impaired as well, i.e. in idiopathic Parkinson's disease and in complex parkinsonian syndromes such as progressive supranuclear palsy (*see below*).

Mechanisms of compensation after lesion of dopaminergic neurones

Pre- and postsynaptic adjustments of dopaminergic neurotransmission are observed after denervation: (*a*) presynaptically, the activity of the surviving dopaminergic neurones may be estimated indirectly from the HVA/dopamine ratio, HVA being considered as an indication of the amount of dopamine released with respect to the degree of innervation represented by the dopamine concentrations. Although the HVA/dopamine ratio may increase partly because of the postmortem degradation of dopamine, if the biochemical data are obtained from groups of carefully matched control and pathological patients, this ratio also provides an indication of the rate of amine turnover in the remaining dopaminergic nerve terminals. (*b*) Postsynaptically, changes may be estimated by determining the characteristics (density and affinity) of D-1 and D-2 receptors (Kebabian and Calne, 1979). The reliability of such investigations has been assessed: receptors are relatively resistant to postmortem conditions.

Increased activity of surviving dopaminergic neurones

In most dopamine-containing areas of the parkinsonian brain, the decrease in DOPAC and HVA content is consistently less severe than the reduction in dopamine concentrations, probably because metabolite formation is increased.

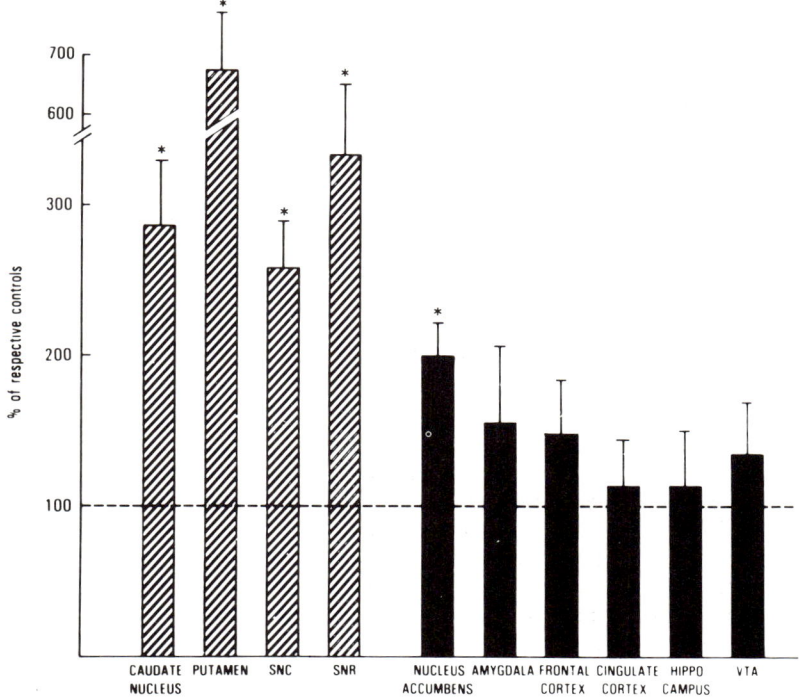

Figure 10.5 HVA/dopamine ratio in brain areas of parkinsonian patients. Results are the mean ± s.e.m. of data obtained on 17–21 control and 10–22 parkinsonian brains, and are expressed as percentage of respective control values (= 100). * Statistically significant when compared to controls. (Figure reproduced from Scatton *et al.*, 1984, with permission)

This accounts for the increased HVA/dopamine ratio (*Figure 10.5*) and is interpreted as the consequence of a functional overactivity of the surviving nigrostriatal dopamine neurones (Hornykiewicz, 1966, 1979b). The hypothesis has been confirmed by experimental lesions in animals. Indeed, an increase in the synthesis and turnover of striatal dopamine is observed after partial destruction of the nigrostriatal dopaminergic pathway in the rat (Agid, Javoy and Glowinski, 1973; Hefti, Melamed and Wurtman, 1980; Zigmond *et al.*, 1984). The amplitude of presynaptic compensation varies as a function of the severity of the lesion: (*a*) small lesions of the substantia nigra causing limited destruction of the nigrostriatal neurones do not change the rates of dopamine synthesis or release in the striatum, suggesting that the amount of neurotransmitter released by the remaining striatal dopaminergic nerve terminals is sufficient to maintain adequate neurotransmission. (*b*) When nigral lesions affect 50–60% of the dopaminergic neurones, dopamine turnover in the remaining striatal terminals increases. (*c*) When denervation reaches 70–90%, despite a marked increase in the amine turnover, the overall dopamine release from the surviving dopamine terminals is no longer sufficient to counterbalance the deficiency and to restore normal striatal dopaminergic transmission. (*d*) When lesions exceed 90%, and only for such severe lesions, postsynaptic dopamine receptors become hypersensitive (Creese and Snyder, 1979), and important behavioural changes are observed (Melamed, Hefti and Wurtman, 1982).

In Parkinson's disease, the magnitude of the change in activity of surviving dopaminergic neurones differs among the dopaminergic systems, and between areas containing nerve terminal or cell bodies.

COMPENSATORY HYPERACTIVITY OF STRIATAL BUT NOT CORTICAL DOPAMINERGIC NERVE TERMINALS

The HVA/dopamine ratio is significantly increased in the putamen, caudate nucleus and the nucleus accumbens, but not in the hippocampus and the frontal cortex of parkinsonian brains (*Figure 10.5*). The hyperactivity observed in the striatum, but not in the remaining cortical and hippocampal neurones, may indicate that the lesion of the mesocortical pathway is not severe enough to induce compensatory metabolic changes. Alternatively, these neurones may not have the capacity to increase their metabolic rate. The high HVA/dopamine ratio in the hippocampus and cerebral cortex compared to the striatum in the control human brain supports the latter hypothesis. In addition, it suggests that the cortical neurones cannot increase their metabolic rate, which may be maximal under normal conditions (Javoy-Agid *et al.*, 1984b).

HYPERACTIVITY OF THE REMAINING DOPAMINERGIC NEURONES IN THE SUBSTANTIA NIGRA

The HVA/dopamine ratio is also increased to a greater extent in the substantia nigra pars reticulata, where the dendrites of the nigrostriatal cells are concentrated, than in the pars compacta, where the cell bodies are located (*Figure 10.5*) (Bokobza *et al.*, 1984). The marked reduction in HVA content compared to controls indicates however, that nigral dopaminergic transmission is not restored to normal and may cause further abnormalities: (*a*) the metabolism of striatal dopamine may be modified. In the rat, dendritic release of dopamine inhibits dopamine release from ipsilateral striatal dopamine terminals and striatonigral afferents, which in turn modulate the activity of the nigrostriatal dopamine system (Cheramy, Leviel and Glowinski, 1981). (*b*) A change in nigral dopamine transmission may influence the function of other systems such as those in the thalamus and the tectum since the dopamine neurones of the substantia nigra also project to these areas (Rinvik, Grofova and Ottersen, 1976).

Hypersensitivity of dopamine receptors

Experiments in animals suggest that, in the striatum, D-1 and D-2 receptors are located on intrinsic neurones and on afferents, in particular from the cerebral cortex. In the substantia nigra, D-2 receptors are present on dopamine neurones, and D-1 receptors on terminals of fibres originating in the striatum (*see* Kebabian and Calne, 1979). Pharmacological (Ungerstedt, 1971), electrophysiological (Ohye *et al.*, 1970) and biochemical (Creese and Synder, 1979; Guerin *et al.*, 1985) studies suggest that after prolonged denervation, dopamine receptors may become hypersensitive.

Modifications of the characteristics of dopamine receptors may be a key element for understanding the pathophysiology of Parkinson's disease, since antiparkinsonian therapy is based essentially on the administration of dopamine agonists. However, there is no clear consensus as to the state of dopamine receptors in this disease, in particular in the striatum.

DOPAMINE RECEPTORS IN THE NIGROSTRIATAL SYSTEM

The density of D-2 receptors in the striatum of parkinsonians has been reported to increase (Lee *et al.*, 1978), or decrease (Reisine *et al.*, 1977). No significant modification in the density (or in the affinity constant) of the receptors was observed by Rinne, Lönnberg and Koskinen (1981), although some patients had hypersensitivity and others hyposensitivity of striatal D-2 receptors. Hypersensitivity of D-2 dopamine receptors may develop in relation to the severity of the dopamine denervation. Indeed, it is detected in the putamen (where the dopamine deficiency usually exceeds 85% and not in the caudate nucleus and nucleus accumbens where the deficit ranges from 60 to 80% (Bokobza *et al.*, 1984). Pooled together, the data suggest that the density of D-2 receptors increases in the putamen, but not in the nucleus accumbens or in the caudate nucleus (*Figures 10.6* and *10.7*). In the substantia nigra, the absence of modification of the density of D-2

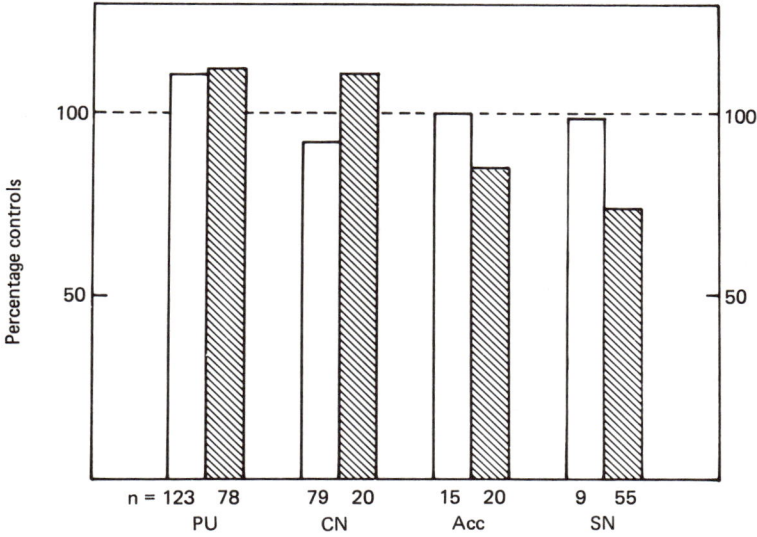

Figure 10.6 Dopamine receptors in Parkinson's disease. The density of D-1 (▨) (labelled with [^{3}H]flupenthixol or ^{3}H-labelled SCH 23390) and D-2 (□) (labelled with [^{3}H]spiperone or [^{3}H]haloperidol) dopamine receptors in parkinsonian brains, is expressed as percentage of respective control. Values are the mean data obtained from: Reisine *et al.*, 1977; Lee *et al.*, 1978; Quik *et al.*, 1979; Rinne, Lönnberg and Koskinen, 1981; Bokobsa *et al.*, 1984; Pimoule *et al.*, 1985; Raisman *et al.*, 1985; Rinne *et al.*, 1985b; Cash, R., Raisman, R., Agid, Y., personal communication. The density in receptor is statistically different from controls for D-2 receptors in the putamen from controls (Bokobsa *et al.*, 1984) and for D-1 receptors in the substantia nigra (Rinne *et al.*, 1985b; Cash R., Raisman R. and Agid Y., personal communication) and putamen (Raisman *et al.*, 1985; Rinne *et al.*, 1985b). n = number of brains. For abbreviations *see Figure 10.1*

178 Biochemistry of neurotransmitters in Parkinson's disease

Figure 10.7 D-2 receptors labelled with [³H]spiperone binding in subjects with Parkinson's disease (▨), and progressive supranuclear palsy (■). Results are the mean ± s.e.m. of data obtained on 20 brains with Parkinson's disease (Bokobsa *et al.*, 1984) and 9 with progressive supranuclear palsy (Ruberg *et al.*, 1985). * Significant difference compared to controls. For abbreviations *see Figure 10.1*

receptors should be regarded with caution, since the precision of the biochemical data is limited by the low density of receptor sites. Density of D-2 receptors does not seem to change with duration of disease (Guttman *et al.*, 1986).

The data concerning D-1 receptors are also controversial. When measured by the activity of the dopamine-sensitive adenylate cyclase, both decreased (Riederer *et al.*, 1978a; Shibuya, 1979) and increased (Nagatsu *et al.*, 1978) activities of the enzyme have been reported. The data obtained by binding studies with radioactive ligands such as ³H-labelled SCH 23390 (Pimoule *et al.*, 1985; Raisman *et al.*, 1985) or [³H]flupenthixol (Rinne *et al.*, 1985b), specific for the D-1 receptor, are equally contradictory. D-1 receptors in the putamen of parkinsonian patients are reported unchanged (Pimoule *et al.*, 1985) or increased in number (Raisman *et al.*, 1985; Rinne *et al.*, 1985b). The increase was reported to be both reversed (Raisman *et al.*, 1985) or potentiated (Rinne *et al.*, 1985b) by levodopa treatment. In the substantia nigra, the density of D-1 receptors decreases (Rinne *et al.*, 1985b) (*Figure 10.6*), as do the concentrations of DARPP-32 (a protein phosphorylated in response to stimulation of the D-1 receptor) (Cash R. and Agid Y., personal communication).

CLINICAL CONSEQUENCES
(1) The number of D-1 and D-2 receptor sites is high in the striatum of parkinsonians considering the marked dopamine denervation. Preservation of a normal density in dopamine receptors may not be surprising since the striatal neurones, and thus the dopaminoceptive cells, seem to be intact (Greenfield and Bosanquet, 1953). Taking into account the suspected presence of D-2

autoreceptor sites, i.e. located presynaptically on degenerated dopaminergic nerve terminals, the presence of normal or slightly increased striatal density of dopamine receptors may indicate that D-2 receptors are in fact markedly increased postsynaptically. This may explain the sustained efficacy of levodopa and/or dopaminergic agonists observed in most patients after several years of evolution of the disease (Birkmayer, 1974; Barbeau, 1980; Bonnet et al., 1986b).

(2) The decrease in D-1 receptors in the substantia nigra would be compatible with loss of striatonigral neurones, but is discordant if the striatum is preserved. It is evident that the localization, regulation and physiological role of the dopamine receptors is still not understood in man. Their role should not be underestimated, since activation of both D-1 and D-2 receptors seems to be necessary to restore normal locomotor behaviour in rats treated with reserpine (Gershanik, Heikkila and Duvoisin, 1983).

(3) An increased density of D-2 receptors is observed in the most severely disabled patients, those who respond well to dopamine replacement therapy, and those who tend to develop dyskinesias and fluctuations in response (on–off effects) (Rinne, Lönnberg and Koskinen, 1981). The increased density is observed preferentially in untreated patients (Lee et al., 1978) or after long evolution of the disease (Bokobza et al., 1984). It seems to be reversed by long-term treatment with levodopa (Lee et al., 1978; Rinne, Lönnberg and Koskinen, 1981) or dopamine agonists (Riederer et al., 1983), although this is contested (Bokobza et al., 1984).

(4) It would obviously be useful for the clinician to be able to measure a marker in the periphery which reflects the state of central dopamine receptors. The binding of [^{3}H]spiperone to lymphocytes (Le Fur et al., 1980) was found to be below normal in patients with Parkinson's disease, and to return to normal after levodopa treatment (Le Fur et al., 1981). The characteristics of [^{3}H]spiperone binding to human lymphocytes differ, however, from those obtained with membrane preparations from the striatum (Bloxham et al., 1981; Maloteaux, Waterkeyn and Laduron, 1981; Fleminger, Jenner and Marsden, 1982), and may reflect labelled ligand that is trapped in the lymphocytes, presumably in lysozomes, rather than ligand which is bound to membrane receptors. Moreover, the increase in [^{3}H]spiperone binding induced by levodopa can be produced by other types of drugs and does not correlate with the improvement of any particular symptom (Maloteaux, Waterkeyn and Laduron, 1983). Although [^{3}H]spiperone binding to lymphocytes may not identify a dopamine receptor, the changes observed in the parkinsonian subjects may point to an abnormality of cell membranes or lysozomes.

(5) The increase in the number of striatal D-2 receptor sites observed in patients with Parkinson's disease is not observed in all parkinsonian syndromes. For example, in progressive supranuclear palsy, the density of D-2 receptors is reduced by 40% in the caudate nucleus and putamen both postmortem (Bokobza et al., 1984) and in vivo (Baron et al., 1985). This reduction is most likely the consequence of the degeneration of dopaminoceptive cholinergic neurones in the striatum (Ruberg et al., 1985). This might also explain why most, if not all, patients with progressive supranuclear palsy are insensitive to levodopa treatment. Interestingly, striatal D-1 receptor sites seem to be intact in this disease (Raisman, R. and Agid, Y., personal communication). The preservation of the D-1 receptors may, in the future, provide the basis for effective treatment.

Dopaminergic lesions and parkinsonian symptoms

MOTOR SYMPTOMS

It is unanimously agreed that the massive dopamine deficiency in the nigrostriatal system plays a major role in the genesis of motor symptoms (akinesia, tremor and rigidity). It is less clear, however, whether it alone is responsible for all the symptoms. The notion that the nigrostriatal lesion is directly responsible for akinesia derives from two observations: in monkeys, electrolytic lesions of the substantia nigra produce a severe contralateral akinesia (Poirier and Sourkes, 1965); in parkinsonian patients, a striking correlation is observed between the severity of akinesia, the decrease in striatal dopamine content and neuronal loss in the substantia nigra (Bernheimer et al., 1973) (*Figure 10.2*). Interestingly, akinesia is primarily observed on the side contralateral to the most severely affected substantia nigra (Bernheimer et al., 1973). Whether the striatal dopamine deficiency is the cause of the other symptoms is less clear. It may contribute to tremor, which can be produced in monkeys by lesioning simultaneously the rubro-olivocerebellorubral loop and the nigrostriatal dopaminergic system (Larochelle et al., 1970; Jenner and Marsden, 1984). Finally, whether rigidity, thought to result from hyperactive alpha-motoneurones of supraspinal origin, is directly and exclusively related to the striatal dopamine deficiency is debatable (Marsden, 1982; Ellenbroek et al., 1985).

Examination of cases of parkinsonism produced in man by MPTP intoxication (Langston et al., 1983) should help to understand the pathophysiology of this triad of symptoms. The clinical picture of this drug-induced parkinsonian syndrome is dominated by severe akinesia, but rigidity and parkinsonian-type tremor also develop. The clinical picture in these patients is all the more interesting, since MPTP is thought to selectively destroy the nigrostriatal dopaminergic neurones in man (Davis et al., 1979) and monkeys (Burns et al., 1983). The selectivity of the lesion, however, is not unequivocally established. Depending on the dose of MPTP absorbed and the age of the patient when intoxicated, other dopaminergic systems (mesocortical, mesolimbic) may also be damaged and, therefore, implicated in the symptomatology (Langston, 1985b). It is noteworthy that other classical neurotransmitter systems (cholinergic, GABAergic in particular) seem to be unaffected by the toxin.

In summary, these observations indicate that the dopaminergic nigrostriatal lesion plays a major, if not exclusive, role in the genesis of motor symptoms observed to varying degrees in patients with Parkinson's disease. The variability of the clinical picture of this disease may reflect differences in the severity of the lesions affecting the dopaminergic systems, as well as dysfunctions of other neurotransmitter systems implicated in the expression of each of the symptoms.

COGNITIVE DISORDERS

Does the central dopaminergic deficiency contribute to the development of cognitive disorders in parkinsonian patients? This hypothesis is controversial. A correlation between akinesia and impaired performance on tests of visuospatial reasoning and psychomotor speed has been reported (Mortimer et al., 1982). Furthermore, the neuropsychological disabilities of parkinsonian patients may be improved by levodopa (Loranger et al., 1972), especially at early stages of the disease (Beardsley and Puletti, 1971). Though open to discussion (Marsden, 1982), the notion that the decrease in nigrostriatal dopaminergic transmission might be

autoreceptor sites, i.e. located presynaptically on degenerated dopaminergic nerve terminals, the presence of normal or slightly increased striatal density of dopamine receptors may indicate that D-2 receptors are in fact markedly increased postsynaptically. This may explain the sustained efficacy of levodopa and/or dopaminergic agonists observed in most patients after several years of evolution of the disease (Birkmayer, 1974; Barbeau, 1980; Bonnet et al., 1986b).
(2) The decrease in D-1 receptors in the substantia nigra would be compatible with loss of striatonigral neurones, but is discordant if the striatum is preserved. It is evident that the localization, regulation and physiological role of the dopamine receptors is still not understood in man. Their role should not be underestimated, since activation of both D-1 and D-2 receptors seems to be necessary to restore normal locomotor behaviour in rats treated with reserpine (Gershanik, Heikkila and Duvoisin, 1983).
(3) An increased density of D-2 receptors is observed in the most severely disabled patients, those who respond well to dopamine replacement therapy, and those who tend to develop dyskinesias and fluctuations in response (on–off effects) (Rinne, Lönnberg and Koskinen, 1981). The increased density is observed preferentially in untreated patients (Lee et al., 1978) or after long evolution of the disease (Bokobza et al., 1984). It seems to be reversed by long-term treatment with levodopa (Lee et al., 1978; Rinne, Lönnberg and Koskinen, 1981) or dopamine agonists (Riederer et al., 1983), although this is contested (Bokobza et al., 1984).
(4) It would obviously be useful for the clinician to be able to measure a marker in the periphery which reflects the state of central dopamine receptors. The binding of [^{3}H]spiperone to lymphocytes (Le Fur et al., 1980) was found to be below normal in patients with Parkinson's disease, and to return to normal after levodopa treatment (Le Fur et al., 1981). The characteristics of [^{3}H]spiperone binding to human lymphocytes differ, however, from those obtained with membrane preparations from the striatum (Bloxham et al., 1981; Maloteaux, Waterkeyn and Laduron, 1981; Fleminger, Jenner and Marsden, 1982), and may reflect labelled ligand that is trapped in the lymphocytes, presumably in lysozomes, rather than ligand which is bound to membrane receptors. Moreover, the increase in [^{3}H]spiperone binding induced by levodopa can be produced by other types of drugs and does not correlate with the improvement of any particular symptom (Maloteaux, Waterkeyn and Laduron, 1983). Although [^{3}H]spiperone binding to lymphocytes may not identify a dopamine receptor, the changes observed in the parkinsonian subjects may point to an abnormality of cell membranes or lysozomes.
(5) The increase in the number of striatal D-2 receptor sites observed in patients with Parkinson's disease is not observed in all parkinsonian syndromes. For example, in progressive supranuclear palsy, the density of D-2 receptors is reduced by 40% in the caudate nucleus and putamen both postmortem (Bokobza et al., 1984) and in vivo (Baron et al., 1985). This reduction is most likely the consequence of the degeneration of dopaminoceptive cholinergic neurones in the striatum (Ruberg et al., 1985). This might also explain why most, if not all, patients with progressive supranuclear palsy are insensitive to levodopa treatment. Interestingly, striatal D-1 receptor sites seem to be intact in this disease (Raisman, R. and Agid, Y., personal communication). The preservation of the D-1 receptors may, in the future, provide the basis for effective treatment.

CONCLUSION

Since the density of D-1 and D-2 receptors is not markedly affected in the striatum of patients with Parkinson's disease (*Figure 10.6*), the lack of responsiveness to levodopa in some parkinsonians does not result from receptor loss. In most patients improved by levodopa at the onset of Parkinson's disease, the drug remains efficacious after years of evolution of the disease (Bonnet *et al.*, 1986a).

In some patients, however, the efficacy of the dopamine therapy obviously decreases in the course of the disease. This might be related to a reduction in the density of dopamine receptors as, for example, in patients with progressive supranuclear palsy. Alternatively, efferent projections from the basal ganglia may become damaged in the course of the disease.

Functional relevance of dopaminergic compensation

In the striatum, pre- and postsynaptic compensation seem to develop in sequence as a function of the severity of the lesion: receptors become hypersensitive when the surviving neurones can no longer compensate for cell loss by an increase in activity. These mechanisms may underlie the evolution of the symptoms of the disease through phases of functional compensation and decompensation (Hornyckiewicz, 1966, 1979b; Agid, Javoy and Glowinski, 1973) (*Figure 10.8*).

COMPENSATION

When less than 70% of the dopaminergic neurones are lost, the increased activity of the surviving dopamine neurones probably suffices to maintain normal dopaminergic transmission in the striatum. Parkinsonian symptoms are latent, but not manifest. Dopamine-dependent limbic and hypothalamic functions may be effectively protected by this compensatory mechanism, since the dopaminergic neurones innervating these structures are usually only moderately damaged even at advanced stages of the disease. During the phase of physiological adaptation, dopamine-related symptoms may emerge, probably when dopaminergic transmission is transiently decompensated, for example after stress (Snyder, Stricker and Zigmond, 1985) or by short-term administration of neuroleptic drugs in otherwise asymptomatic patients (Rajput *et al.*, 1982).

PARTIAL DECOMPENSATION

When the pathological process affects 70–90% of the dopamine neurones, the first symptoms appear. Though the surviving neurones are hyperactive, normal dopaminergic transmission is not maintained, but dopamine receptors are not hypersensitive. This is commonly observed postmortem in the caudate nucleus of patients (*Figures 10.1* and *10.8*). Soon after the onset of levodopa therapy, smooth fluctuations of performance will occur. These reflect the pharmacokinetics of the drug. However, at this stage of the disease, no levodopa-related abnormal involuntary movements are observed, probably because receptors are not yet hypersensitive (Agid *et al.*, 1985).

TOTAL DECOMPENSATION

When more than 90% of the dopaminergic innervation of the striatum is destroyed, dopaminergic transmission is not restored to normal despite presynaptic hyperactivity of the spared neurones. As a consequence, postsynaptic D-2

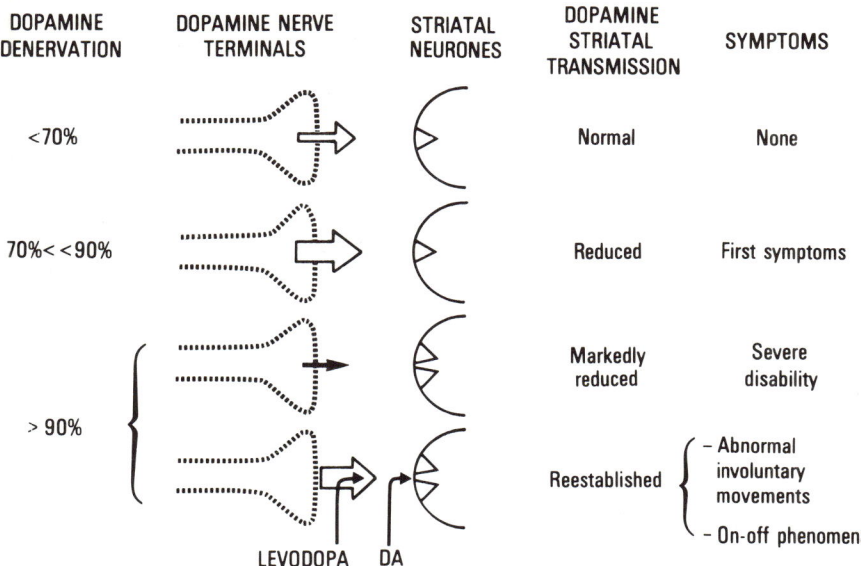

Figure 10.8 Hypothetical role of the nigrostriatal dopamine denervation on the genesis of motor symptoms in Parkinson's disease. Degeneration of dopamine nerve terminals (broken lines), presynaptic dopaminergic activity (arrow) in the surviving neurones, dopamine receptors (triangles) on the striatal dopaminoceptive neurones. Three phases related to the severity of the dopamine denervation (estimated by the percentage decrease in striatal dopamine concentrations compared to control levels) can be considered: (*a*) phase of compensation – the dopamine deficit affects less than 70% of the neurones. The increased activity in the surviving neurones maintains a normal dopamine transmission. No symptoms expressed. (*b*) phase of partial decompensation – 70–90% of the dopamine neurones degenerate. The presynaptic hyperactivity is not sufficient to support normal transmission, the first symptoms appear. (*c*) phase of total decompensation – more than 90% of the dopamine innervation is destroyed. Dopamine transmission is dramatically reduced. As a consequence, postsynaptic dopamine receptors become hypersensitive. Patients are disabled. Dopamine transmission is re-established by levodopa or dopamine agonists (DA). The clinical improvement may be associated with levodopa-induced fluctuations of performance or abnormal involuntary movements

receptors become hypersensitive. At this stage, parkinsonian symptoms are fully expressed. They can be attenuated if striatal dopamine transmission is re-established by administration of levodopa or dopamine agonists. The marked clinical disability is associated with severe fluctuations of performance and abnormal involuntary movements induced by levodopa (*see below*).

Role of the central dopaminergic deficiency in parkinsonian symptoms

In Parkinson's disease, the clinical expression of the central dopaminergic deficiency is different in untreated patients (symptoms) and in those receiving levodopa or dopamine agonists (adverse reactions).

Dopaminergic lesions and parkinsonian symptoms

MOTOR SYMPTOMS

It is unanimously agreed that the massive dopamine deficiency in the nigrostriatal system plays a major role in the genesis of motor symptoms (akinesia, tremor and rigidity). It is less clear, however, whether it alone is responsible for all the symptoms. The notion that the nigrostriatal lesion is directly responsible for akinesia derives from two observations: in monkeys, electrolytic lesions of the substantia nigra produce a severe contralateral akinesia (Poirier and Sourkes, 1965); in parkinsonian patients, a striking correlation is observed between the severity of akinesia, the decrease in striatal dopamine content and neuronal loss in the substantia nigra (Bernheimer et al., 1973) (*Figure 10.2*). Interestingly, akinesia is primarily observed on the side contralateral to the most severely affected substantia nigra (Bernheimer et al., 1973). Whether the striatal dopamine deficiency is the cause of the other symptoms is less clear. It may contribute to tremor, which can be produced in monkeys by lesioning simultaneously the rubro-olivocerebellorubral loop and the nigrostriatal dopaminergic system (Larochelle et al., 1970; Jenner and Marsden, 1984). Finally, whether rigidity, thought to result from hyperactive alpha-motoneurones of supraspinal origin, is directly and exclusively related to the striatal dopamine deficiency is debatable (Marsden, 1982; Ellenbroek et al., 1985).

Examination of cases of parkinsonism produced in man by MPTP intoxication (Langston et al., 1983) should help to understand the pathophysiology of this triad of symptoms. The clinical picture of this drug-induced parkinsonian syndrome is dominated by severe akinesia, but rigidity and parkinsonian-type tremor also develop. The clinical picture in these patients is all the more interesting, since MPTP is thought to selectively destroy the nigrostriatal dopaminergic neurones in man (Davis et al., 1979) and monkeys (Burns et al., 1983). The selectivity of the lesion, however, is not unequivocally established. Depending on the dose of MPTP absorbed and the age of the patient when intoxicated, other dopaminergic systems (mesocortical, mesolimbic) may also be damaged and, therefore, implicated in the symptomatology (Langston, 1985b). It is noteworthy that other classical neurotransmitter systems (cholinergic, GABAergic in particular) seem to be unaffected by the toxin.

In summary, these observations indicate that the dopaminergic nigrostriatal lesion plays a major, if not exclusive, role in the genesis of motor symptoms observed to varying degrees in patients with Parkinson's disease. The variability of the clinical picture of this disease may reflect differences in the severity of the lesions affecting the dopaminergic systems, as well as dysfunctions of other neurotransmitter systems implicated in the expression of each of the symptoms.

COGNITIVE DISORDERS

Does the central dopaminergic deficiency contribute to the development of cognitive disorders in parkinsonian patients? This hypothesis is controversial. A correlation between akinesia and impaired performance on tests of visuospatial reasoning and psychomotor speed has been reported (Mortimer et al., 1982). Furthermore, the neuropsychological disabilities of parkinsonian patients may be improved by levodopa (Loranger et al., 1972), especially at early stages of the disease (Beardsley and Puletti, 1971). Though open to discussion (Marsden, 1982), the notion that the decrease in nigrostriatal dopaminergic transmission might be responsible for some intellectual changes in parkinsonian patients has been put forward: even if moderate, the pattern of mental deficits in MPTP-induced parkinsonism is very similar to that observed in the idiopathic disease (Stern and Langston, 1985). The contention that lesions of the mesocortical and limbic dopaminergic neurones are involved in the neuropsychological alterations is supported by the effects of experimental lesions in animals: for example, delayed alternation in the rat is disrupted by selective lesions of the dopaminergic mesocorticolimbic pathway (Le Moal et al., 1977) and in monkeys by injections of 6-hydroxydopamine in the prefrontal cortex (Brozoski, Brown and Goldman, 1979). However, a number of neuropsychological studies of parkinsonian patients have failed to demonstrate the existence of dopamine-dependent cognitive symptoms (Brown et al., 1984; see Ruberg and Agid, 1986). It may be that the cognitive disorders appear only when the dopaminergic systems are massively destroyed, in particular when nigrostriatal and mesocorticolimbic lesions are associated (Koob et al., 1984). In sum, there is at present no definite evidence that reduced dopaminergic transmission plays a specific role in the genesis of intellectual impairment in patients. The beneficial effect of levodopa in some patients suggests that this brain dopamine deficit might, however, contribute to the reduction of alertness (Brown et al., 1984) and to some aspects of bradyphrenia (see below) (Lees and Smith, 1983; see Agid et al., 1984) and depression (Celesia and Wanamaker, 1972; see Mayeux et al., 1984b), particularly at the onset of the disease, although this assumption is discussed (Gotham, Brown and Marsden, 1986).

ENDOCRINE DISORDERS

Endocrine abnormalities are observed in some parkinsonian patients and may result from the hypothalamic dopamine deficiency (Javoy-Agid et al., 1984a). At the present time, it is not known whether all three sources of dopamine in the hypothalamus are affected (tubero-infundibular, incertohypothalamic). Tubero-infundibular dopamine is itself the major prolactin inhibiting factor. Prolactin levels have been measured in parkinsonian patients, but the data remain controversial: basal levels have been reported to be reduced (Murri et al., 1980), normal (Hyyppa, Langvik and Rinne, 1978; Eisler et al., 1981; Laihinen and Rinne, 1986), or elevated in severely affected patients (Agnoli et al., 1980), probably those with the greatest dopamine deficiency. In spite of a moderate decrease in hypothalamic dopamine (60%), hyperactivity of unlesioned neurones may maintain normal dopaminergic transmission in the hypothalamus.

Autonomic abnormalities that are often observed in patients, such as sweating, can be improved by levodopa treatment (Goetz, Lutge and Tanner, 1986), suggesting that they too may be due to a central dopamine deficiency.

SENSORY DISORDERS

Disabling sensory symptoms are sometimes observed in parkinsonian patients (Snider et al., 1976). They have been assumed to result from a dopamine deficiency in the spinal cord since they are improved by levodopa treatment (Nutt and Carter, 1984). However, dopamine concentrations in the spinal cord of parkinsonian patients have been found to be normal (Scatton et al., 1986). The beneficial effect of levodopa may, therefore, result from a more subtle mechanism, conceivably at the level of the basal ganglia.

Dopaminergic lesions and adverse reactions to L-dopa

Nausea and vomiting, often caused by levodopa at the onset of treatment, may result from a sudden overstimulation of dopamine receptors in the area postrema, a region rich in D-2 receptors, located outside the blood–brain barrier (Schwartz et al., 1986). It is now possible to avoid this side-effect by associating levodopa with a peripheral DOPA-decarboxylase inhibitor, which prevents the production of dopamine outside the blood–brain barrier (Bartholini and Pletscher, 1969), or by administrating dopamine agonists with domperidone, a dopamine receptor antagonist which does not cross the blood–brain barrier (Agid et al., 1979a).

Levodopa-induced abnormal involuntary movements which develop in the course of the disease seem to occur only in patients with marked degeneration of the nigrostriatal dopaminergic system (Barbeau, Mars and Gillio-Joffroy, 1971; Agid et al., 1979b; Marsden, Parkes and Quinn, 1982): (a) they are provoked by medications which stimulate dopamine transmission and are reduced by dopamine D-2 receptor antagonists (Klawans and Weiner, 1974). Drugs which interact with other neurotransmitters are more or less ineffective, although benzodiazepines have sometimes proved useful. (b) They develop at critical plasma dopa concentrations, i.e. beyond a certain threshold of stimulation of central dopamine receptors (Peaston and Bianchine, 1970; Lhermitte et al., 1977b; Muenter et al., 1977). (c) They are observed in patients with severe akinesia who respond dramatically to levodopa, i.e. those with a severe central dopamine deficiency (Agid et al., 1985). The topography of levodopa-induced abnormal movements is related to impairment of dopaminergic transmission in brain structures controlling movement in the corresponding part of the body. This is probably why parkinsonian patients with predominantly unilateral signs develop dyskinesias on the more severely affected side (Mones, Elizan and Seigel, 1971). The reason why the clinical picture of the movements differs from patient to patient is still debated. A choreic, dystonic, or ballic pattern may result from selective dysfunction in the caudate nucleus, the putaminopallidal complex and the subthalamic area, respectively. The timing of these dyskinesias varies. 'Mid-dose', also called 'peak dose', dyskinesias, the most frequently observed, occur during the period of maximum relief of parkinsonian disability, i.e. when levodopa concentrations in plasma are the highest (Muenter and Tyce, 1971). 'Onset and end-of-dose' dyskinesias, less frequent but more disabling, are observed at the beginning and at the end of the period when levodopa is effective, i.e. when plasma levodopa concentrations are increasing or decreasing (Lhermitte et al., 1977a; Muenter et al., 1977). The former most likely result from overstimulation of striatal dopaminergic receptors (*Figure 10.6*), whereas the latter result from inadequate stimulation of the dopamine receptors or from selective stimulation of a subgroup of dopamine receptors (Agid et al., 1985). 'Mid-dose' dyskinesias (monophasic) can be improved through diminution and fractionation of the daily dose of levodopa. 'Onset and end-of' dose dyskinesias (biphasic) can be suppressed in some cases by increasing and fractionating the doses of levodopa (Lhermitte, Agid and Signoret, 1978). This therapeutical approach is difficult to manage, however, because of the risk of exacerbating mid-dose dyskinesias and of triggering intellectual–psychiatric deterioration.

In the course of long-term levodopa treatment, fluctuations of performance develop (Fahn, 1974; McDowell and Sweet, 1976; Marsden and Parkes, 1976). These fluctuations take various forms, two of which are particularly important:

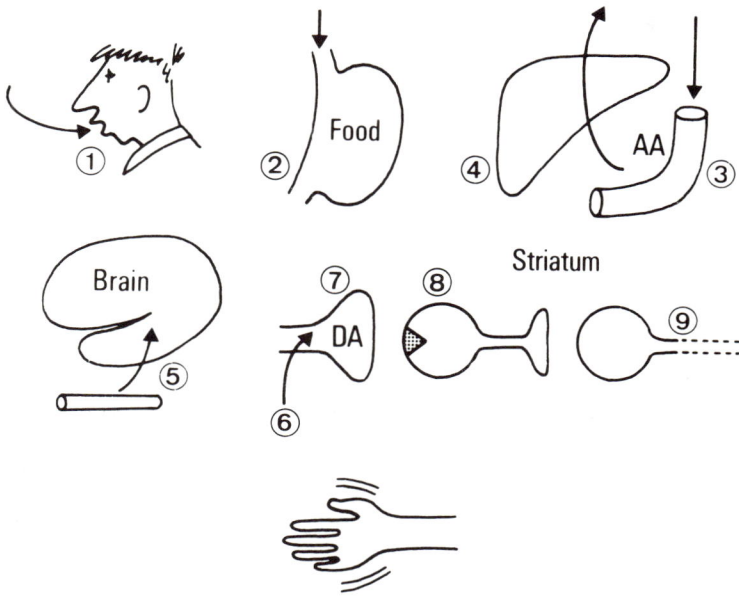

Figure 10.9 Levodopa in Parkinson's disease. The arrows schematize the course of levodopa: (1) oral ingestion; (2) the drug mixes with the alimentary bolus; (3) from the gut to (4) the liver; the drug is transported from the blood (5) to the brain through the blood–brain barrier; (6) uptake of levodopa in dopaminergic nerve terminals; the drug is metabolized to dopamine (7); the newly synthesized dopamine stimulates the dopamine receptors located (8) on the dopaminoceptive cells; restoration of the dopaminergic transmission and reactivation of the striatal output (9). Finally, parkinsonian symptoms are improved. Fluctuations of performance can result from anomalies occurring at any one of these different steps during long-term administration of levodopa

'end-of-dose' or 'wearing-off' phenomena, characterized by smooth disappearance of clinical benefit within 3–5 hours after administration of a single dose of levodopa, observed in most patients after three years of levodopa treatment; disabling 'on–off' phenomena, with abrupt onset and disappearance, not always evidently related to levodopa intake, observed after several years of high dose levodopa therapy. Most, if not all, types of response swings are related to the timing of the dose of the drug (Quinn, Marsden and Parkes, 1982). To prevent these fluctuations it is necessary to control the amount of levodopa reaching its site of action, the striatal dopaminergic receptors (*Figure 10.9*). Delivery of the drug may be hampered by absorption deficits or dilution of the alimentary bolus, peripheral abnormalities such as competition of the drug with other amino acids for uptake by the gut, competition between levodopa and its metabolites, in particular methoxylated metabolites with long half-lives, at the level of the blood–brain barrier. Within the brain, fluctuations of performance most probably result from a decreased capacity for storing the newly formed dopamine because of the progressive degeneration of dopaminergic nerve terminals (Marsden and Parkes, 1976). Reduced accumulation of 18-fluoro-dopa in the striatum, measured by PET scan in brains of parkinsonian patients with 'on–off' phenomena compared to other patients (Leenders *et al.*, 1986) suggests, indeed, that the capacity to restore dopamine transmission is diminished in these parkinsonians. The hypothesis that 'on–off' phenomena occur because striatal dopamine receptors are desensitized by prolonged levodopa treatment (Fahn, 1982) seems unlikely since they disappear after intravenous infusion of levodopa (Shoulson, Glaubiger and Chase, 1975; Hardie, Lees and Stern, 1984; Nutt *et al.*, 1984; Quinn, Parkes and Marsden, 1984). In most patients 'end-of-dose' deteriorations shift with time to 'on–off' phenomena. The reason for this is not fully understood. Assuming that reduced storage of dopamine synthesized from exogenous levodopa is the essential cause for fluctuations of performance, the 'on–off' phenomena may result from a loss in the 'buffer capacity' of the dopaminergic neurones. Consequently, these on–off phenomena (and the severe dyskinesias present during the 'on' period) should appear when the subtle pre- and postsynaptic mechanisms of compensation are overcome, i.e. when the severity of the dopamine denervation produces a marked increase in the sensitivity of postsynaptic dopaminergic receptors (*Figure 10.8*).

Mental disturbances, such as delirium and hallucinations, are the most disabling side-effects. They are most frequently observed in older patients after prolonged treatment with high daily doses of dopamine agonists (Barbeau, 1976; Presthus, 1980; Grimes and Hassan, 1983; Rondot *et al.*, 1984). The cause of these iatrogenic psychic disorders is unclear. It has been postulated that 'bradyphrenia' results from deficient striatal and corticolimbic dopaminergic transmission. If the dopamine deficiencies induce hypersensitivity of the dopamine receptors in the striatum and regions of the cortex and limbic system, stimulation of the hypersensitive receptors in overtreated patients may cause the observed psychiatric reactions, in the same way that abnormal involuntary movements observed in patients treated with dopamine agonists are thought to result from stimulation of hypersensitive receptors in the striatum. The hypothesis is not unreasonable, but is an oversimplification since dysfunction of other neuronal pathways seems also to be involved, in particular the noradrenergic, serotoninergic, cholinergic systems (*see below*), and probably many others yet unknown.

DEGENERATION OF THE OTHER ASCENDING SYSTEMS

The anatomical lesions which characterize Parkinson's disease are mainly confined to brainstem nuclei: the ventral mesencephalon (substantia nigra, ventral tegmental area), the locus ceruleus, areas of the reticular formation (raphe nuclei), and the nucleus basalis of Meynert (Jellinger, 1986). These nuclei are the sites of origin of the long ascending noradrenergic, serotoninergic and cholinergic systems. Neurones in the basal ganglia and cerebral cortex are, in principle, not affected, but they may lose essential input following lesion of the noradrenergic, serotoninergic and cholinergic neurones which project to these regions.

Noradrenergic systems

In rat brain, two ascending noradrenergic pathways have been identified: a dorsal system originating in the locus ceruleus and projecting to the whole of the neocortex and the limbic forebrain (amygdala, septum, hippocampus); a ventral system extending essentially from the lower brainstem to the hypothalamus and the nucleus interstitialis striae terminalis. In addition, a descending noradrenergic pathway innervates the spinal cord (Lindvall and Bjorklund, 1978). The locus ceruleus provides the major input to the ventral and dorsal horns, whereas the cell groups in lower brainstem most probably contribute to the innervation of the zona intermedia. In human brain, the regional distribution of noradrenaline (Farley and Hornykiewicz, 1976) parallels that reported in rat brain (undetectable in the striatum, low levels in cortical areas, highest levels in the nucleus accumbens and hypothalamus). The organization of the central noradrenergic systems seems, therefore, to be similar in human and animal brain.

Degeneration of the ceruleo-corticolimbic neurones

Noradrenaline concentrations are 40–70% below normal in the neocortex and limbic areas (nucleus accumbens, amygdala and hippocampus) of parkinsonian subjects (*Figure 10.10*). In limbic regions, levels of 3-methoxy-4-hydroxyphenylglycol (MHPG), the main metabolite of noradrenaline (Riederer *et al.*, 1977) and, in the hippocampus, the activity of dopamine β-hydroxylase (DBH) (Allen *et al.*, 1985), an enzyme specific for the synthesis of noradrenaline, are reduced as well. In the locus ceruleus, a decrease in noradrenaline concentrations and evidence of neuronal loss, suggest that the noradrenergic neurones of the dorsal system degenerate in this disease. Neuronal damage is accompanied by changes in adrenergic receptors in the frontal cortex. β_1 receptor sites increase in number while α_2 receptors decrease. β_2 and α_1 receptor sites are not affected (Cash *et al.*, 1984). The increase in β_1 receptors may reflect postsynaptic hypersensitivity in reaction to degeneration of the noradrenergic afferents, whereas the decrease in

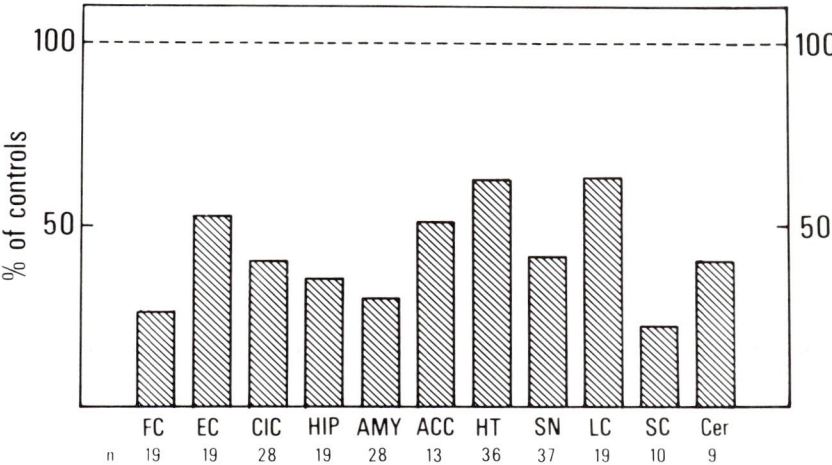

Figure 10.10 Noradrenaline levels in Parkinson's disease. Values are expressed as percentage of controls. *n* represents the number of patients. Data are the mean obtained from references: Hornykiewicz, 1963; Rinne and Sonninen, 1973; Farley and Hornykiewicz, 1976; Riederer *et al.*, 1977; Scatton *et al.*, 1983, 1986; Javoy-Agid *et al.*, 1984a; Kish *et al.*, 1984; Conte-Devolx *et al.*, 1985; Cash *et al.*, 1986. For abbreviations see *Figure 10.1*

cortical α_2 receptors is compatible with a presynaptic localization of some of these receptors on the noradrenergic terminals. Whether the reported decrease in α_2 receptors on platelets from untreated patients (Villeneuve *et al.*, 1985) represents a peripheral index of the reduced density of central adrenergic receptors remains to be demonstrated.

Degeneration of the noradrenergic ceruleocortical neurones may be implicated in the intellectual deterioration observed in some patients with Parkinson's disease: (*a*) in experimental animals, massive destruction of these neurones impairs a number of functions involved in cognition, in particular attention (Iversen, 1984). (*b*) In parkinsonian patients, the deficit in cortical noradrenaline cannot be correlated with global semiquantitative estimates of intellectual deterioration, but is more severe in some cortical areas of demented subjects (Ruberg and Agid, 1986). This is compatible with the observation that, in the locus ceruleus, noradrenergic cell loss is detectable mainly in patients with intellectual impairment (Cash *et al.*, 1986). (*c*) In Alzheimer's disease, a paradigm for cortical dementia, a noradrenergic deficiency is also observed in the cerebral cortex, as are lesions of the locus ceruleus (*see* Hardy *et al.*, 1985).

The relationship between the ceruleocortical noradrenaline deficiency and the severity of mental deterioration may not be direct, but may depend on a common third factor, such as the severity of the disease. However, if the ascending noradrenergic systems modulate cognitive functions residing in the cerebral cortex, lesion of these neurones may contribute to the development of cognitive defects in patients. The depressive states observed in about 50% of the parkinsonian population (Mayeux *et al.*, 1984b) may also be related to the central noradrenergic deficiency since administration of imipramine-like drugs [noradrenaline uptake blockers (Jouvent, Bonnet and Agid, 1986)] and of selective β-adrenergic agonists (Lecrubier *et al.*, 1980) improve depression in these patients.

Other noradrenergic systems

Subnormal noradrenaline levels have been detected in a number of subcortical areas possibly involved in the control of sensory-motor function: the basal ganglia (the substantia nigra), the cerebellar cortex and the spinal cord (particularly the lumbar segment) (*Figure 10.10*). The reported reductions in MHPG concentrations and dopamine β-hydroxylase activity in the CSF (Nagatsu *et al.*, 1982) are consistent with the observation of decreased noradrenaline innervation in the spinal cord, although they may simply reflect the noradrenergic deficiency in the brain.

Lesion of these noradrenergic systems which modulate the activity of other neuronal systems, dopaminergic for example (Hornykiewicz, 1982a), may indirectly aggravate certain symptoms of Parkinson's disease, but may also be directly accountable for other clinical signs. For example, 'freezing episodes' might result from deficient noradrenergic transmission in the regions of the brain implicated in the control of motor behaviour: this symptom may be alleviated by administration of dihydroxyphenylserine (DOPS), a specific noradrenaline precursor (Narabayashi *et al.*, 1981). These observations are contested, however (Quinn *et al.*, personal communication).

The noradrenergic innervation of the hypothalamus may also be slightly affected in Parkinson's disease, where subnormal levels of noradrenaline are observed in some (*Figure 10.10*), though not all, patients (Javoy-Agid *et al.*, 1984a). The dual origin of noradrenergic afferents to the hypothalamus may account for some discrepancies in the biochemical data. Neurones in the locus ceruleus provide a fraction of the noradrenergic input to the hypothalamus, whereas cells in the lower brainstem project massively to the structure. The former are lesioned, but the latter are most likely spared since dopamine β-hydroxylase activity does not decrease, but may even increase, in noradrenergic cells of the lower brainstem in parkinsonian patients (Kopp *et al.*, 1982).

In the periphery, tyrosine hydroxylase activity has been reported to decrease in the adrenal medulla of parkinsonian patients (Riederer *et al.*, 1978b), suggesting that fibres from the sympathetic ganglia innervating this region are damaged. Anatomopathological evidence of cell damage (Lewy bodies) in the sympathetic ganglia of patients (Escourolle, De Recondo and Gray, 1970) are consistent with this assumption.

Conclusion

The central noradrenaline pathways are not uniformly affected in Parkinson's disease. Noradrenergic cell loss probably varies from one patient to another. The dorsal noradrenergic bundle is severely damaged, whereas the ventral system is moderately affected, if at all (*Figure 10.11*). Despite this diffuse although moderate

Figure 10.11 Schematic representation of noradrenergic ascending systems in Parkinson's disease. Broken lines: the systems are damaged in the parkinsonian brain. Hatches represent brain areas with subnormal noradrenaline concentrations. Dark areas correspond to normal levels of noradrenergic markers. For abbreviations *see Figure 10.1*

noradrenergic deficiency, CSF levels of MHPG do not differ from those of controls (Chase, Gordon and Ng, 1973), conceivably because outflow of this metabolite into the CSF is small. The noradrenergic systems seem to be more severely affected in patients with intellectual deterioration, but data are still limited. The clinical consequences of the cortical noradrenergic deficiency are unclear, although it may be implicated in attentional disabilities which develop in many patients (Rogers, 1986).

Serotoninergic systems

On the basis of immunohistochemical and biochemical data obtained in animals, two major serotoninergic systems have been delineated in the mammalian central nervous system: an ascending pathway from the mesencephalic raphe nuclei to the forebrain, and a descending pathway from the pontine raphe nuclei to the spinal cord (Steinbusch, 1984). In man, the organization of the central serotoninergic innervation seems to be similar, given the regional distribution of serotonin and its metabolite, 5-hydroxyindole acetic acid (5-HIAA). As in other mammalian species, the highest concentrations in the brain are found in the substantia nigra, the striatum, the amygdala and the spinal cord. The levels are lower in the neocortex and hippocampus (Riederer and Wuketich, 1976; Mackay et al., 1978; Scatton et al., 1984).

In Parkinson's disease (*Figure 10.12*), serotonin concentrations are reduced in several areas of the forebrain (basal ganglia, hippocampus, cerebral cortex), in some raphe nuclei (Riederer and Wuketich, 1976), in the lumbar spinal cord

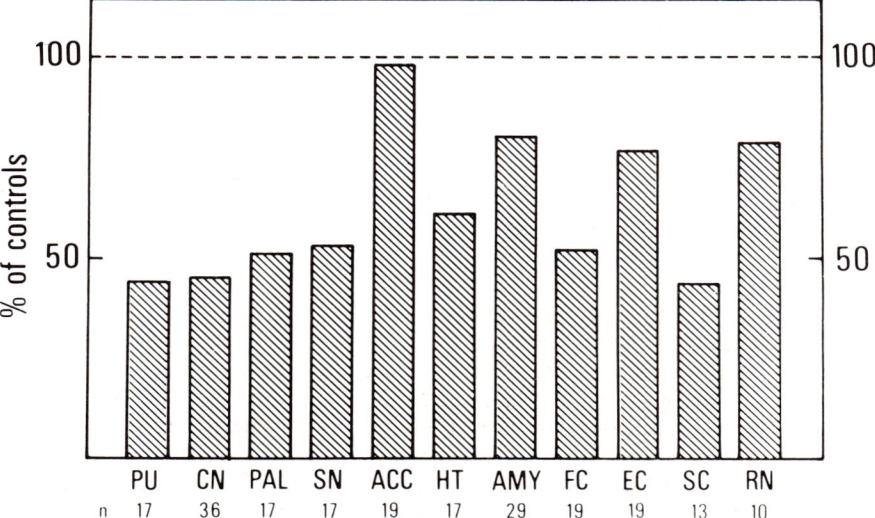

Figure 10.12 Serotonin levels in Parkinson's disease. Values are expressed as percentage of controls. *n* represents the number of patients. Data are the mean of determinations obtained from references: Bernheimer, Birkmayer and Hornykiewicz, 1961; Fahn, Libsch and Cutler, 1971; Riederer and Wuketich, 1976; Scatton et al., 1983, 1984, 1986; Conte-Devolx et al., 1985. For abbreviations see Figure 10.1

(Scatton *et al.*, 1986), and in the hypothalamus (Bernheimer, Birkmayer and Hornykiewicz, 1961), although this is debated (Conte-Devolx *et al.*, 1985). In areas such as the amygdala, nucleus accumbens, ventral tegmental area of the mesencephalon, substantia nigra pars reticulata, cingulate and entorhinal cerebral cortex, serotonin concentrations do not differ from control values (Scatton *et al.*, 1984). Therefore, the ascending and the descending serotoninergic systems must be considered to be only moderately and non-homogeneously affected in Parkinson's disease (*Figure 10.13*). The biochemical alterations probably reflect selective

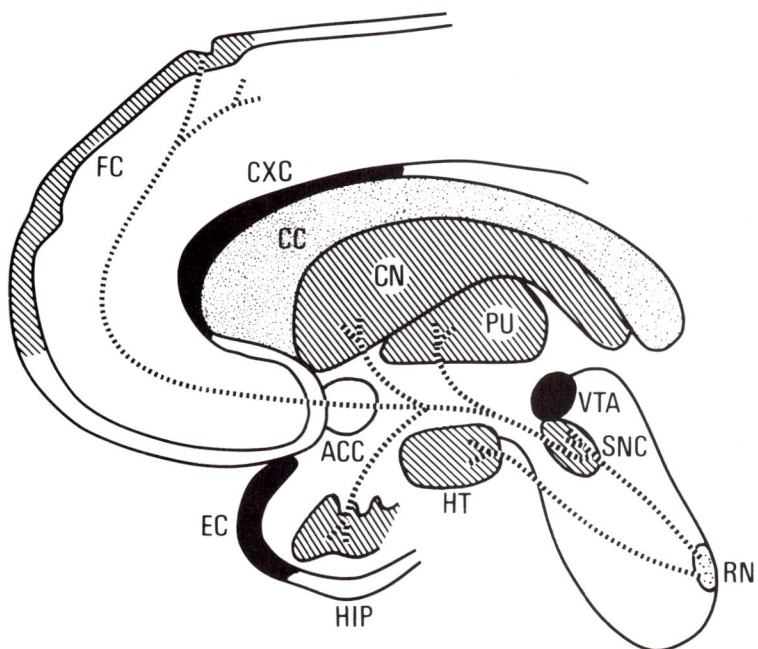

Figure 10.13 Schematic representation of the serotoninergic innervation in the parkinsonian brain. Broken lines: the system degenerates in the disease. Subnormal (hatched areas) and normal (dark areas) serotonin concentrations. For abbreviations *see Figure 10.1*

damage to cell groups in the raphe nuclei (Forno, 1982). In the caudate nucleus and frontal cortex, the levels of 5-HIAA (an index of serotonin metabolism) decrease, to a lesser extent, however, than serotonin itself (a marker for serotoninergic terminals). The resulting increase in the 5-HIAA/serotonin ratio may indicate an activation of serotonin turnover in the surviving serotoninergic terminals. The central serotoninergic deficiency observed in parkinsonian brains postmortem may account for the reduced 5-HIAA concentrations in the CSF of patients (Chase, 1974). Serotonin receptors do not seem markedly affected in the cerebral cortex and striatum. The densities of striatal and cortical 5HT1 receptors (Rinne, Koskinen and Lönneberg, 1980) and 5HT2 receptors (Perry *et al.*, 1984; Maloteaux *et al.*, 1985) are similar in parkinsonian subjects and in controls. A small decrease in the density of cortical receptors has, however, also been reported (Kienzl *et al.*, 1981). The serotonin deficit, which does not exceed 50–60% of normal values according to the biochemical estimations, may not be severe enough to alter receptor levels.

There is at present no evidence of a relationship between parkinsonian symptoms and lesions of descending or ascending serotoninergic projections. Locomotor activity in animals can be affected by serotoninergic lesions because dopamine transmission in both the substantia nigra and the striatum are under inhibitory control of ascending serotoninergic systems. A reduction in serotonin transmission in parkinsonian patients should, therefore, decrease inhibition on the surviving dopaminergic neurones, helping to counteract subnormal dopamine transmission. However, the implication of serotoninergic systems in motor disorders is speculative. Indeed, serotoninergic drugs do not affect motor symptoms (Chase, 1972), even tremor which has been claimed to be serotonin dependent (Goldstein et al., 1969). Since serotonin has been shown to play a role in learning behaviour in animals (Green and Heal, 1985), the central serotoninergic deficiency may contribute to some cognitive disorders, all the more so since this lesion is observed in brains from patients with Alzheimer's disease (see Hardy et al., 1985). The deficit may also play a part in depressive symptoms: (a) altered serotonin metabolism is thought to be a feature of depression in general (Van Praag, 1982); (b) 5-HIAA concentrations in the CSF are lower in depressed parkinsonian patients than in non-depressed patients (Mayeux et al., 1984a); (c) imipramine binding sites, thought to be partly localized on serotoninergic nerve terminals, are reduced in number in the putamen and frontal cortex of parkinsonian patients (Cash et al., 1985; Raisman, Cash and Agid, 1986). This confirms the lesion of serotoninergic fibres and incidently suggests that decreased serotoninergic transmission plays a role in depression. Tricyclic antidepressants (imipramine derivatives), which effectively alleviate depression in patients, very likely act by increasing the availability of serotonin in the synapse by inhibiting reuptake of the amine.

Cholinergic systems

The topography of cholinergic systems in rat brain is becoming increasingly well known (Fibiger, 1982; Mesulam et al., 1983; Kimura, McGeer and Pena, 1984). These systems can be divided into groups of short neurones intrinsic to brain nuclei (particularly in the basal ganglia, but also in the cerebral cortex) and long fibre systems extending from the basal forebrain and brainstem to cortical and subcortical areas. The cholinergic neurones in the striatum are thought to represent less than 1% of the total neuronal population of the structure. Their interconnections with striatal afferents and efferents remains largely unknown. However, studies in animals indicate that the nigrostriatal dopaminergic neurones make synaptic contact with choline acetyltransferase(CAT)-containing dendritic spines (Hattori et al., 1976), inhibiting the activity of the cholinergic neurones (see Agid et al., 1975). The major cholinergic projections to forebrain areas, i.e. olfactory bulb, cerebral cortex, hippocampus, amygdala, and thalamus, originate from large neurones with long, relatively unbranched dendritic trees, concentrated in the basal forebrain. The axon collaterals innervate widely divergent regions in a topographically ordered manner. The fibres innervating the neocortex are located in large part in the substantia innominata, in particular in the nucleus basalis of Meynert but also in mesencephalic nuclei (the pedunculopontine nucleus), whereas those innervating the hippocampus are located in the septum and part of the diagonal band of Broca.

Cholinergic innervation of the basal ganglia and parkinsonian motor disorders

There is some controversy concerning the cholinergic innervation of the basal ganglia in parkinsonian patients. CAT activity, a cholinergic marker, does not seem to be affected in the striatum or substantia nigra (McGeer and McGeer, 1976; Javoy-Agid and Agid, 1980; Dubois *et al.*, 1983), although a decrease was observed in some early investigations (Lloyd *et al.*, 1975; Reisine *et al.*, 1977). Intact striatal cholinergic innervation, indicated by normal CAT activity (*Figure 10.14*), is compatible with the neuropathological observations that the striatum of

Figure 10.14 Choline acetyltransferase (CAT) activity in demented and non-demented parkinsonian patients compared to controls. Values are the mean ± s.e.m. Columns: black = controls; white = non-demented parkinsonians; dots = demented parkinsonian patients. For abbreviations *see Figure 10.1*. Statistically significant from controls (*a*) and non-demented parkinsonians (*b*). (Reproduced from Ruberg and Agid, 1986, with permission)

parkinsonian patients is generally free of lesions, in spite of massive denervation due to degeneration of the afferent nigrostriatal dopaminergic neurones. Data concerning the muscarinic cholinergic receptors are also discordant. In the striatum, the density of the receptors is similar to that found in control brains according to some authors (Ruberg *et al.*, 1982; Dubois *et al.*, 1985a) (*Figure 10.16*), although others have observed a decrease in the parkinsonian brain compared to controls (Rinne, Koskinen and Lönnberg, 1980).

Integrity of the striatal cholinergic innervation associated with the dramatic dopaminergic denervation is remarkable considering the functional relationships between the two neuronal systems observed in rat brain, and may help with the understanding of the neurochemical basis of anti-parkinsonian therapy. Indeed, it may be hypothesized, and is widely admitted, that in Parkinson's disease, the striatal cholinergic neurones are released from the tonic inhibitory dopaminergic input, and consequently develop a functional hyperactivity. The resulting symptoms may thus be corrected either by counteracting the increase in cholinergic transmission (administration of anti-cholinergic medication) or by restoring a presynaptic dopaminergic inhibitory influence (with compounds stimulating

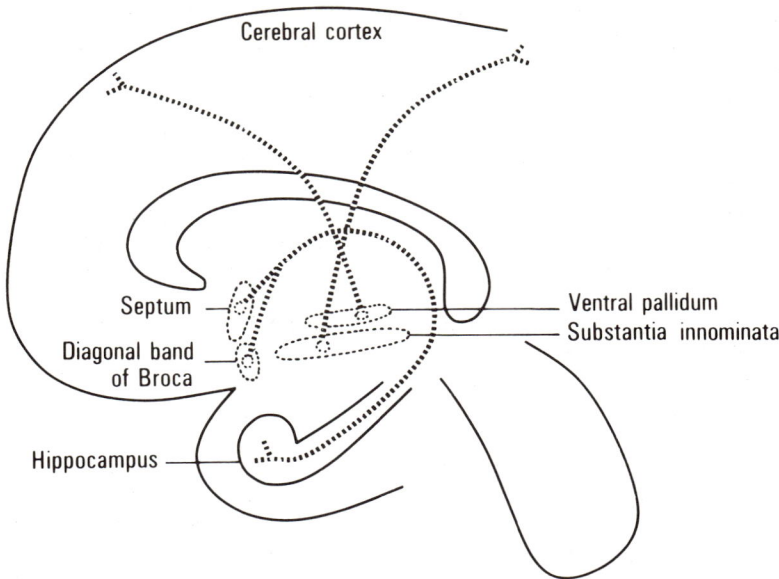

Figure 10.15 Subcorticocortical cholinergic systems in parkinsonian patients with intellectual deterioration. The cortical cholinergic innervation originating in the cholinergic cell groups of the basal forebrain degenerates (broken lines)

dopamine transmission such as levodopa and derivatives). However, such treatments may cause adverse reactions, i.e. levodopa-induced dyskinesias, because cholinergic activity in the striatum is reduced too much by the drug-induced increase in available dopamine.

Cholinergic lesions in the basal forebrain and intellectual deterioration

CHOLINERGIC MARKERS IN THE CEREBRAL CORTEX

Choline acetyltransferase (Figure 10.15) CAT activity decreases in several areas of the cerebral cortex (frontal, entorhinal, cingular and occipital) in patients, indicating damage to cholinergic afferents (Ruberg *et al.*, 1982). The cortical cholinergic deficiency and severe neuronal loss (Arendt *et al.*, 1983; Candy *et al.*, 1983; Whitehouse *et al.*, 1983; Gaspar and Gray, 1984; Rogers, Broggan and Mira, 1985) associated with subnormal CAT activity (Dubois *et al.*, 1983, 1985a) in the substantia innominata (in particular, in the nucleus basalis of Meynert) support the contention that the innominatocortical cholinergic system is lesioned in these subjects. The greatest neocortical cholinergic deficit is detected in brains from patients with evident intellectual impairment (Ruberg *et al.*, 1982; Dubois *et al.*, 1983, 1985a; Perry *et al.*, 1983a, 1985), suggesting that lesion of the innominatocortical cholinergic pathway may be related to dementia in Parkinson's disease. Interestingly, in parkinsonian patients with no intellectual deterioration, a cortical cholinergic deficiency (particularly in the frontal and occipital lobes)

(Dubois *et al.*, 1983, 1985a; Perry *et al.*, 1985) and neuronal loss in the substantia innominata (Nakano and Hirano, 1984), indicate that the innominatocortical cholinergic system is already in the process of degenerating. This lesion might, then, be a general feature of the disease rather than a characteristic of a subpopulation of patients. The septohippocampal cholinergic neurones appear to degenerate as well in Parkinson's disease, as shown by the low CAT activity observed in the hippocampus of patients (Ruberg *et al.*, 1982). Subnormal enzyme activity is also observed in the nucleus interpeduncularis (Javoy-Agid and Agid, 1980) and may result from damage to cholinergic neurones in the diagonal band of Broca. In short, all the cholinergic neurones in the basal forebrain of parkinsonian patients seem subject to degeneration.

Acetylcholinesterase The activity of acetylcholinesterase (AChE), the degradative enzyme for acetylcholine, is low in the cerebral cortex of demented patients when compared to controls (Perry *et al.*, 1985; Ruberg *et al.*, 1986a), and to a lesser degree in subjects with no evident intellectual decline. The changes in CAT activity and in the 10-S form of AChE (the major molecular form of the enzyme) are similar in magnitude and significantly correlated. The functional relevance of these observations is not yet clear. However, since AChE activity decreases to the same extent in the white matter adjacent to the cortex which contains the cholinergic afferents from the substantia innominata, the reduction probably reflects nerve degeneration, originating in the subcortical nucleus. AChE activity, abundant in CSF, has been thought to represent a peripheral indicator of the state of central cholinergic neurones, unlike CAT activity which is undetectable. However, no marked change in AChE activity can be found in the cerebrospinal fluid of

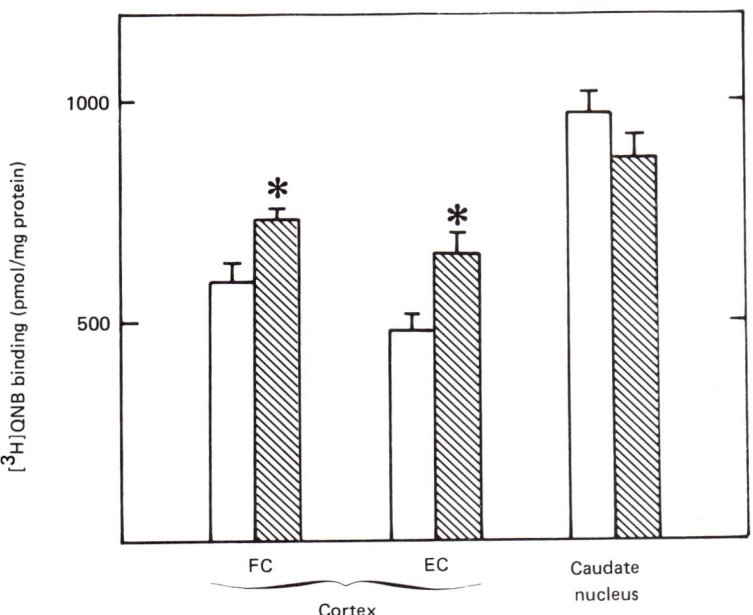

Figure 10.16 Muscarinic receptors (labelled with ^{3}H-labelled QNB) in Parkinson's disease. (□) Control; (▨) Parkinson's disease. * Statistically significant compared to controls. (Redrawn after the results of Dubois *et al.*, 1983)

parkinsonian patients compared to controls, although mean concentrations of the enzyme are increased in those who are demented (Ruberg et al., 1986b).

Muscarinic receptors The density of muscarinic cholinergic receptors is increased in the cerebral cortex of parkinsonians, but not in the caudate nucleus (Ruberg et al., 1982; Dubois et al., 1985a) (*Figure 10.16*). The receptor hypersensitivity results, in part, from anti-cholinergic treatments administered prior to death (Westlind et al., 1981), but it is also detectable in the cortex (frontal and entorhinal) of patients who did not receive such drugs, and may therefore reflect denervation hypersensitivity as well. If this is so, cholinergic denervation hypersensitivity develops following less severe lesions than the observed dopaminergic denervation hypersensitivity (*see above*), suggesting that regulation of neurotransmission in the two systems may differ. It is noteworthy, however, that receptor supersensitivity is not invariably associated with a cortical cholinergic deficit, since it is not observed in patients with Alzheimer's disease (Davies and Verth, 1978; Lang and Henke, 1983; Rinne et al., 1985a).

THE CORTICAL CHOLINERGIC DEFICIENCY AND INTELLECTUAL IMPAIRMENT
An exact figure for the prevalence of dementia in Parkinson's disease is difficult to establish (Brown and Marsden, 1984). About 30% of parkinsonian patients are reported to be affected in most studies, but the figure varies from 10 to 90%. There are at least three reasons for these discrepancies: the structure of the epidemiological study (prospective, retroprospective, in- or out-patients etc.); the difficulty in assessing intellectual deterioration in severely handicapped and often depressed patients (impressions, formal testing, which tests?); the choice of diagnostic criteria. Generally speaking, aphasia, apraxia, or agnosia are not observed (Mayeux and Stern, 1983a), but bradyphrenia (slowness of thinking and difficulty in programming) (De Ajuriaguerra, 1970; Agid et al., 1984; Rogers, 1986) and memory disorders are associated with subtle frontal lobe-like symptoms and deficits in language, visuospatial or perceptuomotor functions (*see* Ruberg and Agid, 1986). In addition, anti-parkinsonian medications, in particular anti-cholinergic drugs, may be responsible for some cognitive disorders. This factor must be taken into account in the evaluation of intellectual impairment. This is relatively easy when confusional states associated with hallucinations are observed, but is less so when deficits (particularly memory impairment) are moderate, or are disregarded by the patient or his family.

Four lines of evidence suggest that the cortical cholinergic deficiency is responsible for some aspects of intellectual deterioration in parkinsonian patients: (*a*) the cholinergic innominatocortical pathway is more severely affected in intellectually deteriorated patients (*Figure 10.14*). It is noteworthy that it is also damaged, but to a lesser degree, in cortical areas and in the hippocampus of patients with no clinical signs of dementia, suggesting that degeneration of subcorticocortical cholinergic systems precedes the appearance of intellectual deterioration. In some patients, subtle and minor cognitive defects may be present, especially at advanced stages of the disease. In others, the cholinergic deficit might not be fully expressed because compensatory mechanisms maintain a sufficient level of cholinergic transmission. (*b*) Anti-cholinergic drugs are known to interfere with memory processes. This has been observed in normal subjects, and the specificity of the effect on cholinergic transmission confirmed (Drachman, 1977). Both therapeutic and subthreshold doses of anti-cholinergic drugs also cause memory disorders in parkinsonian patients (Sadeh, Brahim and Modan, 1982;

Dubois *et al.*, 1986). The data support the hypothesis that non-demented parkinsonian patients have lesions of those cholinergic systems implicated in memory-related cognitive functions, that are masked by effective compensatory mechanisms. In demented parkinsonian subjects characterized by a severe cholinergic deficiency, the administration of anti-cholinergics results in confusional states (De Smet *et al.*, 1982), as if the deficit in cortical cholinergic transmission, due to the nerve damage, was exacerbated by the drug-induced blockade of muscarinic receptors (Agid *et al.*, 1984; *Figure 10.17*). (c) Experiments with rats show that a subcorticocortical cholinergic deficiency is associated with profound disorganization of cognitive functions (Dubois *et al.*, 1985b; Knowlton *et al.*, 1985). For example, lesion of the innominatocortical cholinergic system alters exploratory and feeding behaviour, spatial memory, and the ability to suppress previously learned responses (Dubois *et al.*, 1985b); lesion of the septohippocampal system

Figure 10.17 Hypothetical role of the cortical cholinergic deficit in the genesis of intellectual deterioration and confusional states in patients untreated or treated (Ach-) with anti-cholinergic drugs, respectively. Arrow = presynaptic cholinergic activity; triangles = postsynaptic cholinergic receptors; broken lines = cholinergic nerve terminals degenerating in Parkinson's disease

impairs new memory formation (Deutsch, 1983). (*d*) The innominatocortical and septohippocampal cholinergic systems also degenerate in patients with senile dementia of the Alzheimer type where the cortical cholinergic deficiency (assessed by CAT activity) has been related to intellectual impairment (Perry *et al.*, 1978).

Relationship between intellectual deterioration in Parkinson's and Alzheimer's diseases

Similar neuropathological changes and biochemical abnormalities in the brain are associated with intellectual impairment in most patients with Parkinson's and Alzheimer's diseases.

CLINICAL AND ANATOMOPATHOLOGICAL CONSIDERATIONS
The cognitive disorders observed in patients with Parkinson's disease and Alzheimer's disease are difficult to differentiate with simple neuropsychological tests (Mayeux *et al.*, 1983), although verbal memory disorders seem to predominate in the former, whereas symptoms reminiscent of the frontal lobe syndrome are more characteristic of the latter (Pillon *et al.*, 1986). The memory disorders and other cognitive defects more specific to Alzheimer's disease (aphasia, apraxia, agnosia), are attributed to lesions of the temporo-parieto-occipital association cortex (Brun and Englund, 1981; Terry *et al.*, 1981). In Parkinson's disease, however, neuronal loss is mainly confined to subcortical areas, particularly the basal ganglia and nuclei diffusely innervating the whole of the cerebral cortex, and may underlie bradyphrenia and frontal lobe-like symptoms observed in the patients.

The neuropathological stigmata of Alzheimer's disease (neurofibrillary tangles, senile plaques, granulovacuolar degeneration) are also observed in one-third of the parkinsonian population, in particular in subjects with intellectual deterioration (Hakim and Mathieson, 1979; Boller *et al.*, 1980). This estimation is much higher than that expected in the age-matched elderly population and raises the question whether demented parkinsonians have Alzheimer's disease as well. Quinn, Rosser and Marsden (1986) have recently suggested that there is 'a probability of coincidence and summation of the pathology of Parkinson's disease with subclinical pathology of Alzheimer's disease, and vice versa'. For these authors, analysis of the available literature indicates that there is an overlap of histopathological changes found in Parkinson's disease and Alzheimer's disease insufficient to result in intellectual deterioration by themselves but which could be superimposed to produce 'demented parkinsonians' and 'parkinsonian dements' in addition to the rare coincidence of established Alzheimer's and Parkinson's disease. This interpretation remains to be confirmed, however, since the histopathological criteria (which are part of the definition of a given disease) are not necessarily correlated with nerve cell loss (assumed to cause symptoms). One way to resolve this important issue is to undertake studies where meticulous analysis of cell loss and Alzheimer changes in cortical and subcortical areas will be compared with detailed neuropsychological assessments of patients performed before death.

Dementia may also be clinically evident in the absence of cortical changes characteristic of Alzheimer's disease. In fact, 15–20% of the brains from patients with degenerative dementia of both the parkinsonian (Perry *et al.*, 1983a; Dubois *et al.*, 1985a) and the Alzheimer type (Rossor *et al.*, 1982a) are free of morphological

Figure 10.18 Schematic representation of the two hypothetical types of dementias in Parkinson's disease. Neurofibrillary tangles and neuritic plaques, the histopathological stigmata of Alzheimer's disease, are present (dots) or absent (open) in the cerebral cortex. Broken lines schematize the degeneration of the innominatocortical cholinergic system. (According to the pathological and clinical reports from Perry *et al.*, 1983b and Dubois *et al.*, 1985a)

abnormalities. It has, therefore, been postulated that two types of intellectual deterioration can be found in parkinsonian patients (*Figure 10.18*): a dementia of the 'Alzheimer type' where the cortical cholinergic denervation is associated with the characteristic histopathological abnormalities; a 'non-Alzheimer type' dementia where the damage of the cholinergic afferents to the cerebral cortex is not associated with 'Alzheimer-type' histological abnormalities. In both cases, intellectual deterioration would result from cholinergic denervation of the cortex, although the causes of the cell degeneration might be different.

BIOCHEMICAL ABNORMALITIES

Subcorticocortical cholinergic deficiency is a common feature of both Parkinson's and Alzheimer's diseases. However, in the latter, degeneration of cholinergic fibres is severe and is observed in all patients (*see* Hardy *et al.*, 1985), whereas in Parkinson's disease damage is variable and the cortical cholinergic deficiency ranges from severe to normal (*see above*). Furthermore, intellectual impairment of patients with Alzheimer's disease appears to be more severe than that of parkinsonian subjects with equivalent cholinergic deficiences (Perry *et al.*, 1985). In addition to the cholinergic lesion, the ascending noradrenergic and serotoninergic systems also degenerate in both diseases (Adolffsson *et al.*, 1979; Windblad *et al.*, 1982), as do intracortical somatostatin-containing cells (*see below*). The cognitive disorders observed in patients with Alzheimer's disease that are not found in parkinsonian patients are, therefore, most probably due to substantial loss of neurones in selective cortical areas that are still biochemically undefined. The extrapyramidal symptoms which are characteristic of parkinsonian patients are mostly due to degeneration of the nigrostriatal dopaminergic neurones, a lesion not generally found in patients with Alzheimer's disease. The differences between the diseases are summarized in *Table 10.2*.

Table 10.2 Neurotransmitters in cerebral cortex of patients with Parkinson's and Alzheimer's disease

	Parkinson's disease	Alzheimer's disease
Classical neurotransmitters		
Dopamine (and HVA)	↓	=
Acetylcholine (CAT)	↓ [a]	↓↓
Noradrenaline	↓	↓
Serotonin	↓	↓
GABA (and GAD)	=[b]	=
Histidine decarboxylase	=	?
Glutamate	=	?
Peptides		
Somatostatin	↓ [a]	↓
VIP	=	=
CCK-8	=	=
Met-enkephalin	=	?
Leu-enkephalin	=	?
Substance P	=	=
Neurotensin	=	=
NPY	=	= or ↓
Receptors		
Muscarinic	= or ↑	↓
Serotonin-2	=	↓
Somatostatin	?	↓
Adrenergic α_1	↑	=
α_2	↓	=

= Absolute values in parkinsonians not significantly different from controls. Statistically significant decrease (↓) or increase (↑) when compared to control values.
? Not determined.
[a] Mainly in demented parkinsonian patients.
[b] Although debated.

THERAPEUTIC CONSEQUENCES

In Parkinson's disease, replacement therapy to overcome cortical deafferentation should theoretically be beneficial since most of the cortical target cells are probably intact. Indirect cholinergic agonists (choline, lecithin) have been administered, unsuccessfully, to patients with Alzheimer's disease in an attempt to improve cognitive function (*see* Bartus et al., 1982). There are two possible reasons for this failure: these 'precursors' are not effectively converted to acetylcholine where needed or the target cells in the cortex of patients with Alzheimer's disease may well be lesioned. Since damage to intrinsic cortical neurones is less severe in parkinsonian patients, this type of therapy may have a greater chance of success, although there is a risk of aggravating motor disorders (Duvoisin, 1967). A less problematic therapeutic strategy in these patients may be based on the administration of a combination of drugs which stimulate dopaminergic, noradrenergic, serotoninergic, and perhaps cholinergic transmission in the cortex, since intellectual deterioration in these patients may not result from the destruction of a single neuronal system, i.e. cholinergic, but rather from the combined dysfunction of all these afferent pathways.

Conclusion

In Parkinson's disease, damage to the subcorticocortical cholinergic systems (septohippocampal and innominatocortical) contrasts with the integrity of the cholinergic interneurones of the basal ganglia. The cortical cholinergic abnormality may contribute to the intellectual deterioration observed in a number of parkinsonian patients. However, this does not mean that parkinsonian 'dementia' is a direct consequence of the cortical cholinergic deficiency. Noradrenergic, serotoninergic and somatostatinergic cells also degenerate in demented parkinsonians, as in patients with Alzheimer's disease.

GABAERGIC SYSTEMS

It is generally agreed that about 10% of brain neurones are GABAergic (McGeer, Staines and McGeer, 1984). The long GABAergic striatopallidal, striatonigral, pallidothalamic pathways (Fonnum, Gottesfeld and Grofova, 1978), and the intrinsic striatal neurones (McGeer and McGeer, 1975) have been identified by assay of the activity of the GABA-synthesizing enzyme, L-glutamate decarboxylase (GAD) in conjunction with localized brain lesions in experimental animals. In addition, several classes of cortical interneurones have been visualized by immunocytochemistry with an antibody directed against the enzyme. Some of these neurones contain a neuropeptide (somatostatin, cholecystokinin) as well (Hendry et al., 1984). In the human brain, the distribution of the enzyme is similar (Mackay et al., 1978) although assays are more problematic since the enzyme is fragile and its activity decreases rapidly in response to pre- and postmortem conditions (Bowen et al., 1976; Spokes, Garett and Iversen, 1979; Monfort et al., 1985), whereas the tissue concentrations of the neurotransmitter itself increase postmortem (Perry et al., 1983b). Biochemical data concerning GABAergic systems under pathological conditions must, therefore, be regarded with caution. The changes in markers of GABAergic neurones in patients with Parkinson's disease may indicate disease-related cell loss, but may also reflect non-specific changes due to pre- or postmortem conditions. In spite of the difficulty of the enterprise, it is essential to determine the state of the GABAergic systems in Parkinson's disease given their widespread distribution in brain. In addition, the dopaminergic and GABAergic systems interact, particularly in the striatum where dopamine regulates GABA release (Lehmann and Langer, 1983) and the substantia nigra where the pallido- and striatonigral afferents inhibit the nigrostriatal dopaminergic neurones (Gale, 1984).

In most studies on patients with Parkinson's disease, GAD activity is found to be reduced in the basal ganglia (striatum and substantia nigra) and the cerebral cortex (Bernheimer and Hornykiewicz, 1962; McGeer, McGeer and Wada, 1971; Lloyd and Hornykiewicz, 1973; Rinne et al., 1974; Lloyd et al., 1975; McGeer and McGeer, 1976; Gaspar et al., 1980; Javoy-Agid, Ploska and Agid, 1982). In a study of 55 patients and 38 control subjects, the activity of the enzyme was significantly reduced from 20 to 40% in many brain structures, but not in the putamen (Rinne *et al.*, 1974). In other studies (Kopp *et al.*, 1983; Perry *et al.*, 1983b), however, no change in GAD activity could be detected in the nigrostriatopallidal complex. Since parkinsonian patients in terminal stages of the disease are under intensive care, an obvious cause of anoxia, the reduced GAD activity observed by many authors may reflect, to some extent, the vulnerability of the enzyme to premortem conditions.

Figure 10.19 Glutamic acid decarboxylase activity in brain areas from parkinsonian patients. GAD activity is estimated in various areas of control (open columns) and parkinsonian (hatched columns) brains. * Statistically significant when compared with control values. For abbreviations *see Figure 10.1*. Medial (M.PAL) and lateral (L.PAL) pallidum. (Figure reproduced from Monfort *et al.*, 1985 with permission)

Indeed, if brain samples are carefully matched for age, pre- and postmortem conditions (*Figure 10.19*), no significant differences between parkinsonian and control subjects are observed in most structures, particularly when assayed in groups of control and parkinsonian subjects who died with minimum brain suffering, i.e. in a situation close to sudden death (Monfort *et al.*, 1985). These biochemical data strongly suggest that GABAergic neurones are spared in the cortex and striatum of parkinsonian patients. The stage of the nigral neurones is less clear.

Tissue levels of GABA have been reported to be in the normal range in parkinsonian subjects (Laaksonen *et al.*, 1975; Perry *et al.*, 1983b; Kish *et al.*, 1986), although, on the whole, they are quite consistently above normal in the putamen and below normal in cortical areas (*Figure 10.20*). Normal GABA concentrations have also been found in the CSF of patients (Bonnet *et al.*, 1986b), but subnormal levels have more frequently been reported (Manyam, 1982; Teychenne *et al.*, 1982; De Long, Lakke and Teelken, 1984).

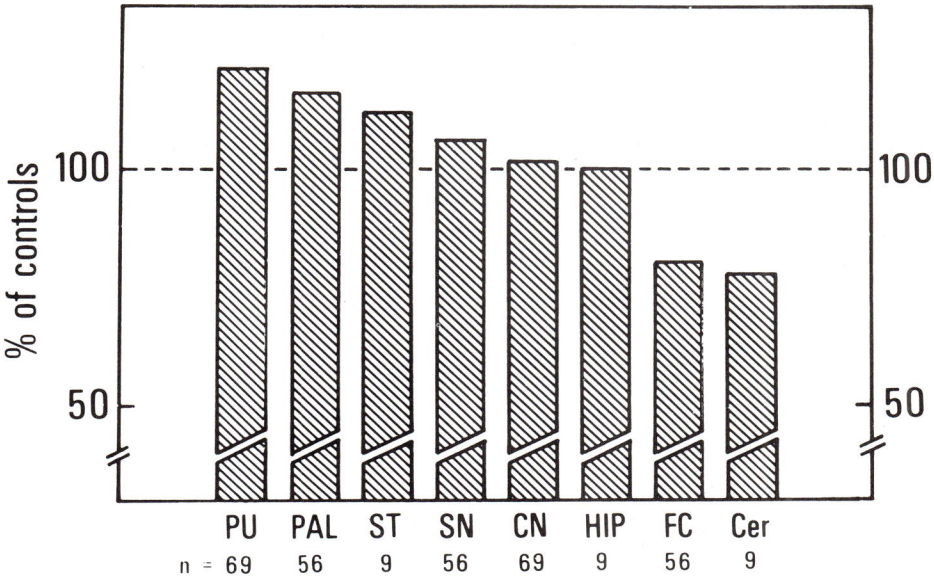

Figure 10.20 GABA levels in Parkinson's disease. Values, expressed as percentage of controls, are the mean of data obtained, from Hornykiewicz, Lloyd and Davison, 1976; Rinne *et al.*, 1979; Perry *et al.*, 1983b; Kish *et al.*, 1986. *n* represents the number of patients. For abbreviations *see* legend to *Figure 10.1*

Figure 10.21 ^{3}H-labelled GABA binding in parkinsonian brain. Data, redrawn after the results from Rinne *et al.*, 1978, are expressed as percentage of control values. $P<0.05$.
* Statistical significance when compared to controls. For abbreviations *see Figure 10.1*

The density of GABA receptors measured with [^{3}H]GABA, the distribution of which differs from that of the neuronal marker GAD activity, is not significantly affected in most areas of the parkinsonian brain (*Figure 10.21*). A marked reduction is observed in the substantia nigra (Lloyd, Shemen and Hornykiewicz, 1977; Reisine *et al.*, 1977; Rinne *et al.*, 1978), however, probably due to loss of GABA-sensitive dopaminergic nigrostriatal neurones.

The biochemical data concerning GAD activity, GABA levels and [^{3}H]GABA binding in the brain of parkinsonian patients raise several questions:

(*a*) What mechanisms underlie the changes in GABA content in the brain of patients? If GABAergic neurones are unaffected by the disease, as the normal levels of GAD activity in many areas of the parkinsonian brain suggest, the modifications in GABA levels may reflect a change in the activity of GABAergic neurones to compensate the deficit in nigrostriatal dopamine transmission (Lloyd, Davidson and Hornykiewicz, 1975). Destruction of dopaminergic input to the striatum in experimental animals decreases the activity of GABAergic neurones increasing striatal GABA concentrations (Perry *et al.*, 1983b). This would reduce the GABA-mediated inhibition of the nigrostriatal dopaminergic neurones, allowing them to fire more rapidly.

(*b*) Does long-term levodopa treatment restore deficient dopaminergic regulation of striatal GABAergic neurones? This would seem to be the case since striatal GAD activity is greater in levodopa-treated patients and is positively correlated with the duration of the drug treatment (Lloyd and Hornykiewicz, 1973). These results and the observation that GABA concentrations in the CSF of patients are significantly greater after long-term anti-parkinsonian therapy (Manyam, 1982; De Jong *et al.*, 1984), are compatible with the hypothesis that altered GABAergic activity in the striatum is reversed by levodopa treatment (Hornykiewicz, Lloyd and Davidson, 1976). However, GAD activity was found to be normal in recent studies on postmortem brain (Monfort *et al.*, 1985) and CSF from patients (Bonnet *et al.*, 1986b).

(*c*) What are the clinical and therapeutic consequences? It has been hypothesized that the putative GABAergic deficiency in the basal ganglia might play a role in the occurrence of tremor and rigidity by disinhibiting the nigrostriatal dopaminergic neurones (Hornykiewicz, 1975). Moreover, GABA agonists seem to decrease levodopa-induced fluctuations of performance whereas dyskinesias provoked by the drug become more severe (Bergmann *et al.*, 1984). Inhibition of striatal cholinergic neurones by these drugs, as observed in animal studies (Scatton and Bartholini, 1980), may explain their efficacy. However, if GABAergic systems are spared in the parkinsonian brain, it is unlikely that GABAergic replacement therapy would be markedly effective.

NEUROPEPTIDES IN PARKINSON'S DISEASE

Neuropeptides, which are stable for several hours after death, can be assayed biochemically and visualized immunohistochemically postmortem. Since both techniques rely upon antibodies to identify the peptides, what is measured is prudently termed 'peptide-like immunoreactivity'. The data concerning the peptides discussed below should be understood in this sense.

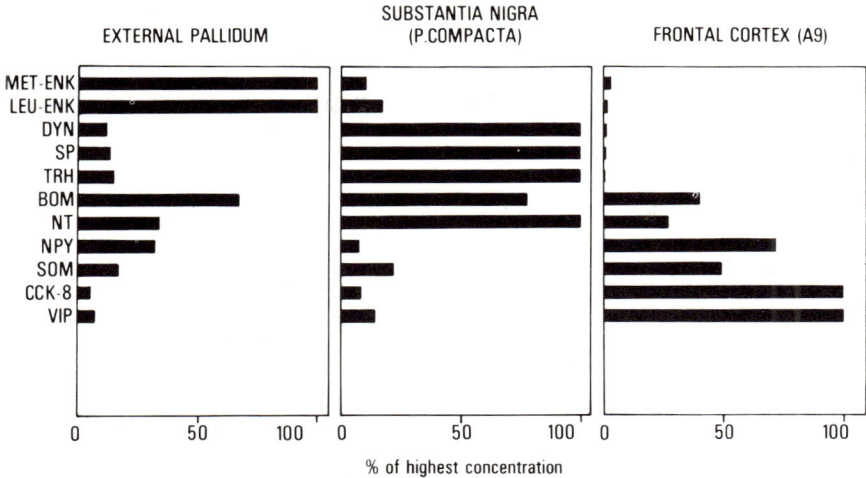

Figure 10.22 Distribution of neuropeptides in human brain. Neuropeptide concentrations are expressed as a percentage of the highest (100%) extrahypothalamic brain concentrations. (BOM) bombesin; (CCK-8) cholecystokinin-8; (DYN) dynorphin; (Leu-Enk) leucine-enkephalin; (Met-Enk) methionine-enkephalin; (NPY) neuropeptide Y; (NT) neurotensin; (SOM) somatostatin; (SP) substance P; (TRH) thyrotropin-releasing hormone; (VIP) vasointestinal polypeptide

In human as in rat brain the distribution of neuropeptides is heterogeneous. Cholecystokinin-8 (CCK-8) and vasointestinal peptide (VIP) are most abundant in cortical areas, whereas methionine- and leucine-enkephalin, substance P, and thyrotropin-releasing factor (TRH) (*Figure 10.22*) are more prevalent in the basal ganglia. Behavioural studies in animals suggest that neuropeptides may be implicated in the parkinsonian symptomatology: (*a*) some neuropeptides have been observed to regulate motor and cognitive functions; (*b*) high concentrations of a number of peptides are found in dopaminergic areas, suggesting that they may interact with dopaminergic systems as co-transmitters (Bartfai, 1985); their role may be to modulate dopamine receptor sensitivity as well (Fuxe *et al.*, 1983). One might thus expect to improve parkinsonian symptoms with drugs manipulating the peptidergic systems which modulate the activity of dopaminergic systems, thereby reactivating in part the deficient dopaminergic transmission.

Neuropeptide deficiencies in Parkinson's disease

Subnormal concentrations of several neuropeptides have been observed in various regions of the brains of patients with Parkinson's disease.

Cholecystokinin-8

In the human brain as in the rat, CCK-8 is most highly concentrated in the amygdala and cerebral cortex, but is also found in dopamine-rich structures such as the striatum (*Figure 10.22*) (Vanderhaegen *et al.*, 1980). In the rat striatum, CCK-8 is contained in nerve terminals distributed in patches close to the median line, and in some dopaminergic nerve terminals in the medial and posterior part of the nucleus accumbens. CCK-8 is found in cell bodies in the mesencephalon and in some dopaminergic cells of the ventral tegmental area, and the external and medial substantia nigra pars compacta (Hökfelt et al., 1980).

CCK-8 levels decrease by 30% in the substantia nigra (pars compacta and reticulata) of parkinsonian subjects, although levels are normal in other structures such as the caudate nucleus, putamen, amygdala, cerebral cortex and hippocampus (Studler et al., 1982) (Table 10.3). The decrease in the substantia nigra may result from degeneration of CCK-8-containing cell bodies within the structure and/or CCK-8-containing afferents of unknown origin. No decrease in CCK-8 concentrations could be detected in the ventral tegmental area. This does not exclude the possibility that some CCK-8–dopamine neurones degenerate since this subpopulation of neurones is small and its loss may be undetectable by biochemical measurement. It is also possible that dopaminergic neurones which contain the peptide as well, might somehow be protected from the degenerative process (Agid and Javoy-Agid, 1985). Some dopaminergic neurones are indeed spared in the ventral tegmental area of parkinsonian patients, possibly those containing the peptide.

Table 10.3 Neuropeptides in brains from parkinsonian patients

Neuropeptide	Pallidum	Caudate nucleus	Pallidum (external)	Nucleus accumbens	Frontal cortex	Substantia nigra pars compacta	References
CCK-8	120 (9)	118 (9)	89 (8)	134 (7)	88 (9)	64* (10)	a
Substance P	80 (55)	85 (53)	53* (13)	125 (18)	108 (32)	68* (54)	d,f
Met-enkephalin	63* b (13)	100 (26)	51* (12)	93 (17)	90 (17)	33* (21)	b,g
Leu-enkephalin	57* (14)	92 (14)	67* (15)	84 (13)	121 (14)	81 (12)	e
Dynorphin	83 (14)	91 (14)	94 (14)	–	92 (14)	94 (14)	j
TRH	86 (9)	93 (9)	100 (6)	69 (13)	ND	95 (7)	c
Bombesin	94 (21)	85* (21)	86* (21)	78 (16)	94 (21)	106 (16)	h
Neurotensin	111 (21)	116 (21)	92 (21)	112 (16)	102 (21)	107 (16)	h
VIP	129 (18)	100 (16)	110 (15)	–	96 (23)	–	i,k

Values are expressed as percentage of respective controls.
Numbers in parentheses represent the number of patients. Frontal cortex accounts for Brodmann area 9.
ND = non-detectable; * statistically significant when compared to controls. Data obtained from: (a), Studler et al., 1982; (b), Taquet et al., 1982; (c), Javoy-Agid et al., 1983; (d), Mauborgne et al., 1983; (e), Taquet et al., 1983; (f), Tenovuo et al., 1984; (g), Rinne et al., 1984; (h), Bissette et al., 1985; (i), Jegou et al., 1985a; (j), Taquet et al., 1985; (k), Jegou et al., 1985b.

The functional consequences of the nigral CCK-8 deficiency is not known. Pharmacological studies in animals show that the peptide has an excitatory effect on nigral dopaminergic neurones (Skirboll et al., 1981). Therefore, the development of putative CCK-8 analogues (not yet available), assumed to increase the activity of nigrostriatal dopamine neurones, should theoretically improve symptoms thought to result from the striatal dopamine deficiency. This hypothesis is questionable, however, since CCK-8 also decreases dopamine release in the striatum (Markstein and Hökfelt, 1984).

Substance P

In human brain, substance P is highly concentrated in the substantia nigra and the internal pallidum (*Figure 10.22*). In the substantia nigra, the peptide is most likely found in nerve terminals of the striatonigral substance P-containing neurones (Kanazawa, Emson and Cuello, 1977), which are thought to modulate the activity of the nigrostriatal dopaminergic neurones (Glowinski, Michelot and Cheramy, 1980).

In Parkinson's disease, substance P levels decrease in the substantia nigra (Mauborgne et al., 1983; Tenovuo, Rinne and Viljanen, 1984) and in the pallidum (Mauborgne et al., 1983), suggesting that striatonigral and striatopallidal substance P-containing neurones may be lesioned (Emson et al., 1980) (*Table 10.3*), although this is still speculative. According to classical neuropathological data, there is little or no neuronal loss in the striatum of patients (Blackwood and Corsellis, 1977), nor has loss of substance P-containing fibres been clearly detected immunohistochemically in the substantia nigra (Grafe, Forno and Eng, 1985). The observed decrease in substance P concentrations may, therefore, indicate a change in turnover rate due to loss of regulatory input rather than loss of the substance P-containing neurones.

Since substance P is known to have an excitatory effect on dopamine neurones (Glowinski, Michelot and Cheramy, 1980), the peptide deficiency in the substantia nigra of parkinsonians may influence dopamine-dependent symptoms.

Methionine-enkephalin

Met-enkephalin is unevenly distributed in the human brain (Gramsch et al., 1979), the pallidum containing the highest concentrations. The distribution of the peptide closely parallels that of dopamine (Ploska et al., 1982). In the striatum, the striosomes, areas of low acetylcholine esterase activity, partly innervated by the nigrostriatal dopaminergic neurones (Gerfen, 1986), contain high concentrations of Met-enkephalin (Graybiel, 1984). In the substantia nigra, the patterns of distribution of dopamine and the peptide are superimposable (Taquet et al., 1982). The dopaminergic neurones (pigmented, tyrosine hydroxylase-positive cells) are surrounded by Met-enkephalin-containing nerve terminals (Gaspar et al., 1983). These data suggest that there is a functional relationship between the two systems (*see* Javoy-Agid et al., 1982).

Met-enkephalin concentrations in patients with Parkinson's disease are similar to those found in controls in many brain areas (nucleus accumbens, caudate nucleus, amygdala, cerebral cortex, hippocampus) (Taquet et al., 1982, 1983; Rinne et al.,

1984). They are reduced by 70% in the substantia nigra and ventral tegmental area, and 30–40% in the putamen and pallidum (*Table 10.3*). The putative putaminopallidal enkephalin system (Cuello and Paxinos, 1978), may therefore be damaged, although alteration of striatal Met-enkephalin neurones (Pickel *et al.*, 1980) cannot be excluded. The marked decrease in Met-enkephalin in the ventral mesencephalon might be due to degeneration of neurones containing both dopamine and the peptide. There is, however, no evidence to support this hypothesis (Gaspar *et al.*, 1983). Enkephalinergic neurones, probably located in the mesencephalon, innervating the substantia nigra and/or nerve terminals might degenerate, as suggested by the decrease in the density of Met-enkephalin-containing fibres in the substantia nigra of a subject with Parkinson's disease (Hunt, Peck and Rossor, 1983), although this result has not been confirmed (Grafe, Forno and Eng, 1985). Consequently, a modification in the metabolism of the peptide, perhaps due to loss of dopaminergic neurones, must also be considered.

The activity of the dopamine neurones in the mesencephalon is thought to be regulated by Met-enkephalin since opiate receptors are most likely located on the nigral dopaminergic cell bodies. In accordance with this hypothesis, the density of these receptors is decreased in the substantia nigra of parkinsonian patients (Llorens-Cortes *et al.*, 1984). In the striatum, however, the density of the receptors is normal (Llorens-Cortes *et al.*, 1984) and may even increase (Rinne *et al.*, 1983). If the mesencephalic Met-enkephalinergic neurones regulate the activity of the nigrostriatal dopaminergic neurones, a change in this regulation may affect parkinsonian dopamine-dependent symptomatology.

Leucine-enkephalin and dynorphin

The distribution of Leu-enkephalin in the human brain is essentially the same as that of Met-enkephalin (Kubek and Wilber, 1980) (*Figure 10.22*). The ratio of the peptides, differs, however, throughout the brain (Taquet *et al.*, 1983) suggesting that they are not located in the same neurones.

In Parkinson's disease, Leu-enkephalin concentrations are reduced (30–40%) only in the pallidum and putamen (*Table 10.3*), indicating that the Leu-enkephalin putaminopallidal pathway (Cuello and Paxinos, 1978) may be affected, whereas in the substantia nigra and the ventral tegmental area, the concentrations of the peptide are similar to controls (Taquet *et al.*, 1983). Therefore, the Leu-enkephalin-containing neurones of the ventral mesencephalon unlike the Met-enkephalinergic innervation, do not seem to be affected in parkinsonians, although alteration of a subpopulation of Leu-enkephalin neurones may be masked. It has recently been shown that there are two populations of Leu-enkephalin-containing neurones which can be distinguished by the precursor molecule from which the peptide is derived. Neurones which contain pro-enkephalin A (the precursor of Met- and Leu-enkephalin) predominate in the striatum and would seem to degenerate, whereas those containing pro-enkephalin B (the precursor of neo-endorphin/dynorphin and Leu-enkephalin) (Kakidani *et al.*, 1982) very likely do not degenerate in the disease. Like Leu-enkephalin, dynorphin levels in the substantia nigra (which contains the highest concentrations of this peptide in the brain) are unchanged in patients (Taquet *et al.*, 1985) (*Table*

10.3). The Leu-enkephalin from pro-enkephalin B neurones may prevent detection of a decrease in Leu-enkephalin due to loss of pro-enkephalin A neurones.

An increase in the density of Leu-enkephalin receptors in the putamen, limbic cortex and hippocampus of parkinsonian brains (Rinne et al., 1983) suggests that the disease is associated with changes in Leu-enkephalin transmission.

Somatostatin

The greatest concentrations of somatostatin in the brain are observed in the hypothalamus, but substantial amounts are found elsewhere, including the cerebral cortex (*Figure 10.22*). Somatostatin-containing neurones which may contain other neurotransmitters as well, in particular neuropeptide Y (NPY) (Hendry et al., 1984), are present in all layers of the cortex.

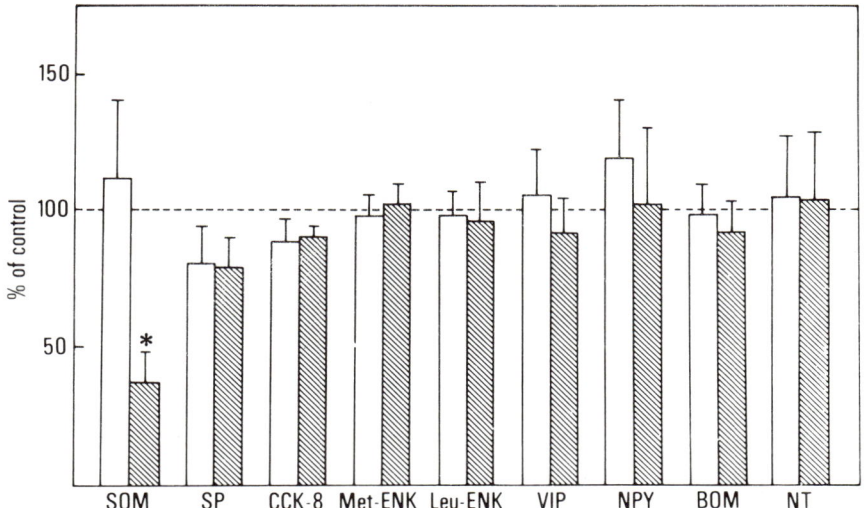

Figure 10.23 Peptides in frontal cortex of patients with Parkinson's disease: (□) non-demented and (▨) demented. Peptide levels ± s.e.m. are expressed as a percentage of control values. * Statistical significance when compared to controls and non-demented parkinsonians. For abbreviations *see* legend to *Figure 10.22*. (Figure reproduced from Agid and Javoy-Agid, 1985, with permission)

Concentrations of the peptide decrease only in the frontal cortex and hippocampus of parkinsonian patients, and only in those with intellectual impairment (*Figure 10.23*) (Epelbaum et al., 1983). The decrease is not observed in other cortical areas (Rinne et al., 1984), nor in the caudate nucleus or hypothalamus (Epelbaum et al., 1983). It is possible that only a subpopulation of cortical somatostatinergic neurones are affected. Those containing NPY as well seem to be spared since the concentrations of this peptide does not decrease in parkinsonian patients whether demented or not (Allen et al., 1985). The decrease in somatostatin tends to parallel the decrease in CAT activity in certain areas of the cortex (Epelbaum et al., 1983), although no anatomical relationship between cortical somatostatin neurones and cholinergic afferents has been demonstrated. A reduction in somatostatin concentrations has also been detected in the cerebrospinal fluid of parkinsonian patients (Dupont et al., 1982), particularly those who are demented (Jolkonen et al., 1986), although this might be related to the severity of the disease (Volicer et al., 1986).

These data suggest that intellectual deterioration is associated with a cortical somatostatin deficiency. Since somatostatin is located in intrinsic neurones in human cerebral cortex (Sorensen, 1982), it may be hypothesized that mental disorders in Parkinson's disease may have a 'cortical' as well as a 'subcortical' component.

Other neuropeptides

Not all peptide-containing neurones are damaged in the parkinsonian brain. Normal concentrations have been found of TRH (Javoy-Agid et al., 1983), bombesin (though a slight decrease in the pallidum has been reported (Bissette et al., 1985), VIP (Jegou et al., 1985a), vasopressin (at least in the substantia nigra, peri-aqueductal grey matter, locus ceruleus and pallidum) (Rossor et al., 1982b), NPY (in particular in the cerebral cortex) (Allen et al., 1985). Neurotensin concentrations are also unchanged in parkinsonian brains, apart from a moderate but significant reduction in the hippocampus (Bissette et al., 1985). Nevertheless a dramatic decrease in neurotensin receptors is observed in the substantia nigra of patients (Sadoul et al., 1984) due to loss of the dopaminergic neurones.

Significance of peptide deficiencies

The abnormal peptide concentrations detected in parkinsonian brains should be considered with caution until they are confirmed and the reason for the abnormalities understood. Do the abnormalities reflect degeneration of the corresponding neurones or metabolic changes possibly related to the degeneration of other neuronal systems? How do they relate to parkinsonian symptoms?

Neuronal damage or metabolic change?

The subnormal peptide concentrations found in various areas of the parkinsonian brain may result from changes in peptide turnover, following alteration of other neuronal systems, dopaminergic included, as has been observed after experimental lesions in the rat (Costa et al., 1978). The effect of lesion of the nigrostriatal dopaminergic neurones on neuropeptide concentrations has also been studied in MPTP-treated monkey thought to represent an animal model of Parkinson's disease (Burns et al., 1983). The lesion has no gross effect on peptide levels (Zamir et al., 1984; Allen et al., 1986; Jenner et al., 1986), suggesting that the abnormally low concentrations of peptides observed in parkinsonian patients are not caused by dopaminergic deficiency. However, the data remain discordant: decreased Met-enkephalin (Zamir et al., 1984) and increased substance P (Allen et al., 1986) concentrations in the substantia nigra and increased somatostatin concentrations in the cortex (Allen et al., 1986) of lesioned animals have been reported. The inconsistencies in the data may be related to differences in the timing (acute or subacute studies) of the experiments. These observations should therefore be confirmed in animals with long-term lesions of the nigrostriatal dopaminergic pathway, a situation which more closely resembles Parkinson's disease. Finally, if the peptide abnormalities correspond to metabolic changes consequent on the dopamine lesions, it is unknown whether the decreased peptide concentrations result from an increase or a decrease in turnover rate and whether the effect of the change would be to palliate or aggravate dopamine-dependent symptoms.

Some of the peptide deficits observed in Parkinson's disease may be indicative of neuronal damage. Morphological evidence in support of this hypothesis has not been forthcoming, but these studies are not yet sufficiently quantitative to permit an unequivocal conclusion to be drawn.

Peptides and parkinsonian symptoms

The only existing evidence for a direct relationship between a change in peptide concentrations and a symptom is the decrease in somatostatin alone in the cerebral cortex of demented patients with Parkinson's disease (*Figure 10.23*) and Alzheimer's disease (Davies, Katzman and Terry, 1980; Rossor *et al.*, 1980). All attempts to correlate this or other peptide deficiencies with parkinsonian motor symptoms, drug treatment, duration or severity of the disease have failed.

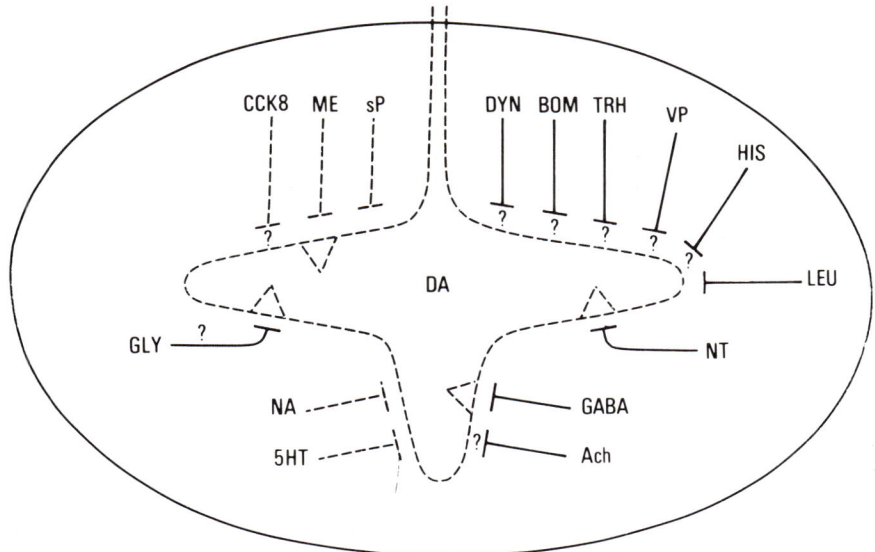

Figure 10.24 Neurochemistry of the substantia nigra in Parkinson's disease. Neurotransmitter systems putatively modulating dopamine cells in the substantia nigra. Broken lines indicate the systems damaged in the disease. Broken triangles correspond to a loss in the neurotransmitter receptor sites. For abbreviations *see* legend to *Figure 10.22;* Ach, acetylcholine; DA, dopamine; GLY, glycine; GLU, glutamate; HIS, histamine; 5HT, serotonin; LEU, leucine-enkephalin; ME, methionine-enkephalin; NA, noradrenaline; sP, substance P; VP = vasopressin

Peptidergic abnormalities might interfere with other neuronal systems thereby modulating their physiological function. The decreases in nigral CCK-8, Met-enkephalin and substance P, all of which have excitatory effects on the nigrostriatal dopaminergic neurones, would theoretically decrease dopaminergic transmission (*Figure 10.24*) still further. Modulation of dopaminergic transmission via therapeutic manipulation of the peptidergic neurones may be envisaged.

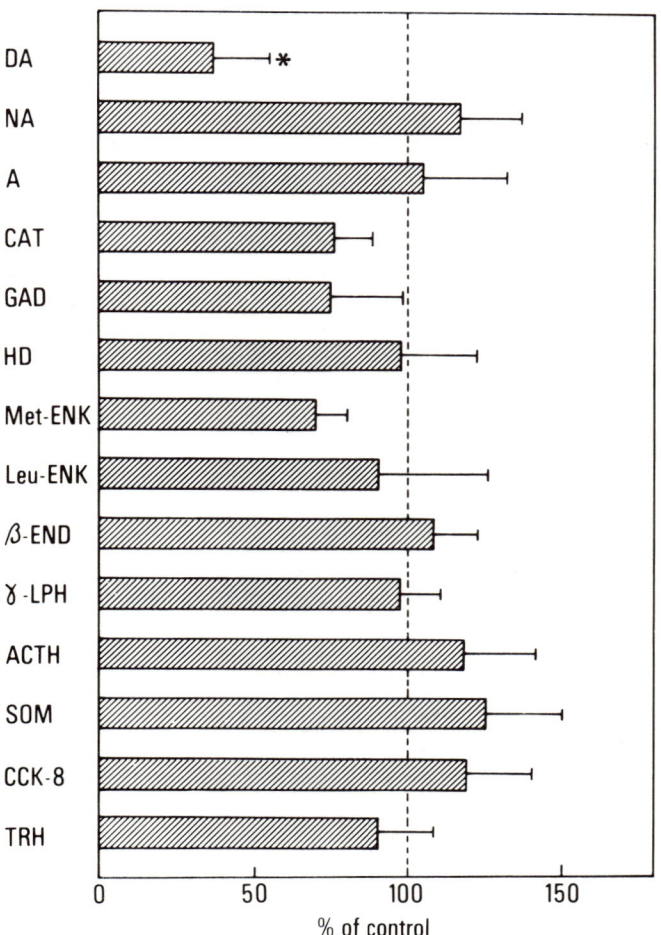

Figure 10.25 Neuromediators and enzyme activities in hypothalamus of parkinsonian patients. Data ± s.e.m. are expressed as a percentage of control values. * Statistical significance when compared with respective control. (DA) dopamine; (NA) noradrenaline; (A) adrenaline; (CAT) choline acetyltransferase; (GAD) glutamic acid decarboxylase; (HD) histidine decarboxylase; (Met-ENK) methionine-enkephalin; (Leu-ENK) leucine-enkephalin; (β-END) β-endorphin; (γ-LPH) γ-lipotropin; (ACTH) corticotropin; (SOM) somatostatin; (CCK-8) cholecystokinin-8; (TRH) thyrotropin-releasing hormone. (Reproduced from Agid and Javoy-Agid, 1985 with permission)

The peptides may also be responsible for clinical signs, indirectly, via other neuronal pathways. For example, a functional imbalance may occur when normal peptidergic transmission is associated with subnormal transmission of a lesioned system as in the hypothalamus where peptide levels are normal, but dopamine concentrations are decreased (*Figure 10.25*).

CONCLUDING REMARKS

Although considerable biochemical data have accumulated, it is not yet possible to completely explain the pathophysiology of Parkinson's disease.

The main biochemical features in the brain of patients with Parkinson's disease

The main features are shown in *Figure 10.26*:

(*a*) Central dopaminergic systems are lesioned, but to different degrees. Massive destruction of the nigrostriatal dopaminergic pathway, a fundamental link between the basal ganglia structures, is responsible by itself for most of the

Figure 10.26 Neurotransmitter systems in Parkinson's disease. Damaged systems are schematized by broken lines. For abbreviations *see* legends to *Figures 10.1* and *10.24;* GLU, glutamate

motor disorders. Preservation (still uncertain) of the dopaminergic innervation of the spinal cord suggests that not all dopaminergic neurones are sensitive to the pathogenic process or that some dopaminergic systems may be more resistant.

(b) The main ascending pathways are damaged by about 50%: the noradrenergic ceruleocortical system, the serotoninergic neurones from the raphe nuclei to the basal ganglia and cerebral cortex, the dopaminergic mesocorticolimbic neurones, the innominatocortical and the septohippocampal cholinergic systems. Dysfunction of these subcorticocortical isodendritic core neurones might contribute to the disruption of the smooth and subtle modulation of cognitive and motor programmes which seem to be intact in most patients.

(c) Alteration of subcorticocortical systems (essentially cholinergic but also noradrenergic) and of intracortical systems (somatostatinergic) might contribute to the intellectual disorders which develop in some patients.

(d) A number of neuronal systems seem preserved, since the neurotransmitter (or its specific synthesizing enzyme) content is within the normal range: the intrastriatal cholinergic neurones; the overall GABAergic (although this is still questionable) and histaminergic (Garbarg *et al.*, 1983) systems; peptidergic systems such as TRH- and most enkephalin-, CCK-8-, substance P-, neurotensin-, bombesin-, somatostatin-containing systems; striatal amino acids (glutamic acid, aspartic acid) (Perry *et al.*, 1983b; Kish *et al.*, 1986).

(e) The peptide abnormalities in the striatopallidonigral complex of patients remain uninterpretable. For example, whether the decrease in Met-enkephalin, substance P and CCK-8 concentrations in the substantia nigra reflects the degeneration of the corresponding peptide-containing neurones, or results from a trans-synaptic effect on metabolism, possibly consequent on dopamine denervation, is not understood.

(f) At receptor sites, changes concern the density of receptors rather than their affinity. Decreases in the density of receptors have usually been related to a loss of target cells. For example, in the substantia nigra, the dramatic decrease in high affinity neurotensin-binding sites (Sadoul *et al.*, 1984) and the reduction in the number of glycinergic, GABAergic, and opiate receptors (Lloyd, Shemen and Hornykiewicz, 1977; De Montis *et al.*, 1982; Llorens-Cortes *et al.*, 1984) (*Figure 10.24*) is most likely due to degeneration of dopamine neurones. Increases (usually not exceeding 20%) of receptor density seem to reflect denervation supersensitivity. For example, the increase in β_1 adrenergic receptors in the cerebral cortex (Cash *et al.*, 1984) and in D-2 dopaminergic receptors in the putamen (*Figure 10.6*) is most likely due to the degeneration of afferent noradrenergic and dopaminergic innervation, respectively. However, the characteristics of most receptors are unaffected despite denervation of the corresponding brain areas. This is the case for D-1 and D-2 dopamine receptors in the caudate nucleus and for muscarinic receptors in several areas of the cerebral cortex.

(g) Degeneration of the nigrostriatal dopamine pathway is also a prominent feature of progressive supranuclear palsy, another parkinsonian syndrome characterized, in addition, by a severe dementia of subcortical origin (Albert, 1978). Despite this striking similarity, several major differences distinguish the two diseases: (i) The subcorticocortical neuronal systems are mildly (cholinergic) or not at all (dopaminergic, noradrenergic, serotoninergic) damaged (*Figure 10.27*), suggesting that intellectual impairment in this disease

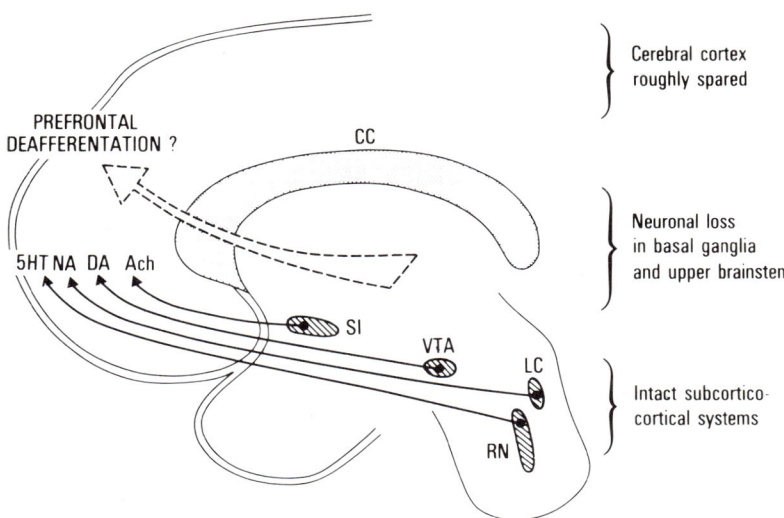

Figure 10.27 Progressive supranuclear palsy: pathological and neurochemical data. For abbreviations *see Figures 10.1* and *10.24*

does not result from subcortical lesions in the basal forebrain and brainstem. The marked 'frontal lobe-like syndrome' observed in such patients (Cambier *et al.*, 1985; Maher, Smith and Lees, 1985; Pillon *et al.*, 1986) is most likely provoked by the frontal deafferentation consequent to disruption of output from the basal ganglia to the frontal cortex (Agid *et al.*, 1986). The poor performance of progressive supranuclear palsy patients on neuropsychological tests sensitive to dysfunction of the parieto-occipitotemporal lobe may be due to a lack of activation of these perceptive areas by the deactivated frontal lobes. (ii) the density of striatal dopamine D-2 receptors is markedly decreased in these patients (Bokobza *et al.*, 1984, Baron *et al.*, 1985) in contrast to the increase found in patients with Parkinson's disease. This may account for the unresponsiveness of patients to levodopa. Striatal D-1 receptors are intact, however (Cash R., Raisman R. and Agid Y., personal communication). (iii) Neuropeptide-containing systems (substance P, CCK-8, Met-enkephalin, Leu-enkephalin), in particular those in the basal ganglia, seem to be spared in patients with progressive supranuclear palsy. This suggests that the peptide deficiencies observed in striatum and substantia nigra of parkinsonians do not result from degeneration of the nigrostriatal dopamine neurones which are dramatically affected in progressive supranuclear palsy as well. Somatostatin-14 concentrations are normal in the cerebral cortex of these patients although they are intellectually deteriorated (Epelbaum J., Javoy-Agid F., personal communication, 1986). This contrasts with the subnormal somatostatin levels found in Parkinson- and Alzheimer-type dementia, and is compatible with neuropathological data indicating that the cerebral cortex is intact in these patients. Furthermore, this observation indicates that the cortical somatostatin deficiency is not a general feature of dementia.

Finally, the biochemical map of progressive supranuclear palsy and idiopathic Parkinson's disease, supports the notion that the nigrostriatal dopamine deficiency is the 'common denominator' of parkinsonian syndromes.

A number of questions remain uncertain from a biochemical, histopathological and clinical standpoint

(a) Despite the original and fundamental observation that depletion of striatal dopamine is the major characteristic of parkinsonism, knowledge of the biochemical abnormalities in Parkinson's disease remains partial. At present, neurochemical data concern a limited number of parameters and brain areas. Their interpretation must be prudent due to possible pitfalls related to postmortem delay, premortem treatments, agonal states, characteristics of the control brains. The development of quantitative immunocytochemical and autoradiographic techniques should bring further insights and help to detect selective anomalies within restricted brain areas (for example in defined cortical layers or in localized striatal areas, e.g. striosomes).

(b) The morphological description of macroscopic and microscopic lesions in Parkinson's disease remains restricted for a pathophysiological approach, since it has mainly been used to confirm diagnoses. In particular, little is known about the cerebral cortex, thalamic nuclei, or many discrete nuclei of the brainstem in this disease. Cell counts combined with biochemical analysis should refine the pathophysiological interpretations of the past, but may also produce evidence of new anatomobiochemical anomalies.

(c) At present, the approach based on anatomobiochemical and clinical correlations remains limited, mainly because the analysis of clinical data obtained for the patients studied postmortem is difficult. The reason is not that clinical records analysed retrospectively are not adequate, but rather that the nosology of parkinsonian syndromes is defective. The point has been in most cases to distinguish between idiopathic Parkinson's disease (characterized by the presence of Lewy bodies) and other parkinsonian syndromes such as olivopontocerebellar atrophy and progressive supranuclear palsy. It now seems necessary to consider the existence of subgroups of patients with Parkinson's disease, some with relatively selective damage to dopamine neurones, others with additional lesions. Might this approach be sufficient to fill in the gaps in our understanding of symptoms as mysterious as intellectual impairment, postural instability and dysautonomia?

Finally, investigation of neurotransmitter systems in parkinsonian brain postmortem has tended to establish the nature and the biochemical consequences of neuronal damage. Considering the tremendous progress in biochemical techniques, the trend should now be to look for biochemical abnormalities which are at the origin of the degenerative process. Various attempts have already been made to explain the destruction of nigral neuromelanin-containing neurones selectively damaged in parkinsonian syndromes (Marsden, 1983; Langston, 1985b; D'Amato, Lipman and Snyder, 1986; Duvoisin et al., 1986; Kopin et al., 1986) and to characterize Lewy bodies (Goldman and Yen, 1984; Nakashima and Ikuta, 1984; Hirsch et al., 1985) which seem to be specific to idiopathic Parkinson's disease. Molecular biology will no doubt contribute to future approaches to the pathogenesis of this disease.

References

ADOLFFSSON, R., GOTTFRIES, C. G., ROOS, B. E. and WINDBLAD, B. (1979) Changes in the brain catecholamines in patients with dementia of Alzheimer type. *British Journal of Psychiatry*, **135**, 216–223

AGID, Y., BONNET, A. M., RUBERG, M. and JAVOY-AGID, F. (1985) Pathophysiology of levodopa induced abnormal involuntary movements. In *Dyskinesia, Research and Treatment. Psychopharmacology*, Supplementum 2, Eds. D. Casey, T. N. Chase, V. Christensen and J. Gerlach, pp. 145–159. Berlin: Springer-Verlag

AGID, Y., BONNET, A. M., SIGNORET, J. L. and LHERMITTE, F. (1979b) Clinical, pharmacological and biochemical approach of 'onset and end of dose' dyskinesias. In *The Extrapyramidal System and Its Disorders*. Eds. L. J. Poirier, T. L. Sourkes and P. J. Bedard. *Advances in Neurology*, Vol. 24. pp. 401–409. New York: Raven Press

AGID, Y., JAVOY, F. and GLOWINSKI, J. (1973) Hyperactivity of remaining dopaminergic neurons after partial destruction of the nigrostriatal dopaminergic system in the rat. *Nature New Biology*, **245**, 150–151

AGID, Y., JAVOY, F., GUYENET, P., BEAUJOUAN, J. C. and GLOWINSKI, J. (1975) Effects of surgical and pharmacological manipulations of the dopaminergic nigrostriatal neurons on the activity of the neostriatal cholinergic system in the rat. In *Neuropsychopharmacology*. Eds. J. R. Boissier, H. Hippius and P. Pichot, pp. 480–486. Amsterdam: Excerpta Medica

AGID, Y. and JAVOY-AGID, F. (1985) Peptides and Parkinson's disease. *Trends in Neurosciences*, **8**, 30–35

AGID, Y., JAVOY-AGID, F., RUBERG, M., PILLON, B., DUBOIS, B., DUYCKAERTS, C. *et al.*, (1986) Progressive supranuclear palsy: anatomoclinical and biochemical considerations. *Advances in Neurology*, **45**, 191–206

AGID, Y., POLLAK, P., BONNET, A. M., SIGNORET, J. L. and LHERMITTE, F. (1979a) Bromocriptine associated with a peripheral dopamine blocking agent in treatment of Parkinson's disease. *Lancet*, **i**, 570–572

AGID, Y., RUBERG, M., DUBOIS, B. and JAVOY-AGID, F. (1984) Biochemical substrates of mental disturbances in Parkinson's disease. *Advances in Neurology*, **40**, 211–218

AGNOLI, A., RUGGIERI, S., FALASCHI, P. *et al.* (1980) A neuropharmacological and neuroendocrine study on idiopathic and chronic pharmacological parkinsonism. *Advances in Biochemistry and Psychopharmacology*, **24**, 551–557

ALBERT, M. L. (1978) Subcortical dementia. In *Alzheimer's Disease: Senile Dementia and Related Disorders*. Eds. R. Katzman, R. D. Terry and K. L. Bick. *Aging*, vol. 7, pp. 173–180. New York: Raven Press

ALLEN, J. M., CROSS, A. J., CROW, T. J., JAVOY-AGID, F., AGID, Y. and BLOOM, S. R. (1985) Dissociation of neuropeptide Y and somatostatin in Parkinson's disease. *Brain Research*, **337**, 197–200

ALLEN, J. M., CROSS, A. J., YEATS, J. C., GHATEL, M. A., McGREGOR, G. P., CLOSE, S. P. *et al.* (1986) Neuropeptides and dopamine in the marmoset – Effect of treatment with l-methyl-4-phenyl-1,2,3,6-tetrahydropyridine (MPTP): an animal model for Parkinson's disease? *Brain*, **109**, 143–157

ARENDT, T., BIGL, V., ARENDT, A. and TENNSTEDT (1983) Loss of neurones in the nucleus basalis of Meynert in Alzheimer's disease, paralysis agitans, and Korsakoff's disease. *Acta Neuropathologica (Berlin)*, **61**, 101–108

BARBEAU, A. (1961) Biochemistry of Parkinson's disease. *International Congress Series*, **38**, 152–153

BARBEAU, A. (1969) Parkinson's disease as a systemic disorder. In *Third Symposium on Parkinson's Disease*. Eds. F. J. Gillingham and I. M. L. Donaldson, pp. 66–73. London: E. & S. Livingstone

BARBEAU, A. (1976) Neurological and psychiatric side-effects of L-DOPA. *Pharmacology and Therapeutics*, **1**, 475–494

BARBEAU, A. (1980) High-level levodopa therapy in severely akinetic parkinsonian patients: twelve years later. In *Parkinson's Disease: Current Progress, Problems and Management*. Eds. U. K. Rinne, M. Klinger and G. Stamm, pp. 229–239. Amsterdam: Elsevier, North Holland Press

BARBEAU, A., MARS, H. and GILLIO-JOFFROY, L. (1971) Adverse clinical side effects of levodopa therapy. In *Parkinson's Disease*. Eds. F. H. McDowell and C. H. Markham, pp. 203–237. Philadelphia: F. A. Davis Co.

BARBEAU, A., MURPHY, G. F. and SOURKES, T. L. (1961) Excretion of dopamine in diseases of basal ganglia. *Science*, **133**, 1706–1707

BARBEAU, A., SOURKES, T. L. and MURPHY, G. F. (1962) Les catécholamines dans la maladie de Parkinson. In *Monoamines et Système Nerveux Central*. Symposium Bel Air, Genève. Ed. J. De Ajuriaguerra, pp. 247–262. Paris: Masson

BAROLIN, G. S., BERNHEIMER, H. and HORNYKIEWICZ, O. (1964) Seitenverschiedenes Verhalten des Dopamins (3-Hydroxytyramin) im Gehirn eines Falles von Hemiparkinsonismus. *Schweizer Archiv fuer Neurologie und Psychiatrie*, **94**, 241–248

BARON, J. C., MAZIÈRE, B., LOC'H, C., SGOUROPOULOS, P., BONNET, A. M. and AGID, Y. (1985) Progressive supranuclear palsy: loss of striatal dopamine receptors demonstrated in vivo by positron tomography. *Lancet*, **i**, 1163–1164

BARTFAI, T. (1985) Presynaptic aspects of the coexistence of classical neurotransmitters and peptides. *Trends in Pharmacological Sciences*, **6**(7), 331–334

BARTHOLINI, G. and PLETSCHER, H. (1969) Effect of various decarboxylase inhibitors on the cerebral metabolism of dihydroxyphenylalanine. *Journal of Pharmacy and Pharmacology*, **21**, 323–324

BARTUS, R. T., DEAN, R. L., III, BEER, B. and LIPPA, A. S. (1982) The cholinergic hypothesis of geriatric memory dysfunction. *Science*, **217**, 408–417

BEARDSLEY, J. and PULETTI, F. (1971) Personality (MMPI) and cognitive (WAIS) changes after levodopa treatment. *Archives of Neurology*, **25**, 145–150

BERGER, B., TASSIN, J. P., RANCUREL, G. and BLANC, G. (1980) Catecholaminergic innervation of the human cerebral cortex in presenile and senile dementia. Histochemical and biochemical studies. In *Enzymes and Neurotransmitters in Mental Disease*. Eds. E. Usdin, T. L. Sourkes and B. H. Youdim, pp. 317–328. London: John Wiley

BERGMANN, K. J., LIMONGI, J. C. P., LOWE, Y. H., MENDOZA, M. R. and YAHR, M. D. (1984) Potentiation of the 'DOPA' effect in Parkinsonism by a direct GABA receptor agonist. *Lancet*, **i**, 559

BERNHEIMER, H., BIRKMAYER, W. and HORNYKIEWICZ, O. (1961) Verteilung des 5-hydroxytryptamins (Serotonin) im Gehirn des Menschen und sein Verhalten, bei Patienten mit Parkinson Syndrom. *Klinische Wochenschrift*, **39**, 1056–1059

BERNHEIMER, H., BIRKMAYER, W., HORNYKIEWICZ, O., JELLINGER, K. and SEITELBERGER, F. (1973) Brain dopamine and the syndromes of Parkinson and Huntington – Clinical, morphological and neurochemical correlations. *Journal of the Neurological Sciences*, **20**, 415–455

BERNHEIMER, H. and HORNYKIEWICZ, O. (1962) Das Verhalten einiger Enzyme im Gehirn normaler und Parkinson-kranker Menschen. *Archiv für Experimentelle Pathologie und Pharmakologie*, **243**, 295–299

BIRKMAYER, W. (1974) Twelve-years experience with L-DOPA treatment of Parkinson's disease. In *Current Concepts in the Treatment of Parkinsonism*. Ed. M. Yahr, pp. 141. New York: Raven Press

BIRKMAYER, W. and HORNYKIEWICZ, O. (1961) Der L-3,4-dioxyphenylalanin (L-DOPA) – Effekt bei der Parkinson-Akinese. *Wiener Klinische Wochenschrift*, **73**, 787–788

BIRKMAYER, W. and RIEDERER, P. (1980) *Parkinson's disease – Biochemistry, Clinical Pathology, and Treatment*. Berlin: Springer-Verlag

BISSETTE, G., NEMEROFF, C. B., DECKER, M. W., KIZER, J. S., AGID, Y. and JAVOY-AGID, F. (1985) Alterations in regional brain concentrations of neurotesin and bombesin in Parkinson's disease. *Annals of Neurology*, **17**, 324–328

BLACKWOOD, W. and CORSELLIS, J. A. N. (Eds.) (1977) *Greenfield's Neuropathology*, 3rd edn, pp. 608–650. London: Edward Arnold

BLOXHAM, C. A., CROSS, A. J., CROW, T. J. and OWEN, F. (1981) Characteristics of [^{3}H]spiperone binding to human lymphocytes. *British Journal of Pharmacology*, **74**, 233

BOKOBZA, B., RUBERG, M., SCATTON, B., JAVOY-AGID, F. and AGID, Y. (1984) [^{3}H]spiperone binding, dopamine and HVA concentrations in Parkinson's disease and supranuclear palsy. *European Journal of Pharmacology*, **99**, 167–175

BOLLER, F., MIZUTANI, T., ROESSMANN, U. and GAMBETTI, P. (1980) Parkinson's disease, dementia and Alzheimer disease: clinico pathological correlations. *Annals of Neurology*, **i**, 329–355

BONNET, A. M., DE SMET, Y., TELL, G., SCHECHTER, P. J., SAINT-HILLAIRE, M. H. and AGID, Y. (1986a) Is it useful to measure GABA levels in degenerative diseases of the CNS? Submitted

BONNET, A. M., LORIA, Y., SAINT-HILAIRE, M. H., LHERMITTE, F. and AGID, Y. (1986b) Does long term aggravation of Parkinson's disease result from non-dopaminergic lesions? *Neurology*, in press

BOWEN, D. M., SMITH, C. B., WHITE, P. and DAVISON, A. N. (1976) Neurotransmitter-related enzymes and indices of hypoxia in senile dementia and other abiotrophies. *Brain*, **99**, 459–496

BROWN, R. G. and MARSDEN, C. D. (1984) How common is dementia in Parkinson's disease? *Lancet*, **ii**, 1262–1265

BROWN, R. G., MARSDEN, C. D., QUINN, N. and WYKE, M. A. (1984) Alterations in cognitive performance and affect arousal state during fluctuations in motor function in Parkinson's disease. *Journal of Neurology, Neurosurgery and Psychiatry*, **47**, 454–465

BROZOWSKI, T. J., BROWN, R. M. and GOLDMAN, P. (1979) Cognitive deficit caused by regional depletion of dopamine in prefrontal cortex of rhesus monkey. *Science*, **205**, 929–931

BRUN, A. and ENGLUND, E. (1981) Regional pattern of degeneration in Alzheimer's disease: neuronal loss and histopathological grading. *Histopathology*, **5**, 549–564

BURNS, R. S., CHIVEH, C. C., MARKEY, S. P., EBERT, M. H., JACOBOWITZ, D. M. and KOPIN, I. J. (1983): A primate model of parkinsonism: selective destruction of dopaminergic neurons in the pars compacta of the substantia nigra by *N*-methyl-4-phenyl-1,2,3,6-tetrahydropyridine. *Proceedings of the National Academy of Science of the United States of America,* **80,** 4546–4560

CAMBIER, J., MASSON, M., VIADER, F., LIMODIER, J. and STRUBE, A. (1985) Le syndrome frontal de la maladie de Steele-Richardson-Olszewski. *Revue Neurologique (Paris),* **141,** 528–536

CANDY, J. M., PERRY, R. H., PERRY, E. K., IRVING, D., BLESSED, G., FAIRBAIRN, A. F. and TOMLINSON, B. E. (1983) Pathological changes in the nucleus of Meynert in Alzheimer's and Parkinson's diseases. *Journal of the Neurological Sciences,* **54,** 277–289

CARLSSON, A., LINDQUIST, M. and MAGNUSSON, T. (1957) 3,4-Dihydroxyphenylalanine and 5-hydroxytryptophan as reserpine antagonists. *Nature,* **180,** 1200

CARLSSON, A., LINDQUIST, M., MAGNUSSON, T. and WALDECK, B. (1958) On the presence of [^{3}H]-hydroxytyramine in brain. *Science,* **127,** 471

CASH, R., RAISMAN, R., JAVOY-AGID, F. and SCATTON, B. (1986) Biochemistry of the locus coeruleus in Parkinson's disease. *Neurology* (in press)

CASH, R., RAISMAN, R., PLOSKA, A. and AGID, Y. (1985) High and low affinity [^{3}H]imipramine binding sites in control and parkinsonian patients. *European Journal of Pharmacology,* **117,** 71–80

CASH, R., RUBERG, M., RAISMAN, R. and AGID, Y. (1984) Adrenergic receptors in Parkinson's disease. *Brain Research,* **322,** 269–275

CELESIA, G. G. and WANAMAKER, W. M. (1972) Psychiatric disturbances in Parkinson's disease. *Diseases of the Nervous System,* **33,** 577–583

CHASE, T. N. (1972) Parkinson's disease – Modification by 5-hydroxytryptophan. *Neurology,* **22,** 479–484

CHASE, T. N. (1974) Serotoninergic mechanisms and extrapyramidal function in man. *Advances in Neurology,* **5,** 31–39

CHASE, T. N., GORDON, E. K. and NG, L. K. Y. (1973) Norepinephrine metabolism in the central nervous system of man: studies using 3-methoxy-4-hydroxyphenylethylene glycol levels in cerebrospinal fluid. *Journal of Neurochemistry,* **21,** 581–587

CHERAMY, A., LEVIEL, V. and GLOWINSKI, J. (1981) Dendritic release of dopamine in the substantia nigra. *Nature,* **289,** 537–542

CONTE-DEVOLX, B., GRINO, M., NIEOULLON, A., JAVOY-AGID, F., CASTANAS, E., GUILLAUME, V. et al. (1985) Corticoliberin, somatocrinin, and amine contents in normal and parkinsonian human hypothalamus. *Neuroscience Letters,* **56,** 217–222

COSTA, E., FRATTA, W., HONG, J. S., MORONI, F. and YANG, H. Y. T. (1978) Interactions between enkephalinergic and other neuronal systems. *Advances in Biochemical Psychopharmacology,* **18,** 217–226

CREESE, I. and SNYDER, S. H. (1979) Nigrostriatal lesions enhance striatal [^{3}H]apomorphine and [^{3}H]spiroperidol binding. *European Journal of Pharmacology,* **56,** 277–281

CROSS, A. J., CROW, T. J., JOHNSON, J. A., JOSEPH, M. H., PERRY, E. K., PERRY, R. H. et al. (1983) Monoamine metabolism in senile dementia of Alzheimer type. *Journal of the Neurological Sciences,* **60,** 383–392

CUELLO, A. C. and PAXINOS, G. (1978) Evidence for a long leu-enkephalin striatopallidal pathway in rat brain. *Nature,* **271,** 178–180

D'AMATO, R. J., LIPMAN, Z. P. and SNYDER, S. H. (1986) Selectivity of the parkinsonian neurotoxin MPTP: toxic metabolite MPP+ binds to neuromelanin. *Science,* **231,** 987–989

DAVIES, P. and VERTH, A. H. (1978) Regional distribution of muscarinic acetylcholine receptor in normal and Alzheimer's-type dementia brains. *Brain Research,* **138,** 385–392

DAVIES, P., KATZMAN, R. and TERRY, R. D. (1980) Reduced somatostatin-like immunoreactivity in cerebral cortex from cases of Alzheimer disease and Alzheimer senile dementia. *Nature,* **288,** 279–280

DAVIS, G. C., WILLIAMS, A. C., MARKEY, S. P., EBERT, M. H., CAINE, E. D., REICHERT, C. M. and KOPIN, I. J. (1979) Chronic parkinsonism secondary to intravenous injection of mepedrine analogues. *Psychiatry Research,* **1,** 249–254

DE AJURIAGUERRA, J. (1970) Etude psychopathologique des parkinsoniens. In *Monoamines, Noyaux Gris Centraux et Syndrome de Parkinson.* Eds. J. de Ajuriaguerra and G. Gauthier. Proceedings of the VI Bel-Air Symposium, Geneva, Sept. 1970, pp. 327–351

DE JONG, P. J., LAKKE, J. P. W. F. and TEELKEN, A. W. (1984) CSF GABA levels in Parkinson's disease. *Advances in Neurology,* **40,** 427–430

DE MONTIS, G., BEAUMONT, K., JAVOY-AGID, F., AGID, Y., CONSTANDINIDIS, J., LOWENTHAL, A. and LLOYD, K. G. (1982) Glycine receptors in the human substantia nigra as defined by [^{3}H]strychnine binding. *Journal of Neurochemistry,* **38,** 718–724

DE SMET, Y., RUBERG, M., SERDARU, M., DUBOIS, B., LHERMITTE, F. and AGID, Y. (1982) Confusion, dementia and anticholinergics in Parkinson's disease. *Journal of Neurology, Neurosurgery and Psychiatry,* **45,** 1161–1164

DEUTSCH, J. A. (1983) *Physiological Basis of Memory,* 2nd edn. London: Academic Press

DRACHMAN, D. A. (1977) Memory and cognitive function in man: does the cholinergic system have a specific role? *Neurology,* **27,** 783–790

DUBOIS, B., DANZÉ, F., PILLON, B., CUSIMANO, J., LHERMITTE, F. and AGID, Y. (1986) Cholinergic dependent-cognitive deficits in non-demented parkinsonian patients. Submitted

DUBOIS, B., HAUW, J. J., RUBERG, M., SERDARU, M., JAVOY-AGID, F. and AGID, Y. (1985a) Demence et maladie de Parkinson: correlations biochimiques et anatomo-cliniques. *Revue Neurologique (Paris),* **141**(3), 184–193

DUBOIS, B., MAYO, W., AGID, G., LE MOAL, M. and SIMON, H. (1985b) Profound disturbances of spontaneous and learned behaviors following lesions of the nucleus basalis magnocellularis in the rat. *Brain Research,* **338,** 249–258

DUBOIS, B., RUBERG, M., JAVOY-AGID, F., PLOSKA, A. and AGID, Y. (1983) A subcortico-cortical cholinergic system is affected in Parkinson's disease. *Brain Research,* **288,** 213–218

DUPONT, E., CHRISTENSEN, S. E., HANSEN, A. P., OLIVARIUS, B. F. and HORSKOV, H. (1982) Low cerebrospinal fluid somatostatin in Parkinson's disease: an irreversible abnormality. *Neurology,* **32,** 312–314

DUVOISIN, R. C. (1967) Cholinergic-anticholinergic antagonism in parkinsonism. *Archives of Neurology and Psychiatry,* **17,** 124–136

DUVOISIN, R. C., HEIKKILA, R. E., NICKLAS, W. J. and HESS, A. (1986) Dopaminergic neurotoxicity of MPTP in the mouse: a murine model of parkinsonism. In *Recent Developments in Parkinson's Diseases.* Eds. S. Fahn, C. D. Marsden, P. Jenner and P. Teychenne, pp. 147–154. New York: Raven Press

EHRINGER, H. and HORNYKIEWICZ, O. (1960) Verteilung von Noradrenalin und Dopamin (3-Hydroxytyramin) im Gehirn des Menschen und ihr Verhalten bei Erkrankungen des extrapyramidalen Systems. *Wiener Klinische Wochenschrift,* **38,** 1236–1239

EISLER, T., THORNER, M. O., McLEOD, R. M., KAISER, D. L. and CALNE, D. B. (1981) Prolactin secretion in Parkinson's disease. *Neurology,* **31,** 1356–1359

ELLENBROEK, B., SCHWARZ, M., SONTAG, K. H., JASPERS, R. and COOLS, A. (1985) Muscular rigidity and delineation of a dopamine-specific neostriatal subregion: tonic EMG activity in rats. *Brain Research,* **345,** 132–140

EMSON, P. C., ARREGUI, A., CLEMENT-JONES, V., SANBERG, B. E. B. and ROSSOR, M. (1980) Regional distribution of methionine-enkephalin and substance P-like immunoreactivity in normal human brain and in Huntington's disease. *Brain Research,* **199,** 147–160

EPELBAUM, J., RUBERG, M., MOYSE, E., JAVOY-AGID, F., DUBOIS, B. and AGID, Y. (1983) Somatostatin and dementia in Parkinson's disease. *Brain Research,* **278,** 376–379

ESCOUROLLE, R., DE RECONDO, J. and GRAY, F. (1970) Etude anatomo-pathologique des syndromes parkinsoniens. In *Monoamines et Noyaux Gris Centraux et Syndrome de Parkinson.* Eds J. de Ajuriaguerra and G. Gantier, pp. 173–229. IVè Symposium de Bel Air, Genève, Sept. 1970

FAHN, S. (1974) 'On–off' phenomenon with levodopa therapy in parkinsonism – Clinical and pharmacologic correlations and the effect of intramuscular pyridoxine. *Neurology,* **24,** 431–441

FAHN, S. (1982) Fluctuation of disability in Parkinson's disease: Pathophysiological aspects. In *Movement Disorders.* Eds. C. D. Marsden and S. Fahn. *Neurology 2:* pp. 123–145. London: Butterworths

FAHN, S., LIBSCH, L. R. and CUTLER, R. W. (1971) Monoamines in the human neostriatum: Topographic distribution in normals and in Parkinson's disease and their role in akinesia, rigidity, chorea and tremor. *Journal of the Neurological Sciences,* **14,** 427–455

FARLEY, I. J. and HORNYKIEWICZ, O. (1976) Noradrenaline in subcortical brain regions of patients with Parkinson's disease and control subjects. In *Advances in Parkinsonism.* Eds. W. Birkmayer and O. Hornyckiewicz, pp. 178–185. Basel: Roche

FIBIGER, H. C. (1982) The organization and some projections of cholinergic neurons of the mammalian forebrain. *Brain Research Review,* **4,** 327–388

FLEMINGER, S., JENNER, F. and MARSDEN, C. D. (1982) Are dopamine receptors present on human lymphocytes? *Journal of Pharmacy and Pharmacology,* **34,** 658–663

FONNUM, F., GOTTESFELD, Z. and GROFOVA, I. (1978) Distribution of glutamate decarboxylase, choline acetyltransferase and aromatic amino acid decarboxylase in the basal ganglia of normal and operated rats. Evidence for striatopallidal, striatoentopeduncular and striatonigral Gabaergic fibers. *Brain Research,* **143,** 125–138

FORNO, L. S. (1982) Pathology of Parkinson's disease. In *Movement Disorders.* Eds. C. D. Marsden and S. Fahn. *Neurology 2,* pp. 25–40. London: Butterworths

FUXE, K., AGNATI, L. F., BENFENATI, F., CELANI, M., ZINI, I., ZOLI, M. and MUTT, V. (1983) Evidence for the existence of receptor-receptor interactions in the central nervous system. Studies on the regulation of monoamine receptors by neuropeptides. *Journal of Neural Transmission,* Suppl. 18, 165–179

GALE, K. (1984) Neurotransmitter interactions in the basal ganglia: 'GABA-GABAcology' versus

'DA-DAism'. In *Dynamics of Neurotransmitter Function.* Ed. I. Hanin, pp. 189–209. New York: Raven Press
GARBARG, M., JAVOY-AGID, F., SCHWARTZ, J. C. and AGID, Y. (1983) Histidine decarboxylase activity in brains of patients with Parkinson's disease. *Lancet,* **i,** 74–75
GASPAR, P., BERGER, B., GAY, M., HAMON, M., CESSELIN, F., VIGNY, A. *et al.* (1983) Tyrosine hydroxylase and methionin-enkephalin in the human mesencephalon: immunohistochemical localization and relationships. *Journal of the Neurological Sciences,* **58,** 247–267
GASPAR, P. and GRAY, F. (1984) Dementia in idiopathic Parkinson's disease: a neuropathological study of 32 cases. *Acta Neuropathologica,* **64,** 43–52
GASPAR, P., JAVOY-AGID, F., PLOSKA, A. and AGID, Y. (1980) Regional distribution of neurotransmitter specific enzymes in the basal ganglia of human brain. *Journal of Neurochemistry,* **34,** 278–283
GERFEN, C. R. (1986) The neostriatal mosaic: the reiterated processing unit. In *Neurotransmitter Interactions in the Basal Ganglia.* Eds. C. Feuerstein, B. Scatton and M. Sandler. New York: Raven Press (in press)
GERSHANIK, O., HEIKKILA, R. E. and DUVOISIN, R. C. (1983) Behavioral correlations of dopamine receptor activation. *Neurology,* **33,** 1489–1492
GLOWINSKI, J., MICHELOT, R. and CHERAMY, A. (1980) Role of striatonigral substance P in the regulation of the activity of the nigrostriatal dopaminergic neurones. In *Neural Peptides and Neuronal Communication.* Eds. E. Costa and M. Trabucchi, pp. 51–63. New York: Raven Press
GOETZ, C. G., LUTGE, W. and TANNER, C. M. (1986) Autonomic dysfunction in Parkinson's disease. *Neurology,* **36,** 73–75
GOLDMAN, J. and YEN, S. (1984) Lewy bodies in Parkinson's disease contain neurofilament antigens. *Science,* **221,** 1082–1083
GOLDSTEIN, M., BATTISTA, A. F., ANAGNOSTE, B. and NAKATANI, S. (1969) Tremor production and striatal amines in monkeys. In *Third Symposium on Parkinson's Disease.* Eds. F. J. Gillingham and I. L. M. Donaldson, pp. 37–40. London: E. & S. Livingstone
GOTHAM, A. M., BROWN, R. G. and MARSDEN, C. D. (1986) Depression in Parkinson's disease: a quantitative and qualitative analysis. *Journal of Neurology, Neurosurgery and Psychiatry,* **49,** 381–389
GOTTFRIES, C. G., GOTTFRIES, I. and ROOS, B. E. (1969) Homovanillic acid and 5-hydroxy-indoleacetic acid in the cerebrospinal fluid of patients with senile dementia, presenile dementia and parkinsonism. *Journal of Neurochemistry,* **16,** 1341–1345
GRAFE, M. R., FORNO, L. S. and ENG, L. F. (1985) Immunocytochemical studies of substance P and Met-enkephalin in the basal ganglia and substantia nigra in Huntington's, Parkinson's and Alzheimer's diseases. *Journal of Neuropathology and Experimental Neurology,* **44,** 47–59
GRAMSCH, C., HOLLT, V., MEHRAEIN, P., PASI, A. and HERZ, A. (1979) Regional distribution of methionine-enkephalin and beta-endorphin like immunoreactivity in human brain and pituitary. *Brain Research,* **171,** 261–270
GRAYBIEL, A. M. (1984) Neurochemically specified subsystems in the basal ganglia. In *Functions of the Basal Ganglia,* Ciba Foundation Symposium 107, pp. 114–119. London: Pitman Press
GREEN, A. R. and HEAL, D. J. (1985) The effects of drugs on serotonin-mediated behavioural model. In *Neuropharmacology of Serotonin.* Ed. A. R. Green, pp. 326–365. Oxford: Oxford University Press
GREENFIELD, J. G. and BOSANQUET, F. D. (1953) The brain stem lesions in parkinsonism. *Journal of Neurology, Neurosurgery and Psychiatry,* **16,** 213–226
GRIMES, J. D. and HASSAN, M. N. (1983) Bromocriptine in the long-term management of advanced Parkinson's disease. *Canadian Journal of Neurological Sciences,* **10,** 86–90
GUERIN, B., SILICE, C., MOUCHET, P., FEUERSTEIN, C. and DEMENGE, P. (1985) Changes of the striatal [^{3}H]spiperone binding 3-6 weeks after nigrostriatal denervation and after two years. *Life Sciences,* **37,** 955–961
GUTTMAN, M., SEEMAN, P., REYNOLDS, G. P., RIEDERER, P., JELLINGER,K. and TOURTELOTTE, W. W. (1986) Dopamine D_2 receptor density remains constant in treated Parkinson's disease. *Annals of Neurology,* **19,** 487–492
HAKIM, A. M. and MATHIESON, G. (1979) Dementia in Parkinson disease: a neuropathologic study. *Neurology,* **29,** 1209–1214
HARDIE, R. J., LEES, A. J. and STERN, G. M. (1984) On–off fluctuations in Parkinson's disease. A clinical and neuropharmacological study. *Brain,* **107,** 487–506
HARDY, J., ADOLFSSON, R., ALAFUZOFF, I., BUCHT, G., MARCUSSON, J., NYBERG, P. *et al.* (1985) Transmitter deficits in Alzheimer's disease. *Neurochemistry International,* 7(4), 545–563
HASSLER, R. (1953) Extrapyramidal-motorische systeme und erkrankungen. In *Handbuch der Innerin Medezin,* Vol. 3, pp. 676–904. Berlin: Springer Verlag

HATTORI, T., SINGH, V. K., McGEER, E. G. and McGEER, P. L. (1976) Immunohistochemical localization of choline acetyltransferase containing neostriatal neurons and their relationship with dopaminergic synapses. *Brain Research*, **102**, 164–173

HEFTI, F., MELAMED, E. and WURTMAN, R. J. (1980) Partial lesions of the dopaminergic nigrostriatal system in rat brain: Biochemical characterization. *Brain Research*, **195**, 95–101

HENDRY, S. H. C., JONES, E. G., DE FELIPE, J., SCHMECHEL, D., BRANDON, C. and EMSON, P. C. (1984) Neuropeptide-containing neurons of the cerebral cortex are also GABAergic. *Proceedings of the National Academy of Sciences of the United States of America*, **81**, 6526–6530

HIRSCH, E., RUBERG, M., JAVOY-AGID, F., AGID, Y., DARDENNE, M. and BACH, J. F. (1985) Monoclonal antibodies raised against Lewy bodies in brains from subjects with Parkinson's disease. *Brain Research*, **345**, 374–378

HÖKFELT, T., ELDE, R., FUXE, K. et al. (1978) Aminergic and peptidergic pathways in the nervous system with special reference to the hypothalamus. In *The Hypothalamus*. Research Publications: Association for Research in Nervous and Mental Disease, Vol. 56. Eds. S. Reichlin, R. J. Baldessarini and J. B. Martin, pp. 69–135. New York: Raven Press

HÖKFELT, T., SKIRBOLL, L., REHFELD, J. F., GOLDSTEIN, M., MARKEY, K. and DANN, O. (1980) A subpopulation of mesencephalic dopamine neurones projecting to limbic areas contains a cholecystokinin-like peptide: evidence from immunohistochemistry combined with retrograde tracing. *Neuroscience*, **5**, 2093–2124

HORNYKIEWICZ, O. (1963) Die topische Lokalization und das Verhalten von Noradrenalin und Dopamin (3-Hydroxytyramin) in der Substantia nigra des normalen und Parkinsonkranken Menschen. *Wiener Klinischer Wochenschrift*, **75**, 309–312

HORNYKIEWICZ, O. (1966) Dopamine (3-hydroxytyramine) and brain function. *Pharmacological Reviews*, **18**, 925–964

HORNYKIEWICZ, O. (1972) Dopamine and extrapyramidal motor function and dysfunction. In *Neurotransmitters*, Research Publications: Association for Research in Nervous and Mental Disease, Vol. 50, pp. 390–415. New York: Raven Press

HORNYKIEWICZ, O. (1975) Parkinson's disease and its chemotherapy. *Biochemical Pharmacology*, **24**, 1061–1065

HORNYKIEWICZ, O. (1979a) Brain dopamine in Parkinson's disease and other neurological disturbances. In *Neurobiology of Dopamines*. Eds. A. S. Horn, J. Korf and B. H. C. Westerink, pp. 633–654. London: Academic Press

HORNYKIEWICZ, O. (1979b) Compensatory biochemical changes at the striatal dopamine synapse in Parkinson's disease – Limitation of L-DOPA therapy. *Advances in Neurology*, **24**, 275–281

HORNYKIEWICZ, O. (1982a) Parkinson's disease. In *Disorders of Neurohumoral Transmission*. Ed. T. J. Crow, pp. 121–143. London: Academic Press

HORNYKIEWICZ, O. (1982b) Brain neurotransmitter changes in Parkinson's disease. In *Movement Disorders*. Eds. C. D. Marsden and S. Fahn. *Neurology 2*, pp. 41–58. London: Butterworths

HORNYKIEWICZ, O., LLOYD, K. G. and DAVIDSON, L. (1976) The GABA system, function of the basal ganglia and Parkinson's disease. In *GABA in Nervous System Function*. Eds. E. Roberts, T. N. Chase and D. B. Tower, pp. 479–485. New York: Raven Press

HUNT, S. P., PECK, R. W. and ROSSOR, M. N. (1983) Patterns of neuropeptide immunoreactivity in the human brain: changes associated with Huntington's chorea and Parkinson's disease. *Peptides and Neurological Diseases*. August, 7–10, Cambridge (abstract)

HYYPPA, M. T., LANGVIK, V. and RINNE, U. K. (1978) Plasma pituitary hormones in patients with Parkinson's disease treated with bromocriptine. *Journal of Neural Transmission*, **42**, 151–157

IVERSEN, S. D. (1984) Cortical monoamines and behavior. In *Monoamine Innervation of Cerebral Cortex*, Vol. VII (5) No. 4, 5th Symposium of the 'Centre de Recherche en Sciences Neurologiques of the University de Montreal', Eds. L. Descarries, T. R. Reader and H. H. Jasper, pp. 321–349. New York: Alan R. Liss

JAVOY-AGID, F. and AGID, Y. (1980) Is the mesocortical dopaminergic system involved in Parkinson's disease? *Neurology*, **30**, 1326–1330

JAVOY-AGID, F., GROUSELLE, D., TIXIER-VIDAL, A. and AGID, Y. (1983) Thyrotropin releasing hormone in brain of patients with Parkinson disease. *Neuropeptides*, **3**, 405–410

JAVOY-AGID, F., PLOSKA, A. and AGID, Y. (1982) Microtopography of TH, CAT, and GAD activity in the substantia nigra and ventral tegmental area of control and parkinsonian human brain. *Neurochemistry*, **37**, 1221–1227

JAVOY-AGID, F., RUBERG, M., HIRSCH, E., CASH, R., RAISMAN, R., TAQUET, H. et al. (1986) Recent progress in the neurochemistry of Parkinson's disease. In *Recent Developments in Parkinson's Disease*. Eds. S. Fahn et al., pp. 67–83. New York: Raven Press

JAVOY-AGID, F., RUBERG, M., PIQUE, L., BERTAGNA, X., TAQUET, H., STUDLER, J. M. *et al.* (1984a) Biochemistry of the hypothalamus in Parkinson disease. *Neurology,* **34,** 672–676

JAVOY-AGID, F., RUBERG, M., TAQUET, H., BOKOBZA, B., AGID, Y., GASPAR, P. *et al.* (1984b) Biochemical neuropathology of Parkinson disease. *Advances in Neurology,* **40,** 189–198

JAVOY-AGID, F., TAQUET, H., BERGER, B., GASPAR, P., MOREL-MAROGER, A., MONTASTRUC, J. L. *et al.* (1982) Relation between dopamine and methionine-enkephalin systems in control and parkinsonian brains. Kyoto, Sept. 20–25, 1981. *Excerpta Medica Neurology,* **568,** 187–202

JAVOY-AGID, F., TAQUET, H., PLOSKA, A., CHERIF-ZAHAR, C., RUBERG, M. and AGID, Y. (1981) Distribution of catecholamines in the ventral mesencephalon of human brain with special reference to Parkinson disease. *Journal of Neurochemistry,* **36,** 2101–2105

JEGOU, S., DELBENDE, C., TRANCHAND-BUNEL, D., VAUDRY, H., JAVOY-AGID, F. and AGID, Y. (1985a) Regional distribution of vasoactive peptide in human brain – Cortical VIP is unchanged in Parkinson's brain. Second International Symposium on VIP and related Peptides. *Regulatory Peptides,* Supplement 3, S24

JEGOU, S., JAVOY-AGID, F., DELBENDE, C., RUBERG, M., VAUDRY, H. and AGID, Y. (1985b) Cortical vasoactive intestinal peptide in relation to dementia in Parkinson's disease. *Journal of Neurology, Neurosurgery and Psychiatry,* **48**(8), 842–843

JELLINGER, K. (1986) Pathology of Parkinsonism. In *Recent Developments in Parkinson's Disease.* Eds. S. Fahn, C. D. Marsden, P. Jenner and P. Teychenne, pp. 33–66. New York: Raven Press

JELLINGER, K. and RIEDERER, P. (1984) Dementia in Parkinson's disease and (pre) senile dementia of Alzheimer type: morphological aspects and changes in the intracerebral MAO activity. *Advances in Neurology,* **40,** 199–210

JENNER, P. and MARSDEN, C. D. (1984) Neurochemical basis of parkinsonian tremor. In *Movement Disorders: Tremor.* Eds. L. J. Findley and R. Capildeo, pp. 305–319. London: Macmillan

JENNER, P., TAQUET, H., BENOLIEL, J. T., MAUBORGNE, A., CESSELIN, F., SALVAGE, S. *et al.* (1986) Lack of change in basal ganglia neuropeptide content following acute MPTP treatment of the common marmoset. *Neurochemistry* (in press)

JOLKKONEN, J., SOININEN, H., HALONEN, T., YLINEN, A., LAULUMAA, V., LAAKSO, M. and RIEKKINEN, P. (1986) Somatostatin-like immunoreactivity in the cerebrospinal fluid of patients with Parkinson's disease and its relation to dementia. *Journal of Neurology, Neurosurgery and Psychiatry,* in press

JOUVENT, R., BONNET, A. M. and AGID, Y. (1986) Heterogeneity of depression in parkinsonism. 1st E.N.E.A. Symposium Basel, March, 4–7, 1984. New York: Raven Press (in press)

KAKIDANI, H., FURUTANI, Y., TAKAHASHI, H., NODA, M., MORIMOTO, Y., HIROSE, T. *et al.* (1982) Cloning and sequence analysis of cDNA for porcine beta-neo-endorphin/dynorphin precursor. *Nature,* **298,** 447–453

KANAZAWA, I., EMSON, P. C. and CUELLO, A. C. (1977) Evidence for the existence of substance P-containing fibres in striato-nigral and pallido-nigral pathways in rat brain. *Brain Research,* **119,** 447–453

KEBABIAN J. W. and CALNE, D. B. (1979) Multiple receptors for dopamine. *Nature,* **277,** 93–96

KIENZL, E., RIEDERER, P., JELLINGER, K. and WESEMANN, W. (1981) Transitional states of central serotonin receptors in Parkinson's disease. *Journal of Neural Transmission,* **51,** 113–122

KIMURA, H., McGEER, P. L. and PENG, J. H. (1984) Choline acetyltransferase-containing neurons in the rat brain. In *Classical Transmitters and Transmitter Receptors in the CNS. Part II – Handbook of Chemical Neuroanatomy,* Vol. 3. Eds. A Bjorklund, T. Hokfelt and M. J. Kuhar, pp. 51–67. Amsterdam: Elsevier

KISH, S. J., CHANG, L. J., MIRCHANDANI, L., SHANNAK, K. and HORNYKIEWICZ, O. (1985) Progressive supranuclear palsy: relationship between extrapyramidal disturbances, dementia and brain neurotransmitter markers. *Annals of Neurology,* **18,** 530–536

KISH, S. J., RAJPUT, A., GILBERT, J., ROZDILSKY, B., CHANG, L. J., SHANNAK, K. and HORNYCKIEWICZ, O. (1986) GABA is elevated in striatal but not extrastriatal brain regions in Parkinson's disease: correlation with striatal dopamine loss. *Annals of Neurology,* **20,** 26–31

KISH, S. J., SHANNAK, K. S., RAJPUT, A. H., GILBERT, J. J. and HORNYCKIEWICZ, O. (1984) Cerebellar norepinephrine in patients with Parkinson's disease and control subjects. *Archives of Neurology,* **41,** 612–614

KLAWANS, H. L. and WEINER, W. J. (1974) Attempted use of haloperidol in the treatment of L-DOPA induced dyskinesias. *Journal of Neurology, Neurosurgery and Psychiatry,* **37**(1), 427–430

KNOWLTON, B. J., WENK, G. L., OLTON, D. S. and COYLE, J. T. (1985) Basal forebrain lesions produce a dissociation of trial-dependent and trial-independent memory performance. *Brain Research,* **345,** 315–321

KOOB, G. F., SIMON, H., HERMAN, J. P. and LE MOAL, M. (1984) Neuroleptic-like disruption of the conditioned avoidance response requires destruction of both the mesolimbic and nigrostriatal dopamine systems. *Brain Research*, **303**, 319–329

KOPIN, I. J., MARKEY, S. P., BURNS, R. S., JOHANNESSEN, J. N. and CHIUEH, C. C. (1986) Mechanisms of neurotoxicity of MPTP. In *Recent Developments in Parkinson's Disease*. Eds. S. Fahn, C. D. Marsden, P. Jenner and P. Teychenne, pp. 165–173. New York: Raven Press

KOPP, N., DENOROY, L., THOMASI, M., GAY, N., CHAZOT, G. and RENAUD, B. (1982) Increase in noradrenaline synthesizing enzyme activity in medulla oblongata in Parkinson's disease. *Acta Neuropathologica (Berlin)*, **56**, 17–21

KOPP, N., JORDAN, D., MICHEL, J. P., PIALAT, J., VEISSEIRE, M., CHAZOT, G. and TOMMASI, M. (1983) Etude topographique et chimique de l'enzyme de synthèse du GABA dans les syndromes parkinsoniens. *Annals de Pathologie*, **3**(4), 327–331

KUBEK, M. J. and WILBER, J. F. (1980) Regional distribution of leucine-enkephalin in hypothalamic and extrahypothalamic loci of the human nervous system. *Neuroscience Letters*, **18**, 155–161

LAAKSONEN, H., RIEKKINEN, P., RINNE, U. K. and SONNINEN, V. (1975) Brain glutamic acid decarboxylase and gamma-aminobutyric acid in Parkinson's disease. In *Advances in Parkinsonism*. Eds. W. Birkmayer and O. Hornykiewicz, pp. 205–210. Roche Scientific Service

LAIHINEN, A. and RINNE, U. K. (1986) Function of dopamine receptors in Parkinson's disease: prolactin responses. *Neurology*, **36**, 393–395

LANG, W. and HENKE, M. (1983) Cholinergic receptor binding and autoradiography in brains of non-neurological and senile dementia of Alzheimer-type patients. *Brain Research*, **267**, 271–280

LANGSTON, J. W. (1985a) MPTP and Parkinson's disease. *Trends in Neurological Sciences*, **8**(2), 79–83

LANGSTON, J. W. (1985b) Mechanism of MPTP toxicity: more answers, more questions. *Trends in Pharmacological Sciences*, **6**(9), 375–378

LANGSTON, J. W., BALLARD, P., TETRUD, J. W. and IRWIN I. (1983) Chronic parkinsonism in humans due to a product of mepedrine analogue synthesis. *Science*, **219**, 979–980

LANGSTON, J. W. and FORNO, L. S. (1978) The hypothalamus in Parkinson's disease. *Annals of Neurology*, **3**, 129–133

LAROCHELLE, L., BÉDARD, P., BOUCHER, R. and POIRIER, L. J. (1970) The rubro-olivo-cerebello-rubral loop and postural tremor in the monkey. *Journal of the Neurological Sciences*, **11**, 53–64

LE FUR, G., MEININGER, V., BAULAC, M., PHAN, T. and UZAN, A. (1981) Récepteurs dopaminergiques lymphocytaires et maladie de Parkinson idiopathique. *Revue Neurologique, (Paris)*, **137**, 89–96

LE FUR, G., MEININGER, V., PHAN, T., GERARD, D., BAULAC, M. and UZAN, A. (1980) Decrease in lymphocyte [^{3}H]-spiroperidol binding sites in parkinsonism. *Life Sciences*, **27**, 1587–1591

LE MOAL, M., STINUS, L., SIMON, H., TASSIN, J. P., THIERRY, A. M., BLANC, G. *et al.* (1977) Behavioral effects of a lesion in the ventral mesencephalic tegmentum: evidence for involvement of A10 dopaminergic neurones. *Advances in Biochemical Psychopharmacology*, **16**, 237–245

LECRUBIER, Y., PUECH, A. J., JOUVENT, R., SIMON, P. and WIDLOCHER, D. (1980) A beta-adrenergic stimulant salbutamol vs clomipramine in depression: a controlled study. *British Journal of Psychiatry*, **136**, 354–358

LEE, T., SEEMAN, P., RAJPUT, A., FARLEY, I. J. and HORNYKIEWICZ, O. (1978) Receptor basis for dopaminergic supersensitivity in Parkinson disease. *Nature*, **273**, 59–60

LEENDERS, K., PALMER, A., TURTON, D., QUINN, N., FIRNAU, G., GARNETT *et al.* (1986) DOPA uptake and dopamine receptor binding visualized in the human brain in vivo. In *Recent Developments in Parkinson's disease*. Eds. S. Fahn, C. D. Marsden, P. Jenner and P. Teychenne, pp. 103–113. New York: Raven Press

LEES, A. J. and SMITH, E. (1983) Cognitive deficits in the early stages of Parkinson's disease. *Brain*, **106**, 257–270

LEHMANN, J. and LANGER, S. Z. (1983) The striatal cholinergic interneuron: synaptic target of dopaminergic terminals? *Neuroscience*, **10**, 1105–1120

LEWY, F. H. (1912) Paralysis agitans. I. Pathologische Anatomie. In *Handbuch der Neurologie*. Ed. M. Lewandowski, pp. 920–933. Berlin: Springer

LHERMITTE, F., AGID, Y., FEUERSTEIN, C., SERRE, F., SIGNORET, J. L., STUDLER, J. M. and BONNET, A. M. (1977a) Mouvements anormaux provoqués par la L-DOPA dans la maladie de Parkinson: corrélation avec les concentrations plasmiques de DOPA et de O-méthyl-DOPA. *Revue Neurologique, (Paris)*, **133**, 445–454

LHERMITTE, F., AGID, Y. and SIGNORET, J. L. (1978) Onset and end-of-dose levodopa-induced dyskinesias, possible treatment by increasing the daily doses of levodopa. *Archives of Neurology*, **35**, 261–263

LHERMITTE, F., AGID, Y., SIGNORET, J. L. and STUDLER, J. M. (1977b) Les dyskinesies de 'debut et fin de dose' provoquées par la L-DOPA. *Revue Neurologique (Paris)*, **133**(5), 297–308

LINDVALL, O. and BJORKLUND, A. (1978) Organization of catecholamine neurons in the rat central nervous system. In *Handbook of Psychopharmacology*. Eds. L. L. Iversen, S. D. Iversen and S. H. Snyder, Vol. 9, pp. 139–231. New York: Plenum Press

LLORENS-CORTES, C., JAVOY-AGID, F., AGID, Y., TAQUET, H. and SCHWARTZ, J. C. (1984) Enkephalinergic markers in substantia nigra and caudate nucleus from parkinsonian subjects. *Journal of Neurochemistry*, **43**(3), 874–877

LLOYD, K. G. (1977) Neurochemical compensation in Parkinson's disease. In *Parkinson's Disease*. Eds. J. P. Lakke, J. Korf and H. Wesseling, pp. 61–77. Amsterdam: Excerpta Medica

LLOYD, K. G., DAVIDSON, L. and HORNYKIEWICZ, O. (1975) The neurochemistry of Parkinson's disease: effect of L-DOPA therapy. *Journal of Pharmacology and Experimental Therapeutics*, **195**, 453–464

LLOYD, K. G. and HORNYKIEWICZ, O. (1973) L-Glutamic acid decarboxylase in Parkinson's disease: effect of L-DOPA therapy. *Nature*, **243**, 521–523

LLOYD, K. G., MOHLER, H., HEITS, P. and BARTHOLINI, G. (1975) Distribution of choline-acetyltransferase and glutamate decarboxylase within the substantia nigra and in other brain regions from control and parkinsonian patients. *Journal of Neurochemistry*, **25**, 789–795

LLOYD, K. G., SHEMEN, L. and HORNYCKIEWICZ, O. (1977) Distribution of high affinity sodium-independent [^{3}H]gamma-aminobutyric acid ([^{3}H]gaba) binding in the human brain: alterations in Parkinson's disease. *Brain Research*, **127**, 269–278

LORANGER, A. W., GOODELL, H., McDOWELL, F. H., LEE, J. E. and SWEET, R. D. (1972) Intellectual impairment in Parkinson's syndrome. *Brain*, **95**, 405–412

McDOWELL, F. H. and SWEET, R. D. (1976) The 'on–off' phenomenon. In *Advances in Parkinsonism*. Eds. W. Birkmayer and O. Hornykiewicz, pp. 603–612. Roche Basle Edition

McGEER, P. L. and McGEER, E. G. (1975) Evidence for glutamic acid decarboxylase containing interneurons in the neostriatum. *Brain Research*, **91**, 331–335

McGEER, P. L. and McGEER, E. G. (1976) Enzyme associated with the metabolism of catecholamines, acetylcholine and GABA in human controls and patients with Parkinson's disease and Huntington chorea. *Journal of Neurochemistry*, **26**, 65–76

McGEER, P. L., McGEER, E. G. and WADA, J. A. (1971) Glutamic acid decarboxylase in Parkinson's disease and epilepsy. *Neurology (Minneapolis)*, **21**, 1000–1007

McGEER, E. G., STAINES, W. A. and McGEER, P. L. (1984) Neurotransmitters in the basal ganglia. *Canadian Journal of Neurological Sciences*, **11**, 89–99

MACKAY, A. V. P., YATES, C. M., WRIGHT, A., HAMILTON, P. and DAVIES, P. (1978) Regional distribution of monoamines and their metabolites in the human brain. *Journal of Neurochemistry*, **30**, 841–848

MAHER, E. R., SMITH, E. M. and LEES, A. J. (1985) Cognitive deficits in the Steele–Richardson–Olszewski syndrome (progressive supranuclear palsy). *Journal of Neurology, Neurosurgery and Psychiatry*, **48**, 1234–1239

MALOTEAUX, J. M., LATERRE, C. E., HENS, L. and LADURON, P. M. (1983) Failure of a peripheral dopaminergic marker in Parkinson's disease. *Journal of Neurology, Neurosurgery and Psychiatry*, **46**, 1146–1148

MALOTEAUX, J. M., LYABEYA, M. K., LATERRE, E. C., JAVOY-AGID, F., AGID, Y. and LADURON, P. M. (1985) S2-serotonin receptors in frontal cortex of parkinsonian patients. VIIIth World Congress of Neurology. Hamburg, September 1–6, 1985. *Journal of Neurology*, Suppl. 32, 108

MALOTEAUX, J. M., WATERKEYN, C. and LADURON, P. M. (1981) Absence of dopamine and muscarinic receptors on human lymphocytes. *British Journal of Pharmacology*, **74**, 233P

MANN, D. M. A., LINCOLN, J., YATES, P. O., STAMP, J. E. and TOPER, S. (1980) Changes in monoamine containing neurons of the human CNS in senile dementia. *British Journal of Psychiatry*, **136**, 533–541

MANYAM, N. V. B. (1982) Low CSF gamma-aminobutyric acid levels in Parkinson's disease, effect of levodopa and carbidopa. *Archives of Neurology*, **39**, 391–392

MARKSTEIN, R. and HÖKFELT, T. (1984) Effects of cholecystokinin-octopeptide on dopamine release from slices of cat caudate nucleus. *Journal of the Neurosciences*, **4**, 570–575

MARSDEN, C. D. (1982) The mysterious motor function of the basal ganglia: The Robert Wartenberg lecture. *Neurology*, **32**, 514–539

MARSDEN, C. D. (1983) Neuromelanin and Parkinson's disease. *Journal of Neural Transmission*, Suppl. **19**, 121–141

MARSDEN, C. D. and PARKES, J. D. (1976) 'On–off' effects in patients with Parkinson's disease on chronic levodopa therapy. *Lancet*, **i**, 292–296

MARSDEN, C. D., PARKES, J. D. and QUINN, N. (1982) Fluctuations of disability in Parkinson's disease – clinical aspects. In *Movement Disorders*. Eds. C. D. Marsden and S. Fahn, *Neurology 2*, pp. 96–122. London: Butterworths

MATZUK, M. M. and SAPER, C. B. (1985) Preservation of hypothalamic dopaminergic neurons in Parkinson's disease. *Annals of Neurology*, **18**, 552–555

MAUBORGNE, A., JAVOY-AGID, F., LEGRAND, J. C., AGID, Y. and CESSELIN, F. (1983) Decrease of substance P-like immunoreactivity in the substantia nigra and pallidum of parkinsonian brains. *Brain Research*, **268**, 167–170

MAYEUX, R. and STERN, Y. (1983) Intellectual dysfunction and dementia in Parkinson's disease. In *The Dementias*. Eds. R. Mayeux and W. G. Rosen, pp. 211–227. New York: Raven Press

MAYEUX, R., STERN, Y., COTE, L. and WILLIAMS, J. B. W. (1984a) Altered serotonin metabolism in depressed patients with Parkinson's disease. *Neurology*, **34**, 642–646

MAYEUX, R., STERN, Y., ROSEN, J. and BENSON, D. F. (1983) Is 'subcortical dementia' a recognizable clinical entity? *Annals of Neurology*, **14**, 278–283

MAYEUX, R., WILLIAMS, J. B. W., STERN, Y. and COTE, L. (1984b) Depression and Parkinson's disease. *Advances in Neurology*, **40**, 241–250

MELAMED, E., HEFTI, F. and WURTMAN, R. J. (1982) Compensatory mechanisms in the nigrostriatal dopaminergic system in Parkinson's disease: studies in an animal model. *Israel Journal of Medical Sciences*, **18**(1), 159–163

MESULAM, M. M., MUFSON, E. J., LEVEY, A. I. and WAINER, B. H. (1983) Cholinergic innervation of cortex by the basal forebrain: cytochemistry and cortical connections of the septal area, diagonal band nuclei, nucleus basalis (substantia innominata), and hypothalamus in the rhesus monkey. *Journal of Comparative Neurology*, **214**, 170–197

MONFORT, J. C., JAVOY-AGID, F., HAUW, J. J., DUBOIS, B. and AGID, Y. (1985) Brain glutamate decarboxylase and 'premortem severity index', with a special reference to Parkinson's disease. *Brain*, **108**(2), 301–313

MONES, R. J., ELIZAN, T. S. and SEIGEL, G. (1971) Analysis of L-DOPA induced dyskinesias in 51 patients with parkinsonism. *Journal of Neurology, Neurosurgery and Psychiatry*, **34**, 668–673

MORTIMER, J. A., PIROZZOLO, F. J., HANSCH, E. C. and WEBSTER, D. D. (1982) Relationship of motor symptoms to intellectual deficits in Parkinson disease. *Neurology*, **32**, 133–137

MUENTER, M. D., SHARPLESS, N. S., TYCE, G. M. and DARLEY, F. L. (1977) Patterns of dystonia ('I-D-I' and 'D-I-D') in response to L-DOPA therapy for Parkinson's disease. *Mayo Clinic Proceedings*, **52**, 163–174

MUENTER, M. D. and TYCE, G. M. (1971) L-DOPA therapy of Parkinson's disease: plasma L-DOPA concentration, therapeutic response and side effects. *Mayo Clinic Proceedings*, **46**, 231–239

MURRI, L., INDICE, A., MURATORIO, A., POLLERRE, A., BARRECA, T. and MURIALDO, G. (1980) Spontaneous nocturnal plasma prolactin and growth hormone secretion in patients with Parkinson's disease and Huntington's chorea. *European Neurology*, **19**, 198–206

NAGATSU, T., KANAMORI, T., KATO, T., IIZUKA, R. and NARABAYASHI, H. (1978) Dopamine stimulated adenylate cyclase activity in the human brain changes in Parkinsonism. *Biochemical Medicine*, **19**, 360–365

NAGATSU, T., WAKUI, Y., KATO, T., FUJITA, K., KONDO, T., YOKOCHI, F. and NARABAYASHI, H. (1982) Dopamine beta-hydroxylase activity in cerebrospinal fluid of parkinsonian patients. *Biomedical Research*, **3**, 395–398

NAKANO, I. and HIRANO, A. (1984) Parkinson's disease: neuron loss in the nucleus basalis without concomitant Alzheimer's disease. *Annals of Neurology*, **15**, 415–418

NAKASHIMA, S. and IKUTA, F. (1984) Tyrosine hydroxylase protein in Lewy bodies of parkinsonian and senile brains. *Journal of the Neurological Sciences*, **66**, 91–96

NARABAYASHI, H., KONDO, T., HAYASHI, A., SUZUKI, T. and NAGATSU, T. (1981) L-*threo*-3,4-Dihydroxyphenylserine treatment for akinesia and freezing of parkinsonism. *Proceedings of the Japan Academy*, **57B**, 351–354

NOBIN, A. and BJORKLUND, A. (1973) Topography of the monoamine neuron systems in the human brain as revealed in foetuses. *Acta Physiologica Scandinavica Supplementum*, **388**, 1–40

NUTT, J. G. and CARTER, J. H. (1984) Sensory symptoms in parkinsonism relate to central dopaminergic function. *Lancet*, **ii**, 456–457

NUTT, J. G., WOODWARD, W. R., HAMMERSTAD, J. P., CARTER, J. H. and ANDERSON, J. L. (1984) The 'on–off' phenomenon in Parkinson's disease; Relation to levodopa absorption and transport. *New England Journal of Medicine*, **310**, 483–488

NUTT, J. G., WOODWARD, W. R. and HAMMERSTAD, J. P. (1986) Pharmacokinetics of intravenous levodopa: implications for mechanisms of therapeutic actions of levodopa and carbidopa. In *Recent Developments in Parkinson's Disease*. Eds. S. Fahn, C. D. Marsden, P. Jenner and P. Teychenne, pp. 239–245. New York: Raven Press

NYBERG, P., NORDBERG, A., WEBSTER, P. and WINBLAD, B. (1983) Dopaminergic deficiency is more pronounced in putamen than in nucleus caudatus in Parkinson's disease. *Neurochemical Pathology*, **1**, 193–202

OHYE, C., BOUCHARD, R., BOUCHER, R. and POIRIER, L. J. (1970) Spontaneous activity of the putamen after chronic interruption of the dopaminergic pathway: effect of L-DOPA. *Journal of Pharmacology and Experimental Therapeutics,* **175,** 700–708

OLSON, R. and ROOS, B. E. (1968) Concentrations of 5-hydroxyindolacetic acid and homovanillic acid in the cerebrospinal fluid after treatment with probenecid in patients with Parkinson's disease. *Nature,* **219,** 502–503

PEASTON, M. J. T. and BIANCHINE, J. R. (1970) Metabolic studies and clinical observations during L-DOPA treatment of Parkinson's disease. *British Medical Journal,* **1, 5693,** 400–403

PERRY, E. K., CURTIS, M., DICK, D. J., CANDY, J. M., ATACK, J. R., BLOXHAM, C. A. et al. (1985) Cholinergic correlates of cognitive impairment in Parkinson's disease: comparisons with Alzheimer's disease. *Journal of Neurology, Neurosurgery and Psychiatry,* **48,** 413–421

PERRY, E. K., PERRY, R. H., CANDY, J. M., FAIRBAIRN, A. F., BLESSED, G., DICK, D. J. and TOMLINSSON, B. E. (1984) Cortical serotonin-S2 receptor binding abnormalities in patients with Alzheimer's disease: comparisons with Parkinson's disease. *Neuroscience Letters,* **51,** 353–357

PERRY, E. K., TOMLINSON, B. E., BLESSED, G., BERGMANN, K., GIBSON, P. H. and PERRY, R. H. (1978) Correlation of cholinergic abnormalities with senile plaques and mental test scores in senile dementia. *British Medical Journal,* **2,** 1457–1459

PERRY, R. H., TOMLINSON, B. E., CANDY, J. M., BLESSED, G., FOSTER, J. F., BLOXHAM, C. A. and PERRY, E. K. (1983a) Cortical cholinergic deficit in mentally impaired parkinsonian patients. *Lancet,* **ii,** 789–790

PERRY, T. L., JAVOY-AGID, F., AGID, Y. and FIBIGER, H. C. (1983b) Is striatal GABAergic neuronal activity reduced in Parkinson's disease? *Journal of Neurochemistry,* **40,** 1120–1123

PICKEL, V. M., SUMAL, K. K., BECKLEY, S. C., MILLER, R. J. and REIS, D. J. (1980) Immunocytochemical localization of enkephalin in the neostriatum of rat brain: a light and electron microscopic study. *Journal of Comparative Neurology,* **189,** 721–740

PILLON, B., DUBOIS, B., LHERMITTE, F. and AGID, Y. (1986) Heterogeneity of intellectual impairment in progressive supranuclear palsy, Parkinson's and Alzheimer's diseases. *Neurology,* in press

PIMOULE, C., SCHOEMAKER, H., REYNOLDS, G. P. and LANGER, S. Z. (1985) [^{3}H]SCH 23390 labeled D1 dopamine receptors are unchanged in schizophrenia and Parkinson's disease. *European Journal of Pharmacology,* **114,** 235–237

PIQUE, L., JEGOU, S., BERTAGNA, X., JAVOY-AGID, F., SEURIN, D., PROESCHEL, M. F. et al. (1985) Pro-opiomelanocortin peptides in the human hypothalamus – comparative study between normal subject and Parkinson patients. *Neuroscience Letters,* **54,** 141–146

PLOSKA, A., TAQUET, H., JAVOY-AGID, F., GASPAR, P., CESSELIN, F., BERGER, B. et al. (1982) Dopamine and methionine-enkephalin in human brain. *Neuroscience Letters,* **33,** 191–196

POIRIER, L. J. and SOURKES, T. L. (1965) Influence of the substantia nigra on the catecholamine content of the striatum. *Brain,* **88,** 181–192

PRESTHUS, J. (1980) Psychiatric side-effects occurring in parkinsonism during long-term treatment with levodopa alone and in combination with other drugs. In *Parkinson's Disease: Current Progress, Problems and Management.* Eds. U. K. Rinne, M. Klinger and G. Stamm, pp. 255–270. Amsterdam: Elsevier North Holland Press

PRICE, K. S., FARLEY, I. J. and HORNYKIEWICZ, O. (1978) Neurochemistry of Parkinson's disease: relation between striatal and limbic dopamine. *Advances in Biochemical Psychopharmacology,* **19,** 293–300

QUIK, M., SPOKES, E. G., MACKAY, A. V. P. and BANNISTER, R. (1979) Alterations in ^{3}H-spiperone binding in human caudate nucleus, substantia nigra and frontal cortex in Shy–Drager syndrome and Parkinson's disease. *Journal of the Neurological Sciences,* **43,** 429–437

QUINN, N., MARSDEN, C. D. and PARKES, J. D. (1982) Complicated response fluctuations in Parkinson's disease: response to intravenous infusion of levodopa. *Lancet,* **ii,** 412–415

QUINN, N., PARKES, J. D. and MARSDEN, C. D. (1984) Control of on/off phenomena by continuous intravenous infusion of levodopa. *Neurology,* **34,** 1131–1136

QUINN, N., ROSSOR, M. N. and MARSDEN, C. D. (1986) Dementia and Parkinson's disease – Pathological and neurochemical considerations. *British Medical Bulletin,* **42**(1), 86–90

RAISMAN, R., CASH, R. and AGID, Y. (1986) Parkinson's disease: decreased density of [^{3}H]-imipramine and [^{3}H]paroxetin binding-sites in putamen. *Neurology,* in press

RAISMAN, R., CASH, R., RUBERG, M., JAVOY-AGID, F. and AGID, Y. (1985) Binding of [^{3}H]SCH 23390 to D-1 receptors in the putamen of control and parkinsonian subjects. *European Journal of Pharmacology,* **113,** 467–468

RAJPUT, A. H., ROZDILSKY, B., HORNYKIEWICZ, O., SHANNAK, K., LEE, T. and SEEMAN, P. (1982) Reversible drug-induced parkinsonism: clinicopathologic study of two cases. *Archives of Neurology,* **39,** 644–646

REISINE, T. D., FIELDS, J. Z., YAMAMURA, H. I., BIRD, E. D., SPOKES, E., SCHREINER, P. S. and ENNA, S. J. (1977) Neurotransmitter receptor alterations in Parkinson's disease. *Life Sciences,* **21,** 335–344

RIEDERER, P., BIRKMAYER, W., SEEMANN, D. and WUKETICH, S. (1977) Brain-noradrenaline and 3-methoxy-hydroxyphenylglycol in Parkinson's syndrome. *Journal of Neural Transmission*, **41**, 241–251

RIEDERER, P., RAUSCH, W. D., BIRKMAYER, W., JELLINGER, K. and DANIELCZYK, W. (1978a) Dopamine-sensitive adenylate cyclase activity in the caudate nucleus and metabolic encephalopathies. *Journal of Neural Transmission*, Suppl. 14, 153

RIEDERER, P., RAUSCH, W. D., BIRKMAYER, W., JELLINGER, K. and SEEMANN, D. (1978b) CNS modulation of adrenal tyrosine hydroxylase in Parkinson's disease and metabolic encephalopathies. *Journal of Neural Transmission*, Suppl. 14, 121

RIEDERER, P., REYNOLDS, G. P., DANIELCZYK, W., JELLINGER, K. and SEEMANN, D. (1983) Desensitization of striatal spiperone-binding sites by dopaminergic agonists in Parkinson's disease. In *Lisuride and Other Dopamine Agonists*. Eds. D. B. Calne *et al.*, pp. 375–381. New York: Raven Press

RIEDERER, P. and WUKETICH, S. (1976) Time course of nigrostriatal degeneration in Parkinson's disease. *Journal of Neural Transmission*, **38**, 277–301

RINNE, J. O., LAAKSO, K., LÖNNBERG, MÖLSÄ, P., PALJÄRVI, L., RINNE, J. K. *et al.* (1985a) Brain muscarinic receptors in senile dementia. *Brain Research*, **336**, 19–25

RINNE, J. O., RINNE, J. K., LAAKSO, K., LÖNNBERG, P. and RINNE, U. K. (1985b) Dopamine D-1 receptors in the parkinsonian brain. *Brain Research*, **359**, 306–310

RINNE, U. K., KOSKINEN, V., LAAKSONEN, H., LÖNNBERG, P. and SONNINEN, V. (1978) GABA receptor binding in the parkinsonian brain. *Life Sciences*, **22**, 2225–2228

RINNE, U. K., KOSKINEN, V. and LÖNNBERG, P. (1980) Neurotransmitter receptors in the parkinsonian brain. In *Parkinson's Disease: Current Progress, Problems and Management*. Eds. U. K. Rinne, M. Klinger and G. Stamm, pp. 93–107. Amsterdam: Elsevier North Holland Press

RINNE, U. K., LAAKSONEN, H., RIEKKINEN, P. and SONNINEN, V. (1974) Brain glutamic acid decarboxylase activity in Parkinson's disease. *European Neurology*, **12**, 13–19

RINNE, U. K., LÖNNBERG, P. and KOSKINEN, V. (1981) Dopamine receptors in the parkinsonian brain. *Journal of Neural Transmission*, **51**, 97–106

RINNE, U. K., RINNE, J. K., RINNE, J. O., LAAKSO, K., TENOVUO, O., LÖNNBERG, P. and KOSKINEN, V. (1983) Brain enkephalin receptors in Parkinson's disease. *Journal of Neural Transmission*, Suppl. 19, 163–171

RINNE, U. K., RINNE, J. O., RINNE, J. K., LAAKSO, K. and LÖNNBERG, P. (1984) Brain neurotransmitters and neuropeptides in Parkinson's disease. *Acta Physiologica Latinoamericana*, **34**, 287–299

RINNE, U. K. and SONNINEN, V. (1973) Brain catecholamines and their metabolites in parkinsonian patients. *Archives of Neurology*, **28**, 107–110

RINNE, U. K., SONNINEN, V. and LAAKSONEN, H. (1979) Responses of brain neurochemistry to levodopa treatment in Parkinson's disease. *Advances in Neurology*, **24**, 259–274

RINNE, U. K., SONNINEN, V. and MARTTILA, R. (1977) Brain dopamine metabolism and the relief of parkinsonism. In *Parkinson's Disease – Concept and Prospects*. Eds. J. P. W. F. Lakke, J. Korf and H. Wesseling, pp. 73–83. Amsterdam: Excerpta Medica

RINVIK, E., GROFOVA I. and OTTERSEN, O. P. (1976) Demonstration of nigrotectal and nigroreticular projections in the cat by axonal transport of proteins. *Brain Research*, **112**, 388–394

ROGERS, J. D., BROGAN, D. and MIRRA, S. S. (1985) The nucleus basalis of Meynert in neurological disease: A quantitative morphological study. *Annals of Neurology*, **17**(2), 163–170

ROGERS, D. (1986) Bradyphrenia in Parkinsonism. *Psychological Medicine*, in press

RONDOT, P., DE RECONDO, J., COIGNET, A. and ZIEGLER, M. (1984) Mental disorders in Parkinson's disease after treatment with L-DOPA. *Advances in Neurology*, **40**, 259–269

ROSSOR, M. N. (1981) Parkinson's disease and Alzheimer's disease as disorders of the isodendritic core. *British Medical Journal*, **283**, 1588–1590

ROSSOR, M. N., EMSON, P. C., MOUNTJOY, C. Q., ROTH, M. and IVERSEN, L. L. (1980) Reduced amounts of immunoreactive somatostatin in the temporal cortex in senile dementia of Alzheimer type. *Neuroscience Letters*, **20**, 373–377

ROSSOR, M. N., GARRETT, N. J., JOHNSON, A. L., MOUNTJOY, C., ROTH, M. and IVERSEN, L. L. (1982a) A postmortem study of the cholinergic and GABA systems in senile dementia. *Brain*, **105**, 313–330

ROSSOR, M. N., HUNT, S. P., IVERSEN, L. L., BANNISTER, R., HAWTHORN, J., ANG, V. T. Y. and JENKINS, J. S. (1982b) Extrahypothalamic vasopressin is unchanged in Parkinson's disease and Huntington's disease. *Brain Research*, **253**, 341–343

RUBERG, M. and AGID, Y. (1986) Dementia in Parkinson's disease. In *Handbook of Psychopharmacology*, Vol. 20: *Psychopharmacology of the Ageing Nervous System*. Eds. L. Iversen, S. D. Iversen and S. H. Snyder. New York: Plenum Press (in press)

RUBERG, M., BONNET, A. M., VILLAGEOIS, A., PILLON, B., RIEGER, F. and AGID, Y. (1986b) CSF acetyl- and butyryl-cholinesterases in various neurological diseases. *Journal of Neurology, Neurosurgery and Psychiatry,* (in press)

RUBERG, M., JAVOY-AGID, F., HIRSCH, E., SCATTON, B., LHEUREUX, R., HAUW, J. J. et al. (1985) Dopamineric and cholinergic lesions in progressive supranuclear palsy. *Annals of Neurology,* **18,** 523–529

RUBERG, M., PLOSKA, A., JAVOY-AGID, F. and AGID, Y. (1982) Muscarinic binding and choline acetyltransferase activity in Parkinson subject with reference to dementia. *Brain Research,* **232,** 129–139

RUBERG, M., RIEGER, F., VILLAGEOIS, A., BONNET, A. M. and AGID, Y. (1986a) Acetylcholinesterase and butyrylcholinesterase in frontal cortex and cerebrospinal fluid of demented and non-demented patients with Parkinson's disease. *Brain Research,* **362,** 83–91

SADEH, M., BRAHIM, J. and MODAN, M. (1982) Effects of anticholinergic drugs on memory in Parkinson's disease. *Archives of Neurology,* **39,** 666–667

SADOUL, J. L., CHECLER, F., KITABGI, P., ROSTÈNE, W., JAVOY-AGID, F. and VINCENT, J. P. (1984) Loss of high affinity neurotensin receptors in substantia nigra from parkinsonian subjects. *Biochemical and Biophysical Research Communications,* **125**(1), 395–404

SCATTON, B. and BARTHOLINI, G. (1980) Modulation by GABA of cholinergic transmission in the striatum. *Brain Research,* **183,** 211–216

SCATTON, B., DENNIS, T., LHEUREUX, R., MONFORT, J. C., DUYCKAERTS, C. and JAVOY-AGID, F. (1986) Degeneration of noradrenergic and serotoninergic but not dopaminergic neurons in the lumbar spinal cord of parkinsonian patients. *Brain Research,* in press

SCATTON, B., JAVOY-AGID, F., ROUQUIER, L., DUBOIS, B. and AGID, Y. (1983) Reduction of cortical dopamine, noradrenaline, serotonin and their metabolites in Parkinson's disease. *Brain Research,* **275,** 321–328

SCATTON, B., MONFORT, J. C., JAVOY-AGID, F. and AGID, Y. (1984) Neurochemistry of monoaminergic neurones in Parkinson's disease. In *Catecholamines: Neuropharmacology and Central Nervous System. Therapeutic Aspects,* pp. 43–52. New York: Alan R. Liss Inc.

SCATTON, B., ROUQUIER, L., JAVOY-AGID, F. and AGID, Y. (1982) Dopamine deficiency in the cerebral cortex in Parkinson disease. *Neurology,* **32,** 1039–1040

SCHOEMAKER, H., PIMOULE, C., ARBILLA, S., SCATTON, B., JAVOY-AGID, F. and LANGER, S. Z. (1985) Sodium dependent [^{3}H]cocaine binding associated with dopamine uptake sites in the rat striatum and human putamen decrease after dopaminergic denervation and in Parkinson's disease. *Naunyn Schmiedebergs Archives of Pharmacology,* **329,** 227–235

SCHWARTZ, J. C., AGID, Y., JAVOY-AGID, F., MARTRES, M. P., POLLARD, H., BOUTHENET, M. L. et al. (1986) Neurochemical investigations into the human area postrema. In *Nausea and Vomiting: Mechanisms and Treatment.* Eds. D. Grahame-Smith, C. J. Davis and C. Lake-Bakaaz. Berlin: Springer Verlag (in press)

SHARPE, J. A., REWCASTLE, N. B., LLOYD, K. G., HORNYKIEWICZ, O., HILL, M. and TASKER, R. R. (1973) Striatonigral degeneration. Response to levodopa therapy with pathological and neurochemical correlation. *Journal of the Neurological Sciences,* **19,** 275–286

SHIBUYA, M. (1979) Dopamine sensitive adenylate cyclase activity in the striatum of Parkinson's disease. *Journal of Neural Transmission,* **44,** 287

SHOULSON, I., GLAUBIGER, G. A. and CHASE, T. N. (1975) On-off response – Clinical and biochemical correlations during oral and intravenous levodopa administration in parkinsonian patients. *Neurology,* **25,** 1144–1148

SKAGERBERG, G. and LINDVALL, O. (1985) Organization of diencephalic dopamine neurones projecting to the spinal cord in the rat. *Brain Research,* **342,** 340–351

SKIRBOLL, L. R., GRACE, A. A., HOMMER, D. W., REHFELD, J. F., GOLDSTEIN, M., HOKFELT, T. and BUNNEY, B. S. (1981) Peptide-monoamine coexistence: studies of the actions of cholecystokinin-like peptide on the electrical activity of mid-brain dopamine neurons. *Neuroscience,* **6,** 2111–2124

SLOVITER, R. S. and CONNOR, J. D. (1977) Postmortem stability of norepinephrine, dopamine and serotonin in rat brain. *Journal of Neurochemistry,* **28,** 1129–1131

SNIDER, S. R., FAHN, S., ISGREEN, W. P. and COTE, L. J. (1976) Primary sensory symptoms in parkinsonism. *Neurology,* **26,** 423–429

SNYDER, A. M., STRICKER, E. M. and ZIGMOND, M. J. (1985) Stress-induced neurological impairments in an animal model of parkinsonism. *Annals of Neurology,* **18,** 544–551

SORENSEN, K. V. (1982) Somatostatin: localization and distribution in the cortex and sub-cortical white matter of human brain. *Neuroscience,* **7,** 1227–1232

SPOKES, E. G. S., GARETT, N. J. and IVERSEN, L. L. (1979) Differential effects of agonal status on measurements of GABA and glutamate decarboxylase in human post-mortem brain tissue from control and Huntington's chorea subjects. *Journal of Neurochemistry,* **33,** 773–778

STEINBUSCH, H. W. M. (1984) Serotonin-immunoreactive neurons and their projections in the CNS. In *Classical Transmitters and Transmitter Receptors in the CNS. Part II. Handbook of Chemical Neuroanatomy*, Vol. 3. Eds. A. Björklund, T. Hökfelt and M. J. Kuhar, pp. 68–126. Amsterdam: Elsevier

STERN, Y. and LANGSTON, J. W. (1985) Intellectual changes in patients with MPTP-induced parkinsonism. *Annals of Neurology*, in press

STUDLER, J. M., JAVOY-AGID, F., CESSELIN, F., LEGRAND, J. C. and AGID, Y. (1982) CCK-8 immunoreactivity distribution in human brain: selective decrease in the substantia nigra from parkinsonian patients. *Brain Research*, **243**, 176–179

TAQUET, H., JAVOY-AGID, F., CESSELIN, F., HAMON, M., LEGRAND, J. C. and AGID, Y. (1982) Microtopography of methionine-enkephalin dopamine and noradrenaline in the ventral mesencephalon of human control and parkinsonian brains. *Brain Research*, **235**, 303–314

TAQUET, H., JAVOY-AGID, F., HAMON, M., LEGRAND, J. C., AGID, Y. and CESSELIN, F. (1983) Parkinson's disease affects differently Met^5 and Leu^5-enkephalin in the human brain. *Brain Research*, **280**, 379–382

TAQUET, H., JAVOY-AGID, F., GIRAUD, P., LEGRAND, J. C., AGID, Y. and CESSELIN, F. (1985) Dynorphin levels in parkinsonian patients: Leu^5-enkephalin production from either proenkephalin A or prodynorphin in human brain. *Brain Research*, **341**, 390–392

TENOVUO, O., RINNE, U. K. and VILJANEN, M. K. (1984) Substance P immunoreactivity in the post-mortem parkinsonian brain. *Brain Research*, **303**, 113–116

TERRY, R. D., PECK, A., DETERESA, R., SCHECHTER, R. and HOROUPIAN, D. S. (1981) Some morphometric aspects of the brain in senile dementia of the Alzheimer type. *Annals of Neurology*, **10**, 184–192

TEYCHENNE, P. F., ZIEGLER, M. G., LAKE, R. C. and ENNA, S. J. (1982) Low CSF GABA in parkinsonian patients who respond poorly to therapy or suffer from the 'on-off' phenomenon. *Annals of Neurology*, **11**, 76–79

TRETIAKOFF, C. (1919) Contribution à l'étude de l'anatomie pathologiquee du locus niger de Soemmering avec quelques déductions relatives à la pathogénie des troubles du tonus musculaire et de la maladie de Parkinson. Thèse Médecine, Paris

UHL, G. R., HEDREEN, J. C. and PRICE, D. L. (1985) Parkinson's disease: loss of neurons from the ventral tegmental area contralateral to therapeutic surgical lesions. *Neurology*, **35**, 1215–1218

UNGERSTEDT U. (1971) Postsynaptic supersensitivity after 6-hydroxydopamine induced-degeneration of the nigrostriatal dopamine system. *Acta Physiologica Scandinavica Supplementum*, **367**, 69–93

VANDERHAEGHEN, J. J., LOSTRA, F., DE MEY, J. and GILLES, C. (1980) Immunohistochemical localization of cholecystokinin- and gastrin-like peptides in the brain and hypophysis of the rat. *Proceedings of the National Academy of Sciences of the United States of America*, **77**, 1190–1194

VAN PRAAG, H. M. (1982) Depression. *Lancet*, **ii**, 1259–1264

VILLENEUVE, A., BERLAN, M., LAFONTAN, M., CARANOBE, C., BONEU, B., RASCOL, A. and MONTASTRUC, J. L. (1985) Platelet alpha-2 adrenoceptors in Parkinson's disease: decreased number in untreated patients and recovery after treatment. *European Journal of Clinical Investigation*, **15**, 403–407

VOLICER, L., BEAL, M. F., DIRENFELD, L. K., MARQUIS, J. K. and ALBERT, M. L. (1986) CSF cyclic nucleotides and somatostatin in Parkinson's disease. *Neurology*, **36**, 89–92

WEIL-MALHERBE, H. and VAN BUREN, J. M. (1969) The excretion of dopamine and dopamine metabolites in Parkinson's disease and the effect of diet thereon. *Journal of Laboratory and Clinical Medicine*, **74**, 305–318

WESTLIND, A., GRYNFARB, M., HEDLUND, B., BARTFAI, T. and FUXE, K. (1981) Muscarinic supersensitivity induced by septal lesion or chronic atropine treatment. *Brain Research*, **225**, 131–141

WHITEHOUSE, P. J., HEDREEN, J. C., WHITE, C. L. and PRICE, D. L. (1983) Basal forebrain neurons in the dementia of Parkinson's disease. *Annals of Neurology*, **13**, 243–248

WINDBLAD, B., ADOLFSSON, R., CARLSSON, A. and GOTTFRIES, C. G. (1982) Biogenic amines in brains of patients with Alzheimer's disease. In *Alzheimer's disease: a Report of Progress*. Eds. S. Lorkin et al., pp. 25–33. New York: Raven Press

YONG, V. W. and PERRY, T. L. (1986) Monoamine oxidase B, smoking and Parkinson's disease. *Journal of the Neurological Sciences*, **72**, 265–272

ZAMIR, N., SKOFITSCH, G., BANNON, M. J., HELKE, C. J., KOPIN, I. J. and JACOBOWITZ, D. M. (1984) Primate model of Parkinson's disease: alteration in multiple opioid systems in the basal ganglia. *Brain Research*, **322**, 356–360

ZIGMOND, M. J., ACHESON, A. L., STACHOWIAK, M. K. and STRICKER, E. M. (1984) Neurochemical compensation after nigrostriatal bundle injury in an animal model of preclinical parkinsonism. *Archives of Neurology*, **41**, 856–861

11
Pharmacokinetics of levodopa
G. Frederick Wooten

Parkinsonism is a symptom complex characterized by tremor at rest, brady- and hypokinesia, cogwheel rigidity, and loss of postural reflexes. Parkinsonism may be produced by drugs that interfere with dopamine neurotransmission, by environmental toxins (e.g. 1-methyl-4-phenyl-1,2,3,6-tetrahydropyridine, MPTP) that selectively destroy nigral dopamine neurones, by poisoning with heavy metals (e.g. manganese) that interfere with dopamine-synthesizing neurones, by infections that result in damage to nigrostriatal dopaminergic neurones and by structural lesions (e.g. micro-infarcts and tumours) that damage the nigrostriatal pathway. The vast majority of cases of parkinsonism result from the idiopathic, selective death of dopamine neurones in the substantia nigra that produces a marked reduction in the dopamine concentration of the striatum (Hornykiewicz, 1972). This clinical–pathological entity is known as Parkinson's disease. Thus, with few exceptions, parkinsonism occurs as the result of a deficiency of dopamine neurotransmission in the striatum. The most effective means currently available for correcting this deficiency, and thereby ameliorating the signs and symptoms of parkinsonism, is to increase brain dopamine levels by the administration of the dopamine precursor, levodopa (Cotzias, Papavasiliou and Gellene, 1969).

Levodopa (L-3,4-dihydroxyphenylalanine) is a large neutral amino acid that is a naturally occurring intermediate in the synthetic pathway of catecholamines from the amino acid, L-tyrosine. Levodopa is synthesized endogenously in dopaminergic neurones from L-tyrosine by the catalytic action of the enzyme, tyrosine hydroxylase. This enzyme is the rate-limiting enzyme in the biosynthesis of dopamine and is highly localized in brain neurones that are specialized to synthesize and release dopamine. Because the exogenous administration of levodopa to patients with parkinsonism bypasses this step in dopamine synthesis, tyrosine hydroxylase activity has little effect on the efficacy of treatment with levodopa. Both exogenously administered and naturally synthesized levodopa is converted to dopamine by the action of the enzyme L-aromatic amino acid decarboxylase (L-AAAD), sometimes referred to as dopa decarboxylase. Unlike tyrosine hydroxylase, L-AAAD is a rather ubiquitous enzyme that is present not only in very high concentrations in dopamine- and other catecholamine- and indoleamine-synthesizing neurones, but also in kidney, liver, gut, and cerebral endothelial cells. There is compelling evidence from studies in experimental animals that a significant proportion of administered levodopa may be converted to dopamine in non-aminergic neuronal sites in the brain (Melamed, Hefti and Wurtman, 1980). Another potential route of metabolism of levodopa is by O-methylation due to the enzymatic action of catechol-*O*-methyltransferase (COMT). COMT is present in high concentrations in the liver and red blood cells and a significant portion of each oral dose of levodopa is metabolized to 3-*O*-methyldopa in these tissues. The enzymatic inactivation of dopamine is catalysed by two proteins, monoamine oxidase and COMT. Monoamine oxidase activity may be separated into two forms (types A and B). Type A has high substrate specificity for serotonin and is selectively inhibited by clorgyline, while type B has high substrate specificity for β-phenylethylamine and is selectively inhibited by deprenyl (Pearce and Roth, 1984). Recent immunocytochemical studies with monoclonal antibodies to monoamine oxidase types A and B indicate that type A is localized in nigrostriatal dopamine-containing neurones while type B is distributed primarily in serotoninergic neurones and glial cells (Denny *et al.*, 1982; Levitt, Pintar and Breakfield, 1982). Both forms of monoamine oxidase are primarily, if not exclusively, associated with mitochondria. In contrast, brain COMT is localized extraneuronally in glial cells (Kaplan, Hartman and Creveling,

Figure 11.1 Major metabolic pathways for levodopa. Abbreviations: L-AAAD, L-aromatic amino acid decarboxylase (or dopa decarboxylase); DBH, dopamine-β-hydroxylase; COMT, catechol-*O*-methyltransferase; MaO, monoamine oxidase; DOPAC, dihydroxyphenylacetic acid. Norepineprine = noradrenaline

1979). Dopamine is O-methylated by COMT to form 3-methoxytyramine or oxidized by monoamine oxidase to form dihydroxyphenylacetic acid. Homovanillic acid is the final product of the inactivation of dopamine. The major metabolic pathways for levodopa are depicted in *Figure 11.1*. (For a general review of catecholamine metabolism *see* Moskowitz and Wurtman, 1975.)

After exogenously administered levodopa is converted to dopamine in the cytoplasm of dopaminergic neurones, storage vesicles accumulate the newly synthesized compound against a concentration gradient. Intravesicular dopamine is protected from inactivation by monoamine oxidase and is released in these vesicular packets from the dopamine neurone by depolarization of the cell. The depolarization-induced release of dopamine from dopaminergic neurones is calcium dependent. Some recent experimental evidence suggests that a significant portion of dopamine synthesized from exogenous levodopa is released from extravesicular cytoplasmic pools or merely diffuses out of neurones or glial cells from which it is synthesized (Melamed et al., 1985). Once in the extracellular space of the striatum, dopamine stands a statistically high likelihood of coming into contact with dopamine receptors on other neuronal surfaces, binding to the receptor, and producing a pharmacological effect.

The definition and classification of subtypes of dopamine receptors has undergone numerous revisions in recent years and would require extensive discussion to review fully. Most of the studies of the molecular properties of dopamine receptors have been carried out in tissues that are less complex than striatum, e.g. goldfish retina and intermediate lobe of pituitary. Extrapolating from these studies to the striatum is obviously dangerous. Currently, however, there appears to be possibly two types of dopamine receptors termed D-1 and D-2. The D-1 receptor is positively linked to adenylate cyclase via a stimulatory (Ns) guanyl nucleotide-dependent subunit. In contrast, the D-2 receptor site appears to be negatively linked to adenylate cyclase via Ni, an inhibitory guanyl nucleotide-dependent subunit (Stoof and Kebabian, 1984). The relative roles of D-1 and D-2 receptors in mediating the anti-Parkinson effects of dopamine synthesized from levodopa are not currently clear, but are the subject of intense investigation. Once dopamine exits from the receptor site, the majority of the extracellar dopamine molecules re-enter dopamine neurones via a carrier-mediated high affinity re-uptake mechanism at the nerve cell membrane. Dopamine, having re-entered

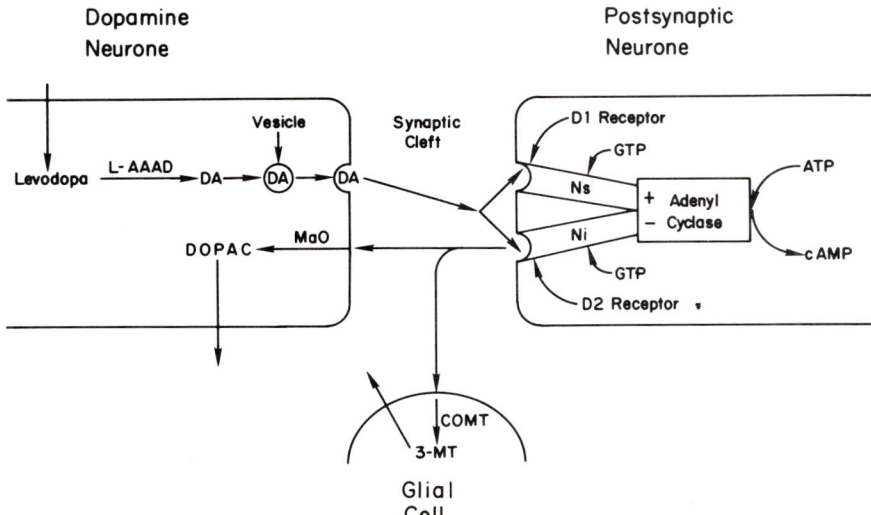

Figure 11.2 Cellular localization of sites of dopamine synthesis, release, receptor transduction, re-uptake, and metabolism. Abbreviations: Ns, stimulatory subunit of receptor complex; Ni, inhibitory subunit of receptor complex; GTP, guanosine triphosphate; ATP, adenosine triphosphate; cAMP, cyclic adenosine monophosphate

the neurone, may then either be concentrated in storage vesicles or oxidized by monoamine oxidase to form dihydroxyphenylacetic acid. A small amount of released dopamine which escapes the synaptic cleft may then enter glial cells and be O-methylated by COMT to form 3-methoxytyramine. The life cycle of brain dopamine synthesized from levodopa is depicted in *Figure 11.2* at the cellular level.

EXTRACEREBRAL PHARMACOKINETICS OF LEVODOPA

For levodopa to be effective in the treatment of Parkinson's disease, appropriate striatal concentrations must be attained. The amount of levodopa reaching the striatum after a single oral dose is a function of the amount of levodopa administered. But, in addition, the striatal concentrations of levodopa that are attained also depend on the rate and extent of levodopa absorption from the gut, the extent of distribution in and binding to extrastriatal tissues, the degree of extrastriatal biotransformation, and the rate of levodopa excretion. The absorption, distribution, biotransformation and excretion of levodopa (*Figure 11.3*) represent a bewildering array of variables that ultimately determine the amount of

1. Variations in gut motility, gastric pH, and emptying rate
2. Conversion to DA (dopamine) by L-AAAD in gut wall
3. Absorption from gut by saturable amino acid transport system
4. Conversion to DA by hepatic L-AAAD activity
5. Conversion to 3-OMD (3-O-methyldopa) by hepatic COMT activity
6. Distribution into red blood cells
7. Conversion to 3-OMD in RBC's by COMT
8. Distribution into muscle
9. Blood-brain barrier: saturable, carrier-mediated, large neutral amino acid transport system

Figure 11.3 Extracerebral transport, distribution, and metabolism of levodopa each oral dose of levodopa that enters the brain. An understanding of the extracerebral pharmacokinetics of levodopa is crucial both to the effective use of this drug in the treatment of Parkinson's disease and, particularly, in developing a rational approach to the management of levodopa-related fluctuations in response.

Absorption

Levodopa is absorbed primarily in the proximal small intestine (Sasahara et al., 1981b) by a carrier-mediated, saturable transport system (Wade, Mearrick and Morris, 1973). Thus the rate of gastric emptying is chronologically the first major variable to affect the rate of levodopa absorption.

Gastric emptying

Several important factors affect the rate of gastric emptying. There exists an inverse relationship between gastric acidity and the rate of gastric emptying (Pocelinko, Thomas and Solomon, 1972). Excessive gastric acidity was shown to reduce levodopa absorption and diminish the clinical response (Rivera-Calimlim et al., 1970). Conversely, the administration of antacids increased levodopa absorption and enhanced the clinical response (Rivera-Calimlim et al., 1970). Several investigators have demonstrated that, the lower the gastric pH, the larger the time to peak plasma concentrations and the lower the peak plasma concentrations attained after an oral dose of levodopa (Bianchine et al., 1971).

It is well known that meals concomitant with oral levodopa will reduce and delay plasma levels of levodopa (Nutt et al., 1984). This phenomenon may be due in part to the capacity of meals to delay gastric emptying. Anticholinergic drugs that are often co-administered with levodopa may contribute to slowed gastric emptying (Fermaglich and O'Doherty, 1972). Likewise dopaminergic drugs may contribute to slowed gastric emptying, as suggested by the observation that metoclopramide, a dopamine antagonist, when co-administered with levodopa, increased the bioavailability and reduced the erratic absorption of levodopa (Mearrick et al., 1974).

Perhaps the most dramatic evidence that the rate of gastric emptying is an important pharmacokinetic variable comes from the observations of extremely rapid levodopa absorption in gastrectomized patients (Rivera-Calimlim, Dujovne and Morgan, 1971) and following direct duodenal administration (Sasahara et al., 1981a). While little levodopa absorption from the stomach occurs (Bianchine et al., 1971), the rate of gastric emptying is an important potential factor in the subsequent rate and extent of levodopa absorption.

Absorption in small intestine

The intestinal absorption of levodopa in the dog is most efficient in the duodenum and becomes progressively less in the course of the small intestines (Sasahara et al., 1981b). Unlike most drugs that are absorbed from the gut by passive diffusion, levodopa is absorbed via a saturable, stereospecific transport system that appears to be highly specific for neutral amino acids (Wade, Mearrick and Morris, 1973).

The properties of this transport system are quite similar to those of the levodopa transport system at the blood–brain barrier. The major clinical significance of this mode of absorption is that neutral amino acids contained in the normal diet may compete with levodopa for this transport system. Investigators have shown that the administration of low protein diets results in a reduction in the required dose of levodopa for a therapeutic response (Mena and Cotzias, 1975). Furthermore, co-administration of levodopa with tryptophan reduced the subsequent blood levels of levodopa attained compared to levodopa alone (Weitbrecht, Nuber and Sandritter, 1976). Thus, there is solid evidence that the transport of levodopa from the small intestine into the portal vein is a critical, potentially rate-limiting, step in the absorption of levodopa.

Distribution

After absorption through the gut wall into the portal system and passage through the liver, levodopa enters the systemic circulation. As with most drugs, the clearance of levodopa from plasma is a biphasic function (Nutt, Woodward and Anderson, 1985). The initial, rather short phase (less than 30 min) is termed the 'distribution phase'. Essentially all levodopa in plasma is free drug because levodopa is apparently not significantly bound to plasma proteins (Hinterberger and Andrews, 1972). The principal net change that occurs during the distribution phase is the transfer of levodopa from the plasma compartment into various tissue reservoirs, such as red blood cells and skeletal muscle. The most important portion of the distribution phase for the anti-Parkinson effects of levodopa is the transfer of levodopa from blood to brain across the blood–brain barrier.

Blood–brain barrier

As with levodopa absorption from the gut, levodopa crosses the blood–brain barrier via a saturable stereospecific, bidirectional transport system (Pardridge and Oldendorf, 1977). Additionally, the transport system is specific for neutral (both aromatic and branched-chain) amino acids (Wade and Katzman, 1975b; Pardridge, 1977). The affinity of this transport system is similar to the normally occurring plasma concentrations of neutral amino acids; therefore, the rate of transport of levodopa is a function of the levodopa plasma concentration as well as the plasma concentrations of the other neutral amino acids that compete for the same finite number of transport sites (Pardridge, 1977; Pardridge and Oldendorf, 1977). The competition between levodopa and other neutral amino acids for entry into brain has been demonstrated both in man (Nutt *et al.*, 1984) and in laboratory animals (Oldendorf, 1971; Wade and Katzman, 1975b; Daniel, Moorhouse and Pratt, 1976). In a series of elegant studies in parkinsonian patients, Nutt *et al.* (1984) demonstrated that administration of neutral amino acids during a constant intravenous infusion of levodopa resulted in transient clinical worsening without affecting levodopa blood levels (*Figure 11.4*). Similarly, ingestion of high protein meals during an intravenous levodopa infusion caused transient clinical deterioration without altering plasma levodopa levels (*Figure 11.5*) (Nutt *et al.*, 1984). Thus, the therapeutic efficacy of levodopa may be significantly modified by competition with other neutral amino acids for entry into the brain across the blood–brain barrier.

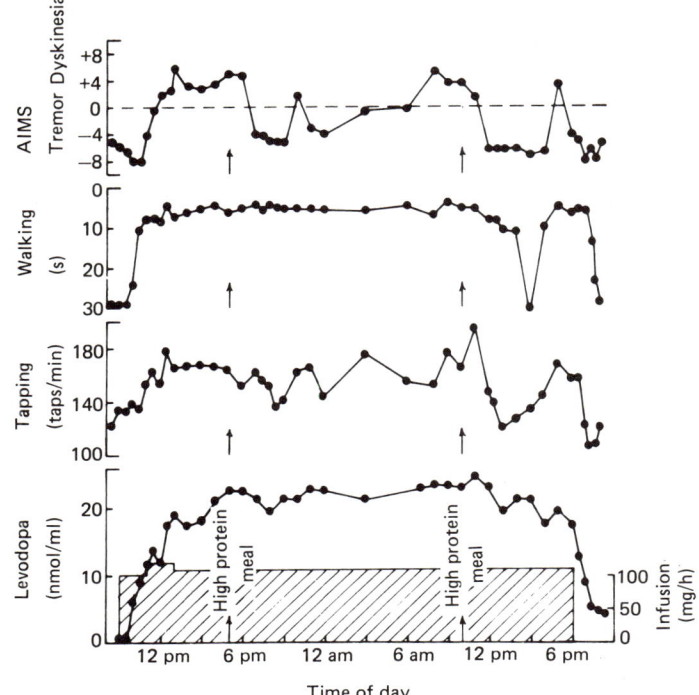

Figure 11.4 Effects of high protein meals on the plasma levodopa concentration and the clinical response during intravenous infusion of levodopa in one patient. The patient was receiving carbidopa 25 mg by mouth every two hours. AIMS denotes the algebraic sum of involuntary movement scores (positive values indicate dyskinesia and negative values indicate tremor). (Reproduced from Nutt *et al.*, 1984, *New England Journal of Medicine* with permission of the Authors and Publishers)

Another potential barrier to the passage of levodopa from blood to brain is the presence of L-AAAD activity in cerebral capillary endothelial cells (Hardebo *et al.*, 1980). Dopamine thus formed would be unlikely to cross the vascular basement membrane and would be subject to further metabolism, particularly by monoamine oxidase, in endothelial cells. The practical clinical relevance of this 'enzymatic barrier' was questioned by the recent observations that the plasma concentration of levodopa producing the optimum clinical response was the same whether or not carbidopa was co-administered (Fahn, 1974; Nutt, Woodward and Anderson, 1985).

Biotransformation

Decarboxylation

The biotransformation or metabolism of levodopa occurs at multiple sites and affects both the rates of absorption and elimination. For a given oral dose of

Figure 11.5 Effects of ingestion of amino acids on the plasma levodopa concentration and the clinical response during intravenous infusion of levodopa in one patient. Amino acids (100 mg/kg) were administered in solution at the times indicated by the arrows. No carbidopa was administered during the infusion. AIMS denotes the algebraic sum of involuntary movement scores. (Reproduced from Nutt *et al.*, 1984, *New England Journal of Medicine* with permission of the Authors and Publishers)

levodopa the first and perhaps quantitatively most important site of biotransformation is in the gastric mucosa. The enzyme, L-AAAD, which catalyses the conversion of levodopa to dopamine, is present in high activity in the gastric and small intestinal mucosa (Rivera-Calimlim *et al.*, 1970; Rivera-Calimlim, Dujovne and Morgan, 1971; Sasahara *et al.*, 1981a). Studies in dogs suggest that over half of an orally administered dose of levodopa is decarboxylated in the gut wall prior to entry into the systemic circulation (Cotler *et al.*, 1976; Sasahara *et al.*, 1981a). In studies in parkinsonian patients which compared the decarboxylated metabolites of levodopa after oral and intravenous administration, similar conclusions were drawn (Andersson *et al.*, 1975). Because of the activity of L-AAAD in gut mucosa, slow gastric emptying rates would predispose towards more gut biotransformation of levodopa, thereby reducing its bioavailability.

Despite the high activity of L-AAAD in liver (Tyce, 1971), this organ appears to be much less important than the gut as a site for levodopa decarboxylation, because the areas under time–action curves for levodopa were similar in dogs after portal and systemic venous administration (Sasahara *et al.*, 1981a). In addition to gut mucosa and liver, L-AAAD activity is present in many other peripheral tissues including kidney. Because of the ubiquitous presence of this enzyme in peripheral tissues, approximately two-thirds of the urinary metabolites of an oral levodopa dose occur as dopamine or its metabolites (Morgan et al., 1971).

O-Methylation

The other major enzymatic pathway for levodopa biotransformation is the conversion to 3-O-methyldopa by the catalytic action of the enzyme, catechol-O-methyltransferase (COMT) (Axelrod, Albers and Clemente, 1959). This step probably occurs primarily in the liver where COMT activity is very high; but other tissues such as red blood cells also contain significant COMT activity (Axelrod, Albers and Clemente, 1959). Approximately 10% of an injected dose of levodopa appeared in the urine as 3-O-methyldopa or related metabolites (Goodall and Alton, 1972). This percentage may be larger when levodopa is co-administered with decarboxylase inhibitors.

The enzymatic production of 3-O-methyldopa may be very relevant to the clinical efficacy of levodopa. The plasma half-life of 3-O-methyldopa is approximately 15 hours; thus this metabolite will accumulate during chronic levodopa dosing (Sharpless et al., 1972). Most relevant is the observation that 3-O-methyldopa has a higher affinity than levodopa for the blood–brain barrier neutral amino acid transport system (Wade and Katzman, 1975a). Furthermore, the concentration of 3-O-methyldopa in plasma of patients taking levodopa chronically is usually higher than that of levodopa (Sharpless et al., 1972). This may be particularly true in patients taking levodopa in combination with decarboxylase inhibitors. In experimental animals, 3-O-methyldopa reduces the accumulation of co-administered levodopa and its metabolites in the brain (Reches and Fahn, 1982). In both man and experimental animals, 3-O-methyldopa reduces the central pharmacological effects of levodopa (Chase and Ng, 1972; Muenter et al., 1973; Reches, Mielke and Fahn, 1982). Finally, several groups of investigators have reported that parkinsonian patients who are poor responders to levodopa tend to have higher circulating 3-O-methyldopa levels (Muenter, Sharpless and Tyce, 1972; Rivera-Calimlim et al., 1977) and greater red blood cell COMT activity (Reilly, Rivera-Calimlim and Van Dyke, 1980) than patients with good responses to levodopa. One is tempted to speculate that the lower optimal therapeutic doses of levodopa required after drug holidays (Sweet et al., 1972) may be due in part to the clearance of 3-O-methyldopa during the drug holidays.

Other routes of levodopa metabolism

Up to 20% of an administered dose of levodopa did not appear in the urine within five days (Goodall and Alton, 1972). Some portion of the dose may have been excreted in the faeces. Perhaps as much as 2% of an oral dose may be excreted unchanged and unabsorbed in the faeces (Peaston and Bianchine, 1970). In addition, after intravenous administration of radiolabelled levodopa, up to 10% of the radioactivity has been recovered in intestinal tissue, a portion of which may be excreted in the faeces (Tyce and Owen, 1979). Even accounting for the elimination of levodopa and metabolites in the faeces, a small, but significant, portion of an administered dose of levodopa cannot be accounted for by decarboxylated and O-methylated metabolites.

One additional potential route of metabolism of levodopa is oxidation to form the dopaquinone polymer, melanin. Another relatively minor route of levodopa biotransformation is via transamination. A variety of cytosolic and mitochondria-associated transaminases exist that will transaminate levodopa (Fellman and Roth, 1971). Several of the principal end-products of levodopa transamination have been identified in the urine after pharmacological doses of levodopa (Wada and Fellman, 1973; Sandler *et al.*, 1974), but the significance of the role that transamination plays in practical terms is yet to be determined.

Elimination

The elimination of levodopa occurs primarily by decarboxylation with smaller percentages of a given dose being O-methylated or transaminated. About 75% of an oral dose appears in the urine within 24 hours, primarily in the form of dopamine metabolites (Morgan *et al.*, 1971; Goodall and Alton, 1972). The clearance or elimination of levodopa from plasma is very rapid. Though the rate of elimination varies among individuals, the plasma half-life of levodopa is on the average about 1.3 hours (Nutt, Woodward and Anderson, 1985).

Effects of decarboxylase inhibitors on levodopa pharmacokinetics

The introduction of peripheral L-AAAD inhibitors such as carbidopa and benserazide provided a significant advance in the therapy of Parkinson's disease. Currently most parkinsonian patients take fixed combinations of levodopa and peripheral decarboxylase inhibitors. In the usual therapeutic doses these compounds do not penetrate the blood–brain barrier, but act peripherally to inhibit the conversion of levodopa to dopamine. Thus a greater percentage of an administered dose of levodopa eventually enters the brain. The co-administration of levodopa with peripheral decarboxylase inhibitors decreases the daily requirements for levodopa by 75–80% (Reid *et al.*, 1972; Mars, 1973). A major consequence of this strategy is to reduce the circulating levels of dopamine resulting from levodopa decarboxylation, thereby reducing the gastrointestinal and cardiac rhythm side-effects of levodopa. The incidence of other side-effects such as dopa-induced dyskinesias and psychiatric disturbances are little affected by the co-administration of decarboxylase inhibitors with levodopa.

The increased bioavailability of levodopa when co-administered with a peripheral decarboxylase inhibitor may occur as a result of several mechanisms. When oral levodopa dosage is held constant, the co-administration of decarboxylase inhibitors with levodopa results in much higher peak plasma levels than when levodopa alone is given (Tissot, Bartholini and Pletscher, 1969; Dunner, Brodie and Goodwin, 1971). Therefore, one of the principal mechanisms of action of decarboxylase inhibitors must be to decrease levodopa metabolism to dopamine in the gut during absorption and during the first pass through the liver, thereby improving bioavailability (Nutt, Woodward and Anderson, 1985). Recent studies by Nutt and colleagues demonstrated that carbidopa administration significantly prolonged both the distribution (0.09 h without carbidopa to 0.19 h with carbidopa) and elimination (1.31 h without carbidopa to 2.22 h with carbidopa) phases of levodopa pharmacokinetics (Nutt, Woodward and Anderson, 1985). Thus, the therapeutic effects of carbidopa with levodopa result from both increasing bioavailability of levodopa and reducing levodopa plasma clearance rates. Nevertheless, the effect of decarboxylase inhibitors on plasma half-life of levodopa did not materially affect the clinical duration of action of levodopa in patients with Parkinson's disease (Fahn, 1974).

Co-administration of decarboxylase with levodopa affects the routes of metabolism of levodopa in several ways. First, there is a reduction in the percentage of an administered dose of levodopa that is converted to the dopamine metabolites, dihydroxyphenylacetic acid and homovanillic acid (Bianchine, Messiha and Hsu, 1972); second, there is an increase in the amount of transaminated products of levodopa metabolism (Sandler *et al.*, 1974); third, there is a relative increase in the percentage of an administered dose of levodopa that is metabolized to 3-*O*-methyldopa.

The optimal daily dose of the decarboxylase inhibitor, carbidopa, has been the subject of several studies. It would appear that approximately 100 mg/day of carbidopa in divided doses is an optimal amount (Preziosi *et al.*, 1972; Kremzer *et al.*, 1973). No further reduction in the daily requirements for levodopa was found when daily carbidopa doses were increased beyond this level.

For additional information on the extracerebral pharmacokinetics of levodopa, *see* Nutt and Fellman (1984).

CEREBRAL PHARMACOKINETICS OF LEVODOPA

The desired end-product of the extracerebral pharmacokinetics of a dose of levodopa is the achievement of an adequate striatal concentration of levodopa. But to be effective in the alleviation of Parkinson symptoms, levodopa must be converted to dopamine in the striatum in adequate amounts by the enzyme L-AAAD and the newly synthesized dopamine must interact with striatal dopamine receptors in sufficient quantity to produce a dopaminergic, anti-Parkinson effect. The temporal relationship between peak plasma levels of levodopa and optimal clinical response would suggest that between 45 and 90 min is required for levodopa transport across the blood–brain barrier, conversion to dopamine, and interaction of newly synthesized dopamine with dopamine receptors in the striatum to produce a therapeutic effect (*see Figure 11.6*; Shoulson, Glaubiger and Chase, 1975).

The principal cerebral pharmacokinetic variables that affect the therapeutic efficacy of a dose of levodopa are the rate and extent of conversion of levodopa to dopamine, the rate of movement of newly synthesized dopamine from the compartment in which it is synthesized to dopamine receptors, and the rate of inactivation of newly synthesized dopamine. None of these variables are currently accessible to direct study in patients with Parkinson's disease. Studies in experimental animal models of Parkinson's disease, however, may provide some insight into these variables.

The level of striatal L-AAAD activity is the principal determinant of the rate and extent of conversion of levodopa to dopamine in the striatum. L-AAAD activity in the striatum is localized primarily in the terminals of nigrostriatal dopamine neurones. In a postmortem study of 13 parkinsonian brains, Lloyd, Davidson and Hornykiewicz (1975) found an approximately 90% reduction in L-AAAD activity in striatum compared to appropriate controls. A similar profound degree of

242   Pharmacokinetics of levodopa

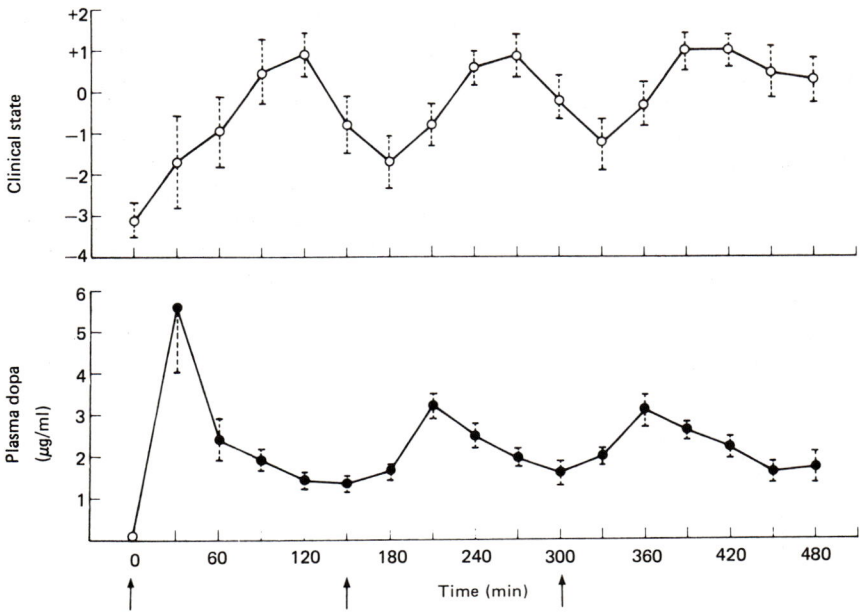

Figure 11.6 Relationship between plasma dopa level and clinical state in seven parkinsonian patients receiving sequential oral doses of levodopa in combination with carbidopa. Arrows indicate time of levodopa administration. (Reproduced from Shoulson, Glaubiger and Chase, 1975, *Neurology* with permission of the Authors and Publishers)

reduction in striatal L-AAAD activity is found in rats after extensive 6-hydroxydopamine lesions of ipsilateral nigral dopaminergic neurones (Melamed *et al.*, 1980). Following the administration of levodopa plus carbidopa to rats with extensive unilateral nigral lesions, dopamine levels increased much less, and remained elevated for a shorter time in the ipsilateral striatum than in the contralateral control striatum (Spencer and Wooten, 1984). This finding cannot be explained by reduced delivery of levodopa to the dopamine-deficient striatum (Horne, Cheng and Wooten, 1984). These data would suggest that the rate and extent of the conversion of levodopa to dopamine in the striatum of patients with Parkinson's disease is reduced, and that the reduction in the rate of conversion of levodopa to dopamine is proportional to the degree of loss of the nigrostriatal innervation of the striatum.

Furthermore, following the administration of levodopa plus carbidopa to rats with unilateral nigral lesions, the ratio of dopamine to its metabolites (i.e. dihydroxyphenylacetic acid, 3-methoxytyramine and homovanillic acid) is lower at all subsequent time points in the ipsilateral striatum compared to the contralateral side (Spencer and Wooten, 1984). This finding suggests that the rate of turnover of dopamine in the striatum deprived of its dopamine innervation is greater than in control striatum. One factor that may contribute to this more rapid turnover and biotransformation is the loss of the storage capacity for dopamine due to the reduction of re-uptake sites and storage vesicles attendant with the death of dopamine neural terminals in the striatum. Postmortem studies of parkinsonian brains indicated that there was no significant reduction in monoamine oxidase

Cerebral pharmacokinetics of levodopa

activity and only an approximately 25% reduction in COMT activity in the striata of patients with Parkinson's disease (Lloyd, Davidson and Hornykiewicz, 1975). Thus the enzymatic machinery for biotransformation of dopamine remains intact while the synthetic capacity, i.e. L-AAAD activity, is drastically reduced. Based on these animal studies, one might predict that the cerebral pharmacokinetics of levodopa are affected in the parkinsonian brain in two ways: the rate and extent of conversion of levodopa to dopamine are reduced and the rate of biotransformation of dopamine is increased. Both changes should vary in proportion to the degree of pathology (*see Figure 11.7*). No conclusions can be made about the rate of movement of newly synthesized dopamine from the compartment in which it is synthesized to dopamine receptors. Hopefully, in the future the cerebral pharmacokinetics of levodopa can be studied directly *in vivo* in parkinsonian patients, using positron emission tomography technology with radiolabelled levodopa.

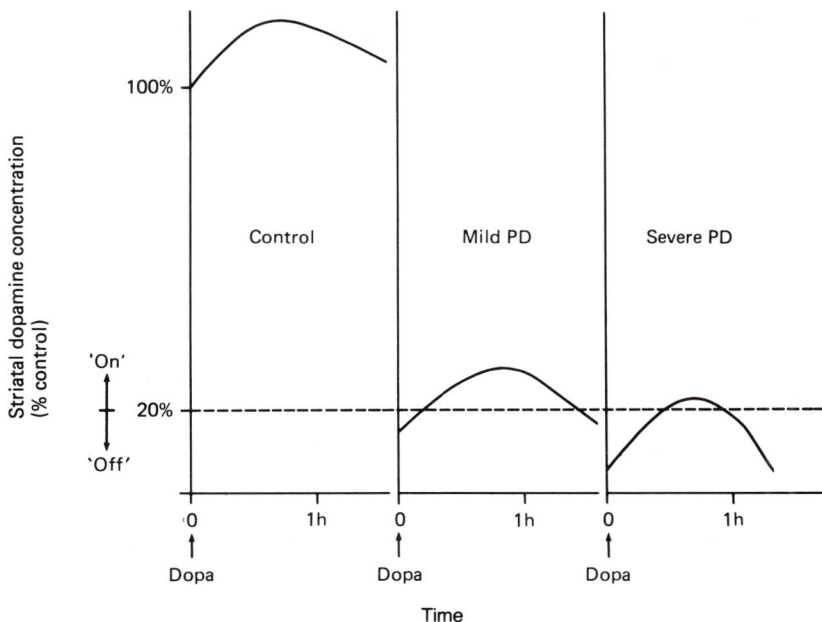

Figure 11.7 Hypothetical summary of the effects of levodopa administration on striatal dopamine concentration and clinical state ('on' or 'off') in control patients and in patients with mild and severe Parkinson's disease (PD). (Reproduced from Spencer and Wooten, 1984, *Neurology*, with permission of the Publishers)

Role of levodopa pharmacokinetics in treatment-related fluctuations and failure to respond

During the course of chronic treatment of parkinsonism with levodopa (with or without decarboxylase inhibitors), several types of complications frequently emerge. The two most common are the development of fluctuations (previously referred to as 'end-of-dose deterioration' or 'wearing-off') and failure to respond (either to random doses or all doses).

Fluctuations

The response to levodopa treatment is usually reasonably stable for the first 2–5 years of therapy. Subsequently, as many as 50% or more of patients begin to develop fluctuations (Marsden and Schachter, 1981). These treatment-related fluctuations begin to become apparent with an accentuation of what Fahn and Marsden have termed the 'medium duration response' (Fahn, 1982; Marsden, Parkes and Quinn, 1982). The 'medium duration response' appears to vary with changes in plasma levodopa levels such that rapid clinical improvement appears from 15 min to 1 hour after an oral dose, with the gradual reappearance of parkinsonian symptoms 3–4 hours later. The problematic fluctuations gradually emerge as the duration of action of each levodopa dose progressively shortens from four hours to as little as one.

There is no known change in the extracerebral metabolism of levodopa with chronic treatment. Based on current evidence, neither the peak plasma levels nor duration of plasma levels of levodopa are significantly altered by chronic levodopa administration (Fellman and Roth, 1971; Nutt and Fellman, 1984). Other than alterations in cerebral pharmacokinetics or pharmacodynamics, the only potential extracerebral mechanism to explain the emergence of the 'wearing-off' phenomenon might be a consequence of 3-O-methyldopa competition with levodopa transport across the blood–brain barrier. As 3-O-methyldopa plasma levels accumulate, less plasma levodopa might be transported into the central nervous system, thereby reducing peak dose brain levels of levodopa and shortening of the duration of elevation in brain levodopa concentration. It is not currently possible to entirely exclude this mechanism as a factor in shortening of response duration.

A seemingly more likely basis for the emergence of the 'wearing-off' phenomenon is the progressive alteration of the cerebral pharmacokinetics of levodopa. As detailed in a previous section, work in experimental animal models of Parkinson's disease would suggest that the basis for 'wearing-off' occurs as a direct consequence of the progressive loss of dopaminergic nigrostriatal terminals in the caudate-putamen of patients with Parkinson's disease (Spencer and Wooten, 1984). The attendant drastic reduction in striatal L-AAAD activity results in a reduction in the rate of conversion of levodopa to dopamine. Furthermore, the turnover of dopamine is more rapid than in control striatum, probably due to the progressive loss of the storage capacity for dopamine. The ultimate effect, then, of disease progression is to reduce both the amount of dopamine formed and the duration of increased dopamine levels in the striatum after each dose of levodopa (Spencer and Wooten, 1984). End-of-dose deterioration most likely occurs, then, as a consequence of recurring striatal dopamine deficiency following the initial response to each levodopa dose. This contention is supported by the observations that 'wearing-off' correlates temporally with falling levodopa blood levels (Shoulson, Glaubiger and Chase, 1975), that administration of the direct acting dopamine agonist, apomorphine, can rapidly reverse 'end-of-dose deterioration' (Duby et al., 1972) and that continuous intravenous infusion of levodopa sufficient to maintain constant therapeutic blood levels will produce a sustained reduction in clinical fluctuations (Shoulson, Glaubiger and Chase, 1975; Nutt et al., 1984). The very early emergence of the levodopa 'wearing-off' phenomenon in patients with severe MPTP-induced parkinsonism (Langston and Ballard, 1984) would suggest that the prerequisites for these fluctuations are moderate to severe parkinsonian symptoms (associated with profound loss of nigrostriatal neurones and L-AAAD activity) and the clear capacity to respond favourably when single doses of levodopa are administered. Thus, based on current evidence, the progressive alteration in the rate of synthesis and inactivation of dopamine in the parkinsonian striatum appears to be the principal mechanism underlying the emergence of progressive shortening of response duration to levodopa.

Failure to respond

The failure of patients with idiopathic Parkinson's disease to respond to levodopa may take several forms. One rather common problem is the occurrence of erratic responses to the same levodopa/carbidopa dose during the course of a day. The first morning dose may produce clear improvement in symptoms for several hours, while subsequent doses may either be randomly or progressively more ineffective. This type of failure to respond may occur as a consequence of pharmacokinetic factors. The progressive global failure to respond to levodopa even at very high doses, usually seen in elderly parkinsonian patients, is more likely to result from pharmacodynamic changes, e.g. loss of dopamine receptors with ageing (Wong *et al.*, 1984).

In approaching the patient with inconsistent or erratic responses to individual levodopa doses, virtually every step of the absorption, distribution, metabolism, and excretion of levodopa must be considered as the potential culprit. The rate of gastric emptying may vary considerably in the course of a day in which patients take many doses of levodopa. Thus, meals, changes in gastric acidity, and effects of concomitant anticholinergic drugs must be considered. The small intestinal absorption of levodopa doses taken with, or shortly after, meals may be compromised by competition with neutral amino acids for transport from gut to portal system (Nutt *et al.*, 1984). Accumulation of 3-*O*-methyldopa during each day may progressively compete with each subsequent levodopa dose in the course of a day for transport across the blood–brain barrier. Likewise, levodopa doses taken after high protein meals may be less effective due to blood–brain barrier transport competition with the circulating amino acids. Only careful attention to recurrent patterns of erratic failure to respond will allow for judicious changes in levodopa dose and dosing interval. Thus, a thorough knowledge of the daily habits of each patient that may have an impact on the extracerebral pharmacokinetics of levodopa is required for the successful management of erratic failures to respond.

References

ANDERSSON, I., GRANERUS, A. K., JAGENBURG, R. and SVANBORG, A. (1975) Intestinal decarboxylation of orally administered L-dopa. *Acta Medica Scandinavia*, **198**, 415–420
AXELROD, J., ALBERS, W. and CLEMENTE, C. D. (1959) Distribution of catechol-*O*-methyltransferase in the nervous system and other tissues. *Journal of Neurochemistry*, **5**, 68–72
BIANCHINE, J. R., CALIMLIM, L. R., MORGAN, J. P., DUJOVNE, C. A. and LASAGNA, L. (1971) Metabolism and absorption of L-3,4-dihydroxyphenylalanine in patients with Parkinson's disease. *Annals of the New York Academy of Sciences*, **179**, 126–140
BIANCHINE, J. R., MESSIHA, F. S. and HSU, T. H. (1972) Peripheral aromatic L-amino acid decarboxylase inhibitor in parkinsonism. II: Effect on the metabolism of L-2-^{14}C-DOPA. *Clinical Pharmacology and Therapeutics*, **13**, 584–594
CHASE, T. N. and NG, L. K. Y. (1972) *O*-Methyldopa in parkinsonism. *Neurology*, **22**, 417

COTLER, S., HOLAZO, A., BOXENBAUM, H. G. and KAPLAN, S. A. (1976) Influence of route of administration on physiological availability of levodopa in dogs. *Journal of Pharmaceutical Sciences*, **65**, 822–827

COTZIAS, G. C., PAPAVASILIOU, P. S. and GELLENE, R. (1969) Modification of parkinsonism: chronic treatment with L-dopa. *New England Journal of Medicine*, **280**, 337–345

DANIEL, R. M., MOORHOUSE, S. R. and PRATT, O. E. (1976) Do changes in blood levels of other aromatic amino acids influence levodopa therapy? *Lancet*, **i**, 95

DENNY, R. M., FRITZ, R. R., PATEL, N. T. and ABELL, C. W. (1982) Human liver MAO-A and MAO-B separated by immunoaffinity chromatography with MAO-B-specific monoclonal antibody. *Science*, **215**, 1400–1403

DUBY, S. E., COTZIAS, G. C., PAPAVASILIOU, P. S. and LAWRENCE, W. H. (1972) Injected apomorphine and orally administered levodopa in parkinsonism. *Archives of Neurology*, **27**, 474–480

DUNNER, D. L., BRODIE, H. K. H. and GOODWIN, F. K. (1971) Plasma dopa response to levodopa administration in man: effects of a peripheral decarboxylase inhibitor. *Clinical Pharmacology and Therapeutics*, **12**, 212–217

FAHN, S. (1974) "On–off" phenomenon with levodopa therapy in parkinsonism. *Neurology*, **24**, 431–441

FAHN, S. (1982) Fluctuations of disability in Parkinson's disease: pathophysiology. In *Movement Disorders*. Eds. C. D. Marsden and S. Fahn, pp. 123–145. London: Butterworth Scientific

FELLMAN, J. H. and ROTH, E. S. (1971) Inhibition of tyrosine amino-transferase activity by L-3,4-dihydroxyphenylalanine. *Biochemistry*, **10**, 408–414

FERMAGLICH, J. and O'DOHERTY, D. S. (1972) Effect of gastric motility on levodopa. *Diseases of the Nervous System*, **33**, 624–625

GOODALL, M. C. and ALTON, H. (1972) Metabolism of 3,4-dihydroxyphenylalanine (L-dopa) in human subjects. *Biochemical Pharmacology*, **21**, 2401–2408

HARDEBO, J. E., ERNSON, P. C., FALCK, B., OWMAN, C. and ROSENGREN, E. (1980) Enzymes related to monoamine transmitter metabolism in brain microvessels. *Journal of Neurochemistry*, **35**, 1388–1393

HINTERBERGER, H. and ANDREWS, C. J. (1972) Catecholamine metabolism during oral administration of levodopa. *Archives of Neurology*, **26**, 245–252

HORNE, M. K., CHENG, C. H. and WOOTEN, G. F. (1984) The cerebral metabolism of L-dihydroxyphenylalanine: an autoradiographic and biochemical study. *Pharmacology*, **28**, 12–26

HORNYKIEWICZ, O. (1972) Neurochemistry of parkinsonism. *Handbook of Neurochemistry*, **7**, 465–501

KAPLAN, G. P., HARTMAN, B. K. and CREVELING, C. R. (1979) Immunohistochemical demonstration of catechol-*O*-methyltransferase in mammalian brain. *Brain Research*, **167**, 241–250

KREMZER, L. T., BERL, S., MENDOZA, M. and YAHR, M. D. (1973) Cerebrospinal fluid levels of DOPA and 3-*O*-methyldopa in parkinsonism during treatment with L-DOPA and MK-486. *Advances in Neurology*, **2**, 79–89

LANGSTON, J. W. and BALLARD, P. (1984) Parkinsonism induced by 1-methyl-4-phenyl-1,2,3,6-tetrahydropyridine (MPTP): implications for treatment and the pathogenesis of Parkinson's disease. *Canadian Journal of Neurological Science*, **11** (Suppl. 1), 160–165

LEVITT, P., PINTAR, J. E. and BREAKFIELD, X. O. (1982) Immunocytochemical demonstration of monoamine oxidase B in brain astrocytes and serotonergic neurons. *Proceedings of the National Academy of Sciences of the United States of America*, **79**, 6385–6389

LLOYD, K. G., DAVIDSON, L. and HORNYKIEWICZ, O. (1975) The neurochemistry of Parkinson's disease: effect of L-DOPA therapy. *Journal of Pharmacology and Experimental Therapeutics*, **195**, 453–464

MARS, H. (1973) Modification of levodopa effect by systemic decarboxylase inhibition. *Archives of Neurology*, **28**, 91–95

MARSDEN, C. D., PARKES, J. D. and QUINN, N. (1982) Fluctuations of disability in Parkinson's disease – clinical aspects. In *Movement Disorders*. Eds. C. D. Marsden and S. Fahn, pp. 96–122. London: Butterworth Scientific

MARSDEN, C. D. and SCHACHTER, M. (1981) Assessment of extrapyramidal disorders. *British Journal of Clinical Pharmacology*, **11**, 129–151

MEARRICK, P. T., WADE, D. N., BIRKETT, D. J. and MORRIS, J. (1974) Metoclopramide, gastric emptying and L-dopa absorption. *Australian and New Zealand Journal of Medicine*, **4**, 144–148

MELAMED, E., GLOBUS, M., UZZAN, A. and ROSENTHAL, J. (1985) Is dopamine formed from exogenous L-dopa stored within vesicles in striatal dopaminergic nerve terminals? Implications for L-dopa's mechanism of action in Parkinson's disease. *Neurology*, **35** (Suppl. 1), 188

MELAMED, E., HEFTI, F., LIEBMAN, J. and WURTMAN, R. J. (1980) Serotonergic neurons are not involved in action of L-DOPA in Parkinson's disease. *Nature*, **283**, 722–774

MELAMED, E., HEFTI, F. and WURTMAN, R. J. (1980) Nonaminergic striatal neurons convert exogenous L-dopa to dopamine in parkinsonism. *Annals of Neurology*, **8**, 558–563

MENA, I. and COTZIAS, G. C. (1975) Protein intake and treatment of Parkinson's disease with levodopa. *New England Journal of Medicine*, **292**, 181–184

MORGAN, J. P., BIANCHINE, J. R., SPIEGEL, H. E., RIVERA-CALIMLIM, L. and HERSEY, R. M. (1971) Metabolism of levodopa in patients with Parkinson's disease. *Archives of Neurology,* **25,** 39–44
MOSKOWITZ, M. A. and WURTMAN, R. J. (1975) Catecholamines and neurologic diseases. *New England Journal of Medicine,* **293,** 274–280; 332–338
MUENTER, M. D., DINAPOLI, R. P., SHARPLESS, N. S. and TYCE, G. M. (1973) 3-O-Methyldopa, L-DOPA, and trihexyphenidyl in the treatment of Parkinson's disease. *Mayo Clinic Proceedings,* **48,** 173–183
MUENTER, M. D., SHARPLESS, N. S. and TYCE, G. M. (1972) Plasma 3-O-methyldopa in L-dopa therapy of Parkinson's disease. *Mayo Clinic Proceedings,* **47,** 389–395
NUTT, J. G. and FELLMAN, J. H. (1984) Pharmacokinetics of levodopa. *Clinical Neuropharmacology,* **7,** 35–49
NUTT, J. G., WOODWARD, W. R. and ANDERSON, J. L. (1985) Effect of carbidopa on pharmacokinetics of intravenously administered levodopa: implications for mechanism of action of carbidopa in the treatment of parkinsonism. *Annals of Neurology* (in press)
NUTT, J. G., WOODWARD, W. R., HAMMERSTAD, J. P., CARTER, J. H. and ANDERSON, J. L. (1984) "On–off" phenomenon in Parkinson's disease: relationship to L-dopa absorption and transport. *New England Journal of Medicine,* **310,** 483–488
OLDENDORF, W. H. (1971) Brain uptake of radiolabeled amino acids, amines, and hexoses after arterial injection. *American Journal of Physiology,* **221,** 1629–1639
PARDRIDGE, W. M. (1977) Kinetics of competitive inhibition of neutral amino acid transport across the blood–brain barrier. *Journal of Neurochemistry,* **28,** 103–108
PARDRIDGE, W. M. and OLDENDORF, W. H. (1977) Transport of metabolic substrates through the blood–brain barrier. *Journal of Neurochemistry,* **28,** 5–12
PEARCE, L. B. and ROTH, J. A. (1984) Monoamine oxidase: separation of the type A and B activities. *Biochemical Pharmacology,* **33,** 1809–1811
PEASTON, M. J. T. and BIANCHINE, J. R. (1970) Metabolic studies and clinical observations during L-dopa treatment of Parkinson's disease. *British Medical Journal,* **1,** 400–403
POCELINKO, R., THOMAS, G. B. and SOLOMON, H. M. (1972) The effect of an antacid on the absorption and metabolism of levodopa. *Clinical Pharmacology and Therapeutics,* **13,** 149a
PREZIOSI, T. J., BIANCHINE, J. R., HSU, T. H. and MESSIHA, F. S. (1972) L-Methyldopa hydrazine (MK-486) and L-DOPA: a double blind study in parkinsonism. *Transactions of the American Neurological Association,* **97,** 321–322
RECHES, A. and FAHN, S. (1982) 3-O-Methyldopa blocks DOPA metabolism in rat corpus striatum. *Annals of Neurology,* **12,** 267–271
RECHES, A., MIELKE, L. R. and FAHN, S. (1982) 3-O-Methyldopa inhibits rotations induced by levodopa in rats after unilateral destruction of the nigrostriatal pathway. *Neurology,* **32,** 887–888
REID, J. L., CALNE, D. B., VAKIL, S. D., ALLEN, J. G. and DAVIES, C. A. (1972) Plasma concentration of levodopa in parkinsonism before and after inhibition of peripheral decarboxylase. *Journal of Neurological Sciences,* **17,** 45–51
REILLY, D. K., RIVERA-CALIMLIM, L. and VAN DYKE, D. (1980) Catechol-O-methyltransferase activity: a determinant of levodopa response. *Clinical Pharmacology and Therapeutics,* **28,** 278–286
RIVERA-CALIMLIM, L., DEEPAK, T., ANDERSON, R. and JOYNT, R. (1977) The clinical picture and plasma levodopa metabolite profile of parkinsonian non-responders. *Archives of Neurology,* **34,** 228–232
RIVERA-CALIMLIM, L., DUJOVNE, C. A. and MORGAN, J. P. (1971) Absorption and metabolism of L-dopa by the human stomach. *European Journal of Clinical Investigation,* **1,** 313–320
RIVERA-CALIMLIM, L., DUJOVNE, C. A., MORGAN, J. P., LASAGNA, L. and BIANCHINE, J. R. (1970) L-Dopa treatment failure: explanation and correction. *British Medical Journal,* **4,** 93–94
RIVERA-CALIMLIM, L., MORGAN, J. P., DUJOVNE, C. A., BIANCHINE, J. R. and LASAGNA, L. (1971) L-3,4-Dihydroxyphenylalanine metabolism by the gut *in vitro. Biochemical Pharmacology,* **20,** 3051–3057
SANDLER, M., JOHNSON, R. D., RUTHVEN, C. R. J., REID, J. L. and CALNE, D. B. (1974) Transamination is a major pathway of L-DOPA metabolism following peripheral decarboxylase inhibition. *Nature,* **247,** 364–366
SASAHARA, K., NITANAI, T., HABARA, T., MOROIKA, T. and NAKAJIMA, E. (1981a) Dosage form design for improvement of bioavailability of levodopa. IV: Possible causes of low bioavailability of oral levodopa in dogs. *Journal of Pharmaceutical Sciences,* **70,** 730–733
SASAHARA, K., NITANAI, T., HABARA, T., MOROIKA, T. and NAKAJIMA, E. (1981b) Dosage form design for improvement of bioavailability of levodopa. V: Absorption and metabolism of levodopa in intestinal segments of dogs. *Journal of Pharmaceutical Sciences,* **70,** 1157–1160
SHARPLESS, N. S., MUENTER, M. D., TYCE, G. M. and OWEN, C. A. (1972) 3-Methoxy-4-hydroxyphenylalanine (3-O-methyldopa) in plasma during oral L-dopa therapy of patients with Parkinson's disease. *Clinica Chemica Acta,* **37,** 359–369

SHOULSON, I., GLAUBIGER, G. A. and CHASE, T. N. (1975) On–off response: clinical and biochemical correlations during oral and intravenous levodopa administration in parkinsonian patients. *Neurology,* **25,** 1144–1148

SPENCER, S. E. and WOOTEN, G. F. (1984) Altered pharmacokinetics of L-dopa metabolism in rat striatum deprived of dopaminergic innervation. *Neurology,* **34,** 1105–1108

STOOF, J. C. and KEBABIAN, J. W. (1984) Two dopamine receptors: biochemistry, physiology, and pharmacology. *Life Sciences,* **35,** 2281–2296

SWEET, R. D., LEE, J. E., SPIEGEL, H. E. and McDOWELL, F. (1972) Enhanced response to low doses of levodopa after withdrawal from chronic treatment. *Neurology,* **22,** 520–525

TISSOT, R., BARTHOLINI, G. and PLETSCHER, A. (1969) Drug-induced changes in extracerebral dopa metabolism in man. *Archives of Neurology,* **20,** 187–190

TYCE, G. M. (1971) Metabolism of 3,4-dihydroxyphenylalanine by isolated perfused rat liver. *Biochemical Pharmacology,* **20,** 3447–3462

TYCE, G. M. and OWEN, C. A. (1979) Administration of L-3,4-dihydroxyphenylalanine to rats after complete hepatectomy. I: Metabolites in tissue. *Biochemical Pharmacology,* **28,** 3271–3278

WADA, G. M. and FELLMAN, J. H. (1973) 2,3,5-Trihydroxyphenylacetic acid: a metabolite of L-3,4-dihydroxyphenylalanine. *Biochemistry,* **12,** 5212–5217

WADE, L. A. and KATZMAN, R. (1975a) 3-*O*-Methyldopa uptake and inhibition of L-dopa at the blood–brain barrier. *Life Sciences,* **17,** 131–136

WADE, L. A. and KATZMAN, R. (1975b) Synthetic amino acids and the nature of L-dopa transport at the blood–brain barrier. *Journal of Neurochemistry,* **25,** 837–842

WADE, D. N., MEARRICK, P. T. and MORRIS, J. L. (1973) Active transport of L-dopa in the intestine. *Nature,* **242,** 463–465

WEITBRECHT, W. U., NUBER, B. and SANDRITTER, W. (1976) Der einflus von L-tryptophan auf die L-dopa resorption. *Deutsche Medizinische Wochenschrift,* **101,** 20–22

WONG, D. F., WAGNER, H. N., DANNALS, R. F., LINKS, J. M., FROST, J. J., RAVERT, H. T. *et al.* (1984) Effects of age on dopamine and serotonin receptors measured by positron tomography in the living human brain. *Science,* **226,** 1393–1396

12
The olivopontocerebellar atrophies
Roger C. Duvoisin

HISTORICAL BACKGROUND

The term 'olivopontocerebellar atrophy' was employed descriptively by Dejerine and Thomas (1900) to denote a disorder they had observed in two middle-aged patients who suffered from a chronic apparently non-familial progressive degenerative disorder of the cerebellum. The chief manifestations were a broad-based short-stepped gait, slowness and hesitation in bodily movements, awkwardness of the hands, minimal action tremor and a slow scanning speech. There was also impairment of ocular motility and the tendon reflexes were hyperactive. One patient was studied postmortem.

They distinguished this disorder from Friedreich's ataxia and from the heterogeneous group of cases of adult onset, labelled 'hereditary cerebellar ataxia' by Marie (1893), but noted its similarity to the familial cases reported previously by Menzel (1891). The latter differed clinically, however, in having a familial pattern consistent with autosomal dominant inheritance, a younger age of onset and choreiform movements in the early stages of the illness.

The pathology in both Menzel's familial cases and in the sporadic case studied anatomically by Dejerine and Thomas was similar. It comprised symmetric atrophy of the cerebellum affecting the hemispheres more than the vermis, severe atrophy of the middle cerebellar peduncle, basis pontis and inferior olive, and partial atrophy of the restiform body. The dentate nucleus was involved in Menzel's cases but was spared in the Dejerine–Thomas case. The pyramids and cerebral peduncles appeared grossly smaller than normal, but degenerating fibres were not demonstrated.

Reports of similar cases studied postmortem gradually accumulated over the subsequent decades and the term 'olivopontocerebellar atrophy or degeneration' (OPCA or OPCD) gained general acceptance. Greenfield (1954) in his classic monograph on the spinocerebellar degenerations divided the reported cases of OPCA into two major categories, the dominantly inherited Menzel type and a sporadic type illustrated by the cases of Dejerine and Thomas. Berciano (1982) was able to collect 117 reported cases studied postmortem in a review published recently.

Many cases, however, differed in the extent of the atrophic process and in their clinical manifestations. Additional clinical features observed included spasticity, dementia, chorea, parkinsonism, myoclonic seizures, retinal degeneration, optic nerve atrophy, dysautonomia and amyotrophy. The distribution of neuronal degeneration gradually broadened to include the substantia nigra, locus ceruleus, substantia innominata, the dentate, anterior horn cells, striatum and other regions. Eadie (1975) accommodated some of the more variant cases in a third 'atypical' group in his extensive review of the subject.

Konigsmark and Weiner (1970) sought to recognize the heterogeneity of OPCA by classifying previously reported cases into the following five types, taking into account clinical as well as morphological features:

I   The Menzel type.
II   Autosomal recessive type comprising the families reported by Fickler and by Winkler.
III   Dominant ataxia with retinal degeneration.
IV   The Schut–Sweir kindred.
V   Dominant ataxia with progressive ophthalmoplegia, dementia and extrapyramidal manifestations.

A brave attempt to bring order out of chaos, this classification has not proved useful for reasons clearly outlined by Harding (1982) among others. It was limited to inherited disorders and completely ignored the much more common 'sporadic cases' usually of later onset. Some authors (e.g. Koeppen and Barron, 1984) would exclude the cases comprising type II as examples of OPCA, leaving only a brief listing of dominantly inherited OPCA. A fundamental problem in the classification of dominantly inherited OPCA is the enormous variation found within the same kindreds, which has been documented when several individuals have been carefully studied. For example, Ferguson and Critchley (1929) noted a broad range of variation in the Drew family of Walworth afflicted with a dominantly inherited ataxia extending from cases who were 'almost indistinguishable from Parkinson's disease' at one extreme to cases 'simulating disseminated sclerosis' at the other. Similar variation has also been noted in other families, and Konigsmark and Weiner themselves inadvertently assigned different members of the Schut–Sweir kindred to separate categories. They placed the cases of Gray and Oliver (1941) in type I and the family reported by Schut and Haymaker (1951) and by Schut (1950) in type IV. Dominant cases subsequently described do not fit within the categories as defined. For example, the childhood-onset cases of Colan, Snead and Ceballos (1981) overlap types III and IV, and neither Joseph's disease (Rosenberg, 1984) nor the cases with slow eye movement and peripheral neuropathy (Wadia and Swami, 1971; Wadia, 1984) correspond to any of these types. The failure of this classification has discouraged further attempts at classifying the OPCAs. Kondo, Hirota and Katagari (1981) commented that such efforts at nosological classification at present 'are more likely to add further controversy to the nosological debate, . . . than to solve the problem'. It seems that, in the dominantly inherited disorders, the most secure diagnosis is the identification of the specific kindred to which a given patient belongs. Ultimately, rational nosological classification of these disorders will depend on the identification of the specific genetic defect.

A number of families apparently representing different morbid entities have been reported under the label OPCA since Konigsmark and Weiner attempted their classification. In addition to the cases with slow eye movements and peripheral neuropathy and the childhood cases cited above, one may note among others the families with urinary glycolipid reported by Berenberg et al. (1984), a family with dementia, peripheral neuropathy and intrafascicular calcification in sympathetic nerve fibres and ganglia (Staal et al., 1981) and others distinguished on biochemical grounds. A dominant kindred with a distinctive defect in glutamate dehydrogenase was reported by Finocchiaro, Taroni and Di Donato (1985). Another was reported with an abnormal pattern of urinary organic acids (Rosenberg, Robinson and Partridge, 1975). Perry (1984) noted different patterns of change in brain neurotransmitter content in five kindreds of dominant OPCA suggesting four different entities in his material. Although the significance of these various pathological and biochemical abnormalities remains uncertain pending further research, it clearly indicates that the dominant OPCAs comprise a large number of distinct morbid entities.

OPCA may occur infrequently as one of the various phenotypic expressions of recognized inherited disorders, for example, type II Joseph disease (Rosenberg, 1984). It has also been identified as an unusual or rare phenotypic expression of hexoseaminidase deficiency (Oonk, ven der Helm and Martin, 1979; Johnson, 1981) and of adrenoleucodystrophy (Ohno et al., 1984). Finally, OPCA may occur as a dysgenesis in association with extraneural congenital and genetic defects as in the cases with ectodermal dysplasia, short stature and hypogonadism (Rushton and Genel, 1981) and in the DIDMOAD syndrome of OPCA with diabetes insipidus, diabetes mellitus, optic nerve atrophy and deafness (Kehl and Keller, 1982).

THE CLINICAL PERSPECTIVE

In the last decade, OPCA has increasingly been recognized on clinical grounds. The CT scan has greatly facilitated clinical diagnosis. As Savoiardo et al. (1983), Abe et al. (1983) and Huang and Plaitakis (1984) have shown, it provides an elegant, effective and non-invasive means of confirming the anatomical diagnosis. Recent biochemical investigations have offered promise of unraveling the underlying pathogenetic mechanisms, while a beginning has been made in defining the underlying molecular genetics. The resulting increased interest in OPCA has changed it from a rare pathological entity to a familiar, if uncommon, clinical disorder. The large clinical literature, dealing chiefly with the apparently sporadic forms, that has accumulated in the last decade makes it clear that OPCA is far more prevalent than had previously been recognized and presents a rather different clinical spectrum of manifestations than had been indicated by the earlier literature based primarily on autopsied cases.

Three perspectives have dominated the subject. First, OPCA has been seen as one of the more common forms of late onset abiotrophic cerebellar ataxia, i.e. of Marie's hereditary ataxia. Patients so diagnosed on clinical grounds comprise a large portion of the adult onset cerebellar ataxias. Kondo and Sobue (1980) and Kondo, Hirota and Katagari (1981) identified 180 cases of OPCA among 844 probands with spinocerebellar degeneration collected in a national collaborative survey of heritable ataxias recently conducted in Japan. These workers defined OPCA as a cerebellar syndrome of adult onset accompanied by two or more of the following features: dementia, rigidity or dystonia, involuntary movements or tremor, and dysautonomia. They also relied on CT scan evidence of pontine and cerebellar atrophy. Among 36 patients with sporadic late onset cerebellar ataxia, Harding (1981) found 18 individuals 'clinically similar to patients previously reported as sporadic examples of olivopontocerebellar atrophy'. In both these studies, the distinction between OPCA and other cases of late onset cerebellar ataxia was relative and Harding challenges the usefulness of distinguishing OPCA as a distinct morbid entity.

In another study, Harding (1982) examined 36 individuals with dominantly inherited cerebellar ataxia from 11 families including the 'Drew family of Walworth' cited above and noted only occasional extrapyramidal features, such as an 'impassive face', cogwheel rigidity or chorea. Of interest, one case had been erroneously thought to have Huntington's chorea.

The second perspective arises from studies of patients presenting with prominent dysautonomia such as the cases of Shy and Drager (1960). Actually, one of the cases of striatonigral degeneration (SND) reported by Adams, van Bogaert and van der Ecken (1964) cited above also had orthostatic syncope, and both of Shy and Drager's cases had cerebellar manifestations. The patient they studied postmortem had marked loss of Purkinje cells as well as nigral degeneration. A number of similar patients have since been described; Oppenheimer (1983) has recently reviewed the subject. Typically, impotence, orthostatic hypotension and neurogenic urinary incontinence may dominate the clinical scene in the earlier phases of the disease to be followed later by ataxia, dysarthria, and a progressive primarily bradykinetic Parkinson syndrome with rigidity and usually minimal parkinsonian and/or cerebellar types of tremor. Oppenheimer (1983) found OPCA in 20 of 41 cases of autonomic failure with multiple system atrophy; 18 of the 20 were also classified as SND. Dysautonomia occurs in several different disorders including Parkinson's disease, SND and several types of OPCA. Chokroverty (1984) feels that a subset of patients in whom dysautonomia precedes the cerebellar and striatal manifestations merits distinction from other cases of OPCA or SND complicated by dysautonomia. The interesting case of OPCA with orthostatic hypotension reported by Evans *et al.* (1972), in which unusual eosinophilic neuronal inclusions different from the Lewy body were found, serves to emphasize the heterogeneity of the Shy–Drager syndrome.

The third perspective derives from the increased interest in parkinsonism stimulated by the advent of levodopa therapy and from studies of familial parkinsonism. OPCA is now diagnosed with increasing frequency in patients who previously would have been simply labelled 'idiopathic parkinsonian'. A quarter of a century ago, OPCA would have been recognized in these patients only as a surprise finding at autopsy. Such patients presenting with parkinsonian features and reporting strongly positive family histories have been reported as examples of familial parkinsonism and have been misinterpreted as evidence that Parkinson's disease is hereditary (Duvoisin, 1984). Today, they comprise by far the most common form of OPCA encountered in clinical practice and account for as much as 5–6% of the Parkinson patient population under the present author's observation. Goetz, Tanner and Klawans (1984) recently collected 24 cases from their Parkinson clinic.

THE SYNDROME OF CEREBELLAR PARKINSONISM

The clinical features of OPCA are shown in *Table 12.1*. The prototype cases of Dejerine and Thomas presented features, notably slowness and hesitation in movement, facial hypomimia, walking with short steps and fatigue, which today

Table 12.1 Clinical features of olivopontocerebellar atrophy

Essential features
  Cerebellar dysfunction and/or atrophy
  Extrapyramidal dysfunction

Features usually or often present
  Corticospinal tract manifestations
  Peripheral neuropathy
  Cerebellar eye signs

Features of variable occurrence
  Positive family history
  Supranuclear ophthalmoplegia
  Optic nerve atrophy
  Retinal degeneration
  Orthostatic hypotension
  Incontinence
  Impotence
  Anhidrosis
  Palatal myoclonus
  Myoclonus
  Amyotrophy
  Dementia

Certain features seen in PSP but not in OPCA
  Hyperextensor posturing of head
  Involuntary levator inhibition
  Epileptic seizures
  Inappropriate laughter
  Hypersexuality

would be recognized as parkinsonian. Subsequent case reports documented the occurrence of rigidity and parkinsonian manifestations and of nigral degeneration in OPCA. Rosenhagen (1943) in an early review of the OPCAs noted parkinsonism in 25 of 45 cases and confirmed the correlation of parkinsonism with the nigral lesion. A number of additional cases with parkinsonism and nigral degeneration were reported later, for example the cases reported by Critchley and Greenfield (1948), Geary, Earle and Rose (1956) and Sigwald *et al.* (1964). Some of these were sporadic, others familial. The most recent comprehensive review of the subject, that of Berciano (1982) comprising 117 autopsy-confirmed cases, found that parkinsonism had been noted in slightly over half the sporadic patients and in 21 of 54 familial cases. However, as in the case of Dejerine and Thomas (1900), parkinsonism may have been overlooked in many and one suspects that it is actually present in the great majority.

  Approaching the subject from the perspective of the pathologist studying the anatomical substrate of parkinsonism, Escourolle, De Recondo and Gray (1971) found that OPCA was the third most common disorder in their pathological material, exceeded only by Parkinson's disease and post-encephalitic parkinsonism. It differed from these in having neither neurofibrillary tangles nor Lewy bodies and in addition exhibited a different pattern of nigral cell loss. They found that the severity of nigral degeneration in their nine cases of OPCA was greater in those patients whose parkinsonism had been clinically more severe.

In many patients, a primarily bradykinetic parkinsonian syndrome with little or no tremor dominates the clinical scene. Usually, the initial manifestation is a gait disturbance. The disorder may slowly progress in the form of an akinetic–rigid Parkinson syndrome for several years before overt cerebellar manifestations make their appearance. Cerebellar dysfunction then combines with parkinsonism to form what may be called the syndrome of 'cerebellar parkinsonism'. Cerebellar atrophy may, however, be seen on CT or magnetic resonance imaging (MRI) scans long before cerebellar signs are clinically evident.

In other patients, the cerebellar syndrome may be prominent initially, presenting with unsteadiness in walking. It is gradually replaced by bradykinesia and extrapyramidal rigidity over a period of years. This temporal sequence has been emphasized by Hirayama (1980) who suggests that the extrapyramidal rigidity masks the cerebellar features. Narabayashi (1984) has presented electrophysiological evidence in support of that view. In either case, however, the patient may present quite different aspects at different times in the evolution of the morbid process. An example is the first case of Plaitakis, Nicklas and Desnick (1980), who presented initially as a case of juvenile parkinsonism responsive to levodopa therapy but eight years later exhibited primarily cerebellar dysfunction.

MULTIPLE SYSTEM ATROPHY

Adams, van Bogaert and van der Ecken (1961, 1964) drew attention to a group of patients who had been clinically diagnosed as 'idiopathic parkinsonian' but, on postmortem study, had findings very different from those of Parkinson's disease. There was pronounced atrophy associated with tan pigmentation of the striatum affecting particularly the putamen, as well as degeneration of the substantia nigra. They termed this condition 'striatonigral degeneration'. Numerous reviews and additional reports indicate that this is not a rare disorder. It accounted for 6% of the cases of parkinsonism in the pathological material available to Takei and Mirra (1973). Escourolle, De Recondo and Gray (1971) had found one among 50 cases identified clinically as parkinsonism.

SND patients respond poorly to levodopa therapy and are apt to exhibit a paradoxical response. Indeed, failure of response to levodopa therapy may comprise, along with absence of tremor and striatal atrophy demonstrated by neuro-imaging techniques, a clinically useful diagnostic triad (Rajput, Kazi and Rozdilski, 1972). Presumably, the lack of response reflects loss of the striatal neurones bearing dopamine receptors.

The clinical distinction of SND from Parkinson's disease can be quite difficult clinically; its distinction from OPCA is even more problematical. As Hirayama (1980) and, more recently, Gossett *et al.* (1983) and Oppenheimer (1983) have noted, most cases of SND also have atrophy of the olive, pons and cerebellum. This was true of case 3 of Adams, van Bogaert and van der Ecken (1964), but Gosset *et al.* concluded from their review of 35 cases that the pontocerebellar atrophy is relatively mild.

The differentiation of SND from OPCA may seem obvious on purely clinical grounds, the former presenting a pure akinetic–rigid Parkinson syndrome with no sign of cerebellar dysfunction even though some degree of cerebellar atrophy may be present on anatomical study, and the latter being distinguished by overt cerebellar features early in the course of the disease. However, this distinction is difficult to apply in clinical practice because cerebellar features may be absent early on but appear later in the course of the illness. Solitary signs of cerebellar dysfunction may easily be overlooked. For example, the illustration of an SND patient used by Hirayama (1980) in support of this view shows a broad-based gait. One also wonders whether minor ocular signs of pontine or cerebellar origin, such as square wave jerks or supranuclear gaze defects, would suffice to make the distinction. Many cases of SND will be found to have some degree of cerebellar atrophy on CT or MRI brain scanning and will thus be labelled OPCA.

The frequent concurrence of OPCA and SND in the same patient led Graham and Oppenheimer (1969) to suggest that they be lumped together under the rubric *multiple system atrophy* (MSA). Oppenheimer (1980, 1983, 1984) includes under this designation the Shy–Drager syndrome, but it is not clear whether it may properly be applied to the many other types of OPCA which have no relationship to SND, especially the dominantly inherited cases or the OPCA phenotypes which occasionally appear in kindreds of hereditary ataxia. For example, should type II Joseph disease be termed 'multiple system atrophy' since Rosenberg *et al.* (1976) referred to one of their Joseph disease patients as a case of 'autosomal striatonigral degeneration'? The value of this new term has unfortunately been compromised by the frequent practice of applying it in a non-specific manner to progressive supranuclear palsy and other disorders which are entirely different morbid entities. Despite these uncertainties, the term is useful in clinical practice in thinking about patients presenting an akinetic–rigid syndrome with minor oculomotor dysfunction and minimal or equivocal 'cerebellar' signs and one hopes that it may be used in the more restricted sense its authors probably intended.

OPCA WITH GLUTAMATE DEHYDROGENASE DEFICIENCY

Deficiency of the enzyme glutamate dehydrogenase in fibroblasts, platelets or leucocytes, in certain patients presenting OPCA syndromes, first reported by Plataikis, Nicklas and Desnick (1980) has now been confirmed by several other groups of investigators (Yamaguchi *et al.*, 1982; Duvoisin *et al.*, 1983; Finocchario, Taroni and Di Donato, 1985). There seems to be good agreement that deficiency of the enzyme is found in a chronic progressive neurodegenerative disorder which presents a variable mixture of cerebellar and extrapyramidal features, usually with mild supranuclear dysfunction in ocular motility, a mild peripheral mainly sensory neuropathy and sometimes widespread motor neurone involvement. In the later stages of the condition, tendon reflexes tend to become depressed and extensor plantar reflexes may appear. Dysarthria has been severe and some cases have progressed to anarthria.

The predominant clinical feature may change over the course of several years. For example, a patient may present a cerebellar syndrome initially, then several years later an akinetic–rigid Parkinson syndrome and subsequently severe widespread amyotrophy with fasciculations resembling amyotrophic lateral sclerosis. Thus, considerable variability may be seen from one case to another and in the same case at different times, but it is not unlimited. All adequately studied cases to date have shown evidence of a peripheral neuropathy on electrophysiological study whereas, in contrast, sporadic cases with normal glutamate dehydrogenase (GDH) activity have not. On the other hand, many features encountered in other OPCAs – spasticity, myoclonus, chorea, athetosis, scoliosis, dysautonomia, retinal degeneration, optic nerve atrophy and dementia – have not thus far been encountered in the GDH-deficiency syndrome. The clinical spectrum observed (Duvoisin and Chokroverty, 1984) suggests that GDH deficiency accounts for a particular subset of the patients clinically diagnosed as OPCA in contemporary practice.

Plaitakis, Berl and Yahr (1982) have presented evidence of impaired glutamate tolerance in GDH-deficient patients. This important observation awaits independent confirmation. It would support the hypothesis that dysfunction of the enzyme is not merely a marker, but underlies the pathogenesis of the disorder. According to this hypothesis, deficiency of GDH could allow toxic amounts of glutamate, an excitotoxic neurotransmitter, to accumulate in the nervous system and produce gradual death of neurones with glutamate receptors. The possibility that excitatory amino acid neurotransmitters may play a significant pathogenetic role in certain circumstances has been reviewed by Olney (1978) and more recently by Coyle (1982). One may further suggest that dysregulation of glutamate metabolism may result from a variety of abnormalities in the enzyme and may be the final common pathway determining the clinical expression of a variety of disorders with similar clinical manifestations. The only patient with GDH deficiency studied postmortem at the time of writing was found to have lipofuscinosis (Chokroverty *et al.*, 1984). It seems unlikely that this rare disorder will be found in other cases, and thus this case suggests that the enzyme defect is probably not specific to a single entity.

GENETIC ASPECTS

A beginning has been made in exploring the genetic basis of the dominantly inherited OPCAs. Evidence of HLA linkage was first noted by Yakura *et al.* (1974) in a family with a dominant ataxia which they considered to be an example of 'Marie's ataxia'. A number of linkage studies have since been reported but the results have been conflicting. Morton *et al.* (1980) found significant though loose linkage in nine pedigrees of 'typical' OPCA which they characterized as type I of Konigsmark and Weiner, but no evidence of linkage in four other 'atypical' kindreds. Koeppen *et al.* (1981) were unable to confirm HLA linkage in the five families they studied and Van Rossum, Veneema and Went (1981) similarly found negative lod scores for a number of genetic markers including HLA linkage in two families with dominant OPCA (type IV) comprising 15 affected individuals. More recently Haines *et al.* (1984) found 'strong' evidence of HLA linkage in the Schut kindred and have concluded that the abnormal gene lies between the HLA-A and HLA-B loci on chromosome 6. Pedersen *et al.* (1980) found one HLA A/B recombinant in a Dutch kindred in which the gene appeared to follow HLA-B.

It is difficult to draw firm conclusions but this data may suggest a locus on chromosome 6 in some OPCA kindreds. The pathogenetic significance of a gene defect at that site, if confirmed by further work, remains to be established. The clinical and pathological correlations in these studies are not clear. This is unfortunate for, in view of the strong clinical and pathological evidence that the clinical spectrum of OPCA comprises many distinct disorders, one cannot expect to find a general sort of 'ataxia gene'. Meanwhile, in those kindreds in which HLA linkage can be established, this finding may have important applications at least with regard to genetic counselling.

More recently, evidence has been presented for a primary gene mutation underlying Joseph disease on chromosome 1 (Rosenberg, 1986). Absence of clinical disease in the Joseph disease families appears to correlate with the presence of the BA isoenzyme of erythrocyte acid phosphatase. Since this enzyme maps to chromosome 2, it has been postulated that a modifier gene determining penetrance is located on that chromosome. One may speculate that modifier genes may also determine clinical expression, i.e. whether a given affected individual develops an OPCA phenotype, a spastic paraplegia or a predominantly spinocerebellar phenotype. Ultimately, of course, the problem of classifying the OPCAs can only be solved by molecular genetics; the specific genotype will be the diagnosis.

A number of cases of OPCA studied pathologically were thought to be recessively inherited, e.g. type II of Konigsmark and Weiner, but Koeppen and Barron (1984) argue that the diagnosis in these cases, with the possible exception of the apparently sex-linked recessive cases of Malamud and Cohen (1958), is incorrect and conclude that the evidence for a recessively transmitted pathologically confirmed OPCA is presently insufficient. Nevertheless, it must be admitted that recessive inheritance may be difficult to detect, especially in disorders of late adult onset with low penetrance. The possibility of recessive inheritance in many of these cases remains a serious consideration awaiting further study.

SND appears to be a sporadic disorder. Thus far, no pathologically confirmed familial cases have been noted. The case reported under that rubric by Rosenberg *et al.* (1976) was, in fact, a case of type II Joseph disease, had significant cerebellar degeneration and was more appropriately regarded as an OPCA phenotype. Those presenting with prominent dysautonomia as illustrated by the case of Shy and Drager (1960), have also appeared to be sporadic. However, an affected brother and sister were personally observed and Lewis (1964) had reported a family with an apparently dominantly inherited disorder presenting ataxia, parkinsonian tremor and rigidity and orthostatic hypotension which he believed to represent the Shy–Drager syndrome. It seems likely that it represents still another kindred of dominant OPCA.

The experience with GDH deficiency illustrates the difficulty of assessing the role of heredity in apparently sporadic or recessive disorders. For example, the proband in the kindred of GDH-deficient OPCA illustrated in *Figure 12.1* could only be considered as a sporadic case from the clinical data. However, two of his four offspring were also found to be GDH deficient although clinically normal. Thus, without knowledge of the biochemical defect, the hereditary basis of his disorder would not be suspected. Many other apparently sporadic cases of OPCA may reflect a similar genetic aetiology.

The genetic basis of GDH deficiency remains unclear. Plaitakis (1984) believes it to be recessively inherited and this appears consistent with the observation of Duvoisin and Chokroverty (1984) that one-quarter of the first degree relatives they studied were GDH deficient or clinically affected. However, there are problems with this formulation. The enzyme deficiency is only partial with a 50–60% decrease in its activity. A nearly complete absence of the enzyme and a heterozygous state would be expected in a genetic disorder, but neither has been demonstrated. One possible explanation is that only one of two isoenzymes is

258 *The olivopontocerebellar atrophies*

☷ symptomatic, not examined
◩ GDH deficient asymptomatic
■ GDH deficient symptomatic

Figure 12.1 Genealogy of a family with GDH-deficient OPCA. Proband is II-6. Two of his children are GDH deficient but clinically normal. Proband's brother, II-2, may also have been affected. (Reprinted from Duvoisin *et al.* (1983) with permission of the publishers)

defective. Plaitakis, Berl and Yahr (1984) have suggested, on the basis of thermolability data, that GDH activity resides in two isoenzymes and that it is the heat-labile isoenzyme which is deficient. However, other workers have not confirmed a consistent loss of the thermolabile fraction of enzyme activity in GDH deficient cases.

Both the proband and her unaffected identical twin sister whose genealogy is shown in *Figure 12.2* had offspring who were either clinically affected or GDH deficient. This observation suggests that the enzyme defect is inherited in a

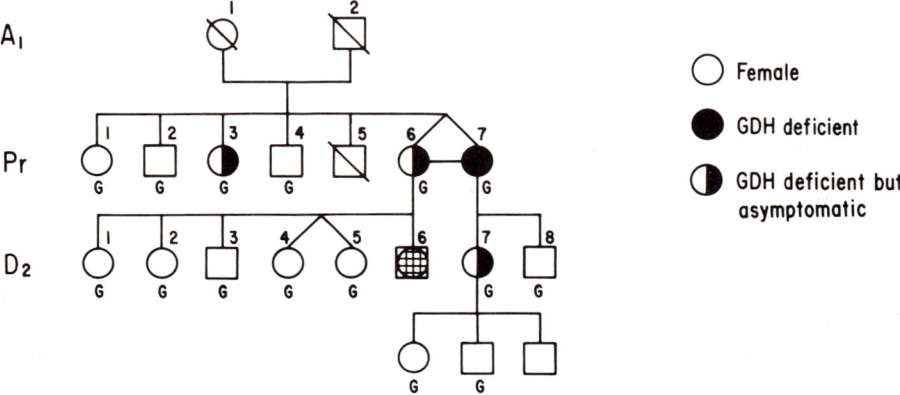

Figure 12.2 Genealogy of a family with GDH-deficient OPCA. Proband is Pr-7. Her monozygotic twin sister is clinically unaffected but GDH deficient. Offspring D-6 is clinically affected. Proband's daughter, D-7, is GDH deficient but clinically normal. (Reprinted from Duvoisin and Chokroverty (1984) with permission of the publishers Raven Press, New York)

dominant pattern, for it is unlikely that both sisters would have married carriers for a rare recessive disorder. If this reasoning is correct, then the failure to find the enzyme deficient in more than one-quarter of the first degree relatives studied may reflect underascertainment of cases due to limitations in the reliability of the enzyme assay, or incomplete penetrance of the enzyme defect itself. Clearly, more work needs to be done to clarify this subject.

OCULOMOTOR DYSFUNCTION

A disturbance in ocular motility (*see Table 12.2*) had been noted by Dejerine and Thomas (1900) in their patients. One had complained of diplopia. Upward gaze was accomplished in several steps and rapid eye movements were described as 'uncertain'. Perhaps these remarks refer to hypometric saccades and saccadic or 'jerky' pursuit in contemporary terminology. Wadia and Swami (1971) had noted a particularly striking abnormality in their patients consisting of a severe loss of saccadic movement. Saccadic velocity was found to be reduced on quantitative electro-oculography to one-sixth to one-eighth that recorded in control subjects. These patients employed a quick head thrust as a strategy to bring their eyes onto a desired target, the eyes following in a slow drift. There was no nystagmus, ptosis, diplopia or pupillary defect. There was a full range of eye movement. This striking abnormality is not unique, however, and has been noted in a number of other dominant kindreds, for example in the dominant families reported by Koeppen and Hans (1976) and others recently reviewed by Wadia (1984).

Table 12.2 Comparison of oculomotor deficits found in Parkinson's disease, progressive supranuclear palsy and olivopontocerebellar atrophy

Abnormality	Parkinson's disease	PSP	OPCA
Nystagmus	0	+	++
Jerky pursuit	+	+++	++
Fixation instability	0	+++	+++
Ocular dysmetria	0	0	+
Hypometric saccades	+†	++	++
Faulty suppression of VORs	+	+++	+++
Loss of OKNs	0	++++	++
Slowing of saccades	+†	++++	++*
Lateropulsion	+	0	0
Levator inhibition	+ (rare)	+++	?
Loss of Bell's phenomenon	0	+++	0
Supranuclear ophthalmoplegia			
Vertical	0	++++ (down>up)	+ (up>down)
Horizontal	0	++++	+

+   Uncommon or minimal.
++   Common or moderate.
+++   Frequent or marked.
++++ Present in nearly all cases or severe.
*   Seen only in familial cases and accompanied by head thrusting.
†   Seen on oculography but not clinically evident.

Lepore (1984) has recently reviewed the remarkable range of abnormalities in eye movement which have been described in 108 previously reported cases of OPCA. These include, in addition to the supranuclear defects, all the expected cerebellar disorders of ocular motility: gaze-evoked nystagmus, fixation instability (square-wave jerks), ocular dysmetria, jerky pursuit, faulty suppression of vestibulo-ocular responses and, albeit rarely, down-beating nystagmus. Hypometric saccades, impairment of upward gaze and loss of opticokinetic responses appear to be the most common findings. Nuclear and internuclear ophthalmoplegia are unusual.

These abnormalities are not specific for OPCA and have been seen in all varieties of spinocerebellar degeneration. They are clinically useful in distinguishing OPCA from Parkinson's disease but complicate the clinical differentiation of sporadic OPCA from progressive supranuclear palsy (*see* Chapter 13).

The pathological substrate of the ocular motility defects remains undefined. One would expect involvement of the paramedian pontine reticular formation where the neurones responsible for generating saccades are believed to be located, but postmortem confirmation has not yet been established.

NEURO-IMAGING

The anatomical features of OPCA are demonstrable on pneumoencephalography, but this procedure has rarely been used to aid in establishing the diagnosis. Although the resolution provided by the early models was not sufficient to provide good visualization of posterior fossa structures and the images were often obscured by Hounsfield artefact, the CT scan quickly showed promise as a non-invasive means of documenting infratentorial atrophy (Pedersen and Gyldenstad, 1978; Allen, Martin and McLain, 1979). The later generations of CT scanners have had a major impact on the clinical diagnosis of OPCA (Savoiardo *et al.*, 1983; Huang and Plaitakis, 1984).

(a) (b)

Figure 12.3 CT scan of patient with GDH-deficient OPCA showing prominent cerebellar folia, enlargement of the cisterna ambiens, widened interpeduncular fossa, some atrophy of the cerebral peduncles and an enlarged third ventricle. (Reprinted from Duvoisin *et al.* (1983) with permission of the publishers)

The 10-mm sections commonly employed in the routine screening CT scan may not suffice. Scanning should preferably be done without contrast in 5-mm sections through the posterior fossa to the foramina of Munro. One can readily see the cerebellar cortical and vermal atrophy with enlargement of the fourth ventricle, and also enlargement of the cisterna ambiens reflecting brainstem atrophy. With good imaging, atrophy of the basis pontis and cerebral peduncles can also be seen. The interpeduncular fossa is widened, the cerebral peduncles are small and exhibit an angular rather than the normal rounded outline (*Figure 12.3*). Moreover, different patterns of cerebellar atrophy can be recognized, which Huang and Plaitakis (1984) recently showed may be correlated with different clinical entities.

Magnetic resonance imaging promises to be even more helpful.

NEUROPHYSIOLOGICAL STUDIES

Electroencephalography may show minor non-specific changes in OPCA. Physiological studies of sleep have shown various abnormalities. Neil *et al.* (1980) in all-night sleep studies in two cases found reduced REM activity, decreased to absent delta sleep, large spindles during stage II sleep, increased stage I sleep and a disproportionate decrease of phasic eye movements. They suggested that these findings were consistent with the lesions of the locus ceruleus and pontine tegmentum described in OPCA. Adelman *et al.* (1984) found in their case mixed central and obstructive sleep apnea. Chokroverty, Sachdeo and Masdeu (1984) similarly found sleep apnea with a mixture of central and upper airway obstructive features in five of the 10 cases they studied. They also noted in three of these cases noctural myoclonus and periodic leg movements. Presumably, the observed sleep-related disturbances reflect neuronal degeneration in the brainstem regions where hypnogenic and respiratory control mechanisms are located. Chokroverty *et al.* (1984) have suggested that the cerebellar lesions, notably degeneration of the fastigial nucleus, may also contribute to dysregulation of respiration during sleep.

In view of the occasional involvement of the afferent visual system observed clinically and pathologically, it is not surprising that prolonged latencies and interocular differences in latencies of visual evoked potentials have been recorded in a broad variety of cerebellar degenerations (Bird and Crill, 1981; Hammond and Wilder, 1983), including occasional cases of OPCA, even in the absence of clinically evident visual dysfunction or optic nerve atrophy.

Brainstem auditory evoked responses (BAERs) have frequently been abnormal in OPCA. Gilroy and Lynn (1978) suggested that abnormal BAERs combined with CT evidence of posterior fossa atrophy suffices to establish the diagnosis of OPCA in patients with a suggestive history and appropriate physical findings. Nuwer *et al.* (1983) found the BAERs abnormal in all five OPCA patients but normal in all 21 Freidreich's ataxia patients they studied and agreed that BAERs might be useful in diagnosing OPCA. Satya-Murti, Cacace and Hanson (1980), however, found normal BAERs in the two patients they studied. More recently, Chokroverty *et al.* (1985) found prolonged latency of wave I but normal interwave latencies in waves I to V in three of five GDH-deficient OPCA patients; they found no abnormality in eight OPCA patients who were not GDH deficient. Clearly, the BAERs are not consistently abnormal in OPCA, but the variable results reported may reflect the heterogeneity of the OPCAs. Whether the BAERs may be useful in distinguishing different types or in monitoring the progress of the disorder remains to be determined in future work.

As would be expected from the known occurrence of amyotrophy and anterior horn cell loss in some cases of OPCA, electromyography has shown evidence of denervation in occasional cases. Motor and sensory nerve conduction velocities and the amplitudes of sensory potentials have repeatedly been found reduced in dominantly inherited OPCA (McLeod and Evans, 1981; Subramony and Currier, 1983; Carenini *et al.*, 1984) and also in the GDH-deficiency syndrome (Chokroverty *et al.*, 1985). The latter workers suggest that electrophysiological evidence of peripheral neuropathy may help distinguish the GDH-deficiency syndrome from other non-dominant OPCAs and use it as a measure of progression of disease and response to treatment.

THERAPEUTICS

Treatment opportunities in the OPCAs were recently reviewed by Goetz, Tanner and Klawans (1984). The parkinsonian features may respond, often quite well, to dopaminergic agents but the cerebellar features are not altered. A good response may also be seen in dominantly inherited OPCA with parkinsonian features. The expected side-effects of dopaminergic therapy may occur, including chorea, hallucinations and sleep disturbances. However, some patients do not respond well or rapidly lose an initial response as their disease progresses. Presumably, this reflects loss of striatal receptors.

Cholinergic treatment with oral physostigmine, reported to be slightly helpful in alleviating ataxia, has not gained general acceptance. It would, of course, be expected to aggravate the parkinsonian features present in so many patients. Propranolol, the beta-adrenergic antagonist, has been moderately useful in alleviating prominent intention tremor, but has no effect on ataxia and titubation. Goetz, Tanner and Klawans (1984) found baclofen ineffective; in four of five patients, there were complaints of weakness and increased difficulty walking. More recently, Trauner (1985) reported a favourable response to baclofen in members of an OPCA kindred manifesting dementia, blindness and chorea of youthful onset.

Involvement of the locus ceruleus in some cases of OPCA with loss of cerebellar noradrenaline (Kish, Shannak and Hornykiewicz, 1984) suggests the use of noradrenergic agents. Shimamoto, Murase and Numans (1976) had claimed improvements in speech, and coordination in four patients treated with phthalazinol, but no further data has been reported. Narabayashi *et al.* (1981) reported improvement of the 'freezing phenomenon' in gait, speech and writing with dihydroxyphenylserine (DOPS) in two patients with pure akinesia. Clinical descriptions of one of these patients plus three other similar patients reported earlier by Narabayashi *et al.* (1976) include evidence of cerebellar atrophy on pneumoencephalography and thus one may suspect that they were cases of OPCA or of SND with OPCA. These observations await confirmation from other investigators.

Because the branched-chain amino acid leucine activates GDH, treatment with a leucine-rich diet or dietary supplementation with a mixture of the branched-chain amino acids leucine, valine and isoleucine which will deliver 10 g L-leucine daily has been attempted in GDH-deficient cases. Apparent arrest of progression was observed in four patients by Plaitakis, Berl and Yahr (1983). The present author has noted sustained partial improvement in one patient over a period of three years, apparent arrest of progression in two and failure in two other patients on such dietary treatment. These data can only be considered anecdotal and suggestive at present, but perhaps sufficiently provocative to merit further evaluation.

The orthostatic hypotension encountered in some cases of OPCA may present a formidable therapeutic challenge and is discussed by Bannister and Oppenheimer (1982) in the previous volume.

TOWARD A CLINICAL DEFINITION OF OPCA

The great diversity of specific morbid entities to which the term 'OPCA' is presently applied calls for an attempt to define the syndrome in clinical terms. The essential and common features of OPCA are listed in *Table 12.1*. Clearly, the essential feature is cerebellar involvement, whether reflected in clinical manifestations of cerebellar dysfunction not attributable to sensory deficit or demonstrated on CT or MRI scanning, showing atrophy of the pons and cerebellum. OPCA was originally defined by its gross anatomical pathology and this can now be demonstrated by modern high-resolution CT scanning or MRI. Secondly, there should be evidence of involvement of the extrapyramidal system. Usually, this is bradykinesia and rigidity; occasionally there is chorea or even dystonia; exceptionally, extrapyramidal features may be lacking or masked by prominent cerebellar signs. Additional neuronal systems are often involved, especially the pyramidal, autonomic and peripheral nervous systems. Dementia, myoclonus, palatal myoclonus and amyotrophy may also occur but are less distinctive manifestations.

The sequence in which different systems are affected during the course of the illness may vary and the differential diagnosis will differ according to the sequence followed in a particular case. In a patient previously presenting a Parkinson syndrome, usually atypical because of the predominance of bradykinesia and rigidity, the advent of cerebellar manifestations raises the possibility of OPCA. The gait may be broad-based, the speech dysarthric and scanning in quality as well as monotone, and the plantar reflexes may be extensor, though care must be taken to avoid confusing the Babinski sign with the striatal toe or what Hunt (1917) called the 'pseudo-Babinski sign' often seen in extrapyramidal disease. There may also be some 'cerebellar' eye signs such as fixation instability, jerky pursuit and hyperactive vestibulo-ocular reflexes. These minor disturbances of ocular motility may be detected in Parkinson's diseases with appropriate instrumentation as White *et al.* (White, Saint-Cyr and Sharpe, 1983; White *et al.*, 1983) have reported, but they are not, in the writer's experience, prominent in Parkinson's disease on ordinary clinical examination except in its advanced stages. These features serve to distinguish OPCA from Parkinson's disease, but they may not suffice to exclude progressive supranuclear palsy (PSP).

The differentiation of early PSP prior to the development of the characteristic supranuclear ophthalmoplegia from OPCA of the sporadic type with parkinsonian features and minimal cerebellar signs can be very difficult, and the two conditions are often confused. A major difficulty is that the ophthalmoplegia of PSP may not appear until several years after the initial symptoms and in some cases not until 7–8 years later. Thus the diagnosis of PSP is made, on average, 3–4 years after the onset (Kristensen, 1985). As Dubas, Bergeron and McLachlan (1983) and Davis,

Gray and Escourolle (1985) have noted, rare patients with PSP may fail to develop ophthalmoplegia altogether. The diagnosis in their cases was established on postmortem study.

Certain features may, nevertheless, assist in distinguishing the two conditions early in the course. The distribution of muscular rigidity tends to be more sharply confined to the nuchal and shoulder girdle musculature in PSP. Indeed, one may find very marked nuchal rigidity but hypotonia at the wrist and elbow. Such striking rigidity so sharply localized is not seen in OPCA. Posturing of the head with the neck hyperextended, if present, points very strongly to PSP. The facial expression suggesting surprise or astonishment with elevated brows and furrowed forehead as Jankovic (1984) has recently pointed out is a useful clue to PSP. Involuntary levator inhibition (Lepore and Duvoisin, 1984), inappropriate laughter, hypersexuality, and partial complex seizures (Nygaard et al., 1986) are rarely seen in Parkinson syndromes other than PSP.

These features individually have only relative value, but if several are present together, the probability that PSP is the diagnosis is greatly increased. On the other hand, other features are rare in PSP but common in OPCA. For example, a confirmed positive family history argues against PSP. A peripheral neuropathy not otherwise explained essentially excludes the possibility of PSP. With the doubtful exception of Weinman's patient with folate deficiency (1976), peripheral neuropathy has not thus far been found in PSP. In contrast, it is not uncommon in OPCA. Similarly, dysautonomia occurs with extreme rarity in PSP, but is not uncommon in OPCA.

Ultimately, the characteristic defect of vertical downgaze establishes the clinical diagnosis of PSP. A variety of oculomotor abnormalities may occur in OPCA (Lepore, 1984), including a distinctive form of supranuclear ophthalmoplegia in some dominantly inherited OPCAs (Wadia, 1984) with extremely slow saccades for which the patients compensate with head thrusting. Head thrusting has not been observed in PSP. Other OPCA cases have some limitation of ocular excursions on voluntary gaze or pursuit and a normal range of eye movement on oculocephalic manoeuvres, but the defects are milder than those seen in PSP and there is not the predilection for vertical downgaze. There is considerable overlap in the oculomotor deficits observed in OPCA and in PSP (*Table 12.2*) and differentiation may be difficult when the deficits are minor. When they are pronounced, however, they are helpful in distinguishing the two entities.

Cerebellar manifestations are not prominent in PSP and do not occur, if at all, until late in the course of the illness. Significant truncal and limb ataxia with a broad-based gait, dysmetria, coarse intention tremor, hypotonia, exaggerated rebound and loss of check, renders OPCA the more likely diagnosis. Thus the syndrome of cerebellar parkinsonism with prominent cerebellar features is essentially diagnostic of OPCA, barring some accidental association of two separate pathological processes.

CT and MRI scans may assist in the differentiation of OPCA from PSP. In the former, these will demonstrate atrophy of the basis pontis, mid-brain and cerebellum (Huang and Plaitakis, 1984). In contrast, the cerebellum is not affected until late in the course of PSP if at all, the brunt of the atrophy falling on the tegmentum of the pons and mid-brain (Abe et al., 1983; Schonfield et al., 1986). The aqueduct and quadrigeminal cisterns are dilated while the basis pontis is spared. In cases presenting with relatively mild extrapyramidal manifestations and minimal or equivocal cerebellar signs, the anatomical demonstration of atrophy of the basis pontis and cerebellum provides strong confirmation and may clinch the diagnosis of OPCA.

Finally, electrophysiological studies may be of some assistance. For example, peripheral nerve conduction studies may document the presence of a peripheral neuropathy when clinical findings are minimal or equivocal. Prolonged latency of wave I of the BAER with normal interpeak latencies for the remaining waves would be more consistent with OPCA than with PSP. The finding of bitemporal paroxsysmal activity on the EEG favours the diagnosis of PSP.

In sporadic cases presenting initially a pure cerebellar syndrome, classification as OPCA is typically suggested by the development of extrapyramidal features. Again, involvement of other systems also frequently occurs. In familial cases, the features presented by other family members may help define the syndrome.

In patients presenting initially with dysautonomia and sometimes classified as idiopathic orthostatic hypotension, the advent of extrapyramidal features – almost invariably akinesia and rigidity – changes the diagnosis to the Shy–Drager syndrome or, according to one's preference, *multiple system atrophy*. The additional presence of cerebellar manifestations and/or the finding of pontine and cerebellar atrophy on neuro-imaging usually justifies classifying these patients as examples of OPCA.

CONCLUSION

The increasing clinical recognition of OPCA since the introduction of levodopa in the treatment of parkinsonism and the advent of the CT scanner has broadened and altered our concepts of this entity. Formerly a rare pathological entity considered a distinctive form of ataxia, OPCA has become a clinical syndrome comprising a large heterogeneous group of disorders, some dominantly inherited and others sporadic or recessively inherited, which share clinical and morphological features with the hereditary ataxias on the one hand and with Parkinson's disease and the hereditary choreas on the other, yet stands apart from both these general groups of degenerative disorders. The clinical syndrome includes patients whose histopathology differs from that of the historical prototype cases. A beginning has been made through biochemistry and biochemical genetics in elucidating pathogenetic factors and identifying underlying genetic defects. A rational classification must await further progress in these areas. Meanwhile, OPCA represents a useful diagnostic category into which the clinician may place patients presenting combined involvement of cerebellar and extrapyramidal systems with clear implications for diagnostic study and therapy.

References

ABE, S., MIYASAKI, K., TASHIRO, K., TAKEI, H., ISU, T. and ISORI, M. (1983) Evaluation of the brainstem with high-resolution CT in cerebeller atrophic processes. *American Journal of Neuroradiology*, **4**, 446–449

ADAMS, R., VAN BOGAERT, L. and VAN DER ECKEN, H. (1961) Dégénérescences nigro-striées et cerebéllo-nigro-striées. *Psychiatria et Neurologia*, **142**, 219–259

ADAMS, R., VAN BOGAERT, L. and VAN DER ECKEN, H. (1964) Striatonigral degeneration. *Journal of Neuropathology and Experimental Neurology* (Basel), **23**, 219–259

ADELMAN, S., DINNER, D. S., GOREN, H., LITTLE, J. and NICKERSON, P. (1984) Obstructive sleep apnea in association with posterior fossa neurologic disease. *Archives of Neurology*, **41**, 509–510

ALLEN, J. H., MARTIN, J. T. and McLAIN, J. W. (1979) Computed tomography in cerebellar atrophic processes. *Radiology*, **130**, 379–382

BANNISTER, R. and OPPENHEIMER, D. (1982) Parkinsonism, system degeneration and autonomic failure. In *Movement Disorders*, Eds. C. P. Marsden and S. Fahn, pp. 174–190. London: Butterworth

BERCIANO, J. (1982) Olivopontocerebellar atrophy. *Journal of the Neurological Sciences*, **53**, 253–272

BERENBERG, R. A., MELEN, O., HOWARD III, G. F. and HARTER, D. H. (1984) Dominantly inherited ataxia with abnormal urinary glycolipid content. *Advances in Neurology*, **41**, 195–204

BIRD, T. D. and CRILL, W. E. (1981) Pattern-reversal evoked potentials in the hereditary ataxias and spinal degenerations. *Annals of Neurology*, **9**, 243–250

CARENINI, L., FINOCCHIARO, G., DI DONATO, S., VISCIANI, A. and NEGRI, S. (1984) Electromyography and nerve conduction study in autosomal dominant olivopontocerebellar atrophy. *Journal of Neurology (Berlin)*, **231**, 34–37

COLAN, R. V., SNEAD, O. C. and CEBALLOS, R. (1981) Olivopontocerebellar atrophy in children: a report of seven cases in two families. *Annals of Neurology*, **10**, 355–363

COYLE, J. T. (1982) Neurotoxic amino acids in human degenerative disorders. *Trends in Neuroscience*, **5**, 287–288

CHOKROVERTY, S. (1984) Autonomic dysfunction in olivopontocerebellar atrophy. *Advances in Neurology*, **41**, 105–142

CHOKROVERTY, S., DUVOISIN, R. C., SACHDEO, R., SAGE, J., LEPORE, F. E. and NICKLAS, W. (1985) Neurophysiologic study of olivopontocerebellar atrophy with or without glutamate dehydrogenase deficiency. *Neurology*, **35**, 652–659

CHOKROVERTY, S., KHEDEKAR, R., DERBY, B., SACHDEO, R., YOOK, C., LEPORE, F. E. et al. (1984) Pathology of olivopontocerebellar atrophy with glutamate dehydrogenase deficiency. *Neurology*, **34**, 1451–1455

CHOKROVERTY, S., SACHDEO, R. and MASDEU, J. (1984) Autonomic dysfunction and sleep apnea in olivopontocerebellar degeneration. *Archives of Neurology*, **41**, 926–932

CRITCHLEY, M. and GREENFIELD, J. G. (1948) Olivo-ponto-cerebellar atrophy. *Brain*, **71**, 343–364

DAVIS, P. H., BERGERON, C. and MCLACHLAN, D. A. (1985) Atypical presentation of progressive supranuclear palsy. *Annals of Neurology*, **17**, 337–343

DEJERINE, J. and THOMAS, A. (1900) L'atrophie olivo-ponto-cerebelleuse. *Nouv. Iconogr. Salpet.*, **13**, 330–370

DUBAS, F., GRAY, F. and ESCOUROLLE, R. (1983) Maladie de Steele–Richardson–Olszewski sans opthalmoplegie. Six cas anatomoclinicques. *Revue Neurologique*, **139**, 407–416

DUVOISIN, R. C. (1984) Is Parkinson's disease acquired or inherited? *Canadian Journal of Neurological Sciences*, **11**, (Suppl. 1), 151–155

DUVOISIN, R. C. and CHOKROVERTY, S. (1984) Clinical expression of glutamate dehydrogenase deficiency. *Advances in Neurology*, **41**, 267–279

DUVOISIN, R. C., CHOKROVERTY, S., LEPORE, F. and NICKLAS, W. (1983) Glutamate dehydrogenase deficiency in patients with olivopontocerebellar atrophy. *Neurology*, **33**, 1322–1326

EADIE, M. J. (1975) Olivopontocerebellar atrophy (atypical forms). In *Handbook of Clinical Neurology*, Vol. 21. Eds. P. J. Vinken and G. W. Bruyn, pp. 457–472. Amsterdam: North Holland

ESCOUROLLE, R., DE RECONDO, J. and GRAY, F. (1971) Etude anatomo-pathologique des syndromes parkinsoniens. In *Monoamines, Noyaux Gris Centraux et syndrome de Parkinson*. Eds. J. de Ajuriaguerra and G. Gauthier, pp. 173–229. Geneva: Georg & Co.

EVANS, D. J., LEWIS, P. D., MALHOTRA, O. and PALLIS, C. (1972) Idiopathic orthostatic hypotension: report of autopsied case with histochemical and ultrastructural studies of the neuronal inclusions. *Journal of the Neurological Sciences*, **17**, 209–218

FERGUSON, F. T. and CRITCHLEY, M. (1929) A clinical study of an heredo-familial disease resembling disseminated sclerosis. *Brain*, **52**, 203–225

FINOCCHIARO, G., TARONI, F. and DI DONATO, S. (1985) Glutamate dehydrogenase activity in leukocytes and muscle mitochondria in olivopontocerebellar atrophies. *Neurology (Suppl. 1)*, **35**, 193

GEARY, J. R., EARLE, K. M. and ROSE, A. S. (1956) Olivopontocerebellar atrophy. *Neurology*, **6**, 218–224

GILROY, J. and LYNN, G. E. (1978) Computed tomography and auditory evoked potentials. Use in the diagnosis of olivo-ponto-cerebellar degeneration. *Archives of Neurology*, **35**, 143–147

GOETZ, C. G., TANNER, C. M. and KLAWANS, H. L. (1984) The pharmacology of olivopontocerebellar atrophy. *Advances in Neurology*, **41**, 143–148

GOSSETT, A., PELLISSIER, J. F., DELPUECH, F. and KHALIL, R. (1983) Degenerescence striato-nigrique associee a une atrophie olivo-ponto-cerebelleuse. *Revue Neurologique (Paris)*, **139**, 125–139

GRAHAM, J. C. and OPPENHEIMER, D. R. (1969) Orthostatic hypotension in a case of multiple system atrophy. *Journal of Neurology, Neurosurgery and Psychiatry*, **32**, 28–34

GRAY, R. C. and OLIVER, C. P. (1941) Marie's hereditary cerebellar ataxia (olivopontocerebellar atrophy). *Minnesota Medicine*, **24**, 327–335

GREENFIELD, J. G. (1954) *The Spinocerebellar Degenerations*. Springfield: Illinois, Charles C. Thomas

HAINES, J., SCHUT, L., WEITKAM, P. L. and THAYER, M. (1984) Spinocerebellar ataxia in a large kindred: age at onset, reproduction and genetic linkage studies. *Neurology*, **34**, 1542–1548

HAMMOND, E. J. and WILDER, B. J. (1983) Evoked potentials in olivopontocerebellar atrophy. *Archives of Neurology,* **40,** 366–369
HARDING, A. E. (1981) 'Idiopathic' late onset cerebellar ataxia. *Journal of the Neurological Sciences,* **51,** 259–271
HARDING, A. E. (1982) The clinical features and classification of the late onset autosomal dominant cerebellar ataxias. *Brain,* **105,** 1–28
HIRAYAMA, K. (1980) Analysis of clinical features in cerebello-extrapyramidal system degeneration. In *Spinocerebellar Degeneration.* Ed. I. Sobue. Baltimore: University Park Press
HUANG, Y. P. and PLAITAKIS, A. (1984) Morphological changes of olivopontocerebellar atrophy in computed tomography and comments on its pathogenesis. *Advances in Neurology,* **41,** 39–85
HUNT, J. R. (1917) Progressive atrophy of the globus pallidum. *Brain,* **40,** 40–58–98
JANKOVIC, J. (1984) Progressive supranuclear palsy; clinical and pharmacological update. *Neurology Clinics,* **2,** 473–486
JOHNSON, W. G. (1981) The clinical spectrum of hexoseaminidase deficiency diseases. *Neurology,* **31,** 1453–1456
KEHL, O. and KELLER, U. (1982) DIDMOAD syndrom (diabetes insipidus, diabetes mellitus, optic atrophy, deafness) mit zerebellar-pontiner atrophie. *Schweizerische Medizinische Wochenschrift,* **112,** 348–352
KISH, S. J., SHANNAK, K. S. and HORNYKIEWICZ, O. (1984) Reduction of noradrenaline in cerebellum of patients with olivopontocerebellar atrophy. *Journal of Neurochemistry,* **42,** 1476–1478
KOEPPEN, A. H. and BARRON, K. D. (1984) The neuropathology of olivopontocerebellar atrophy. *Advances in Neurology,* **41,** 13–38
KOEPPEN, A. H., GOEDDE, H. W., HILLER, C., HIRTH, L. and BENKMAN, H. G. (1981) Hereditary ataxia and the sixth chromosome. *Archives of Neurology,* **38,** 158–164
KOEPPEN, A. H. and HANS, M. B. (1976) Supranuclear ophthalmoplegia and olivo-ponto-cerebellar degeneration. *Neurology,* **26,** 764–768
KONIGSMARK, B. W. and WEINER, L. P. (1970) The olivopontocerebellar atrophies: a review. *Medicine,* **49,** 227–241
KONDO, K., HIROTA, K. and KATAGARI, T. (1981) Genetic and clinical patterns of heritable cerebellar ataxias in adults. II Clinical manifestations. *Journal of Medical Genetics,* **18,** 276–284
KONDO, K. and SOBUE, I. (1980) Genetic and clinical patterns of heritable cerebellar ataxias in adults. I Genetic analyses. *Journal of Medical Genetics,* **17,** 416–423
KRISTENSEN, M. O. (1985) Progressive supranuclear palsy – 20 years later. *Acta Neurologica Scandinavica,* **71,** 177–189
LEPORE, F. E. (1984) Disorders of ocular motility in the olivopontocerebellar atrophies. *Advances in Neurology,* **41,** 97–104
LEPORE, F. and DUVOISIN, R. C. (1985) 'Apraxia' of eyelid opening. An involuntary levator inhibition. *Neurology,* **35,** 423–427
LEWIS, P. (1964) Familial orthostatic hypotension. *Brain,* **87,** 719–728
McLEOD, J. G. and EVANS, W. A. (1981) Peripheral neuropathy in spinocerebellar degenerations. *Muscle Nerve,* **4,** 51–61
MALAMUD, N. and COHEN, P. (1958) Unusual form of cerebellar ataxia with sex-linked inheritance. *Neurology,* **8,** 261–266
MARIE, P. (1893) Sur l'heredo-ataxie cerebelleuse. *Semana Medica,* **13,** 444–447
MENZEL, P. (1891) Beitrag zur Kenntniss der hereditaren Ataxie und Kleinhirnatrophie. *Archiv fuer Psychiatrie und Nervenkrankheiten,* **22,** 160–190
MORTON, N. E., LALOUEL, J-M., JACKSON, J. F., CURRIER, R. D. and YEE, S. (1980) Linkage studies in spinocerebellar ataxia. *American Journal of Medical Genetics,* **6,** 251–257
NARABAYASHI, H. (1984) Cerebellodiencephalic interactions in olivopontocerebellar atrophy. *Advances in Neurology,* **41,** 87–96
NARABAYASHI, H., IMAI, H., YOKOCHI, M., HIRAYAMA, K. and NAKAMURA, R. (1976) Cases of pure akinesia without rigidity and tremor and with no effect by L-DOPA therapy. In *Advances in Parkinsonism.* Eds. W. Birkmayer and O. Hornyckiewicz, pp. 335–342. Basle: Editions (Roche)
NARABAYASHI, H., KONDO, T., HAYASHI, A., SUZUKI, T. and NAGATSU, T. (1981) L-Threo-3,4-dihydroxyphenylserine treatment for akinesia and freezing of parkinsonism. *Proceedings of the Japan Academy,* **57,** Series B, 351–354
NEIL, J. F., HOLZER, B. C., SPIKER, D. G., COBLE, P. A. and KUPFER, D. J. (1980) EEG sleep alteration in olivopontocerebellar degenerations. *Neurology,* **30,** 660–662
NUWER, M. R., PERLMAN, S. L., PACKWOOD, J. W. and KARK, R. A. P. (1983) Evoked potential abnormalities in the various inherited ataxias. *Annals of Neurology,* **13,** 20–27
NYGAARD, T., DUVOISIN, R. C., CHOKROVERTY, S. and MANOCHA, M. (1986) Epileptic seizures in progressive suppranuclear palsy. *Neurology,* **36** (Suppl. 1), 341

OLNEY, J. W. (1978) Neurotoxicity of excitatory amino acids. In *Kainic Acid as a Tool in Neurobiology*. Eds. E. G. McGeer, J. W. Olney and P. L. McGeer, pp. 95–121. New York: Raven Press

OHNO, T., TSUCHIDA, H., FUKUHARA, N., YUASA, T., HARAYAMA, H., TSUJI, S. and MIYATAKE, T. (1984) Adrenoleukodystrophy: a clinical variant presenting as olivopontocerebellar atrophy. *Journal of Neurology*, **231**, 167–169

OONK, J. G. W., VAN DER HELM, H. J. and MARTIN, J. J. (1979) Spinocerebellar degeneration: hexosaminidase A and B deficiency in two adult sisters. *Neurology*, **29**, 380–384

OPPENHEIMER, D. R. (1980) Multiple system atrophy and the Shy–Drager syndrome. In *Spinocerebellar Degenerations*. Ed. I. Sobue, pp. 165–170. Baltimore: University Park Press

OPPENHEIMER, D. R. (1983) Neuropathology of progressive autonomic failure. In *Autonomic Failure*. Ed. R. Bannister, pp. 267–283. New York: Oxford University Press

OPPENHEIMER, D. R. (1984) Diseases of the basal ganglia, cerebellum and motor neurons. In *Greenfield's Neuropathology*, 4th ed. Eds. J. H. Adams, J. A. N. Corsellis and L. W. Duchen, pp. 699–747. London: Edward Arnold

PEDERSEN, L. and GYLDENSTED, C. (1978) Computerized tomography in hereditary ataxia. *Acta Neurologica Scandinavica*, **58**, 81–88

PEDERSEN, L., PLATZ, P., RYDER, L. P., LARSON, L. V. and DISSING, J. (1980) A linkage study of hereditary ataxia and related disorders; evidence of heterogeneity of dominant cerebellar ataxia. *Human Genetics*, **54**, 371–383

PERRY, T. L. (1984) Four biochemically different types of dominantly inherited olivopontocerebellar atrophy. *Advances in Neurology*, **41**, 205–216

PLAITAKIS, A. (1984) Abnormal metabolism of neuroexcitatory amino acids in olivopontocerebellar atrophy. *Advances in Neurology*, **41**, 245–266

PLAITAKIS, A., BERL, S. and YAHR, M. D. (1982) Abnormal glutamate metabolism in an adult onset degenerative neurological disorder. *Science*, **216**, 193–196

PLAITAKIS, A., BERL, S. and YAHR, M. D. (1983) The treatment of GDH-deficient olivopontocerebellar atrophy with branched chain amino acids. *Neurology*, **33** (Suppl. 2), 78

PLAITAKIS, A., BERL, S. and YAHR, M. D. (1984) Neurological disorders associated with deficiency of glutamate dehydrogenase. *Annals of Neurology*, **15**, 144–153

PLAITAKIS, A., NICKLAS, W. and DESNICK, R. J. (1980) Glutamate dehydrogenase deficiency in three patients with spinocerebellar syndrome. *Annals of Neurology*, **7**, 297–303

RAJPUT, A. H., KAZI, K. G. and ROZDILSKI, B. (1972) Striatonigral degeneration. Response to levodopa therapy. *Journal of the Neurological Sciences*, **16**, 331–341

ROSENBERG, R. N. (1984) Joseph disease: an autosomal dominant motor system degeneration. *Advances in Neurology*, **41**, 179–193

ROSENBERG, R. N. (1986) *Neurogenetics: Principles and Practice*, pp. 119–124. New York: Raven Press

ROSENBERG, R. N., NYHAN, W. L., BAY, C. and SHORE, P. (1976) Autosomal dominant striatonigral degeneration. *Neurology*, **26**, 703–714

ROSENBERG, R. N., ROBINSON, A. B. and PARTRIDGE, D. (1975) Urine vapor pattern for olivopontocerebellar degeneration. *Clinical Biochemistry*, **8**, 365–368

ROSENHAGEN, H. (1943) Die Primare atrophie des Bruckenfuss und der unteren oliven. *Archiv fuer Psychiatrie und Nervenkrankheiten*, **116**, 163–228

RUSHTON, A. R. and GENEL, M. (1981) Hereditary ectodermal dysplasia, olivopontocerebellar atrophy, short status and hypogonadism. *Journal of Medical Genetics*, **18**, 335–339

SAVOIARDO, J. W., BRACCHI, M., PASSERINI, A., VISCIANI, A., DIDONATO, S. and COCCHINNI, F. (1983) Computed tomography of olivopontocerebellar degeneration. *American Journal of Neuroradiology*, **4**, 509–512

SATYA-MURTIS, S., CACACE, A. T. and HANSON, P. A. (1980) Auditory dysfunction in Freidreich's ataxia: results of spiral ganglion degeneration. *Neurology*, **30**, 1047–1053

SCHONFIELD, S. M., SAFER, J. N., SAGE, J. and DUVOISIN, R. C. (1986) Computed tomographic findings in progressive supranuclear palsy. *Movement Disorders*, (in press)

SCHUT, J. W. (1950) Hereditary ataxia. Clinical study through six generations. *Archives of Neurology Psychiatry*, **63**, 535–567

SCHUT, J. W. and HAYMAKER, W. (1951) Hereditary ataxia: a pathological study of 5 cases of common ancestry. *Journal of Neuropathology and Clinical Neurology*, **1**, 183–213

SHIMAMOTO, T., MURASE, H. and NUMANS, F. (1976) Treatment of senile dementia and cerebellar disorders with phthalazinol. *Mechanisms of Ageing and Development*, **5**, 241–250

SHY, G. M. and DRAGER, G. A. (1960) A neurological syndrome associated with hypotension: a clinical pathological study. *Archives of Neurology*, **2**, 511–527

SIGWALD, J., LAPRESLE, J., RAVERDY, P. and RECONDO, J. (1964) Atrophie cerebelleause familiale avec association de lesions nigeriennes et spinales. *Presse Medicales*, **72**, 557–562

STAAL, A., STEFANKO, S. Z., BUSCH, H. F. M., JENNEKENS, F. G. I. and DE BRUIJN, W. C. (1981) Autonomic nerve calcification and peripheral neuropathy in olivopontocerebellar atrophy. *Journal of the Neurological Sciences*, **51**, 383–394
SUBRAMONY, S. H. and CURRIER, R. D. (1983) Peripheral nerve involvement in late-onset ataxias. *Muscle Nerve*, (Abstract), **6**, 537-A
TAKEI, Y. and MIRRA, S. S. (1973) Striato-nigral degeneration: a form of multiple system atrophy with clinical parkinsonism. *Progress in Neuropathology*, **21**, 26–32
TRAUNER, D. A. (1985) Olivopontocerebellar atrophy with dementia, blindness and chorea. Response to baclofen. *Archives of Neurology*, **42**, 757–758
VAN ROSSUM, J., VEENEMA, H. and WENT, L. N. (1981) Linkage investigations in two families with hereditary ataxia. *Journal of Neurology, Neurosurgery and Psychiatry*, **44**, 516–522
WADIA, N. H. (1984) A variety of olivopontocerebellar atrophy distinguished by slow eye movements and peripheral neuropathy. *Advances in Neurology*, **41**, 149–178
WADIA, N. H. and SWAMI, R. K. (1971) A new form of heredo-familial spinocerebellar degeneration with slow eye movements. *Brain*, **94**, 359–374
WEINMAN, R. L. (1976) Heterogenous system degeneration of the central nervous system associated with peripheral neuropathy. *Neurology*, **17**, 597–603
WHITE, O. B., SAINT-CYR, J. A. and SHARPE, J. A. (1983) Ocular motor deficits in Parkinson's disease. I. The horizontal vestibulo-ocular reflex and its regulation. *Brain*, **106**, 555–570
WHITE, O. B., SAINT-CYR, J. A., TOMLINSON, R. D. and SHARPE, J. A. (1983) Ocular motor deficits in Parkinson's disease. II. Control of the saccadic and smooth pursuit systems. *Brain*, **106**, 571–587
YAKURA, H., WAKISAKA, A., FUJIMOTO, S. and ITAKORA, I. (1974) Hereditary ataxia and HLA genotype. *New England Journal of Medicine*, **291**, 154–155
YAMAGUCHI, T., HAYASHI, K., MURAKAMI, H., OTA, K. and MARUYAMA, S. (1982) Glutamate dehydrogenase, deficiency in spinocerebellar degenerations. *Neurochemical Research*, **7**, 627–636

Commentary: Olivopontocerebellar atrophy is not a useful concept
A. E. Harding

The pathological entity of OPCA

Olivopontocerebellar atrophy (OPCA) is a pathological syndrome comprising degeneration of the pontine, arcuate and olivary nuclei and middle cerebellar peduncles, together with loss of white matter and Purkinje cells in the cerebellar hemispheres. This constellation of pathological features is rarely isolated; associated degenerative changes in the basal ganglia, dentate nuclei, cerebral cortex, spinal cord, or peripheral nerves are the rule rather than the exception, and may be more prominent (Berciano, 1982). Thus OPCA is not complete in describing even the pathological features to which it has been ascribed. Analysis of the confusing literature on this subject is complicated by the fact that several authors have disagreed in their interpretation of autopsy findings (Koeppen and Barron, 1984).

OPCA is not specific to a single disease, but may be found in a number of aetiological distinct degenerative ataxic disorders, as well as in cases of progressive autonomic failure and striatonigral degeneration. It has been described in patients with more than one type of dominantly inherited ataxia, distinguished either clinically or on the basis of genetic linkage studies (van Rossum, Veenema and Went, 1981; Harding, 1982; Hains et al., 1984). There is scanty evidence for the existence of a recessive form of OPCA, as discussed by Koeppen and Barron (1984). Slightly over half of the reported cases of pathologically proven OPCA did not have similarly affected relatives, and it is unlikely that the majority of such patients have a genetically determined disease (Harding, 1981; Berciano, 1982). Conversely, even within families with dominantly inherited ataxic disorders,

OPCA may be found at autopsy in some members but not others, and therefore this pathological syndrome does not closely reflect the effects of a single mutant gene (Schut and Haymaker, 1951; Pogacar et al., 1978).

The clinical features of patients with pathologically proven OPCA are enormously variable. Cerebellar dysfunction is the commonest manifestation and occurs in 90%. Parkinsonism, involuntary movements, dementia, ophthalmoplegia, optic atrophy, retinal degeneration, peripheral neuropathy, pyramidal signs, autonomic failure, bulbar and pseudobulbar palsy, have all been described in various combinations. Clinicopathological correlation is not high. Marked intrafamilial variation is seen in dominantly inherited OPCA (Berciano, 1982; Harding, 1984).

To summarize the above points, most of which are conceded by Roger Duvoisin, OPCA incompletely describes a heterogeneous group of degenerative neurological disorders pathologically, is an inconsistent morphological marker for more than one disease, and gives rise to a diverse group of neurological syndromes which few clinicians would categorize under a single diagnostic label. For these reasons the present author concurs with Oppenheimer's (1984) view that the OPCAs should be included under the broader pathological rubric of the multiple system degenerations.

The clinical entity of OPCA

If OPCA is to be used as a diagnostic label in clinical practice, a natural assumption is that it will be applied to patients with clinical features similar to those seen in autopsy proven cases. As these are so variable, this implies making the same diagnosis in a parkinsonian patient with cerebellar atrophy on CT scan, as in another with late-onset cerebellar ataxia, dementia and optic atrophy. Although the protagonists of this approach may stress that OPCA is heterogeneous, the use of such a specific sounding label for both cases seems inappropriate, even if only instinctively.

Many patients with identical clinical syndromes to those seen in the OPCAs do not have OPCA at autopsy. These include those with Joseph disease, adrenoleucodystrophy, and hexosaminidase deficiency included in Roger Duviosin's review. Nosologically, this is a retrograde step which leads to a series of teleological arguments. The purported radiological features of OPCA have not been verified histologically in more than a few cases and, in the author's experience, patients with a variety of degenerative ataxic syndromes, including those with recognizable metabolic cause, have CT evidence of cerebellar and brainstem atrophy of indistinguishable type.

OPCA has been increasingly diagnosed (not recognized) on clinical grounds in the last decade. The reasons for the increasing popularity of this label are complex. 'However uninformative the name of his illness may be a patient feels his foe is partly vanquished once he knows its name' (Asher, 1972). More disturbingly, this feeling may be shared by his physician.

Objections to using a pathological diagnosis in clinical practice may reasonably be thought pedantic and rejected. Inappropriate terms which stand the test of time and are easily understood by all who use them are both acceptable and useful as long as they are mishandled consistently. This does not appear to be true of OPCA, with serious implications in defining prognosis, deriving genetic counselling data, setting up therapeutic trials, and investigating aetiology. The Humpty Dumpty approach ('it means just what I choose it to mean, neither more nor less') is not a useful nosological tool. Most clinicians' view of what constitutes OPCA will be defined by the patients that they see. I would disagree with Roger Duvoisin's diagnostic criteria for OPCA, particularly the requirement for involvement of the extrapyramidal system which is not borne out by previous reviews of its clinical features (Berciano, 1982). This difference of opinion is almost certainly due to variation in referral practice.

The term 'OPCA' may fill a diagnostic need in the difficult area of degenerative neurological disorders, but the present author feels that Roger Duvoisin's alternative is preferable. The disorders often referred to as 'OPCA' should be included in an expanded group of multiple system degenerations divisible on the basis of the clinical presentation (progressive autonomic failure, atypical parkinsonism, or cerebellar ataxia). The presence of heterogeneity is more explicit and the terminology less precise, as it should be.

References

ASHER, R. (1972) Making sense. In *Richard Asher Talking Sense*, Ed. F. Avery Jones. London: Pitman Medical
BERCIANO, J. (1982) Olivopontocerebellar atrophy. *Journal of the Neurlogical Sciences*, **53**, 253–272
HAINS, J., SHUT, L., WEITKAM, P. L. and THAYER, M. (1984) Spinocerebellar ataxia in a large kindred: age at onset, reproduction and genetic linkage studies. *Neurology*, **34**, 1542–1548
HARDING, A. E. (1981) 'Idiopathic' late-onset cerebellar ataxia. A clinical and genetic study of 36 cases. *Journal of the Neurological Sciences*, **51**, 259–271
HARDING, A. E. (1982) The clinical features and classification of the late onset autosomal dominant cerebellar ataxias; a study of eleven families, including descendants of the 'Drew family of Walworth'. *Brain*, **105**, 1–28
HARDING, A. E. (1984) *The Hereditary Ataxias and Related Disorders*. Edinburgh: Churchill Livingstone
KOEPPEN, A. H. and BARRON, K. D. (1984) The neuropathology of olivopontocerebellar atrophy *Advances in Neurology*, **41**, 13–38
OPPENHEIMER, D. R. (1984) Diseases of the basal ganglia, cerebellum and motor neuron. In *Greenfield's Neuropathology*, 4th edn. Eds J. H. Adams, J. A. N. Corsellis and L. W. Duchen, pp. 699–747. London: Edward Arnold
POGACAR, S., AMBLER, M., CONKLIN, W. J., O'NEIL, W. A. and LEE, H. Y. (1978) Dominant spinopontine atrophy: report of two additional members of family W. *Archives of Neurology*, **35**, 156–162
SHUT, J. W. and HAYMAKER, W. (1951) Hereditary ataxia: a pathological study of 5 cases of common ancestry. *Journal of Neuropathology and Clinical Neurology*, **1**, 183–213
VAN ROSSUM, J., VEENEMA, H. and WENT, L. N. (1981) Linkage investigations in two families with hereditary ataxia. *Journal of Neurology, Neurosurgery and Psychiatry*, **44**, 516–522

13
The Steele–Richardson–Olszewski syndrome (progressive supranuclear palsy)

A. J. Lees

In 1963, at the American Neurological Association meeting in Atlantic City, Richardson described nine men all of whom had presented in their fifties or sixties with a progressive brainstem degeneration which was characterized by supranuclear ophthalmoplegia, axial dystonia, severe dysarthria, pseudobulbar palsy and a mild dementia. Cerebellar, parkinsonian and corticospinal signs were also noted in some of the patients and death occurred within five to seven years of the first symptoms, usually from bronchopneumonia (Richardson, Steele and Olszewski, 1963). A detailed pathological examination was carried out on four of these patients and less complete histological data were available in three of the others. Globose and, less frequently, flame-shaped neurofibrillary tangles and neuronal loss with gliosis, were found in a number of brainstem structures, but there was a predilection for the subthalamic nucleus, the globus pallidus, substantia nigra, peri-aqueductal grey matter, superior colliculus, locus ceruleus and the dentate, pontine and raphe nuclei. The red nucleus, the pontine tegmentum, the nucleus cuneiformis and subcuneiformis, oculomotor nucleus and superior cerebellar peduncles were also frequently involved, whereas the cerebral and cerebellar cortices were strikingly spared. In their seminal paper published the following year, the Canadian authors expressed surprise that a disorder with such a distinctive clinical and pathological picture should have escaped the eye of previous generations of neurologists (Steele, Richardson and Olszewski, 1964). Having said this, however, they themselves were able to find one or two similar cases within the earlier literature and subsequent excavations unearthed at least 15 reasonably convincing cases, the first being reported by the American ophthalmologist Campbell Posey in 1904. In addition to these sporadic reports, probably many other cases were buried erroneously as arteriosclerotic Parkinson's syndrome, post-encephalitic disease, multisystem degeneration and 'unusual Parkinson's disease'. There are also close similarities with the pyramidopallidal syndrome described by L'Hermitte, Jakob's disease and some cases of normal pressure hydrocephalus.

Steele, Richardson and Olszewski felt that the disorder was probably not excessively rare and might be caused by a postviral degeneration akin to post-encephalitic Parkinson's syndrome and the Parkinson–dementia syndrome of Guam. They also affirmed that further observations would almost certainly enlarge the clinical spectrum of the disease. By 1979, Brusa and his colleagues were able to review 75 histologically verified cases and Kristensen, in her recent survey, included 202 well-described clinical reports (Kristensen, 1985). Fifty-two additional cases fulfilling accepted clinical criteria were admitted to the National Hospitals for Nervous Diseases, London, between 1971 and 1984 (Maher and Lees, 1986) and Mastaglia and colleagues (1973) estimated the incidence to be four per million in Western Australia. The condition has now been reported from many different countries and the original marked male preponderance has been shown to be artefactual, the probable ratio being more like three males to two females. The median age at onset of the Steele–Richardson–Olszewski syndrome is 60 years, three-quarters of all cases beginning between 50 and 65 years; the median survival time is 5.9 years (Maher and Lees, 1986).

THE CLINICAL PICTURE

A diagnostic paradox comparable to that which arises in Parkinson's disease is present. The earliest complaints are vague, non-specific and often frankly misleading; the early signs may embrace multiple neuronal systems and again, in isolation, are not diagnostic. As the disease progresses, however, the appearance of most patients is so singular that recognition may be possible from the end of the ward. A characteristic supranuclear ophthalmoplegia affecting down-gaze is the only diagnostic prerequisite as the other manifestations, although sometimes suggestive of the disease, are less than specific. However, the ophthalmoplegia may, on occasion, occur late in the course of the illness (Pfaffenbach, Layton and Kearns, 1972; Perkin *et al.*, 1978) and indeed a few cases have been reported with typical pathology who did not have eye movement abnormalities at all in life (Dubas, Gray and Escourolle, 1983). The issue is further complicated by the fact that there are a number of other progressive non-familial neurological diseases, which may have a supranuclear ophthalmoplegia as part of the clinical picture (*see Table 13.1*). A minimum of two of a further five cardinal features should also be present before the diagnosis is considered clinically definite. A large number of other physical signs are compatible with the diagnosis of Steele–Richardson–Olszewski syndrome and are listed together with the diagnostic criteria in *Table 13.2*.

Unsteadiness with poor balance and unexplained falls is the commonest initial complaint, occurring in about two-thirds of patients. A spastic, low volume

Table 13.1 Multisystem degenerative disorders in which a supranuclear ophthalmoplegia has been reported

(1) Creutzfeldt–Jakob disease (Ross-Russell, 1980)
(2) Olivopontocerebellar degeneration (Koeppen and Hans, 1976)
(3) Corticobasal degeneration (personal unpublished cases)
(4) Dentato-pallido-nigro-luysian atrophy (Iizuka, Hirayama and Maehara, 1984)
(5) Subcortical gliosis of Neumann (personal unpublished case)
(6) Dystonic lipidosis (adult onset Niemann–Pick) (Nevill *et al.*, 1973)
(7) Joseph's disease (Rosenberg *et al.*, 1976)
(8) Young onset familial neurofibrillary tangle disorder (Mata *et al.*, 1983)
(9) Young onset tangle disorder in mentally retarded (Jellinger, Riederer and Tomonaga, 1980)

dysarthria is another early symptom and articulatory difficulties are occasionally compounded by the emergence of an acquired stutter, palilalia or even echolalia. Neurobehavioural disturbances are also seen early in at least half the patients and include depression, irascibility and uncharacteristic aggressiveness, emotional lability, apathy and slowness of thinking with forgetfulness. Many patients are misdiagnosed as having a dementia or psychotic illness. Blurred vision, reading difficulties, problems looking down while eating, double vision, photophobia and dry eyes are the commonest of a large number of ocular symptoms. Other fairly frequent early symptoms are swallowing difficulties, explosive coughing, a slowing up or clumsiness, stiffness of the limbs or face and bladder disturbances. A median delay of 3.9 years occurs before the clinical picture is sufficiently clearcut for the diagnosis to be made (Maher and Lees, 1986). Although the earliest symptoms differ quite strikingly from those which occur in Parkinson's disease, there are a small number of patients, possibly a benign variant, who present with a bradykinetic–rigid syndrome without ophthalmoplegia and may be misdiagnosed for a number of years as having Parkinson's disease. Indeed, most of the long-term follow-up series on the value of L-dopa in the treatment of Parkinson's disease have been obliged to exclude a few patients who have responded poorly or not at all to the drug initially, and who eventually developed a supranuclear down-gaze palsy and other signs of Steele–Richardson–Olszewski syndrome (Shaw, Lees and Stern,

Table 13.2 Diagnostic criteria for the clinical diagnosis of Steele–Richardson–Olszewski syndrome

Definition
A progressive non-familial disorder beginning in middle or old age with a supranuclear ophthalmoplegia including down-gaze abnormalities and at least two more of the following five cardinal features:
  (*a*) Axial dystonia and rigidity
  (*b*) Pseudobulbar palsy
  (*c*) Bradykinesia and rigidity
  (*d*) Frontal lobe signs (bradyphrenia, perseveration, forced grasping and utilization behaviour)
  (*e*) Postural instability with falls backwards

Other signs
Rest tremor
Chorea
Dystonia of the limbs and face
Cerebellar ataxia
Muscle wasting, fasciculation and weakness
Dysphasia and dyspraxia
Respiratory dyskinesias (inspiratory gasps, tachypnoea)
Depression
Schizophreniform psychoses
Echolalia and palilalia
Myoclonus
Perceptive deafness
Sleep disturbances
Other ocular abnormalities (*see text*)

1980). Jackson, Jankovic and Ford (1983) in a series of 450 patients with Parkinson's disease found that 16 (3.9%) really had the Steele–Richardson–Olszewski syndrome. Helpful features in distinguishing these cases from brainstem Lewy body Parkinson's disease are shown in Table 13.3.

Table 13.3 Clinical features helpful in distinguishing the bradykinetic–rigid presentation of Steele–Richardson–Olszewski syndrome from Parkinson's disease

Symmetrical onset
Presents frequently with gait disturbance
Rest tremor extremely rare
Rigidity in extension may be present
Different facial appearance (deeper lines, brisk jerks, blinking more frequent)
Early neurobehavioural symptoms
Unresponsive or at best weakly responsive to L-dopa

CARDINAL FEATURES

Neuro-ophthalmological and neuro-otological abnormalities

The onset of ophthalmoplegia is usually gradual with a progressive slowing down of willed eye movements before the appearance of a supranuclear paresis. The velocity of the saccades declines before their magnitude, but eventually hypometric refixations, sometimes with square-wave jerks, are seen (Troost and Daroff, 1977). Upward gaze and convergence are usually the first ocular movements to be impaired. It is not, however, until impairment of down-gaze appears that the diagnosis can be considered, as the former disturbances occur in other basal ganglia disorders and may occur to some degree in normal old age. Ultimately supranuclear down-gaze paresis may be more severe than the abnormality on looking upwards. Classically, movements to command are more deranged than those to pursuit, with doll's eye movements by definition being preserved. Damage to the superior colliculi and the pretectal area are probably responsible for these abnormalities.

Neuro-otological examination reveals an absence or severe disturbance of the fast component of nystagmus in the caloric and optokinetic responses which may occur even before the presence of a directionally corresponding gaze palsy. The nystagmus elicited by the caloric test is replaced by a tonic conjugate ocular deviation in the direction of the anticipated slow component, and similar tonic ocular deviations up or down can be obtained by simultaneous hot and cold stimulation (Dix, Harrison and Lewis, 1971). A small number of patients develop an internuclear ophthalmoplegia (Mastaglia and Grainger, 1975) and periodic alternating nystagmus has also been reported (Perkin et al., 1978). Perceptive deafness has been reported in a few patients, but, perhaps rather surprisingly in view of the extensive nature of the brainstem lesions, auditory evoked potentials are usually normal (Tolosa and Zeese, 1979).

Complete supranuclear ophthalmoplegia with eventual involvement of lateral gaze appears in at least half the patients. A small number of patients finally develop a nuclear ophthalmoplegia with loss of oculocephalic responses (Blumenthal and

Miller, 1969). The visual acuities and visual fields remain normal. Other late findings in some patients include an absent Bell's phenomenon and impaired pupillary light reflexes. The ophthalmoplegia, together with frequent occurrence of lid retraction, gives the patient a fixed, staring, somewhat astonished expression and the need to turn the neck in order to fixate presents an eerie reptilian appearance, with the impression that the patient's eyes are following one round the room, rather like the Mona Lisa. Eyelid abnormalities are also by no means rare and include ptosis and blepharospasm which may be severe. A number of patients exhibit a supranuclear levator palpebrae inhibition (apraxia of eyelid opening) with vigorous frontalis contraction, but no orbicularis oculi contraction. Others have apraxia of eyelid closure with complete inability to close the eyes to command, but with preservation of reflex closure on blinking to menace and on falling asleep.

Dystonia

In contrast to the flexed posture of the limbs, neck and trunk in Parkinson's disease, the neck is held stiffly in extension with the head pointing skywards. Often the neck is so stiff that it is quite impossible to flex or extend it, whereas tone on rotation or lateral flexion may be normal. While standing the patient assumes a striking hyperlordotic erect posture which, when combined with impairment of righting reflexes, leads to a proclivity to topple backwards. A painful opisthotonus when the patient is lying in bed is another common late feature and at this stage the limbs may also be stiff and dystonic. Behrman *et al.* (1969) suggested that the neck posture might be a manifestation of decerebrate rigidity due to damage to the interneurones in the upper cervical cord. A similar mechanism has been implicated in the pathogenesis of spinal encephalomyelitis with rigidity ('stiff man syndrome') (Howell, Lees and Toghill, 1979). Alternatively, a lesion in the striatopallidothalamic complex may be responsible, but the susceptibility of the axial musculature is unexplained.

Pseudobulbar palsy

This is present to some degree in almost all patients and may be the earliest symptom, when a diagnosis of motoneurone disease may be made in error. The spastic dysarthria may be compounded by a parkinsonian speech disturbance and, in the terminal stages, many patients are completely anarthric. Difficulty with swallowing both fluids and solids may lead ultimately to a diet of semi-liquid food, administered by a nasogastric tube. Tongue movements are often slow and facial and jaw jerks pathologically brisk. The face is frozen and deeply furrowed as a result of spasticity and dystonia. Bilateral Babinski signs are a common late finding. Forced laughter and crying are common, although this was not reported in the original cases reported by Steele, Richardson and Olszewski. Damage to the corticobulbar and corticospinal tracts is responsible for these clinical findings.

Neurobehavioural and neuropsychological abnormalities

Although a particular type of dementia is not infrequently a presenting feature of the disorder, this is an inconstant finding even in the terminal phase (Steele, 1972). Some authors have suggested in fact that neuropsychological impairments are restricted to non-verbal tasks requiring visual scanning ability (Kimura, Barnett and Burkhart, 1981). Furthermore, Fisk *et al.* (1982) failed to find significant differences between verbal IQs in a small number of patients compared with controls, and it is a recognized clinical fact that, although forgetfulness is a common complaint, the majority of patients can in fact remember if given sufficient time. Nevertheless, Albert, Feldman and Willis (1974) pinpointed a number of difficulties which they believed to be frequent and characteristic. These included an impaired ability to manipulate acquired knowledge, apathy and irritability and a slowing of thought processes. Albert considered that this spectrum of symptoms might be due to damage to ascending frontolimbic connections. In a much larger, neuropsychological study on 27 patients with the Steele–Richardson–Olszewski syndrome, 18 were found to be demented at the time of first hospital referral. The dementia was moderate in nine patients and severe in the other nine, and of 10 patients tested seven had particular difficulties with tests believed to be relatively specific for frontal lobe function (verbal fluency, Weigl test). 'Frontal lobe signs' were also seen in some patients including forced grasping, utilization behaviour and marked motor perseveration (Maher, Smith and Lees, 1985). Cambier *et al.* (1985) obtained similar results in 10 patients, but with an even greater incidence of abnormalities seen with frontal lobe syndromes. Mental slowing, impaired attention, poor abstract thinking and reasoning, reduced verbal fluency, mild to moderate memory loss and impaired elaborated linguistic abilities were found with a high incidence of frontal lobe signs on examination. Pillon *et al.* (1986) have compared the neuropsychological abnormalities in Steele–Richardson–Olszewski syndrome with those occurring in both Parkinson's disease and Alzheimer's disease, as well as in controls. No differences were detectable between the three disease groups on language tests, calculation, apraxia and visuomotor activity. However, tests believed to be sensitive to frontal lobe function were more abnormal in the Steele–Richardson–Olszewski patients (word fluency and imitation), whereas tests of verbal and logical memory were more affected in the Alzheimer's disease cases. Severe dysphasia, however, may occur rarely in the Steele–Richardson–Olszewski syndrome (Perkin *et al.,* 1978) so that this distinction between a 'frontolimbic' dementia in Steele–Richardson–Olszewski syndrome and a 'temporoparietal' dementia in Alzheimer's disease may not be clearcut. Present evidence raises the possibility that the cognitive impairments occurring in the Steele–Richardson–Olszewski syndrome might occur as a result of primary damage to the caudate nucleus or functional de-activation of the complex loop to prefrontal cortex. Support for the view that functional abnormalities occur in the frontal lobes also comes from recent work using position emission tomography and [18-F]fluorodeoxyglucose to explore regional glucose metabolism. A significant reduction in frontal glucose utilization was shown in six patients with probable Steele–Richardson–Olszweski syndrome compared with eight controls. Some inter-patient variability was evident and glucose utilization was down in all brain regions, but only reached functional significance in the frontal areas (D'Antona *et al.,* 1985). In studies on four patients in London this finding was broadly confirmed with a global cortical decrease in tissue oxygen demand ($CMRO_2$) and cerebral blood flow (CBF), but with the most severe change occurring in the frontal regions. The oxygen extraction ratio (OER) was also found to be higher in the patients because the fall of cerebral blood flow was greater than the decrease in tissue oxygen demand. This, however, does not necessarily suggest that the Steele–Richardson–Olszewski syndrome is a vascular disorder; it might be explained by disturbances in the innervation of the cerebral vasculature. Similar findings have been reported in Parkinson's disease. A comparison of frontal activity with the psychological test results on these patients failed to disclose any obvious relationship (Linders, Frackowiak and Lees, 1986).

NEUROPATHOLOGICAL ABNORMALITIES

The histological lesions

On naked eye examination of the brain, the only detectable abnormalities may be some bleaching of substantia nigra, slight dilatation of the third and lateral ventricles and a pale shrunken globus pallidus with some general atrophy of the brain. At the light microscopical level, the disorder is distinguished by nerve cell loss, gliosis and numerous neurofibrillary tangles in a specific distribution. Broadly, three main areas of damage can be distinguished in the majority of cases: the pallidosubthalamic complex with particular destruction of the internal segment of the pallidum at the origin of the pallidothalamofrontal pathway; the zona compacta of the substantia nigra which is the source of striatal dopaminergic neurones; and the superior colliculus, peri-aqueductal grey matter and pre-tectal areas which are

Table 13.4 The distribution of cell loss and neurofibrillary tangles in Steele–Richardson–Olszewski syndrome

Severe almost constant involvement	*Moderate inconstant involvement*	*Areas never or exceptionally rarely affected*
Globus pallidus (especially inner segment)	Dentate nucleus	Amygdala
	Red nucleus	Cerebellar cortex
Subthalamic nucleus	Locus ceruleus	Temporal neocortex
Substantia nigra (compacta and reticulata)	Corpus striatum	Parietal neocortex
Superior colliculi	Thalamus	Occipital neocortex
Pretectal area	Olive	
Peri-aqueductal grey matter	Nucleus cuneiformis	
Nuclei pontis	Nucleus subcuneiformis	
	Septum	
	Hippocampus	
	Frontal cortex	
	Nuclei of III, IV, VI, XII cranial nerves	
	Spinal cord	
	Posterior hypothalamus	

Table 13.5 Other neurological disorders characterized by neurofibrillary tangle formation

Alzheimer's disease
  Severe involvement of pyramidal neurones of neocortex, nuclei pontis, locus ceruleus, n.dorsalis raphe, nigra compacta, posterior hypothalamus, nucleus magnocellularis, n.supratrachlearis

Post-encephalitic Parkinson's syndrome
  Extensive brainstem involvement but less involvement of superior colliculus and dentate nucleus, cerebral cortex not commonly involved

Parkinson–dementia of Guam
  Hippocampus, substantia nigra, anterior horn cells, globus pallidus

Down's syndrome
  As for Alzheimer's disease

Dentato-pallido-luysian atrophy

Motoneurone disease
  Rare, usually familial cases

Dementia pugilistica
  Hippocampus, substantia nigra, brainstem tegmentum

Subacute sclerosing panencephalitis

Juvenile neurovisceral lipid storage disease
  Dystonic lipidosis

known to be involved in the control of ocular movements. The amygdala, most areas of the cerebral neocortex and the cerebellar cortex are, for the most part, spared from damage.

The neurofibrillary tangles are strongly argyrophilic and mainly of globose type, although a few flame-shaped varieties are also usually seen. These morphological differences may, in any case, merely reflect the type of cell in which the pathological process originates. In general, the degree of nerve cell loss is inversely proportional to the extent of neurofibrillary degeneration. The characteristic distribution of the lesions in Steele–Richardson–Olszewski syndrome is shown in Table 13.4 and it is this which enables the disorder to be distinguished pathologically from other disease states characterized by neurofibrillary tangles (see Table 13.5). The gliosis is mainly fibrillary astrocytosis, although increases in microglia have also been seen in a few patients. Gemistocytic astrocytes are not present, implying that the pathological process is proceeding relatively slowly. Perivascular lymphocytic cuffing and neuronophagia have only exceptionally been seen. Although Steele, Richardson and Olszewski stressed the presence of granulovacuolar degeneration in the red nucleus and nucleus pontis; this is an inconstant finding. Argyrophilic fibrillary inclusions resembling Pick bodies have been reported and Lewy bodies are seen in about 5% of cases. Demyelination is seen, due to a loss of nerve cells from which the affected tract originates.

Ultrastructural abnormalities

The large majority of neurofibrillary tangles in Steele–Richardson–Olszewski syndrome have been shown under the electron microscope to be made up of clusters of straight filaments arranged in circling and interlacing bundles (Tellez-Nagel and Wisniewski, 1973; Powell, London and Lampert, 1974; Roy et al., 1974; Bugiani et al., 1979). They have an average diameter of 15 nm, are of indeterminate length with a central region which is seldom electron lucent. Narrowing up to 9–11 nm may be seen, giving an irregular outline; a variable number of dense granules are also usually visible. These filaments are characteristically stable to postmortem change and to formaldehyde fixation. Originally, it was proposed that straight filament neurofibrillary tangles were pathognomonic for Steele–Richardson–Olszewski syndrome and indicated a distinct neurotubule defect. However, it is now known that these straight filaments are not unique and occur in Alzheimer's disease, post-encephalitic Parkinson's syndrome and the Parkinson–dementia of Guam. Moreover, pairs of 10-nm helical filaments with regular constrictions at 70–90-nm intervals have also been reported, together with the straight filaments (Tomonaga, 1977; Ghatak, Nochlin and Hadfield, 1980).

Both these types were seen separately in brainstem neurones and only very few straight filaments were mixed with paired helical filaments in the cortical tangles (Yagishita et al., 1979). Ishii and Ito (1979) have reported a patient who had only twisted tubules at postmortem, and Probst (1977) described an even more intriguing case with fine straight filaments of 10-nm diameter mixed with twisted 20-nm tubules. Although no definite transitional forms have been found, the distribution of straight and paired helical filaments suggests that the same neurones must be capable of making different types of fibrillary protein in different pathological states. It is also conceivable that the two types merely represent different stages in a similar pathological process.

Biochemical and immunological methods are now being used to examine the molecular structures of neurofibrillary tangles. Antiserum raised against human brain microtubule fractions and which binds specifically to the paired helical filaments of senile dementia of Alzheimer's type, also react positively with 15-nm straight fibres in the Steele–Richardson–Olszewski syndrome (Dickson et al., 1985). This suggests that both types of tangle share immunological properties with components in the microtubule fraction of human brain (Yen, Horoupian and Terry, 1983). A monoclonal antibody raised to neurofilament protein also stains the straight fibres in the Steele–Richardson–Olszewski syndrome (Brownell et al., 1983). Nakazato and colleagues (1984), using antisera raised against each of the subunit fractions of neurofilament in a patient with 12-nm straight fibrils, also found occasional positive immunoreactivity. The fact that antibodies which bind to Alzheimer neurofibrillary tangles have also been shown to bind to the straight fibres in the Steele–Richardson–Olszewski syndrome suggests that there may be shared amino acid sequences in the two diseases. Immunoelectron microscopy has confirmed that the binding sites for anti-Alzheimer neurofibrillary tangle antibodies are located on 15-nm straight filaments. This would support the two structures being morphological variants constructed from the same or related polypeptides. It remains unclear, however, why a predominance of straight fibres occurs in Steele–Richardson–Olszewski syndrome, whereas paired helical filaments are the usual cytoskeletal abnormality in Alzheimer's disease.

Neurochemical abnormalities

Jellinger, Riederer and Tomonaga (1980) reported a severe reduction in tyrosine hydroxylase, the biosynthetic rate-limiting enzyme of dopamine synthesis, in two patients which was more pronounced than that normally found in Parkinson's disease in all areas of the brainstem except the globus pallidus. These authors also reported a decrease in both spiperone and ADTN binding in the corpus striatum and nucleus accumbens. A 50% reduction of D-2 receptors in the corpus striatum was subsequently confirmed, whereas D-1 receptors are normal (Bokobza et al., 1984). In a further more extensive study on nine patients with Steele–Richardson–Olszewski syndrome, all of whom had psychomotor retardation as part of their symptomatology, and 27 controls, the Pitié-Salpêtrière group reported a reduction in [^{3}H]spiperone binding in the putamen (42%), caudate nucleus (48%), nucleus accumbens (44%), frontal cortex (34%) and substantia innominata (67%). A significant negative correlation was found between the numbers of neurofibrillary tangles and the number of [^{3}H]spiperone binding sites. Dopamine levels were reduced by more than 85% and homovanillic acid levels (HVA) by 50% in the caudate nucleus and putamen, but, intriguingly, in contrast to Parkinson's disease, no reduction was observed in the nucleus accumbens or frontal cortex. Significant correlations were found for homovanillic acid, [^{3}H]spiperone binding and choline acetyltransferase activity in both the caudate and putamen (Ruberg et al., 1985). It seems probable, therefore, that in contradistinction to Parkinson's disease, the striatal cholinergic interneurones are damaged as well as the nigrostriatal dopaminergic pathway, although the possibility that there is simply a defective synthesis or down-regulation of dopaminergic receptors as a result of chronic dopaminergic agonist therapy cannot be excluded. Kish et al. (1985) found a comparable 75–80% loss of dopamine and 50% loss of homovanillic acid to that found in Parkinson's disease in five pathologically verified cases of the Steele–Richardson–Olszewski syndrome, three of whom had not had a supranuclear gaze palsy in life and two of whom had severe Alzheimer-type dementia. However, there was a slightly greater loss of dopamine in the caudate than in the putamen, which is the reverse of what is normally found in Parkinson's disease. Dopamine and homovanillic acid levels were also normal in this study in the nucleus accumbens, hypothalamus and temporal cortex, although a 33% reduction of dopamine occurred in the para-olfactory cortex. Taken together these two studies bring into considerable doubt the view that the neuropsychiatric impairment seen in Parkinson's disease and the Steele–Richardson–Olszewski syndrome is due to lesions in the dopaminergic mesocorticolimbic pathway.

Demonstration *in vivo* of nigrostriatal dopamine decrease in this disorder has recently been demonstrated in five of the author's patients by the MRC Cyclotron Unit at the Hammersmith Hospital, London, using radioactive fluorodopa. Striatal dopamine uptake varied considerably from patient to patient but was always lower than the controls (*see Figure 13.1*) and in three of the five was at the level seen in Parkinson's disease. The nigrostriatal dopamine decrease paralleled the degree of frontal decline of $CMRO_2$ and CBF (Linders, Frackowiak and Lees, 1986). A loss of striatal D-2 receptors has also been demonstrated using [^{11}C]spiperone ligands and positron emission tomography (Baron et al., 1985).

Both Agid's group and Kish and colleagues measured choline acetyltransferase (CAT) in several brain regions, but here marked discrepancies occurred between the two studies. The French group found CAT to be decreased slightly in the

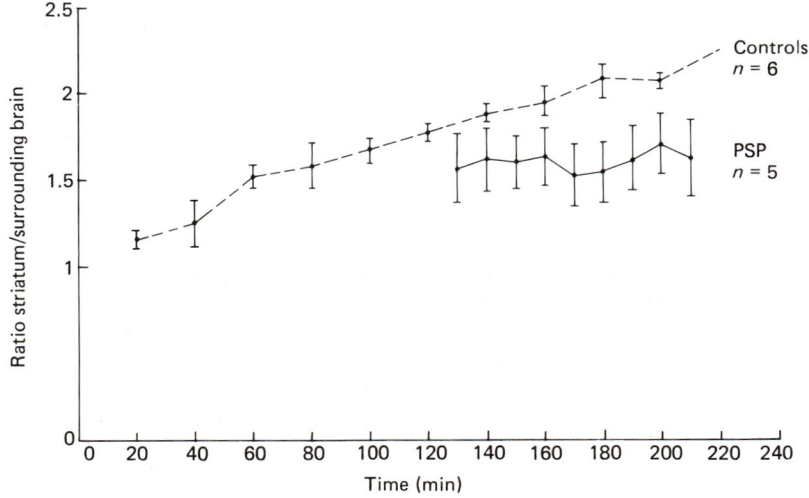

Figure 13.1 Position emission tomography findings using L-[^{18}]fluorodopa in the Steele–Richardson–Olszewski syndrome (PSP).

cerebral cortex (20%), moderately in the caudate, putamen and nucleus accumbens (40–60%) and severely in the substantia innominata (70%), the latter structure being the presumed source of the cortical cholinergic afferents. [^{3}H]Quinoclidynyl benzylate ([^{3}H]QNB) was also measured as an indicator of cholinergic transmission potential. Only in the substantia innominata, where a non-significant 26% was observed, were differences from controls detected with this ligand. Ruberg *et al.* (1985) interpret these findings as possibly due to loss of cholinergic afferents to the substantia innominata from other brainstem structures. Kish *et al.* (1985), however, found normal CAT levels in all neocortical areas in four patients and modest reductions in the striatum, temporal cortex and hippocampus in the other case. CAT levels were normal in both patients with severe dementia. These differences will need to be resolved by further studies, but neuropathological evidence would point to at least modest cell loss in the substantia innominata in some patients with Steele–Richardson–Olszewski syndrome (Tagliavini *et al.*, 1984). Neither group found changes approaching the decreases in cerebral CAT found in Alzheimer's disease, suggesting that the neuropsychological abnormalities in Steele–Richardson–Olszewski syndrome are unlikely to be primarily caused by cortical cholinergic deficits.

Kish and colleagues also reported increased glutamic acid levels in three of their five patients in the temporal and occipital cerebral cortex, the corpus striatum and medial globus pallidus, but there was no correlation between the degree of elevation of this excitatory transmitter and the severity of the histological lesions. Gamma-aminobutyric acid (GABA) levels were reduced only in the subthalamic nucleus (Kish *et al.*, 1985) and Javoy-Agid and colleagues reported decreased glutamic acid decarboxylase (GAD) levels in the putamen, external pallidum, subthalamic nucleus and the hippocampus (Ruberg *et al.*, 1985). Normal 5-hydroxytryptamine (5-HT), 5-hydroxyindoleacetic acid (5-HIAA) and noradrenaline (NA) levels were found in the basal ganglia, hypothalamus and temporal cortex, again a finding which contrasts with Parkinson's disease (Kish *et al.*, 1985).

Recent progress has therefore been achieved in understanding the biochemical abnormalities which might underly the L-dopa refractory parkinsonian symptoms of the Steele–Richardson–Olszewski syndrome and the caudate dopamine loss might also be of functional relevance with respect to the neurobehavioural disturbances. However, the chemical lesions causing the ophthalmoplegia, the pseudobulbar palsy and axial dystonia with rigidity remain unknown.

DIAGNOSTIC INVESTIGATIONS

Problems of diagnosis are likely to arise when the ophthalmoplegia shows unusual features or is absent altogether. In this situation, detailed neuro-otological examination may pick up early suggestive subclinical abnormalities. Computerized tomography and magnetic resonance imaging reveal enlargement of the third ventricle, enlargement of the interpeduncular cistern and cistern magna with brainstem atrophy and no cerebellar atrophy. Mild cortical atrophy may also occur, particularly in pre-frontal regions (Haldeman et al., 1981; Masucci et al., 1985). The electroencephalogram is normal in 50% of cases, but recorded abnormalities include non-specific diffuse slowing, bilateral theta or asymmetrical theta activity (Maher and Lees, 1986). Polygraphic sleep EEG telemetry may reveal marked, but non-specific, disturbances including disorganization of non-REM sleep patterns, reduced or absent REM sleep and a reduction in the total number of hours of sleep (Leygonie et al., 1976; Gross, Spehlmann and Daniels, 1978). Sleep apnoea also occurs in some patients (Perret and Jouvet, 1980) which might explain the common clinical observation that death usually occurs at night in this disorder. Positron and photon emission tomography and magnetic resonance imaging combined with spectroscopy may prove useful diagnostic tools in the future. The distribution of iron in the brain using high field strength magnetic resonance imaging may prove an even more sensitive diagnostic tool (Drayer et al., 1986). At present, however, the diagnosis remains a clinical one.

MANAGEMENT

Drug treatment has so far proved extremely disappointing, probably because multiple neurotransmitter systems are deranged as a result of the extensive brainstem pathology. Even the parkinsonian features which one might have expected to be responsive to dopamine replacement therapy are only exceptionally improved and, when this occurs, the response tends to be shortlived and occur in the early stages of the illness. The dopamine receptor agonists, such as bromocriptine, pergolide and lisuride, are even less effective than L-dopa, a finding which would be in keeping with the notion that cholinergic striatal neurones are also damaged. Jackson, Jankovic and Ford (1983) have recently reviewed the available literature on drug treatment in 91 patients in 179 trials. They obtained the following percentage figures of the number of patients improved: L-dopa 46% (74 trials), bromocriptine 50% (18 trials), pergolide 50% (4 trials), lisuride 13% (8 trials), anti-cholinergics 32% (28 trials) and amantadine 22% (23 trials). These authors concluded that dopamine replacement therapy was the most effective available treatment. The author's own experience, however, indicates that these figures, selectively culled from the literature and their own work, are unrepresentative and that, if one excludes placebo effect, the therapeutic response is much poorer than this to all these drugs. Twenty-one of 26 patients failed to respond at all to L-dopa, the others only experiencing slight benefit; only one of six patients improved at all on bromocriptine and only one of eight patients responded to anti-cholinergic drugs (Maher and Lees, 1986). Exceptional reports have occurred in the literature of striking improvement, however, in both parkinsonian signs and eye movements to L-dopa (Mendell, Chase and Engel, 1970) and bromocriptine (Williams et al., 1979). Methysergide, a 5-hydroxytryptamine antagonist, has also been reported to improve some of the disabilities seen in the Steele–Richardson–Olszewski syndrome when given either alone or combined with anti-parkinsonian drugs (Rafal and Grimm, 1981), but the author's group and others have been unable to confirm this (Paulson, Lowery and Taylor, 1981; Duncombe and Lees, 1985).

There have also been two encouraging reports of the use of amitriptyline (Kvale, 1982; Newman, 1985) which need to be followed up. At the very least, this drug may prove useful in the control of the emotional incontinence and psychomotor retardation. It is believed that the striatopallidal and striatothalamic pathways and also those from the substantia nigra reticulata to the superior colliculus are gabaminergic. The development of safe and effective drugs which enhance gamma-aminobutyric acid transmission might be of value.

Physical and speech therapy, involvement of an occupational therapist and social worker, and antibiotic treatment for intercurrent chest infections, are all important measures in the early stages of the disease. Nasogastric feeding may eventually become necessary and a cricopharyngeal myotomy may also help dysphagia if there is dystonia of the cricopharynx muscle. An elective tracheotomy for sleep apnoea is occasionally indicated and repeated injections of the orbicularis oculi with botulinus toxin is sometimes helpful for refractory blepharospasm.

COURSE

Despite drug treatment, the malady progresses relentlessly in every case to an invariably fatal outcome, usually as a direct consequence of the complications of the disease process. Although the exact order in which the different neurological systems become involved varies greatly from case to case, by the terminal stages the patient presents a tragic and distinctive picture.

The patient becomes chair or bedbound, unable to feed, bathe or dress, and cannot even turn in bed without considerable assistance. The eyes become fixed centrally and the patient is obliged to move the whole head to look at things. Speech becomes impossible apart from guttural croaks, and severe swallowing problems cause inanition and cachexia with considerable risk of aspiration pneumonia. Severe emotional lability may be evident with uncontrollable crying or, less often, laughter. Eventually the patient lies locked in with severe opisthotonus and double hemiplegia. Marked bradykinesia and rigidity are also present in the limbs and dystonic contractures develop. Even at this late stage the patient is often well aware of his/her surroundings with only modest weakness of intellect and memory.

Kristensen (1985) reported the median survival time in 73 patients reviewed in the literature to be five years with a range of 1–23 years, death usually occurring from intercurrent chest infection. Maher and Lees (1986) followed 52 consecutive patients and reported a similar figure of median duration of onset to death of 5.9 years in 30 of the patients (range 1.2–10.3 years). No significant difference in survival rates was found for those older or younger than 65 years, those with or without dysphagia and those with or without severe cognitive deficits. In 21 of the 30 cases for whom death certificates were available, the certified cause of death was felt to be pneumonia. Death certificates, however, would have been an unreliable source of ascertaining the incidence of Steele–Richardson–Olszewski syndrome as only 13 of the 30 mentioned the disorder and eight were misclassified as Parkinson's disease.

CONCLUSIONS

The Steele–Richardson–Olszewski syndrome is an acquired multisystem degenerative condition of middle and old age which affects the subthalamic nucleus, the globus pallidus, substantia nigra and superior colliculi, and frequently a number of other brainstem nuclei. The cerebellar cortex and cerebral cortex, with the exception of the frontal lobes and hippocampus, are characteristically spared. There are no pathognomonic clinical or pathological features, but the distribution of the lesions in the fully established case, combined with the relentless and relatively rapid progression, is characteristic. The aetiology is unknown, but a toxin or slow virus are the most attractive hypotheses.

References

ALBERT, M. L., FELDMAN, R. G. and WILLIS, A. L. (1974) The 'subcortical dementia' of progressive supranuclear palsy. *Journal of Neurology, Neurosurgery and Psychology,* **37,** 121–130

BARON, J. C., MAZIÈRE, B., LOC'H, C., SCOUROPOULOS, P., BONNET, A.-M. and AGID, Y. (1985) Progressive supranuclear palsy: loss of striatal dopamine receptors *in vivo* by positron tomography. *Lancet,* **i,** 1163–1164

BEHRMAN, S., CARROLL, J. D., JANOTA, I. and MATTHEWS, W. B. (1969) Progressive supranuclear palsy. Clinico-pathological study of four cases. *Brain,* **92,** 663–678

BLUMENTHAL, H. and MILLER, C. (1969) Motor nuclear involvement in progressive supranuclear palsy. *Archives of Neurology,* **20,** 362–367

BOKOBZA, B., RUBERG, M., SCATTON, B., JAVOY-AGID, F. and AGID, Y. (1984) [^{3}H]Spiperone binding, dopamine and HVA concentrations in Parkinson's disease and supranuclear palsy. *European Journal of Pharmacology,* **99,** 167–175

BROWNELL, B., GARSON, J., ANDERTON, B. H. and KAHN, J. (1983) Progressive supranuclear palsy: observations on nine cases using a monoclonal antibody to neurofilaments. *Neuropathology and Applied Neurobiology,* **9,** 334 (Abstract)

BRUSA, A., MANCARDI, G. L. and BUGIANI, O. (1979) Progressive supranuclear palsy 1979: an overview. *Italian Journal of Neurological Science,* **i,** 205–222

BUGIANI, O., MANCARDI, G. L., BRUSA, A. and EDERLI, A. (1979) The fine structure of subcortical neurofibrillary tangles in progressive supranuclear palsy. *Acta Neuropathologica,* **45,** 147–152

CAMBIER, J., MASSON, M., VIADER, F., LIMODIN, J. and STRUBE, A. (1985) Le syndrome frontal de la paralysie supranucléaire progressive. *Revue Neurologique (Paris),* **141,** 528–536

D'ANTONA, R., BARON, J. C., SAMSON, Y., SERDARU, M., VIADER, F., AGID, Y. and CAMBIER, J. (1985) Subcortical dementia: frontal cortex hypometabolism detected by positron tomography in patients with progressive supranuclear palsy. *Brain,* **108,** 785–799

DICKSON, D. W., KRESS, Y., CROWE, A. and YEN, S-H. (1985) Monoclonal antibodies to Alzheimer neurofibrillary tangles (ANT). Demonstration of a common antigenic determinant between ANT and neurofibrillary degeneration in progressive supranuclear palsy. *American Journal of Pathology,* **120,** 292–303

DIX, M. R., HARRISON, M. J. G. and LEWIS, P. D. (1971) Progressive supranuclear palsy (the Steele–Richardson–Olszewski syndrome). A report of 9 cases with particular reference to the mechanism of the oculomotor disorder. *Journal of the Neurological Sciences,* **13,** 237–256

DRAYER, B. P., OLANOW, W., BURGER, P., JOHNSON, G. A., HURFKENS, R. and RIEDERER, S. (1986) Parkinson plus syndrome: diagnosis using high field MR imaging of brain iron. *Radiology,* **159,** 493–498

DUBAS, F., GRAY, F. and ESCOUROLLE, R. (1983) Maladie de Steele–Richardson–Olszewski sans ophththalmoplegie. *Revue Neurologique (Paris)*, **139**, 407–416

DUNCOMBE, A. S. and LEES, A. J. (1985) Methysergide in progressive supranuclear palsy. *Neurology*, **35**, 936–937

FISK, J. D., GOODALE, M. Z., BURKHART, G. and BARNETT, H. J. M. (1982) Progressive supranuclear palsy: the relationship between ocular motor dysfunction and psychological test performance. *Neurology*, **32**, 698–705

GHATAK, N. R., NOCHLIN, D. and HADFIELD, M. G. (1980) Neurofibrillary pathology in progressive supranuclear palsy. *Acta Neuropathologica*, **52**, 73–76

GROSS, R. A., SPEHLMANN, R. and DANIELS, J. C. (1978) Sleep disturbances in progressive supranuclear palsy. *Electroencephalography and Clinical Neurophysiology*, **45**, 16–25

HALDEMAN, S., GOLDMAN, J. W., HYDE, J. and PRIBRAM, H. F. W. (1981) Progressive supranuclear palsy. Computed tomography and response to anti-parkinsonian drugs. *Neurology*, **31**, 442–445

HOWELL, D. A., LEES, A. J. and TOGHILL, P. J. (1979) Spinal internuncial neurones in progressive encephalomyelitis with rigidity. *Journal of Neurology, Neurosurgery and Psychology*, **42**, 773–785

IIZUKA, R., HIRAYAMA, K. and MAEHARA, K. (1984) Dentato-rubro-pallido-luysian atrophy: a clinicopathological study. *Journal of Neurology, Neurosurgery and Psychiatry*, **47**, 1288–1298

ISHII, Y. and ITOH, T. (1979) An autopsy case of progressive supranuclear palsy. *Clinical Neurology (Tokyo)*, **19**, 187

JACKSON, J. A., JANKOVIC, J. and FORD, J. (1983) Progressive supranuclear palsy: clinical features and response to treatment in 16 patients. *Annals of Neurology*, **13**, 273–278

JELLINGER, K., RIEDERER, P. and TOMONAGA, M. (1980) Progressive supranuclear palsy: clinico-pathological and biochemical studies. *Journal of Neural Transmission*, Suppl. 16, 111–128

KIMURA, D., BARNETT, H. J. M. and BURKHART, G. (1981) The psychological test pattern in progressive supranuclear palsy. *Neuropsychologia*, **19**, 301–306

KISH, S. J., CHANG, L. J., MIRCHANDANI, L., SHANNAK, K. and HORNYKIEWICZ, O. (1985) Progressive supranuclear palsy: relationship between extrapyramidal disturbances, dementia and brain neurotransmitter markers. *Annals of Neurology*, **18**, 530–536

KOEPPEN, A. H. and HANS, M. B. (1976) Supranuclear ophthalmoplegia in olivopontocerebellar degeneration. *Neurology*, **26**, 764–768

KRISTENSEN, M. O. (1985) Progressive supranuclear palsy – 20 years later. *Acta Neurologica Scandinavica*, **71**, 177–189

KVALE, J. N. (1982) Amitriptyline in the management of progressive supranuclear palsy. *Archives of Neurology*, **39**, 387–388

LEYGONIE, F., THOMAS, J., DEGOS, J. D., BOUCHAREINE, A. and BARBIZET, J. (1976) Troubles du sommeil dans la maladie de Steele–Richardson–Olszewski. Etude polygraphique de 3 cas. *Revue Neurologique (Paris)*, **132**, 125–136

LINDERS, K. L., FRACKOWIAK, R. S. J. and LEES, A. J. (1986) Progressive supranuclear palsy: brain energy metabolism, blood flow and fluorodopa uptake measured by positron emission tomography. Submitted for publication

MAHER, E. R., SMITH, E. M. and LEES, A. J. (1985) Cognitive deficits in the Steele–Richardson–Olszewski syndrome (progressive supranuclear palsy). *Journal of Neurology, Neurosurgery and Psychology*, **48**, 1234–1239

MAHER, E. R. and LEES, A. J. (1986) The clinical features and natural history of the Steele–Richardson–Olszewski syndrome (progressive supranuclear palsy). *Neurology* (in press)

MASTAGLIA, F. L. and GRAINGER, K. M. R. (1975) Internuclear ophthalmoplegia in progressive supranuclear palsy. *Journal of the Neurological Sciences*, **25**, 303–308

MASTAGLIA, F. L., GRAINGER, K., KEE, F., SADKA, M. and LEFROY, R. (1973) Progressive supranuclear palsy: the Steele–Richardson–Olszewski syndrome: clinical and electrophysiological observations in eleven cases. *Proceedings of the Australian Association of Neurologists*, **10**, 35–44

MASUCCI, E. F., BORTS, F. T., SMIRNIOTOPOULOS, J. G. and KURTZKE, J. F. (1985) Thin section CT of midbrain abnormalities in progressive supranuclear palsy. *American Journal of Neuroradiology*, **6**, 767–772

MATA, M., DOROVINI-ZIS, K., WILSON, M. and YOUNG, A. B. (1983) New form of familial Parkinson-dementia syndrome: clinical and pathological findings. *Neurology*, **33**, 1439–1443

MENDELL, J. R., CHASE, T. N. and ENGEL, W. K. (1970) Modification by L-dopa of a case of progressive supranuclear palsy. *Lancet*, **i**, 593–594

NEVILL, B. G. R., LAKE, B. A., STEPHENS, R. and SANDERS, M. D. (1973) A neurovisceral storage disease with vertical supranuclear ophthalmoplegia and its relation to Niemann–Pick disease. *Brain*, **96**, 97–120

NEWMAN, G. C. (1985) Treatment of progressive supranuclear palsy with tricyclic antidepressants. *Neurology*, **35**, 1189–1193

PAULSON, G. W., LOWERY, H. W. and TAYLOR, G. C. (1981) Progressive supranuclear palsy: pneumoencephalography, electronystagmography and treatment with methysergide. *European Neurology*, **20**, 13–16

PERKIN, G. D., LEES, A. J., STERN, G. M. and KOCEN, R. S. (1978) Problems in the diagnosis of progressive supranuclear palsy (Steele–Richardson–Olszewski syndrome). *Canadian Journal of Neurological Science*, **5**, 167–173

PERRET, J. L. and JOUVET, M. (1980) Sleep study of progressive supranuclear palsy. *Electroencephalography and Clinical Neurophysiology*, **49**, 323–329

PFAFFENBACH, D. D., LAYTON, O. D. and KEARNS, T. P. (1972) Ocular manifestations in progressive supranuclear palsy. *American Journal of Ophthalmology*, **74**, 1179–1184

PILLON, B., DUBOIS, B., L'HERMITTE, F. and AGID, Y. (1986) Heterogeneity of intellectual impairment in progressive supranuclear palsy, Parkinson's disease and Alzheimer's disease. *Neurology* (in press)

POSEY, W. C. (1904) Paralysis of upward movement of the eyes. *Annals of Ophthalmology*, **13**, 523–529

POWELL, H. C., LONDON, G. W. and LAMPERT, P. W. (1974) Neurofibrillary tangles in supranuclear palsy: electron microscopic observations. *Journal of Neuropathology and Experimental Neurology*, **33**, 98–106

PROBST, A. (1977) Dégénerescence de neurofibrillaire sous-corticale sénile avec présence de tubule contournes et de filaments droits. Forme atypique de la paralysie supranucléaire progressive. *Revue Neurologique (Paris)*, **15**, **133**, 417–428

RAFAL, R. D. and GRIMM, R. J. (1981) Progressive supranuclear palsy: functional analysis of the response to methysergide and anti-parkinsonian agents. *Neurology*, **31**, 1507–1518

RICHARDSON, J. C., STEELE, J. and OLSZEWSKI, J. (1963) Supranuclear opthalmoplegia, pseudobulbar palsy, nuchal dystonia and dementia. *Transactions of the American Neurological Association*, **88**, 25–27

ROSENBERG, B., NYHAN, W. L., DAY, C. and SHORE, P. (1976) Autosomal dominance strionigral degeneration. *Neurology*, **26**, 703–714

ROSS-RUSSELL, R. (1980) Supranuclear palsy of eyelid closure. *Brain*, **103**, 71–82

ROY, S., DATTA, O. K., HIRANO, A., GHATAK, N. R. and ZIMMERMAN, H. M. (1974) Electron microscopic study of neurofibrillary tangles in Steel–Richardson–Olszewski syndrome. *Acta Neuropathologica*, **29**, 175–179

RUBERG, M., JAVOY-AGID, F., HIRSCH, E., SCATTON, B. et al. (1985) Dopaminergic and cholinergic lesions in progressive supranuclear palsy. *Annals of Neurology*, **18**, 523–529

SHAW, K. M., LEES, A. J. and STERN, G. M. (1980) The impact of treatment with levodopa on Parkinson's disease. *Quarterly Journal of Medicine*, **49**, 283–293

STEELE, J. C. (1972) Progressive supranuclear palsy. *Brain*, **95**, 693–704

STEELE, J. C., RICHARDSON, J. C. and OLSZEWSKI, J. (1964) Progressive supranuclear palsy. A heterogeneous degeneration involving the brain stem, basal ganglia and cerebellum with vertical gaze and pseudobulbar palsy, nuchal dystonia and dementia. *Archives of Neurology*, **10**, 333–358

TAGLIAVINI, F., PILLERI, G., BOCIRAS, C. and CONSTANTINIDIS, J. (1984) The basal nucleus of Meynert in patients with progressive supranuclear palsy. *Neuroscience Letters*, **44**, 37–42

TELLEZ-NAGEL, I. and WISNIEWSKI, H. M. (1978) Ultrastructure of neurofibrillary tangles in Steele–Richardson–Olszewski syndromes. *Archives of Neurology*, **29**, 324–327

TOLOSA, E. S. and ZEESE, J. A. (1979) Brain stem auditory evoked responses in progressive supranuclear palsy. *Annals of Neurology*, **6**, 369

TOMONAGA, M. (1977) Ultrastructure of neurofibrillary tangles in progressive supranuclear palsy. *Acta Neuropathologica*, **37**, 177–181

TROOST, B. T. and DAROFF, R. B. (1977) The ocular motor defects in progressive supranuclear palsy. *Annals of Neurology*, **2**, 397–403

WILLIAMS, A. C., NUTT, J., LAKE, C. R., PFEIFFER, R., TEYCHENNE, P. E., EBERT, M. et al. (1979) Actions of bromocriptine in the Shy–Drager and Steele–Richardson–Olszewski syndromes. In *Dopaminergic Ergot Derivatives and Motor Function*. Eds. K. Fuxe and D. B. Calne, pp. 271–283. Oxford: Pergamon Press

YAGISHITA, S., ITOH, Y., AMANO, N., NAKANO, T. and SAITOH, A. (1979) Ultrastructure of neurofibrillary tangles in progressive supranuclear palsy. *Acta Neuropathologica*, **48**, 27–30

YEN, S-H., HOROUPIAN, D. S. and TERRY, R. D. (1983) Immunocytochemical comparison of neurofibrillary tangles in senile dementia of Alzheimer type, progressive supranuclear palsy and post-encephalitic Parkinsonism. *Annals of Neurology*, **13**, 172–175

14
Wilson's disease
Irmin Sternlieb, Denis R. Giblin and I. Herbert Scheinberg

INTRODUCTION

In 1912, S.A.K. Wilson described a unique, progressive, familial syndrome of cirrhosis of the liver and a disturbance of the motor system, later characterized by F.M.R. Walshe as a combination of multiple sclerosis and parkinsonism (Walshe, F.M.R. and Walshe, J.M., personal communication). For decades, what Wilson described was considered to be a rare medical curiosity of only academic interest ('I saw a case in medical school'), and of no practical clinical significance – since its course was always relentless and fatal.

This state of affairs has been revolutionized in the last 35 years. The disease has been shown to be caused by an inherited defect in the excretion of copper that leads to the accumulation of toxic amounts of the metal in liver and brain, almost always accompanied by a deficiency of a specific copper protein of plasma – ceruloplasmin (Scheinberg and Gitlin, 1952; Scheinberg and Sternlieb, 1984). Diagnostic application of this pair of biochemical criteria has simplified nosology: what Wilson termed 'progressive lenticular degeneration', now generally referred to as the classical dystonic form of the disease, is now known to be aetiologically the same as the pseudosclerosis of Westphal–Strümpell, torsion dystonia of Thomalla–Wilson, a variety of psychiatric disorders, a number of liver diseases with no disturbance of the central nervous system at all, certain reproductive problems of young women and, indeed, the same as the totally asymptomatic state exhibited by individuals still in the latent phase of their copper toxicosis.

Diagnosis, which until 1952 was made antemortem only on the basis of a physical examination, can now be unequivocally confirmed or excluded biochemically even in patients in whom no clinical manifestations are apparent (Sternlieb and Scheinberg, 1968). Specific drug therapy can prolong indefinitely the asymptomatic state, and can significantly ameliorate the symptomatology and prevent death from the disease in almost all other patients. No other crippling and fatal movement disorder is as susceptible to diagnosis, therapy and prophylaxis as is Wilson's disease. As a consequence it has become an illness of the greatest clinical import since it is disastrous to the patient, and to his neurologist, when it is overlooked.

Copyright © 1985 by The Foundation for the Study of Wilson's Disease, Inc.

GENETICS AND PREVALENCE

Nine years after Wilson had noted the familial character of his disease, Hall (1921) reported family studies that strongly suggested that the disorder was inherited as a mendelian autosomal recessive trait, and this was confirmed 30 years later by Bearn (1960). In the last decade three sets of epidemiological data, from Europe, the United States and Japan, have indicated a worldwide prevalence of the homozygously abnormal patient (with a pair of 'Wilson's disease genes') of about 30 per million of the general population (Scheinberg and Sternlieb, 1984): the probability of a patient with a movement disorder having Wilson's disease is considerably greater. The corresponding prevalence of carriers (individuals with one Wilson's disease gene, in whom no clinical manifestations of the disease have ever been reported) is approximately 1.1% (Scheinberg and Sternlieb, 1984).

BIOCHEMISTRY

In his initial publication, Wilson (1912) suspected that the neurological disorder was the result of a toxin that was associated with the cirrhosis of the liver present in all his patients. Several hints appear in the literature of the next 35 years that copper or silver might play aetiological roles. In 1948, following the discovery of a fatal demyelinating disease of new-born lambs due to copper deficiency, Mandelbrote and his colleagues analysed the urine of a dozen patients with a variety of neurological diseases, including one with Wilson's disease whose urine contained significantly more copper than that of any of the other patients (Mandelbrote *et al.*, 1948). The investigations of several researchers, notably Cumings (1948), that followed yielded the unexpected finding that the excessive cupriuria that was present in all patients with Wilson's disease did not cause copper deficiency but reflected abnormally high concentrations of free copper in serum, derived from the high concentrations of hepatic copper, which were filtered at the glomerulus. Rather than being analogous to the ovine disease, Wilson's disease was soon shown to be its opposite: copper toxicosis of the liver and brain – a conclusion that led Cumings to suggest that removal of the excess copper might arrest the progression of the disease. Injections of British anti-lewisite (BAL, 2,3-dimercaptopropanol) proved to be capable of removing copper from patients and, used by Denny-Brown and Porter (1951), resulted in significant clinical improvement. In 1955, Walshe found that penicillamine (dimethylcysteine) more effectively promoted the excretion of copper than did BAL, and had the great advantage of being administrable orally (Walshe, 1956).

In 1952 deficiency of serum ceruloplasmin (one of about a dozen human copper proteins) was discovered to be an almost constant finding in patients with Wilson's disease (Scheinberg and Gitlin, 1952). Though of great diagnostic value, no pathogenetic relation between the large excesses of tissue copper and the deficiency of ceruloplasmin, which together characterize the disease biochemically, has yet been discovered.

Copper is as essential to life as are iron and zinc. Heritable homeostatic mechanisms normally protect the organism from variations of dietary content that might otherwise result in deficiency or toxicosis of these metals – but the existence of these processes is apparent only in the genetically abnormal individuals who have a defect in one or other mechanism. In Wilson's disease, there appears to be defective excretion of that portion of metabolized copper normally excreted from hepatic lysosomes into bile (Sternlieb, 1980).

PATHOLOGY

The hepatic defect in biliary copper excretion causes copper to accumulate in the liver and produce pathological changes years or decades before the metal diffuses, with toxic effects, to extrahepatic tissues (Sternlieb, 1980).

The earliest changes in the liver are ultrastructural: alterations of mitochondrial membranes, cristae and matrix which are associated with hepatic steatosis. This lesion may evolve, with no clinical evidence of liver disease, into a mixed macro- and micronodular cirrhosis (a finding in virtually every patient with neurological symptomatology) which sooner or later will cause illness or death. In other patients, there may be acute, subacute or chronic toxic hepatitis with light-microscopical findings that are non-specific (fat, inflammation, increase in fibrous tissue, lipofuscin deposits, necrotic hepatocytes), but present in all patients to some degree (Sternlieb, 1980; Scheinberg and Sternlieb, 1984).

Early in the disease, the excess copper is diffusely distributed throughout the hepatic cytoplasm. Later copper is concentrated in lysosomes where, although less toxic to the liver, it finally exceeds the capacity of these organelles and enters the blood, whence it can cross the blood–brain barrier in toxic amounts. Even in patients without overt neurological disturbances (patients dying from the hepatic effects of Wilson's disease), there may be a ten-fold or more increase in copper concentration compared to normal values, ubiquitously in the brain.

Grossly, the commonest pathological result of copper toxicity in the brain is softening, atrophy, pigmentation and cystic degeneration of the basal ganglia, particularly the putamen. There may also be degeneration of cortical white matter, ventricular dilatation, degeneration and spongy changes in the cerebellar folia and dentate nucleus, and central pontine myelinolysis (Scheinberg and Sternlieb, 1984).

Microscopically, Alzheimer types I and II cells, and the more specific (for Wilson's disease) Opalski cells are seen. Deeper layers of cerebral white matter may show spongy changes, diffuse gliosis, and loss of myelinated fibres. Loss of white matter may result in contact between the dorsal and ventral laminae of the dentate nucleus. Cavitation, liquefaction and total loss of structure can occur – but this is usually severe only in the basal ganglia.

Although copper has been shown experimentally to (*a*) interfere with the polymerization of tubulin, the depolymerization of microtubules, and the accumulation of monoamines by rat-brain synaptosomes, (*b*) inhibit microsomal Na^+-K^+ ATPase *in vitro*, and (*c*) inhibit dopamine-β-hydroxylase in the hypothalamus (Nagatsu *et al.*, 1979), it is not known how, or even if, these findings relate to the pathological histology, ultrastructure, or physiology of the brain in Wilson's disease.

What is remarkable in Wilson's disease is the lack of correlation between the pathology of both the liver and brain and the patient's clinical condition. Frank cirrhosis may not be reflected in any clinical or chemical abnormality; gross cerebral atrophy, demonstrated by computerized axial tomography (Williams and Walshe, 1981; Dettori *et al.*, 1984), may be present in an individual with a high level of intellectual functioning who is free of neurological or psychiatric symptoms.

CLINICAL MANIFESTATIONS

Neurological

In about 40% of patients with Wilson's disease, the first clinical manifestation of the illness is a neurological abnormality. The onset of neurological symptoms usually occurs in the second or third decade; the appearance of symptoms before adolescence or after the age of 40 is unusual (Scheinberg and Sternlieb, 1984) (*Figure 14.1*). Yet isolated reports of patients becoming neurologically symptomatic in their early fifties exist (Czlonkowska and Rodo, 1981; Ross *et al.*, 1985).

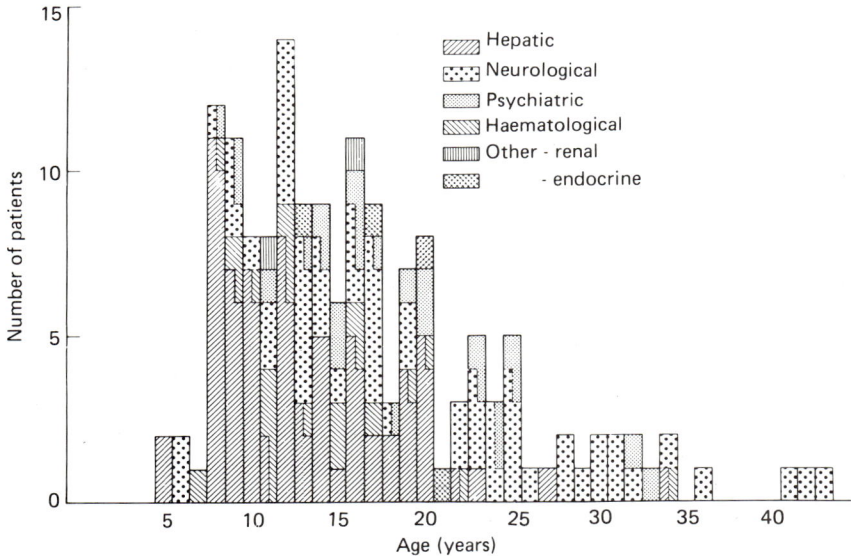

Figure 14.1 Initial mode of clinical onset of Wilson's disease as a function of age in a group of 151 symptomatic patients. The bars referring to patients presenting with two modes are divided into vertical halves. (From Scheinberg and Sternlieb, 1984, with permission)

Despite the widespread toxic concentrations of copper in the brain, the neurological disorders which are seen are virtually confined to the motor systems of the brain, and consist primarily of abnormal involuntary movements of various types together with incoordination and abnormalities of muscle tone. There is a striking predilection for involvement of facial and bulbar muscles. While motor disability can become very severe, significant weakness of either lower motor neurone or long-tract type is not a feature of the disease. Muscle stretch reflexes may be altered and Babinski plantar responses may be present, but the syndrome of progressive spastic para- or quadriparesis, with prominent disturbance of sphincter function, is not encountered in Wilson's disease. Likewise, disorders of vision and somatosensory function are never seen on clinical examination, a circumstance of obvious importance in differential diagnosis of patients presenting with incoordination or other motor disorders.

292   Wilson's disease

A single symptom, which may persist alone virtually unchanged for years, may herald the onset of the neurological phase of the illness. The abnormality, perhaps a change in speech or gait, may be appreciated by relatives, friends or by a physician during a routine examination before the patient is aware that something is wrong. Alternatively, the patient may complain of a functional disability at a time when the findings on neurological examination are quite subtle and not taken seriously even by a neurologist.

Inevitably the initial symptom worsens and others appear, not uncommonly with a rapidly progressive course from the onset. Alternatively, exacerbations can be abrupt and dramatic, often associated with emotional stress. Without appropriate de-coppering treatment, progression to total neurological incapacity and, ultimately, death is certain (Walshe, 1976, 1982; Dobyns, Goldstein and Gordon, 1979; Scheinberg and Sternlieb, 1984).

The earliest neurological symptoms and findings in patients with Wilson's disease are, as one would expect, those seen most frequently in patients in advanced stages of the disorder. They include dysarthrias of various types – generally in association

Figure 14.2 Severe dystonia developed in this dysarthric 17-year-old boy. Over one year it progressed to this stage of rigidity of the upper extremities with contractures and deformities of the fingers of both hands, introversion and contractures of both feet and poor posture, contributing to his difficulties in walking and in maintaining his balance. The pathological changes in the central nervous system have become largely irreversible and his response to treatment was disappointing

with drooling of excess saliva, clumsiness and loss of dexterity often affecting handwriting, tremors of several types, and disturbances of gait.

Abnormality of the facial and bulbar musculature is especially common in patients with Wilson's disease: dysarthria is its most frequent manifestation and may be the sole presenting symptom as well as a prominent feature of the advanced case. Different pathophysiological mechanisms can be involved, producing disturbances that include, in one group of patients, the monotonous, hypophonic speech of patients with masked facies and other manifestations of the parkinsonian syndrome, or the scanned speech of those with signs of cerebellar dysfunction. The dysarthria due to dystonia of facial and bulbar muscles is more frequent, and more disabling, becoming progressively unintelligible until the patient is anarthric. Articulation is impaired by dystonia of the face as well as of the muscles directly involved in speech; visible movement of the lips may be so limited that the patient appears to be a ventriloquist – although a poor one. Impaired control of respiratory muscles may be involved in causing hypophonia which becomes diminuendo at the end of a single short phrase. Examination of such patients usually shows that they are unable to whistle, and may show failure of elevation of the soft palate and impairment of tongue movements that are restricted in range and remarkably slowed. Dystonia of these muscles is also responsible for two features almost uniquely characteristic of Wilson's disease: the inappropriate, and eventually fixed, pseudo-smile (risus sardonicus), and the prolonged, high-pitched or gargling inspiratory whine or cry that is distressing to patient and listener.

This type of patient may also exhibit abnormal involuntary movements – quick dystonic ones, or more sustained dystonic posturing (*Figure 14.2*). Examples observed include intermittent or sustained dorsiflexion of the big toe, and dystonic movements of the fingers, hands, elbows or shoulders. These may be elicited by attempts to perform voluntary movements. In one such patient, walking evoked dystonic posturing of one arm which was carried behind the body, extended at the elbow, flexed at the wrist and fully pronated. In one form of the disease, severe sutained dystonic contractions of limb and axial muscles predominate, with fixed contractures such as extreme degrees of equinovarus deformity. This was, indeed, the picture exhibited by most of Wilson's original patients.

Abnormalities of tone are most commonly of the type associated with extrapyramidal disorders rather than spasticity. Increased resistance to passive stretch of flexor and extensor muscles may have a ratchety or cogwheel quality as in parkinsonism and, as in that disorder, may be augmented if the patient is asked to alternate opening and closing of the contralateral fist.

As the dystonic dysarthria worsens, difficulty in swallowing develops. Ingestion of food becomes inordinately slow and eventually the patient requires feeding by a nasogastric tube. The profuse drooling that is so common is an early manifestation of the dysphagia due to a loss of automatic swallowing.

Although, in many respects, patients with this dystonic form of facial and bulbar involvement due to Wilson's disease resemble patients with pseudobulbar palsy caused by multiple infarcts or motor neurone disease and, like them, may exhibit an exaggeration or disinhibition of emotional expression and an abnormal explosive or braying laugh, it is probable that the lesions responsible involve the basal ganglia rather than predominantly the corticobulbar pathways. Thus, while a prominent snout reflex is common in these patients, an abnormally brisk jaw jerk and contraction of facial muscles to stretch are not – suggesting hypertonus on an extrapyramidal basis rather than spasticity.

There can be few more pitiable patients than those with the advanced form of dystonic Wilson's disease. Unable to express themselves by speech or writing, facies fixed in a vacuous smile, drooling copiously, and making only animal-like sounds, to the untrained (and, alas, occasionally to the trained) observer, they are thought to be mentally impaired, imbecilic, addicted to drugs or acting out psychological problems. Ironically, most often there is imprisoned in this neurological catastrophe an individual with an intact intellect who is fully aware of his predicament and, consequently, angrily frustrated in the extreme.

In a form of Wilson's disease that resembles parkinsonism, motor abnormalities of limb and axial muscles consist primarily of abnormal involuntary movements, incoordination, gait disturbances and, to a relatively minor degree compared to the dystonic patient, abnormalities in tone. Most common are tremors. Resting tremors may closely resemble those seen in the parkinsonian syndrome: slow, predominantly distal, increased by emotional stress; at least transiently attenuated by initiation of voluntary movement; disappearing during sleep. Other features of parkinsonism may be present to some extent but only rarely do these dominate the clinical picture with masked facies, decreased blink frequency, hypophonia, bradykinesia and plastic rigidity. Micrographia is occasionally striking. Although not a common sign, some patients exhibit a continuous wing-beating tremor of the arms of such large amplitude and force as to cause injury to, and even ecchymoses on, the anterior chest. Postural tremors, both proximal and distal, are also common; they may at times be initiated by gently tapping the outstretched arm, resulting in a prolonged rhythmic oscillation of the limb.

Finally, cerebellar findings may predominate in the form of Wilson's disease termed 'pseudosclerotic' because of its resemblance to disseminated sclerosis. Prominent findings in these patients include: dysmetria accompanied by intention tremor made evident on finger-to-nose or heel–knee–shin testing; difficulty in using a fork or knife, and drinking from a glass or cup; inability to light a cigarette or, indeed, to perform almost any skilled act. Such patients may exhibit a typical ataxia of gait – broad-based, unsteady, staggering with steps of uneven length. Typically, too, the speech of these patients is scanned, and easily understood, and there is titubation of the head. It is not common for a patient to exhibit purely cerebellar signs (just as it is uncommon for one to suffer solely from extrapyramidal symptomatology) so that most patients manifest a neurological picture of mixed aetiology.

Chorea or choreo-athetoid movements are seen in Wilson's disease, but rarely. When severe they may disable the patient so that he is confined to a bed-and-chair existence.

Disturbances of the extra-ocular motor nerves are not uncommon but do not usually produce symptoms – just as, incidentally, Kayser–Fleischer rings never interfere with vision. There may be loss of smooth pursuit movements which become ratchety or saccadic in character. Loss of convergence may occur. One of our patients, who had lost both voluntary and pursuit upward gaze, regained these abilities after a year of treatment with penicillamine, suggesting that her gaze palsy was due to Wilson's disease. Similarly, in another patient (who could move his eyes conjugately but was unable to maintain eccentric gaze for more than a second or two) these abnormalities resolved with treatment. An occasional patient shows impaired pupillary light reflexes. Surprisingly, nystagmus is not a frequent finding even in patients with evidence of brainstem or cerebellar dysfunction.

Psychiatric

Psychiatric disturbance, present to some degree in almost all patients, precedes neurological and hepatic illness in about 20% of cases. Disturbances range from a severe psychosis, dementia or socially unacceptable behavioural abnormalities to psychoneuroses. Paranoid delusions, manic depressive psychosis and severe depression may be so little, if at all, different from idiopathic schizophrenia or cyclothymic disease, that Wilson's disease is not suspected unless the physician is alerted by finding a neurological or hepatic manifestation.

Dementia, which is not common, may first be noted in learning disability, often manifest in a rather abrupt deterioration of schoolwork of adolescents, an inability to concentrate or read, memory loss, or confusion about life and its activities.

Anxiety (chronic or as acute attacks; hypochondria, usually misdirected rather than referring to the real, subliminal catastrophe that is brewing; preoccupation

Figure 14.3 Retraction of upper lip and drooling in an untreated 38-year-old woman with neurological Wilson's disease of eight years' duration

with sexuality or death; depression) occasionally leading to suicidal attempts, insomnia, or compulsive, obsessive or phobic behaviour and thoughts are (particularly if unaccompanied by neurological signs but, alas, often in the presence of them), almost always interpreted as psychoneurosis.

Perhaps most common is impulsive, and often grossly antisocial, behaviour, exemplified by assault, tantrums, exhibitionism, sexual promiscuity, lying and thievery. Behavioural changes may take the form of frequent, prolonged day-dreaming; intense interpersonal friction, notably between adolescent patients and their parents; poor judgement, not uncommonly to do with money matters; alcoholism, sometimes triggered by the patient's awareness that any tremulousness that has developed is lessened by a drink or two; or an ill-defined (but all too obvious) personality change. Patients with this kind of mental symptomatology are often diagnosed as psychopathic personalities with the recommendation that they be institutionalized – as indeed some are.

In some patients devastating psychiatric disease is clearly the result of the neurological symptomatology because of the profound effects Wilson's disease produces on the patients' sexual attractiveness (*Figure 14.3*). The open-mouthed drooling, mask-like face, usually accompanied by halitosis, and the ill-kempt appearance and dirtiness of the entire body, often stemming from the dystonia or tremulousness that makes them unable to care for or groom themselves effectively, all too frequently produce a sexually and socially grimly repulsive individual. The frustrations of a patient who cannot talk, walk, eat or kiss become all the more overwhelming because their intellectual capacities and emotional sensitivities are generally little, if at all, diminished. It is often difficult to know whether the patient's disabilities and appearance have deceived the physician into interpreting neurological dysfunction as mental illness. On the other hand, in the 40% or so of patients who first present with neurological manifestations, these may be so severe that accompanying psychiatric disturbances are overlooked until neurological improvement, induced by de-coppering therapy, unmasks the mental symptoms.

It is the authors' belief that the emotional and mental disturbances of Wilson's disease are the direct and indirect results of copper toxicity: directly, from the effects of the widespread cerebral deposits of copper on higher integrative brain centres – occasionally complicated by hepatic encephalopathy in patients with significant portosystemic shunts or profound hepatic dysfunction; indirectly, from the patient's reactions to the neurological and hepatic effects of copper toxicosis.

Other modes of clinical presentation of Wilson's disease are listed in *Table 14.1*.

DIAGNOSIS

The possibility of Wilson's disease must be considered in every patient with a movement disorder. If it is not, and the patient has Wilson's disease, he will worsen and die until, and unless, it *is* thought of, the diagnosis is confirmed and de-coppering treatment is instituted. In particular, patients below the age of 40 presenting as a case of juvenile parkinsonism, multiple sclerosis, typical or atypical dystonia with or without a history of liver disease, may be suffering from Wilson's disease.

In such patients, the eyes should be examined with a slit-lamp by an ophthalmologist who has seen Kayser–Fleischer rings. A definite determination that these rings (visible deposits of copper in Descemet's membrane) are present or

Table 14.1 Clinical syndromes of Wilson's disease other than those related to dysfunction of the central nervous system

Hepatic	Asymptomatic persistent transaminasaemia 'Acute hepatitis', 'infectious mononucleosis' 'Chronic active hepatitis' 'Fulminant hepatitis' Cirrhosis
Haematological	Bruisability, excessive bleeding, epistaxis Hypersplenism Haemolytic anaemia
Renal	Proximal tubular dysfunction (aminoaciduria, hyperphosphaturia, hypercalciuria, glycosuria) Distal tubular dysfunction (K^+ wasting, concentration defect) Combined proximal and distal tubular dysfunction (uricosuria, acidification defect, bicarbonate wastage) Calculi Nephrocalcinosis
Skeletal	Vitamin D-resistant rickets Osteoporosis, spontaneous fractures Osteomalacia Osteo-arthritis Osteochondritis dissecans Premature degenerative arthritis
Skin	Pigmentation on the shins Spider angiomas Azure lunulae

absent, confirms, or rules out, respectively, the diagnosis of Wilson's disease. A recent paper states that Kayser–Fleischer rings were not seen in a patient with neurologically manifest Wilson's disease and bilateral arcus senilis (Ross *et al.*, 1985). The latter lipid deposits in Bowman's and Descemet's membranes may interfere with the formation of, and the examiner's ability to visualize, Kayser–Fleischer rings (Scheinberg, Sternlieb and Walshe, 1986). To the authors' knowledge there is no indubitable report of the absence of these rings in a patient with neurological signs of Wilson's disease.

The concentration of ceruloplasmin (the copper-containing protein of plasma) should also be determined in such a patient. Ninety-six per cent of patients with Wilson's disease will have less than 20 mg/dl of serum (*Table 14.2*), corresponding to less than 56 µg/dl of ceruloplasmin–copper. For this critical determination to be reliable, it should be performed by a laboratory that does ceruloplasmin and copper analyses regularly and routinely.

Measurement of total serum copper, frequently included in the work-up of a patient suspected of having Wilson's disease, is not only of no value, but may be misleadingly normal because of the abnormally high concentration of non-ceruloplasmin copper characteristic of untreated Wilson's disease. The confirmed presence or absence of Kayser–Fleischer rings, and the concentration of serum ceruloplasmin, will almost always establish or exclude the diagnosis in a patient

Table 14.2 Concentrations of ceruloplasmin in serum of symptomatic patients with Wilson's disease

Ceruloplasmin (mg/100 ml)	Patients	
	No.	%
0–<1	92	25
1– 4.9	98	27
5– 9.9	91	25
10–14.9	45	12
15–19.9	26	7
20–29.3	15	4
Total	367	100

Normal: 20–40 mg/100 ml.

with a movement disorder without needle hepatic biopsy of the liver. The latter procedure may, however, occasionally resolve uncertainties regarding the diagnosis and is helpful in determining the nature and the severity of the suspected liver disease. Two needle biopsy specimens should be obtained with copper-free instruments: one whole needle core should be processed for copper analysis in a specialized laboratory, and the second should be fixed in formalin and examined for morphological abnormalities by light microscopy. In contrast to diseases associated with hepatic iron overload, histochemical studies for copper deposits on liver biopsy specimens from patients with Wilson's disease may be misleading (Goldfischer, Popper and Sternlieb, 1980; Sternlieb, 1980; Scheinberg and Sternlieb, 1984).

In untreated patients with Wilson's disease the hepatic copper concentration is generally markedly in excess of 250 μg/g dry tissue (normal, less than 50 μg/g) (Sternlieb and Scheinberg, 1968). With overt neurological disease, however, mobilization of copper from the liver to other organs including the brain may have reduced the hepatic copper concentration to as little as 100 μg/g. Consequently, values below 250 μg/g do not necessarily exclude Wilson's disease in patients who fulfil other diagnostic criteria.

It is important to note that an elevated hepatic copper concentration in a patient with an elevated serum ceruloplasmin concentration and histological findings indicative of cholestasis (e.g. primary biliary cirrhosis, sclerosing cholangitis) is not diagnostic of Wilson's disease, even in the presence of Kayser–Fleischer rings. Such cholestatic syndromes can be differentiated from Wilson's disease clinically, biochemically and serologically (Goldfischer, Popper and Sternlieb, 1980).

Urinary copper excretion is generally in excess of 100 μg/24 h in almost all patients with neurological symptoms and signs. Unless measures are taken to prevent contamination, this determination is likely to be misleading. The 'penicillamine loading test' is of no diagnostic value (Scheinberg and Sternlieb, 1984).

In a patient with neurological signs, Kayser–Fleischer rings and a low normal ceruloplasmin concentration (20–30 mg/dl) (and otherwise healthy, not pregnant, and not receiving oestrogens) and in whom liver biopsy cannot safely be performed, a radiocopper loading test may resolve the diagnostic dilemma. A standardized dose of radiocopper administered orally to a fasting subject and the appearance of the radioisotope in the subject's serum is determined at five intervals in the next 48 hours. The concentration of ^{64}Cu in serum reaches a maximum within one or two hours, and then falls in any subject. Beginning in the next few hours, in individuals without Wilson's disease, the serum concentration of ^{64}Cu rises again, as the radiocopper is incorporated into ceruloplasmin, generally exceeding the initial maximum, at 48 hours. In patients with Wilson's disease, this secondary rise in serum radiocopper is absent even in the presence of a normal ceruloplasmin concentration (Sternlieb *et al.*, 1961; Sternlieb and Scheinberg, 1979). This test is of no value in subjects exhibiting ceruloplasmin deficiency. All siblings (each having, *a priori*, one chance in four of being a patient), and cousins and children of known patients should be screened for Wilson's disease by performing physical and slit-lamp examinations and by measuring the concentrations of ceruloplasmin and transaminases (AST and ALT) in serum (Sternlieb and Scheinberg, 1968). Finding a ceruloplasmin concentration below 20 mg/dl in one of these individuals obligates the physician to obtain a liver biopsy in order to establish whether the subject is a homozygote in whom Wilson's disease will develop (hepatic copper in excess of 250 µg/g dry tissue *and* abnormal liver histology), or a heterozygous carrier (hepatic copper concentration below 250 µg/g dry tissue *and* normal liver histology) in whom Wilson's disease will never develop and who should not be treated. Finding a ceruloplasmin concentration above 20 mg/dl, and persistent transaminasaemia for which no other certain cause is proven, requires the same investigations. A child older than two years with no physical abnormality, normal ceruloplasmin and transaminase values does not have Wilson's disease.

Ancillary tests

Cranial computed tomography may reveal hypodensity of the basal ganglia, cerebellar nuclei, brainstem and cerebral white matter, as well as ventricular dilatation and cortical and brainstem atrophy. Correlation of these findings with clinical manifestations is variable (Williams and Walshe 1981; Dettori *et al.*, 1984).

Magnetic resonance imaging may reveal symmetrical abnormal signals in the lenticular, thalamic, caudate and dentate nuclei and asymmetric focal white-matter lesions (Lawler *et al.*, 1983). In one recent study only 15 of 23 patients demonstrated one or more of these abnormalities (Aisen *et al.*, 1985).

Brainstem auditory evoked responses may be abnormal in some patients with Wilson's disease and normal in others, particularly in the absence of neurological manifestations (Roach *et al.*, 1985).

Treatment

Treatment consists of removing the excess of copper in the brain and liver. In the great majority of patients this is accomplished by the administration, on an empty stomach, of one gram of penicillamine (Walshe, 1956; Scheinberg and Sternlieb, 1984), in four doses of 0.25 g daily, together with a daily dose of 25 mg pyridoxine (because of a possible anti-pyridoxine effect of penicillamine). In the absence of irreversible and serious intolerance to penicillamine, this regimen must be continued indefinitely. Although severe restriction of dietary intake of copper is not necessary, patients should be advised to limit their intake of foods known to contain large amounts of copper, notably liver, mushrooms, nuts, chocolate, oysters, clams, shrimps and lobster.

The progress of therapy is best monitored by clinical evaluation of the patient. It is also helpful to compare the 24-hour urinary excretion of copper while the patient is taking penicillamine with the excretion determined immediately before penicillamine administration is begun. Patients will excrete 2 or more mg of copper a day on penicillamine and usually only several hundred µg without penicillamine. With time, the urinary excretion of copper will decrease but indications of clinical improvement, including fading or disappearance of Kayser–Fleischer rings, indicate that there is no need to increase the dose of the drug. Curiously, worsening of neurological signs and symptoms occurs during the first weeks or months of penicillamine therapy in about 10–20% of cases. Patients must be warned of this possibility before therapy is begun, and told that eventually improvement will almost always occur while continuing the drug. Six months or longer may pass before noticeable improvement takes place.

Allergic reactions to penicillamine may occur in the first three to six weeks of therapy, commonly producing fever or rash and, less frequently, leucopenia or thrombocytopenia. Patients should be appropriately monitored for these reactions, and the drug temporarily withdrawn, in the face of a reaction, until it subsides. Reinstitution of therapy, perhaps at 0.25 g daily initially, with gradual increase to 1 g over a week or two, is usually successful in overcoming these reactions. The temporary administration of 20 mg of prednisone daily, in instances of fever or rash, may more certainly avoid a recurrent reaction of this type. This dosage is progressively tapered over a few weeks (Scheinberg and Sternlieb, 1984).

Reactions to penicillamine of a more serious nature may occur later in therapy. Patients must, therefore, be seen at intervals not only to evaluate the state of their neurological and hepatic manifestations but also to ascertain that proteinuria, the commonest of serious late toxic reactions, or another side-effect, such as lupus, pemphigus, myasthenia or Goodpasture's syndrome, has not appeared.

In a small percentage of patients, particularly if Wilson's disease is severe when treatment is instituted, improvement does not occur after months of adequate penicillamine treatment. In these patients we have occasionally seen improvement begin if a course of 10–20 injections of BAL (0.3 g in 3.0 ml of peanut oil) are given daily, intramuscularly. Most patients tolerate this drug, but reactions (flushing, hypertension, tachycardia, weakness) may require its discontinuation.

In patients who are intolerant to penicillamine, or in whom BAL has not been effective in improving therapeutic response, triethylene tetramine (trien) is available as an oral chelating agent (Walshe, 1982a,b). It is also given in an average dose of one gram daily, in four divided doses, on an empty stomach.

It appears that the daily administration of 100–200 mg of elemental zinc, as the sulphate, acetate or gluconate, daily can inhibit the absorption of copper from the gastrointestinal tract (Brewer et al., 1983; Hoogenraad, van der Hamer and van Hattum, 1984). Several groups of investigators are presently investigating whether zinc alone can maintain an already de-coppered (by penicillamine or trien) patient in that state, and whether zinc can be used as initial treatment of a patient with Wilson's disease.

References

AISEN, A. M., MARTELL, W., GABRIELSEN, T. O., GLAZER, G. M., BREWER, G., YOUNG, A. B. and HILL, G. (1985) Wilson's disease of the brain: MR imaging. *Radiology,* **157,** 137–141

BEARN, A. G. (1960) A genetical analysis of thirty families with Wilson's disease (hepatolenticular degeneration). *Annals of Human Genetics,* **24,** 33–43

BREWER, G. J., HILL, G. M., PROSAD, A. S., COSSACK, Z. T. and RABBANI, P. (1983) Oral zinc therapy for Wilson's disease. *Annals of Internal Medicine,* **99,** 314–320

CUMINGS, J. N. (1948) The copper and iron content of brain and liver in the normal and in hepatolenticular degeneration. *Brain,* **71,** 410–415

CZLONKOWSKA, A. and RODO, M. (1981) Late onset of Wilson's disease. *Archives of Neurology,* **38,** 729–730

DENNY-BROWN, D. and PORTER, H. (1951) The effect of B.A.L. (2,3-dimercaptopropanol) on hepatolenticular degeneration (Wilson's disease). *New England Journal of Medicine,* **245,** 915–917

DETTORI, P., RACHELE, M. G., DEMELIA, L., PELAGHI, A. E., NURCHI, A. M., AROMANDO, P. and GIAGHEDDU, M. (1984) Computerized cranial tomography in presymptomatic and hepatic form of Wilson's disease. *European Neurology,* **23,** 56–63

DOBYNS, W. B., GOLDSTEIN, N. P. and GORDON, H. (1979) Clinical spectrum of Wilson's disease (hepatolenticular degeneration). *Mayo Clinic Proceedings,* **54,** 35–42

GOLDFISCHER, S., POPPER, H. and STERNLIEB, I. (1980) The significance of variations of copper in liver disease. *American Journal of Pathology,* **99,** 715–730

HALL, H. C. (1921) *La Degenerescence Hepato-Lenticulaire. Maladie de Wilson – Pseudo-Sclerose.* Paris: Masson

HOOGENRAAD, T. U., VAN DEN HAMER, C. J. A. and VAN HATTUM, J. (1984) Effective treatment of Wilson's disease with oral zinc sulphate: two case reports. *British Medical Journal,* **289,** 273–276

LAWLER, G. A., PENNOCK, J. M., STEINER, R. E., JENKINS, W. J., SHERLOCK, S. and YOUNG, I. R. (1983) Nuclear magnetic resonance (NMR) imaging in Wilson's disease. *Journal of Computer Assisted Tomography,* **7,** 1–8

MANDELBROTE, B. M., STANIER, M. W., THOMPSON, R. H. S. and THRUSTON, M. N. (1948) Studies on copper metabolism in demyelinating diseases of the central nervous system. *Brain,* **17,** 212–228

NAGATSU, T., KATO, T., NAGATSU, I., KONDO, Y., INAGAKI, S., IIZUKA, R. and NARABAYASHI, H. (1979) Catecholamine-related enzymes in the brain of patients with Parkinsonism and Wilson's disease. In *Advances in Neurology.* Eds L. J. Poirier, T. S. Sourkes and P. J. Bedard, pp. 283–292. New York: Raven Press

ROACH, E. S., FORD, C. S., SPUDIS, E. V., RIELA, A. R., McLEAN, JR, W. T., GILLIAM, J. and BALLA, M. R. (1985) Wilson's disease: evoked potentials and computed tomography. *Journal of Neurology,* **232,** 20–23

ROSS, M. E., JACOBSON, I. M., DIENSTAG, J. L. and MARTEN, J. B. (1985) Late-onset Wilson's disease with neurological involvement in the absence of Kayser–Fleischer rings. *Annals of Neurology,* **17,** 411–413

SCHEINBERG, I. H. and GITLIN, D. (1952) Deficiency of ceruloplasmin in patients with hepatolenticular degeneration (Wilson's disease). *Science,* **116,** 484–485

SCHEINBERG, I. H. and STERNLIEB, I. (1984) *Wilson's Disease.* Philadelphia: Saunders

SCHEINBERG, I. H., STERNLIEB, I. and WALSHE, J. M. (1986) Wilson's disease and Kayser–Fleischer rings. *Annals of Neurology* (in press)

STERNLIEB, I. and SCHEINBERG, I. H. (1979) The role of radiocopper in the diagnosis of Wilson's disease. *Gastroenterology,* **77,** 138–142

STERNLIEB, I. (1980) Copper and the liver. *Gastroenterology,* **78,** 1615–1628

STERNLIEB, I., MORELL, A. G., BAUER, C. D., COMBES, B., DE BOBES-STERNBERG, S. and SCHEINBERG, I. H. (1961) Detection of the heterozygous carrier of the Wilson's disease gene. *Journal of Clinical Investigation,* **40,** 707–715

STERNLIEB, I. and SCHEINBERG, I. H. (1968) Prevention of Wilson's disease in asymptomatic patients. *New England Journal of Medicine,* **278,** 352–359

WALSHE, J. M. (1956) Wilson's disease. New oral therapy. *Lancet,* **i,** 25–26

WALSHE, J. M. (1976) Wilson's disease (hepatolenticular degeneration). In *Handbook of Clinical Neurology, Metabolic and Deficiency Diseases of the Nervous System.* Eds P. J. Vinken, G. W. Bruyn and H. L. Klawans, Vol. 27, Part I, pp. 379–414. New York: American Elsevier

WALSHE, J. M. (1982a) Copper and the brain. In *Metabolic Disorders of the Nervous System*. Ed. F. Rose, pp. 352–358. London: Pitman Press
WALSHE, J. M. (1982b) Treatment of Wilson's disease with trientine (triethylene tetramine) dihydrochloride. *Lancet,* **i,** 643–647
WILLIAMS, F. J. B. and WALSHE, J. M. (1981) Wilson's disease: an analysis of the cranial computerized tomographic appearances found in 60 patients and the changes in response to treatment with chelating agents. *Brain,* **104,** 735–752
WILSON, S. A. K. (1912) Progressive lenticular degeneration. A familial nervous disease associated with cirrhosis of the liver. *Brain,* **34,** 295–309

Part III
Dyskinesias

15
Problems in the dyskinesias
C. D. Marsden and Stanley Fahn

INTRODUCTION

In the last volume we selected certain dyskinesias for review, and these will not be considered in detail in this edition. The editors, with Mark Hallett, discussed the nosology and pathophysiology of myoclonus; since then the proceedings of a recent major international symposium on myoclonus has been published (Fahn, Marsden and Van Woert, 1986). Clinical and experimental aspects of tardive dyskinesia were reviewed by Angus Mackay, and Christopher Goetz and Harold Klawans, respectively. Again there have been recent major publications on tardive dyskinesia (Jeste and Wyatt, 1982; Casey *et al.*, 1985), to which the interested reader can refer. The management of patients and families with Huntington's disease was discussed by Ira Shoulson in the previous volume, and a series of chapters dealt with surgical approaches to the dyskinesias.

This time we have chosen different topics. The aetiology, nosology and management of dystonia are given full coverage. John Rothwell and Jose Obeso review what is known of the anatomy and pathophysiology of dystonia in Chapter 16. The editors with Donald Calne discuss the classification and investigation of dystonia in Chapter 17. The editors review the treatment of dystonia in Chapter 18. Tics and essential tremor also receive special treatment. Joe Jankovic reviews the neurology of tics in Chapter 19, and Michael Trimble the psychiatry of tics in Chapter 20. Bob Lee discusses the pathophysiology of essential tremor in Chapter 21, and Leslie Findley the pharmacology of essential tremor in Chapter 22. Wilson's disease, which may present with dyskinesias as well as an akinetic–rigid syndrome, is reviewed in Chapter 14.

This has left many topics in dyskinesias untouched. In what follows in this chapter, we discuss briefly a number of areas in which advances have occurred recently, or which pose particular problems to the practitioner.

CHOREA

Increased attention has been given to the differential diagnosis of hereditary chorea, particularly to conditions other than Huntington's disease. Benign hereditary chorea has been recognized for some time, although there have been difficulties in distinguishing it from benign hereditary myoclonus (*see* later). Hereditary chorea-acanthocytosis, perhaps more correctly termed 'neuroacanthocytosis', has been recognized to be more common outside Japan than had been appreciated. Choreic movements in this condition are less severe than in Huntington's disease. Indeed, many patients exhibit other types of abnormal movements rather than chorea; these include myoclonic jerks, tics, and vocalizations such as humming sounds or tongue-clicking noises. The characteristic severe bulbar dystonia causing great difficulty with eating, often with mutilation of the lips, along with areflexia and other signs of axonal peripheral neuropathy, and an elevated serum creatine kinase concentration, provide clues to diagnosis. This is established by finding acanthocytes (spikes on erythrocytes) in a peripheral blood film. The blood smear must be made with a freshly drawn sample; acanthocytes can be found in normal subjects if the smear is taken from blood left sitting in a test-tube for too long!

Research in Huntington's disease has proceeded apace (Martin, 1984) with the spectacular discovery of genetic linkage to the G8 marker, localizing the gene to the short arm of chromosome 4 (*see* Chapter 4). The clinical significance of this outstanding application of recombinant DNA technology will be considerable. For the first time, there is a powerful marker for the disease, which can be applied to those at risk or their progeny. At present it seems that G8 linkage is about 95% accurate, providing sufficient generations and family members are available to establish linkage to a specific haplotype. The discovery of flanking markers has proved more difficult than expected, possibly because the gene sits right at the end of the chromosome, and the gene itself has not been identified yet. It is important to emphasize that existing methods are only informative in families in which sufficient members (affected and unaffected) from more than one generation are available for study. This means that it is crucial to take blood from existing patients with Huntington's disease, and from their available blood relatives, for DNA extraction and storage. Availability of such material will enable subsequent generations to benefit from linkage analysis.

The ethical and social problems of how to use a marker of the Huntington's disease gene have been widely debated in recent years by physicians, families and other professionals. The stage is now set for the application of predictive testing to those at risk provided appropriate genetic and psychiatric counselling is available before and after testing.

The diagnosis of Huntington's disease in a patient with a clear family history of a similar illness in previous generations is relatively straightforward, provided other hereditary autosomal dominant conditions can be excluded (for example, benign hereditary chorea, hereditary essential myoclonus, neuroacanthocytosis, and hereditary spinocerebellar degenerations). However, the sporadic case of chorea, with or without mental changes, continues to pose a difficult problem. Metabolic and endocrine disorders can be identified in a few patients. These include hepatocerebral degenerations, thyrotoxicosis and chorea gravidarum or its counterpart induced by the contraceptive pill or hormone replacement therapy. Polycythaemia rubra vera and systemic lupus erythematosus should be looked for; the latter may be difficult to diagnose for occasionally tests for serum antinuclear antibodies and specific DNA antibodies may be negative, although the serum lupus anticoagulant may be found.

However, the major problems occur in (*a*) those with a psychiatric illness treated with neuroleptics who develop choreic dyskinesias (is this Huntington's disease, tardive dyskinesia, or a combination of the two?) and (b) elderly patients with sporadic chorea with or without some degree of mental change (is this Huntington's disease, but we can't trace the relatives, or is it senile chorea, whatever that is?).

There are clinical clues to distinguish tardive dyskinesias from Huntington's disease. Prominent repetitive orobuccolingual movements are typical of tardive dyskinesia, as are rocking movements of the trunk and akathisia; the gait is relatively normal. In Huntington's disease, the choreic movements are not repetitive, but random – they flow from one body part to another; the gait is abnormal with interruptions, stuttering and halting, and balance is impaired.

In the case of senile chorea, there is insufficient pathological evidence to be certain that this is an entity separate from Huntington's disease. Some such cases turn out to have the pathological changes of Alzheimer's disease or multi-infarct cerebrovascular disease.

What is required to resolve these dilemmas is some test specific for Huntington's disease. The CT scan does not give a clear answer. The editors have first-hand experience of normal CT scans in those with undoubted Huntington's disease, and of flattening of the caudate bulge in those with other degenerations, such as the strionigral variant of multiple system atrophy, Pick's disease, and neuroacanthocytosis. However, positron emission scanning (PET) using ^{18}F-labelled deoxyglucose may provide an answer to this problem. The profound reduction in striatal glucose utilization shown by PET scanning in Huntington's disease (Kuhl et al., 1982) may be seen even in those with normal CT scans, and may even antedate the clinical onset of the disease. The same PET scan appearance, however, may be seen in benign hereditary chorea (Suchowersky et al., 1986).

Sooner or later the gene for Huntington's disease will be precisely localized, sequenced and cloned, but this has not yet been achieved. Even then it may be a major problem to determine what the gene programmes, and thereby get a clue as to the cause of the disease. At present, the best hypothesis concerns the actions of the amino acid glutamate in the striatum. Glutamate is believed to be the neurotransmitter in corticostriate fibres. Under certain experimental conditions, glutamate can be neurotoxic. A number of analogues of glutamate, including kainic acid and the naturally occurring substance quinolinic acid, when injected into the striatum of animals, can produce profound destruction of the striatal structures with striking similarities to those found in Huntington's disease. This has led to the suggestion that reduction of glutamate neurotransmission might slow or halt progression of the illness. Baclofen is one such drug which reduces glutamatergic activity, and is currently under trial. Until the results of this investigation are available, we prescribe baclofen to our patients with Huntington's disease, in the hope that it may slow functional decline.

Another issue in the therapeutics of Huntington's disease has also become clearer. The most effective drugs for controlling chorea remain the neuroleptics, such as phenothiazines, haloperidol, reserpine or tetrabenazine. However, all too frequently it is apparent that such drugs, while improving chorea, actually make the patients functionally worse. We have therefore become far more conservative in their use, employing these agents only in those in whom chorea causes substanital physical disability. In some patients, the benzodiazepines can reduce choreic movements as well as calming behaviour.

Another important issue that has emerged is the quality of care required for those with Huntington's disease who have reached the stage of long-term admission to hospital. Such patients often are not demented in the sense that those with Alzheimer's disease are. Patients with Huntington's disease may preserve insight, memory and individuality until the end, but this may be difficult to perceive in the face of their grotesque movement disorder and severe dysarthria or anarthria. It is important to recognize the special needs of this group of patients.

TARDIVE DYSKINESIA

The variety of movement disorders that may appear in about 20% of those on long-term neuroleptic treatment still poses formidable management problems. Tardive dyskinesias are being seen with increasing frequency in those taking metoclopramide for gastrointestinal disorders and phenothiazines for vertigo, as well as in schizophrenia. Whilst the typical stereotyped orobuccolingual dyskinesia is the most common variety, especially in the elderly, it is now apparent that tardive dystonia is not uncommon in the younger patient. Tardive dystonia (*see* Chapter 17) often causes considerable functional disability, which is frequently persistent and resistant to therapeutic approaches.

Another major component in many with tardive dyskinesias is an accompanying akathisia or motor restlessness, which can cause great discomfort. Such a distressing tardive akathisia occurs in about 25% of patients with tardive dyskinesia. It can be generalized or limited to focal parts of the body. Besides the subjective symptoms of restlessness ('I feel as if I am going to jump out of my skin'), objective signs of tardive akathisia may be detected. These include continual shifting of position or squirming while sitting, crossing and uncrossing of the legs, rubbing the scalp or limbs, arising from the chair, pacing around the room, or even running from place to place.

Obviously, the best management of tardive dyskinesias is to withdraw the offending drug, if this is practical. Sadly, in our experience a large proportion of those who develop tardive dyskinesia and akathisia have been treated with neuroleptics for conditions which did not require such drugs in the first place. Withdrawal of neuroleptics in such patients is the first measure. However, the problem is much greater in those with schizophrenia.

The risks of schizophrenic relapse, with all the consequent social and occupational disasters that this may entail, has to be weighed against the disability caused by the tardive dyskinesia. If neuroleptics can be withdrawn, there is a substantial chance (perhaps about 40% or more) of the dyskinesia disappearing, although it may take up to five years for this to occur. It is important to recognize that tardive dyskinesias may get worse in the initial weeks after neuroleptic withdrawal. Indeed, they may appear for the first time when neuroleptic drugs are stopped (so-called 'withdrawal dyskinesias').

If it is judged on psychiatric grounds that neuroleptic treatment must be continued, then the question is often asked as to which neuroleptic should be employed. Unfortunately, there is no easy answer. All of the neuroleptics in worldwide use carry the risk of provoking tardive dyskinesias and there is no hard evidence that one group of neuroleptics is less likely to be associated with this problem than any other. It is to be hoped that the next generation of neuroleptic drugs may be designed to avoid this problem, but at present the best advice is to use the minimum dose of the neuroleptic required to control the schizophrenia.

Treatment of tardive dyskinesia and akathisia is difficult. Mild dyskinesias are often ignored by the patient and cause no functional deficit. More severe dyskinesias may cause unacceptable social or functional disability, demanding therapy. The dopamine depletors, reserpine and tetrabenazine, can suppress the rapid, repetitive movements and associated motor manifestations of akathisia. These drugs can be used in severe cases, or to control worsening of dyskinesias when neuroleptics are stopped until a remission occurs. Unfortunately, however, adverse effects such as parkinsonism, depression (sometimes suicidal) and postural hypotension may be the price that has to be paid for this relief.

If dystonia is the major problem, anti-cholinergic drugs such as trihexyphenidyl (Artane) may give benefit in less than half the patients, particularly when used in high doses. However, anti-cholinergics make orobuccolingual dyskinesias worse rather than better.

Finally, there are some patients with severe disabling and intractable tardive dyskinesia, particularly those with severe tardive dystonia, who do not respond to the measures described above. In these cases, one may be forced to utilize neuroleptics to control their muscular spasms and abnormal postures. Obviously, one is reluctant to employ this strategy, which is difficult to explain to the patient and relatives, except as a last resort. However, it is our impression that the tardive dyskinesias in these patients may be controlled for many years without any obvious deterioration in the severity or extent of their movement disorder.

MYOCLONUS

The long list of conditions associated with myoclonus that was presented in our chapter on this topic in the previous volume has been expanded since then by the recognition of a number of other diseases that enter into the differential diagnosis.

Of particular importance is the approach to investigation of patients with myoclonus and a progressive encephalopathy. Investigations are required to exclude a variety of neuronal storage diseases, including the sphingolipidoses, sialidoses, ceroid-lipofuscinosis, and Lafora's disease. To this list must now be added Whipple's disease and malabsorption syndrome (which necessitates jejunal biopsy) (Lu et al., 1986), mitochondrial encephalomyopathies (for which measurement of serum lactate and pyruvate, and muscle biopsy to search for 'ragged-red' fibres and biochemical abnormalities of mitochondrial function are required) (Hopkins and Rosing, 1986), and biotin-responsive encephalopathy associated with multiple carboxylase deficiencies (Bressman et al., 1986).

The area of progressive myoclonic syndromes associated with cerebellar ataxia continues to cause debate. We believe it useful to employ the 'Ramsay Hunt syndrome' to describe this clinical problem. There are many pathological causes of the Ramsay Hunt syndrome, which should prompt further full investigation (including search for the conditions described above). Patients with a progressive myoclonic cerebellar syndrome may also exhibit a mild to moderate degree of intellectual deterioration late in the course of their illness. Some may have no epilepsy, but others may develop seizures. Here lies the source of the confusion, for such patients are often described as having 'progressive myoclonic epilepsy', as initially introduced by Unverricht and Lundborg to describe the familial form of this illness, which is common in Nordic countries, hence the contemporary designation of this condition as Baltic myoclonus (Koskiniemi, 1986). Patients with

Baltic myoclonus have grand mal seizures and epileptic abnormalities in the electroencephalogram; over a course of one or two decades they become increasingly disabled by myoclonus and ataxia, and their intellect shows a modest deterioration; pathologically there is a diffuse loss of Purkinje cells. To begin with, Baltic myoclonus was confused with Lafora body disease (and other neuronal storage diseases), but patients with these latter conditions exhibit not only myoclonus and severe seizures, but also a rather rapidly progressive dementia relatively early in the course of the illness. Thus, within this group of progressive myoclonic encephalopathies, there is a spectrum of associations with cerebellar ataxia, epilepsy and dementia.

In an attempt to resolve this nosological confusion, we would suggest that two syndromes of progressive myoclonic encephalopathy should be delineated: (a) the Ramsay Hunt syndrome in which myoclonus and ataxia dominate, with seizures, if present, being mild, and dementia occurring late if at all, and (b) progressive myoclonic dementia, in which dementia and severe epilepsy are early and dominant manifestations. In this light, Baltic myoclonus would be viewed as one of the causes of the Ramsay Hunt syndrome, while Lafora body and related neuronal storage diseases would be considered as progressive myoclonic dementias.

Focal myoclonus presents the difficult diagnostic problem of where its source lies in the nervous system. Myoclonic jerking of the arm, for example, may be due to epilepsia partialis continua arising in cerebral cortex, brainstem or cerebellar lesions (when it may be associated with the palatal myoclonus syndrome), damage to the spinal cord, or even to the spinal roots or brachial plexus. Investigation of such patients requires extensive physiological and neuroradiological studies to define the source of their focal myoclonus. Even then one may be left in doubt. Such patients may be classified as cases of sporadic idiopathic or essential myoclonus (Bressman and Fahn, 1986), but probably are distinct from the entity of hereditary essential myoclonus.

Hereditary essential myoclonus, itself, is turning out to be less clearcut as a distinct single entity. Many of the families described in the literature under this title exhibit two other features, namely dystonia and sensitivity to alcohol. This entity of 'myoclonic dystonia' or 'dystonia with lightning jerks sensitive to alcohol' is a distinctive condition with autosomal dominant inheritance (*see* Chapter 17) separate from true isolated hereditary essential myoclonus which, in our experience, is rare.

Advances have been made in the treatment of various myoclonic syndromes. The mainstay of therapy remains the use of sodium valproate and clonazepam, but newer agents which have proved of benefit in some cases include lisuride, serotonin uptake inhibitors such as paroxetine and fluoxetine, and the curious drug piracetam. Often a combination of agents is required to produce maximum benefit.

THE RESTLESS LEGS AND PERIODIC MOVEMENTS OF SLEEP SYNDROME

Since the topic of myoclonic jerks during sleep was written about in the previous volume, the status of the conditions to be considered has been clarified. Lugaresi *et al.* (1986) distinguish a number of physiological phenomena that may occur during sleep, or in the transition from sleep to wakefulness or *vice versa:* (a) partial myoclonic jerks, consisting of very short (10–100 ms) localized jerks occurring irregularly, particularly in distal muscles, and particularly in light (stage 1) and REM sleep; (b) massive myoclonic jerks ('sleep-starts'), which are longer (more than a second), affect simultaneously the axial and proximal limb muscles, occur while falling asleep or during light sleep (stages 1 and 2), often are precipitated by sudden noise, and are similar to the startle reaction during wakefulness; and (c) periodic movements of sleep (which are called nocturnal myoclonus), which consist of stereotyped repetitive dorsiflexions of the big toe and/or foot, sometimes also involving flexion of the knee and hip, affecting one or both legs, each contraction lasting one or two seconds, and occurring every 20–40 seconds for many minutes, associated with electroencephalographic evidence of arousal (K complexes) during light sleep (stages 1 and 2). Periodic movements of sleep increase in prevalence with age; it is rare below 30 years, occurs in 5% of those aged 30–50, and in 29% of those over 50.

Any of these conditions may lead the sleeping partner to complain of being kicked in bed! However, periodic movements of sleep may also occur in association with the restless legs syndrome. Such patients complain not only of discomfort in the legs at rest or when trying to sleep, but also of periodic flexor leg jerks at the same time, and of disturbed night sleep due to these movements. This association of the restless legs syndrome and periodic movements of sleep is often familial, with a suggestion of autosomal dominant inheritance. The distressing symptoms are difficult to treat, but may be helped by clonazepam or baclofen, and Walters et al. (1986) have reported benefit from opiates.

STARTLE SYNDROMES

A pathological response to sudden unexplained noises or visual stimuli may cause patients to have a seizure (startle epilepsy) or to exhibit a massive generalized body jerk without loss of consciousness (startle myoclonus). Both may cause the patient to drop to the floor, often with injury. Wilkins, Hallett and Wess (1986) have reviewed the basis of physiological and pathological startle reactions.

The normal response to a sudden unexpected noise such as a pistol shot is invariably a bilateral blink (latency 30–50 ms), often with neck flexion (55–85 ms) and sometimes limb movements (arms 85–100 ms, legs 100–140 ms). Whether there is an associated initial electroencephalographic correlate of this startle response is uncertain. Repetition of the stimulus leads to rapid habituation. Animal experiments suggest that the physiological startle response is of brainstem origin, perhaps originating in the nucleus reticularis pontis caudalis and transmitted to bulbar and spinal motoneurones by way of reticulobulbar and reticulospinal pathways.

Pathological startle syndromes may either be due to exaggeration of normal startle responses at their usual latencies, or to the appearance of pathological startle response at different timings. The syndrome of hyperekplexia appears to fall into the latter category. Familial hyperekplexia (Suhren, Bruyn and Tuynman, 1966) is dominated by sudden muscle spasms provoked by external stimuli, often leading to falls to the ground without loss of consciousness. Affected individuals are abnormal from an early age, with infantile hypertonia and hyper-reflexia, and the development of a wide-based stiff gait. The latencies of muscle responses to sudden loud noise in those patients are shorter than those of the normal startle response.

Problems in the dyskinesias

The startles may be helped by clonazepam. In our experience, sporadic cases of this disorder are more common than familial examples.

Exaggeration of the physiological startle response is also encountered. In such cases, the response is greater and fails to habituate. Such a condition may be seen in some with epilepsy, or diffuse brain damage.

The relation of startle diseases to the various syndromes of jumping described in Maine and Quebec, latah in Malaysia, and myriachit in Siberia is discussed by Andermann and Andermann (1986).

References

ANDERMANN, F. and ANDERMANN, E. (1986) Excessive startle syndromes: Startle disease, jumping and startle epilepsy. In *Myoclonus*. Eds. S. Fahn, C. D. Marsden and M. Van Woert, pp. 321–328. New York: Raven Press

BRESSMAN, S. and FAHN, S. (1986) Essential myoclonus. In *Myoclonus*. Eds. S. Fahn, C. D. Marsden and M. Van Woert, pp. 287–294. New York: Raven Press

BRESSMAN, S., FAHN, S., EISENBERG, M., BRIN, M. and MALTESE, W. (1986) Biotin-responsive encephalopathy with myoclonus, ataxia and seizures. In *Myoclonus*. Eds. S. Fahn, C. D. Marsden and M. Van Woert, pp. 119–125. New York: Raven Press

CASEY, D. E., CHASE, T. N., CHRISTENSEN, A. V. and GERLACH, J. (Eds) (1985) Dyskinesia: research and treatment. *Psychopharmacology Supplementum* **2**, 1–230

FAHN, S., MARSDEN, C. D. and VAN WOERT, M. (Eds) (1986) *Advances in Neurology*, Vol. 43, *Myoclonus*. New York: Raven Press

HOPKINS, L. C. and ROSING, H. S. (1986) Myoclonus and Mitochondrial myopathy. In *Myoclonus*. Eds. S. Fahn., C. D. Marsden and M. Van Woert, pp. 105–117. New York: Raven Press

JESTE, D. V. and WYATT, R. J. (1982) *Understanding and Treating Tardive Dyskinesias*. New York: Guilford Press

KOSKINIEMI, M. L. (1986) Baltic myoclonus. In *Myoclonus*. Eds. S. Fahn, C. D. Marsden and M. Van Woert, pp. 57–64. New York: Raven Press

KUHL, D. E., PHELPS, M. E., MARKHAM, C. H., METTER, E. J., RIEGE, W. H. and WINTER, J. (1982) Cerebral metabolism and atrophy in Huntington's disease determined by ^{18}FDG and computed tomographic scan. *Annals of Neurology,* **12**, 425–434

LU, C-S., THOMPSON, P. D., QUINN, N. P., PARKES, J. D. and MARSDEN, C. D. (1986) Ramsay Hunt syndrome and coeliac disease: A new association. *Movement Disorders* (in press).

LUGARESI, E., CIRIGNOTTA, F., COCCAGNA, G. and MONTAGNA, P. (1986) Nocturnal myoclonus and restless legs syndrome. In *Myoclonus*. Eds. S. Fahn, C. D. Marsden and M. Van Woert, pp. 295–307. New York: Raven Press

MARTIN, J. B. (1984) Huntington's disease: New approaches to an old problem. *Neurology,* **34**, 1059–1072

SUCHOWERSKY, O., HAYDEN, M. R., MARTIN, W. R. W., STOESSL, A. J., HILDE-BRAND, A. M. and PATE, B. D. (1986) Cerebral metabolism of glucose in benign hereditary chorea. *Movement Disorders,* **1**, 33–44

SUHREN, O., BRUYN, G. W. and TUYNMAN, J. A. (1966) Hyperekplexia. A hereditary startle syndrome. *Journal of the Neurological Sciences,* **3**, 577–605

WALTERS, A., HENNING, W., COTE, L. and FAHN, S. (1986) Dominantly inherited restless legs with myoclonus and periodic movements of sleep: A syndrome related to the endogenous opiates. In *Myoclonus*. Eds. S. Fahn, C. D. Marsden and M. Van Woert, pp. 309–319. New York: Raven Press

WILKINS, D. E., HALLETT, M. and WESS, M. (1986) Audiogenic startle reflex of man and its relationship to startle syndromes. A review. *Brain,* **109**, 561–573

16
The anatomical and physiological basis of torsion dystonia
John C. Rothwell and Jose A. Obeso

INTRODUCTION

Torsion dystonia is characterized by sustained and forceful muscle contractions which twist the body and/or limbs into characteristic postures. Attempted voluntary movement exacerbates the dystonia, producing an 'overflow' of activity to distant muscles during action (Oppenheim, 1911; Foerster, 1921). Tendon jerks are normal and in spite of abnormal muscle activity most patients with dystonia are capable of carrying out a wide variety of voluntary movements with reasonable accuracy (Rothwell et al., 1983).

The term 'dystonia' (used alone, without the prefix 'torsion') sometimes has been used in a more general sense to describe any fixed abnormal posture (Denny-Brown, 1968). Such conditions include decerebrate rigidity, spastic dystonia following lesions of the corticospinal motor pathways and the flexion dystonia of Parkinson's disease. However, torsion dystonia as defined above is quite distinct from any of these phenomena. Patients with torsion dystonia may also show characteristics of other movement disorders in addition to dystonia. Examples of these are the rapid, shock-like muscle jerks of 'myoclonic dystonia' (Obeso et al., 1983), repetitive and rhythmic muscle contractions for which the term myorhythmia may be apt (Herz, 1944) and postural tremor of the limbs (Yanigasawa and Goto, 1971).

Torsion dystonia is a syndrome which may be divided aetiologically into primary (or idiopathic) and secondary forms (Fahn and Eldridge, 1976). Idiopathic torsion dystonia may be hereditary or sporadic. The hereditary form usually starts in childhood, first affecting one leg and later spreading to involve all four limbs and trunk (generalized dystonia). Sporadic forms include the focal primary dystonias (writer's cramp, torticollis, blepharospasm etc.) of adult onset which are often non-progressive and are usually limited to adjacent muscle groups (segmental dystonia). Hemidystonia is very often secondary to a focal brain lesion or cerebral hemi-atrophy (Marsden et al., 1985; Pettigrew and Jankovic, 1985).

The biochemical and pathological basis of primary torsion dystonia is as yet unknown. Response to drug therapy is very variable from one patient to another, so that pharmacological studies have given few clues as to possible biochemical mechanism(s) of the disease. There has been no detailed biochemical analysis of brains from patients with idiopathic torsion dystonia which might reveal any underlying biochemical pathology. In this chapter the available data on the anatomical and neurophysiological basis of dystonia are discussed.

PATHOLOGICAL ANATOMY

Torsion dystonia generally is considered to be a disease of the basal ganglia but the evidence is rather sparse and relatively recent. The reason for this is that conventional pathological studies have found no definite abnormality in brains of patients with generalized idiopathic torsion dystonia (Zeeman and Dyken, 1968). Distinctive brain damage is seen in patients with generalized dystonia secondary to other pathological conditions, such as Wilson's disease, 'état marbré' following birth anoxia or carbon monoxide intoxication. However, the damage often is not restricted to the basal ganglia. In these instances, dystonia might have been caused by damage to other non-basal ganglia structures. Cases of focal idiopathic torsion dystonia which have been studied pathologically are very rare in the literature. Garcia-Albea *et al.* (1981) reported normal findings in their study of a patient with cranial dystonia (Meige's disease). However, Altrocchi and Forno (1983), who also studied a patient with cranial dystonia, found neuronal cell loss and severe gliosis with a mosaic pattern distribution, limited to the dorsal halves of the caudate and putamen. Recently, the authors had the chance to carry out a detailed pathological analysis (unpublished), including cell counts and immunochemistry, of an adult patient with hereditary focal (hand) dystonia of late onset. No abnormality was demonstrated.

In order to establish the anatomo-pathological basis of dystonia, the authors therefore turned to the study of patients with focal or hemidystonia which was identical clinically to that seen in patients with idiopathic torsion dystonia, but in whom CT scan or pathological study had revealed a single focal lesion affecting discrete zones of the brain (Marsden *et al.*, 1985). In this chapter previous data have been expanded by including examples from a selected number of similar cases reported in the literature.

Anatomical basis of symptomatic focal and hemidystonia

The main characteristics of nine patients reported in the literature who had pathologically verified focal brain lesions are summarized in *Table 16.1*. The most recently published case, an eight-year-old boy with a low grade astrocytoma (Narbona *et al.*, 1984), is particularly illustrative. For a few months, dystonia was limited to the left forearm and hand during action, and spread later to the arm and foot when walking. *Figure 16.1* (top) shows the tumour with damage mainly to the right inferolateral putamen, although perivascular tumour infiltration was also detected in the globus pallidus, hypothalamus, and roof of the third ventricle (*Figure 16.1* (bottom)). The case is interesting in that it may reveal a correlation between the topography of the lesion and the distribution of dystonia. Animal data show that there is a gross somatotrophic arrangement of input to the putamen such that the leg area is anterodorsal, the face area postero-inferior and the arm area in the middle (Kunzle, 1975). This organization roughly coincides with the distribution of dystonia in this patient and the topography of the lesion. In the other

Table 16.1 Discrete focal lesions causing dystonia studied pathologically in the literature

Author	Type of dystonia	Aetiology	Thalamus	Topography int. capsule	Striatum	Globus pallidus
Steck (1921)	Left hand	Cystic lesion	No	No	Right putamen	No
Bouttier, Bertrand and Marie (1922)	Left forearm and hand, fixed dystonia	Fibroma	Right posterolateral	No	No	No
Urechia, Dragomir and Usinievia (1942)	Right hemidystonia	Glioblastoma	No	No	Left lenticular and caudate	
Barraquer-Bordas and van Bogaert (1954)	Left hand, mobile dystonia	Tuberculoma	Right ventrolateral	Yes	No	External segment
Garcin (1955)	Left hand	Infarction	Right posterolateral	No	No	No
Lopez-Aydillo and Sanz-Ibanez (1956)	Left forearm and hand, mobile dystonia	Infarction	No	No	Right putamen and head of caudate	No
Denny-Brown (1962)	Right hemidystonia mobile	Infarction	Atrophy on left side	No	Left two-thirds putamen; one-third caudate	No
Oppenheimer (1967)	Left fixed hemidystonia	Infarction	No	No	Right putamen and body of caudate	No
Narbona et al. (1984)	Left hemidystonia	Glioma	No	No	Right inferolateral putamen	External segment

Figure 16.1 Top, coronal section at the level of the mamillary body studied by Narbona *et al.* (1984). An area of cystic necrosis in the inferolateral region of the putamen and infiltration of the surrounding area is shown. A small tumoral mass also can be seen in the right hypothalamus. Bottom, reconstruction of the histological distribution of the tumour in coronal sections at the level of the anterior commissure (left) and infundibulum (right). The white area indicates cystic necrosis. The solid black corresponds to solid tumour and dotted black zones indicate perivascular infiltration. (Reproduced from Narbona *et al.*, 1984, with permission)

cases of *Table 16.1*, lesions were found in the putamen, caudate and the ventralis posterolateralis thalamic nucleus, but precise clinicopathological correlation was not attempted.

Cases lacking pathological correlation but with CT scan evidence of focal brain lesions are summarized in *Table 16.2*. Since it is difficult to distinguish the boundaries of lesions affecting the putamen and the globus pallidus in CT scans,

Table 16.2 Clinicopathological correlation in 21 patients with discrete focal lesions demonstrated by CT scan

Type of dystonia	Topography		
	Lenticular	Caudate	Thalamus
Hemidystonia	10	2	1
Arm	1	0	0
Hand	1	0	3
Torticollis	0	3	0

Figure 16.2 Dystonic posture of the left arm (*a*) secondary to a putamenal infarction shown in the CT scan (*b*)

these nuclei are combined in the table as the lentiform nucleus. Only cases with well-defined, very small lesions have been included. Patients with limb or hemidystonia secondary to relatively large caudo-capsulolenticular lesions were omitted.

The aetiology of the lesion was infarction (13 cases), arteriovenous malformation (6 cases), and haemorrhage (2 cases). More than half the patients included in *Table 16.2* had a lesion of the lentiform nucleus, mainly producing hemidystonia. In nine of these patients the putamen was thought to be predominantly (or exclusively) involved (*Figure 16.2*), but only one example of a lesion of the globus pallidus sparing the putamen has been found (case No. 7 of Pettigrew and Jankovic, 1985). Focal lesions of the caudate or posterolateral thalamic nuclei also produced dystonia in an important proportion of patients (*Figure 16.3*).

As with the pathological material, it is difficult to establish any precise correlation between the topography of a lesion and the type of dystonia. However, it is interesting to note that in three patients with torticollis there was a lesion in the ipsilateral head of the caudate nucleus and in four of six patients with hand dystonia a thalamic lesion was present. It is also of note that neither in the authors' own series (Marsden *et al.*, 1985) nor in the literature is there a case of limb(s) or generalized dystonia secondary to an isolated cortical lesion. There is only a single report of a patient with torticollis following head trauma, which disappeared after resection of a frontal cortical scar (David, Hecaen and Constans, 1952). Well-localized brainstem lesions have not been found in association with dystonia, except in Jankovic and Patel's (1983) cases of blepharospasm in patients with upper brainstem lesions.

Bilateral lenticular lesions (particularly putamenal), with relative sparing of other brain areas, have sometimes been associated with generalized dystonia in patients with presumed Leigh's disease (Burton *et al.*, 1984; Gallego *et al.*, 1986), and infantile striatal necrosis (Goutiere and Aicardi, 1982). Pallidal necrosis with minimal cortical damage has been reported in a few patients with carbon monoxide intoxication (Denny-Brown, 1962). These bilateral lesions typically produced a flexion posture of the upper limb, and extension of the lower limb, accompanied by rigidity.

In summary, the available data indicate that symptomatic dystonia may be produced by isolated lesions in the putamen, caudate, thalamus and globus pallidus (rarely) or their connecting pathways. This conclusion confirms previous suggestions that lesions of the striatum with sparing of the globus pallidus are the primary cause of symptomatic dystonia (Dooling and Adams, 1975). We believe that detailed neurochemical analysis of the putamen in patients with idiopathic torsion dystonia may yield essential information as to the biochemical pathology of dystonia and provide a rational basis for its drug therapy.

PHYSIOLOGICAL STUDIES IN TORSION DYSTONIA

Conventional electrophysiological investigations have revealed no abnormalities in patients with idiopathic torsion dystonia. EMG, nerve conduction, EEG, and evoked potential studies are all normal. Using the new technique of high voltage stimulation of the human brain through the intact scalp (Merton and Morton, 1980) the authors have also been able to extend this to examine corticospinal tract function in dystonia. Central conduction times for biceps and thenar muscle

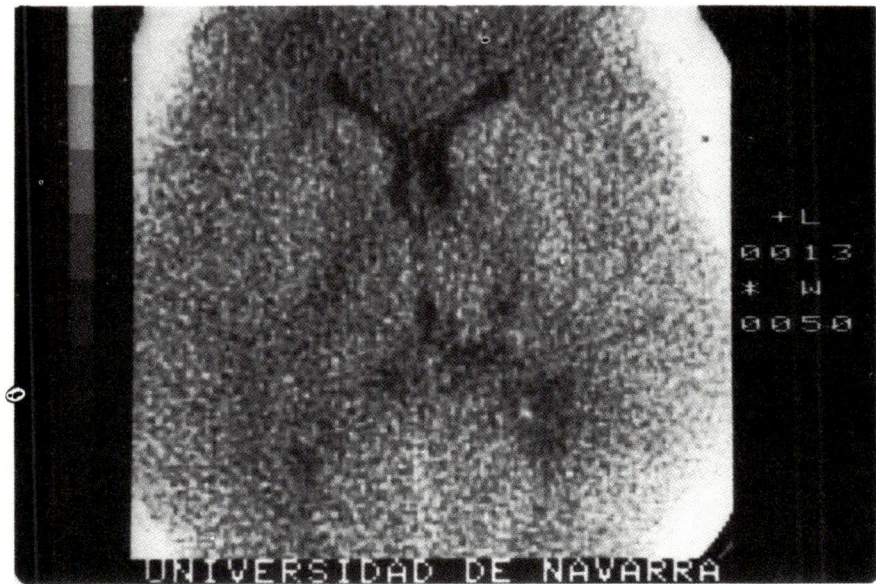

Figure 16.3 Top: action dystonia of the left hand. Bottom: CT scan without contrast showing a small, low-density, lesion in right posterolateral thalamic nucleus. (Reproduced from Marsden *et al.*, 1985, with permission)

Table 16.3 Corticospinal tract latencies in dystonia

	Normals (n=10)	Dystonic (n=5)
Cortex-biceps	10.0 ± 0.8	10.0 ± 0.8
Cortex-thenar	19.6 ± 1.0	19.0 ± 1.2

Values (in ms) are mean ± 1 s.d.

activation were assessed by subtracting the latency of muscle activation produced by segmental stimulation over the spinal cord from that seen following stimulation of the scalp over the motor cortex. *Table 16.3* shows that conduction times in patients with dystonia were the same as those in normal individuals. This suggests that large diameter corticospinal tract axons are functioning normally. In addition to these conventional techniques, there are several more specialized physiological techniques now available which shed some light on the possible pathophysiological mechanisms involved in dystonia.

EMG patterns in dystonia

Rest

Polymyographic analysis has been performed in patients with torsion dystonia of the limbs and trunk, torticollis and blepharospasm (Herz, 1944; Yanagisawa and Goto, 1971; Rothwell, Obeso and Marsden, 1983; Berardelli *et al.*, 1985). It confirms and extends the clinical impression of the muscle contractions referred to above. In mildly affected patients there is no involuntary muscle activity when at complete rest. In this state, the patients appear indistinguishable from normals. Moderately and severely affected individuals have continuous, involuntary muscle activity even during attempted complete relaxation, which disappears only during sleep. Characteristically this involuntary EMG activity does not follow the normal pattern of reciprocal innervation. Antagonist muscle groups at a joint are active simultaneously and the EMG is described as co-contracting.

Involuntary EMG activity in dystonia can be classified into three types, depending on the length of the EMG bursts:

(1) Almost continual spasms of muscle activity lasting many seconds and terminated by relatively short periods of silence (*Figure 16.4* (top)).
(2) Shorter (up to 2 s) EMG bursts, sometimes repetitive and rhythmical, separated by similar periods of silence (*Figure 16.4* (middle)). This pattern of EMG bursting was termed 'myorhythmia' by Herz in 1944.
(3) Brief (less than 500 ms) bursts of activity resembling those seen in myoclonus. The combination of relatively long spasms of EMG activity in some muscles, with brief myoclonic-like bursts in other muscles, is sometimes termed 'myoclonic dystonia' (*Figure 16.4* (bottom)).

This range of EMG patterns is seen in all forms of torsion dystonia. For example, patients with blepharospasm may have prolonged spasms of eye closure (type 1) or relatively regular, repetitive, but short-lasting bursts of closure (type 2) (Berardelli *et al.*, 1985). Similarly, eye closure in blepharospasm not only involves contraction of the agonist muscle, orbicularis oculi, but also of one of its antagonists, the frontalis muscle. Recording from the main muscle involved in eye opening, the elevator palpebrae, is extremely difficult because of the extreme thinness of the muscle and its location within the eyelid.

Figure 16.4 Three types of involuntary muscle activity in different individuals with generalized dystonia. Top: continuous periods of muscle activity lasting from 2 to 30 s. Middle: repetitive, rhythmical, and co-contracting spasms lasting only 1–2 s each ('myorhythmia'). Bottom: rapid, irregular and brief jerks lasting only some 100 ms. Muscles are left sternocleidomastoid (L.SCM), right biceps (R.Bic), triceps (Tri), wrist and finger flexors (FF) and wrist and finger extensors (FE). (From Rothwell, Obeso and Marsden, 1983, with permission)

Active

Any attempt at voluntary movement, either in sustaining a posture, such as standing, or performing some task with the hand and arms, exacerbates the number and severity of involuntary muscle spasms in all patients with dystonia. In mildly affected patients, dystonic contractions can be seen only when certain types of voluntary movement are made. The most striking examples of this are the occupational cramps, a form of focal dystonia (Marsden, 1976). A person with writer's cramp may be able to use his affected hand to feed and drink for himself. Excessive involuntary muscle activity only becomes noticeable in the performance of the most delicate manual tasks such as writing or typing or playing a musical instrument.

The excessive involuntary contractions (which are co-contracting in antagonist muscles like those seen at rest), appear in muscles that may normally be uninvolved in the task. The activity is sometimes described as 'overflow', suggesting that voluntary effort cannot be directed effectively to the appropriate muscle groups. However, despite excessive activity in some muscle groups, activity in the prime moving muscles sometimes may be relatively spared. For example, in all the patients who have been examined by the authors, even those with gross generalized dystonia, there has been alternating activity in flexor and extensor muscles during rapid waving of the wrist or elbow (*Figure 16.5*). Slower, or more delicate, movements, however, show relative degrees of inappropriate activity in antagonist muscles depending upon the severity of the patient's clinical symptoms.

Dystonia, therefore, is mainly characterized by excessive muscle activity, in spite of which patients can usually carry out a great variety of motor tasks. These clinical

Figure 16.5 Normal reciprocal activation of wrist flexors and extensors during waving (left), and resumption of typical co-contraction when the subject stops to pick up a pen and write his name (right). (From Rothwell, Obeso and Marsden, 1983, with permission)

observations indicate that patients with dystonia are perfectly capable of generating and conceiving the idea and motor plan to move, but either (a) the selection and/or quality of the motor programmes is abnormal, or (b) the physiological mechanism(s) responsible for executing motor programmes are altered. In the following section these possibilities are examined in the light of newer physiological techniques.

Specialized physiological investigations

In view of the constant existence of co-contraction and frequent observation of abnormal postures in patients with dystonia, abnormalities of the stretch reflex and reciprocal inhibition have been first considered as the possible pathophysiological basis of dystonia.

Stretch reflexes

Stretch reflexes have been examined in the flexor muscles of the thumb, wrist and elbow by two groups of workers (Rothwell, Obeso and Marsden, 1983; Tatton et al., 1984). The technique involves the subject exerting a constant background contraction of the appropriate flexor muscle against a small force offered by a low inertia electric motor. At irregular and random intervals, the force supplied by the motor is suddenly increased so as to extend the joint and stretch the flexor muscle. A reflex EMG response to the stretch can be recorded in averaged records beginning with a latency of some 20 ms or so following the disturbance. The response consists of two main components: the first is a short latency (or M1) response of about 20-ms duration which probably reflects activity in the same neuronal pathways as are responsible for the tendon jerk. The second part of the response, which has a latency of about 50 ms and a duration of 30–40 ms, is known as the long latency (or M2) component. It may represent activity traversing a transcortical (or long loop) reflex pathway.

Both Rothwell, Obeso and Marsden (1983) and Tatton et al. (1984) found that the sizes of both short and long latency components of the stretch reflex EMG response were within the normal range in patients with dystonia. Rothwell, Obeso and Marsden (1983) used relatively rapid muscle stretches and concluded that there was no change in the duration of either component of the reflex. Tatton et al. (1984), who used a much wider range of stretch velocities, found this to be true only at high velocities. At lower rates of stretch the duration of the long latency component of the EMG was prolonged in dystonic patients, even though its size remained within the normal range.

There is a further abnormality in the stretch reflex which is reminiscent of the EMG activity seen in attempted voluntary movements. In normal subjects, the stretch reflex activity is fairly well localized to the agonist and synergist muscles involved in the stretch. However, in dystonia, there is a conspicuous 'overflow' of reflex activity to muscles distant from the joint being studied (Rothwell, Obeso and Marsden, 1983).

Finally, stretch of one muscle will always be accompanied by passive shortening of the antagonist muscle. In normal individuals, this produces a reflex reduction in activity of the shortened muscle, at about the same latency as the agonist stretch reflex. However, in patients with dystonia, there is sometimes a paradoxical activation of the shortened antagonist muscle. This is particularly clear in the tibialis anterior muscle in the leg during passive dorsiflexion of the ankle. It is not so readily obtainable in muscles of the arm. This response is presumably the same as the shortening reaction (or Westphal's phenomenon) seen in the same muscle in patients with Parkinson's disease. In tibialis anterior, a small shortening reaction is sometimes seen even in normal individuals. The mechanism of the shortening reaction has been investigated in some detail (Berardelli and Hallett, 1984). Anaesthetic block of afferents in the stretched (triceps surae) muscle does not change the size of the reflex, so that afferents from the joint and/or the shortened muscle are thought to be involved. One possibility is the removal of some tonic Ib inhibitory influence from Golgi tendon organs when the muscle is shortened.

H-reflex studies

Although the tendon jerks and the M1 component of the stretch reflex are normal in dystonia, an abnormality has been described in the H-reflex recovery curve by Matsuoka *et al.* (1966). Using paired H-reflex testing with a stimulus intensity of 1.1 times the H-reflex threshold, there was a facilitation of the recovery curve from 100 ms onwards (phases IV and V) which was similar to that seen in Parkinson's disease and which is also seen in spastic patients. Such changes are not easy to interpret. The H-reflex recovery curve is believed to reflect activity in both spinal and supraspinal neuronal pathways. At present such 'changes in excitability curves signify only that the reactivity of interneuronal circuits is altered' (Delwaide, 1984).

Reciprocal inhibition

Some of the mechanisms responsible for reflex inhibition of antagonist muscles can be examined at rest in the flexor and extensor muscles of the forearm (Day *et al.*, 1984). Animal studies have suggested that two mechanisms operate to produce the normal reciprocal inhibition of antagonist muscles during voluntary activation of the agonist. These are shown in *Figure 16.6*. The descending command activates the agonist motoneurones and at the same time excites the group of Ia inhibitory interneurones within the grey matter of the spinal cord. These interneurones inhibit the motoneurones of the antagonist muscle. In addition to this, when movement begins, contraction of the agonist muscle, particularly during slow movements, may be accompanied by an increase in discharge from agonist muscle spindle afferents, due to alpha-gamma linkage. Activity in the primary afferent Ia fibres also feeds on to the spinal Ia inhibitory interneurone to produce further inhibition of the antagonist motoneurones. This latter action of the agonist spindle afferents can be referred to as peripheral antagonist inhibition, whilst the initial action of the descending command is known as central antagonist inhibition. Since the principal EMG deficit in dystonia is a lack of reciprocal inhibition, it is of some interest to investigate any possible abnormalities in the system.

In the relaxed arm, a single electrical stimulus given to the radial nerve at submotor threshold intensity will excite only the largest afferent fibres in the nerve. These are predominantly muscle afferents from the extensor muscles, together with a proportion of large diameter cutaneous afferents from the back of the forearm.

Physiological studies in torsion dystonia 325

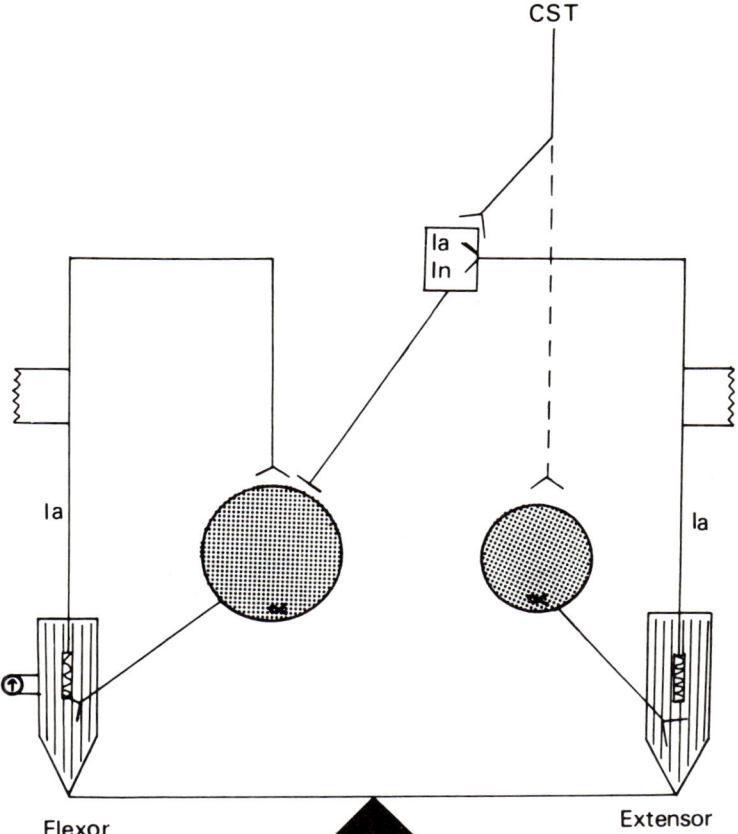

Figure 16.6 Diagrammatic summary of the central and peripheral components of reciprocal inhibition. Both the direct corticospinal tract (CST) projection to the extensor muscles of the wrist (central inhibition) and the Ia afferent fibres from extensor muscle spindles (peripheral inhibition) send branches to the Ia inhibitory interneurones (IaIN) of the spinal cord. These then project monosynaptically to inhibit the flexor motoneurone pool. The excitability of the α-motoneurones can then be tested by eliciting H-reflexes in flexor muscles at different times after a conditioning shock has been applied to the extensor afferents in the radial nerve. (From Rothwell, Obeso and Marsden, 1983, with permission)

Any inhibition directed towards the flexor muscles can be detected with monosynaptic testing, using H-reflexes in the forearm flexor muscles. The experimental arrangement is, therefore, to give a single submotor threshold conditioning stimulus to the radial nerve in the spinal groove. At different times before and after this conditioning volley, a single submotor threshold stimulus is given to the median nerve in the cubital fossa to elicit monosynaptic H-reflexes in the flexor muscles in the forearm. By comparing the size of a series of conditioned flexor H-reflexes with the size of control H-reflexes obtained without a radial nerve shock, the depth of flexor inhibition can be calculated. *Figure 16.7* illustrates the technique and timing convention used.

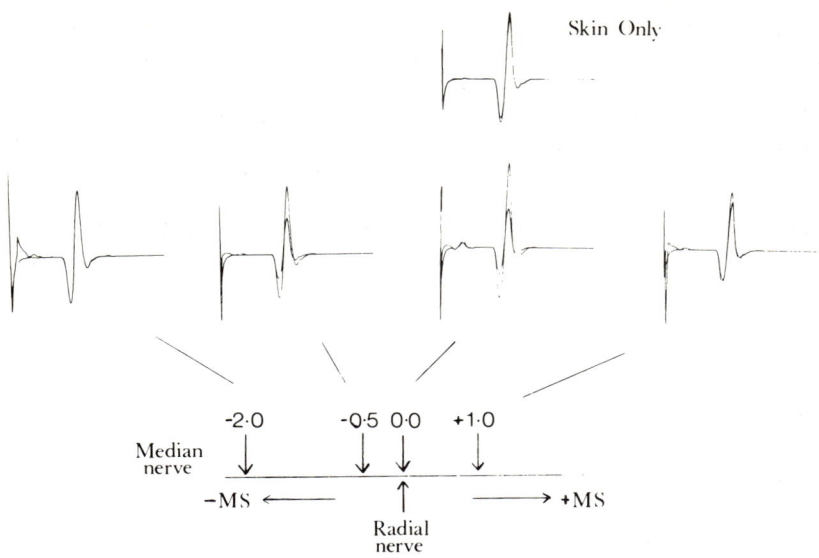

Figure 16.7 Summary of the timing convention used in testing reciprocal inhibition between the extensor and flexor muscles in the forearm. The occurrence of the median nerve test shock was expressed relative to that of the radial nerve conditioning shock (time line at bottom of the figure). Above the time line are some representative averages (10) of control and test H-reflexes from the forearm flexors of a normal subject, superimposed at four different time intervals. Maximum inhibition is seen at −0.5 and 0.0 ms. If the conditioning radial nerve test shock is applied to the surrounding skin alone, then no effect is seen on the flexor H-reflex (top traces). (From Rothwell, Obeso and Marsden, 1983, with permission)

If the radial and median nerve stimuli are given at about the same time, the radial nerve volley evokes a strong (>50%) inhibition of the flexor H-reflex. Previous studies have suggested very strongly (Day *et al.*, 1984) that this inhibition is produced via the classical disynaptic Ia reciprocal inhibitory pathway in the spinal cord. This period of inhibition lasts only some 2–4 ms, but is followed by two equally deep but much longer lasting phases of inhibition from about 10 to 40 ms and 60 to 500 (or more) ms. The mechanisms responsible for these later phases of inhibition are unclear at present. However, they can be evoked in the forearm muscles by submotor threshold stimuli of the radial nerve, suggesting that the same large diameter afferents are responsible as for the disynaptic phase of inhibition. It has been suggested (Berardelli *et al.*, 1985) that, in the arm, the later phases of inhibition in the H-reflex testing curve are produced by presynaptic influences on the terminals of the flexor Ia afferents. The reason for this is that only the early and short-lasting disynaptic inhibition can be seen in the EMG if the flexor muscles are activated by a descending voluntary command rather than by H-reflex testing. The same is true if high voltage cortical stimulation is used to activate corticospinal inputs to the motoneurone: radial nerve stimulation fails to evoke late periods of inhibition of cortically evoked flexor activity (Berardelli *et al.*, 1985). Presynaptic inhibition might therefore be directed preferentially to the Ia terminals from peripheral receptors and not to the terminals of descending tracts from the brain.

Testing reciprocal inhibition between forearm muscles with this technique reveals no abnormality of the early disynaptic inhibition in idiopathic torsion dystonia. However, the later phases of inhibition are greatly reduced, and there is a period of frank excitation at 50 ms or so (*Figure 16.8*). We have also been able to confirm that the reciprocal inhibition curve shows similar abnormalities in a patient with symptomatic hemidystonia secondary to an arteriovenous malformation in the basal ganglia.

Unfortunately we are uncertain of the mechanism underlying this change in peripheral reciprocal inhibition. It is tempting to suggest that it represents a

Figure 16.8 Time course of first (top) and later (bottom) phases of reciprocal inhibition in eight normal (continuous line) and eight dystonic (dotted line) subjects. Average values are plotted ± 1 s.e. There is no difference between normal and dystonic subjects in the first (disynaptic) phase of reciprocal inhibition. However, the second phase of inhibition (from 10 to 50 ms) is much reduced in the patients

decrease in the effectiveness of presynaptic inhibitory mechanisms in the spinal cord. However, it is equally possible that, in dystonia, the radial nerve stimulation produces some excess of excitation from some other source which obscures the normal reciprocal inhibitory curve at 50 ms or so.

'BALLISTIC' MOVEMENTS AT A SINGLE JOINT

Abnormalities of movement control in dystonia are described clinically in terms of difficulties with complex movements such as writing, eating or walking. Such movements are made up of many subunits, the timing and scaling of which must be carefully controlled to produce an accurate outcome. From the physiological viewpoint errors might therefore arise from defects in (*a*) the production of the simple subunits of each complex task, (*b*) the relative timing of the subunits or (*c*) the relative amplitudes of the units. The study of ballistic single joint movements provides a method of analysing the simple subunits which might be involved in more complex tasks.

Rapid limb movements from one position to another are characterized in man by a bi- or triphasic pattern of EMG activity in antagonist muscles acting about the joint. There is an initial burst of activity in the agonist muscle, which provides the propulsive force for the movement. This is followed by a burst of activity in the antagonist muscle, which serves to halt the movement at the appropriate position. The relative size, duration and timing of these bursts of EMG activity is remarkably precise and adjusted carefully to the speed and amplitude of the required movement. The EMG pattern can even be observed in deafferented patients (Hallett, Shahani and Young, 1975; Rothwell *et al.*, 1982), indicating its independence of afferent feedback. Thus study of this type of movement can provide insights into how the brain executes internally planned movements.

In the authors' own experiments patients with dystonia affecting the arm were asked to make rapid elbow extension or flexion movements through an angle of 10–60° as rapidly as possible in their own time. One of the surprising findings of this study was that, despite their clinical difficulties, almost all the patients were able to perform the task. Most patients could perform movements of different amplitudes when required, although their accuracy was more variable than usual. However, the EMG pattern responsible for the movement often showed differences from normal. There was a wide range of variation in the pattern of muscle activity, ranging from normal to unrecognizable. In the most severely affected patients the EMG bursts tended to be longer than normal and there was often inappropriate co-contraction of the antagonist, rather than the precisely timed burst seen in normals. In addition, recording from other muscles of the arm, usually used as fixators or synergists, reveals that, in many patients with dystonia, there is an 'overflow' of EMG activity. Whereas in normal subjects postural and fixator muscles are activated briefly at the same time as the prime movers, in dystonia there is a tendency for there to be excessive and prolonged activity in the same muscles (*Figure 16.9*). Such observations suggest that, even in the simplest of movements about a single joint, errors in size and timing of muscle activity are present, as seen when more complex movements are performed.

Figure 16.9 Average (of eight) position, velocity and rectified EMG traces recorded during a rapid, self-paced elbow flexion through 30 degrees. Data are from a patient with segmental dystonia affecting the neck and right arm (left-hand traces), and a normal subject (right-hand traces). Muscles are biceps (Bic), triceps (Tri), wrist and finger flexor (FF) and extensor (FE) muscles, pectoralis major (PM) and anterior deltoid (Delt). Note the co-contracting pattern of EMG activity in the prime moving muscles, biceps and triceps, and the massive 'overflow' to the postural fixators, pectoralis and deltoid in the patient

CONCLUSIONS

A general feature of all the physiological tests described above is a lack of inhibition (or excess excitation) in both reflex and voluntary movement. There is an increase in duration of both the long latency stretch reflex, and the first burst of agonist EMG activity in ballistic arm movements. There is excessive co-contraction of antagonist muscles during voluntary movement, and abnormalities in the time course of reciprocal inhibition between wrist flexors and extensors. There is overflow of activity to non-prime moving muscles in both voluntary and reflex movements and the shortening reaction is enhanced.

Even though the physiological deficits seen in these tests are very similar, it is unlikely that they result from abnormalities at a low level of the motor system. This conclusion rests on clinical observation. In many patients with dystonia there are muscles usually involved in dystonic spasms which can, on occasion, be activated almost normally. The extreme example is dystonic writer's cramp where the muscles of the forearm and hand may be well controlled in many tasks, but produce a dystonic posture when the patient attempts to write. At the other extreme are patients with generalized dystonia who may be unable to walk forwards, but can run, climb stairs or walk backwards relatively easily. Indeed, one young man with generalized dystonia, studied by the authors, was unable to stand or walk without assistance yet could drive his own car and shoot with remarkable accuracy on the local pistol range. If the deficit in dystonia lay at a low level in the CNS, then one would expect it to be evident in all types of movement. Since this is not the case, we must assume that dystonia represents a high-level disorder of movement control.

The conclusion is consistent with the anatomical findings of damage to structures of the basal ganglia. The major output of the striopallidal complex ends, via the thalamus, in the supplementary motor area. Stereotaxic surgery causing lesions of the ventrolateral thalamic nuclei may sometimes ameliorate dystonia. This suggests that the erroneous selection and modulation of motor programmes occurring in dystonia may arise as a consequence of inappropriate information being delivered to the supplementary motor cortex. Why the same apparent lesion of the basal ganglia may produce different types of dystonia or even no motor disturbance at all is still unresolved. Equally obscure is the frequently observed time-delay between the cerebral insult responsible for a basal ganglia lesion and the final appearance of dystonia. Prospective studies, with detailed clinical analysis of motor function, are needed to correlate different types of dystonia, with the topography and evolution of lesions recognized by CT and NMR scan.

References

ALTROCCHI, P. H. and FORNO, L. S. (1983) Spontaneous oro-facial dyskinesia: neuropathology of a case. *Neurology*, **33**, 802–805

BARRAQUER-BORDAS, L. and VAN BOGAERT, L. (1954) Sur l'evolution tardive de certaines hemiplegie cerebrales infantiles. *Monatsschrift fuer Psychiatrie und Neurologie*, **127**, 31–39

BERARDELLI, A., DAY, B. L., MARSDEN, C. D. and ROTHWELL, J. C. (1985). Observations on the mechanism of long-lasting reciprocal inhibition in the human forearm. *Journal of Physiology*, **365**, 24P

BERARDELLI, A. and HALLETT, M. (1984) Shortening reaction of tibialis anterior. *Neurology*, **34**, 242–246

BERARDELLI, A., ROTHWELL, J. C., DAY, B. L. and MARSDEN, C. D. (1985) Pathophysiology of blepharospasm and oromandibular dystonia. *Brain*, **108**, 593–608

BOUTTIER, H., BERTRAND, I. and MARIE, A. P. (1922) Sur un cas anatomo-clinique de syndrome thelamique dissocie. *Revue Neurologique*, **38**, 1492–1502

BURTON, K., FARRELL, J., LI, D. and CALNE, D. B. (1984) Lesions of the putamen and dystonia: CT and magnetic resonance imaging. *Neurology*, **34**, 962–965

DAVID, M., HECAEN, H. and CONSTANS, J. (1952) Torticollis spasmodique consecutif a une lesion corticale traumatique. Discussion de resultat favorable obtenu apres excision de la lesion corticale. *Revue Neurologique*, **86**, 57–61

DAY, B. L., MARSDEN, C. D., OBESO, J. A. and ROTHWELL, J. C. (1984) Reciprocal inhibition between the muscles of the human forearm. *Journal of Physiology*, **349**, 519–534

DELWAIDE, P. J. (1984) Contribution of human reflex studies to the understanding and management of the pyramidal syndrome. In *Electromyography in CNS Disorders*. Ed. by B. T. Shahani, pp. 77–110. London: Butterworths

DENNY-BROWN, D. (1962) *The Basal Ganglia and their Relation to Disorders of Movement*. London: Oxford University Press

DENNY-BROWN, D. (1968) Clinical symptomatology of diseases of the basal ganglia. In *Handbook of Neurology*, Vol. 6. Ed. by P. J. Vinken and G. W. Bruyn, pp. 133–172. Amsterdam: North Holland

DOOLING, E. C. and ADAMS, R. D. (1975) The pathological anatomy of posthemiplegic athetosis. *Brain*, **98**, 29–48

FAHN, S. and ELDRIDGE, R. (1976) Definitions of dystonia and classification of the dystonic states. *Advances in Neurology*, **14**, 1–5

FOERSTER, O. (1921) Zur analyse and pathophysiologie der striaren Bewegungstorungen. *Zeitschrift für de Gesamte Neurologie und Psychiatrie*, **73**, 1–169

GALLEGO, J., OBESO, A., DELGADO, G. and VILLAMURA, J. A. (1986) Enfermedad de Leigh con distonia de torsion como unica manifestacions clinica. *Archives de Neurobiologia* (in press)
GARCIA-ALBEA, E., FRANCH, O., MUNOZ, D. and RICAY, J. R. (1981) Breughel's syndrome: report of a case with post-mortem studies. *Journal of Neurology, Neurosurgery and Psychiatry*, **44**, 437–440
GARCIN, R. (1955) Syndrome cerebello-thalamique par lesion localisee du thalamus. *Revue Neurologique*, **93**, 143–149
GOUTIERE, F. and AICARDI, J. (1982) Acute neurological dysfunction associated with destructive lesions of the basal ganglia in children. *Annals of Neurology*, **12**, 328–332
HALLETT, M., SHAHAMI, B. T. and YOUNG, R. R. (1975) EMG analysis of stereotyped voluntary movements in man. *Journal of Neurology, Neurosurgery and Psychiatry*, **38**, 1154–1162
HERZ, E. (1944) Dystonia I. Historical review; analysis of dystonic symptoms and physiological mechanisms. *Archives of Neurology and Psychiatry*, **51**, 305–318
JANKOVIC, J. and PATEL, S. C. (1983) Blepharospasm associated with brainstem lesions. *Neurology*, **33**, 1237–1240
KUNZLE, H. (1975) Bilateral projections from precentral motor cortex to the putamen and other parts of the basal ganglia. An autoradiographic study in Macaca fasicularis. *Brain Research*, **88**, 195–210
LOPEZ AYDILLO, N. R. and SANZ-IBANEZ, I. (1956) A proposito de un caso de distonia de torsion (variente miostatica o paralitica) en una diabetica glucosurica. *Trabajos de Instituto Cajal de Investigaciones Biologicas*, **48**, 81–108
MARSDEN, C. D. (1976) The problem of adult-onset idiopathic torsion dystonia and other isolated dyskinesias in adult life (including blepharospasm, oromandibular dystonia, dystonic writers' cramp, torticollis and axial dystonia). *Advances in Neurology*, **14**, 259–276
MARSDEN C. D., OBESO, J. A., ZARRANZ, J. J. and LANG, A. E. (1985) The anatomical basis of symptomatic hemidystonia. *Brain*, **108**, 463–483
MATSUOKA, S., WALTZ, J. M., TERADA, C., IKEDA, T. and COOPER, I. S. (1966) A computer technique for evaluation of recovery cycle of the H-reflex in abnormal movement disorders. *Electroencephalography and Clinical Neurophysiology*, **21**, 496–500
MERTON, P. A. and MORTON, H. B. (1980) Stimulation of the cerebral cortex in the intact human subject. *Nature*, **285**, 227
NARBONA, J., OBESO, J. A., TUNON, T., MARTINEZ-LAGE, J. M. and MARSDEN, C. D. (1984) Hemi-dystonia secondary to a localised basal ganglia tumour. *Journal of Neurology, Neurosurgery and Psychiatry*, **47**, 707–709
OBESO, J. A., ROTHWELL, J. C., LANG, A. E. and MARSDEN, C. D. (1983) Myoclonic dystonia. *Neurology*, **33**, 825–830
OPPENHEIM, H. (1911) Uber eine ergenartige Krampfkrankheit des Kindlichen und jugendlichen Alters (Dystonia tardotica progressiva, Dystonia musculorum deformans). *Neurologisches Zentralblatt*, **30**, 1090–1107
OPPENHEIMER, D. R. (1967) A case of striatal hemiplegia. *Journal of Neurology, Neurosurgery and Psychiatry*, **30**, 134–139
PETTIGREW, L. C. and JANKOVIC, J. (1985) Hemidystonia: a report of 22 patients and a review of the literature. *Journal of Neurology, Neurosurgery and Psychiatry*, **48**, 650–657
ROTHWELL, J. C., OBESO, A. and MARSDEN, C. D. (1983) Pathophysiology of dystonias. In *Advances in Neurology*, Vol. 39. Ed. by J. E. Desmedt, pp. 851–863. New York: Raven Press
ROTHWELL, J. C., TRAUB, M. M., DAY, B. L., OBESO, J. A., THOMAS, P. K. and MARSDEN, C. D. (1982) Manual motor performance in a deafferented man. *Brain*, **105**, 515–542
STECK, H. (1921) Zur pathologischen Anatomie der echten posthemipegischen athetose. *Schweizer Archiv für Neurologie und Psychiatrie*, **8**, 75–83
TATTON, W. G., REDINGHAM, W., VERRIER, M. C. and BLAIR, R. D. G. (1984) Characteristic alterations in responses to imposed wrist displacements in parkinsonian rigidity and dystonia musculorum deformans. *Canadian Journal of the Neurological Sciences*, **11**, 281–287
URECHIA, C.-I., DRAGOMIR, L. and USINIEVIA, G. (1942) Spasme de torsion unilateral cause par une tumeur cerebrale. *Confinia Neurologica*, **5**, 271–280
YANAGISAWA, N. and GOTO, A. (1971) Dystonia musculorum deformans. *Journal of Neurological Science*, **13**, 39–65
ZEEMAN, W. and DYKEN, P. (1968) Dystonia musculorum deformans. In *Handbook of Neurology*, Vol. 6. Ed. by P. J. Vinken and G. W. Bruyn, pp. 517–543. Amsterdam: North Holland

17
Classification and investigation of dystonia

Stanley Fahn, C. David Marsden and Donald B. Calne

INTRODUCTION

Oppenheim (1911) originally introduced and defined the term 'dystonia' in 1911 to indicate the 'muscle tone was hypotonic at one occasion and in tonic muscle spasm at another, usually but not exclusively elicited upon volitional movements'. Oppenheim was impressed with this variation in muscle tone seen in the neurological syndrome that had recently been described in the doctoral dissertation thesis of Schwalbe. Schwalbe (1908) described a family with three affected siblings, which he labelled 'chronic cramp syndrome with hysterical symptoms'. However, whereas Schwalbe, a psychiatric trainee, considered the problem to be due to psychological factors, Oppenheim, who described six new cases, disagreed and argued for an organic aetiology. Oppenheim, in addition to describing coexisting hypo- and hypertonia, noted other features in this syndrome. These were twisted postures associated with the muscle spasms and affecting limbs and trunk; bizarre walking with bending and twisting of the torso; rapid, sometimes rhythmic, jerking movements; and progression of symptoms leading eventually to sustained fixed postural deformities (for review of historical details, *see* Zeman (1976) and Fahn (1984)).

Oppenheim used two different names for this syndrome, each emphasizing different features. 'Dysbasia lordotica progressiva' was coined to describe the progressive nature of the disorder and the abnormal dromedary gait with twisted truncal posturing. 'Dystonia musculorum deformans' was designed to refer to the altering muscle tone and the ultimate postural deformities that develop with time. The latter term was adopted by the neurological community and has remained to this day. In the same year as Oppenheim's publication, Flatau and Sterling (1911) described two boys with the disorder, emphasizing not only its organic nature, but also that it is probably an inherited disease. They disagreed with the term 'dystonia' because they did not believe that altering muscle tone was the clinical hallmark of the condition. Rather, they emphasized torsion spasms, and suggested the name for the disorder be progressive torsion spasm. The influence of Oppenheim, a widely respected neurologist, prevailed and the term 'dystonia' was accepted. However, since it is not a disease of muscles and because not all patients necessarily progress to have fixed postural deformities (Marsden, 1976; Fahn and Jankovic, 1984), objections have been raised over the use of the term 'dystonia musculorum deformans' (Eldridge, 1970). Indeed, patients themselves may dislike the term because of the implication of deformity. Many neurologists have simply shortened the name to 'dystonia', and others use 'torsion dystonia' which emphasizes the twisting nature of the abnormal movements. Some use the term 'dystonia musculorum deformans' (DMD) to indicate childhood onset that has progressed to generalized dystonia. The definition of DMD will be more extensively discussed in the section on Classification.

Over the years, the term 'dystonia' has evolved to mean more than just abnormal muscle tone or fluctuations in muscle tone as originally used by Oppenheim. It has come to represent the specific neurological syndrome described by Oppenheim (1911), Flatau and Sterling (1911), and other neurologists of that period (for historical review, see Fahn (1984)). Moreover, the term is also used to describe the abnormal movements characteristically seen in this disorder. These abnormal movements are diverse, with a wide range in speed, amplitude, rhythmicity, torsion, forcefulness, distribution in the body, and relationship to rest or voluntary activity. Thus, 'dystonia' refers to both a neurological disorder (syndrome and disease entity) and to certain types of abnormal involuntary movements.

DEFINITIONS

Since the introduction of electromyographic analysis of dystonic movements (Herz, 1944), emphasis has been placed on sustained simultaneous contractions of agonists and antagonists in this syndrome (Yanagisawa and Goto, 1971; see Chapter 16). Clinically, emphasis on the types of abnormal movements that characterize this entity have varied widely over the years. Most authors noted the range of abnormal movements encountered, and prior to and after the introduction of the term 'dystonia', they used phrases such as tetanoid chorea, tic-like, myoclonia, tonic spasms, and myorhythmia to describe the types of abnormal movements present in this disorder (*Table 17.1*).

As the term 'dystonia' was adopted to identify the clinical entity, the definition originally coined by Oppenheim (1911) was no longer accepted. Flatau and Sterling (1911) did not consider alternating muscle tone to be the clinical hallmark of the disorder, and emphasized twisting sustained movements. Other authorities considered different aspects of the clinical features to be crucial for dystonia (*Table 17.2*). Herz (1944), from analysis of cinematographic and electromyographic recordings, regarded slow, sustained postures as the best definition for dystonia. Denny-Brown (1962) subsequently expanded upon this definition and defined dystonia as a fixed or relatively fixed attitude.

One problem with using only sustained postures for the definition of dystonia is that it allows all types of abnormal postures to be called dystonia. Another problem is that these definitions do not take into account the other types of abnormal movements seen in the disorder. Herz (1944) attempted to solve this problem by creating another term for the rapid rhythmical movements so commonly seen, and called this 'myorhythmia'. Clearly, the ideal definition of dystonia should (*a*) emphasize the type of sustained posture seen only in this disorder; (*b*) exclude all other fixed postures; (*c*) include other highly characteristic abnormal movements present in most patients with the condition. In order to adopt a useful and acceptable definition of 'dystonia', a committee (*Ad Hoc* Committee, 1984)

Table 17.1 Clinical descriptions of abnormal movements in torsion dystonia described by investigators before and after the introduction of the term 'dystonia' by Oppenheim (1911)

Year	Authors	Clinical characteristics emphasized	Terminology
1893	Gowers	Continued tonic spasms and attacks of more intense spasms	Tetanoid chorea
1901	Destarac	Sustained postures when sitting; spasms with specific action, including writer's cramp	Functional spasms; foot tic; gait cramp; clonic agitations
1903	Leszynsky	Abnormal posturing when walking	Hysterical gait
1908	Hunt	Rapid trunk movements	Myoclonia of the trunk
1908	Schwalbe	Truncal twisting; arms thrown behind back when walking	Maladie des tics; tonic cramps
1911	Ziehen	Twisting tonic leg spasms, lordosis, peculiar movements of arm	Torsion neurosis; chorea; athetosis
1911	Oppenheim	Sustained posturing, tonic and clonic spasms, activated by voluntary movement, dromedary gait, fluctuating muscle tone, rapid movements, tremor with writing	Dysbasia lordotica progressiva; dystonia musculorum deformans; clonic, rhythmic movements; tremor; mobile spasms; chronic chorea; athetosis
1911	Flatau and Sterling	Jerky movements of arms, increasing with voluntary motor activity, repetitive pattern	Tremor; hemiballism; choreic; progressive torsion spasms
1912	Fraenkel	Rapid, twisting and sustained movements	Tortipelvis
1916	Hunt	Slow, torsion, twisting spasms of trunk and extremities, more with active movements	Restlessness of chorea and athetosis; clonic rhythmic movements
1919	Mendel	Twisting axial postures	Torsion dystonia
1920	Taylor	Spasmodic sustained opisthotonus, violent twisting of the body	Choreic and athetoid
1922	Wechsler and Brock	Hyperkinetic form and a postural tonic form with rigidity, coarse rhythmic tremor	Kinetic form; myostatic form
1926	Davidenkow	Rapid movements, tic-like	Myoclonic dystonia
1940	Benedek and Rakonitz	Rapid movements	Myoclonic torsion dystonia
1940	Wilson	Waxing and waning, irregularly repetitive, rapid movements	Clonic or tic-like spasms, choreic and athetoid
1944	Herz	Slow, long-sustained turning movements; rapid involuntary movements; alternating with flexion and extension	Dystonia; myorhythmia
1965	Denny-Brown	Labile attitudes that gradually become more fixed	Dystonia
1983	Obeso et al.	Brief shock-like contractions plus slow, twisting spasms, plus repetitive or rhythmic contractions	Myoclonic dystonia

consisting of members of the Scientific Advisory Board of the Dystonia Medical Research Foundation met, deliberated and developed the following definition: *Dystonia is a syndrome of sustained muscle contractions, frequently causing twisting and repetitive movements, or abnormal postures.*

Table 17.2 Clinical definitions of dystonia

Year	Authors	Clinical definitions emphasized
1911	Oppenheim	Alternating muscle tone
1911	Flatau and Sterling	Progressive torsion spasms
1922	Wechsler and Brock	Hyperkinetic and tonic forms
1944	Herz	Slow, long-sustained turning movements
1962	Denny-Brown	Fixed or relatively fixed attitude
1976	Fahn and Eldridge	Sustained, involuntary, twisting movements; may be fast or slow
1982c	Fahn	Abnormal involuntary movements that are usually twisting; the peak of the movement is sustained for a second or longer
1982	Marsden	Continuous contractions forcing limbs and trunk into sustained postures, or intermittent to cause repetitive, sometimes rhythmic abnormal movements
1984	Fahn	Abnormal movements usually of a twisting nature, ranging in speed from rapid to slow, and usually being sustained for a second or longer at the height of the contraction
This chapter		A syndrome dominated by sustained muscle contractions, frequently causing twisting and repetitive movements, or abnormal postures

Dystonic movements can be present in virtually any part of the body, when that body part is 'at rest' or engaged in voluntary motor activity. As originally described by Destarac (1901) and independently by Oppenheim (1911), the dystonic movements are almost always aggravated during voluntary movement. The appearance of dystonic movements with voluntary movement is referred to as 'action dystonia'. Idiopathic dystonia commonly begins with a specific action dystonia, i.e. the abnormal movements appear with a special action and are not present at rest. To give an example, a person who develops idiopathic dystonia may have the initial symptom in one arm, but only when writing. It could be absent when tying shoelaces, buttoning, cutting food, or brushing teeth. As the dystonic condition progresses, less specific actions of the affected arm may activate the dystonia, e.g. when buttoning or combing hair. With further evolution, actions in other parts of the body can induce dystonic movements of the involved arm, so-called 'overflow'. With still further worsening, the affected limb can develop dystonic movements while it is at rest, and eventually display sustained posturing. Thus, dystonia at rest is usually a more severe form than pure action dystonia.

From the above descriptions, the syndrome of dystonia consists of either dystonic movements, dystonic postures, or a combination, as pointed out by Zeman and Dyken (1968). The speed of the dystonic movements can range from slow to rapid; they can be rhythmic or unpatterned, but usually repetitive to some extent; they are influenced by the placement of the affected body parts into specific postures; they tend to be increased with fatigue, stress and emotional states; they tend to be suppressed with relaxation, hypnosis and sleep; and they can be reduced by 'sensory tricks' which are frequently tactile or proprioceptive. Dystonia usually is present continually throughout the day whenever the affected body part is in use, or in more severe cases at rest, and disappears with deep sleep. However, there are three conditions that can be considered as distinct entities or variants of torsion dystonia in that the abnormal movements are intermittent and/or variable: dystonic tics, paroxysmal dystonia, and diurnal dystonia.

Tics, which can be simple or complex patterned movements, are not continual unless they are severe; rather the tics appear as a sudden abnormal movement on a background of normal motor behaviour. Usually they are very rapid and transient. But sometimes the movements are longer, sustained posturing, as originally described by Meige and Feindel (1907) who called these prolonged posturings 'tonic tics', in contrast to the more common clonic tics. Such tonic tics may transiently twist the body into dystonic posturing. Today, the tendency is to use the term 'dystonic tics' to refer to such tonic tics (Fahn, 1982b). Dystonic tics are more appropriately classified in the tic category of abnormal involuntary movements than in the category of dystonia, particularly as they can be suppressed voluntarily (with mounting inner tension). In support of this notion is the presence of phonations, complex patterned movements, and clonic tics in these same patients with dystonic tics.

When dystonic movements or postures occur as paroxysmal bursts (without the presence of other clinical phenomenology of tics), followed by a return to normality with no neurological deficit between attacks, these are referred to as paroxysmal dystonic choreoathetosis or preferably as paroxysmal dystonia. The duration of these bursts last minutes to hours. Many are familial (Lance, 1977), although non-familial cases have also been described (Fahn and Bressman, 1983). These types of paroxysmal dyskinesias are not induced by sudden voluntary movement, in contrast to the entity referred to as paroxysmal kinesigenic choreoathetosis. In the latter type, the abnormal movements last seconds to minutes, and are usually easy to control with anti-convulsants (Lance, 1977). Although these kinesigenic dyskinesias are usually choreic or ballistic in type, we have seen patients in whom the abnormal movements were sustained and twisting in nature, thus satisfying the criteria of dystonic movements. Paroxysmal dyskinesia is a subject beyond the scope of this chapter and will not be discussed further.

Some patients, who otherwise satisfy the criteria of dystonia, may be relatively free of dystonic movements and postures in the morning, but are afflicted severely in the late afternoon, evening and night. This temporal pattern has been considered a variant of dystonia and referred to as dystonia with marked diurnal variation by Segawa and colleagues (1976). Although there were earlier reports of dystonia with such diurnal variations (Corner, 1952; Burns, 1959), it was Segawa who emphasized that this pattern may be a distinct clinical entity. There are two other clinical features that highlight this disorder: many have features of parkinsonism (Sunohara *et al.*, 1985; Nygaard and Duvoisin, 1986; Segawa *et al.*, 1987) and these patients respond remarkably well to low-dosage levodopa (Segawa *et al.*, 1976;

Nygaard and Duvoisin, 1986), bromocriptine (Sabouraud *et al.*, 1978) or anti-cholinergics (Corner, 1952; Burns, 1959). One of us (SF) has seen four patients with this entity, and all four had complete relief of symptoms with low dosage anti-cholinergics.

The designation of this entity as dystonia with marked diurnal fluctuations does not cover the full spectrum of the condition and fails to account for its distinctive pharmacological response. In fact, patients with this type of pharmacological response and without diurnal fluctuations should also be considered within this subgroup of dystonia. Nygaard, Duvoisin and Marsden (1987), reviewing their own experience and the 80 or more cases reported in the literature, found that a substantial number of patients with the syndrome of onset of gait dystonia in childhood and adolescence with dramatic responsiveness to low doses of levodopa do not report diurnal fluctuations. They support the term 'dopa-responsive dystonia' to designate this important subgroup. The spectrum of dopa-responsive dystonia includes not only those presenting with dystonia of gait in that age group, but others with what appears to be a dystonic paraplegia, or a bizarre gait with unexplained falls. This entity is probably more common than generally appreciated, particularly amongst the non-Jewish population. Further discussion of the condition of dopa-responsive dystonia is beyond the scope of this chapter.

CLASSIFICATION

Torsion dystonia is classified in three ways: by age at onset, by aetiology, and by body distribution of the abnormal movements (*Table 17.3*).

Classification by age at onset

Classification by age at onset is desirable because this is the most important single factor related to prognosis of idiopathic dystonia. Marsden, Harrison and Bundey (1976) analysed 72 cases of idiopathic dystonia and found that, in general, the younger the age at onset, the more likely that the dystonia would become severe and also spread to involve multiple parts of the body. This pattern was seen by Cooper, Cullinan and Riklan (1976) and more recently confirmed in the patient population reported by Fahn (1986). The *Ad Hoc Committee* (1984) set up categories by age at onset as follows: childhood (0–12 years); adolescent (13–20 years); adult (>20 years).

Classification by aetiology

The aetiological classification divides the causes of dystonia into two major categories: idiopathic (or primary) and symptomatic (or secondary). The idiopathic group is subdivided into familial and non-familial (sporadic) patterns. Whether the natural history of dystonia or the pattern of genetic transmission differs among different ethnic groups are questions that remain to be answered definitively. Although most patients with torsion dystonia have a negative family history for this disorder, Zeman and Dyken (1967) have emphasized the importance of personal examination of family members to be absolutely certain about the presence or absence of dystonia. These investigators have clearly shown that a pattern of autosomal dominant transmission exists in many families (Zeman and Dyken, 1968). An X-linked inheritance pattern has also been found, but only in the Philippines on the Island of Panay (Lee et al., 1976).

Eldridge (1970) suggested that autosomal recessive inheritance is the genetic pattern for dystonia affecting the Ashkenazi Jewish population. This ethnic group has a higher prevalence rate than the non-Jewish and Sephardic Jewish populations and there is a low frequency of involvement in successive generations in the Ashkenazi population. However, this postulate has been questioned by Korczyn et al. (1980) and Zilber et al. (1984), since they found a few families in Israel with dystonia present in two successive generations. They believed that this could best be accounted for by an autosomal dominant hereditary pattern with incomplete penetrance. On the other hand, Eldrige (1981) argues that the few Ashkenazi families with dystonia in two generations could be explained by the phenomenon of pseudo-dominance (or quasi-dominance). In an autosomal recessively inherited disorder, if there is a high gene frequency in an in-bred population, a reasonable likelihood exists that an affected individual could marry a carrier of the gene. The offspring from this marriage would have the statistical chance of being affected in a pattern that is identical to that of autosomal dominant inheritance. Thus, the question remains open as to the nature of the hereditary pattern of dystonia in the Ashkenazi Jewish population, and further population studies are required before this issue can be settled conclusively.

Eldridge (1970) has also described a different course of progression of dystonia in the Ashkenazi population compared to the non-Jewish autosomal dominant population. These analyses have not yet been repeated by other investigators, but there is some evidence from the preliminary data presented by Burke and his colleagues (1985) that the two populations may not differ as much as previously suggested. In a review of the patient population seen at the Dystonia Clinical Research Center in New York, Fahn (1987) observed that, proportionately, the Jewish patients tended to have an earlier onset of dystonia than the non-Jewish

Table 17.3 Classification of dystonia

(I) *By cause*
    (a) Idiopathic
        Sporadic
        Familial
    (b) Symptomatic (*see Table 17.7*)

(II) *By age at onset*
    (a) Childhood-onset: 0–12 years
    (b) Adolescent-onset: 13–20 years
    (c) Adult-onset: >20 years

(III) *By distribution* (*see Table 17.4*)
    (a) Focal
    (b) Segmental
    (c) Multifocal
    (d) Generalized
    (e) Hemidystonia

patients, but for any given age at onset, the progressive course of dystonia was similar. In other words, it was the age at onset, rather than the ethnic origin, that determined the natural history of the illness.

Zeman and Dyken (1967) reviewed their own cases of generalized dystonia, and estimated the gene frequency to be 1 in 200 000 for the non-Jewish population of Indiana, but this figure may be an underestimate because it does not include the much larger number of cases of focal dystonia (see below), such as torticollis and blepharospasm. From the literature's reported cases, they calculated the gene frequency in the Jewish population to be 1 in 38 000. More recently Eldridge and Gottlieb (1976), based on literature reports and their own knowledge of affected patients, estimated the disease frequency in the Jewish population of the United States to be 1 in 17 000. Zilber et al. (1984), who surveyed patients with dystonia in Israel, calculated a frequency of 1 in 23 000 for the Ashkenazi population.

The symptomatic group is subdivided into those conditions associated with various hereditary neurological disorders, those due to environmental causes, dystonia associated with parkinsonism, and psychogenic dystonia. A major portion of the clinical investigation of dystonia (see below) concerns the tests required to uncover the aetiology of symptomatic dystonia. The categorization of symptomatic dystonia is, therefore, covered in a later part of this chapter.

Classification by distribution

Dystonia can affect different parts of the body. Marsden, Harrison and Bundey (1976) proposed a simple terminology to classify the bodily distribution of dystonia. *Focal dystonia* referred to the involvement of a single region, *segmental dystonia*, for involvement of two or more contiguous regions, and *generalized dystonia*, for involvement of multiple parts of the body. To this should be added *hemidystonia*, for involvement of one side of the body. This simple classification suffices for everyday needs, but does not cover the many variations seen in practice. A more extensive, although inevitably more complex, classification is required for accurate documentation, as is necessary, for example, for research purposes. The *Ad Hoc* Committee (1984) expanded upon the Marsden classification; this new classification by distribution is presented in *Table 17.4*.

Table 17.4 Classification of dystonic movements according to distribution of parts of the body affected

---

(1) Focal dystonia: a single body part is affected, e.g. eyelids (blepharospasm), mouth (oromandibular dystonia), larynx (dystonic adductor dysphonia), neck (torticollis), arm (writer's cramp)
(2) Segmental dystonia
  (a) Cranial – two or more parts of cranial and neck musculature are affected
  (b) Axial – neck and trunk are affected
  (c) Brachial – one arm and axial; both arms ± neck ± trunk
  (d) Crural – one leg and trunk; both legs ± trunk
(3) Generalized dystonia: a combination of segmental crural dystonia and any other segment
(4) Multifocal dystonia: two or more non-contiguous parts are affected
(5) Hemidystonia: ipsilateral arm and leg are affected

Focal dystonia indicates that only a single area of the body is affected. Frequently seen types of focal dystonia tend to have specific labels (*Table 17.5*). As a general rule, idiopathic dystonia begins as a focal dystonia. The disorder can remain as a focal dystonia, or it can spread to involve other parts of the body. The age at onset is a major factor associated with the progression of dystonia (*Figure 17.1*). When it does spread, it most commonly does so by next affecting a contiguous body part. When dystonia affects two or more contiguous parts of the body, it is then referred to as segmental dystonia.

Table 17.5 Commonly used names for dystonia affecting specific parts of the body

Common name	*Muscles contracting involuntarily*
Blepharospasm	Orbicularis occuli and neighbouring facial muscles
Lingual dystonia	Glossal muscles
Oromandibular dystonia	Muscles innervated by cranial nerve V, VII, X and XII, when jaw, lower face, or mouth area is involved
Dystonic adductor dysphonia	Laryngeal muscles, with vocal spasms to produce constricted speech with interrupting pauses
Dystonic dysphagia	Pharyngeal muscles, to produce difficulty with swallowing
Torticollis	Sternocleidomastoid, trapezius, and other nuchal muscles to cause rotation, tilting, extension, flexion, shifting, or displacement of the head; can be tonic or associated with head tremor or irregular jerking movements
Writer's cramp	Muscles of hand, forearm and arm
Soliosis, lordosis, kyphosis, or tortipelvis	Muscles of back
Leg dystonia	Muscles of foot, leg and thigh

Only when any of the above types of dystonia is pure and isolated, without other parts of the body being affected, can the designation of focal dystonia be used. The above terms can also be used to refer to the type of disorder affecting a specific region of the body, even when it is part of more widespread dystonia. For example, a patient can have torticollis and writer's cramp; this combination would be a form of segmental dystonia. *See Table 17.4* for the listings of the various types of segmental dystonias.

The *Ad Hoc* Committee recommended terminology for the various patterns of segmental dystonia encountered (*Table 17.4*). 'Segmental cranial dystonia' is the term for involvement of musculature of the head and neck region. Examples include a combination of blepharospasm and oromandibular dystonia, a common enough state to have its own eponym, Meige's syndrome (Paulson, 1972; Tolosa and Klawans, 1979). Other examples of segmental cranial dystonia would include torticollis plus spastic dysphonia, oromandibular dystonia plus torticollis, blepharospasm plus oromandibular dystonia plus spastic dysphonia, etc. As an aside, some neurologists prefer the term 'spasmodic dysphonia' over the term 'spastic dysphonia' to refer to dystonic spasm of the vocal cord adductors. The argument is that the term 'spasmodic' links the dysphonia with dystonia, particularly spasmodic torticollis, and that the term 'spastic' suggests the condition of spasticity. Unfortunately, the term 'spasmodic' indicates intermittent contractions, which can sometimes apply to those with torticollis who have intermittent increased spasms of the neck muscles. But such intermittency is not commonly seen with dystonic dysphonia. Thus, neither term is entirely satisfactory. Perhaps calling it 'dystonic adductor dysphonia', although clumsy, may be the best choice.

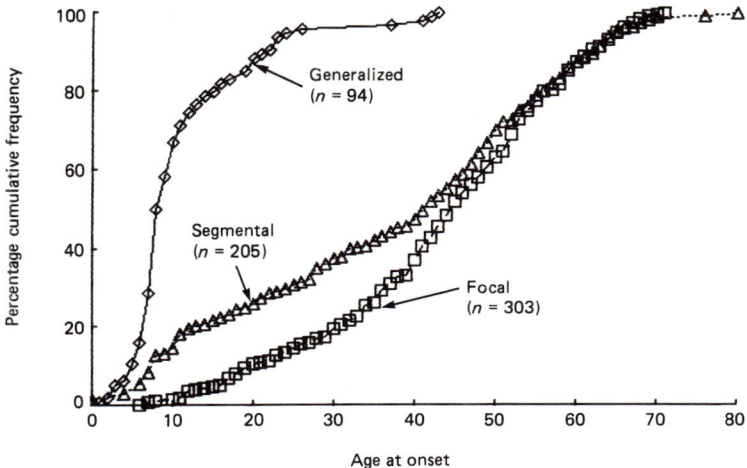

Figure 17.1 The distribution of dystonia as a function of age at onset. The curves show the percentage cumulative frequency of patients with generalized, segmental (plus multifocal), and focal dystonias evaluated at the Dystonia Clinical Research Center in New York through March 1986 according to the age at onset

Segmental axial dystonia represents involvement when both neck and trunk are affected, without involvement elsewhere. Segmental brachial dystonia refers to dystonia affecting both arms only, or one arm plus a contiguous axial structure (neck, trunk, or both), or both arms plus contiguous axial region (neck, trunk, or both). Segmental crural dystonia indicates that there is dystonia of both legs (with or without the trunk also being affected) or one leg plus the trunk. To avoid ambiguity and any gaps in this nomenclature, two other types of segmental dystonia need to be listed: segmental cranial plus brachial dystonia and segmental cranial plus axial dystonia. Some examples for the former would include the following patterns of involvement: jaw, neck, and at least one arm; face, neck, arm, and trunk; tongue, jaw, and both arms. Examples for the latter would include the following patterns of involvement: jaw, neck, and trunk; face, tongue, vocal cords, neck, and trunk.

Some areas of the body can be assigned to more than one region, namely those borderline areas: shoulder and hips. The ambiguity can be resolved by the company kept by dystonia in these regions. For example, shoulder involvement in the presence of torticollis would place the shoulder as part of the neck; shoulder involvement with arm dystonia would place the shoulder as part of the arm. Analogous associations of the hip to the trunk or to the leg would be equally applicable.

The revision of the Marsden classification by the *Ad Hoc* Committee defines generalized dystonia as affecting at least one or both legs plus some other region of the body. If only one leg is affected, the trunk must also be involved to qualify as generalized dystonia. Thus, generalized dystonia represents a combination of segmental crural dystonia plus involvement of any other area of the body. The following examples would be applicable for generalized dystonia: trunk, one leg, and the opposite arm; trunk, one leg, and neck; trunk, two legs, and one arm; two legs and one arm; two legs and neck; both legs, trunk, both arms, neck, larynx, jaw, and face.

The term 'multifocal dystonia' fills a gap in the above designations. It applies to the involvement of two or more non-contiguous parts of the body. Examples include one leg and the opposite arm, one leg and neck, one arm and jaw.

Dystonia affecting one-half of the body is called 'hemidystonia'. Examples include involvement of one leg and the ipsilateral arm; one leg, trunk, and ipsilateral arm; one leg, ipsilateral arm, and ipsilateral face. Almost always, hemidystonia indicates that the dystonia is symptomatic rather than idiopathic (Narbona et al., 1984; Marsden et al., 1985; Pettigrew and Jankovic, 1985).

To understand the relative frequencies of the idiopathic and symptomatic focal, segmental and generalized dystonias, *Table 17.6* lists the numbers of patients in each category seen at the Dystonia Clinical Research Center located in the Neurological Institute of New York. It is clear that adult-onset focal dystonias are much more common than generalized dystonias. The most common focal dystonia is torticollis. If these data are analysed for differences between Jewish and non-Jewish patients with dystonia, one finds that those with the same distribution of dystonia had a similar pattern of age at onset (*Figure 17.2*). This is another argument that dystonia is similar in different ethnic groups.

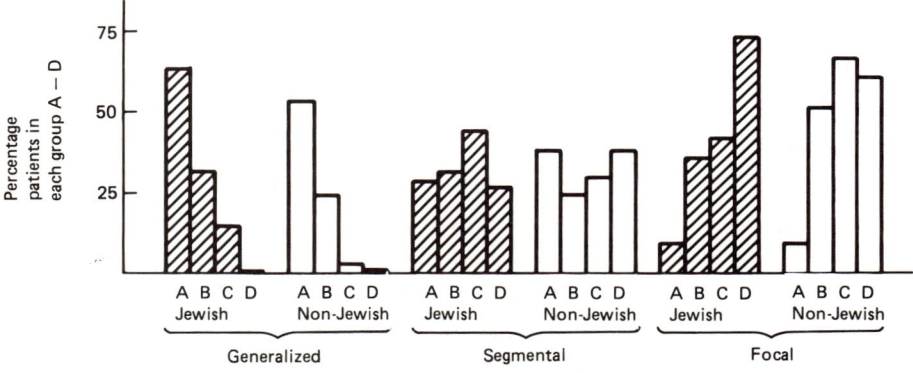

Figure 17.2 The age at onset for Ashkenazi Jewish and non-Jewish patients, according to the development of generalized, segmental or focal dystonia. The bars indicate the percentage of Jewish (hatched bars) and non-Jewish (open bars) patients at each age at onset who developed generalized, segmental (plus multifocal), and focal dystonias evaluated at the Dystonia Clinical Research Center in New York through March 1986. (A) Childhood-onset (ages 0–12); (B) adolescent-onset (ages 13–20); (C) young adult-onset (ages 21–40); (D) older adult-onset (ages greater than 40). The percentages are calculated by using the total number of subjects belonging to each category of age at onset as the denominator. Thus, group A for Jewish patients are divided into generalized, segmental and focal dystonias; their sum equals 100%. Each of the eight groups (A through D; Jewish and non-Jewish) will comprise a set whose value is 100%. When viewed in this manner, little difference is seen between Jewish and non-Jewish patients

Table 17.6 Distribution pattern of patients with dystonia

Category of patient	Idiopathic		Symptomatic	
	Number	Percentage	Number	Percentage
Childhood-onset				
Focal	11	1.2	5	0.5
Segmental	34	3.7	10	1.1
Multifocal	6	0.6	3	0.3
Generalized	70	7.5	54	5.8
Unilateral	2	0.2	15	1.6
Subtotal	123	13.2	87	9.3
Adolescent-onset				
Focal	21	2.3	3	0.3
Segmental	8	0.9	10	1.1
Multifocal	5	0.5	2	0.2
Generalized	13	1.4	5	0.5
Unilateral	3	0.3	3	0.3
Subtotal	50	5.4	23	2.4
Adult-onset				
Focal	271	29.1	33	3.5
Segmental	150	16.1	11	1.2
Multifocal	2	0.2	6	0.6
Generalized	11	1.2	9	1.0
Unilateral	1	0.1	8	0.9
Subtotal	435	46.7	67	7.2
Paroxysmal dystonia	17	1.8	16	1.7
Tardive dystonia			90	9.6
Psychogenic dystonia			24	2.6
TOTAL	625	67.1	307	32.8

A total of 932 patients with dystonia were seen by the Movement Disorder Group between September 1, 1973, and March 31, 1986, at the Dystonia Clinical Research Center located at Columbia-Presbyterian Medical Center, New York City. The categories of paroxysmal, tardive and psychogenic dystonia were removed from the idiopathic and symptomatic dystonias in order to list them as separate entities; their definitions are explained in the text; no distinction was made as to age at onset for these last three categories. Three patients with diurnal fluctuations are included among childhood-onset idiopathic dystonia.

Relationship between generalized, segmental and focal dystonias

From the reports of Marsden, Harrison and Bundey (1976) and Fahn (1986), patients with generalized dystonia usually had their onset in childhood or adolescence, and always by age 43, whereas those with focal dystonia usually had onset after the age of 40, although about 30% had an earlier onset. The question is:

Are generalized, segmental and focal dystonias the same disorder with a difference only in distribution in the body with the final distribution reflecting predominantly the age at onset, or are these groups (particularly generalized versus focal dystonias) distinct and separate entities, without any connection other than that they each have dystonic movements? If they are the same disorder, but only differ in extent of the disease, one can consider focal and segmental dystonias to be formes frustes of generalized dystonia as originally suggested by Zeman, Kaelbling and Pasamanick (1960). If generalized and focal dystonias are separate and distinct from each other, how does segmental dystonia fit into the picture? Is it also separate, is it a forme fruste of generalized dystonia, or is it a progression of focal dystonia? Moreover, how does one focal dystonia (such as blepharospasm) relate to another type of focal dystonia (such as writer's cramp)? One can fairly easily relate blepharospasm with other focal cranial dystonias such as oromandibular dystonia, dystonic dysphonia and torticollis, because often a focal cranial dystonia progresses to a segmental cranial dystonia. The other questions raised cannot be answered with absolute certainty at this time. Arguments in favour of the concept that generalized, segmental and focal dystonias are related include:

(a) Idiopathic and hereditary generalized dystonia almost always begin as a focal dystonia before it spreads to involve other parts of the body. It is possible that in some individuals, for unknown reasons (age at onset being the most important relevant factor), the spread may not take place or may be limited and then plateau; the dystonia may remain as a focal dystonia or as a segmental dystonia.
(b) In families with dystonia, various members may have generalized, segmental or focal dystonia, suggesting that they are related, giving rise to the concept that the less involved individuals are formes frustes of generalized dystonia (Zeman, Kaelbling and Pasamanick, 1960).
(c) Sensory tricks often ameliorate dystonic movements and postures and this manoeuvre can be effective in different parts of the body (Fahn, 1985a). Such a common phenomenology suggests a common pathophysiology.

More definitions

Three more terms can now be defined. Dystonia musculorum deformans (DMD) can be considered as equivalent to idiopathic generalized dystonia. Although DMD was originally used to describe patients with childhod onset, it seems reasonable to exclude age from the definition. As seen in *Figure 17.1*, few patients develop generalized dystonia with onset after the age of 20, but for those who do so, why arbitrarily exclude them from the label of DMD? We prefer to avoid the term 'DMD' for several reasons.

(a) One could just as easily define DMD to be less restrictive. For example, two siblings become affected with dystonia in childhood, but only one progresses to have generalized dystonia, while the other plateaus at segmental brachial dystonia. Why should the first be labelled as DMD, but not the second? In other words, the definition is arbitrary and does not really add to the overall concept of dystonia. It seems preferable to label these two individuals as having

childhood-onset idiopathic generalized dystonia and childhood-onset idiopathic segmental brachial dystonia, respectively. These labels give a clearer picture of the degree of involvement.
(b) Most physicians continue to use DMD in an ambiguous and inconsistent manner, e.g. for idiopathic generalized, idiopathic childhood-onset generalized, idiopathic childhood-onset generalized and segmental, idiopathic childhood-onset generalized, segmental or focal etc.
(c) Finally, as expressed by many authors, dystonia is not always deforming and it is not a disease of muscle.

The term 'torsion dystonia' can be used to refer to the syndrome of dystonia, rather than to dystonic movements or postures. For reasons stated above, the focal and segmental dystonias are considered as strongly related to generalized dystonia. Thus, in this chapter, the term 'torsion dystonia' will be applied to any type of dystonic syndrome, whether idiopathic or symptomatic, regardless of age at onset, and regardless of the distribution of the dystonic movements and postures.

The term 'formes frustes of dystonia' requires elaboration. Zeman, Kaelbling and Pasamanick (1960) used the term to describe incomplete forms of fully developed, generalized torsion dystonia. Based on clinical findings observed in relatives of patients with generalized dystonia, they listed action dystonia, speech defects, postural abnormalities such as pes equinovarus and kyphoscoliosis, blepharospasm and tremor as formes frustes of dystonia. Subsequently, Zeman and Dyken (1968) questioned the validity of speech defects and congenital club foot, and emphasized action dystonia as the major type of forme fruste. Marsden and Harrison (1974) also argued that focal dystonias, such as blepharospasm and torticollis, are formes frustes. Marsden (1976) added to the evolution of the concept by pointing out that adult-onset torticollis, blepharospasm, oromandibular dystonia, and writer's cramp are focal dystonias. A more detailed review of patients with writer's cramp by Sheehy and Marsden (1982) also emphasized the focal action dystonias, referred to by some as occupational cramps, to be part of the spectrum of dystonia.

Thus, today we no longer consider the focal dystonias as formes frustes of dystonia; they are accepted as milder expressions of torsion dystonia compared to generalized dystonia. Instead, the term 'formes frustes' may be more appropriately applied to manifestations that are not clearly dystonic movements or postures; it should not be applied to well-recognized and accepted dystonic movements, such as action dystonia and the focal dystonias. What motor manifestations, then, can be considered a forme fruste of dystonia? At present, more detailed clinical descriptions are needed. The authors suggest that stuttering, clumsiness, and tremor should be studied in family members and controls to determine if these motor symptoms could be present in a higher proportion of patients with dystonia and in their families. It is clear that the concept of formes frustes of dystonia is continuing to evolve.

CLINICAL FEATURES

Although many aspects of the clinical features have been discussed above, some additional points should be made here to be complete.

Myoclonic dystonia

Shock-like movements are common in dystonia. To the casual observer these look like myoclonus. Unless the accompanying dystonia is also recognized, such patients may be, and often are, incorrectly designated as cases of myoclonus. In our experience, this is one of the commonest causes of confusion in the diagnosis of patients with movement disorders. It was for this reason that Obeso et al. (1983) drew attention to the problem and re-introduced the term 'myoclonic dystonia' (originally employed by Davidenkow (1926)) to describe such patients. As pointed out by Fahn (1984) and Obeso et al. (1983), these patients have dystonia, not myoclonus. Indeed, the electrophysiology of their shock-like movements shows prolonged EMG bursts typical of dystonia, not the short-duration EMG bursts characteristic of myoclonus.

This matter was complicated further by the recognition of a subgroup of patients with idiopathic dystonia who exhibit the combination of shock-like jerks with dystonic spasms and postures, occurring in families with apparent autosomal dominant inheritance, and characteristically showing dramatic benefit with alcohol (Quinn and Marsden, 1984; Kurlan et al., 1985). A possible designation of this entity might be 'hereditary dystonia with lightning jerks, responsive to alcohol'. There is a complex relationship of this condition to other movement disorders, such as hereditary essential myoclonus, which is beyond the scope of this chapter (Quinn and Marsden, 1987).

Sensory tricks

One feature of dystonia that is unique, and is therefore helpful in diagnosis, is that often the severity of dystonic posturing can be reduced by various sensory 'tricks', i.e. certain tactile or proprioceptive stimuli can often lessen or eliminate the abnormal posturing. Two common examples illustrate this point. The patient with spasmodic torticollis often obtains relief by bringing a hand to his chin or touching the back of his head. The patient with blepharospasm often obtains relief by touching the skin around the orbit or by talking. Similar tricks are sometimes employed by those with other dystonias elsewhere. However, with increasing severity of dystonia, the ability to respond to these selective stimuli diminishes. While the term 'sensory tricks' is a convenient way of describing these phenomena, their mechanism is unknown. They may invoke afferent feedback from the periphery, or central corollary discharge provoked by the motor output that generates the trick movement (in which case, 'sensory' is inappropriate).

Onset and progression of dystonia

Usually the onset of idiopathic dystonia is confined to a single part of the body. In a series of 72 patients with idiopathic dystonia Marsden, Harrison and Bundey (1976) reported that the site of onset of dystonia is most often in one leg (approximately 68%) when the disorder begins before the age of 11. It starts in the arm in about 24% of these patients, and in the remaining 8% it begins in the axial musculature. With onset during the second decade, the initial site is in the leg, arm or trunk almost equally. With age at onset greater than 20, no patient in Marsden's series had the initial site in the leg. The majority of such patients had onset in an arm.

With progression over time, not only does the dystonia in that affected part worsen, but there is a tendency for the dystonia to spread to involve other body parts. The most important prognostic factor for patients with idiopathic dystonia is the age at onset. As a general rule, the younger the age at onset, the more likely that the legs be affected, the severity worsens, and the dystonia becomes generalized; with older age at onset, the more likely that the legs be spared, the severity be less, and the distribution of the dystonia be limited. In the series of 72 patients reported by Marsden, Harrison and Bundey (1976), generalized dystonia developed in approximately 85% of all patients with onset below the age of 11; 60%, with onset between 11 and 20; 16%, with onset between 21 and 40; and not at all when the onset was greater than age 40. The adult-onset group divided almost equally between progression to segmental dystonia and remaining as a focal dystonia. The dystonia in this adult-onset group remained mild in more than 50% of cases, and only 14% progressed to become severe. In contrast, 50% of cases with onset below the age of 11 developed severe dystonia, and 27% with onset during the second decade did so.

Details of patients with generalized and focal idiopathic dystonias were recently reviewed (Marsden and Harrison, 1974; Fahn, 1986). Of the 560 patients reported by Fahn (1986a), 90 had developed generalized torsion dystonia, 183 segmental dystonia, and 287 focal dystonia. These three groups were analysed as a function of age at onset. When plotted as percentage cumulative frequency, each group was found to have a distinct curve. The percentage cumulative frequency rose rapidly for patients with generalized dystonia, and much more slowly for those with segmental and focal dystonia. Moreover, no patient with generalized dystonia had an onset age greater than 43 years, similar to the findings of Marsden, Harrison and Bundey (1976), whereas onset above age 70 years was seen in patients with segmental and focal dystonia. The median age at onset was 8 years for generalized dystonia, 40 years for segmental dystonia, and 45 years for focal dystonia.

The peak time of onset for generalized dystonia was between ages 6 and 10 years. In contrast, the sixth decade was the peak for focal and segmental dystonia, and these showed a much broader range. Segmental dystonia had a bimodal onset, with a small curve in the younger ages and a more broad curve later in life (Fahn, 1986). This supports the concept that some patients with segmental dystonia may be 'aborted' cases of generalized dystonia.

SYMPTOMATIC DYSTONIA

Approximately one-third of all patients with dystonia have symptomatic dystonia (Table 17.6). In the idiopathic dystonias, the only neurological abnormality is the presence of dystonic postures and movements. There is no associated amyotrophy, weakness, spasticity, ataxia, reflex change, abnormality of eye movements, disorder of retina, dementia or seizures, except where they may be the result of a concomitant problem such as a complication from a neurosurgical procedure undertaken to correct the dystonia, or the presence of some other incidental neurological disease. Since many of the symptomatic dystonias have additional neurological abnormalities, the presence of any of these findings in a patient with dystonia immediately suggests that one is dealing with symptomatic dystonia. However, the absence of such neurological findings does not necessarily exclude the possibility of a symptomatic dystonia, which may present as a pure dystonia (Lang et al., 1985; Pettigrew and Jankovic, 1985).

Table 17.7 Aetiological classification of torsion dystonia

(I) Idiopathic (primary)
    (*a*) With hereditary pattern
        Autosomal dominant
        Autosomal recessive
        X-linked recessive
    (*b*) Without hereditary pattern

(II) Symptomatic
    (*a*) Associated with other hereditary neurological syndromes
        Wilson's disease (Scheinberg and Sternlieb, 1984)
        Huntington's disease (Bruyn, 1968)
        Hallervorden–Spatz disease (Gilman and Barrett, 1973)
        Progressive pallidal degeneration (Jellinger, 1968)
        Juvenile neuronal ceroid-lipofuscinosis (Pettigrew and Jankovic, 1985)
        Metachromatic leucodystrophy (Case Records, 1984; Lang *et al.*, 1985)
        GM_1 and GM_2 gangliosidosis (Goldman, *et al.*, 1981; Meek *et al.*, 1984; Nakano *et al.*, 1985)
        Hexosamidase A and B deficiency (Goldie, Holtzman and Suzuki, 1977)
        Glutaric acidaemia (Leibel *et al.*, 1980)
        Homocystinuria (Davous and Rondot, 1983)
        Methylmalonic aciduria (observed by CDM)
        Lesch–Nyhan syndrome (Watts *et al.*, 1982)
        Ataxia–telangiectasia (Bodensteiner, Goldblum and Goldman, 1980)
        Leigh's syndrome (Marsden *et al.*, 1986)
        Infantile bilateral striatal necrosis (Goutieres and Aicardi, 1982)
        Leber's disease (Novotny *et al.*, 1986)
        Joseph's disease (Rosenberg and Fowler, 1981)
        Hartnup's disease (Tahmoush *et al.*, 1976)
        Intraneuronal inclusion disease (Yerby, Shaw and Watson, 1986)
        Familial basal ganglia calcifications (Aicardi and Gontieres, 1984; Larsen *et al.*, 1985)
        Dystonic lipidosis (sea-blue histiocytosis) (de Leon *et al.*, 1969; Neville *et al.*, 1973; Longstreth *et al.*, 1982; Ashwal *et al.*, 1984)
        Rett's syndrome (Philippart and Brown, 1984)
        Triosephosphate isomerase deficiency (Poll-The *et al.*, 1985)
    (*b*) Due to known environmental cause
        Perinatal cerebral injury
            Athetoid cerebral palsy (Bruyn and Kyllerman, 1979)
            Delayed onset dystonia (Burke *et al.*, 1985)
        Encephalitis and postinfectious (Benda, 1949; Aronson and Aronson, 1965)
            Reye's syndrome (observed by SF)
            Subacute sclerosing leucoencephalopathy (observed by CDM)
            Wasp sting (observed by CDM)
        Head trauma (Mauro, Fahn and Russman, 1980; Brett, Sheehy and Marsden, 1981; Grimes *et al.*, 1982)
        Thalamotomy (Pettigrew and Jankovic, 1985)
        Brainstem lesion (Jankovic and Patel, 1983)
        Focal cerebral vascular injury (Dooling and Adams, 1975; Demierre and Rondot, 1983; Obeso *et al.*, 1984)
        Brain tumour (Narbona *et al.*, 1984)
        Multiple sclerosis (Bachman, Lao-Velez and Estanol, 1976; Heath and Nightingale, 1982; Jankovic and Patel, 1983)
        Cervical cord injury (Subczynski *et al.*, 1969; Berardelli *et al.*, 1986)

Table 17.7 cont.

> Peripheral injury (Marsden, Harrison and Bundey, 1976; Sheehy and Marsden, 1980, 1982; Schott, 1985; Brin et al., 1986)
> Drugs
> > D-2 receptor antagonists (Burke et al., 1982)
> > Levodopa (Melamed, 1979)
> > Ergotism (Quinn, 1983)
> > Anti-convulsants (Chadwick, Reynolds and Marsden, 1976; Crosley and Swender, 1979; Jacome, 1979)
> Toxins
> > Mn, CO, carbon disulphide (Franke and Neu, 1977; Barbeau, 1984)
> > Methanol (LeWitt, 1986)
> Metabolic – hypoparathyroidism (Muenter and Whisnant, 1968)
> (c) Dystonia associated with parkinsonism
> (d) Psychogenic dystonia (Fahn et al., 1983; Batshaw et al., 1985)

The references cited are a selection only, and are not complete. They serve as a guide for those desiring further study of the symptomatic dystonias.

There are many environmental and metabolic disorders that can present as torsion dystonia (Table 17.7). The major purpose of the investigation of patients with dystonia is to determine if symptomatic, rather than idiopathic, dystonia is present. Most of the symptomatic dystonias are not amenable to specific therapies at present, but the most important exception is Wilson's disease, which is reviewed in Chapter 14.

Clinical clues suggesting that a patient may have symptomatic dystonia come both from the history and the physical findings. Exposure to drugs known to cause dystonia is obviously relevant. Anti-psychotic agents are the most common drugs causing acute dystonic reactions and tardive dystonia (Burke et al., 1982). Previous head trauma, encephalitis, birth injury, stroke, or toxin exposure can all cause dystonia, often with a delay before manifestation of the dystonic symptoms (Burke, Fahn and Gold, 1980; Mauro, Fahn and Russman, 1980; Brett, Sheehy and Marsden, 1981; Grimes et al., 1982).

Certain features on examination also point to the likelihood that one is dealing with symptomatic dystonia. Hemidystonia usually implies a structural lesion in the contralateral putamen or its afferent or efferent connections (Burton et al., 1984; Narbona et al., 1984; Marsden et al., 1985; Pettigrew and Jankovic, 1985). The patient with idiopathic dystonia who has a hemidystonia is almost certainly in the process of developing generalized dystonia; most of the cases with hemidystonia in Table 17.6 have symptomatic dystonia.

Onset of the syndrome of dystonia as a resting, rather than as an action, dystonia appears to be more likely with symptomatic dystonias. The presence of risus sardonicus is uncommon in idiopathic dystonia and suggests a symptomatic disorder. Early involvement of speech with dysarthria or hypophonia (but not dystonic adductor dysphonia) also suggests symptomatic dystonia. The most clearcut clinical indicator of symptomatic dystonia is the presence of non-dystonic neurological signs, such as a cognitive defect, pyramidal signs, a cerebellar or sensory deficit, and oculomotor or retinal abnormalities. Dystonia of ocular muscles, such as oculogyric crises, are a feature of symptomatic, particularly post-encephalitic and neuroleptic-induced dystonia, and not idiopathic dystonia. Seizures and cognitive deficits also imply symptomatic dystonia or an additional neurological problem. Loss of postural reflexes, which occurs in parkinsonism and Huntington's disease, is exceptional in idiopathic dystonia.

The clinical course can often differentiate between idiopathic and symptomatic dystonia. The former begins insidiously, usually with action dystonia, and tends to be a slowly and irregularly progressive disorder with plateaus and, rarely, partial remissions with subsequent recurrence (Marsden and Harrison, 1974; Friedman and Fahn, 1986). Dystonic postures do not develop for several years. In contrast, most symptomatic dystonias begin with dystonia at rest and sustained postures are seen at an early stage. Some symptomatic dystonias have an obvious sudden beginning, for example on recovery from acute encephalitis. Others may have a delayed, insidious onset after the encephalopathic event (Burke, Fahn and Gold, 1980). The symptomatic dystonias associated with metabolic diseases (e.g. Wilson's disease, Leigh's disease) tend, at least initially, to have a more rapidly progressive course than the idiopathic dystonias (*see* Chapter 14). Many of the symptomatic dystonias due to environmental causes, such as head trauma, encephalitis, and exposure to toxins, run a course that stabilizes after the completion of the intracranial lesion.

Drugs that block the dopamine D-2 receptor (anti-psychotics and the substituted benzamides, such as metoclopramide) can induce two types of dystonia: acute dystonic reactions (Christian and Paulson, 1958; Casteels-Van Daele *et al.*, 1970) and delayed, persistent dystonia, so-called 'tardive dystonia' (Burke *et al.*, 1982). The latter is a variant of the more classical tardive dyskinesia.

The acute dystonic reaction is self-limiting, and can be reversed readily by parenteral administration of diphenhydramine, anti-cholinergics (Paulson, 1960), or diazepam (Korczyn and Goldberg, 1972). Tardive dystonia may not only be persistent, but also frequently unresponsive to therapy (Kang, Burke and Fahn, 1986). The clinical appearance of tardive dystonia can resemble pure primary dystonia; the major diagnostic clue is the development of dystonia while the patient is receiving a D-2 receptor-blocking drug or has recently stopped such a drug. Children can develop tardive dystonia, whereas they rarely develop more classical tardive dyskinesia. Tardive dystonia in a child or adolescent can be a generalized dystonia, with the legs involved, or it can be segmental or focal dystonia, whereas adults tend to have focal and segmental dystonias only. These patterns of involvement are similar to the distribution of idiopathic dystonia.

Aside from the juvenile dystonia–parkinsonism syndrome mentioned earlier in the discussion on diurnal variations, dystonic features are common in parkinsonism. Patients with Parkinson's disease can have dystonic postures as part of the illness. It is very common for those with advanced Parkinson's disease to have sustained postures, such as an ulnar deviated hand, flexion of the head (anterocollis), a postured foot (Duvoisin *et al.*, 1972), kyphosis, and lateral tilt of the trunk. The parkinsonian syndrome of progressive supranuclear palsy is commonly associated with retrocollis and with the deep nasolabial folds and wrinkled forehead of facial dystonia; some patients also have blepharospasm (Jankovic, 1984; *see also* Chapter 13). An occasional patient with idiopathic parkinsonism may have a sustained dystonic posture of a limb that is more pronounced than usual, and appears to be part of the illness; the disorder may even begin with foot dystonia or torticollis. In contrast to these three types of dystonia occurring as part of the parkinsonian disorder, there are also three varieties that are the result of levodopa treatment of parkinsonism: peak-dose dystonia, diphasic dystonia, and 'off-effect' dystonia (e.g. early morning dystonia) (Melamed, 1979; Fahn, 1982a; Marsden, Parkes and Quinn, 1982).

At one time it was fairly common for patients with dystonia to be misdiagnosed as having a psychiatric disorder (Lesser and Fahn, 1978). A rebound reaction to correct this error probably led to an underdiagnosis of psychogenic dystonia (Fahn and Eldridge, 1976). Although psychiatric-induced dystonia occurs, it is relatively uncommon (*Table 17.6*) and should be diagnosed only if there is clearcut evidence of a conversion reaction or malingering. Fahn *et al.* (1983) described 10 patients with psychogenic dystonia, conclusively established because the dystonic movements and postures resolved with appropriate psychiatric treatment, emotionally supportive therapy, or placebo therapy. Such improvement implies non-organic dystonia because only some types of torticollis show complete spontaneous improvement (Tsai *et al.*, 1983; Friedman and Fahn, 1986), whereas other forms of dystonia do not. Findings that are suspicious for psychogenic dystonia are the presence of any of the following: false weakness, false sensory complaints, multiple somatizations, obvious psychiatric disturbances such as self-inflicted injuries, and incongruous and inconsistent dystonic movements and postures (such as exacerbation when the child does not get his/her way and disappearing when the parents give in to the child). Care is required to avoid misinterpreting normal variations of dystonia as psychiatric phenomena. Relief with sensory tricks or variations with change of posture or voluntary motor activity are common in the idiopathic dystonia. Psychogenic dystonia can be severe enough to lead to fixed permanent contractures (Fahn, personal observations) and to surgical procedures (Batshaw *et al.*, 1985).

INVESTIGATION

Following the history and examination, it is useful to quantitate the severity of the dystonia and to obtain a videotape recording as a means of following the course of the illness and the response to treatment. The degree of involvement can be assessed with the Fahn–Marsden rating scale (Burke *et al.*, 1985) which was designed to evaluate generalized dystonia in the absence of other neurological problems. This scale is less sensitive for the focal dystonias, where more detailed information on the affected region is desirable (Fahn, 1985b). The Fahn–Marsden rating scale evaluates both the factors which precipitate the dystonic movements (provoking factor) and the severity of the movements in each part of the body. The provoking factor assessment designates whether dystonia is present with specific action, multiple actions, with overflow, or at rest. The definitions for measuring severity (severity factor) differs for each section of the body, depending on the functional use of each specific body part. As an example, the main function of the leg is for walking; if the dystonia of the leg is severe enough to prevent walking, the severity score is maximum. The quantitative score is less with increasing functional use of the leg. To obtain a total score for generalized dystonia, the product of provoking and severity factors for each part of the body is calculated and the sum of these products for all body parts yields the final score. In addition to quantitating dystonic movements, the Fahn–Marsden scale also generates a functional disability score on a separate scale.

Laboratory tests are normal in the idiopathic dystonias. If anything is abnormal, such as the EEG, CSF, or CT scan, symptomatic dystonia must be considered. Most patients with dystonia that is clinically compatible with idiopathic torsion dystonia rarely need an extensive laboratory work-up. However, children and young adults, even if they appear to have typical primary dystonia, should undergo laboratory tests to exclude Wilson's disease since this is a treatable condition, that would otherwise progress (*see* Chapter 14). Serum ceruloplasmin and a slit lamp examination by an ophthalmologist experienced in detecting Kayser–Fleischer rings constitute adequate screening, but if any doubt exists, determination of 24-hour urinary copper excretion and a liver biopsy for histology and copper content are required.

On the other hand, all patients, adult and children, who have clinical features atypical for primary dystonia, need laboratory evaluation, not only for Wilson's disease, but also for the other disorders listed in *Table 17.7*. A procedure for this investigation was evolved by the staff of the Dystonia Clinical Research Center in New York and is presented in *Table 17.8*. A similar evaluation is undertaken in

Table 17.8 Investigation of dystonia

(I) Patients with typical clinical features of idiopathic dystonia with onset before the age of 35
 Videotape
 Quantitate dystonia on Fahn–Marsden rating scale
 CBC, SMAC, uric acid, ESR, serology
 Lysosomal enzymes on peripheral blood
 Serum ceruloplasmin
 Slitlamp examination
 EEG
 CT scan and MR scan

(II) Patients with typical clinical features of idiopathic dystonia with onset after the age of 34
 Videotape
 Quantitate dystonia on Fahn–Marsden rating scale
 CT scan and MR scan (not required, but may be valuable)
 Serum ceruloplasmin and slitlamp examination if generalized or progressive dystonia is present

(III) Patients with clinical features atypical for idiopathic dystonia regardless of age at onset
 Videotape
 Quantitate dystonia on Fahn–Marsden rating scale
 CBC, SMAC, uric acid, ESR, serology
 Urinalysis, T3RU/T4
 ANA, latex fixation, immunoglobulins, alpha-fetoprotein
 Fresh blood smear for acanthocytes
 Lysosomal enzymes on peripheral blood
 Arterial blood: gases, pH, lactate, pyruvate
 Electron microscopy of leucocytes and skin and conjunctival biopsy
 Urine for oligosaccharides and mucopolysaccharides
 Urine for quantitative organic acids
 Urine for quantitative amino acids
 CSF: lactate, pyruvate
 EMG, nerve conduction
 Evoked potentials
 Electroretinogram
 Bone marrow aspiration to include electron microscopy
 Nerve and muscle biopsy, with electron microscopy (indicated if EMG or nerve conduction studies suggest abnormalities)

Part B – Visitors to Canada

All visitors identified in Part A must be included in Part B.

You can bring in **personal goods** without paying duty or tax, as long as you do not leave them in Canada. You can also bring the amounts of alcohol and tobacco listed in Table 1 without paying duty or tax.

You can bring in **gifts** without paying duty or tax, as long as they are not alcohol or tobacco or business goods, and they have a value of CAN$60 or less per gift. Gifts valued at more than CAN$60 each are subject to duty and tax on the amount of their value that exceeds CAN$60.

Citizenship and Immigration Canada advises you that all visitors admitted to Canada will be permitted to stay for a maximum of six months, unless otherwise notified in writing by an examining officer.

Part C – Residents of Canada

Each resident must complete Part C in the **same order** as listed in Part A.

Your declaration must include the total value of all goods (including gifts) that you have purchased, received, or acquired abroad or at duty-free shops and that you are bringing into Canada.

The following table lists the available exemptions.

Table 2 – Personal exemptions for residents of Canada		
Minimum absence from Canada	Exemption limit – CAN$	Alcohol and tobacco
24 hours	$50	No
48 hours	$200	Yes – see Table 1
7 days	$750	Yes – see Table 1

Each traveller is allowed only **one** of these exemptions per trip.

The $50 exemption does not apply if the total value of your goods is more than $50. The $750 exemption can include goods (other than alcohol and tobacco) you acquired during your trip, which are not accompanying you. To calculate the number of days absent, do not count the day you left Canada, but include the day you return.

For residents of Canada only, effective October 1, 2001, you must pay duty on cigarettes, tobacco sticks, and manufactured tobacco that you include in your personal exemption entitlement, unless they are marked "CANADA-DUTY PAID • DROIT ACQUITTÉ".

Part D – Signatures

Each traveller must sign the declaration in the **same order** as listed in Part A.

Information from this declaration will be used for customs control purposes, and may be shared with other government departments to enforce Canadian law. Details are available in the Treasury Board of Canada publication called *Infosource*, under the reference number RC PPU 043. *Infosource* is available at public libraries, Government public reading rooms, and on the Internet at: http://infosource.gc.ca

Each person 16 years of age and older must sign.
Have your detached declaration card and your proof of citizenship ready to hand to a customs officer.

Partie B – Visiteurs au Canada

Tous les visiteurs identifiés dans la partie A doivent être compris dans la partie B.

Vous pouvez apporter des **effets personnels** sans payer de droits ni de taxes, à condition de ne pas les laisser au Canada. Vous pouvez aussi apporter les quantités d'alcool et de tabac indiquées dans le tableau 1 sans payer de droits ni de taxes.

Vous pouvez apporter des **cadeaux** sans payer de droits ni de taxes, à condition qu'il ne s'agisse pas d'alcool, de tabac ni de marchandises à usage commercial. Si un cadeau a une valeur de plus de 60 $CAN, des droits et des taxes s'appliqueront au montant de leur valeur qui dépasse 60 $CAN.

Citoyenneté et Immigration Canada vous informe que les visiteurs admis au Canada auront le droit de rester au pays durant six mois au plus, à moins d'indication contraire par écrit d'un agent examinateur.

Partie C – Résidents du Canada

Chaque résident doit remplir la partie C **dans l'ordre de présentation** de la partie A.

Votre déclaration doit inclure la valeur totale de toutes les marchandises (y compris les cadeaux) que vous avez achetées, reçues ou acquises à l'étranger ou dans des boutiques hors taxes et que vous apportez au Canada.

Le tableau suivant indique les différentes exemptions.

Tableau 2 – Exemptions personnelles pour les résidents du Canada		
Absence minimale du Canada	Limite de l'exemption – $CAN	Alcool et tabac
24 heures	50 $	Non
48 heures	200 $	Oui – voir tableau 1
7 jours	750 $	Oui – voir tableau 1

Un voyageur peut demander **une seule** de ces exemptions par voyage.

Vous ne pouvez pas bénéficier de l'exemption de 50 $ si la valeur totale de vos marchandises dépasse 50 $. L'exemption de 750 $ peut inclure des marchandises (sauf l'alcool et le tabac) que vous avez acquises durant votre voyage, mais qui ne vous accompagnent pas. Pour calculer le nombre de jours où vous avez été absent du Canada, tenez compte de la date de retour mais non de la date de départ.

Pour les résidents du Canada seulement, à compter du 1er octobre 2001, vous devrez payer des droits sur les cigarettes, les bâtonnets de tabac et le tabac fabriqué que vous inclurez dans votre droit d'exemption personnelle, à moins qu'il ne soit mentionné «"CANADA-DUTY PAID • DROIT ACQUITTÉ» sur ces articles.

Partie D – Signatures

Chaque voyageur doit signer la déclaration **dans l'ordre de présentation** de la partie A.

Les renseignements fournis dans cette déclaration serviront à des fins de contrôle douanier et pourront être partagés avec d'autres ministères gouvernementaux afin de faire respecter les lois canadiennes. Vous trouverez des détails à ce sujet dans la publication du Conseil du Trésor du Canada intitulée *Infosource*, sous le numéro de référence RC PPU 043. *Infosource* est disponible dans les bibliothèques publiques, les salles de lecture publiques du gouvernement et sur Internet à l'adresse suivante : **http://infosource.gc.ca**

Chaque voyageur âgé de 16 ans et plus doit signer.
Détachez votre carte de déclaration et préparez-vous à la présenter avec votre preuve de citoyenneté à un agent des douanes.

| AX | | ÉQUIP | IMM | AR | REF | DIP | MILT |

Carte de déclaration douanière

Partie A – Tous les voyageurs (doivent vivre à la même adresse domiciliaire)

Nom de famille, prénom et initiales

Date de naissance | Citoyenneté

Nom de famille, prénom et initiales

Date de naissance | Citoyenneté

Nom de famille, prénom et initiales

Date de naissance | Citoyenneté

Nom de famille, prénom et initiales

Date de naissance | Citoyenneté

Adresse domiciliaire – n°, rue | Ville ou village domiciliaire

Province ou État | Pays | Code postal/Zip

Arrivée par	But du voyage	En provenance de
Compagnie aérienne	études	É.-U. seulement
	personnel	autre pays (vol direct)
N° de vol	affaires	autre pays via les É.-U.

J'apporte (nous apportons) au Canada :   Oui   Non

- des armes à feu ou autres armes
- des biens reliés à ma (notre) profession ou des marchandises commerciales, destinés ou non à la revente (p. ex. échantillons, outils, équipement)
- des aliments (des fruits, des légumes, de la viande, des œufs, des produits laitiers), des animaux, des oiseaux, des insectes, des plantes, des boutures, de la terre, des organismes vivants, des vaccins
- des articles fabriqués à partir ou provenant d'espèces menacées d'extinction

J'ai (nous avons) expédié des marchandises, qui ne m' (nous) accompagnent pas.

Je visiterai (nous visiterons) une ferme ou une foire agricole au Canada dans les 14 prochains jours.

J'ai (nous avons) visité une ferme dans un pays autre que le Canada dans les 14 derniers jours.

(Si vous avez répondu oui, veuillez indiquer dans quel(s) pays)

4

5

6

Partie B – Visiteurs au Canada

Durée du séjour au Canada (jours)	Valeur complète de chaque cadeau qui excède 60 $CAN	Précisez les quantités	
		Alcool	Tabac

Partie C – Résidents du Canada *(remplissez dans l'ordre de présentation de la partie A)*

Date de départ du Canada	Valeur des marchandises – $CAN (cadeaux, alcool et tabac compris)	Précisez les quantités	
A M J		Alcool	Tabac

Partie D – Signatures (16 ans et plus)

| | 3 |
| | 4 |

Government of Canada   Gouvernement du Canada

Welcome to Canada
Your Customs Declaration Card – Completion Guide

This guide gives you information about rules and exemptions that may apply to you and the goods you are bringing into Canada. The following information corresponds to the sections on the attached Customs Declaration Card.

Part A – All travellers

All travellers must be identified on a Customs Declaration Card. You may list up to four family members living at the **same address** on one declaration card. Please ensure that each traveller's answers are included on the card. **Each traveller is responsible for his or her own declaration.**

You must declare all goods that you are bringing into Canada, whether or not they are part of your exemption. A customs officer may examine your goods. It is important to note that the value of goods that do not qualify for a personal exemption may be subject to duties, taxes, and/or fees.

Customs officers may seize any goods you do not declare or any goods you falsely declare. You may also face prosecution.

Goods like the following ones may be **restricted, controlled, or prohibited** in Canada, or you may need a **special admission permit.** Failure to declare all of these items could result in fines, arrest, and prosecution:
- Firearms or other weapons (e.g., mace, switchblades, fireworks);
- Drugs;
- Endangered species (live specimens or products made from wild plants or animals, e.g., ivory, corals, reptile skin products); and
- Cultural property (e.g., antiquities, cultural objects).

Under Canadian law, as administered by the **Canadian Food Inspection Agency**, you have to declare all animals and plants and their products. Failure to do so could result in fines and prosecution.

There are specific personal exemption limits for importing alcohol and tobacco into Canada. Determine your limit from the following table.

Table 1 – Personal exemption limits for importing alcohol and tobacco		
Minimum age	Province or territory	Alcohol and tobacco
18 years	Alberta, Manitoba, Quebec	1.5 L of wine or 1.14 L of liquor **or** 24 x 355 mL (12 oz.) bottles/cans of beer or ale (8.5 L)
19 years	All others	
18 years	Alberta, Manitoba, Quebec, Saskatchewan, Yukon Territory, Northwest Territories, Nunavut	200 cigarettes, 200 tobacco sticks, 50 cigars or 50 cigarillos, **and** 200 grams manufactured tobacco
19 years	All others	

During your travels, you may have been exposed to infectious diseases not common in Canada. While the risks posed by most of these illnesses are low, some, such as malaria, may be life threatening. If you develop a fever or flu-like illness within three months of travel to a tropical country, **Health Canada** advises you to get immediate medical attention, inform your doctor of your travel history, and ask for a blood test to rule out malaria.

(Français au verso)

E311 (01/11)

London and Vancouver. Haematological work-up, including bone marrow examination, may detect a lipid storage disease, as may the electron microscopic examination of skin and conjunctival biopsies (Pettigrew and Jankovic, 1985). Properly prepared peripheral lymphocytes may reveal vacuolation on light microscopy and inclusions on electron microscopy (Swaiman et al., 1983). Lysosomal enzymes measured in skin fibroblasts or white blood cells may indicate hexosaminidase, beta-gangliosidase or arylsulphatase A deficiency. Urine should be assayed for organic acids, for example to detect glutaric acid, and amino acids, for example to detect homocystinuria. Severe dystonic movements may increase serum creatine kinase activity and rarely can cause myoglobinuria (Jankovic and Penn, 1982). Caudate atrophy on CT scan would suggest Huntington's disease or neuroacanthocytosis. The CT scan can demonstrate basal ganglia calcifications (Aicardi and Goutieres, 1984; Burton et al., 1984) and can also detect lucencies in the basal ganglia (Nelson et al., 1979; Ropper, Hatten and Davis, 1979; Harik and Post, 1981; Williams and Walshe, 1981), thalamus (Selekler, Kansku and Zileli, 1981), cerebral white matter (Takano et al., 1983), and grey matter (Haenggeli, Hauser and Paunier, 1981) in Wilson's disease and a variety of other conditions. Atrophic changes occur in Hallervorden–Spatz disease (Dooling, Richardson and Davis, 1980) and in Wilson's disease.

An abnormality in the EEG, the evoked responses, or electroretinogram indicates some disease not compatible with idiopathic dystonia. But since these alterations generally lack specificity for any particular condition, they are only needed in patients with findings atypical for idiopathic dystonia. The presence of basal ganglia calcifications in a patient with dystonia suggests one is dealing with a symptomatic dystonia. However, since such calcifications can be found in normal individuals, it is not yet clear what they signify in patients who otherwise would be regarded as having idiopathic dystonia. There is, however, a specific familial syndrome of basal ganglia calcification with torsion dystonia (Larsen et al., 1985).

There is no laboratory test to diagnose idiopathic dystonia. The diagnosis depends on a history free of any of the environmental and disease factors listed in *Table 17.7* and clinical findings without other neurological findings. A positive family history strongly suggests idiopathic dystonia. Dystonia in an Ashkenazi Jewish individual, although commonly idiopathic, can just as easily be symptomatic (*Table 17.6*).

References

AD HOC COMMITTEE (1984) *Ad Hoc* Committee of the Dystonia Medical Research Foundation met in February 1984. Its members included Drs A. Barbeau, D. B. Calne, S. Fahn, C. D. Marsden, J. Menkes and G. F. Wooten

AICARDI, J. and GOUTIERES, F. (1984) A progressive familial encephalopathy in infancy with calcifications of the basal ganglia and chronic cerebrospinal fluid lymphocytosis. *Annals of Neurology*, **15**, 49–54

ARONSON, S. M. and ARONSON, B. E. (1965) Clinical Neuropathological Conference. *Diseases of the Nervous System*, **26**, 245–250

ASHWAL, S., THRASHER, T. V., RICE, D. R. and WENGER, D. A. (1984) A new form of sea-blue histiocytosis associated with progressive anterior horn cell and axonal degeneration. *Annals of Neurology*, **16**, 184–192

BACHMAN, D. S., LAO-VELEZ, C. and ESTANOL, B. (1976) Dystonia and choreoathetosis in multiple sclerosis. *Archives of Neurology*, **33**, 590

BARBEAU, A. (1984) Manganese and extrapyramidal disorders. *Neurotoxicology*, **5**, 13–36

BATSHAW, M. L., WACHTEL, R. C., DECKEL, A. W., WHITEHOUSE, P. J., MOSES, H. III., FOCHTMAN L. J. et al. (1985) Munchausen's syndrome simulating torsion dystonia. *New England Journal of Medicine*, **312**, 1437–1439

BENDA, C. E. (1949) Chronic rheumatic encephalitis, torsion dystonia and Hallervorden–Spatz disease. *Archives of Neurology and Psychiatry*, **61**, 137–163

BENEDEK, L. and RAKONITZ, E. (1940) Heredopathic combination of a congenital deformity of the nose and of myoclonic torsion dysonia. *Journal of Nervous and Mental Disease*, **91**, 608–624

BERARDELLI, A., THOMPSON, P. D., DAY, B. L., ROTHWELL, J. C., O'BRIEN, M. D. and MARSDEN, C. D. (1986) Dystonia of the legs induced by walking or passive movement of the big toe in a patient with cerebellar ectopia and syringomyelia. *Neurology*, **36**, 40–44

BODENSTEINER, J. B., GOLDBLUM, R. M. and GOLDMAN, A. S. (1980) Progressive dystonia masking ataxia in ataxia-telangectasia. *Archives of Neurology*, **37**, 464–465

BRETT, E. M., SHEEHY, M. P. and MARSDEN, C. D. (1981) Progressive hemi-dystonia due to focal basal ganglia lesion after mild head trauma. *Journal of Neurology, Neurosurgery and Psychiatry*, **44**, 460

BRIN, M. F., FAHN, S., BRESSMAN, S. B. and BURKE, R. E. (1986) Dystonia precipitated by peripheral trauma. *Neurology*, **36** (Supplement 1), 119

BRUN, A. and KYLLERMAN, M. (1979) Clinical, pathogenetic and neuropathological correlates in dystonic cerebral palsy. *European Journal of Pediatrics*, **131**, 93–104

BRUYN, G. W. (1968) Huntington's chorea: Historical, clinical and laboratory synopsis. In *Handbook of Clinical Neurology*. Eds P. J. Vinken and G. W. Bruyn, Volume 6, pp. 298–378. Amsterdam: North-Holland Publishing Co.

BURKE, R. E., FAHN, S., BRIN, M. F., BRESSMAN, S. and MOSKOWITZ, C. (1985) The clinical course of autosomal dominant torsion dystonia. *Neurology*, **35** (Supplement 1), 273

BURKE, R. E., FAHN, S. and GOLD, A. P. (1980) Delayed onset dystonia in patients with 'static' encephalopathy. *Journal of Neurology, Neurosurgery and Psychiatry*, **43**, 789–797

BURKE, R. E., FAHN, S., JANKOVIC, J., MARSDEN, C. D., LANG, A. E., GOLLOMP, S. et al. (1982) Tardive dystonia: Late-onset and persistent dystonia caused by antipsychotic drugs. *Neurology*, **32**, 1335–1346

BURKE, R. E., FAHN, S., MARSDEN, C. D., BRESSMAN, S. B., MOSKOWITZ, C. and FRIEDMAN, J. (1985) Validity and reliability of a rating scale for the primary torsion dystonias. *Neurology*, **35**, 73–77

BURNS, C. L. C. (1959) The treatment of torsion spasm in children with trihexyphenidyl (Artane). *The Medical Press*, **241**, 148–149

BURTON, K., FARRELL, K., LI, D. and CALNE, D. B. (1984) Lesions of the putamen and dystonia: CT and magnetic resonance imaging. *Neurology*, **34**, 962–965

CASE RECORDS OF THE MASSACHUSETTS GENERAL HOSPITAL (1984) Case 7–1984. *New England Journal of Medicine*, **310**, 445–455

CASTEELS-VAN DAELE, M., JAEKEN, J., VAN DER SCHUEREN, P., ZIMMERMAN, A. and VAN DEN BON, P. (1970) Dystonic reactions in children caused by metoclopramide. *Archives of Disease in Childhood*, **45**, 130–133

CHADWICK, D., REYNOLDS, E. H. and MARSDEN, C. D. (1976) Anticonvulsant-induced dyskinesias: a comparison with dyskinesias induced by neuroleptics. *Journal of Neurology, Neurosurgery and Psychiatry*, **39**, 1210–1218

CHRISTIAN, C. D. and PAULSON, G. (1958) Severe motility disturbance after small doses of prochlorperazine. *New England Journal of Medicine*, **259**, 828–830

COOPER, I. S., CULLINAN, T. and RIKLAN, M. (1976) The natural history of dystonia. *Advances in Neurology*, **14**, 157–169

CORNER, B. D. (1952) Dystonia musculorum deformans in siblings treated with Artane (trihexyphenidyl). *Proceedings of the Royal Society of Medicine*, **45**, 451–452

CROSLEY, C. J. and SWENDER, P. T. (1979) Dystonia associated with carbamazepine administration: Experience in brain-damaged children. *Pediatrics*, **63**, 612–615

DAVIDENKOW, S. (1926) Auf hereditar-abiotrophischer Grundlage akut auftretende, regressierende und episodische Erkrankungen des Nervensystems und Bemerkungen uber die familiare subakute, myoklonische Dystonie. *Zeitschrift gesamte für Neurologie und Psychiatrie*, **104**, 596–622

DAVOUS, P. and RONDOT, P. (1983) Homocystinuria and dystonia. *Journal of Neurology, Neurosurgery and Psychiatry*, **46**, 283

DE LEON, G. A., KABACK, M. M., ELFENBEIN, I. B., PERCY, A. K. and BRADY, R. O. (1969) Juvenile dystonic lipidosis. *Johns Hopkins Medical Journal*, **125**, 62–77

DEMIERRE, B. and RONDOT, P. (1983) Dystonia caused by putamino-capsulo-caudate vascular lesions. *Journal of Neurology, Neurosurgery and Psychiatry*, **46**, 404–409

DENNY-BROWN, D. (1962) *The Basal Ganglia and their Relation to Disorders of Movement*, p. 78. London: Oxford University Press

DENNY-BROWN, D. (1965) The nature of dystonia. *Bulletin of the New York Academy of Medicine*, **41**, 858–869

DESTARAC. (1901) Torticolis spasmodique et spasmes fonctionnels. *Revue Neurologique,* **9,** 591–597
DOOLING, E. C. and ADAMS, R. D. (1975) The pathological anatomy of posthemiplegic athetosis. *Brain,* **98,** 29–48
DOOLING, E. C., RICHARDSON, E. P. JR, and DAVIS, K. R. (1980) Computed tomography in Hallervorden–Spatz disease. *Neurology,* **30,** 1128–1130
DUVOISIN, R. C., YAHR, M. D., LIEBERMAN, J., ANTUNES, J. and RHEE, S. (1972) The striatal foot. *Transactions of the American Neurological Association,* **97,** 267
ELDRIDGE, R. (1970) The torsion dystonias: Literature review and genetic and clinical studies. *Neurology,* **20,** No. 11(2), 1–78
ELDRIDGE, R. (1981) Inheritance of torsion dystonia in Jews. *Annals of Neurology,* **10,** 203–204
ELDRIDGE, R. and GOTTLIEB, R. (1976) The primary hereditary dystonias: Genetic classification of 768 families and revised estimate of gene frequency, autosomal recessive form, and selected bibliography. *Advances in Neurology,* **14,** 457–474
FAHN, S. (1982a) Fluctuations of disability in Parkinson's disease: pathophysiological aspects. In *Movement Disorders.* Eds C. D. Marsden and S. Fahn, pp. 123–145. London: Butterworths
FAHN, S. (1982b) The clinical spectrum of motor tics. *Advances in Neurology,* **35,** 341–344
FAHN, S. (1982c) Torsion dystonia: Clinical spectrum and treatment. *Seminars in Neurology,* **2,** 316–323
FAHN, S. (1984) The varied clinical expressions of dystonia. *Neurologic Clinics,* **2,** 541–554
FAHN, S. (1985a) Blepharospasm: a focal dystonia. *Advances in Ophthalmic Plastic and Reconstructive Surgery,* **4,** 87–91
FAHN, S. (1985b) Rating scales for blepharospasm. *Advances in Ophthalmic, Plastic and Reconstructive Surgery,* **4,** 97–101
FAHN, S. (1986) Generalized dystonia: concepts and treatment. *Clinical Neuropharmacology,* in press
FAHN, S. (1987) The twists and turns of torsion dystonia. The Robert Wartenberg Lecture. *Neurology,* in press
FAHN, S. and BRESSMAN, S. (1983) Sporadic paroxysmal dystonic choreoathetosis. *Neurology,* **33** (Supplement 2), 131
FAHN, S. and ELDRIDGE, R. (1976) Definition of dystonia and classification of the dystonic states. *Advances in Neurology,* **14,** 1–5
FAHN, S. and JANKOVIC, J. (1984) Practical management of dystonia. *Neurologic Clinics,* **2,** 555–569
FAHN, S., WILLIAMS, D., RECHES, A., LESSER, R. P., JANKOVIC, J. and SILBERSTEIN, S. D. (1983) Hysterical dystonia, a rare disorder: report of five documented cases. *Neurology,* **33** (Supplement 2), 161
FLATAU, E. and STERLING, W. (1911) Progressiver Torsionspasms bie Kindern. *Zeitschrift Gesamte für Neurologie und Psychiatrie,* **7,** 586–612
FRAENKEL, J. (1912) Dysbasia lordotica progressiva, dystonia musculorum deformans – tortipelvis. *Journal of Nervous and Mental Disease,* **39,** 361–374
FRANKE, A. and NEU, I. (1977) Ein Fall von Torsions-Dystonie nach Kohlenmonoxydvergiftung. *Nervenarzt,* **48,** 345–347
FRIEDMAN, A. and FAHN, S. (1986) Spontaneous remissions in spasmodic torticollis. *Neurology,* **36,** 398–400
GILMAN, S. and BARRETT, R. E. (1973) Hallervorden–Spatz disease and infantile neuroaxonal dystrophy. *Journal of the Neurological Sciences,* **19,** 189–205
GOLDIE, W. D., HOLTZMAN, D. and SUZUKI, K. (1977) Chronic hexosaminidase A and B deficiency. *Annals of Neurology,* **2,** 156–158
GOLDMAN, J. E., KATZ, D., RAPIN, I., PURPURA, D. P. and SUZUKI, K. (1981) Chronic GM-1 gangliosidosis presenting as dystonia: I. Clinical and pathological features. *Annals of Neurology,* **9,** 465–475
GOUTIERES, F. and AICARDI, J. (1982) Acute neurological dysfunction associated with destructive lesions of the basal ganglia in children. *Annals of Neurology,* **12,** 328–332
GOWERS, W. R. (1893) *A Manual of Diseases of the Nervous System,* 2nd edn. pp. 709–710. Philadelphia: Blakiston
GOWERS, W. R. (1906) On tetanoid chorea and its association with cirrhosis of the liver. *Review of Neurology and Psychiatry,* **4,** 249–258
GRIMES, J. D., HASSAN, M. H., QUARRINGTON, A. M. and D'ALTON, J. (1982) Delayed-onset posthemiplegic dystonia: CT demonstration of basal ganglia pathology. *Neurology,* **32,** 1033–1035
HAENGGELI, D. A., HAUSER, H. and PAUNIER, L. (1981) CT in Wilson disease. *Neurology,* **31,** 1056
HARIK, S. I. and POST, J. D. (1981) Computed tomography in Wilson disease. *Neurology,* **31,** 107–110
HEATH, P. D. and NIGHTINGALE, S. (1982) Clusters of tonic spasms as an initial manifestation of multiple sclerosis. *Annals of Neurology,* **12,** 494–495
HERZ, E. (1944) Dystonia. I. Historical review: Analysis of dystonic symptoms and physiologic mechanisms involved. *Archives of Neurology and Psychiatry,* **51,** 305–318
HUNT, J. R. (1908) A case of myoclonia of the trunk muscles improved by psychophysical therapeutics. *Journal of Nervous and Mental Disease,* **35,** 656–657

HUNT, J. R. (1916) The progressive torsion spasm of childhood (dystonia musculorum deformans): a consideration of its nature and symptomatology. *Journal of the American Medical Association,* **67,** 1430–1437

JACOME, D. (1979) Carbamazepine-induced dystonia. *Journal of the American Medical Association,* **241,** 2263

JANKOVIC, J. (1984) Progressive supranuclear palsy: clinical and pharmacologic update. *Neurologic Clinics,* **2,** 473–486

JANKOVIC, J. and PATEL, S. C. (1983) Blepharospasm associated with brainstem lesions. *Neurology,* **33,** 1237–1240

JANKOVIC, J. and PENN, A. S. (1982) Severe dystonia and myoglobinuria. *Neurology,* **32,** 1195–1197

JELLINGER, K. (1968) Degenerations and exogenous lesions of the pallidum and striatum. *Handbook of Clinical Neurology,* **6,** 632–693

KANG, U. J., BURKE, R. E. and FAHN, S. (1986) Natural history and treatment of tardive dystonia. *Neurology,* **36** (Supplement 1), 121

KORCZYN, A. D. and GOLDBERG, G. J. (1972) Intravenous diazepam in drug-induced dystonic reactions. *British Journal of Psychiatry,* **121,** 75–77

KORCZYN, A. D., KAHANA, E., ZILBER, N., STREIFLER, M., CARASSO, R. and ALTER, M. (1980) Torsion dystonia in Israel. *Annals of Neurology,* **8,** 387–391

KURLAN, R., BEHR, J., MILLER, C. and SHOULSON, I. (1985) Inherited myoclonic dystonia. *Annals of Neurology,* **18,** 164

LANCE, J. W. (1977) Familial paroxysmal dystonic choreoathetosis and its differentiation from related syndromes. *Annals of Neurology,* **2,** 285–293

LANG, A. E., CLARKE, J. T. R., RESCH, L., STRASBERG, P., SKOMOROSKI, M. A. and O'CONNOR, P. (1985) Progressive long-standing 'pure' dystonia: A new phenotype of juvenile metachromatic leukodystrophy (MLD) *Neurology,* **35** (Supplement 1), 194

LARSEN, T. A., DUNN, H. G., JAN J. E. and CALNE, D. B. (1985) Dystonia and calcification of the basal ganglia. *Neurology,* **35,** 533–537

LEE, L. V., PASCASIO, F. M., FUENTES, F. D. and VITERBO, G. H. (1976) Torsion dystonia in Panay, Philippines. *Advances in Neurology,* **14,** 137–151

LEIBEL, R. L., SHIH, V. E., GOODMAND, S. I., BAUMAN, M. L., McCABE, E. R. B., ZWERDLING, R. G. et al. (1980) Glutaric acidemia: A metabolic disorder causing progressive choreoathetosis. *Neurology,* **30,** 1163–1168

LESSER, R. P. and FAHN, S. (1978) Dystonia: A disorder often misdiagnosed as a conversion reaction. *American Journal of Psychiatry,* **153,** 349–452

LESZYNSKY, W. (1903) Hysterical gait. *Journal of Nervous and Mental Disease,* **30,** 33–34

LEWITT, P. A. (1986) Case demonstration of dystonia secondary to methanol intoxication. Presented at Unusual Movement Disorder Seminar, American Academy of Neurology Meeting

LONGSTRETH, W. T. JR, DAVEN, J. R., FARRELL D. F., BOLEN, J. W. and BIRD, T. D. (1982) Adult dystonic lipidosis: Clinical, histologic and biochemical findings of a neurovisceral storage disease. *Neurology,* **32,** 1295–1299

MARSDEN, C. D. (1976) The problem of adult-onset idiopathic torsion dystonia and other isolated dyskinesias in adult life (including blepharospasm, oromandibular dystonia, dystonic writer's cramp, and torticollis, or axial dystonia). *Advances in Neurology,* **14,** 259–276

MARSDEN, C. D. (1982) The focal dystonias. *Seminars in Neurology,* **2,** 324–333

MARSDEN, C. D. and HARRISON, M. J. G. (1974) Idiopathic torsion dystonia. *Brain,* **97,** 793–810

MARSDEN, C. D., HARRISON, M. J. G. and BUNDEY, S. (1976) Natural history of idiopathic torsion dystonia. *Advances in Neurology,* **14,** 177–187

MARSDEN, C. D., LANG, A. E., QUINN, N. P., McDONALD, I., ABDALLAT, A. and NIMRI, S. (1986) Familial dystonia and visual failure with striatal CT lucencies. *Journal of Neurology, Neurosurgery and Psychiatry,* **49,** 500–509

MARSDEN, C. D., OBESO, J. A., ZARRANZ, J. J. and LANG, A. E. (1985) The anatomical basis of symptomatic hemidystonia. *Brain,* **108,** 461–483

MARSDEN, C. D., PARKES, J. D. and QUINN, N. (1982) Fluctuations of disability in Parkinson's disease – clinical aspects. In *Movement Disorders.* Eds C. D. Marsden and S. Fahn. pp. 96–122. London: Butterworths

MAURO, A. J., FAHN, S. and RUSSMAN, B. (1980) Hemidystonia following 'minor' head trauma. *Transactions of the American Neurological Association,* **105,** 229–231

MEEK, D., WOLFE, L. S., ANDERMANN, E. and ANDERMANN, F. (1984) Juvenile progressive dystonia: A new phenotype of GM2 gangliosidosis. *Annals of Neurology,* **15,** 348–352

MEIGE, H. and FEINDEL, E. C. L. (1907) *Tics and Their Treatment.* Translated from the French by Wilson SAK. London: Appleton

MELAMED. E. (1979) Early-morning dystonia: A late side effect of long term levodopa therapy in Parkinson's disease. *Archives of Neurology,* **36,** 308–310

MENDEL, K. (1919) Torsiondystonie (Dystonia musculorum deformans, Torsionsspasmus). *Monatschrift für Psychiatrie und Neurologie,* **46,** 309–361

MUENTER, M. D. and WHISNANT, J. P. (1968) Basal ganglia calcification, hypoparathyroidism, and extrapyramidal motor manifestations. *Neurology,* **18,** 1075–1083

NAKANO, T., IKEDA, S-I., KONDO, K., YANAGISAWA, N. and TSUJI, S. (1985) Adult GM1-gangliosidosis: Clinical patterns and rectal biopsy. *Neurology,* **35,** 875–880

NARBONA, J., OBESO, J. A., TUNON, T., MARTINEZ-LAGE, J. M. and MARSDEN, C. D. (1984) Hemidystonia secondary to localised basal ganglia tumour. *Journal of Neurology, Neurosurgery and Psychiatry,* **47,** 704–709

NELSON, R. F., GUZMAN, D. A., GRAHOVAC, Z. and HOWSE, D. C. N. (1979) Computerized cranial tomography in Wilson disease. *Neurology,* **29,** 866–868

NEVILLE, B. G. R., LAKE, B. D., STEPHENS, R. and SANDERS, M. D. (1973) A neurovisceral storage disease with vertical supranuclear ophthalmoplegia, and its relationship to Niemann–Pick disease. *Brain,* **96,** 97–120

NOVOTNY, E. J. Jr, SINGH, G., WALLACE, D. C., DORFMANN, L. J., LOUIS, A., SOGG, R. L. et al. (1986) Leler's disease and dystonia: a mitochondrial disease. *Neurology,* **36,** 1053–1060

NYGAARD, T. G. and DUVOISIN, R. C. (1986) Hereditary dystonia–parkinsonism syndrome of juvenile onset. *Neurology,* in press

NYGAARD, T. G., DUVOISIN, R. C. and MARSDEN, C. D. (1987) Dopa-responsive dystonia. *Advances in Neurology,* in press

OBESO, J. A., MARTINEZ-VILA, E., DELGADO, G., VAAMONDE, J., MARAVI, E. and MARTINEZ-LAGE, J. M. (1984) Delayed onset dystonia following hemiplegic migraine. *Headache,* **24,** 266–268

OBESO, J. A., ROTHWELL, J. C., LANG, A. E. and MARSDEN, C. D. (1983) Myoclonic dystonia. *Neurology,* **33,** 825–830

OPPENHEIM, H. (1911) Uber eine eigenartige Krampfkrankheit des kindlichen und jugendlichen Alters (Dysbasia lordotica progressiva, Dystonia musculorum deformans). *Neurologie Centralblatt,* **30,** 1090–1107

PAULSON, G. (1960) Procyclidine for dystonia caused by phenothiazine derivatives. *Diseases of the Nervous System,* **21,** 447–448

PAULSON, G. W. (1972) Meige's syndrome. *Geriatrics,* **27,** 69–73

PETTIGREW, L. C. and JANKOVIC, J. (1985) Hemidystonia: a report of 22 patients and a review of the literature. *Journal of Neurology, Neurosurgery and Psychiatry,* **48,** 650–657

PHILIPPART, M. and BROWN, W. J. (1984) Dystonia and lactic acidosis: New features of Rett's syndrome. *Annals of Neurology,* **16,** 387

POLL-THE, B. T., AICARDI, J., GIROT, R. and ROSA, R. (1985) Neurological findings in triosephosphate isomerase deficiency. *Annals of Neurology,* **17,** 439–443

QUINN, N. P. (1983) Dystonia in epidemic ergotism. *Neurology,* **33,** 1267

QUINN, N. P. and MARSDEN, C. D. (1984) Dominantly inherited myoclonic dystonia with dramatic response to alcohol. *Neurology,* **34** (Supplement 1), 236

QUINN, N. P. and MARSDEN, C. D. (1987) Hereditary dystonia with lightning-like jerks, responsive to alcohol. *Advances in Neurology,* in press

ROPPER, A. H., HATTEN, H. P. JR, and DAVIS, K. R. (1979) Computed tomography in Wilson disease: report of 2 cases. *Annals of Neurology,* **5,** 102–103

ROSENBERG, R. N. and FOWLER, H. L. (1981) Autosomal dominant motor system disease of the Portuguese: A review. *Neurology,* **31,** 1124–1126

SABOURAUD, O., ALLAIN, H., PINEL, J. F. and MENAULT, P. (1978) Famialiale transformee par la bromocriptine. *Nouvelle Presse Medicale,* **7,** 3370

SCHEINBERG, I. H. and STERNLIEB, I. (1984) *Wilson's Disease.* Philadelphia: W. B. Saunders Co.

SCHOTT, G. D. (1985) The relationship of peripheral trauma and pain to dystonia. *Journal of Neurology, Neurosurgery and Psychiatry,* **48,** 698–701

SCHWALBE, W. (1908) *Eine eigentumliche tonische Krampfform mit hysterischen Symptomen.* Inaugural Dissertation, Berlin: G. Schade

SEGAWA, M., HOSAKA, A., MIYAGAWA, F., NOMURA, Y. and IMAI, H. (1976) Hereditary progressive dystonia with marked diurnal fluctuation. *Advances in Neurology,* **14,** 215–233

SEGAWA, M., NOMURA, Y. and KASE, M. (1987) Hereditary progressive dystonia with marked diurnal fluctuation: Clinico-pathophysiological identification in reference to juvenile Parkinson's disease. *Advances in Neurology,* in press

SELEKLER, K., KANSU, T. and ZILELI, T. (1981) Computed tomography in Wilson's disease. *Archives of Neurology,* **38,** 727–728

SHEEHY, M. P. and MARSDEN, C. D. (1980) Trauma and pain in spasmodic torticollis. *Lancet,* **i,** 777–778
SHEEHY, M. P. and MARSDEN, C. D. (1982) Writer's cramp – a focal dystonia. *Brain,* **105,** 461–480
SUBCZYNSKI, J., HAQUE, I., WOLDRING, S. and OWENS, G. (1969) Involuntary movement syndrome after high cervical percutaneous cordotomy. *New York State Journal of Medicine,* **69,** 697–699
SUNOHARA, N., MANO, Y., ANDO, K. and SATOYOSHI, E. (1985) Idiopathic dystonia–parkinsonism with marked diurnal fluctuation of symptoms. *Annals of Neurology,* **17,** 39–45
SWAIMAN, K. F., SMITH, S. A., TROCK, G. L. and SIDDIQUI, A. R. (1983) Sea-blue histiocytes, lymphocytic cytosomes, movement disorder and ^{59}Fe-uptake in basal ganglia: Hallervorden–Spatz disease or ceroid storage disease with abnormal isotope scan? *Neurology,* **33,** 301–305
TAHMOUSH, A. J., ALPERS, D. H., FEIGIN, R. D., ARMBRUSTMACHER, V. and PRENSKY, A. L. (1976) Hartnup disease: Clinical, pathological, and biochemical observations. *Archives of Neurology,* **33,** 797–807
TAKANO, K., KUROIWA, Y., SHIMADA, Y., MANNEN, T. and TOYOKURA, Y. (1983) CT manifestation of cerebral white matter lesion in Wilson disease. *Annals of Neurology,* **13,** 108–109
TAYLOR, E. W. (1920) Dystonia lenticularis (dystonia musculorum deformans). *Archives of Neurology and Psychiatry,* **4,** 417–427
TOLOSA, E. S. and KLAWANS, H. L. (1979) Meige's disease: A clinical form of facial convulsion, bilateral and medial. *Archives of Neurology,* **36,** 635–637
TSAI, N., CHEN, Y., ZHAO, X.-B. and QUIN, Z.-J. (1983) Acute infectious torticollis. *Neurology,* **33,** 1344–1346
WATTS, R. W. E., SPELLACY, E., GIBBS, D. A., ALLSOP, J., McKERAN, R. O. and SLAVIN, G. E. (1982) Clinical, post-mortem, biochemical and therapeutic observations on the Lesch–Nyhan syndrome with particular reference to the neurological manifestations. *Quarterly Journal of Medicine,* **201,** 43–78
WECHSLER, I. S. and BROCK, S. (1922) Dystonia musculorum deformans with especial reference to a myostatic form and the occurrence of decerebrate rigidity phenomena. A study of six cases. *Archives of Neurology and Psychiatry,* **8,** 538–552
WILLIAMS, F. J. B. and WALSHE, J. M. (1981) Wilson's disease: analysis of the cranial computerized tomographic appearances found in patients and the changes in response to treatment with chelating agents. *Brain,* **104,** 735–752
WILSON, S. A. K. (1940) *Neurology,* Vol. II, pp. 834–835. Baltimore: Williams & Wilkins
YANAGISAWA, N. and GOTO, A. (1971) Dystonia musculorum deformans: Analysis with electromyography. *Journal of the Neurological Sciences,* **13,** 39–65
YERBY, M. S., SHAW, C.-M. and WATSON, J. M. D. (1986) Progressive dementia and epilepsy in a young adult: Unusual intraneuronal inclusions. *Neurology,* **36,** 68–71
ZEMAN, W. (1976) Dystonia: an overview. *Advances in Neurology,* **14,** 91–103
ZEMAN, W. and DYKEN, P. (1967) Dystonia musculorum deformans; clinical, genetic and pathoanatomical studies. *Psychiatria Neurologia Neurochirurgia,* **10,** 77–121
ZEMAN, W. and DYKEN, P. (1968) Dystonia musculorum deformans. *Handbook of Clinical Neurology,* **6,** 517–543
ZEMAN, W., KAELBLING, R. and PASAMANICK. B. (1960) Idiopathic dystonia musculorum deformans. II. The formes frustes. *Neurology,* **10,** 1068–1075
ZIEHEN, T. (1911) Ein fall von tonischer Torsionsneurose. *Neurologie Centralblatt,* **30,** 109–110
ZILBER, N., KORCZYN, A. D., KAHANA, E., FRIED, K. and ALTER, M. (1984) Inheritance of idiopathic torsion dystonia among Jews. *Journal of Medical Genetics,* **21,** 13–20

18
The treatment of dystonia
Stanley Fahn and C. David Marsden

INTRODUCTION

Therapeutic approaches to patients with dystonia, like other neurological disorders, can be divided into two categories: specific rational therapy for specific causes of the condition, and non-specific therapy that treats the symptoms but not the cause of the disease. It is obvious that if a specific form of treatment is available for any aetiological form of dystonia, this should be used. Wilson's disease is an excellent example: drugs that deplete the body stores of copper are required. The preceding chapter on classification and investigation of dystonia emphasized the work-up necessary to establish or exclude not only the diagnosis of Wilson's disease, but also other aetiologies of dystonia that require specific rational therapy. Details on the clinical presentation and treatment of Wilson's disease are presented in Chapter 14 by Sternlieb, Giblin and Scheinberg. Thus, no more needs to be said about the treatment of this disorder, other than to point out that if residual dystonia persists despite copper depletion therapy, non-specific therapy, namely anticholinergic drugs, have been reported to be useful in ameliorating such symptoms (Shoulson et al., 1983).

Drug-induced dystonias are another category requiring specific therapy. Those due to anti-convulsants (Kooiker and Sumi, 1974; Chadwick, Reynolds and Marsden, 1976; Lukdorf and Lurd, 1977; Crosley and Swender, 1979; Jacome, 1979) can be treated by discontinuing or reducing the dosage of the anti-convulsant. Acute dystonic reactions secondary to anti-psychotic drugs or other dopamine receptor antagonists such as metoclopramide (Casteels-van Daele et al., 1970; Gatrad, 1976; Pinder et al., 1976; Reasbeck and Hossenbocus, 1979) can respond to parenteral administration of anti-cholinergics or anti-histaminics (Paulson, 1960; Waugh and Metts, 1960; Smith and Miller, 1961). A standard dosage of diphenhydramine is 50 mg by slow intravenous injection. The dose can be repeated if necessary. Intravenous diazepam has also been shown to be effective and can be used as an alternative therapy (Korczyn and Goldberg, 1972; Gagrat, Hamilton and Belmaker, 1978; Rainer-Pope, 1979). There is also a report that intravenous administration of methylphenidate 20–50 mg can produce an immediate relief of symptoms (Fahn, 1966).

Persistent dystonia as a complication of anti-psychotic drugs and other dopamine receptor antagonists has been given the name of tardive dystonia (Burke et al., 1982). This disorder is part of the tardive dyskinesia spectrum, but is more difficult to treat (Fahn, 1984) than 'classical' tardive dyskinesia with stereotypic oral–lingual–buccal movements (Paulson, 1968). Tardive dystonia, like classical tardive dyskinesia, can sometimes remit spontaneously if the offending drug is withdrawn. Similarly, anti-dopaminergic drugs can mask the symptoms, but this approach is not as consistently effective for tardive dystonia as it is for classical tardive dyskinesia. Kang, Burke and Fahn (1986) recently reviewed the treatment outcome in 67 patients with tardive dystonia, evaluating a variety of medications in open-label trials. Anti-dopaminergic drugs were effective in more than 50% of the patients, whereas anti-cholinergics were effective in approximately 40%, benzodiazepines in 26%, and baclofen in 8% of patients. Other drugs reported to be helpful in isolated patients with tardive dystonia are bromocriptine (Luchins and Goldman, 1985), deanol (McLean and Casey, 1978), clonidine (Nishinawa et al., 1984), and lisuride (Quinn et al., 1985). Electroconvulsive therapy has also been reported to be effective (Kwentus, Schulz and Hart, 1984).

Dystonia, whether peak-dose dystonia or diphasic dystonia, can occur in patients being treated with levodopa for Parkinson's disease. Peak-dose dystonia can be relieved by discontinuing or reducing the dosage of levodopa; however, symptoms of parkinsonism reappear, so readjustment of the medication or addition of a dopamine agonist is a more satisfactory approach. Diphasic dyskinesias are more complicated. They disappear if levodopa is withdrawn, but may also be improved by increasing levodopa dosage; however, this usually causes an unacceptable peak-dose dyskinesia. Substituting a dopamine agonist for levodopa may be helpful. Dystonia as a symptom of untreated parkinsonism (see Chapter 17) can sometimes improve or be made worse with anti-parkinsonism drugs.

Dystonia secondary to cerebral arteriovenous malformations, or displacement or compression of the basal ganglia by cerebral tumours or other mass lesions can sometimes be relieved by appropriate surgical therapy.

The great majority of patients with either idiopathic or symptomatic dystonia require non-specific therapy, designed to treat the symptoms rather than the cause. Non-specific therapy of dystonia is basically of three types: (a) physical and behavioural modification techniques, such as sensory biofeedback and other relaxation therapies including self-hypnosis, (b) pharmacotherapy, systemic and local, and (c) surgical procedures. Pharmacotherapy can be divided into two categories, namely, injections of drugs directly into dystonic muscles to act locally, and administration of medication to have widespread effects on the body, particularly the central nervous system (CNS). Surgical approaches can be divided into ablative lesions within the CNS, electrical stimulation of the CNS, ablative lesions of the peripheral neuromuscular system to weaken specific muscles responsible for focal dystonias, and orthopaedic procedures to correct focal postural deformities. Each of these therapeutic strategies will be discussed in this chapter except for the orthopaedic procedures. There is surprisingly little information regarding the value of orthopaedic approaches to dystonia. To the best of our knowledge, no large surveys have been reported on the outcome of various types of orthopaedic operation that have been attempted in patients to correct the deformities of posture produced by dystonia. It is our impression that even simple procedures, such as lengthening the Achilles tendon in those walking on their toes, is doomed to failure. However, it may be that we have not seen those in whom this operation has been a success. Nevertheless, such procedures are cautioned against since a number of patients have been seen whose dystonia has accentuated after such surgery; spasms in the affected limb may increase, or may spread to other parts of the body not previously affected.

This chapter will discuss each of these three major non-specific therapeutic modalities and then conclude with an approach to treatment that has been found useful.

PHYSICAL METHODS AND BEHAVIOURAL MODIFICATION

Non-invasive approaches, if effective, would be the ideal choice of therapy. Since dystonia can increase in severity with fatiguing exercise and stress, and decrease in severity with sleep and relaxation, it is reasonable to try to help patients avoid stress and teach them methods of relaxation. Self-hypnosis was used in one patient by Fahn (unpublished observation), which effectively reduced the augmented dystonic movements due to stress. In fact, any of the methods of relaxation therapy in current vogue (hypnotherapy, aromatherapy etc.) may help dystonia by reducing anxiety and stress-related exacerbation of dystonia, if the patient believes in such approaches and gains relaxation from them. In our experience, the majority of patients welcome the opportunity for discussion of common problems with other sufferers contacted through the self-help lay organizations (Dystonia Medical Research Foundation in North America and The Dystonia Society in the United Kingdom).

Behavioural modification therapy for torticollis was utilized by Brierly (1967) who thought he was dealing with a hysterical disorder. Brierly used an avoidance-conditioning plan by delivering mild cutaneous shock to an arm when the position-sensitive device on the patient's head was activated by head deviation. Cleeland (1973) extended this design by pairing the cutaneous shocks with EMG activity (feedback) of the contracting neck muscles. Within a laboratory setting most patients were able to reduce the severity of the spasms.

Sensory biofeedback coupled with relaxation therapy was employed for spasmodic torticollis by Brudny (Brudny, Grynbaum and Korein, 1974; Brudny et al., 1974). Extensive use of this approach in 48 patients with torticollis was noted to result in improvement in 32 (58%) (Korein et al., 1976). In other forms of focal dystonia and whenever dystonia is more widespread, results have not been so favourable. Although this therapeutic approach is benign and non-invasive, it is time consuming and the best results are obtained when patients are actively monitoring themselves in front of a mirror with sensory EMG feedback to indicate the quantity and severity of contractions of the neck muscles. It is more difficult to keep those muscles relaxed when the patient is not concentrating on the task. Thus, early success with biofeedback therapy is usually not maintained, and many patients abandon this method. Because of the lack of sustained success with this approach, it is not considered to be of much practical value and patients are no longer referred for this form of therapy unless they wish to avoid more active intervention. Nevertheless, it is worth exploring whether well-established methods of psychological shaping and reinforcement may make such approaches more powerful.

As with most medical disorders, supportive psychotherapy is an important adjunct in treating patients. It is helpful for the physician to provide accurate factual explanations and to have a positive approach, especially for a patient who is discouraged by the illness. Unfortunately, too many patients still go through years of uncertainty before they are informed of the diagnosis of dystonia and what this means (Bakshaw and Haslam, 1976). Other than supportive psychotherapy to assist the patient and family to adjust to the disorder, prolonged or intensive psychotherapy is generally of no benefit in treating torsion dystonia, except for cases of psychogenic dystonia. Eldridge, Riklan and Cooper (1969) reported that, of 24 patients who underwent a trial of psychotherapy, seven reported that their general condition was made worse, 12 reported no benefit, and five stated there was benefit in emotional status but not in the dystonia. One should keep in mind that great emotional damage to the patient and the patient's family can arise from misdiagnosing patients as having psychogenic dystonia leading to extensive psychotherapy searching for the emotional 'cause' of the disorder. Cooper (1976) described the breakup of a family because each parent blamed the other for causing the psychological damage that was supposed to have induced the dystonic movements in their child who was incorrectly diagnosed as having hysteria. Similar cases have been encountered by the authors. The error is to assume that the dystonia is caused by a psychological disturbance. On the other hand, formal psychotherapy and psychiatric treatments may be of value to patients with overt secondary psychological disturbances or psychiatric illness, provided the therapist clearly acknowledges the physical basis of the dystonia and concentrates on relieving the secondary emotional consequences. An important, but often overlooked, aspect of dystonia is its effect upon sexual attractiveness. Many young patients have considerable difficulties in forming relationships and experience great emotional disturbances as a result.

Mechanical braces can sometimes be helpful, but also can be harmful. Since certain sensory stimuli (sensory tricks) can frequently reduce the severity of dystonia (*see* Chapter 17), patients with this phenomenon will usually use such tricks to reduce the severity of their dystonia. If a hand on a chin reduces torticollis, the patient will usually sit so that this manoeuvre is utilized. In those patients in whom tactile input on the occiput reduces torticollis, a device sometimes can be constructed so that the sensory input is constant, allowing the patient to keep the head fairly straight. Very often, however, forcefully contracting muscles contract even more actively when splints, braces, and casts are applied in an effort to straighten a twisted body. This can lead to abrasion of the skin and even increasing abnormal posturing. The authors have seen patients whose dystonic limb was more abnormal after a period of being in a cast than before the cast was applied. Even soft cervical collars for torticollis are not usually helpful. Most patients obtain little relief from them unless the sensory input from the collar provides some relief due to the sensory trick phenomenon.

Physiotherapy in the form of exercising to build up strength in antagonist musculature in order to counteract the force of the major muscle involuntarily contracting is usually not helpful and can also lead to aggravation of the dystonic pulling. Hot soaks and whirlpool baths can provide some transient comfort to painful dystonic muscles.

PHARMACOTHERAPY

Systemic administration

Many drugs have been reported to be of some benefit in variable numbers of patients with torsion dystonia (Eldridge, 1970). In contrast to Parkinson's disease and choreic disorders, in which levodopa therapy and anti-dopaminergic drugs, respectively, can rather consistently produce improvement, no such claim can be made for any single drug in the treatment of torsion dystonia. Until a few years ago it was rare to find reports of major drug trials in dystonia. Most reports on efficacy of medications were based on a few cases or just single case reports. In the last few years, however, there have been a number of drug studies in fairly large series of patients. Enough accumulated experience has been gathered about some drugs to summarize these findings and to draw some general conclusions.

Drug treatment could be discussed in terms of therapy for specific focal dystonias (such as blepharospasm, spasmodic torticollis, and writer's cramp), varieties of segmental dystonia, or generalized dystonia. However, there is insufficient evidence to state categorically if pharmacological differences exist among the various focal, segmental, and generalized dystonias. Accordingly, pharmacotherapy of all types of dystonia has been reviewed, organized by classes of drugs.

Anti-cholinergics

Since the introduction of high-dosage anti-cholinergic drugs, these agents have become one of the mainstays of non-specific therapy in dystonia. Based originally on open-label trials (Fahn, 1979, 1983), the efficacy of these drugs given in high dosages has been substantiated by double-blind investigations (Burke, Fahn and Marsden, 1986) and by other open-label trials on large numbers of patients (Duvoisin, 1983; Marsden, Marion and Quinn, 1984; Lang, 1986). In general, all these studies show that approximately 50% of children and 40% of adults with idiopathic dystonia obtain moderate to dramatic benefit from this class of drugs.

Earlier studies using lower dosages of anti-cholinergics also reported benefit, but not in the same high percentage of cases (Marsden and Harrison, 1974; Lal et al., 1979; Tanner et al., 1979; Girotti et al., 1982; Lang, Sheehy and Marsden, 1982; Tanner, Glantz and Klawans, 1982; Marsden, Lang and Sheehy, 1983; Nutt et al., 1987). Tanner and her colleagues (Tanner et al., 1987) reported that the intramuscular injection of scopolamine 0.01 mg/kg can predict the outcome of high-dosage chronic administration of oral trihexyphenidyl in 80% of patients.

It is of historical interest that perhaps the first patient to receive anti-cholinergics for dystonia was Wolf Lewin, a member of the family reported in the first paper on idiopathic generalized dystonia by Schwalbe (1908). Treatment of Wolf with scopolamine resulted in sufficient improvement of his dystonia to allow him to marry and have children (Regensburg, 1930; Jankowska, 1934).

Dose-limiting problems with anti-cholinergics are their peripheral and central adverse effects. Peripheral adverse effects such as dry mouth and blurred vision are fairly common, but can often be ameliorated by co-administration of peripherally acting anti-cholinesterase drugs and eyedrops of pilocarpine, a muscarinic agonist. Central adverse effects, such as forgetfulness, confusion, hallucinations, or behavioural changes, can only be overcome by reducing the dose of the anti-cholinergic which lessens the usefulness of these agents.

Despite the very high doses of anti-cholinergic drugs now employed in many patients with dystonia, no long-term problems have emerged. Children and adults have been treated with doses of trihexyphenidyl of up to 40 mg/day for periods of up to 15 years and doses of 100–130 mg/day for up to 8 years. Naturally, there has been concern about the effects of such treatment on intellect, memory and school performances. However, no obvious adverse effects have emerged, and if short-term memory is affected in individual patients, it is remedied by a reduction of dose. Nevertheless, such concern leads to a conservative use of this approach, with the aim of keeping the dose of anti-cholinergic as low as is required to maintain physical independence, rather than pushing the dose to its limits in the hope of abolishing all evidence of dystonia.

Central adverse effects are more common in adults than in children (Burke and Fahn, 1985a), which could explain, at least in part, the lower percentage of adults who respond compared to children. Serum levels of trihexyphenidyl correlate with total daily dose, but do not correlate with therapeutic response or toxicity (Burke and Fahn, 1985a). The pharmacokinetics of trihexyphenidyl do not change between short-term and long-term treatment; trihexyphenidyl has an initial rapid distribution phase and a later, slower elimination phase (Burke and Fahn, 1985b).

In keeping with the improvement of dystonia seen with anti-cholinergic drugs, dystonia is exacerbated in patients who receive physostigmine, a centrally as well as peripherally acting cholinergic (Tanner et al., 1979; Stahl and Berger, 1982).

In their analysis of 227 patients with dystonia treated with anti-cholinergics in a long-term open-label trial, Greene, Shale and Fahn (1987) confirmed that more than 50% of patients with childhood onset responded with moderate to marked improvement, and approximately 40% of adult-onset patients also responded. When these authors analysed for features that could account for a favourable response, the only factor found to be significant was the duration of the disease before anti-cholinergic medication was initiated. There was a statistically significant likelihood for improvement if the medication was begun within 5 years of onset. Other factors, such as severity of dystonia, gender, ethnic background, and previous thalamotomy, failed to correlate with therapeutic responsiveness. The implications of this finding are that delay of treatment can result in an unfavourable response.

The mechanism as to how anti-cholinergics are effective in the treatment of torsion dystonia is unknown. Similarly, the mechanism whereby these drugs are effective in the treatment of acute dystonic reactions due to anti-psychotic drugs, including tetrabenazine (Burke et al., 1985), is also unknown. Although the striatum and the nucleus accumbens are the richest sites in the brain for acetylcholine and its synthesizing and degrading enzymes, choline acetyltransferase and acetylcholinesterase (Fahn, 1976), it is not certain that these structures are the site of therapeutic action of anti-cholinergic drugs in dystonia. There are numerous other cholinergic pathways in the central nervous system. Nor is it clear why high doses are often required, and why it may take some weeks or months for the greatest benefit to be obtained. Whether large doses and a long time are required to achieve the maximum central anti-cholinergic effect, or whether other changes, such as adaptation of receptors or alterations of other central neurotransmitters, are necessary is not known.

Dopamine agonists

Shortly after the introduction of high-dosage levodopa for Parkinson's disease (Cotzias, Van Woert and Schiffer, 1967), this drug was tried in patients with torsion dystonia. Anecdotal case reports initially described good results (Chase, 1970; Coleman, 1970). At the same time, others failed to discern much benefit from levodopa (Barrett, Yahr and Duvoisin, 1970; Mandell, 1970). Subsequently,

Cooper (1972) reported that the cases previously shown to have benefited from levodopa ultimately worsened. Eldridge, Kanter and Koerber (1973) surveyed 39 patients who had received levodopa: 5% had lasting improvement, and 39% had an initial short-lived benefit. Levodopa worsened the symptoms in 34%. There have been a number of subsequent reports evaluating levodopa and dopamine agonists in generalized and focal idiopathic torsion dystonia. These have been reviewed recently by Lang (1985, 1987). Only a small percentage of patients with dystonia have shown a favourable response to these agents.

However, patients with diurnal fluctuations of dystonia usually obtain a dramatic response to low-dosage levodopa or dopamine agonists (Segawa et al., 1976; Rondot and Ziegler, 1983; Deonna, 1986). Recently, Nygaard, Marsden and Duvoisin (1987) reported that approximately 5–10% of patients with childhood-onset dystonia beginning in the legs, with or without diurnal fluctuations, can respond dramatically to low-dosage levodopa. These authors suggested that the group of levodopa responders, whether with or without diurnal fluctuations, should be considered a pharmacological subset of idiopathic torsion dystonia (see Chapter 17). It is not clear if patients responding to levodopa would also respond to anti-cholinergics. However, it does appear that some patients with diurnal fluctuations of dystonia also respond to low-dosage anti-cholinergics (Corner, 1952; Burns, 1959; Fahn, personal observations). It is difficult to carry out a pharmacological study evaluating responses to a variety of drugs in patients who have a dramatic response to a given drug, because such patients are reluctant to discontinue that drug and participate in other drug trials; nor are physicians eager to embark on such studies if their patients are doing very well. The evidence so far indicates that patients with diurnal fluctuations can respond to either low-dosage levodopa, dopamine agonists, or anti-cholinergics. Because of the potential for anti-cholinergics to interfere with memory (see above), levodopa therapy may be the preferred therapy for these patients.

From various reports, it would appear that dopamine agonists have approximately the same efficacy as levodopa (Stahl and Berger, 1982; Newman et al., 1985; Nutt et al., 1985; Quinn et al., 1985). Although the response rate to these drugs is quite low, there have been no reports comparing the same patients with different dopamine agonists, and also no comparisons with levodopa and anti-cholinergics. In the study reported by Greene, Shale and Fahn (1987), levodopa and dopamine agonists were used predominantly in patients who had failed to obtain adequate response to anti-cholinergics. These authors reported that 12% of 41 patients tested with dopamine agonist therapy had a favourable response. These authors also reported that many patients who had failed previous trials of levodopa responded to anti-cholinergic therapy, Thus, it appears fairly consistently that there is a lower percentage of patients with dystonia who can respond favourably to dopaminergics compared to anti-cholinergics. Nevertheless, in the small number of patients who respond favourably to low-dosage levodopa or dopamine agonists, the response can be dramatic. Thus, as will be discussed further (see below), it is worthwhile trying levodopa for a short period in all patients with childhood-onset dystonia before proceeding to anti-cholinergic therapy.

Dopamine antagonists

It is difficult to understand why one small population of patients with dystonia (approximately 10%) responds favourably to dopamine agonists while another subset of approximately twice that magnitude responds favourably to the oppositely acting dopamine antagonist drugs (dopamine receptor blockers and dopamine storage depletors, such as tetrabenazine and reserpine (Jankovic, 1982; Lang and Marsden, 1982; Jankovic and Ford, 1983; Lang, 1987)). An explanation commonly invoked to explain this apparent incongruity is that torsion dystonia is due to more than one pathophysiological mechanism; patients with one type of dystonia respond to one class of drugs, and those with another type respond to different agents. At least consistent with this proposal is the absence of any description of an individual responding to both dopamine agonists and antagonists.

An early report of the general effectiveness of anti-psychotic drugs in the treatment of dystonia (Gilbert, 1972) was not substantiated by subsequent studies. Lang (1987) recently reviewed the literature on dopamine antagonists in the treatment of idiopathic dystonia. The results of these studies have been highly variable. For example, the frequency of response to these drugs in generalized and segmental dystonias varied from 0% to 78%; for cranial dystonia, from 3% to 34%; for spasmodic torticollis, from 9% to 46%; and no patient with writer's cramp responded.

The most commonly used drugs of this class have been phenothiazines, haloperidol, tetrabenazine, and pimozide. Marsden, Marion and Quinn (1984) recently reported that a triple combination of a dopamine depletor, a dopamine receptor blocker, and an anti-cholinergic may allow greater benefit in some patients than any of these drugs alone. From this study, it is not clear whether both the dopamine receptor blocker and the dopamine depletor are necessary in combination or whether a higher dosage of either one drug would be equally effective. This 'cocktail' was arrived at empirically. Tetrabenazine was kept at low dose (75–150 mg/day) because higher doses caused an unacceptable incidence of depression. Tetrabenazine depletes the brain not only of dopamine, but also of noradrenaline and serotonin, which may be involved with depression. Pimozide (or haloperidol) is a relatively selective dopamine receptor blocking agent, so it was added to increase dopamine antagonism. Trihexyphenidyl was included to prevent drug-induced parkinsonism and for its effect on dystonia.

In the analysis of open-label trials of anti-dopaminergics on patients with idiopathic dystonia by Greene, Shale and Fahn, 1987), 35% of 26 showed moderate to marked benefit to dopamine receptor blockers, whereas 25% of 44 had such benefit from dopamine depletors. Most of these patients were also taking an anti-cholinergic drug. From this study, it appears that anti-dopaminergics are the second most effective class of drugs for the non-specific treatment of idiopathic torsion dystonia in terms of percentage of patients who respond.

Other pharmacological agents

There are only scattered reports on the efficacy of other drugs in the treatment of dystonia. Baclofen in high dosage was found to be beneficial in some patients with blepharospasm (Gollamp et al., 1983; Fahn, et al., 1985a). This drug has now been studied in other forms of dystonia as well. Of 108 patients with a variety of idiopathic dystonias treated with baclofen, 20% of patients had a moderate to marked benefit (Greene, Shale and Fahn, 1987). In the analysis of 58 patients with segmental cranial dystonia who were treated with baclofen, of the 20 who responded favourably, three-quarters had a marked beneficial response. It would appear that in this variety of dystonia, baclofen either fails to produce any beneficial effect or it produces a highly successful response.

The benzodiazepines have occasionally provided some benefit in anecdotal reports (Ziegler, 1981). Greene, Shale and Fahn (1987) reported that clonazepam and other benzodiazepines were effective in 15% of 177 patients with idiopathic dystonia. There is no evidence of superiority of any one benzodiazepine. Jankovic and Ford (1983) reported that clonazepam is sometimes beneficial for Meige's syndrome.

The initial highly enthusiastic reports on the effectiveness of carbamezepine in dystonia (Geller, Kaplan and Christoff, 1974, 1976) could not be substantiated by subsequent studies, which showed that only a small percentage of patients respond to this agent (Isgreen *et al.*, 1976). In the large study by Greene, Shale and Fahn (1987), of the 67 patients treated with carbamazepine, only 11% obtained moderate or greater benefit.

Alcohol has been effective in patients with autosomal dominant dystonia with lightning jerks (Quinn and Marsden, 1984). A study evaluating intravenous infusion of alcohol reported that it can be effective in reducing spasmodic torticollis, but that it had no effect in patients with cranial or generalized dystonia (Biary and Koller, 1985).

Riker *et al.* (1982) reported that clonidine was not effective in four patients with generalized dystonia, but was effective in one out of five with torticollis. None of three patients with idiopathic dystonia tested with clonidine by Greene, Shale and Fahn (1987) responded. These investigators reported that 7% of 14 patients treated with lithium had a favourable response, as did 4% of 25 patients treated with tricyclic antidepressants. Lithium may be helpful in some patients with Meige's syndrome (Jankovic and Ford, 1983).

The experimental drug, gamma-vinyl-GABA is a GABA-mimetic agent, which acts by inhibiting GABA transaminase. When tested in patients with dystonia, there was no benefit (Stahl *et al.*, 1985; Carella *et al.*, 1986).

Comments

It is difficult to interpret 'negative' drug trials because a number of factors could lead to a lack of benefit. Two major factors that have contributed to poor outcome in a number of reported studies are inadequate dosage and inadequate duration of the trial. For example, as Cotzias, Van Woert and Schiffer (1967) showed in the treatment of Parkinson's disease, for dopa to be effective it must be given in high dosage and over a sustained period of time. In torsion dystonia, anti-cholinergics are mainly effective only when given in high dosage, and some patients fail to show benefit unless treated for two months or longer (Fahn, 1983). It is possible that other drugs may be similar, and thus most of the studies carried out on dystonia could have failed to show benefit due to faulty design. It is for this reason that we have deliberately not tabulated every pharmacological study carried out on dystonia, but have concentrated on those agents which have been shown to give appreciable benefit to some patients.

Local administration – botulinum toxin

Botulinum toxin acts presynaptically at peripheral nerve terminals to prevent calcium-dependent release of acetylcholine (Kao, Drachman and Price, 1976).

Scott (1981) injected botulinum toxin into eye muscles to correct strabismus in 1981 and began to use it for the treatment of blepharospasm at the beginning of 1983. Since then several open-label trials on the effectiveness of botulinum toxin in blepharospasm have been reported (Frueh et al., 1984; Elston and Russell, 1985; Mauriello, 1985; Scott, Kennedy and Stubbs, 1985; Shorr, Seiff and Kopelmam, 1985; Tsoy, Buckley and Dutton, 1985; Dutton and Buckley, 1986; Perman et al., 1986; Brin et al., 1987). There have been only two double-blind trials. In one, five patients received unilateral injection of toxin or saline, with the opposite eyelid receiving the other agent (Fahn et al., 1985b). Jankovic (1987) carried out a double-blind study in 12 patients with blepharospasm. All of these studies have consistently shown botulinum toxin to be safe and effective in controlling blepharospasm, giving functional benefit in approximately 70% of patients. The most common adverse effect is ptosis due to weakness of the levator palpebrae muscle.

Tsui et al. (1985), Brin et al. (1987), and Jankovic (1987) reported on the effectiveness of botulinum toxin in the treatment of spasmodic torticollis. All studies showed that muscle pain can be relieved if the toxin is injected directly into the painful site. Furthermore, many of the patients have functional and even cosmetic benefit by weakening of the overly contracting neck muscles. However, two patients have developed antibodies to botulinum toxin (Brin et al., 1987). These were patients with torticollis who received very large doses repeatedly into the neck musculature. In these patients, after the antibodies developed, the toxin became ineffective.

Other musculature involved in various focal dystonias has also been treated with botulinum toxin. Lingual dystonia, adductor dystonic dysphonia, finger dystonia, and toe dystonia were all effectively treated in the series of patients reported by Brin et al. (1987). No serious complications were reported in any of these patients, and botulinum toxin appears to be a promising new treatment strategy for many of the focal dystonias. Long-term effects of the toxin need to be determined.

Although botulinum toxin has been labelled the 'most deadly' poison, these studies showed that small doses can serve as a useful pharmacological agent to cause local muscle weakness, and no major toxicity has been so far reported. Distal effects of the toxin have been detected by single muscle fibre physiological monitoring techniques (Lange et al., 1985; Sanders, Massey and Buckley, 1986), but no distal weakness has been reported, other than a feeling of increased fatigue in one elderly patient with Parkinson's disease and a dystonic toe (Brin et al., 1987).

SURGICAL THERAPY

Brain surgery

Horsley in 1909 was the first to carry out ablative lesions of brain tissue in an attempt to treat hyperkinetic disorders. He excised the motor cortex in a boy with hemi-athetosis, dramatically relieving the involuntary movements. This work was a milestone in understanding motor physiology and anatomy.

A few decades elapsed before this surgical approach was taken up again. Bucy and Case (1939) and Klemme (1940) excised parts of the cerebral cortex for parkinsonian tremor and dystonia. Unfortunately, however, this type of ablative surgery produced a spastic hemiparesis, which was too great a price to pay for relief of dyskinesias. At this time, Putnam (1938) was incising the pyramidal tract in the upper cervical cord, which also produced relief of the dyskinesia, but in addition ipsilateral hemiplegia. The degree of relief correlated with the severity of the hemiplegia. Also noted with this type of surgery was contralateral hypalgesia, bladder difficulties, and impotence (Putnam and Herz, 1950). Incising the cerebral peduncle in the midbrain was developed later by Walker (1952), but this also produced hemiparesis as a substitute for the dyskinesia. The principle of lesioning the corticospinal pathway to relieve dyskinesias indicates that this tract is the 'final' motor pathway coming to the spinal level from the cerebral hemispheres. This physiological understanding is supported by anatomical evidence that the major outflow from the basal ganglia is to the premotor areas of the cortex by way of the thalamus.

Surgical lesioning deep within the cerebral hemispheres for hyperkinetic movement disorders was introduced by Meyers (1940, 1942). He studied the effects of lesions in the caudate nucleus and globus pallidus and found the latter to be superior. Not only was there relief of tremor in approximately 40% of patients with parkinsonism, but for the first time there was also improvement of rigidity. Furthermore, improvement of dyskinesia was not accompanied by the production of spasticity and weakness. Although considerable mortality (16%) occurred with this type of surgery, the observation that pallidal lesions could reduce dyskinesias on the contralateral side was a major advance (Meyers, 1951).

Other surgeons soon adopted Meyer's approach by electrically coagulating efferent fibres from the globus pallidus (Fenelon and Thiebaut, 1950; Guiot and Brion, 1952) or by using a leucotome (Bertrand, 1958). In 1953, Cooper was performing this type of surgery in a patient with parkinsonism when he accidentally cut the anterior choroidal artery, and he was forced to ligate that vessel to prevent an intracerebral haematoma. To Cooper's surprise, the patient had dramatic relief of tremor and rigidity on the contralateral side. Cooper (1954a) subsequently and deliberately ligated the anterior choroidal artery in more than 50 patients and reported relief of contralateral tremor and rigidity without hemiparesis in approximately two-thirds. The mortality rate was 10%.

Stereotactic surgery was developed in animals in 1908 by Horsley and Clark. Several decades passed before Spiegel and his colleagues (1946) were the first to apply the principles of stereotactic surgery to humans. They employed intracerebral ventricular landmarks rather than bony landmarks to locate the target. Their initial operation was performed in 1948 on a patient with Huntington's chorea; they stereotactically made a lesion in the pallidum and obtained a reduction of choreic movements (Spiegel and Wycis, 1950). The operative procedure proved feasible and safe. Spiegel and Wycis (1954, 1958) then applied stereotaxy to electrically coagulate the globus pallidus and its efferent fibres, the ansa lenticularis, for the relief of tremor and rigidity in Parkinson's disease, a technique they referred to as ansotomy.

The anterior choroidal artery supplies blood to the medial globus pallidus and to the lateral ventral nuclear group of the thalamus, among other neighbouring structures. Ligating this vessel results in necrosis of these nuclei. With this understanding and with the introduction of stereotactic surgery in humans by Spiegel and his colleagues, Cooper changed his operative tactics in an effort to avoid the high mortality rate of choroidal artery ligation. He began to perform chemopallidectomy by stereotactically injecting procaine and alcohol (Cooper, 1954b). Despite the marked improvement in mortality with this and with subsequent stereotaxic targets in the thalamus, Cooper (1969) maintained that the most dramatic relief obtained in far advanced, totally helpless patients occurred with choroidal artery ligation.

Based on anatomical awareness that the pallidum projects primarily to the thalamus, Hassler (1955a,b) proposed the concept of ablative surgery on the ventrolateral nucleus of the thalamus. Reichert, working with Hassler, may have carried out the first thalamotomy (see summary by Reichert (1962)). Cooper et al. (1958) then began comparing chemothalamectomy with chemopallidectomy and found superior results with the former target.

Although most stereotactic operations were done predominantly in Parkinson's disease for tremor and rigidity, operations for other dyskinesias were being carried out simultaneously. Cooper (1969) developed the idea of carrying out chemopallidectomies and chemothalamectomies in patients with torsion dystonia based on the observation of relief of a fixed dystonic flexion deformity of the left hand and wrist in a patient with post-encephalitic parkinsonism who had undergone a right anterior choroidal artery ligation. Once he realized that stereotactic lesions in the pallidum and thalamus were preferable to anterior choroidal ligation for the relief of parkinsonian tremor and rigidity, he applied these ablative lesions to patients with torsion dystonia.

By the end of 1966, Cooper (1969) had operated on 144 patients with dystonia. Of these patients, 97 had bilateral surgery; the thalamus was the target in 128 patients and the globus pallidus in 16 patients. Cooper recommended delaying the operation on the second side of the brain until one or more weeks had passed in order to determine the persistence of benefit from the first operation. He reported that 77% of all his patients with dystonia achieved long-standing reversal of dystonic symptoms, even though one-third of cases had recurrence of symptoms sufficient to warrant re-operation (Cooper, 1969). Cooper emphasized that the lesion for dystonia should be centred within the posterior half of the ventral lateral nucleus. Beginning in 1961, he changed from making chemical lesions to producing lesions by freezing the tissue, using liquid nitrogen delivered through a vacuum-insulated cannula (Cooper, 1962). He reported that cryothalamotomy resulted in a lower mortality and morbidity than the previous chemical methods (Cooper, 1965).

Cooper, who has operated on more patients with torsion dystonia than anyone else, summarized his findings near the time of his retirement (Cooper, 1976). Between 1955 and 1974 he had operated on 226 patients. Most of the patients had either one or two operations, but many had more, and two patients had up to seven operations. Cryothalamotomy was the most common procedure. Follow-up data were available in 208 patients for a mean of eight years after surgery. Cooper reported that 25% of the patients had marked improvement, 45% moderate improvement, 18% no change, and 12% were worse (Cooper, 1976). Overall, 70% gained some benefit. Other neurosurgeons have not reported such favourable results for stereotactic thalamotomy in patients with dystonia. Mundinger, Riechert and Disselhoff (1970), reported that 50% of 80 patients with torsion dystonia had good improvement. Andrew, Fowler and Harrison (1983) found benefit in only 4 out of 16 patients with generalized dystonia.

It is generally agreed that this type of surgery is more effective for limb dystonia than for axial dystonia. Andrew, Fowler and Harrison (1983) reported that patients with hemidystonia requiring only a unilateral thalamotomy do better than patients with generalized dystonia requiring bilateral procedures. Dysarthria occurred in

11% of their patients who had unilateral lesions and in 56% of patients with bilateral lesions. Dysphonia has been reported to occur in 18% of cases by Cooper, and 33% of cases by Ojemann and Ward (1982).

Despite the observation that thalamotomy tends to be more successful for dystonia of the limbs compared to involvement of axial musculature, a number of surgeons have performed thalamotomies in patients with spasmodic torticollis. Cooper (1977) reported that 60% of 160 patients with this condition had a satisfactory alleviation of symptoms, although 20% developed dysphonia. Andrew, Fowler and Harrison (1983) found a similar success rate in 16 patients with bilateral thalamotomies, but three out of the 16 patients had a relapse, and 56% had dysphonia. Cooper (1977) found that restricted small bilateral thalamotomies usually were inadequate to relieve torticollis, and that the lesion had to extend into the ventroposteromedial and centrum medianum nuclei to be successful. Bertrand (1982), who originally carried out thalamotomies in patients with spasmodic torticollis, stated that peripheral denervation surgery is a preferred method. He believed that stereotactic surgery for torticollis should be reserved for patients who have torticollis as part of a generalized dystonia, and should not be employed for isolated focal dystonia of the neck.

Today, many surgeons are using sophisticated computerized guided placement of the operating probe, and refined neurophysiological techniques to locate the target accurately. Data from CT scans, magnetic resonance scans, and even arteriography are utilized to compute the direction and depth of the probe insertion to reach the target more accurately and to avoid rupturing blood vessels. Physiological recording of spontaneous and evoked thalamic neuronal activity is employed to determine the exact site of the probe within different thalamic nuclei. Time will tell whether these methods provide more successful results in dystonias and a lower risk of adverse effects.

Peripheral surgery

Theoretically, extirpation or denervation of excessively contracting muscles should prevent their sustained contractions in patients with torsion dystonia. It is reasonable to consider such peripheral surgical methods when dystonia is limited to one region of the body. The two focal dystonias in which peripheral surgery has most often been used are spasmodic torticollis and blepharospasm. These surgical approaches were reviewed in the previous volume of *Movement Disorders* by Maccabe (1982), Bertrand (1982), Battista (1982) and Talbot, Gregor and Bird (1982).

Since publication of that volume, there have been several reviews on myectomy and facial nerve section for the surgical treatment of blepharospasm (Anderson, 1985; Battista, 1985; Callahan, 1985; Fett, Putterman and Weingarten, 1985; Perman and Baylis, 1985; Shorr, 1985; Small, 1985; Wilkins and Byrd, 1985). However, the development and success of local injections of botulinum toxin for the relief of blepharospasm (*see above*) has led to a marked reduction in surgical treatment of blepharospasm. Those in whom botulinum toxin fails to relieve their blepharospam subsequently can be treated by open surgery, either myectomy or facial nerve section, but there is no need to elaborate further on these techniques.

In contrast to blepharospasm, botulinum toxin injections into contracting neck muscles in patients with spasmodic torticollis has been less extensively studied (Tsui *et al.*, 1985; Brin *et al.*, 1987; Jankovic, 1987). More investigations of this approach are required to establish its role in management of patients with torticollis. The large doses of botulinum toxin required to denervate neck muscles may render this strategy impractical, and peripheral surgery may be required in severe intractable cases of torticollis.

Peripheral surgical denervation for torticollis has a long history and is still widely practiced. In 1891, Keen divided the first three cervical nerves in an extraspinal approach to relieve torticollis. Taylor (1915) carried out the first intraspinal operation in 1915. Myotomy was also developed, but is rarely used today (Maccabe, 1982). Bilateral cervical motor root section was introduced by McKenzie (1924) and Dandy (1930). Modifications of their operations have been in use up to the present time. The standard rhizotomy procedure is to section the anterior roots of C1–C3 bilaterally, including a contribution to C1 from the spinal accessory nerve. Using these procedures, a number of surgeons reported benefit in up to 79% of patients (Hamby and Schiffer, 1969; Arseni and Maretsis, 1971). However, Maccabe (1982) pointed out that with such operations, weakness of neck muscles and a feeling of instability of the head are common complications; other problems included difficulty in swallowing and subluxation of the cervical spine; death and quadriparesis have occasionally occurred due to interference with the blood supply to the lower brainstem and cervical cord. Meares (1971) followed 41 cases of spasmodic torticollis and found that the surgical approach often failed to abolish the abnormal movements and that the operated patients tended to fare worse than unoperated patients. Gauthier, Perot and Bertrand (1987) recently reviewed their results of bilateral rhizotomies using a modification of the McKenzie (1955) operation. Sectioning the anterior roots of C1–C4 on the side to which the face turns and C1–C3 and the upper rootlets of the spinal accessory nerve on the opposite side was the usual procedure. Fifty-one patients were operated on, and long-term follow-up was available for 24 of them. The head was considered to be perfectly straight in 10 of these 24 patients. Patients with predominant retrocollis had an unsatisfactory result. Transient weakness, dysphagia, and dysarthria occurred in a few.

Bertrand (1982) and Bertrand and Molina-Negro (1987) emphasized that selective extraspinal peripheral denervation, rather than bilateral intraspinal rhizotomies, is the preferred method. They believe that the bilateral contractions of neck muscles seen on electromyography in patients with spasmodic torticollis are often due to compensatory contractions of antagonist muscles, and that the major abnormal involuntary contractions are unopposed. In other words, in patients with classical rotational torticollis, the trapezius and splenius muscles on the side ipsilateral to the direction of rotation of the chin and sternocleidomastoid on the opposite side are the muscles most commonly involved. However, in patients with retrocollis, the posterior neck muscles bilaterally are involved. Bertrand and Molina-Negro (1987) recommended that electromyography be utilized prior to surgery to be certain which muscles are involved. They also recommended that, prior to the nerve section, nerve block be used to determine what the effect of denervation will be. These authors emphasized that this approach avoids a laminectomy and many of the complications seen with indiscriminate nerve or root section.

With the patient under general anaesthesia, they stimulate the nerves to ascertain their innervation prior to nerve sectioning, and also to ascertain that denervation is complete at the end of the procedure. For rotational torticollis, they section (*a*) branches of the spinal accessory nerve to the sternocleidomastoid muscle contralateral to the direction of turning of the chin and (*b*) on the other side, they section the posterior roots of C1 and C2 and the posterior primary divisions (rami) of C3, C4, C5, and usually C6. With selective peripheral denervation in 111 patients with torticollis, these authors claimed total or marked relief of symptoms in 97 (87%). Moreover, they reported no complications other than atrophy of the denervated muscles and anaesthesia in the territory of the occipital nerves. If such results can be replicated by other neurosurgeons, this approach would be the preferred method of surgical treatment of spasmodic torticollis that is intractable to pharmacotherapy.

Cervical cord stimulation

In the previous volume of *Movement Disorders,* Waltz (1982) reported that he had carried out cervical cord electrical stimulation in 55 patients with generalized torsion dystonia and in 26 patients with toticollis; approximately 70% of patients showed moderate to marked improvement in these two groups. Gutstein and Waltz (1985) subsequently reported on an expanded series of 110 patients with dystonia. They stated that 72% of the patients had a moderate to marked benefit from continuous cervical cord stimulation. Following the earlier report by Waltz (1982), one of us (SF) began to refer patients with intractable torsion dystonia for this surgical procedure. In addition, several patients referred themselves for cervical cord stimulation. In reviewing the results in all 25 patients seen in follow-up, Fahn (1985) found only one who had sustained benefit from cervical cord stimulation, and this was a patient who deteriorated back to baseline if concomitant administration of an anti-cholinergic drug was withdrawn. Fahn concluded that he was unable to support the claim made by Waltz.

Recently Goetz, Penn and Tanner (1987) carried out a double-blind evaluation of 10 patients with dystonia undergoing this procedure. Prior to the 'blinded' evaluations, patients were asked to determine the stimulator setting that they considered to be optimum for relief of dystonia and a setting that they considered to be ineffective. During the double-blind testing phase, the stimulator was set to these predetermined settings in random order. Neither the 'blinded' investigators nor the patients could detect any difference between the two settings. They concluded that all patients failed to show beneficial response to cervical cord stimulation.

In the light of the experiences of Fahn (1985) and Goetz, Penn and Tanner (1987), we must conclude that cervical cord stimulation is a procedure that has not yet been proven to be of benefit and we cannot recommend it for patients with torsion dystonia.

CONCLUSIONS

From the foregoing information, we have developed a therapeutic strategy for the non-specific treatment of our patients with dystonia that seems reasonable in the present circumstances. No single drug is uniformly effective in the treatment of dystonia, nor are surgical approaches uniformly beneficial or without risk. This poses a problem as to what should be the first choice of treatment in any given patient. Enough information is available from both open-label and double-blind drug trials and from surgical experience to draw some conclusions.

374 The treatment of dystonia

One principle that we follow is that it is important to avoid potential harm when searching for effective therapy. Thus, surgical procedures and the use of drugs that can cause irreversible complications are used late in empirical trials of treatments for dystonic patients. We will divide our discussion into the treatment of focal dystonias and the treatment of the segmental and generalized dystonias (*Table 18.1*).

Table 18.1 Order of selecting therapeutic choices for patients with dystonia

---

Focal dystonias

Blepharospasm
    Anti-cholinergics
    Baclofen
    Benzodiazepine
    Tetrabenazine
    Botulinum toxin injections
    Peripheral surgery

Torticollis
    Anti-cholinergics
    Baclofen
    Carbamazepine
    Benzodiazepine
    Tetrabenazine or reserpine
    Dopamine receptor blocker
    Botulinum toxin injections
    Extraspinal selective peripheral denervation

Writer's cramp
    Learn to write with the other arm
    Anti-cholinergics

Segmental and generalized dystonias

    Levodopa
    Anti-cholinergics
    Baclofen
    Carbamazepine
    Benzodiazepine
    Tetrabenazine or reserpine
    Dopamine receptor blocker
    Triple therapy: dopamine depletor, dopamine receptor blocker, and anti-cholinergics
    Thalamotomy

Focal dystonias

The focal dystonias have the therapeutic advantage that local injections of botulinum toxin and peripheral surgical denervation can be effective in many patients with a low risk of serious adverse effects. Since trials of botulinum toxin in patients with blepharospasm have consistently shown that 70% of patients can improve for up to three months' duration and can have continued improvement with subsequent injections, this may turn out to be the first line of treatment for this condition, particularly since drugs have a lower success rate and more adverse effects. However, botulinum toxin is not commercially available and, until it becomes so, most practising physicians will not have access to this agent. Therefore, our recommendation is first to use pharmacological agents that have been shown to have some effectiveness in the treatment of blepharospasm. But when these drugs fail, the patient should be referred to investigators who have access to botulinum toxin. Anti-cholinergic drugs, baclofen, and tetrabenazine appear to be the ones most likely to be effective without producing permanent complications. Anti-psychotic drugs, such as haloperidol and the phenothiazines, although occasionally effective, have the added risk of potentially causing tardive dyskinesia and tardive dystonia, so we recommend avoiding them unless everything else fails. In fact, for blepharospasm we could consider facial nerve section or myectomy to be preferable to the use of anti-psychotic drugs. These open operations can also be used if botulinum toxin injections fail.

Spasmodic torticollis, the most common focal dystonia, can also respond to botulinum toxin, but few studies have been published so far. Furthermore, the high dosages of botulinum toxin needed to induce appropriate weakness of neck muscles and the possibility that such large doses may eventually result in development of antibodies or peripheral adverse effects, leaves serious doubts as to the long-term usefulness of botulinum toxin in the treatment of spasmodic torticollis. One of us (SF) opts for further trials of the toxin before subjecting patients to peripheral denervation surgery; however, the other (CDM) has been favourably impressed by posterior primary ramisectomy in carefully selected cases. But our first choice would be to try drug treatment. Our order of preference of drugs to test is as follows: anti-cholinergics, baclofen, carbamazepine, and a benzodiazepine. If those drugs fail tetrabenazine alone or later in combination with pimozide or haloperidol, together with an anti-cholinergic (Marsden, Marion and Quinn, 1984) can be tried. If medications fail, then botulinum toxin injections or peripheral surgery using the extraspinal selective denervation approach of Bertrand and Molino-Negro (1987) may be indicated. However, it is critical to choose patients with care for either procedure. Total relief of torticollis is rarely achieved and, if the patient's reason for proceeding to such treatments is to overcome social embarrassment, they may be disappointed. On the other hand, if torticollis (or retrocollis) is causing functional disability (inability to read, write, drive or walk safely), then such measures may be of great benefit. Likewise, pain may be relieved by either procedure. It is also worth noting that cervical root pain or myelopathy that can occur in long-standing torticollis may be effectively treated by classical anterior cervical spinal fusion. One of us (CDM) has experience of use of this operation in four patients, with success and without complications.

Writer's cramp is probably the focal dystonia that is most resistant to pharmacological approaches. An occasional patient will respond to anti-cholinergics, but other drugs have not yet been found to be useful in this condition. It is unlikely that either botulinum toxin injections or peripheral surgery will prove helpful for this problem; usually too many muscles in the entire arm are involved, and the abnormal movements are present principally with action. For patients with only one or two muscles affected, then botulinum toxin injections into these muscles can be tried. If writer's cramp is limited to one side, we recommend that the patient learn to write with the other hand. If writer's cramp spreads to the other side (as it will do in about 33% of cases (Sheehy and Marsden, 1982)), then a trial of anti-cholinergics is recommended.

Other focal dystonias can be approached by the principles outlined above.

Segmental and generalized dystonias

Peripheral denervation therapy and botulinum toxin injections cannot be used to treat the segmental and generalized dystonias because of the greater number of muscles involved. Systemic pharmacological agents and stereotactic thalamotomy are the only alternatives. Pharmacological trials are always recommended before considering stereotactic thalamotomies.

Bilateral thalamotomies are required for generalized dystonia. The risk of permanent dysphonia or other serious neurological complications of surgery is high, and the chance for improvement is rather small, so that the risk/benefit ratio is not very good. Thalamotomy should be offered only to patients with generalized dystonia who are desperate with intractable dystonia and are willing to take the risk of permanent complications because their dystonia is so severe.

For those patients with hemidystonia, however, a unilateral thalamotomy may be a reasonable proposition. The chance of success is quite high, and the risk of complications low. Most patients with hemidystonia, however, have some localized symptomatic cause, which must be taken into account in planning surgery. Furthermore, we would always try drug treatment before advising surgery.

Our choice of pharmacological agents is to begin with a short course of levodopa to see if the patient belongs in that small subset of patients who respond to this agent. A dose of levodopa plus carbidopa (Sinemet) 5/50 mg three times daily or 10/100 mg three times daily, can be used. If this dosage fails, it is reasonable to increase the dose to a maximum of 25/250 mg three times daily for 2 months before giving up.

The next drug to be tried is an anti-cholinergic agent. From the studies of Greene, Shale and Fahn (1987), trihexyphenidyl is better tolerated in children than is ethopropazine, whereas the latter is the better tolerated in adults. Thus for children we begin with trihexyphenidyl, 2.5 mg twice daily, and increase the dosage gradually. Our usual regimen is to increase the daily dosage by 2.5 mg every week, and occasionally holding a dose constant for four weeks before increasing the dosage further. Some patients have a delay before they respond. We maintained the minimum dose that provides adequate benefit. If no benefit is seen, the dosage is increased until intolerable adverse effects are encountered. Antidotes for some of the adverse peripheral effects were discussed above. The dosage of ethopropazine is approximately 10 times greater than that of trihexyphenidyl; otherwise the dosing strategy is identical. If anti-cholinergics provide any benefit, but higher doses cannot be used because of intolerable side-effects, then the optimum dose achieved is maintained and a second drug is added. There is little difference between baclofen, benzodiazepine, and carbamazepine. All three drugs should be tested in any order. If those drugs fail, it is reasonable to test an anti-dopaminergic. Again, the concern about producing a tardive dyskinesia on top of idiopathic dystonia by the administration of a dopamine receptor blocker needs to be considered. It is possible that a dopamine depletor like tetrabenazine or reserpine can be used as a substitute for an anti-psychotic drug since the depletors have not been reported to cause tardive dyskinesia or tardive dystonia (Fahn, 1984). If an anti-psychotic drug is needed, the use of one of the dopamine depletors in combination could enhance the effect of the anti-psychotic at a lower dose than would otherwise be needed. This combination may even protect against the development of tardive dyskinesia or tardive dystonia.

Rarely, we have come across patients with life-threatening dystonia. The dystonic spasms are so severe as to embarrass respiration, cause hyperthermia, and even muscle necrosis (Jankovic and Penn, 1982). In this situation, when death seems imminent, we employ muscle paralytics, artificial respiration and sedatives for a period of one to several weeks. During this time, drug therapy with a dopamine depletor, a dopamine receptor blocker, and an anti-cholinergic is introduced in increasing dosage. Paralysis and sedation are reduced at weekly intervals to monitor the state of the dystonia. Successful control of this disastrous and desperate dystonia has been achieved in such cases.

As new centrally acting drugs are developed for other neurological conditions, they should be tested for the treatment of dystonia as well. By empirical trials, an effective therapeutic agent may be discovered.

References

ANDERSON, R. L. (1985) Myectomy for blepharospasm and hemifacial spasm. *Advances in Ophthalmic Plastic and Reconstructive Surgery,* **4,** 313–332

ANDREW, J., FOWLER, C. J. and HARRISON, M. J. G. (1983) Stereotaxic thalamotomy in 55 cases of dystonia. *Brain,* **106,** 981–1000

ARSENI, C. and MARETSIS, M. (1971) The surgical treatment of spasmodic torticollis. *Neurochirurgia,* **14,** 177–180

BARRETT, R. E., YAHR, M. D. and DUVOISIN, R. C. (1970) Torsion dystonia and spasmodic torticollis – results of treatment with L-dopa. *Neurology,* **20,** No. 11, Part 2, 122–130

BATSHAW, M. L. and HASLAM, R. H. A. (1976) Multidisciplinary management of dystonia misdiagnosed as hysteria. *Advances in Neurology,* **14,** 367–373

BATTISTA, A. F. (1982) Surgical approach to blepharospasm: nerve thermolysis. In *Movement Disorders.* Eds. C. D. Marsden and S. Fahn, pp. 319–321. London: Butterworths

BATTISTA, A. F. (1985) Percutaneous thermolytic fractional destruction of branches of the facial nerve for the relief of blepharospam. *Advances in Ophthalmic Plastic and Reconstructive Surgery,* **4,** 369–377

BERTRAND, C. (1958) A pneumotaxic technique for producing localized cerebral lesions and its use in the treatment of Parkinson's disease. *Journal of Neurosurgery,* **15,** 251–264

BERTRAND, C. M. (1982) Peripheral versus central surgical approach for the treatment of spasmodic torticollis. In *Movement Disorders.* Eds. C. D. Marsden and S. Fahn, pp. 315–318. London: Butterworths

BERTRAND, C. M. and MOLINA-NEGRO, P. (1987) Selective peripheral denervation in 111 cases of spasmodic torticollis. *Advances in Neurology,* in press

BIARY, N. and KOLLER, W. (1985) Effect of alcohol on dystonia. *Neurology,* **35,** 239–240

BRIERLY, H (1967) The treatment of hysterical spasmodic torticollis by behaviour therapy. *Behavioral Research Therapy,* **5,** 139

BRIN, M. F., FAHN, S., MOSKOWITZ, C., FRIEDMAN, A., SHALE, H. M., GREENE, P. E. *et al.* (1987) Localized injections of botulinum toxin for the treatment of focal dystonia and hemifacial spasm. *Advances in Neurology,* in press

BRUDNY, J., GRYNBAUM, B. and KOREIN, J. (1974) Spasmodic torticollis: treatment by feedback display of the EMG. *Archives of Physical Medicine and Rehabilitation,* **55,** 403–408

BRUDNY, J., KOREIN, J., LEVIDOW, L., GRYNBAUM, B., LIEBERMAN, A. and FRIEDMAN, L. (1974) Sensory feedback therapy as a modality of treatment in central nervous system disorders of voluntary movement. *Neurology,* **24,** 925–932

BUCY, P. C. and CASE, J. T. (1939) Tremor: Physiologic mechanism and abolition by surgical means. *Archives of Neurology and Psychiatry,* **41,** 721–746

BURKE, R. E. and FAHN, S. (1985a) Serum trihexyphenidyl levels in the treatment of torsion dystonia. *Neurology,* **35,** 1066–1069

BURKE, R. E. and FAHN, S. (1985b) Pharmacokinetics of trihexyphenidyl after short-term and long-term administration to dystonic patients. *Annals of Neurology,* **18,** 35–40

BURKE, R. E., FAHN, S., JANKOVIC, J., MARSDEN, C. D., LANG, A. E., GOLLOMP, S. *et al.* (1982) Tardive dystonia: Late-onset and persistent dystonia caused by antipsychotic drugs. *Neurology,* **32,** 1335–1346

BURKE, R. E., FAHN, S. and MARSDEN, C. D. (1986) Torsion dystonia: A double-blind, prospective trial of high-dosage trihexyphenidyl. *Neurology,* **36,** 160–164

BURKE, R. E., RECHES, A., TRAUB, M. M., ILSON, J., SWASH, M. and FAHN, S. (1985) Tetrabenazine induces acute dystonic reactions. *Annals of Neurology,* **17,** 200–202

BURNS, C. L. C. (1959) The treatment of torsion spasm in children with trihexyphenidyl (Artane). *The Medical Press,* **241,** 148–149

CALLAHAN, A. (1985) Neurectomy of the facial nerve plexus and partial removal of orbicularis muscle for blepharospam. *Advances in Ophthalmic Plastic and Reconstructive Surgery,* **4,** 379–384

CARELLA, F., GIROTTI, F., SCIGLIANO, G., CARACENI, T., JODER-OHLENBUSCH, A. M. and SCHECHTER, P. J. (1986) Double-blind study of oral gamma-vinyl GABA in the treatment of dystonia. *Neurology,* **36,** 98–100

CASTEELS-VAN DAELE, M., JAEKEN, J., VAN DE SCHUEREN, P., ZIMMERMAN, A. and VAN DEN BON, P. (1970) Dystonic reactions in children caused by metoclopramide. *Archives of Diseases in Childhood,* **45,** 130–133

CHADWICK, D., REYNOLDS, E. H. and MARSDEN, C. D. (1976) Anticonvulsant-induced dyskinesias: a comparison with dyskinesias induced by neuroleptics. *Journal of Neurology, Neurosurgery, and Psychiatry,* **39,** 1210–1218

CHASE, T. N. (1970) Biochemical and pharmacologic studies of dystonia. *Neurology,* **20,** Part 2, 122–130

CLEELAND, C. S. (1973) Behavioral technics in the modification of spasmodic torticollis. *Neurology,* **23,** 1241–1247

COLEMAN, M. (1970) Preliminary remarks on the L-dopa therapy of dystonia. *Neurology,* **20,** No. 11, Part 2, 114–121

COOPER, I. S. (1953) Ligation of the anterior choroidal artery for involuntary movements of parkinsonism. *Psychiatric Quarterly,* **27,** 317–319

COOPER, I. S. (1954a) Surgical alleviation of parkinsonism: effects of occlusion of the anterior choroidal artery. *Journal of the American Geriatric Society,* **11,** 691–717

COOPER, I. S. (1954b) Intracerebral injection of procaine into the globus pallidus in hyperkinetic disorders. *Science,* **119,** 417–418

COOPER, I. S. (1962) Cryogenic surgery of the basal ganglia. *Journal of the American Medical Association,* **181,** 600–604

COOPER, I. S. (1965) Clinical and physiologic implications of thalamic surgery for disorders of sensory communication. Part 2: Intention tremor, dystonia, Wilson's disease and torticollis. *Journal of the Neurological Sciences,* **2,** 520–553

COOPER, I. S. (1969) *Involuntary Movement Disorders.* New York: Hoeber Medical Division

COOPER, I. S. (1972) Levodopa-induced dystonia. *Lancet,* , **ii,** 1317–1318

COOPER, I. S. (1976) *The Victim is Always the Same.* New York: Norton

COOPER, I. S. (1976) 20-year followup study of the neurosurgical treatment of dystonia musculorum deformans. *Advances in Neurology,* **14,** 423–452

COOPER, I. S. (1977) Neurosurgical treatment of the dyskinesias. *Clinical Neurosurgery,* **24,** 367–390

COOPER, I. S., BRAVO, G., RIKLAN, M., DAVIDSON, N. and GOREK, E. (1958) Chemopallidectomy and chemothalamectomy for parkinsonism. *Geriatrics,* **13,** 127–147

CORNER, B. D. (1952) Dystonia musculorum deformans in siblings treated with Artane (trihexyphenidyl). *Proceedings of the Royal Society of Medicine,* **45,** 451–452

COTZIAS, G. C., VAN WOERT, M. H. and SCHIFFER, L. M. (1967) Aromatic amino acids and modification of parkinsonism. *New England Journal of Medicine,* **276,** 374–379

CROSLEY, C. J. and SWENDER, P. T. (1979) Dystonia associated with carbamazepine administration: experience in brain-damaged children. *Pediatrics,* **63,** 612–615

DANDY, W. E. (1930) Operation for treatment of spasmodic torticollis. *Archives of Surgery,* **20,** 10–32

DEONNA, T. (1986) DOPA-sensitive progressive dystonia of childhood with fluctuations of symptoms: Segawa's syndrome and possible variants. *Neuropediatrics,* **17,** 81–85

DUTTON, J. J. and BUCKLEY, E. G. (1986) Botulinum toxin in the management of blepharospasm. *Archives of Neurology,* **43,** 380–382

DUVOISIN, R. C. (1983) Meige syndrome: relief on high-dose anticholinergic therapy. *Clinical Neuropharmacology,* **6,** 63–66

ELDRIDGE, R. (1970) The torsion dystonias: Literature review and genetic and clinical studies. *Neurology,* **20,** No. 11, Part 2, 1–78

ELDRIDGE, R., KANTER, W. and KOERBER, T. (1973) Levodopa in dystonia. *Lancet,* **ii,** 1027–1028

ELDRIDGE, R., RIKLAN, M. and COOPER, I. S. (1969) The limited role of psychotherapy in torsion dystonia. Experience with 44 cases. *Journal of the American Medical Association,* **210,** 705–708

ELSTON, J. S. and RUSSELL, R. W. R. (1985) Effect of treatment with botulinum toxin on neurogenic blepharospasm. *British Medical Journal,* **290,** 1857–1859

FAHN, S. (1976) Biochemistry of the basal ganglia. *Advances in Neurology,* **14,** 59–88

FAHN. S. (1979) Treatment of dystonia with high-dosage anticholinergic medication. *Neurology,* **29,** 605

FAHN, S. (1983) High dosage anticholinergic therapy in dystonia. *Neurology*, **33**, 1255–1261
FAHN, S. (1984) The tardive dyskinesias. In *Recent Advances in Clinical Neurology*, Eds. W. B. Matthews and G. H. Glaser, pp. 229–260. Edinburgh: Churchill Livingstone
FAHN, S. (1985) Lack of benefit from cervical cord stimulation for dystonia. *New England Journal of Medicine*, **313**, 1229
FAHN, S., HENING, W. A., BRESSMAN, S., BURKE, R., ILSON, J. and WALTERS, A. (1985a) Long-term usefulness of baclofen in the treatment of essential blepharospasm. *Advances in Ophthalmic Plastic Reconstructive Surgery*, **4**, 219–226
FAHN, S., LIST, T., MOSKOWITZ, C., BRIN, M., BRESSMAN, S., BURKE, R. et al. (1985b) Double-blind controlled study of botulinum toxin for blepharospasm. *Neurology*, **35**, Suppl. 1, 271–272
FANN, W. E. (1966) Use of methylphenidate to counteract acute dystonic effects of phenothiazines. *American Journal of Psychiatry*, **122**, 1293–1294
FENELON, F. and THIEBAUT, F. (1950) Essais du traitement neurochirurgical du syndrome parkinsonism par intervention directe sur les voies extrapyramidales immediatement sous-strio-palldales (anse lenticulaire). *Revue Neurologie*, **83**, 437–440
FETT, D. R., PUTTERMAN, A. M. and WEINGARTEN, C. Z. (1985) Facial nerve avulsion and primary rhytidectomy in the treatment of essential blepharospasm. *Advances in Ophthalmic Plastic and Reconstructive Surgery*, **4**, 349–360
FRUEH, B. R., FELT, T. H., WONJO, T. H. and MUSCH, D. C. (1984) Treatment of blepharospasm with botulinum toxin: a preliminary report. *Archives of Ophthalmology*, **102**, 1464–1468
GAGRAT, D., HAMILTON, J. and BELMAKER, R. H. (1978) Intravenous diazepam in the treatment of neuroleptic-induced acute dystonia and akathisia. *American Journal of Psychiatry*, **135**, 1232–1233
GATRAD, A. R. (1976) Dystonic reactions to metoclopramide. *Developmental Medicine and Child Neurology*, **18**, 767–769
GAUTHIER, S., PEROT, P. and BERTRAND, G. (1987) Role of surgical anterior rhizotomies in the management of spasmodic torticollis. *Advances in Neurology*, in press
GELLER, M., KAPLAN, B. and CHRISTOFF, N. (1974) Dystonic symptoms in children: treatment with carbamazepine. *Journal of the American Medical Association*, **229**, 1755–1757
GELLER, M., KAPLAN, B. and CHRISTOFF, N. (1976) Treatment of dystonia symptoms with carbamazepine. *Advances in Neurology*, **14**, 403–410
GILBERT, G. J. (1972) Treatment of spasmodic torticollis. *New England Journal of Medicine*, **286**, 1161–1162
GIROTTI, F., SCIGLIANO, G., NARDOCCI, N., ANGELINI, L., BROGGI, G., GIOVANNI, P. et al. (1982) Idiopathic dystonia: neuropharmacologic study. *Journal of Neurology*, **227**, 239–247
GOETZ, C. G., PENN, R. D. and TANNER, C. M. (1987) Efficacy of cervical cord stimulation in dystonia. *Advances in Neurology*, in press
GOLLOMP, S. M., FAHN, S., BURKE, R. E., RECHES, A. and ILSON, J. (1983) Therapeutic trials in Meige syndrome. *Advances in Neurology*, **37**, 207–213
GREENE, P. E., SHALE, H. and FAHN, S. (1987) Analysis of a large series of patients with torsion dystonia treated with high dosages of anticholinergic and other drugs. *Advances in Neurology*, in press
GUIOT, G. and BRION, S. (1952) Traitement neurochiurgical de syndromes choreo-athetosiques at Parkinsoniens. *Semaine Hôpital, Paris*, **49**, 2095–2099
GUTSTEIN, H. S. and WALTZ, J. M. (1985) Spinal cord stimulation in the treatment of dystonia. *Neurology*, **35** (Suppl. 1), 273–274
HAMBY, W. B. and SCHIFFER, S. (1969) Spasmodic torticollis results after cervical rhizotomy in 50 cases. *Journal of Neurosurgery*, **31**, 323–326
HASSLER, R. (1955a) The pathological and pathophysiological basis of tremor and parkinsonism. *Proceedings of the Second International Congress of Neuropathology*, Part 1, pp. 29–40. Amsterdam: Excerpta Medica Foundation
HASSLER, R. (1955b) The influence of stimulations and coagulations in the human thalamus on the tremor at rest and its physiopathologic mechanism. *Proceedings of the Second International Congress of Neuropathology*, Part 2, pp. 637–642. Amsterdam: Excerpta Medica Foundation
HORSLEY, V. (1909) The functions of the so-called motor areas of the brain. *British Medical Journal*, **124**, 5–28
HORSLEY, V. and CLARKE, R. H. (1908) The structure and functions of the cerebellum examined by a new method. *Brain*, **31**, 45
ISGREEN, W. P., FAHN, S., BARRETT, R. E., SNIDER, S. R. and CHUTORIAN, A. M. (1976) Carbamazepine in torsion dystonia. *Advances in Neurology*, **14**, 411–416
JACOME, D. (1979) Carbamazepine-induced dystonia. *Journal of the American Medical Association*, **241**, 2263

JANKOVIC, J. (1982) Treatment of hyperkinetic movement disorders with tetrabenazine: A double-blind crossover study. *Annals of Neurology*, **11**, 41–47

JANKOVIC, J. (1987) Blepharospasm and oromandibular–laryngeal–cervical dystonia: a controlled trial of botulinum A toxin therapy. *Advances in Neurology,* in press

JANKOVIC, J. and FORD, J. (1983) Blepharospasm and orofacial–cervical dystonia: clinical and pharmacological findings in 100 patients. *Annals of Neurology*, **13**, 402–411

JANKOVIC, J. and PENN, A. S. (1982) Severe dystonia and myoglobinuria. *Neurology*, **32**, 1195–1197

JANKOWSKA, H. (1934) Przycznek do zagadnienia dziedzicznosci dystonji torsyjnej. *Neurologische Polonskie*, **16–17**, 258–264

KANG, U. J., BURKE, R. E. and FAHN, S. (1986) Natural history and treatment of tardive dystonia. *Movement Disorders*, in press

KAO, I., DRACHMAN, D. B. and PRICE, D. L. (1976) Botulinum toxin: mechanism of presynaptic blockade. *Science*, **193**, 1256–1258

KEEN, W. W. (1891) New operation for wry neck, namely division or exsection of the nerves supplying the superior rotator muscles of the neck. *Annals of Surgery*, **13**, 44

KLEMME, R. M. (1940) Surgical treatment of dystonia, paralysis agitans and athetosis. *Archives of Neurology and Psychiatry*, **44**, 926

KOOIKER, J. C. and SUMI, S. M. (1974) Movement disorder as a manifestation of diphenylhydantoin intoxication. *Neurology*, **24**, 68–71

KORCZYN, A. D. and GOLDBERG, G. J. (1972) Intravenous diazepam in drug-induced dystonic reactions. *British Journal of Psychiatry*, **121**, 75–77

KOREIN, J., BRUDNY, J., GRYNBAUM, B., SACHS-FRANKEL, G., WEISINGER, M. and LEVIDOW, L. (1976) Sensory feedback therapy of spasmodic torticollis and dystonia: results in treatment of 55 patients. *Advances in Neurology*, **14**, 375–402

KWENTUS, J. A., SCHULZ, S. C. and HART, R. P. (1984) Tardive dystonia, catatonia, electroconvulsive therapy. *Journal of Nervous and Mental Disease*, **172**, 171–173

LAL, S., HOYTE, K., KIELY, M. E., SOURKES, T. L., BAXTER, D. W., MISSALA, K. et al. (1979) Neuropharmacological investigations and treatment of spasmodic torticollis. *Advances in Neurology*, **24**, 335–351

LANG, A. E. (1985) Dopamine agonists in the treatment of dystonia. *Clinical Neuropharmacology*, **8**, 38–57

LANG, A. E. (1986) High dose anticholinergic therapy in adult dystonia. *Canadian Journal of Neurological Sciences*, **13**, 42–46

LANG, A. E. (1987) Dopamine agonists and antagonists in the treatment of idiopathic dystonia. *Advances in Neurology,* in press

LANG, A. E. and MARSDEN, C. D. (1982) Alphamethylparatyrosine and tetrabenazine in movement disorders. *Clinical Neuropharmacology*, **5**, 375–387

LANG, A. E., SHEEHY, M. P. and MARSDEN, C. D. (1982) Anticholinergics in adult-onset focal dystonia. *Canadian Journal of Neurological Sciences*, **9**, 313–319

LANGE, D. J., WARNER, C., BRIN, M., LIST, T., FAHN, S. and LOVELACE, R. E. (1985) Botulinum toxin therapy: distant effects on neuromuscular transmission. *Muscle and Nerve*, **8**, 624–625

LUCHINS, D. J. and GOLDMAN, M. (1985) High-dose bromocriptine in a case of tardive dystonia. *Biological Psychiatry*, **20**, 179–181

LUHDORF, K. and LUND, M. (1977) Phenytoin-induced hyperkinesia. *Epilepsia*, **18**, 409–415

MACCABE, J. J. (1982) Surgical treatment of spasmodic torticollis. In *Movement Disorders*, Eds. C. D. Mardsen and S. Fahn, pp. 308–314. London: Butterworths

MANDELL, S. (1970) The treatment of dystonia with L-dopa and haloperidol. *Neurology*, **20**, Part 2: 103–106

MARSDEN, C. D. and HARRISON, M. J. G. (1974) Idiopathic torsion dystonia. *Brain*, **97**, 793–810

MARSDEN, C. D., LANG, A. E. and SHEEHY, M. P. (1983) Pharmacology of cranial dystonia. *Neurology*, **33**, 1100–1101

MARSDEN, C. D., MARION, M.-H. and QUINN, N. (1984) The treatment of severe dystonia in children and adults. *Journal of Neurology, Neurosurgery and Psychiatry*, **47**, 1166–1173

MAURIELLO, J. A. (1985) Blepharospasm, Meige syndrome, and hemifacial spasm: Treatment with botulinum toxin. *Neurology*, **35**, 1499–1500

McLEAN, P. and CASEY, D. E. (1978) Tardive dyskinesia in an adolescent. *American Journal of Psychiatry*, **135**, 969–971

McKENZIE, K. G. (1924) Intrameningeal division of the spinal accessory and roots of the upper cervical nerves for the treatment of spasmodic torticollis. *Surgery, Gynecology and Obstetrics*, **39**, 5–10

McKENZIE, K. (1955) Surgical treatment of spasmodic torticollis. *Clinical Neurosurgery*, **2**, 37–43

MEARES, R. (1971) Natural history of spasmodic torticollis, and effect of surgery. *Lancet*, **ii**, 149–150

MEYERS, R. (1940) Surgical procedure for postencephalitic tremor, with notes on the physiology of premotor fibres. *Archives of Neurology and Psychiatry,* **44,** 455–457

MEYERS, R. (1942) The modification of alternating tremors, rigidity and festination by surgery of the basal ganglia. *Proceedings of the Association of Nervous and Mental Diseases,* **21,** 602–665

MEYERS, R. (1951) Surgical experiments in therapy of certain 'extrapyramidal' diseases: current evaluation. *Acta Psychiatrica et Neurologica, Scandinavica Supplementum,* **67,** 1–42

MUNDINGER, F., RIECHERT, T. and DISSELHOFF, J. (1970) Long-term results of stereotaxic operations on extrapyramidal hyperkinesia (excluding parkinsonism). *Confinia Neurologica,* **32,** 71–78

NEWMAN, R. P., LeWITT, P. A., SHULTS, C., BRUNO, G., FOSTER, N. L., CHASE, T. N. et al. (1985) Dystonia: treatment with bromocriptine. *Clinical Neuropharmacology,* **8,** 328–333

NISHINAWA, T., TANAKA, M., TSUDA, A. et al. (1984) Clonidine therapy for tardive dyskinesia and related syndromes. *Clinical Neuropharmacology,* **7,** 239–245

NUTT, J. G., HAMMERSTAD, J. P., CARTER, J. H. and deGARMO, P. L. (1985) Lisuride treatment of focal dystonias. *Neurology,* **35,** 1242–1243

NUTT, J. G., HAMMERSTAD, J. P., deGARMO, P. and CARTER, J. (1984) Cranial dystonia: double-blind crossover study of anticholinergics. *Neurology,* **34,** 215–217

NYGAARD, T. G., MARSDEN, C. D. and DUVOISIN, R. C. (1987) Dopa-responsive dystonia. *Advances in Neurology,* in press

OJEMANN, G. A. and WARD, A. A. Jr (1982) Abnormal movement disorders. In *Neurological Surgery,* Ed. J. R. Youmans, Vol. 6, pp. 3821–3857. Philadelphia: Saunders

PAULSON, G. (1960) Procyclidine for dystonia caused by phenothiazine derivatives. *Diseases of the Nervous System,* **21,** 447–448

PAULSON, G. W. (1968) 'Permanent' or complex dyskinesias in the aged. *Geriatrics,* **23,** 105–110

PERMAN, K. I. and BAYLIS, H. I. (1985) Facelift and coronal approach to blepharospam surgery. *Advances in Ophthalmic Plastic and Reconstructive Surgery,* **4,** 397–405

PERMAN, K. I., BAYLIS, H. I., ROSENBLUM, A. L. and KIRSCHEN, D. G. (1986) The use of botulinum toxin in the medical management of benign essential blepharospasm. *Ophthalmology,* **93,** 1–3

PINDER, R. M., BROGDEN, R. N., SAWYER, P. R., SPEIGHT, T. M. and AVERY, G. S. (1976) Metoclopramide: A review of its pharmacological properties and clinical use. *Drugs,* **12,** 81–131

PUTNAM, T. J. (1938) Relief from unilateral paralysis agitans by section of the lateral pyramidal tract. *Archives of Neurology and Psychiatry,* **40,** 1049

PUTNAM, T. J. and HERZ, E. (1950) Results of spinal pyramidotomy in the treatment of the parkinsonian syndrome. *Archives of Neurology and Psychiatry,* **63,** 357–366

QUINN, N. P., LANG, A. E., SHEEHY, M. P. and MARSDEN, C. D. (1985) Lisuride in dystonia. *Neurology,* **35,** 766–769

QUINN, N. P. and MARSDEN, C. D. (1984) Dominantly inherited myoclonic dystonia with dramatic response to alcohol. *Neurology,* **34,** (Suppl. 1), 236

RAINER-POPE, C. R. (1979) Treatment with diazepam of children with drug-induced extrapyramidal symptoms. *South Africa Medical Journal,* **55,** 328, 220

REASBECK, P. G. and HOSSENBOCUS, A. (1979) Death following dystonic reaction to oral metoclopramide. *British Journal of Clinical Practice,* **33,** 31–33

REGENSBURG, J. (1930) Zur Klinik des hereditaren torsionsdystonischen Symptomenkomplexen. *Monatsschrift für Psychiatrie und Neurologie,* **75,** 323–345

REICHERT, T. (1962) Long-term follow-up of results of stereotaxic treatment in extrapyramidal disorders. *Confinia Neurologia,* **22,** 356–363

RIKER, D. K., HURTIG, H., LAKE, C. R., COPELAND, P. and ROTH, R. (1982) Open trial of clonidine in dystonia musculorum deformans. *Society of Neuroscience Abstracts,* **8,** 563

RONDOT, P. and ZIEGLER, M. (1983) Dystonia – L-dopa responsive or juvenile parkinsonism? *Journal of Neural Transmission,* Suppl. 19, 273–281

SANDERS, D. B., MASSEY, E. W. and BUCKLEY, E. C. (1986) Botulinum toxin for blepharospasm: single fiber EMG studies. *Neurology,* **36,** 545–547

SCHWALBE, W. (1908) Eine eigentumliche tonische Krampfform mit hysterischen Symptomen. *Inaugural Dissertation,* Berlin, G. Schade

SCOTT, A. B. (1981) Botulinum toxin injection of eye muscles to correct strabismus. *Transactions of the American Ophthalmological Society,* **79,** 734–770

SCOTT, A. B., KENNEDY, R. A. and STUBBS, M. A. (1985) Botulinum toxin injection as a treatment for blepharospasm. *Archives of Ophthalmology,* **103,** 347–350

SEGAWA, M., HOSAKA, A., MIYAGAWA, F., NOMURA, Y. and IMAI, H. (1976) Hereditary progressive dystonia with marked diurnal fluctuation. *Advances in Neurology,* **14,** 215–233

SHEEHY, M. P. and MARSDEN, C. D. (1982) Writer's cramp – a focal dystonia. *Brain,* **105,** 461–480

SHORE, J. W. (1985) Coronal approach to protractor myectomy for essential blepharospasm. *Advances in Ophthalmic Plastic and Reconstructive Surgery,* **4,** 333–347

SHORR, N., SEIFF, S. R. and KOPELMAM, J. (1985) The use of botulinum toxin in blepharospasm. *American Journal of Ophthalmology,* **99,** 542–546

SHOULSON, I., GOLDBLATT, D., PLASSCHE, W. and WILSON, G. (1983) Some therapeutic observations in Wilson's disease. *Advances in Neurology,* **37,** 239–246

SMALL, R. G. (1985) A selective facial neurectomy technique for essential blepharospasm. *Advances in Ophthalmic Plastic and Reconstructive Surgery,* **4,** 385–395

SMITH, M. J. and MILLER, M. M. (1961) Severe extrapyramidal reaction to perphenazine treated with diphenhydramine. *New England Journal of Medicine,* **264,** 396–397

SPIEGEL, A. E. and WYCIS, H. T. (1950) Pallidothalamotomy in chorea. *Archives of Neurology and Psychiatry,* **64,** 295–296

SPIEGEL, E. A. and WYCIS, H. T. (1954) Ansotomy in paralysis agitans. *Archives of Neurology and Psychiatry,* **71,** 598–614

SPIEGEL, E. A., WYCIS, H. T. and BAIRD, H. W. (1958) Long-range effects of electropalliodensotomy in extrapyramidal and convulsive disorders. *Neurology,* **8,** 734–740

SPIEGEL, E. A., WYCIS, H. T., MARKS, M. and LEE, A. J. (1946) Stereotaxic apparatus for operations on the human brain. *Science,* **106,** 349–359

STAHL, S. M. and BERGER, P. A. (1982) Bromocriptine, physostigmine, and neurotransmitter mechanisms in the dystonias. *Neurology,* **32,** 889–892

STAHL, S. M., THORNTON, J. E., SIMPSON, M. L., BERGER, P. A. and NAPOLIELLO, M. J. (1985) Gamma-vinyl-GABA treatment of tardive dyskinesia and other movement disorders. *Biological Psychiatry,* **20,** 888–893

TALBOT, J. F., GREGOR, Z. and BIRD, A. C. (1982) The surgical management of essential blepharospasm. In *Movement Disorders,* Eds. C. D. Marsden and S. Fahn, pp. 322–329. London: Butterworths

TANNER, C. M., GLANTZ, R. H. and KLAWANS, H. L. (1982) Meige disease: acute and chronic cholinergic effects. *Neurology,* **32,** 783–785

TANNER, C. M., GOETZ, C. S., WEINER, W. J., NAUSIEDA, P. A., WILSON, R. and KLAWANS, H. L. (1979) The role of cholinergic mechanisms in spasmodic torticollis. *Neurology,* **29,** 604–605

TANNER, C. M., WILSON, R. S., GOETZ, C. S. and SHANNON, K. M. (1987) The predictive value of acute antimuscarinic drugs for the chronic efficacy of antimuscarinic drugs in adults with focal dystonia. *Advances in Neurology,* in press

TAYLOR, A. S. (1915) Operations on the peripheral and cranial nerves. In *Operative Therapeusis,* Ed. A. B. Johnson. New York: Appleton and Co.

TSOY, E. A., BUCKLEY, E. G. and DUTTON, J. J. (1985) Treatment of blepharospasm with botulinum toxin. *American Journal of Ophthalmology,* **99,** 176–179

TSUI, J. K., EISEN, A., MAK, E., CARRUTHERS, J., SCOTT, A. B. and CALNE, D. B. (1985) A pilot study on the use of botulinum toxin in spasmodic torticollis. *Canadian Journal of Neurological Sciences,* **12,** 314–316

WALKER, A. E. (1952) Cerebral pedunculotomy for the relief of involuntary movements. II. Parkinsonian tremor. *Journal of Nervous and Mental Diseases,* **116,** 766–775

WALTZ, J. M. (1982) Surgical approach to dystonia. In *Movement Disorders,* Eds. C. D. Marsden and S. Fahn, pp. 300–307. London: Butterworths

WAUGH, W. H. and METTS, J. C. Jr (1960) Severe extrapyramidal motor activity induced by prochlorperazine. *New England Journal of Medicine,* **262,** 353–354

WILKINS, R. B. and BYRD, W. A. (1985) Differential section of the seventh nerve. *Advances in Ophthalmic Plastic and Reconstructive Surgery,* **4,** 361–368

ZIEGLER, D. K. (1981) Prolonged relief of dystonic movements with diazepam. *Neurology,* **31,** 1457–1458

19
The neurology of tics
Joseph Jankovic

Over a century ago, George Albert Edouard Brutus Gilles de la Tourette, 28-year-old student of Charcot at the Salpêtrière, described a 'rare' disorder that now bears his name (Gilles de la Tourette, 1885). Among the original nine patients, six of whom he personally examined, all nine had tics, six had involuntary vocalizations, five had coprolalia, five had echolalia, two had echopraxia, and two had family members with similar symptoms. Although Gilles de la Tourette was credited with the first clinical description of the motor and phonic tic syndrome, several individuals with tics were recorded by historians as early as the fifteenth century (Shapiro and Shapiro, 1982a). A French nobleman in the seventeenth century and a French noblewoman in the eighteenth century were reported to have involuntary barking, obscene utterances, and other tics (Itard, 1825; Stevens, 1971).

One of the earliest descriptions of Gilles de la Tourette syndrome (TS) was provided by the friends and acquaintances of Samuel Johnson (1709–1784). At age 7, he was described as 'awkward', and later he exhibited multiple motor tics, including facial grimacing, twirling of fingers, tilting of head, shrugging of shoulders, and other gesticulations. Besides the 'constant agitation' he often shocked his friends with loud vocalizations, such as groaning, blowing, whistling, explosive utterances, and peculiar complex compulsions (Murray, 1982).

In addition to the various accounts of individuals with clinical features of TS, several culture-bound syndromes were described before Gilles de la Tourette's original report. Gilles de la Tourette, himself, saw a resemblance between these syndromes and the disorder he recognized in his patients. These peculiar cultural eccentricities have been described as 'latah' among groups of people in Malaysia and Indonesia (O'Brien, 1883), as 'myriachit' in Siberia (Hammond, 1884), and as the 'jumping Frenchmen' in Maine and Quebec (Beard, 1886). They are characterized by unusual startle response, impulsiveness without inhibition, automatic obedience, and intermittently bizarre and dramatic behaviour (*Table 19.1*). Besides the characteristic startle response, some groups exhibit echolalia and echopraxia (the 'myriachit' and the 'jumping Frenchmen'), and others have coprolalia (the 'latah'). These culture-bound startle syndromes are distributed worldwide and are probably more prevalent than previously recognized (Kenny, Simons and Murphy, 1983; Lees, 1985). Sociologists, epidemiologists, archaeologists, and historians have attributed these interesting psychosocial entities to mass hysteria, religious revivals, and even to ergotism (Yap, 1951; Massey and Massey, 1984).

Table 19.1 Differential diagnosis of 'jerks'

	Culture-bound startle syndrome	Hyperekplexia	Startle epilepsy	Myoclonus	Tourette's syndrome
Startle response	+	+	+	±	±
Spontaneous and during sleep	–	+	+	+	+
Suggestibility	+	–	–	–	–
Coprolalia	±*	–	–	–	+
Echolalia	+	–	–	–	+
Echopraxia	+	–	–	–	+
Loss of consciousness	–	–	+	–	–
Comments	'Jumpers' of Maine and Quebec, 'myriachit' of Russia, 'latah' of Malaysia. *Coprolalia only in 'latah'	Aut. dom. or sporadic hypertonia in infancy, hyper-reflexia, sudden falls, insecure gait, nocturnal > daytime repetitive myoclonus of legs > arms *EEG*: 80–100 ms positive sharp wave followed by delta wave(s), augmented long-loop reflexes *Treatment*: Clonazepam, phenobarbital, valproate, 5-hydroxytryptophan	Onset in first two decades, usually associated with motor and intellectual deficits *EEG*: Epileptiform *Treatment*: Clonazepam, valproate, and carbamazepine	*Physiological class* (1) Cortical (2) Reticular (3) Ballistic movement overflow (4) Segmental *Aetiological class* (1) Physiological (2) Essential (3) Epileptic (4) Symptomatic *Treatment*: Clonazepam, serotonin precursors, valproate	Familial, M:F = 3:1, motor–vocal tics, multifocal, variable frequency, duration and amplitude of tics, compulsive behaviour and sleep disorders *Treatment*: Dopamine blockers and depletors, clonidine

A 'jerk' is defined here as a sudden and brief muscle contraction which occurs spontaneously, or in response to a stimulus. It occurs as a spontaneous tic in TS, and as a startle response in the culture-bound syndromes, in hyperekplexia (Kurczynski, 1983; Markand, Garg and Weaver, 1984; Sáenz-Lope et al., 1984a), in startle epilepsy (Sáenz-Lope, Herranz and Masdey, 1984b), and in myoclonus (Hallet, 1985; Obeso, Rothwell and Marsden, 1985; Pranzatelli and Snodgrass, 1985; Andermann and Andermann, 1986). Despite overlapping clinical features, the pathophysiology of the various 'jerks' is different, and therefore the 'jerk' syndromes should be separated (*Table 19.1*).

PHENOMENOLOGY AND PATHOPHYSIOLOGY OF TICS

Motor tic may occur as a single, isolated, simple event, such as a blink, facial gesture, head jerk, shoulder shrug, and abdominal or respiratory muscle retraction. At the other end of the clinical spectrum there are motor tics characterized by a burst or sequence of repetitive, patterned, coordinated movements, such as shaking of hands, kicking, squatting, jumping, skipping, hitting, touching, scratching, kissing, obscene gesturing. Thus, some tics consist of well-coordinated, complex motor acts and may be difficult to differentiate from voluntary movements.

The repetitive and forceful contractions associated with tics may result in a compressive radiculopathy or neuropathy (Goetz and Klawans, 1980). We studied a 43-year-old man with progressive spastic quadriplegia. When evaluated for the progressive weakness he was observed to have violent, jerk-like movements of the head and other motor and vocal tics. Myelogram revealed spinal stenosis and a cervical block. After decompressive cervical and lumbar laminectomy, his weakness stabilized, but he remained bedridden. Perhaps if the diagnosis of TS had been made during childhood, and the patient was appropriately treated, the severe disability from the compressive myelopathy, aggravated by the tics, would have been prevented.

While most tic patients are still diagnosed not by their primary physicians but by their parents, relatives, friends, and teachers, more and more patients are being referred to neurologists by astute specialists, such as ophthalmologists who recognize the features of TS in patients who blink excessively or roll their eyes, otolaryngologists who see TS patients because of repetitive throat clearing, allergists who correctly diagnose a tic disorder in patients with repetitive sniffing, or psychologists who become impressed with an obsessive–compulsive personality, impulsiveness, attentional deficit, various sleep disturbances and other neurobehavioural abnormalities.

Although a very characteristic symptom, coprolalia, an irresistible urge to utter obscene words, actually occurs in less than half of TS patients. However, mental coprolalia, the thought of obscene words, may be more common. Coprolalia can occur without apparent provocation and often in polite company. However, the four-letter words or other obscene utterances are usually slurred, mispronounced and shortened (e.g. 'sh' or 'f'). Nuwer (1982), using a Markov process and a computer-generated language, contends that coprolalia is a natural linguistic equivalent of a tic. Words used in coprolalia consist of strings of phonemes occurring with high probability out of proportion to other words. Moreover, certain letter sequences are more likely to result in physical obscenities in contrast to religious profanities. Thus, TS patients use words describing sexual or body elimination acts with much greater frequency than words such as 'God', 'Hell' and 'damn'. Other speech and voice problems, such as stuttering, palilalia, echolalia and spasmodic dysphonia, occur in TS, and may be more common than coprolalia (Ludlow et al., 1982; Lang and Marsden, 1983; Lees et al., 1984).

The clinical expression of motor tics in an individual patient is more variable than that of other hyperkinetic movement disorders, such as tremor, chorea, athetosis, ballism, dystonia, myoclonus, and tardive dyskinesia. It is this variability in frequency, duration, amplitude, and location of tics that is often used to differentiate tics from the other hyperkinesias. The irregular, intermittent occurrence of tics is in marked contrast to the continuous movements characteristic of tremor, chorea, athetosis, and tardive dyskinesia. Tics usually consist of spontaneous, sudden, abrupt, unpredictable, brief, unsustained muscle contractions (clonic tics), but sometimes the tics are more sustained and patterned (dystonic or tonic tics). Because myoclonic and dystonic movements commonly occur in patients with TS, it is not necessary to postulate that these movement disorders represent a new 'paroxysmal myoclonic difference (Feinberg, Shapiro and Shapiro, 1986). Thus, some patients with dystonic tics exhibit blepharospasm, oculogyric crises, and dystonic movements of the neck, shoulders and abdominal muscles. While tics are usually multifocal and often migrate from one location to another, they most commonly occur in the face, head and neck regions. The neuro-ophthalmological findings in TS include increased blinking, blepharospasm, involuntary gaze deviation (oculogyric crises), and forced staring (Jankovic, Havins and Wilkins, 1982; Frankel and Cummings, 1984).

Tics usually occur spontaneously without provocation by any particular stimulus. However, they are often exacerbated by stress. The effects of relaxation are more variable. Some patients claim that their tics are less frequent and less intense when they are not under stress; others report increased tics in the privacy of their home. Thus, in a relaxed and familiar environment, or in the company of family members and friends, the patients are less likely to conceal their tics and therefore let them express freely. Generally, the tics are diminished during absorbing activities, such as when playing a musical instrument or during sexual intercourse.

There are three relatively unique features which help differentiate tics from the other hyperkinetic movement disorders. First, tics are often preceded by a peculiar sensation and an irresistible urge to move. The patient feels a crescendo tension culminating in the movement which, when executed, temporarily relieves the urge (Bliss, 1980; Bullen and Hemsley, 1983). This sensory–motor relationship is not associated with the other movement disorders, except for akathisia, phantom dyskinesia, restless legs and painful legs (arms)–moving toes (fingers) syndrome. However, in akathisia the feeling of restlessness is relatively constant and without crescendo buildup prior to each movement. Furthermore, in akathisia the movements are continuous, repetitive and stereotyped, e.g. stamping of feet, pacing, crossing–uncrossing of legs, touching of the face or scalp (Munetz and Cornes, 1982; Burke, 1984). A peculiar sensation of movement also occurs in the phantom limb phenomenon (Jankovic and Glass, 1985) and in the syndrome of restless legs (Schoenen, Gonce and Delwaine, 1984; Montplaisir et al., 1985; Verhagen and Horstink, 1985). Although the pathophysiology of sensory phenomena in association with motor disorders is poorly understood, it is possible that the limbic system is involved in this interaction between the motor and the sensory pathways (Jurgens and Ploog, 1981; Bonnett, 1982; Devinsky, 1983).

The second feature useful in differentiating tics from other movement disorders is the ability of the patient to willfully suppress the tics, albeit only temporarily. Voluntary control of tics leads to a 'build-up' and eventually even a 'rebound' exacerbation. During an interview or a public appearance, the patients may be able to conceal the tics, but later release them, often with exaggerated intensity. Some patients with relatively mild tics often suppress the tics subconsciously without apparent effort, particularly when they are in the company of strangers or when they are being observed, for example in the physician's office. It should be pointed out, however, that suppressibility, although characteristic, is not specific for tics.

Figure 19.1 Time-synchronized EEG and polygraphic recording system showing motor and verbal tics during non-REM sleep. (Reproduced from Glaze, Frost and Jankovic, 1983, with permission of the Editors of *Neurology*)

Some patients with tremors, dystonia, chorea, and ballism are able to voluntarily control the movements by changing position or by using autohypnosis or biofeedback.

Third, in contrast to the other hyperkinesias, tics persist during all stages of sleep (Glaze, Frost and Jankovic, 1983). Using overnight polygraphic sleep studies, which include infrared video monitoring and accelerometry, we demonstrated motor and vocal tics in almost all patients during REM and non-REM stages of sleep (*Figures 19.1* and *19.2*). The recorded tics were similar to those observed during wakefulness. These involuntary movements should be differentiated from

Figure 19.2 Motor tic during REM sleep. (Reproduced from Glaze, Frost and Jankovic, 1983, with permission of the Editors of *Neurology*)

the more stereotypic, periodic movements in sleep (previously referred to as nocturnal myoclonus) (Coleman, Pollack and Weitzman, 1980; Ohana *et al.*, 1985). Disorders of sleep (e.g. somnambulism, nightmares, enuresis) and arousal are common and occasionally are the earliest symptoms of TS. In some relatives of TS patients, the sleep disturbance may be the only manifestation (forme fruste) of TS (Mendelson, Caine and Goyer, 1980; Barabas, Mathews and Ferrari, 1984a). Recent morphological studies suggest that TS patients are able to maintain tonic arousal during psychological tests better than controls (Bock and Goldberg, 1985).

The presence of the characteristic movements during sleep provides evidence that tics indeed are involuntary.

Further evidence for the involuntary origin of tics is the observation that they are not preceded by a pre-movement negative EEG wave (Obeso, Rothwell and Marsden, 1981). When a normal subject is instructed to voluntarily mimic the tic movement, a slow negative EEG wave can be recorded 500–800 milliseconds before the actual movement occurs. Using computerized back-averaging techniques, this pre-movement potential could not be detected in patients before their involuntary tics. Thus, although tics can be voluntarily mimicked and modified, they probably originate in subcortical structures and employ motor pathways which are different from those used in normal voluntary movements.

The neurophysiological studies, including the polygraphic sleep recordings and the measurements of pre-movement EEG potentials, provide support for the neurological origin of tics (*Table 19.2*). Some investigators have demonstrated a 'flattened' wave IV amplitude of visually evoked responses and non-specific EEG abnormalities in some TS patients, However, other reports concluded that these neurophysiological findings did not differ from the results obtained in controls (Bergen, Tanner and Wilson, 1982; Domino *et al.*, 1982; Krumholz *et al.*, 1983).

Table 19.2 Evidence for neurological origin of TS

---

(1) Male-to-female ratio: 3 to 1
(2) Family history of tics or TS in 85% of patients
(3) Identical twins concordant for TS
(4) Soft neurological signs
(5) 'Organicity' on psychological tests
(6) Increased left-handedness and ambidexterity
(7) Association of TS with attentional deficit and learning disorders
(8) Increased blink rates in patients and their relatives
(9) Motor and behavioural abnormalities seen in TS have been observed in disorders with specific pathology in the basal ganglia ('secondary tourettism')
(10) Occurrence of tics during sleep
(11) Absence of normal pre-movement EEG potential suggests that tics are not voluntary
(12) Flattened wave IV amplitude on VER (?)
(13) EEG abnormalities (?)
(14) Decreased CSF homovanillic acid and 5-hydroxyindole acetic acid; increased CSF 3-methoxy-4-hydroxyphenylethylene glycol (?)
(15) Improvement with dopamine blocking or depleting agents and exacerbation with CNS stimulants and dopaminergic drugs
(16) Complex, coordinated, stereotyped movements and species-specific vocalizations can be produced by electrical stimulation of the anterior cingulate and peri-aqueductal grey area

---

Although the electrophysiological studies suggest subcortical origin of TS, the precise anatomical substrate for this complex neurobehavioural disorder is unknown. Electrical stimulation of the human anterior cingulate cortex results in complex, coordinated, stereotyped movements preceded by an 'urge' (Bonnett, 1982; Devinsky, 1982). These movements may be accompanied by involuntary vocalizations (Jurgens and Ploog, 1981). Species-specific vocalizations also can be produced by an electrical stimulation of the midbrain peri-aqueductal grey region

(Devinsky, 1983). Rostral brainstem has been implicated in the pathogenesis of blepharospasm, a common neuro-ophthalmological disorder in TS and in other basal ganglia disorders (Jankovic and Patel, 1983; Jankovic, 1985). These, and other, observations suggest that the midbrain, basal ganglia, and other subcortical structures are involved in the pathogenesis of TS (Devinsky, 1983; Caine, 1985). However, postmortem examinations of three TS brains have not revealed any specific pathological changes (Richardson, 1982; Haber, 1986).

The important role of genetic susceptibility in the pathogenesis of TS has been recognized since the original report of Gilles de la Tourette (Gilles de la Tourette, 1885). Several reports of monozygotic twins concordant for TS provide additional evidence for genetic influence in the pathogenesis of this disorder (Jenkins and Ashby, 1983; Waserman, Lal and Gauthier, 1983; Price et al., 1985). Price and colleagues (1985) reported 77% concordance of tics among 30 pairs of monozygotic twins with one TS co-twin; 23% concordance for 13 dizygotic pairs. Because not all monozygotic twins were fully concordant, non-genetic factors may affect expression of TS. Frequently the affected family members are unaware of their tics or other neurobehavioural symptoms of TS, and the family history of such problems is denied. This is exemplified by the following anecdote. After a detailed questioning of parents failed to reveal the presence of tics in other family members, a TS child remarked, as he was leaving the clinic, that he was going to visit his uncle 'Blinkie'.

The true incidence of familial TS is unknown, but, in our experience, about 85% of patients have at least one affected first-degree relative. However, specific patterns of transmission within families have not been determined. This may be explained by incomplete penetrance and by inaccurate ascertainment of TS findings in relatives of TS patients. Some investigators have attempted to explain the male preponderance in this syndrome by proposing that the female patients have a 'higher genetic loading' before the disorder expresses itself (Baron et al., 1981; Kidd and Pauls, 1982). Furthermore, a single major locus, a multifactorial mode of inheritance, and a vertical transmission from generation to generation have been proposed. Recently identified large kindreds with TS provide an opportunity for the application of recombinant DNA linkage techniques in an attempt to localize a genetic marker (Comings et al., 1984; Kurlan et al., 1986).

The phenotypic polymorphism in some families suggests that a transient tic of childhood, a chronic simple tic, a sleep disorder or a behavioural disturbance, may each represent a forme fruste of TS. Thus, it is possible that almost all cases of TS are inherited and that sporadic mutations are rare. Some studies, however, have concluded that the familial TS is different pathogenetically from the sporadic form. For example, Nee and colleagues (1980) showed that patients with familial TS had a higher occurrence of sleep disturbance and obsessive–compulsive behaviour, and responded better to haloperidol as compared to patients without a family history.

Besides the physiological and genetic findings, there are many other observations which provide support for neurological (rather than psychogenic) origin of TS (*Table 19.2*). For example, hormonal factors play an important, but poorly understood, role in the pathogenesis of TS. Endocrine studies in TS may explain the marked male preponderance and why puberty and menses often exacerbate TS symptoms. Minor neurological signs, organicity on psychological tests, and a higher incidence of left-handedness, ambidexterity, attentional deficit and learning disorders also have been used as evidence of 'organic' origin of TS (Shapiro et al., 1978).

Because behavioural disturbances, such as attentional deficit disorder with hyperactivity, sleep disturbance, coprolalia, copropraxia, and obsessive–compulsive, impulsive, and self-destructive behaviour are frequently associated with TS, the disorder has long been considered a behavioural problem and a psychiatric curiosity. However, during the the last two decades, research into the neurophysiological, neurochemical, neuropharmacological, and neurobehavioural mechanisms of TS has intensified, and important advances have been made in the understanding of this complex disorder (Cohen et al., 1979, 1982; Leckman and Cohen, 1983; Messiha and Carlson, 1983; Brunn, 1984; Butler, 1984; Caine, 1985; Erenberg, Cruse and Rothner, 1985). TS is now regarded as a hereditary neurological disorder characterized by involuntary motor tics, vocalizations, and a variety of behavioural disturbances. As a result of increased awareness of this disorder among the primary care physicians, educators, and the general public, the diagnosis is made more frequently and with less delay. While the prevalence of TS has been estimated at 0.5 per 1000, the true prevalence of the syndrome is yet unknown (Shapiro and Shapiro, 1982b).

DIFFERENTIAL DIAGNOSIS OF TICS

Due to the variable expression and the absence of pathognomonic laboratory tests, the correct diagnosis of TS depends on the recognition of typical clinical features (Jankovic and Fahn, 1985; Lees, 1985). Until the various tic disorders can be differentiated by either neurochemical, neurophysiological or neuropharmacological tests, it is best to view them as a continuum along a spectrum from mild, simple, and suppressible tics on one end to chronic, multiple, complex and non-suppressible tics on the other end of the spectrum (Golden, 1978; Fahn, 1982a). In the mild cases the most difficult diagnostic problem is to differentiate normal mannerisms, which are the individual's motor expressions or habits (physiological tics), and simple tics as the first or the only manifestation of TS (pathological tics). Although most mannerisms disappear after adolescence, they may persist and become incorporated into the individual's characteristic gestures. When the tics are complex, multifocal, and associated with vocalizations, then the diagnosis of TS is obvious. However, up to 15% of children have simple motor tics or vocalizations which last a few weeks or months and then they spontaneously disappear or are replaced by different transient tics. Other children may have chronic simple tics which do not change over a course of years or lifetime. When a tic first appears it is impossible to predict whether it will be acute, subacute, transient, or chronic, and therefore the classification of Shapiro et al. (1978) is not practical. It is not clear whether transient tics of childhood and chronic motor tics are distinct clinical entities, separate from TS, or merely variants of the same syndrome. The occurrence of these conditions in relatives of patients with typical TS favours the notion of a 'continuum' of the various tic disorders within the TS. However, for the purpose of research into the pathogenesis of the tic disorders, it is better to 'split' rather than to 'lump' the various tic syndromes (Cohen, Leckman and Shaywitz, 1984).

Due to the clinical heterogeneity of TS, it is difficult to adhere to strict diagnostic criteria, such as those proposed by Shapiro et al. (1978) and adopted by the *Diagnostic and Statistical Manual of Mental Disorders* (DSMIII) (American

Psychiatric Association, 1980). These criteria, for example, specify that TS symptoms begin between 2 and 15 years of age. While, in most TS patients, tics first occur in early childhood, we and others have observed patients in whom a reliable history revealed the onset during infancy or as late as the fourth decade (Marneros, 1983; Sutula and Hobbs, 1983). TS is generally a lifelong condition, but about 20% of patients achieve permanent remission after the age of 20.

The course of TS is just as variable as its clinical presentation. Waxing and waning in intensity and frequency of symptoms are common. Often, at the beginning of the school year or during a stressful period, tics intensify and migrate from one location to another, or completely new tics and vocalizations appear. Some patients experience remissions lasting up to several months, but most patients experience an acute change in the pattern or location of tics at six-week to three-month intervals. A common problem in the differential diagnosis of tic disorders is the similarity between TS and attentional deficit disorder with hyperactivity. The problem is compounded by the frequent association of the two disorders in the same patient.

Based on a study of 250 patients with TS, Comings and Comings (1984) noted attentional deficit disorder with hyperactivity in 62% of TS patients under 20 years of age. The mean latency from the onset of hyperactivity to the onset of TS symptoms was three years. The authors suggested that the TS gene could be expressed as attentional deficit disorder with hyperactivity, but without tics. This conclusion agrees with other studies, which suggest that genetic predisposition is important in both TS and attentional deficit disorder, but it is not clear whether the two disorders are genetically linked (Pauls *et al.*, 1986).

Behavioural disturbances are commonly associated with TS and present difficulties in separating the various manifestations of TS. About half of all TS patients exhibit various obsessions and compulsions (Frankel, 1986). They frequently ruminate about seemingly insignificant ideas or events, compulsively touch certain objects (e.g. hot plates or stoves, knives, door frames, light posts, floors, 'erotic' textures) or body parts (e.g. genitalia, breasts, face, lips) and some gain weight from excessive compulsive eating. Many patients, and their families, have difficulties differentiating the behavioural manifestations of the underlying TS and 'their own' feelings. As a result of this loss of autonomy and self-control, they lose self-esteem and become frustrated, irritable, impulsive, and argumentative. In one study, marked discipline problems associated with anger and violence were seen in 61% of 250 TS patients; exhibitionism was present in 15.9% of males and 6.1% of females (Cumings and Cumings, 1985). It is tempting to speculate whether these psychological disturbances are a part of the adaptation process or whether they are the neurobehavioural manifestations of the underlying disorder (*see* Chapter 20).

Besides the primary (idiopathic and hereditary) tic disorders, there are many secondary tic disorders. These TS-like disorders, which are due to a variety of identifiable causes, are referred to as 'acquired tourettism' (Sacks, 1982) (*Table 19.3*). Tics and other TS symptoms have been observed after treatment with antipsychotic drugs – 'tardive Tourette' (Klawans *et al.*, 1982). Anticonvulsants, CNS stimulants and dopaminergic drugs also may produce motor tics and vocalizations (Golden, 1977; Lowe *et al.*, 1982; Neglia, Glaze and Zion, 1984). In addition, TS symptoms have been reported after carbon monoxide intoxication (Pulst, Walshe and Romero, 1983), head trauma (Fahn, 1982b), and encephalitis (Sacks, 1982; Devinsky, 1983).

There are reports of two brothers, 46 and 40 years old, who had the onset of motor tics, lip and tongue biting, involuntary vocalizations, and coprolalia at age 36. However, at age 40, they developed progressive parkinsonism, supranuclear ophthalmoparesis, and motor neurone disease (Spitz, Jankovic and Killian, 1985). Both had acanthocytosis, but normal lipoproteins. This form of 'neuro-acanthocytosis' has been associated not only with facial tics and self-mutilating behaviour but also with peripheral neuropathy, high CK, and other abnormalities.

Finally, the authors and others have observed TS in association with various neurological disorders, such as migraine, epilepsy, XYY karyotype, congenital myopathies, and neurocutaneous syndromes (Jankovic, 1986, unpublished results), but a clear pathogenetic relationship between these disorders and TS has not been established (Merskley, 1974; Matthews, 1981; Barabas, Matthews and Ferrari, 1984b).

Table 19.3 Classification of tics

Physiological tics
  Mannerisms ('habit spasms')

Pathological tics
  Primary (idiopathic)
  Hereditary
    Gilles de la Tourette syndrome
    Huntington's disease
    Dystonia musculorum deformans
    Neuroacanthocytosis
  Secondary or aquired 'tourettism'
    Infectious/post-infectious: infectious encephalitis, klazomania, Creutzfeldt–Jakob disease, Sydenham's chorea, other
    Drugs: stimulants, levodopa, antipsychotics (tardive tics), carbamazepine, phenobarbital, phenytoin
    Toxins: carbon monoxide
    Perinatal: static encephalopathy
    Head trauma
    Stroke
    Neurocutaneous syndromes
    Chromosomal abnormality
    Degenerative disorders
    Senile tics

Stereotypic movements may be present in TS, and they are also characteristically seen in autism, mental retardation, Rett's syndrome, Lesch–Nyhan syndrome, schizophrenia, and in tardive dyskinesia (Barabas and Matthews, 1983; Jankovic, 1986a). We have evaluated several patients with Rett's syndrome in whom other diagnostic considerations included possible autism or TS. However, Rett's syndrome occurs only in girls who, in contrast to autistic children, have normal prenatal and perinatal growth and development. Between the ages of 6 and 18 months the development ceases, and there is a progressive regression and a loss of communication, dementia, jerky ataxia of the trunk and gait, clumsiness of the hands and legs, loss of purposeful use of hands, and a development of stereotypic 'hand-washing' movements, teeth grinding, facial grimacing, and other involuntary movements. The patients may have spasticity, intermittent hyperventilation, generalized and partial seizures with abnormal EEG, vasomotor cutaneous disturbances, acquired microcephalia, and cortical atrophy. In a single case of Rett's syndrome studied at autopsy there was evidence of severe reduction of dopamine, noradrenaline, and serotonin and reduced D-2 dopamine receptor activity (Hagberg et al., 1983; Riederer et al., 1985; El-Hibri et al., 1986).

Self-mutilation, stereotypic movements, choreo-athetosis, spasticity, and other motor signs are characteristic of another childhood disorder, the Lesch–Nyhan syndrome (Stein and Morrison, 1985). This X-linked, recessive disorder is associated with a deficiency of the enzyme hypoxanthine–guanine phosphoribosyl transferase (HPRT), which is normally found highly concentrated in the basal ganglia. Despite the clinical similarities there is no abnormality in purine metabolism in TS (Van Woert, Yip and Balis, 1977). Like TS patients the Lesch–Nyhan patients have low cerebrospinal fluid homovanillic acid (Silverstein et al., 1985). However, we found normal cerebrospinal fluid homovanillic acid, but increased cerebrospinal fluid 5-hydroxyindole acetic acid in some patients with Lesch–Nyhan syndrome (Jankovic, 1986, unpublished results). Goldstein and colleagues (1985) have suggested that the self-mutilation in this syndrome is related to dopaminergic denervation and that perturbation of the D-1 dopaminergic receptors may play a role in such behaviour.

Certain non-verbal sounds, such as grunting, throat clearing, snorting, sniffing, belching, moaning, and humming, occur not only in TS but also in Huntington's disease, Parkinson's disease, progressive supranuclear palsy, pseudobulbar palsy, cranial–cervical dystonia (Meige's syndrome), and tardive dyskinesia (Jankovic, 1986b). However, TS patients produce more complex noises, such as squeaking, squealing, barking, coughing, spitting, hissing, whistling, blowing, and obscene utterances (coprolalia). Coprolalia is not unique for TS, and it is seen in other neurological disorders such as dementia, non-fluent aphasia, hemiballism (Marti-Massó and Obeso, 1985) and in klazomania. The latter syndrome is a sequela to encephalitis lethargica characterized by parkinsonism with oculogyric crises and tic-like movements, involuntary vocalizations, echolalia, and coprolalia (Wohlfart, Ingvar and Hellberg, 1961).

NEUROPHARMACOLOGY AND MANAGEMENT OF TS

Before recommending a specific treatment plan, it is wise to determine the range and fluctuations of the baseline symptoms by following the patient for several weeks or months. If the behavioural or motor symptoms interfere with the child's normal development, then pharmacological therapy may be necessary. Drug management is also indicated when the symptoms are occupationally and socially disabling. However, many patients do not require any medications and an educational discussion about the disorder and the available therapeutic options is enough to reassure the patients and their families. Once medical therapy is decided the clinician must constantly monitor, not only the effects of the specific therapy, but also the impact of the symptoms on the development of the child, school performance, family and peer relationships and other psychosocial aspects (Shapiro and Shapiro, 1981; Jankovic, 1986b).

Perhaps the single most important reason for the rising interest in TS has been the demonstration of effective therapy with haloperidol and other pharmacological

Table 19.4 Neurotransmitters in TS

Dopamine
  Symptoms suppressed by dopamine depletors, postsynaptic dopamine receptor blockers and presynaptic (autoreceptor) dopamine agonists and aggravated by levodopa and by postsynaptic dopamine receptor agonists
  Symptoms exacerbated by CNS stimulants
  Decreased CSF homovanillic acid – 'dopamine receptor supersensitivity'
  Normal dopamine binding on PET scans

Serotonin
  Variable effect of serotonin precursors (5-hydroxytryptophan) serotoninergic drugs (clonazepam), serotonin uptake blockers (chlorimipramine) and antiserotonin drugs (methysergide)
  Normal or decreased CSF 5-hydroxyindole acetic acid
  Sleep abnormalities possibly mediated via serotonin system

Noradrenaline
  Improvement with clonidine
  Increased CSF 3-methoxy-4-hydroxyphenylethylene glycol or no change

Acetylcholine
  Variable effect with cholinergic and anticholinergic agents, improvement with intravenous physostigmine?
  Increased red blood cell choline

GABA
  GABA agonists may have a mild beneficial effect

Other
  Decreased dynorphine in dorsal globus pallidus

See *text* for details and references.

agents (Shapiro and Shapiro, 1981; Jankovic, 1986b). However, before discussing the pharmacological approach in TS, it is useful to review the biochemical hypotheses on which some of the pharmacological strategies are based. Despite many attempts to demonstrate neurotransmitter changes, no consistent abnormality has been identified (*Table 19.4*). In the absence of postmortem biochemical data, the cerebrospinal fluid (CSF) studies provide the best, albeit only indirect, evidence for a possible biochemical disturbance (Koslow and Cross, 1982). Some, but not all, CSF studies found low baseline homovanillic acid in untreated TS patients (Cohen *et al.*, 1979; Singer *et al.*, 1982). Because there are no Parkinson's findings in TS and because most patients improve with antidopaminergic drugs, the low CSF homovanillic acid has been interpreted by some to be a reflection of supersensitive dopamine receptors associated with abnormal ontogenic neuronal development (Butler, 1984). Because of this receptor supersensitivity and an enhanced negative feedback, there is, presumably, an inhibition of the presynaptic dopamine synthesis, which results in low CSF homovanillic acid. Whether this postulated mechanism is relevant to the pathogenesis of TS is unknown. Furthermore, the validity and methodology of some of the CSF studies have been challenged (Koslow and Cross, 1982).

The notion of dopamine receptor supersensitivity could not be confirmed by positron emission tomography (PET) or by dopamine receptor ligand binding studies in one autopsied brain (Singer et al., 1986). Only one of seven TS patients studied with PET had dopaminergic binding activity more than expected for controls. The serotoninergic receptor activity was normal in all patients. While the PET and the postmortem study failed to demonstrate a neurotransmitter abnormality in TS, limitations of such studies should be noted. The youngest TS patient studied with PET was 19 years old; thus, increased dopamine receptors may have been demonstrated if younger patients had been included in the study. Moreover, the postmortem chemical analysis was performed on a brain tissue which was disrupted during the fatal head trauma.

Another postmortem study of a TS brain found a striking decrease of the peptide dynorphin in striatal fibres projecting to the pallidum (Haber et al., 1986). In contrast, both enkephaline and substance P were normally distributed in the TS brain. Additional brains have to be analysed to confirm this interesting finding. Thus far, no animal models of TS have been developed on which the various biochemical hypotheses could be tested.

Although a sound understanding of the biochemical mechanisms underlying TS is still lacking, effective therapies are available. Unfortunately, many therapeutic trials in TS are difficult to interpret because of a small number of subjects, a non-random selection, and unreliable methods of assessment. Despite these shortcomings, several medications have been used extensively enough to formulate impressions about their relative efficacy.

Although never tested in a double-blind placebo-controlled trial, the most frequently used drug in the management of TS is haloperidol (Shapiro et al., 1978). Clinical improvement may be achieved in about two-thirds of all patients, but because of tolerance and an emergence of unwanted side-effects, less than one-third continue haloperidol for an extended period of time (Shapiro and Shapiro, 1981). When the dosage is increased slowly by 0.5 mg/week, most of the undesirable side-effects can be prevented, and the dosage may be increased up to 40 mg/day. Despite this slow increase, about 30% of patients experience parkinsonian symptoms, akathisia, drowsiness, depression, phobia, poor attention span, mental dullness, fatiguability, weight gain, allergic reactions, hepatotoxicity, or agranulocytosis. Although high dosages were used in the initial studies, subsequent experience had shown that daily doses higher than 8 mg were rarely necessary. The author and others have observed tardive dyskinesia in TS patients treated with haloperidol or with other dopamine receptor-blocking agents (Mizrahi, Holtzman and Tharp, 1980; Golden, 1984; Jankovic, 1986b). The symptoms of tardive dyskinesia in patients with facial tics may be difficult to detect and this may be the reason for the low incidence of this complication reported in TS.

Other dopamine receptor blocking agents, such as trifluoperazine (Borison et al., 1982), penfluridol (Shapiro, Shapiro and Eisenkraft, 1983a), pimozide (Shapiro and Shapiro, 1984), and fluphenazine (Goetz, Tanner and Klawans, 1984), may offer certain advantages over haloperidol. Of these agents, pimozide and fluphenazine seem to have the lowest incidence of sedation, with efficacy equal or superior to haloperidol. Pimozide is a diphenylbutylpiperidine derivative extensively used in Europe, but only recently approved in the United States. The starting dose is 0.1 mg/day, and the dosage may be increased up to 10 mg/day in children and up to 20 mg/day in adults. Because of its long half-life (55 hours), pimozide may be administered once a day. Besides the usual antidopaminergic and anticholinergic effects, up to 25% of patients taking pimozide have ECG changes, particularly T-wave inversions, U-waves and prolonged Q-T intervals. Therefore, potential cardiotoxicity of pimozide must be monitored by repeat ECGs at three weeks and every three to six months thereafter. While tardive dyskinesia has not yet been reported with pimozide, it does produce an 'extrapyramidal' reaction, and it is likely that permanent tardive dyskinesia as a result of chronic pimozide therapy will occur.

Several studies (Borison et al., 1982; Goetz, Tanner and Klawans, 1984) have shown that fluphenazine, a piperazine phenothiazine, is as effective as haloperidol and in many patients may have a lower incidence of adverse reactions. In the Baylor Movement Disorder Clinic the author's group uses fluphenazine as the first antidopaminergic drug, even before haloperidol and pimozide. The starting dose is 0.5 mg/day, and this is increased weekly until a satisfactory tic control is achieved or adverse effects occur. The average daily dosage is 7 mg with a range of 2-15 mg. The side-effects are similar to the other antidopaminergic drugs, but it seems to be less sedating.

Due to the concern over the risk of tardive dyskinesia with the antipsychotic agents, tetrabenazine, a benzoquinoline derivative which depletes monoamines and blocks both presynaptic and postsynaptic dopamine receptors has been studied (Jankovic, 1983; Reches et al., 1983). Tetrabenazine has been found effective in a variety of hyperkinetic movement disorders, especially Huntington's disease, tardive dyskinesia, and some dystonias. In a double-blind placebo-controlled study of hyperkinetic movement disorders, a patient with dystonic tics due to TS showed a remarkable reduction in frequency and severity of tics (Jankovic, 1983). This observation, coupled with reports of possible effectiveness of tetrabenazine in TS, encouraged further studies of this drug (Sweet et al., 1974). Using global rating scales and polygraphic sleep studies, marked and lasting dose-dependent improvement in four patients, mild or transient improvement in three patients, and a poor response in two patients, both adults, were demonstrated (Jankovic, Glaze and Frost, 1984). Since the initial report additional patients have been studied with similar results; children generally respond to tetrabenazine better than adult TS patients. The side-effects of tetrabenazine include daytime drowsiness, mild tremor, parkinsonian features, and depression. One patient developed oculogyric crises. This neuro-ophthalmological symptom has been reported in untreated TS patients (Frankel and Cumings, 1984) and in four young patients treated with tetrabenazine for various movement disorders (Burke et al., 1985). Despite the occurrence of this acute dystonic reaction, presumably due to postsynaptic blocking action, there has been no case report of tardive dyskinesia attributed to tetrabenazine therapy (Mikkelsen, 1983).

While antidopaminergic drugs ameliorate TS, the dopaminergic agents, e.g. levodopa, bromocriptine, and the CNS stimulants, e.g. dextroamphetamines, methylphenidate and pemoline, seem to exacerbate, or even precipitate, tics and other symptoms of TS (*Table 18.5*) (Golden, 1977; Feinberg and Carroll, 1979; Sleator, 1980; Lowe et al., 1982; Caine et al., 1984). The CNS stimulants may actually trigger tics, but recent reports contend that, when used cautiously, these drugs are safe and beneficial in many patients with the combination of TS and attentional deficit disorder (Erenberg, Cruse and Rothner, 1985).

Due to the CSF studies of monoamine metabolites, supported by the clinical pharmacological studies, major emphasis has been placed on the role of dopamine in TS. CSF measurements of 3-methoxy-4-hydroxyphenylethylene glycol (MHPG), a noradrenaline metabolite, show normal or slightly increased values (Koslow and

Table 19.5 Pharmacological treatment of TS

Drugs	Clinical effect*
Dopamine antagonists	
Haloperidol	+++
Phenothiazines (fluphenazine)	+++
Pimozide, penfluridol	+++
Clozapine	0
Dopamine depletors	
Tetrabenazine	++
α-Methyl-*p*-tyrosine	+
Dopaminergic drugs	
Levodopa, bromocriptine	−
CNS stimulants	−
Serotoninergic drugs	
L-5-Hydroxytryptophan	±
L-Tryptophan	±
Clorimipramine, amitriptyline, imipramine	±
Clonazepam	+
Noradrenergic drugs	
Clonidine	++
Desimipramine	0
Imipramine	−
Anti-noradrenergic drugs	
Propranolol	±
Disulfiram (DBH inhibitor)	−
Cholinergic drugs	
Physostigmine (IV)	+
Lecithin–choline	±
Deanol	0
Anticholinergic drugs	
Benztropine	−
Scopolamine (IM)	+
GABA agonists	
β-Chlorphenyl-GABA	+
Baclofen	+
Muscimol	±
Clonazepam	+
Valproate	±
Other	
Monoamine oxidase inhibitors	0
Lithium	±
Barbiturates	0
Phenytoin	0
Carbamazepine	0
Aprezolam	+
Other benzodiazepines	0

+++ >50% improvement; ++ 20–50% improvement; + <20% improvement; ± improves some, worsens others; − worsening; 0 no effect.
* Clinical effect is a subjective impression based on a review of the reported effects and personal experience.

Cross, 1982; Singer et al., 1982). However, some clinical pharmacological studies have indicated a possible role of noradrenaline. Clonidine, an imidazoline derivative with agonist effect on presynaptic α_2-adrenergic receptors, reduces central noradrenaline turnover (Svensson, Bunney and Aghajanian, 1975). Although not uniform in its effect on TS, at least half of the patients experience satisfactory response with clonidine, particularly with regard to behavioural symptoms (Borison et al., 1982; Shapiro, Shapiro and Eisenkraft, 1982; Leckman et al., 1985). Clonidine has been used as an effective antihypertensive agent, but has not yet been approved for the treatment of TS. When used in treating TS patients, it should be started at a very low dose of 0.05 mg/day and slowly increased over several weeks up to 0.3–0.5 mg/day ($4\,\mu\text{g}\cdot\text{kg}^{-1}\cdot\text{day}^{-1}$). The patients often feel 'calmer' within a few days after starting the drug, but the full effects may not be appreciated for several weeks or months. The side-effects of clonidine include dry mouth, drowsiness, orthostatic lightheadedness and prolongation of the P–R interval on ECG. It is possible that the non-specific anxiolytic and sedating action, rather than specific anti-noradrenergic effect, is primarily responsible for the beneficial effects of clonidine. However, the exact mechanism of action of clonidine in TS is unknown. Desipramine, a noradrenaline re-uptake blocker, has no effect on the symptoms of TS (Caine, 1985).

Except for sleep disturbance, which may be a reflection of central serotonin dysfunction (Glaze, Frost and Jankovic, 1983), there is little evidence for serotonin involvement in the pathogenesis of TS. The CSF 5-hydroxyindoleacetic acid a serotonin metabolite, is either normal or slightly reduced (Koslow and Cross, 1982; Singer et al., 1982). Furthermore, modulation of the serotoninergic system with clonazepam, which increases central serotonin, and with serotonin re-uptake inhibitors, such as chlorimipramine and trazodone, while successful in some, has been disappointing in most patients (Gonce and Barbeau, 1977; Yaryura-Tobias and Neziroglu, 1977; Borison et al., 1983).

The evidence for involvement of the cholinergic system in TS is also weak, and the effects of cholinergic drugs, such as intravenous physostigmine, are inconsistent (Rosenberg and Davis, 1982; Stahl and Berger, 1982; Tanner, Goetz and Klawans, 1982; Singer, Oshida and Coyle, 1984). Despite elevated levels of red blood cell choline, the anticholinergic drugs have not been effective in TS (Hanin et al., 1979).

Since postsynaptic dopamine receptors and presynaptic gamma-aminobutyric acid (GABA) receptors are located on the same striatal neurones, the GABA system has been studied in TS. However, the blood and cerebrospinal fluid GABA levels in TS patients seem normal (Van Woert, Rosenbaum and Enna, 1982). Furthermore, pharmacological modulation of central GABA with β-chlorophenyl-GABA, baclofen, muscimol, clonazepam and valproate, has been essentially ineffective (*Table 19.5*) (Shapiro, Shapiro and Sweet, 1981).

The therapeutic approach in TS must be individualized according to the patient's needs. This is particularly important for patients in whom either the motor or the behavioural manifestations predominate. While there is a marked therapeutic overlap (Borison et al., 1982), the antidopaminergic drugs may be more useful for the treatment of tics, whereas clonidine or clonazepam may be more effective for the control of behavioural problems. In patients with severe attentional deficit disorders, the CNS stimulants may be required despite their potential risk of exacerbating tics (Erenberg, Cruse and Rothner, 1985; Price, 1986). Pharmacological therapy is probably not indicated for patients with a mild and non-disabling disorder.

Besides pharmacological therapy, behavioural therapy, psychotherapy, academic intervention and genetic counselling play an important role in the management of TS (Cohen, Leckman and Shaywitz, 1984). Elimination of certain artificial food additives from a diet (the Feingold diet) has been reported by some patients to be very beneficial and has apparently resulted in remarkable symptom reduction. Lastly, during the First International Tourette's Syndrome Symposium in May 1981, in New York City, Professor Hassler of Germany reported the preliminary results in 16 TS patients treated with thalamotomy of the intralaminar nuclei. However, a detailed long-term follow-up of this unconventional treatment is not known. Using a similar surgical approach in three patients, de Divitis D'Errico and Cerillo (1977) reported only transient improvement.

In order to assess the risk–benefit ratio of any treatment, it is extremely important to develop methods which allow a quantitative assessment of the symptomatic response. A validated multidimensional global rating scale, which measures not only the motor and phonic tics, but also the various behavioural manifestations, is needed (Harcherik *et al.*, 1984). Recording of tics during sleep has certain advantages over recordings during wakefulness because the psychological influence on tics is eliminated (Jankovic, Glaze and Frost, 1984). Because of the variable course of TS, and because of a marked placebo response, all therapeutic trials should be longitudinal and well-controlled.

Although first recognized 100 years ago, most of our current understanding of the neurobiology of TS has been derived from clinical, behavioural, genetic, physiological, neurochemical, and pharmacological research in the last 20 years. As a result of this intense interest in TS, a greater insight has been gained into the mechanisms of this complex neurobehavioural disorder. However, more detailed *in vivo* and postmortem biochemical analyses are needed to formulate more sophisticated pharmacological models of TS. Genetic linkage studies of informative kindreds utilizing the most advanced DNA recombinant technology may provide insight into the molecular biology of TS. When coupled with further characterization of TS by neurophysiological, neuroendocrinological and neurobehavioural techniques, the results of such research should lead to the development of accurate diagnostic tests and specific therapeutic approaches for patients with this curious neurological syndrome.

References

AMERICAN PSYCHIATRIC ASSOCIATION (1980) *Diagnostic and Statistical Manual of Mental Disorders (DSMIII)*, 3rd edn. Washington DC: American Psychiatric Association

ANDERMANN, F. and ANDERMANN, E. (1986) Excessive startle syndromes: Startle disease, jumping and startle epilepsy. In *Myoclonus*. Eds. S. Fahn, C. D. Marsden and M. Van Woert. New York: Raven Press (in press)

BARABAS, G. and MATTHEWS, W. S. (1983) Coincident infantile autism and Tourette syndrome: A case report. *Developmental and Behavioural Pediatrics*, **4**, 180–281

BARABAS, G., MATTHEWS, W. S. and FERRARI, M. (1984a) Disorders of arousal in Gilles de la Tourette's syndrome. *Neurology*, **34**, 815–817

BARABAS, G., MATTHEWS, W. S. and FERRARI, M. (1984b) Tourette's syndrome and migraine. *Archives of Neurology*, **41**, 871–872

BARON, M. E., SHAPIRO, E., SHAPIRO, A. and RAINER, J. D. (1981) Genetic analysis of Tourette syndrome suggesting major gene effect. *American Journal of Human Genetics*, **33**, 765–775

BEARD, G. M. (1886) Experiments with the 'jumpers' or 'jumping' Frenchmen of Maine. *Journal of Nervous and Mental Disease*, **7**, 487–490

BERGEN, D., TANNER, C. M. and WILSON, R. (1982) The electroencephalogram in Tourette syndrome. *Annals of Neurology*, **11**, 382–385
BLISS, J. (1980) Sensory experiences of Gilles de la Tourette syndrome. *Archives of General Psychiatry*, **37**, 1343–1347
BOCK, R. D. and GOLDBERG, L. (1985) Tonic, phasic and cortical arousal in Gilles de la Tourette's syndrome. *Journal of Neurology, Neurosurgery and Psychiatry*, **48**, 535–544
BONNETT, K. A. (1982) Neurobiological dissection of Tourette syndrome: A neurochemical focus on a human neuroanatomical model. In *Gilles de la Tourette Syndrome*. Eds. A. J. Friedhoff and T. N. Chase, pp. 77–82. New York: Raven Press
BORISON, R. L., ANG, L., CHANGE, S., DYSKEN, M., COMATY, J. E. and DAVIS, J. M. (1982) New pharmacological approaches in the treatment of Tourette syndrome. In *Gilles de la Tourette Syndrome*. Eds. A. J. Friedhoff and T. N. Chase. *Advances in Neurology*, Vol. 35, pp. 377–382. New York: Raven Press
BORISON, R. L., HAMILTON, W. J., NICHOLS, F. T. and DIAMOND, B. I. (1983) Trazodone and Tourette's syndrome. *Neurology*, **33** (Suppl. 2), 199 (Abstract)
BRUUN, R. D. (1984) Gilles de la Tourette's syndrome. An overview of clinical experience. *Journal of the American Academy of Child Psychiatry*, **23**, 126–133
BULLEN, J. G. and HEMSLEY, D. R. (1983) Sensory experience as a trigger in Gilles de la Tourette's syndrome. *Journal of Behavioural Therapy and Experimental Psychiatry*, **14**, 197–201
BURKE, R. E. (1984) Tardive dyskinesia: Current clinical issues. *Neurology*, **34**, 1348–1353
BURKE, R. E., RECHES, A., TRAUB, M. M., ILSON, J., SWASH, M. and FAHN, S. (1985) Tetrabenazine induces acute dystonic reactions. *Annals of Neurology*, **197**, 200–202
BUTLER, I. J. (1984) Tourette's syndrome. Some new concepts. In *Movement Disorders*. Ed. J. Jankovic. *Neurologic Clinics*, Vol. 2, pp. 571–580. Philadelphia: W. B. Saunders
CAINE, E. D. (1985) Gilles de la Tourette's syndrome. A review of clinical and research studies and consideration of future directions for investigation. *Archives of Neurology*, **42**, 393–397
CAINE, E. D., LUDLOW, C. L., POLINSKY, R. J. and EBERT, M. H. (1984) Provocative drug testing in Tourette's syndrome: d- and l-amphetamine and haloperidol. *Journal of the American Academy of Child Psychiatry*, **23**, 147–152
COHEN, D. J., DETLOR, J., SHAYWITZ, B. A. and LECKMAN, J. F. (1982) Interaction of biological and psychological factors in the natural history of Tourette syndrome: A paradigm for childhood neuropyschiatric disorders. In *Gilles de la Tourette Syndrome*. Eds. A. J. Friedhoff and T. N. Chase. *Advances in Neurology*, Vol. 35, pp. 31–40. New York: Raven Press
COHEN, D. J., LECKMAN, J. F. and SHAYWITZ, B. A. (1984) Developmental and habit disorders. In *A Clinical Guide to Child Psychiatry*. Eds. A. A. Ehrhardt and L. Greenhill, pp. 3–28. New York: MacMillan Free Press
COHEN, D. J., SHAYWITZ, B. A., YOUNG, J. G., CARBONARE, C. M. *et al.* (1979) Central biogenic amine metabolism in children with the syndrome of chronic multiple tics of Gilles de la Tourette: Noreprinephrine, serotonin and dopamine. *Journal of the American Academy of Child Psychiatry*, **18**, 320–341
COLEMAN, R. M., POLLACK, C. P. and WEITZMAN, E. D. (1980) Periodic movement in sleep (nocturnal myoclonus): Relation to sleep disorders. *Annals of Neurology*, **4**, 416–421
COMINGS, D. E. and COMINGS, B. G. (1984) Tourette's syndrome and attention deficit disorder with hyperactivity: Are they genetically related? *Journal of American Academy of Child Psychiatry*, **23**, 138–146
COMINGS, D. E. and COMINGS, B. G. (1985) Tourette syndrome: Clinical and psychological aspects of 250 cases. *American Journal of Human Genetics*, **37**, 435–450
COMINGS, D. E., COMINGS, B. G., DEVOR, E. J. and CLONINGER, C. R. (1984) Detection of major gene for Gilles de la Tourette syndrome. *American Journal of Human Genetics*, **36**, 586–600
DE DIVITIS, E., D'ERRICO, A. and CERILLO, A. (1977) Stereotactic surgery in Gilles de la Tourette syndrome. *Acta Neurochirurgica*, **73** (Suppl.), 24–28
DEVINSKY, O. (1983) Neuroanatomy of Gilles de la Tourette's syndrome. Possible midbrain involvement. *Archives of Neurology*, **40**, 508–514
DOMINO, E. F., PIGGOTT, L., DEMETRIOU, S. and CULBERT, J. (1982) Visually evoked responses in Tourette syndrome. In *Gilles de la Tourette Syndrome*. Eds. A. J. Friedhoff and T. N. Chase. *Advances in Neurology*, Vol. 35, pp. 115–120. New York: Raven Press.
EL-HIBRI, H. Y., PERCY, A. K., GLAZE, D. G., BUTLER, I. J. and RICCARDI, V. M. (1986) Biogenic amines in Rett syndrome: A possible role in pathogenesis. *New England Journal of Medicine* (in press)
ERENBERG, G., CRUSE, R. P. and ROTHNER, D. A. (1985) Gilles de la Tourette's syndrome: Effects of stimulant drugs. *Neurology*, **35**, 1346–1348
ERENBERG, G., CRUSE, R. P. and ROTHNER, A. D. (1986) Tourette syndrome: An analysis of 200 pediatric and adolescent cases. *Cleveland Clinic Quarterly* (in press)

FAHN, S. (1982a) The clinical spectrum of motor tics. In *Gilles de la Tourette Syndrome*. Eds. A. J. Friedhoff and T. N. Chase. *Advances in Neurology*, Vol. 35, pp. 341–344. New York: Raven Press

FAHN, S. (1982b) A case of post-traumatic tic syndrome. In *Gilles de la Tourette Syndrome*. Eds. A. J. Friedhoff and T. N. Chase. *Advances in Neurology*, Vol. 35, pp. 349–350. New York: Raven Press

FEINBERG, M. and CARROLL, B. J. (1979) Effects of dopamine agonists and antagonists in Tourette's disease. *Archives of General Psychiatry*, **36**, 979–985

FEINBERG, T. G., SHAPIRO, A. K. and SHAPIRO, E. (1986) Paroxysmal myoclonic dystonia with vocalisations: new entity or variant of preexisting syndromes? *Journal of Neurology, Neurosurgery and Psychiatry*, **49**, 52–57

FRANKEL, M. and CUMMINGS, J. L. (1984) Neuro-ophthalmic abnormalities in Tourette's syndrome: Functional and anatomic implications. *Neurology*, **34**, 359–361

FRANKEL, M., CUMMINGS, J. L., ROBERTSON, M. M., TRIMBLE, M. R., HILL, M. A. and BENSON, D. F. (1986) Obsessions and compulsions in Gilles de la Tourette's syndrome. *Neurology*, **36**, 378–382

GILLES DE LA TOURETTE, G. (1885) Étude sur une affection nerveuse caracterisée par de l'incoordination motrice accompagnée d'echolalie et de copralalie. *Archives de Neurologie*, **9**, 19–42, 153–156

GLAZE, D. G., FROST, J. D. and JANKOVIC, J. (1983) Gilles de la Tourette's syndrome. Disorder of arousal. *Neurology*, **33**, 586–592

GOETZ, C. G. and KLAWANS, H. L. (1980) Gilles de la Tourette's syndrome and compressive neuropathies. *Annals of Neurology*, **8**, 453

GOETZ, C. G., TANNER, C. M. and KLAWANS, H. L. (1984) Fluphenazine and multifocal tic disorders. *Archives of Neurology*, **41**, 271–272

GOLDEN, G. S. (1977) The effect of central nervous system stimulants on Tourette syndrome. *Annals of Neurology*, **2**, 69–70

GOLDEN, G. S. (1978) Tics and Tourette's: A continuum of symptoms? *Annals of Neurology*, **4**, 145–148

GOLDEN, G. S. (1984) Tardive dyskinesia in Tourette's syndrome. *Annals of Neurology*, **16**, 390 (Abstract)

GOLDSTEIN, M., ANDERSON, L. T., REUBEN, R. and DANCIS, J. (1985) Self-multilation in Lesch–Nyman disease is caused by dopaminergic denervation. *Lancet*, **i**, 338–339

GONCE, M. and BARBEAU, A. (1977) Seven cases of Gilles de la Tourette's syndrome: Partial relief with clonazepam: A pilot study. *Canadian Journal of Neurological Sciences*, **4**, 279–283

HABER, S. N., KOWELL, N. W., VONSATTEL, J. P., BIRD, E. D. and RICHARDSON, E. P. (1986) Lack of dynorphin, but no enkephalin or substance P, immunoreactivity in the dorsal globus pallidus in Gilles de la Tourette's syndrome. *Journal of the Neurological Sciencies* (in press)

HAGBERG, B., AICARDI, J., DIAS, K. and RAVISO, O. (1983) A progressive syndrome of autism, dementia, ataxia, and loss of purposeful hand use in girls. Rett's syndrome: Report of 35 cases. *Annals of Neurology*, **14**, 411–479

HALLETT, M. (1985) Myoclonus: Relation to epilepsy. *Epilepsia*, **26** (Suppl. 1), S67–S77

HAMMOND, W. A. (1884) Myriachit, a newly described disease of the nervous system and its analogues. *New York Medical Journal*, **39**, 191–192

HANIN, I., MERIKANGAS, J. R., MERIKANGAS, K. R. and KOPP, U. (1979) Red-cell choline and Gilles de la Tourette syndrome. *New England Journal of Medicine*, **301**, 661–662

HARCHERIK, D. F., LECKMAN, J. F., DETLOR, J. and COHEN, D. J. (1984) A new instrument for clinical studies of Tourette's syndrome. *Journal of American Academy of Child Psychiatry*, **23**, 153–160

ITARD, J. M. G. (1825) Memoire sur quelques fonctions involuntaries des appareils de la locomotion de la prehension et de la voix. *Archives of General Medicine*, **8**, 385–402

JANKOVIC, J. (1983) Tetrabenazine in the treatment of hyperkinetic movement disorders. In *Experimental Therapeutics of the Movement Disorders*. Eds. S. Fahn, D. B. Calne and I. Shoulson, *Advances in Neurology*, Vol. 37, pp. 277–289. New York: Raven Press

JANKOVIC, J. (1985) Clinical features, differential diagnosis and pathogenesis of blepharospasm and cranial-cervical dystonia. In *Blepharospasm*. Eds S. L. Bosniak, *Advances in Ophthalmology and Plastic Reconstructive Surgery*, Vol. 4, pp. 67–82. New York: Pergamon Press

JANKOVIC, J. (1986a) Cranial–cervical dyskinesia. In *Current Neurology*. Ed. S. H. Appel, Vol. 6, pp. 153–176. Chicago: Year Book Medical Publishers

JANKOVIC, J. (1986b) Recent advances in the management of tics. *Clinical Neuropharmacology* (in press)

JANKOVIC, J. and FAHN, S. (1986) The phenomenology of tics. In *Movement Disorders*, Eds C. D. Marsden and S. Fahn. Vol. 1, pp. 17–26. London: Butterworth

JANKOVIC, J. and GLASS, J. P. (1985) Metoclopramide-induced phantom dyskinesia. *Neurology*, **35**, 432–435

JANKOVIC, J., GLAZE, D. G. and FROST, J. D. (1984) Effect of tetrabenazine on tics and sleep of Gilles de la Tourette's syndrome. *Neurology*, **34**, 688–692

JANKOVIC, J., HAVINS, W. E. and WILKINS, R. (1982) Blinking and blepharospasm: Mechanism, diagnosis and treatment. *Journal of the American Medical Association,* **248,** 3160–3164
JANKOVIC, J. and PATEL, S. (1983) Blepharospasm associated with brainstem lesions. *Neurology,* **33,** 1237–1240
JENKINS, R. L. and ASHBY, H. B. (1983) Gilles de la Tourette's syndrome in identical twins. *Archives of Neurology,* **40,** 249–251
JURGENS, U. and PLOOG, D. (1981) On the neural control of mammalian vocalization. *Trends in Neurosciences,* **4,** 135–137
KENNY, M. G., SIMONS, R. C. and MURPHY, H. B. M. (1983) A debate on Simmon's 1980 paper: 'Revolution of the Latah Paradox'. *Journal of Nervous and Mental Diseases,* **171,** 159–181
KIDD, K. K. and PAULS, D. L. (1982) Genetic hypotheses for Tourette syndrome. In *Gilles de la Tourette Syndrome.* Eds. A. J. Friedhoff and T. N. Chase. *Advances in Neurology,* Vol. 35, pp. 243–249. New York: Raven Press
KLAWANS, H. L., NAUSIEDA, P. A., GOETZ, C. C., TANNER, C. M. and WEINER, W. J. (1982) Tourette-like symptoms following chronic neuroleptic therapy. In *Gilles de la Tourette Syndrome.* Eds. A. J. Friedhoff and T. N. Chase. *Advances in Neurology,* Vol. 35, pp. 415–421. New York: Raven Press
KOSLOW, S. H. and CROSS, C. K. (1982) Cerebrospinal fluid monoamine metabolites in Tourette syndrome and their neuroendocrine implications. In *Gilles de la Tourette Syndrome.* Eds. A. J. Friedhoff and T. N. Chase. *Advances in Neurology,* Vol. 35, pp. 185–197. New York: Raven Press
KRUMHOLZ, A., SINGER, H. S., NIEDERMEYER, E., BURNITE, R. and HARRIS, K. (1983) Electrophysiological studies in Tourette's syndrome. *Annals of Neurology,* **14,** 638–641
KURCZYNSKI, T. W. (1983) Hyperekplexia. *Archives of Neurology,* **40,** 246–248
KURLAN, R., BEHR, J., MEDVED, L., SHOULSON, I., PAULS, D., KIDD, J. R. and KIDD, K. K. (1986) Familial Tourette syndrome: Report of a large pedigree and potential for linkage analysis. *Neurology,* **36,** 772–776
LANG, A. E. and MARSDEN, C. D. (1983) Spasmodic dysphonia in Gilles de la Tourette's disease. *Archives of Neurology,* **40,** 51–52
LECKMAN, J. F. and COHEN, D. J. (1983) Spasmodic dysphonia in Gilles de la Tourette's syndrome: implications for clinical practice and future research. *Psychiatric Development,* **3,** 301–316
LECKMAN, J. F., DETLOR, J., HARCHERICK, D. F., ORT, S., SHAYWITZ, B. A. and COHEN, D. J. (1985) Short and long-term treatment of Tourette's syndrome with clonidine: A clinical perspective. *Neurology,* **35,** 343–351
LEES, A. J. (1985) *Tics and Related Disorders.* Edinburgh: Churchill Livingstone
LEES, A. J., ROBERTSON, M., TRIMBLE, M. R. and MURRAY, N. M. F. (1984) A clinical study of Gilles de la Tourette syndrome in the United Kingdom. *Journal of Neurology, Neurosurgery and Psychiatry,* **47,** 1–8
LOWE, T. L., COHEN, D. J., DETLOR, J., KREMENITZER, M. W. and SHAYWITZ, B. A. (1982) Stimulant medications precipitate Tourette's syndrome. *Journal of the American Medical Association,* **247,** 1929–1931
LUDLOW, C. L., POLINSKI, R. J., CAINE, E. D., BASSICH, C. J. and EBERT, M. H. (1982) Language and speech abnormalities in Tourette's syndrome. In *Gilles de la Tourette Syndrome.* Eds. A. J. Friedhoff and T. N. Chase. *Advances in Neurology,* Vol. 35, pp. 351–361. New York: Raven Press
MARKAND, O. N., GARG, B. P. and WEAVER, D. D. (1984) Familial startle disease (hyperekplexia). Electrophysiologic studies. *Archives of Neurology,* **41,** 71–74
MARNEROS, A. (1983) Adult onset of Tourette's syndrome: A case report. *American Journal of Psychiatry,* **140,** 924–925.
MARTI-MASSÓ, J. F. and OBESO, J. A. (1985) Coprolalia associated with hemiballismus: Response to tetrabenazine. *Clinical Neuropharmacology,* **8,** 189–190
MASSEY, J. M. and MASSEY, E. W. (1984) Ergot, the 'jerks' and revivals. *Clinical Neuropharmacology,* **7,** 99–105
MATTHEWS, K. L. (1981) Familial Gilles de la Tourette's syndrome associated with tuberous sclerosis. *Texas Medicine,* **77,** 46–49
MENDELSON, W. B., CAINE, E. D. and GOYER, P. (1980) Sleep in Gilles de la Tourette syndrome. *Biological Psychiatry,* **15,** 339–343
MERKSLEY, H. (1974) A case of multiple tics with vocalization (partial syndrome of Gilles de la Tourette) and XYY karyotype. *British Journal of Psychiatry,* **125,** 593–594
MESSIHA, F. S. and CARLSON, J. C. (1983) Behavioural and clinical profiles of Tourette's disease: A comprehensive overview. *Brain Research Bulletin,* **11,** 195–204
MIKKELSEN, B. O. (1983) Tolerance of tetrabenazine during long-term treatment. *Acta Neurologica Scandinavica,* **68,** 57–60

MIZRAHI, E. M., HOLTZMAN, D. and THARP, B. (1980) Haloperidol-induced tardive dyskinesia in a child with Gilles de la Tourette's syndrome. *Archives of Neurology,* **37,** 780

MONTPLAISIR, J., GODBOUT, R., BOGHEN, D., DECHAMPLAIN, J., YOUNG, S. N., LAPIERRE, G. and ING, M. (1985) Familial restless legs with periodic movements in sleep: Electrophysiologic, biochemical and pharmacologic study. *Neurology,* **35,** 130–134

MUNETZ, M. R. and CORNES, C. L. (1982) Akathisia, pseudo-akathisia and tardive dyskinesia: Clinical examples. *Comprehensive Psychiatry,* **23,** 345–352

MURRAY, T. J. (1982) Doctor Samuel Johnson's Tourette Syndrome, In *Gilles de la Tourette Syndrome.* Eds. A. J. Friedhoff and T. N. Chase. *Advances in Neurology,* Vol. 35, pp. 25–30. New York: Raven Press

NEE, L. E., CAINE, E. D., POLINSKY, R. J., ELDRIDGE, R. and EBERT, M. H. (1980) Gilles de la Tourette syndrome: Clinical and family study of 50 cases. *Annals of Neurology,* **7,** 41–49

NEGLIA, J. P., GLAZE, D. G. and ZION, T. E. (1984) Tics and vocalizations in children treated with carbamazepine. *Pediatrics,* **73,** 841–844

NUWER, M. R. (1982) Coprolalia as an organic symptom. In *Gilles de la Tourette Syndrome.* Eds. A. J. Friedhoff and T. N. Chase. *Advances in Neurology,* Vol. 35, pp. 363–368. New York: Raven Press

OBESO, J. A., ROTHWELL, J. C. and MARSDEN, C. D. (1981) Simple tics in Gilles de la Tourette's syndrome are not prefaced by a normal pre-movement potential. *Journal of Neurology, Neurosurgery and Psychiatry,* **44,** 735–738

OBESO, J. A., ROTHWELL, J. C. and MARSDEN, C. D. (1985) The spectrum of cortical myoclonus. From focal reflex jerks to spontaneous motor epilepsy. *Brain,* **108,** 193–224

O'BRIEN, J. A. (1883) Latah. *Journal of the British Asiatic Society,* **1,** 381–429

OHANNA, N., PELED, R., RUBIN, A. H. E., ZOMER, J. and LAVIE, P. (1985) Periodic leg movements in sleep: Effect of clonazepam treatment. *Neurology,* **35,** 408–411

PAULS, D. L., HURST, C. R., KIDD, K. K., KRUGER, S. D., LECKMAN, J. F. and COHEN, D. J. (1986) Evidence against a genetic relationship between Tourette syndrome and attention deficit disorder. *Archives of General Psychiatry* (in press)

PRANZATELLI, M. R. and SNODGRASS, S. R. (1985) The pharmacology of myoclonus. *Clinical Neuropharmacology,* **9,** 99–130

PRICE, R. A., KIDD, K. K., COHEN, D. J., PAULS, D. L. and LECKMAN, J. F. (1985) A twin study of Tourette syndrome. *Archives of General Psychiatry,* **42,** 815–820

PRICE, R. A., LECKMAN, J. F., PAULS, D. L., COHEN, D. J. and KIDD, K. K. (1986) Gilles de la Tourette's syndrome: Tics and central nervous system stimulants in twins and non-twins. *Neurology,* **36,** 232–237

PULST, S. M., WALSHE, T. M. and ROMERO, J. A. (1983) Carbon monoxide poisoning with features of Gilles de la Tourette's syndrome. *Archives of Neurology,* **40,** 443–444

RECHES, A., BURKE, R. E., KUHN, C. M., HASSAN, M. N., JACKSON, V. R. and FAHN, S. (1983) Tetrabenazine, an amine-depleting drug, also blocks dopamine receptors in rat brain. *Journal of Pharmacology and Experimental Therapeutics,* **225,** 515–521

RICHARDSON, E. P. (1982) Neuropathological studies of Tourette's syndrome. In *Gilles de la Tourette Syndrome.* Eds. A. J. Friedhoff and T. N. Chase. *Advances in Neurology,* Vol. 35, pp. 31–40. New York: Raven Press

RIEDERER, P., BRUCKE, T., KIENZL, E., SCHINECKER, K., SCHAY, V. *et al.* (1985) Neurochemistry of Rett syndrome. *Brain and Development,* **7,** 351–360

ROSENBERG, G. S. and DAVIS, K. L. (1982) Precursors of acetylcholine: Considerations underlying their use in Tourette's syndrome. In *Gilles de la Tourette Syndrome.* Eds. A. J. Friedhoff and T. N. Chase. *Advances in Neurology,* Vol. 35, pp. 407–412. New York: Raven Press

SACKS, O. W. (1982) Acquired Tourettism in adult life. In *Gilles de la Tourette Syndrome.* Eds. A. J. Friedhoff and T. N. Chase. *Advances in Neurology,* Vol. 35, pp. 89–92. New York: Raven Press

SÁENZ-LOPE, E., HERRANZ-TANARRO, F. J., MASDEU, J. C. and CHACÓN-PEÑA, J. R. (1984) Hyperekplexia: A syndrome of pathological startle responses. *Annals of Neurology,* **15,** 36–41

SÁENZ-LOPE, E., HERRANZ, F. J. and MASDEY, J. C. (1984) Startle epilepsy: A clinical study. *Annals of Neurology,* **16,** 78–81

SCHOENEN, J., GONCE, M. and DELWAINE, P. J. (1984) Painful legs and moving toes: A syndrome with different physiopathologic mechanisms. *Neurology,* **34,** 1108–1112

SHAPIRO, A. K. and SHAPIRO, E. (1981) The treatment and etiology of tics and Tourette syndrome. *Comparative Psychiatry,* **22,** 193–205

SHAPIRO, A. K. and SHAPIRO, E. (1982a) Tourette syndrome: History and present state. In *Gilles de la Tourette Syndrome.* Eds. A. J. Friedhoff and T. N. Chase. *Advances in Neurology,* Vol. 35, pp. 17–23. New York: Raven Press

SHAPIRO, A. K. and SHAPIRO, E. (1982b) An update on Tourette syndrome. *American Journal of Psychotherapy,* **36,** 379–389

SHAPIRO, A. K. and SHAPIRO, E. (1984) Controlled study of pimozide vs placebo in Tourette's syndrome. *Journal of the American Academy of Child Psychiatry*, **23**, 161–173
SHAPIRO, A. K., SHAPIRO, E. S., BRUUN, R. D. and SWEET, R. D. (1978) *Gilles de la Tourette Syndrome*. New York: Raven Press
SHAPIRO, A. K., SHAPIRO, E. and EISENKRAFT, G. J. (1983a) Treatment of Tourette disorder with penfluridol. *Comparative Psychiatry*, **24**, 327–331
SHAPIRO, A. K., SHAPIRO, E. and EISENKRAFT, G. J. (1983b) Treatment of Tourette's syndrome with clonidine and neuroleptics. *Archives of General Psychiatry*, **40**, 1235–1240
SHAPIRO, A. K., SHAPIRO, E. and SWEET, R. D. (1981) Treatment of tics and Tourette syndrome. In *Disorders of Movement*. Ed. A. Barbeau, pp. 105–132. Lancaster, England: MTP Press
SILVERSTEIN, F. S., JOHNSON, M. V., HUTCHINSON, R. H. and EDWARDS, N. L. (1985) Lesch–Nyhan syndrome: CSF neurotransmitter abnormalities. *Neurology*, **35**, 907–1011
SINGER, H. S., BUTLER, I. J., TUNE, L. E., SEIFERT, W. D. and COYLE, J. T. (1982) Dopaminergic dysfunction in Tourette syndrome. *Annals of Neurology*, **12**, 361–366
SINGER, H. S., OSHIDA, O. and COYLE, J. T. (1984) CSF cholinesterase activity in Gilles de la Tourette's syndrome. *Archives of Neurology*, **41**, 756–757
SINGER, H. S., WONG, D. F., TIEMEYER, M., WHITEHOUSE, P. and WAGNER, H. N. (1986) Pathophysiology of Tourette syndrome: A PET and postmortem analysis. *Annals of Neurology* (in press)
SLEATOR, E. K. (1980) Deleterious effects of drugs used for hyperactivity on patients with Gilles de la Tourette syndrome. *Clinical Pediatrics*, **19**, 453–454
SPITZ, M. C., JANKOVIC, J. and KILLIAN, J. M. (1985) Familial tic disorder, parkinsonism, motor neurone disease, and acanthocytosis – a new syndrome. *Neurology*, **35**, 366–377
STAHL, S. M. and BERGER, P. A. (1982) Cholinergic and dopaminergic mechanisms in Tourette's syndrome. In *Gilles de la Tourette Syndrome*. Eds. A. J. Friedhoff and T. N. Chase. *Advances in Neurology*, Vol. 35, pp. 141–150. New York: Raven Press
STEIN, S. A. and MORRISON, M. R. (1985) The molecular biology of Lesch–Nyman syndrome. *Trends in Neuroscience*, **8**, 148–150
STEVENS, M. (1971) Gilles de la Tourette and his syndrome by serendipity. *American Journal of Psychiatry*, **128**, 489–492
SUTULA, T. and HOBBS, W. R. (1983) Senile-onset vocal and motor tics. *Archives of Neurology*, **40**, 825–826
SVENSSON, T. H., BUNNEY, B. S. and AGHAJANIAN, G. K. (1975) Inhibition of both noradrenergic and serotonergic neurons in brain by the α-adrenergic agonist clonidine. *Brain Research*, **92**, 291–306
SWEET, R. D., BRUUN, R. D., SHAPIRO, E. and SHAPIRO, A. K. (1974) Presynaptic catecholamine antagonists as treatment for Tourette syndrome: Effects of alpha-methyl-para-tyrosine and tetrabenazine. *Archives of General Psychiatry*, **31**, 857–861
TANNER, C. M., GOETZ, C. G. and KLAWANS, H. L. (1982) Cholinergic mechanisms in Tourette syndrome. *Neurology*, **32**, 1315–1317
VAN WOERT, M. H., YIP, L. C. and BALIS, M. E. (1977) Purine phosphoribosyltransferase in Gilles de la Tourette syndrome. *New England Journal of Medicine*, **296**, 210–212
VAN WOERT, M. H., ROSENBAUM, D. and ENNA, S. J. (1982) Overview of pharmacological approaches to therapy for Tourette syndrome. In *Gilles de la Tourette Syndrome*. Eds. A. J. Friedhoff and T. N. Chase. *Advances in Neurology*, Vol. 35, pp. 369–375. New York: Raven Press
VERHAGEN, W. I. M. and HORSTINK, M. W. I. M. (1985) Painful arm and moving fingers. *Journal of Neurology, Neurosurgery and Psychiatry*, **48**, 384–389
WASERMAN, J., LAL, S. and GAUTHIER, S. (1983) Gilles de la Tourette's syndrome in monozygotic twins. *Journal of Neurology, Neurosurgery and Psychiatry*, **46**, 75–77
WOHLFART, G., INGVAR, D. H. and HELLBERG, A. M. (1961) Compulsory shouting (Benedek's 'klazomania') associated with oculogyric spasm in chronic epidemic encephalitis. *Acta Psychiatrica Scandinavica*, **36**, 369–377
YAP, P-M. (1951) Mental diseases peculiar to certain cultures: A survey of comparative psychiatry. *Journal of Mental Science*, **97**, 313–327
YARYURA-TOBIAS, J. A. and NEZIROGLU, F. A. (1977) Gilles de la Tourette syndrome: A new clinico-therapeutic approach. *Progress in Neuro-Psychopharmacology*, **1**, 335–338

20
The psychopathology of tics
M. R. Trimble and M. M. Robertson

LITERATURE BEFORE 1965

There can be no better starting point in discussing the psychopathology of tics than to consider the important work of Meige and Feindel entitled *Tics and their Treatment*. This book, written in the neuropsychiatric climate of the late nineteenth century, and translated into English by Kinnier Wilson (Meige and Feindel, 1907) begins with 'the confessions of a victim to tic'. They describe a patient, who they consider to be the prototype of the tic patient, in great detail. In retrospect, it is clear that this particular patient would now be diagnosed as having the Gilles de la Tourette syndrome. At the time of writing he was 54 years old and his earliest tics, namely facial and head movements, appeared when he was 11. He suffered from echolalia and echopraxia, a wide variety of simple tics and more complicated movements, torticollis and impairment of downward gaze, and 'a tic of phonation dating back to his 15th year'. The latter included soft expiratory noises, clucking and 'an impulse to use slang'.

The authors discuss in detail his psychopathology. They draw attention to 'the fundamental importance of the psychical element that precedes the motor reaction' as they document his impatience and impulsivity, his suicidal tendencies, and his obsessive compulsive behaviour. They note the intimate analogies between tics and obsessions and the obsessional fears of the patient. Their conclusions from this case and from others they studied led them to suggest: 'it has been possible to determine the origin of the tics and to confirm the association with them of a peculiar mental state'.

They then considered the historical background to tic disorders. They noted the confusion with regard to chorea and quote, with approval, Trousseau's definition that 'non-dolorous tic consists of abrupt momentary muscular contractions more or less limited as a general rule, involving preferably the face, but affecting also neck, trunk and limbs'. Trousseau in 1873 had drawn attention to the fact that such movements are not infrequently associated with a characteristic vocalization, although did not distinguish them from chorea. Meige and Feindel noted that Trousseau suggested that the mental state of tic patients was abnormal, but gave credit for demonstrating the significance of psychical factors in tics to Charcot.

The delineation of a separate form of tic disorder, separate from chorea, by Gilles de la Tourette in the 1880s is now well known. Interestingly, in Gilles de la Tourette's original 1885 paper where he described nine cases, little mention is made of associated psychopathology. He commented that amongst the accidental causes frequently found were lively emotions, especially fear, but referred to the determining cause as being of hereditary origin. This has to be seen in the light of theories of neuropsychiatric disease at that time influenced in particular by the concepts of Magnan and Morel's doctrine of degeneration.

It was in the paper of 1899 that Gilles de la Tourette commented most on the associated psychopathology. He noted the hereditary factor, and commented on the anxieties and phobias of his patients. In this paper he acknowledged the contribution of Guinon (1886) who noted that 'tiqueurs' nearly always had associated psychiatric disorders characterized by multiple phobias, arithmomania and agoraphobia. Gilles de la Tourette made the point that the mental stigmata appeared late in the natural history of the disorder, that it was rare for an adult case to be completely free of them, and that they are more pronounced during periods of exacerbation of the tics. A similar view was held by Grasset (1890), who also quoted widely from Guinon's paper.

It was at this time that psycho-analytical speculation emerged as the dominant view to explain the pathogenesis of neuropsychiatric conditions. The Gilles de la Tourette syndrome was no exception, and several analysts attempted interpretation of the symptoms. A good example of this is given by Ferenczi (1921); he felt that tics were closely related to narcissism, although accepted that his hypothesis was very speculative. He discussed the work of Meige and Feindel, and noted that these former authors failed to quote Breuer and Freud. He likened the origin of the tic to that of hysterical conversion symptoms, hinting at past trauma and retrogression of incompletely abreacted affects. Other analysts, including Abraham (1927) and Klein (1925), brought to the subject their own idiosyncratic interpretations, firmly rooted in variations of the psycho-analytical scheme. Some authors discussed the relationship to psychosis, distinguishing single tics (one of a series of neurotic symptoms) from generalized tics which were seen as a defence against becoming psychotic (Heuscher, 1953).

An extension of these ideas comes from Mahler *et al.* (Mahler and Rangell, 1943) who specifically discussed the Gilles de la Tourette syndrome, and acknowledged underlying organic cerebral changes, the somatic nucleus being activated by psychodynamic forces. An analysis of the psychodynamics involved suggested that the tics were an expression of emotional conflict, representing both the partial gratification of repressed instinctual impulses and defences against these impulses. The coprolalia was seen as partly aggressive and partly erotic. Their own attempts at psychotherapy, in the case history presented, were less than successful.

In further papers (Mahler, 1944, 1949), many more case histories are presented and have been reviewed in detail by Shapiro *et al.* (1978). The latter were critical of the selection of patients, many of whom they felt did not have the Gilles de la Tourette syndrome. Further, they were selected from a psychiatric setting and thus the observed psychopathology may have been unrelated to the underlying tic disorder. The conclusions from Mahler's work, particularly with regard to the psychodynamic influences in the psychopathology of the disorder, were criticized by Shapiro *et al.* (1978) as leading to 'the belief that this disorder was predominantly psychological in origin', which apparently held sway for the next 30 years. Shapiro *et al.*, commenting on the whole of the psycho-analytical era, including the papers of Mahler and many single case histories which appeared at around the same time, concluded: 'although the observations, theories, and methods of treatment were unusually diverse, a common thread was the use of psycho-analytic principles, largely Freudian, of unconscious psychosexual conflicts and defences . . . The postulated psychopathology (represents) the disowned psychological conflicts of the clinician.'

In addition to the psycho-analytical data, a number of authors during this period commented on two specific relationships of the tic disorder. The first relates to obsessive compulsive features, a common theme throughout the history of the condition, and the second to the development of a paranoid state or a psychosis.

With regard to obsessions and compulsions these are clearly outlined by Meige and Feindel (1907) and were discussed by Gilles de la Tourette (1899) and Charcot (1889). Meige and Feindel state: 'the frequency with which obsessions, or at least a proclivity for them, and tics are associated, cannot be a simple coincidence'. The obsession they note is irresistible, as is the tic, and they describe case histories of patients with typical features of obsessive compulsive disorder including the relief of anxiety that accompanied the carrying out of a particular motor act. However, in addition to the close link between the motor movement and a compulsion, they noted that often there was no direct connection between a patient's obsessions and the tics, the former occurring in the form of extraordinary scrupulousness, phobias and excessive punctiliousness with their actions. They specifically mentioned arithmomania, onomatomania (the dread of uttering a forbidden word or the impulse to intercollate another) and *folie du pourquoi*, which is the irresistible habit to seek explanations for the most commonplace facts by asking perpetual questions. Of the phobias, they include fear of death or sickness, fear of water, knives, firearms, but also agoraphobia and claustrophobia. Interestingly, they commented that the phobias were often associated with a tendency to melancholia. Guinon (1886) and Grasset (1890) referred to the obsessions and phobias, which were for them an accompaniment of the disease, representing psychical tics.

Another example, this time from the neurologist Kinnier Wilson (1927), is as follows: 'no feature is more prominent in tics than its irresistibility . . . The element of compulsion links the condition intimately to the vast group of obsessions and fixed ideas.' Ascher (1948) noted that all of the five patients he reported had obsessive personalities, and Bockner (1959) commented that the majority of cases described in the literature had obsessive compulsive neurosis.

The potential for patients with the Gilles de la Tourette syndrome to develop psychosis was inherent in the nineteenth century view of degeneration. Gilles de la Tourette himself concurred with the view of 'degeneration', and cases were described who appeared to develop psychosis in the course of their illness (Mahler and Luke, 1946; Ascher, 1948). Heuscher (1953), who had postulated that tics were defences against impending psychosis, described three cases who developed frank psychosis, and during this illness the tics disappeared.

The final theme of psychopathology that runs through this earlier literature relates to aggression. Generally, however, this is couched in analytical language, the tic either representing some form of internalized unexpressed aggression, or being seen as a defence against aggressive impulses, or as an outlet for unmanageable aggressive feelings. One of the few attempts to test this by actual use of psychological techniques was by using the Rorschach projective test. In a single case, Dunlap (1960) reported that 'movements are a method of self-punishment, and are related to feelings of hostility and guilt towards authority figures'. In a further case study, Downing, Comer and Ebert (1964), again using the Rorschach test, commented on the tics being an effective way of allowing the patient to express rebelliousness and hostility.

STUDIES SINCE 1965

The investigations in more recent years have followed two main lines. The first has been the measurement of psychological performance using standardized tests of intelligence, in an attempt to assess areas of generalized or specific abnormality in Gilles de la Tourette patients. Secondly, there have been several investigations into the psychopathology of Gilles de la Tourette syndrome, assessing this using clinical ratings or standardized methods such as rating scales for the collection of data. In this second series there are four types of investigation pursued. Firstly, the association of Gilles de la Tourette syndrome with psychopathology; secondly, the specific links between Gilles de la Tourette syndrome and the obsessive compulsive disorder; thirdly, the influence of stress as a provoking factor on symptoms or methods for stress relief as a form of treatment; finally the possibility that treatments themselves may provoke psychiatric problems.

Gilles de la Tourette syndrome and intellectual performance

It is generally agreed that patients with the Gilles de la Tourette syndrome have a normal span of intellectual abilities. Corbett *et al.* (1969) examined 180 children with tics (only 23% of whom had vocal tics) and reported that the mean IQ was 98.8 for the whole population. The frequency distribution was similar to that obtained from a general population clinic.

With regard specifically to the Gilles de la Tourette syndrome, the largest collection has come from Shapiro *et al.* (1978). The data on 50 subjects were compared to a control group on a variety of tests, in particular the WAIS or WISC, the Bender Gestalt test and the Rorschach test. The full-scale IQ of the patients was 106.4 (standard deviation 13.5), again within the normal range of functioning. There were no significant differences noted between the verbal, performance and full scale IQs. Fifty per cent of the Tourette patients compared to 14% of controls had a 15 point or more difference between the verbal and performance scales of their IQ, a highly significant difference. All of their adult patients had a higher verbal than performance IQ and, when subtests were evaluated, a significant difference was found for the block design and the picture arrangement tests, the Gilles de la Tourette group doing significantly worse. Many of their patients were receiving drugs at the time of testing and so they examined verbal-performance IQ differences between those on medication and those off medication: the difference was not significant. Further, when the dosage of haloperidol was examined for those patients with verbal-performance differences, there was no difference to those without differences, and the dosage of haloperidol did not correlate with the magnitude of the verbal-performance difference scores.

Shapiro *et al.* also used the Bender Gestalt test. Significantly more patients with the Gilles de la Tourette syndrome were rated as having mild to moderate organic changes as reflected in the results of this test, 42% of the sample being judged as having mild or moderate organicity compared to 16% of control subjects. Overall,

68% were reported as having some degree of abnormality on one or other of the psychological tests in their study.

Incagnoli and Kane (1981) reported data on 13 patients with the Gilles de la Tourette syndrome aged from 10 to 13 years who were given the Halstead Neuropsychological tests battery for children, the WISC, the Wide Range Achievement test and Bender Gestalt test. The overall performance was normal for 11 of their subjects, but they reported a significant impairment of visual motor copying noted on the Bender Gestalt test and on coding of the WISC. Four of their patients demonstrated significant verbal-performance deficits. The Halstead and Wide Range Achieving tests were generally within normal limits. Their conclusions on these data were that there was no evidence of generalized cerebral dysfunction in their patients, the main problem being in non-constructional visuopractic abilities.

Hagin et al. (1982) provided data on ten children with the Gilles de la Tourette syndrome, but no control group. The majority had behaviour problems, notably with impulse control and interpersonal relationships. They were given a learning disorders battery which revealed a generally higher WISC than the equivalent standardized results, although the standard deviation of the Gilles de la Tourette sample was also greater. Most of the children were consistent at or above the expected level and, in the few cases where scores were low, the discrepancies were in mathematics, written language and reading abilities. Thus, nine of the ten children had independent reading scores below that expected. They also commented on dexterity problems, again notably with the visuomotor measure on the Bender Gestalt test and equivalents. Their conclusion was that the children tended to have no generalized handicaps, but 'difficulty demonstrating skills on measures requiring independent reading or on tasks requiring sustained handwriting such as mathematics computation and written language'.

Sutherland et al. (1982) examined neuropsychological assessments of children and adults with the Gilles de la Tourette syndrome, comparing data to those with learning difficulties and with schizophrenia. There were 32 index subjects, 31 age and full-scale IQ and handedness matched controls, 47 learning disabled subjects and 30 schizophrenic patients. A comprehensive battery of neuropsychological tests was given, and the profile of the three patient groups was different when compared to controls. Again, deficits of performance IQ were noted in the Gilles de la Tourette sample. Further, copying and drawing from memory, delayed recall of non-verbal memory, verbal fluency and immediate recall of a verbally presented story were all significantly impaired. These deficits reflected more right hemisphere disturbance, in contrast to the learning disabled who had more impairments on tests of left parietal function, and the schizophrenia group who had widespread abnormalities reflecting abnormalities in both hemispheres. Again, in this study, most patients were receiving medication, and the way this may have affected the results is unclear.

Finally, an intensive neuropsychological test battery was given to three patients and the results reported in detail by Joschko and Rourke (1982). This essentially was the Halstead Reiten battery with additional subtests, but, on this very limited sample, they were not able to define a pattern of deficits as suggested by Sutherland et al. (1982).

In conclusion, it seems that most authors are agreed that patients with the Gilles de la Tourette syndrome do not suffer from any overall impairment of intellectual function, scoring within the average range on standardized measures of intelligence. There is a hint, particularly from the study of Hagin *et al.* (1982), of specific areas of deficit relating to reading and writing and arithmetic, although the relationship of these to organic brain syndromes, such as epilepsy (*see* Trimble and Thompson, 1985), is well known, and it is not clear whether they relate to some fundamental aspect of the Gilles de la Tourette syndrome disturbance or more generally reflect organicity. Further, since children with behaviour disorders also display similar deficits, and the majority of their patients had such problems, further work needs to be done in this field before firm conclusions can be drawn.

Psychopathology

Feild *et al.* (1966), in a paper in which they presented seven cases, noted 'mental deterioration, schizophrenia, or some other serious personality disorder developed in 40%' of patients. However, examination of the case histories themselves do not clarify this statement, although where the IQ assessment was recorded it was less than 80 in two of the cases, at variance with information presented above.

A more extensive study, which related to both tics and the Gilles de la Tourette syndrome, was that reported by Corbett *et al.* (1969). Their results were based upon a retrospective examination of case records and follow-up interviews or home visits where necessary. A variety of symptoms of psychopathology were noted in the sample, ranging from over 35% with 'tension habits' and 'tempers and aggression', to a much smaller number with depression, hypochondriasis and sexual disorders. When the tiqueurs were matched to a population of disturbed, but not psychotic, children attending the same hospital, they scored significantly higher on 'disorders of defaecation', 'speech disorders', 'gratification habits' and 'obsessional symptoms'. In particular, tempers and aggression, fighting and depression were significantly less. Their comments were that items under the heading of 'habit disorders' seemed to occur relatively frequently among their tic patients, and that 'relative to the total population of disturbed children, tiqueurs are not characterised by the over-expression of affect, e.g. aggression or depression'. In a follow-up of 30 patients from between one and 18 years following their original attendance to hospital, they commented that generalized anxiety was observed in all patients and 'a general impression of a withdrawn and neurotic pattern was obtained'. Depressive symptoms were reported in 33% of patients and two patients developed schizophrenia. When they compared patients with and without vocal tics, they noted that the latter, who presumably conformed more to a diagnosis of Gilles de la Tourette syndrome, showed the greatest tendency to subsequent anxiety and neurotic symptoms.

An extensive study of the psychopathology of the Gilles de la Tourette syndrome was reported by Shapiro in a number of reports (Shapiro *et al.*, 1972, 1978). In these studies the subjects were rated by two psychologists, but also the Minnesota Multiphasic Personality Inventory (MMPI) was given to those over 16 years of age. No formal rating system was used to assess psychopathology, and the inter-observer reliabilities published were remarkably low (0.29). Three patients were diagnosed as markedly schizophrenic by both psychologists. There were no ratings of other psychoses, although 'underlying psychosis' was commonly reported, as was 'inhibition of hostility' and 'general maladjustment'. When disagreements between raters were taken into account, it was concluded that some 34% of Gilles de la Tourette patients had 'clinically meaningful inhibition of hostility', a similar rate reported for a control psychiatric outpatient group. Similarly, the ratings for maladjustment were equivalent for a control psychiatric group and the Gilles de la Tourette group.

With regard to the MMPI profile, when compared to various psychiatric populations, there were significantly less elevated profiles for the Gilles de la Tourette sample. The only significantly higher subscale for the Gilles de la Tourette patients was increased scoring on the masculinity/femininity factor.

The conclusions of Shapiro, based on these studies and his clinical experience, was that 'most Tourette patients had some degree of maladjustment. Their problems were no more severe, however, than those of a psychiatric out-patient group . . .'

Some authors have specifically studied behaviour disturbance in children. Wilson et al. (1982) examined 21 children with the Gilles de la Tourette syndrome using the behaviour problem check list, which assessed 55 behaviour problems as present or absent, from which three subscales were derived from factor analysis, namely conduct problem, personality problem and inadequacy/immaturity. When compared to controls, the Gilles de la Tourette sample showed considerably more disturbance, their rating scale scores being comparable to those problem children attending special education classes. However, no specific subscale was outstanding. Interestingly, the total number of problems checked on the behaviour rating scale was significantly related to the number of motor symptoms and the number of errors on the Wisconsin Card Sorting test which was also performed. The authors concluded that the behaviour disturbance should be considered as an integral feature of the syndrome, particularly on account of the relationship between the psychopathology and the movement symptoms. Rosenberg, Harris and Singer (1984) used the child behaviour check list in 28 subjects, whose severity of illness was assessed independently. For children over the age of 12 (all subjects were male), again a significant positive relationship was noted between severity of illness and the scores on the behaviour check list. When subscores were analysed the significant associations were with schizoid, obsessive compulsive, social withdrawal, hyperactive, delinquent and internalizing categories.

Several authors have looked for psychopathology in the immediate families of Gilles de la Tourette patients. Corbett et al. (1969) noted that 31% of their tic patients had one or both parents that had attended a psychiatrist, in contrast to 19% of hospital referral controls and 6% of a dental clinic sample. The result was highly significant. Montgomery, Clayton and Friedhoff (1982), in a study of 15 patients whose first degree relatives were also examined, noted psychopathology in 21 first degree relatives, the commonest diagnoses being unipolar depression and obsessive compulsive illness. Finally, in a paper on the Gilles de la Tourette syndrome in the Chinese, Lieh Mak et al. (1982) noted psychiatric disorders in the families of five of 15 patients, two of whom were positive for schizophrenia.

Obsessive compulsive neurosis

The association of Gilles de la Tourette syndrome and obsessive compulsive symptoms was commented on by early authors such as Guinon (1886), Grasset (1890) and Gilles de la Tourette himself. It is a constant feature of the personality of these patients discussed by several authors (e.g. Meige and Feindel, 1907; Ascher, 1948) and further, numerous psycho-analytical references to the anal character immediately interlinks it in their theories with obsessive compulsive disorder.

Unfortunately, the majority of studies have failed to attempt measurement of obsessive compulsive symptoms using the now available check lists, or even to apply standardized research criteria during the investigation. Nonetheless, Corbett *et al.* (1969) noted obsessional symptoms to be significantly greater in their sample of tiqueurs than the control hospital sample, and in their follow-up of 30 patients they reported three who had obsessive compulsive phenomena. Morphew and Sim (1969) presenting six of their own cases and reviewing the literature found obsessional personality in 15 out of 21 cases (71%). Fernando (1967), in his review of the published literature, including four of his own cases, reported obsessionality in 20 out of 65 cases (31%).

Abuzzahab and Anderson (1973) conducted a more extensive worldwide literature review on 430 cases and derived a figure of 33% for the presence of psychopathology, the vast majority of which were classified as obsessive compulsive. They commented on the frequently encountered arithmomania, *folie du doute* and *delire du touche*.

With regard specifically to children, the series of Hagin *et al.* (1982) noted obsessive compulsive symptoms in 60%, considerably higher than that of Corbett *et al.*, although Corbett's study was very much broader and did not specify Gilles de la Tourette patients. Rosenberg, Harris and Singer (1984), using the child behaviour check list, noted a significant association between obsessive compulsive symptoms and severity of the Gilles de la Tourette syndrome ($r = +0.72$).

Shapiro *et al.* (1978) examined obsessive compulsive phenomena in the Gilles de la Tourette syndrome in more detail. In their own series, the inter-rater reliability for the assessment of this condition was only 0.27 and 46.8% of their subjects were rated as 'not obsessive compulsive'. However, only 12.8% were rated by both observers as having such traits. Further, since 14.6% of their controls were also rated as having these traits, they concluded that obsessive compulsive traits did not characterize patients with the Gilles de la Tourette syndrome.

Exacerbating and relieving factors

It is well known that anxiety tends to exacerbate tics and relaxation to relieve them. Interestingly, few authors have studied this in any detail. Corbett *et al.* (1969) reported a few cases where the onset of the disorder followed a single traumatic incident, and Fahn (1982) reported a case of post-traumatic syndrome following a head injury. Interestingly, this patient developed compulsive behaviour and shortly thereafter developed characteristic vocal sounds leading to a diagnosis of the Gilles de la Tourette syndrome. Morphew and Sim (1969) quoted the usual exacerbating factors as psychological stresses, even if they appeared overtly physical; for example, tonsillectomy or other operations. Other authors have pointed out how tics can be relieved by relaxation, the consumption of alcohol, with intense concentration, or with orgasm (*see* Turpin, 1982).

However, most of the work in this field has come from attempts to treat patients with either relaxation or behaviour therapy. Generally these treatments are less than effective, although they may temporarily induce a beneficial effect (Shapiro *et al.*, 1976). Most of the studies have been carried out on single cases and the measurement of tic severity is always problematic. Amongst the techniques used include massed practice, perhaps effective for some monosymptomatic tics, operant conditioning, self-monitoring and feed-back, habit reversal, and desensitization techniques (Turpin, 1982). Abuzzahab and Anderson (1973) compared the efficiency of various treatments in this condition as a result of their international case register, and the list of various treatments given testifies to the wide range of therapies used for the syndrome. The most outstanding finding in management was the dramatic increase in successes following the introduction of major tranquillizers, and the relative inefficiency of most forms of psychological intervention.

Psychopathology as a consequence of treatment

Although there was some concern that patients who had their tics improved by treatment may develop symptom substitution, this does not appear to occur (Shapiro *et al.*, 1978). Of more interest are the reports of psychopathology consequent to the administration of major tranquillizers, particularly haloperidol. Early case reports were those of Penna and Lion (1975) and Caine and Polinsky (1979). Bruun (1982) reported 26 patients who experienced dysphoric symptoms with haloperidol which repeatedly occurred when the dose was raised above a certain threshold level that varied for each patient. In half of the patients the symptoms were severe enough to warrant treatment with antidepressants. None of the patients had a prior history of depression nor any family history of major depressive disorder, and the depression did not immediately resolve following the reduction of the medication. They were seen in some patients in spite of complete relief of the tics with treatment.

The National Hospital studies

At the National Hospitals over 90 patients with the Gilles de la Tourette syndrome have been evaluated in recent years. Information has been prospectively gathered on these patients with regard not only to the pattern and development of their tics, but also information about other abnormalities of motor behaviour, family history of psychopathology and motor disorder, and past and current psychopathology in the patients. Fifty-four adult patients, over the age of 17 years, were specifically studied, using rating scales for psychopathology. In these investigations, a pre-prepared questionnaire was filled out by the subjects and added to by objective collection of evidence by the investigators. All patients were subject to further special investigations including electroencephalography, computerized axial tomography (CAT) and serum copper and ceruloplasmin measurements. For determining psychopathology the following rating scales were employed: the Beck Depression Inventory (Beck *et al.*, 1961); the Spielberger Trait Anxiety Inventory (Spielberger, Gorsuch and Lushene, 1970); the Borderline Syndrome Index (Conte *et al.*, 1980); the Mood Adjective Check List (McNair and Lorr, 1964); the Hysteroid/Obsessoid Questionnaire (Caine and Hope, 1967); the Middlesex Hospital Questionnaire (Crown and Crisp, 1966, 1979); the Hostility and Direction of Hostility Questionnaire (Foulds, Caine and Creasy, 1960; Caine, Foulds and Hope, 1967); the Written Questionnaire Form of the Leyton Obsessional Inventory (Snowdon, 1980) and the Eysenck Personality Inventory (Eysenck and Eysenck, 1964).

In these investigations data were analysed using the chi-squared test and the Fisher's Exact Probability test for contingency tables. Further, the Mann–Whitney U test and Kruskal–Wallis test were used for examining relationships between discrete and continuous variables, and the Spearman Correlation Coefficient for pairs of continuous variables. Non-parametric tests were employed because many of the continuous variables had non-normal distributions. In the analyses of the data, psychopathological variables were related to motor phenomena, and certain hypotheses regarding links between the two tested.

Sixty-six per cent of our sample were males, and the mean full-scale IQ was 100.6 (range 78–128, standard deviation 13.3). The mean depression score, rated on the various scales with equivalent normative data, is given in *Table 20.1*. It can be seen that the Gilles de la Tourette patients report considerably more affective symptoms than expected. Further, on the anxiety rating scales, again much higher levels than expected using normative ranges were noted in our patients, for example, the mean score of the Spielberger Trait Anxiety Scale being 47.0 (range 22–74), and the total hostility score on the Hostility and Direction of Hostility Questionnaire 21.9 (range 5–35), a value considerably elevated from the normal population. The direction of hostility scores indicated high levels of acting out hostility and criticism of others.

Table 20.1 Rating scale results employed to assess depression and obsessionality

Rating scale	TS patients			British normative data	
	Mean	Range	s.d.	Mean	Reference
Beck Depression Inventory	12.6	0–41	9.7	5.4	Metcalfe and Goldman, 1965
Mood Adjective Checklist Depression	4.6	0–27	5.6	1.6	Thompson, 1981
Middlesex Hospital Questionnaire					
Depression	6.3	0–15	4.2	3.3	Crown and Crisp, 1966
Obsessionalism	7.9	0–16	3.7	5.8	
Leyton Obsessional Inventory					
Symptom	20.1	0–50	12.0	12.6	Snowdon, 1980
Trait	9.6	0–20	5.5	5.2	
Total	28.8	0–60	16.3	17.8	

Fifty-four adult TS patients completed the ratings.

With specific reference to obsessionality, the data are shown in *Tables 20.1* and *20.2*. It can be seen that, compared to the normal population means, the Gilles de la Tourette sample score high on the Leyton Obsessional Inventory, and the Obsessional subscale of the Middlesex Hospital Questionnaire. On clinical evaluation patients being questioned as to whether they exhibited obsessive compulsive behaviour or not, 37% admitted to having such behaviours or rituals. A number of other interesting relationships which emerged from this analysis are

Table 20.2 Significant relationships between symptoms, obsessive compulsive phenomena and aggression

Symptoms or demographic details	Obsessive compulsive behaviour	Obsessive compulsive phenomena				Aggression				
		Leyton Obsessional Inventory			MHQ Obsessional Scale	Aggressive behaviour	Hostility and Direction of Hostility Questionnaire			
		Symptom	Trait	Total			Criticism of others	Paranoid hostility	Self criticism	Sum of hostility
Forced to touch	***					*				
Coprophenomena		* (Coprolalia)	*	* (Coprolalia)		** (Copropraxia)	** (Coprolalia)	* (Coprolalia)		* (Coprolalia)
Echophenomena			*		****		*		**	**
Family history	* Family history of TS or tics	With family history of psychiatric illness		With family history of TS or tics						
Tic	** Shoulder shrug									
Medication		*** With butyrophenones	*** With butyrophenones	*** With butyrophenones						

* ≤ 0.05; ** ≤ 0.01; *** ≤ 0.005; **** ≤ 0.001.

shown in *Table 20.2*, particularly with regard to obsessive compulsive behaviour and aggression. The age of onset of the Gilles de la Tourette symptoms was not associated with any psychopathological variable, and the only index which related to duration of illness was that those with a longer history scored higher on the depression rating scales. Echo phenomena were significantly associated with psychopathology in general, but, in particular, with two of the obsessive compulsive measures (Leyton Obsessional Trait Inventory and the Middlesex Hospital Questionnaire Obsessional subscale). Further, they were related to depressive and some of the hostility variables. Coprolalia, one of the hallmarks of the Gilles de la Tourette syndrome, was related to higher scores on the Leyton Obsessional Inventory, and again to a number of hostility variables. Copropraxia appeared to be associated with the clinical presentation of aggressive behaviour.

Clinical assessment of the presence of obsessive compulsive behaviour was associated with being forced to touch, shoulder shrugging, and the family history of either the Gilles de la Tourette syndrome or tics. Further, it was significantly related to the presence of aggressive behaviour and some of the hostility scores on the Mood Adjective Check List and the Hostility and Direction of Hostility Questionnaire.

Interestingly, abnormal serum copper values (Robertson *et al.*, 1985), electroencephalographic or the presence of neurological abnormalities were not associated with any of these psychopathological variables.

Finally, with regard to medication, of note is the fact that a high Mood Adjective Check List fatigue score was significantly related both to the prescription of current and previous medication, and scores on the Leyton Obsessional Inventory were inversely related to the prescription of butyrophenones.

In view of the high frequency of obsessive compulsive phenomena in this study, and the questioning by some as to their link to the Gilles de la Tourette syndrome, a further cross-cultural comparison has been carried out in conjunction with UCLA (Frankel *et al.*, 1986). Thus, a questionnaire was constructed specifically to elicit obsessive compulsive disorder and this was given to five groups of patients. These were, 31 Gilles de la Tourette patients from the United States, 33 from Great Britain, and 12 patients who met DSM 111 criteria for obsessive compulsive disorder *without* the Gilles de la Tourette syndrome. Finally, two control groups were used: one of 17 patients suffering from a wide variety of neuropsychiatric disorders and 41 normal controls. Using this questionnaire, the obsessive compulsive disorder patients had the highest mean score, 83% scoring at or above one standard deviation of the mean. Using this same criteria, 58% and 45% of the USA and British patients with the Gilles de la Tourette syndrome scored above the same level, in comparison to 18% and 12% of the two control groups. These data therefore complement those described above, emphasizing the frequency of obsessive compulsive disorder in association with the Gilles de la Tourette syndrome, using more objective techniques in different cultural settings and comparing them with control samples.

DISCUSSION AND CONCLUSIONS

The literature on the psychopathology of tics has mainly concerned the Gilles de la Tourette syndrome, and most of the data gathered has been with respect to that condition. Review of the early literature emphasizes that, from its original descriptions, psychopathology was included as part of the spectrum of the clinical presentation. Although Gilles de la Tourette in his original paper makes little reference to this, it is clear that later he acknowledges the contributions of other authors who discussed the psychopathology of his syndrome, and generally supported their viewpoints. Most authors who have written on the subject concur, and, in particular, draw attention to obsessive compulsive phenomena and aggressive behaviour. Latterly, some attention has been paid to the concurrent affective symptoms of patients, and the possibility that treatment with, for example, neuroleptic medications may provoke a dysphoria has recently been suggested.

Much of the data discussed in this chapter is clinical, and based on anecdotal evidence or clinical experience. Nonetheless, since 1965, a number of authors have attempted to use more standardized and objective techniques for examining the psychopathology of patients with tic disorders, and generally support the earlier viewpoints. The exception to this comes from the studies of Shapiro *et al.* (1978) to be discussed further below.

Most authors agree that patients with the Gilles de la Tourette syndrome have a normal spectrum of intellectual abilities. In our experience patients who are retarded with this syndrome either have evidence of pervasive developmental disorder, or have some associated and often identifiable chromosomal (Robertson, Hughes and Trimble, unpublished data) or central nervous system disorder. However, there is a suggestion that some patients, in spite of a normal intellectual quotient, have specific areas of cognitive disability, and in assessment of patients, particularly children, attention to writing, reading and arithmetical skills is important. Further, minor motor deficits and problems of visuomotor control may lead to educational problems that require special handling.

Our own studies, and those of several others, would suggest that psychopathology does occur to a greater degree than would be expected in normal patients, although deterioration, particularly to a psychotic state, would appear to be the exception. This is also in keeping with the data of others, such as Shapiro *et al.* (1978) who noted that the level of psychopathology was similar to that found in a psychiatric outpatient population. However, an important consideration is whether this is merely secondary to all of the social problems that may accrue from having this disorder, or whether there are indeed any specific links which can be suggested. The most obvious one is the link to obsessive compulsive symptoms. Shapiro *et al.* (1978) argue most strongly that there is no specific link, referring to their own studies and also to a definition of obsessive compulsive symptoms given in the first edition of the *American Psychiatric Association's Diagnostic and Statistical Manual of Mental Disorders*. According to Shapiro *et al.* the tics are poorly organized *involuntary* acts, only partially modified by external events: compulsions they suggest are *voluntary*. This distinction of motor behaviour into a voluntary/involuntary dichotomy is notoriously fallible, and fails to note that the majority of acts which human beings carry out can neither be classified at one end of the spectrum nor another, but are more or less voluntary or involuntary. The insistence of Shapiro *et al.* that the movements of Gilles de la Tourette syndrome are involuntary does not accord with the recorded experience of sufferers. Thus, in Meige and Feindel's (1907) confessions, we read what elsewhere would be described as a typical description of obsessional behaviour with regard to the patients' symptoms. He states: 'I have been conscious equally of the absurdity and yet of the irresistability of the idea; each time the attempt to withstand it has been

Discussion and conclusions 419

labour lost'. Bliss (1980), a life-long sufferer from the Gilles de la Tourette syndrome, describes his self-observation of his symptoms and comments thus: 'the TS movement is not the whole message. The TS movement is not rhythmic, spasmodic or involuntary. The movement only *seems* involuntary because of the instant capitulation to the unrecognised sensory stimulus. It can be detected and interrupted when in progress and at any stage.' Bliss rails over clinical evaluations which concentrate only on the overt symptoms of the syndrome, noting that 'the movement, even if grotesque and miserable, is not the most important part of TS activity'.

It seems clear that classification of the symptoms along the voluntary/involuntary continuum is, to say the least, a hazardous exercise. The data from our studies, in contradistinction to those reported by Shapiro, but using validated and reliable rating scales for the assessment of psychopathology, not only confirms the extent of the reporting of obsessive compulsive symptoms in our patients, but further shows close links between some of the motor phenomena and these obsessive compulsive features. In particular, coprolalia, echophenomena, and the symptom of being forced to touch are outstanding, although the close relationship to coprolalia, one of the core features of the Gilles de la Tourette syndrome, suggests closer biological links than recognized by Shapiro *et al*. Our data are broadly in keeping with some others already discussed, including those of Rosenberg (1984) who noted the significant association between obsessive compulsive symptoms and the severity of the disorder.

If it is indeed correct, as review of the literature suggests, that between 31 and 71% of patients with the Gilles de la Tourette syndrome also report obsessive compulsive phenomena, as severe in many cases as patients with obsessive compulsive disorder, the underlying biology of this requires explanation. Thus, there is no other disorder of the central nervous system where such a high frequency of obsessive compulsive phenomena is reported, although obsessive compulsive traits have been suggested as accompanying a number of disorders such as Parkinson's disease and encephalitis lethargica (*see* Trimble, 1981, for review). The earlier speculations of the psycho-analysts are of historical interest, and provided a theory which, at the time it was prevalent, may have suited the socioeconomic climate in which it derived, and provided possible hypotheses for testing in a number of neuropsychiatric conditions. As with many theories in medicine, it has been superceded by others and, at the present time, the dominant trend in understanding psychopathology has moved towards attempting to understand brain function and its disturbance in illness based on current knowledge of neuroanatomy and neurochemistry. There are various speculations with regard to possible functional disturbances in the Gilles de la Tourette syndrome, although most of them revolve around the extrapyramidal system. The role of dopamine has become important, particularly with the observations that patients with the syndrome respond well to drugs which block dopamine receptors (Shapiro *et al.*, 1978).

There are, however, many problems with such a theory. For example, although the simple tics often respond to such compounds, more complicated motor phenomena, and the associated behavioural disturbances, have not been shown consistently to do so. In our study, the reduced reporting of obsessional symptoms in patients receiving neuroleptic drugs bears further study, since the relationship of obsessional symptoms to dopamine activity within the central nervous system remains to be clarified. Although much attention has been placed on the striatum in understanding this condition, we would prefer to speculate a possible role for the cingulate gyrus. Thus, the cingular cortex, continuous with the frontal cortex anteriorly, is one of the largest structures within the limbic system and is rich in dopamine fibres. It formed part of the original Papez circuit. Ablation of the cingulate area leads to marked disturbances of behaviour and stimulation leads to vocalizations both in animals and in man (Wieser, 1983; MacLean, 1985). Further, some groups suggest that in neurosurgical studies, improvement following operation is most likely in obsessive compulsive patients after destruction of part of the same region (see Flor-Henry, 1975). This conclusion fits with the data of electrical brain stimulation from Talairach et al. (1975) who noted that electrical stimulation of the anterior cingulate gyrus led to the presentation of integrated motor behaviours that were felt to be forced on the subject, reminiscent of the intrusiveness of obsessive and compulsive symptoms. Thus, the anterior cingulate area, with its corticobulbar projections and links to other areas of the limbic system and ventral pallidum, may be a key anatomical locus for our understanding of some of the complicated relationships between psychopathology, especially obsessive compulsive behaviour, and movements in such disorders as the Gilles de la Tourette syndrome.

Acknowledgements

We would like to acknowledge Dr A. J. Lees for his clinical cooperation; Dr D. Rogers for translating the French manuscripts; The Goldsmith Company, The Raymond Way Trust and Janssen Pharmaceuticals for financial support, and Miss S. J. Presland for typing the manuscript.

References

ABRAHAM, K. (1927) Contributions to a discussion on tic. In *Selected Papers of Karl Abraham MD*. Translated by D. Bryan and A. Strackey (1949). London: Hogarth Press

ABUZZAHAB, F. E. and ANDERSON, F. O. (1973) Gilles de la Tourette's syndrome. International Registry. *Minnesota Medicine*, **56**, 492–496

ASCHER, E. (1948) Psychodynamic considerations in Gilles de la Tourette's disease (maladie des tics): with a report of five cases and discussion of the literature. *American Journal of Psychiatry*, **105**, 267–276

BECK, A. T., WARD, C. H., MENDELSON, M., MOCK, J. and ERBAUGH, J. (1961) An inventory for measuring depression. *Archives of General Psychiatry*, **4**, 561–571

BLISS, J. (1980) Sensory experiences of Gilles de la Tourette syndrome. *Archives of General Psychiatry*, **37**, 1343–1347

BOCKNER, S. (1959) Gilles de la Tourette's disease. *Journal of Mental Science*, **105**, 1078–1081

BRUUN, R. D. (1982) Dysphoric phenomena associated with haloperidol treatment of Tourette syndrome. *Advances in Neurology*, **35**, 433–436

CAINE, E. D. and POLINSKY, R. J. (1979) Haloperidol induced dysphoria in patients with Tourette Syndrome. *American Journal of Psychiatry*, **136**, 1216–1217

CAINE, T. M., FOULDS, G. A. and HOPE, K. (1967) *Manual of the Hostility and Direction of Hostility Questionnaire*. London: University of London Press

CAINE, T. M. and HOPE, K. (1967) *Manual of the Hysteroid–Obsessoid Questionnaire (HOQ)*. London: University of London Press

CHARCOT, J. M. (1889) *Lecons du Mardi a la Salpetriere-Polyclinique, 1888–1889*, **2**, 13–17

CONTE, H. R., PLUTCHIK, R., KARASU, T. B. and JERRETT, I. (1980) A self-report borderline scale. Discriminative Validity and Preliminary Norms. *Journal of Nervous and Mental Disease*, **168**, 428–435

CORBETT, J. A., MATTHEWS, A. M., CONNELL, P. H. and SHAPIRO, D. A. (1969) Tics and Gilles de la Tourette's Syndrome: A follow-up study and critical review. *British Journal of Psychiatry*, **115**, 1229-1241
CROWN, S. and CRISP, A. H. (1966) A short clinical diagnostic self-rating scale for psychoneurotic patients: The Middlesex Hospital Questionnaire (MHQ). *British Journal of Psychiatry*, **112**, 917-923
CROWN, S. and CRISP, A. H. (1979) *Manual of the Crown-Crisp Experiental Index*. Sevenoaks, Kent: Hodder and Stoughton
DOWNING, R. W., COMER, N. L. and EBERT, J. N. (1964) Family dynamics in a case of Gilles de la Tourette's Syndrome. *Journal of Nervous and Mental Disease*, **138**, 548-557
DUNLAP, J. R. (1960) A case of Gilles de la Tourette's Disease (Maladie des Tics): A study of the intrafamily dynamics. *Journal of Nervous and Mental Disease*, **130**, 340-344
EYSENCK, H. J. and EYSENCK, S. B. G. (1964) *Manual of the Eysenck Personality Inventory*. London: University of London Press
FAHN, S. (1982) A case of post-traumatic Tic Syndrome. In *Gilles de la Tourette Syndrome*. Eds A. J. Friedhoff and T. N. Chase, pp. 349-350. New York: Raven Press
FEILD, J. R., CORBIN, K. B., GOLDSTEIN N. P. and KLASS, D. W. (1966) Gilles de la Tourette Syndrome. *Neurology*, **16**, 453-463
FERENCZI, S. (1921) Psycho-analytic observations on tic. *International Journal of Psychoanalysis*, **2**, 1-30
FERNANDO, S. J. M. (1967) Gilles de la Tourette's Syndrome. A report on four cases and a review of published case reports. *British Journal of Psychiatry*, **113**, 607-617
FLOR-HENRY, P. (1975) Psychiatric Surgery, 1935-1973; evolution and current perspectives. *Journal of the Canadian Psychiatric Association*, **20**, 157-167
FOULDS, G. A., CAINE, T. M. and CREASY, M. A. (1960) Aspects of extra and intrapunitive expression in mental illness. *Journal of Mental Science*, **106**, 599-610
FRANKEL, N., CUMMINGS, J. L., ROBERTSON, M. M., TRIMBLE, M. R., HILL, M. A. and BENSON, D. F. (1986) Obsessions and compulsions in Gilles de la Tourette syndrome. *Neurology* (in press)
GILLES DE LA TOURETTE, G. (1885) Etude sur une affection nerveuse caracterisee par de l'incoordination motrice accompagnee d'echolalie et de coprolalie. *Archives de Neurologie*, **9**, 19-42 and 158-200
GILLES DE LA TOURETTE (1899) La Maladie des tics convulsifs. *La Semaine Medicale*, **19**, 153-156
GRASSET, J. (1890) Lecons sur un cas de maladie des tics et un cas de tremblement singulier de la tete et des membres gauches. *Archives de Neurologie*, **20**, 27-45 and 187-211
GUINON, G. (1886) Sur la maladie des tics convulsifs. *Revue de Medicine*, **6**, 50-80
HAGIN, R. A., BEECHER, R., PAGANO, G. and KREEGER, H. (1982) Effects of Tourette Syndrome on learning. In *Gilles de la Tourette Syndrome*. Eds. A. J. Friedhoff and T. N. Chase, pp. 323-328. New York: Raven Press
HEUSCHER, J. E. (1953) Intermediate states of consciousness in patients with generalised tics. *Journal of Nervous and Mental Disease*, **117**, 29-38
INCAGNOLI, T. and KANE, R. (1981) Neuropsychological functioning in Gilles de la Tourette's Syndrome. *Journal of Clinical Neuropsychology*, **3**, 165-169
KLEIN, M. (1925) Zur gerese des tics. *International Journal of Psycho-Analysis*, **11**, 332
JOSCHKO, M. and ROURKE, B. P. (1982) Neuropsychological dimensions of Tourette Syndrome: Test-retest stability and implications for intervention. In *Gilles de la Tourette Syndrome*. Eds. A. J. Friedhoff and T. N. Chase, pp. 297-304. New York: Raven Press
LEIH MAK, F., CHUNG, S. Y., LEE, P. and CHEN, S. (1982) Tourette Syndrome in the Chinese: A follow up of 15 cases. In *Gilles de la Tourette Syndrome*. Eds A. J. Friedhoff and T. N. Chase, pp. 281-283. New York: Raven Press
MACLEAN, P. D. (1985) Brain evolution relating to family, play and the separation call. *Archives of General Psychiatry*, **42**, 405-420
McNAIR, D. M. and LORR, M. (1964) An analysis of mood in neurotics. *Journal of Abnormal and Social Psychology*, **69**, 620-627
MAHLER, M. S. (1944) Tics and impulsions in children: a study of motility. *Psychoanalytic Quarterly*, **13**, 430-444
MAHLER, M. S. (1949) Psychoanalytic evaluation of tics: A sign and symptom in psychopathology. *Psychonalytic Study of the Child*, **3-4**, 279
MAHLER, M. S. and LUKE, J. A. (1946) Outcome of the tic syndrome. *Journal of Nervous and Mental Disease*, **103**, 433-445
MAHLER, M. S. and RANGELL, L. (1943) A psychosomatic study of maladie des tics (Gilles de la Tourette's Disease). *Psychiatric Quarterly*, **17**, 579-603
MEIGE, H. and FEINDEL, E. (1907) *Tics and their Treatment*. Translated and edited by S. A. K. Wilson. New York: William Wood and Co.
METCALFE, M. and GOLDMAN, E. (1965) Validation of an inventory for measuring depression. *British Journal of Psychiatry*, **111**, 240-242

MONTGOMERY, M. A., CLAYTON, P. J. and FRIEDHOFF, A. J. (1982) Psychiatric illness in Tourette Syndrome patients and first-degree relatives. In *Gilles de la Tourette Syndrome.* Eds. A. J. Friedhoff and T. N. Chase, pp. 335–339. New York: Raven Press

MORPHEW, J. A. and SIM, M. (1969) Gilles de la Tourette's Syndrome: a clinical and psychopathological study. *British Journal of Medical Psychology,* **42,** 293–301

PENNA, M. W. and LION, J. R. (1975) Gilles de la Tourette Syndrome and depression: A case report. *Diseases of the Nervous System,* **36,** 41–43

ROBERTSON, M. M., EVANS, K., ROBINSON, A., TRIMBLE, M. R. and LASCELLES, P. (1985) Copper abnormalities in the Gilles de la Tourette syndrome. Presented at the Fourth World Congress of Biological Psychiatry, Philadelphia

ROSENBERG, L. A., HARRIS, J. C. and SINGER, H. S. (1984) Relationship of the child behaviour checklist to an independent measure of psychopathology. *Psychological Reports,* **54,** 427–430

SHAPIRO, A. K., SHAPIRO, E. S., BRUUN, R. D. and SWEET, R. D. (1978) *Gilles de la Tourette's Syndrome.* New York: Raven Press

SHAPIRO, A. K., SHAPIRO, E. S., BRUUN, R. D., SWEET, R., WAYNE, H. and SOLOMON, G. (1976) Gilles de la Tourette's Syndrome: summary of clinical experience with 250 patients and suggested nomenclature for tic syndromes. In *Advances in Neurology.* Eds. R. Eldridge and S. Fahn. Vol. 14. pp. 277–281. New York: Raven Press

SHAPIRO, A. K., SHAPIRO, E., WAYNE, H. L. and CLARKIN, J. (1972) The psychopathology of Gilles de la Tourette's Syndrome. *American Journal of Psychiatry,* **129,** 427–434

SNOWDON, J. (1980) A comparison of written and postbox forms of the Leyton Obsessional Inventory. *Psychological Medicine,* **10,** 165–170

SPIELBERGER, C. D., GORSUCH, R. L. and LUSHENE, R. E. (1970) *Manual for the State-Trait Anxiety Inventory ('Self-Evaluation Questionnaire').* Palo Alto: Consulting Psychologists Press Inc.

SUTHERLAND, R. J., KOLB, B., SCHOEL, W. M., WHISHAW, I. Q. and DAVIES, D. (1982) Neuropsychological assessment of children and adults with Tourette Syndrome: A comparison with learning disabilities and schizophrenia. In *Gilles de la Tourette Syndrome.* Eds. A. J. Friedhoff and T. N. Chase, pp. 311–322. New York: Raven Press

TALAIRACH, J., BANCAUD, J., GEIER, S., BORDAS-FERRER, M., BONNIS, A., SZIKLA, G. and RUSU, M. (1975) The cingulate gyrus and human behaviour. *Electroencephalography and Clinical Neurophysiology,* **34,** 45–52

THOMPSON, P. J. (1981) The effects of anticonvulsant drugs on the cognitive functioning of normal volunteers and patients with epilepsy. *PhD Thesis,* University of London

TRIMBLE, M. R. (1981) *Neuropsychiatry.* Chichester: Wiley and Sons Ltd

TRIMBLE, M. R. and THOMPSON, P. J. (1986) Neuropsychological aspects of epilepsy. In *Neuropsychological Assessment in Neuropsychiatric Disorders.* Eds. I. Grant and K. M. Adams. Oxford University Press (in press)

TURPIN, G. C. H. (1982) Behavioural management of Gilles de la Tourette's and multiple tic syndromes. *MPhil. Thesis,* University of London

WIESER, H. G. (1983) *Electroclinical Features of the Psychomotor Seizure.* London: Butterworths

WILSON, R. S., GARRON, D. C., TANNER, C. M. and KLAWANS, H. L. (1982) Behaviour disturbance in children with Tourette Syndrome. In *Gilles de la Tourette Syndrome.* Eds. A. J. Friedhoff and T. N. Chase, pp. 329–333. New York: Raven Press

WILSON, S. A. K. (1927) Tics and child conditions. *Journal of Neurology and Psychopathology,* **8,** 93–109

21
The pathophysiology of essential tremor
Robert G. Lee

The diagnostic label essential tremor has been used to refer to a group of disorders. Although these share some common clinical features, it is quite likely that more than one underlying mechanism may be responsible for their production. Therefore, before embarking on a discussion of pathophysiology of essential tremor, it is important to clarify what is and what is not included under this term.

Marsden (1984) lists the following clinical criteria for essential tremor: (a) the tremor is absent at rest; (b) it is present on maintaining a posture, particularly of the outstretched arms; (c) it is not made strikingly worse by movement (although it often persists and may be accentuated slightly by manoeuvres, such as the finger–nose test); (d) it is not associated with signs of Parkinson's disease or cerebellar dysfunction.

These criteria are accepted by most neurologists. Some would add other features to the list, including positive family history in up to 50% of cases, suppression of tremor with alcohol and β-adrenoreceptor blocking drugs, and a tremor frequency which is slower than physiological tremor and faster than parkinsonian tremor, usually somewhere between 5 and 8 Hz.

The classification proposed by Marsden, Obeso and Rothwell (1983) is useful in helping identify the various entities which have been lumped together under the term 'essential tremor'. These include: (a) enhanced physiological tremor; (b) classical 'benign' essential tremor; (c) severe essential tremor; (d) symptomatic essential tremor occurring in association with other neurological disorders. Most neurologists would agree that the second category in this list meets the criteria for essential tremor. Whether the other disorders represent parts of a continuous spectrum with a common underlying pathogenesis, or whether they are distinct entities, remains uncertain at this time.

The cause and pathogenesis of essential tremor is unknown. However, there are several clues which may point us in certain directions. This discussion will focus on four areas which seem most likely to provide information concerning the pathophysiology of essential tremor. The anatomical basis for tremor is considered first and then the various physiological investigations which have been carried out, including studies of synchronization of motor unit discharges and methods for resetting tremor by introducing perturbations into peripheral reflex loops. Next, the role of β-adrenoreceptors is briefly reviewed and possible mechanisms of action of drugs which block these receptors. Finally, some of the animal models of tremor produced by CNS lesions or tremogenic agents are discussed.

ANATOMICAL AND PATHOLOGICAL CONSIDERATIONS

In searching for a mechanism to account for a clinical abnormality such as tremor, the traditional approach has been to turn to the pathological literature in an attempt to determine what anatomical structures may be responsible for the abnormality. This approach has not been fruitful in essential tremor, except possibly in a negative sense. Due to the benign nature of the condition, there have been few well-documented pathological studies. Those which have been done have not revealed any consistent pathological changes which could be correlated with the tremor (Hersovits and Blackwood, 1969). This stands in direct contrast to the two other major pathological tremors, parkinsonian tremor and cerebellar intention tremor, both of which are usually associated with clearly identified lesions in the central nervous system involving either the nigrostriatal system or the dentate nucleus and its outflow in the superior cerebellar peduncle.

An alternative starting point might be to consider the various sites in the central nervous system which are known to be associated with tremors or other abnormal oscillations. Some of these are listed in *Table 21.1*. Although the major

Table 21.1 Sites within the central nervous system where lesions or dysfunction may result in tremor or oscillations

	Anatomical structure	*Clinical example*
Humans	Substantia nigra (pars compacta)	Parkinsonian tremor
	Dentate nucleus, superior cerebellar peduncle	'Cerebellar' intention tremor
	Red nucleus	'Rubral' tremor
	Central tegmental tract	Palatal myoclonus
Monkeys	Ventral tegmentum of midbrain	Experimental parkinsonian tremor
	Inferior olive	Harmaline tremor

pathological changes in Parkinson's disease are in the substantia nigra, it is likely that the oscillations which generate the tremor develop within the neural loop which includes basal ganglia, thalamus and cortex, possibly due to loss of some modulating effect which the nigrostriatal dopaminergic system normally exerts on striatal neurones. The other major system which seems capable of generating tremor is the neural loop, which includes cerebellum, red nucleus and inferior olive. There are several examples of abnormal oscillations occurring with lesions in this system. These include intention tremor associated with lesions of the dentate nucleus or superior cerebellar peduncle, rubral tremor, and palatal myoclonus with lesions affecting the central tegmental tract. Experimental parkinsonian tremor in monkeys can be produced by lesions in the ventral tegmentum of the midbrain, involving both the outflow from substantia nigra and part of the cerebellorubral connections (Poirier *et al.*, 1969).

However, none of these conditions closely resemble essential tremor and there is so far no entirely satisfactory animal model for this disorder. The possible role of the inferior olive in generation of tremor will be considered later.

There are a number of reports in the literature of disorders which resemble essential tremor occurring in association with other neurological conditions. Perhaps these can provide some clues to the origin of essential tremor. Some of these disorders are listed in *Table 21.2* (for detailed review *see* Larsen and Calne, 1983). Most cases of this type would now be considered to belong to group 4 in the classification proposed by Marsden, Obeso and Rothwell (1983). They represent a rather diverse group of disorders and, so far, there is no obvious linking thread to suggest why essential tremor should be a feature common to all these conditions.

Table 21.2 Neurological disorders sometimes associated with essential tremor

Parkinson's disease	Barbeau and Pourcher (1982)
	Geraghty *et al.* (1985)
Spasmodic torticollis	Couch (1976)
Torson dystonia	Yanagisawa, Goto and Narabayashi (1972)
	Baxter and Lal (1979)
Essential myoclonus	Korten *et al.* (1974)
Peripheral neuropathies	Said, Bathien and Cesaro (1982)
Friedreich's ataxia	Geoffroy *et al.* (1976)

The most consistent associations have been with Parkinson's disease and dystonias, either focal or generalized. Barbeau and Pourcher (1982) described a subgroup of early onset cases of Parkinson's disease with tremor as a prominent feature. In these patients there was an unusually high incidence of familial essential tremor, usually preceding the onset of parkinsonian symptoms. Other studies, using epidemiological approaches, have failed to demonstrate a significant correlation between essential tremor and Parkinson's disease (Larsson and Sjogren, 1960; Rautakorpi *et al.*, 1982). However, a recent report by Geraghty, Jankovic and Zetusky (1985) describes 130 patients with essential tremor in whom the prevalence of Parkinson's disease was 24 times greater than expected.

The association of essential tremor with spasmodic torticollis and idiopathic torsion dystonia appears to be well established, but neither of these conditions correlates with any consistent central nervous system pathology, and these observations therefore do not shed a great deal of light on the possible anatomical and physiological abnormalities which may be responsible for essential tremor.

Several of the disorders listed in *Table 21.2* are genetically determined, suggesting that the abnormal gene may be located in close proximity to the gene responsible for familial essential tremor. Further genetic linkage studies of families in this category may provide information concerning the underlying genetic abnormality responsible for at least some cases of essential tremor.

PHYSIOLOGICAL CONSIDERATIONS

Tremor of an extremity occurs as a result of complex interactions between the mechanical properties of the limb, segmental and suprasegmental reflex mechanisms, and central oscillators (Stein and Lee, 1981). Mechanical factors play a role in determining the frequency and amplitude of tremor (Joyce and Rack, 1974; Stiles and Pozos, 1976; Vilis and Hore, 1977). The bones, muscles and other soft tissues of a limb comprise a mechanical system which is analogous in some respects to a mass and set of springs. Such a system has a natural frequency at which it will oscillate in response to an appropriate driving force. The frequency will depend partially on the specific mechanical properties of the part of the limb which is affected. For example, tremors involving the fingers are generally faster than those involving more proximal parts of the extremities.

Synchronization of motor units

During most natural movements there is asynchronous activation of the participating motor units, a feature which helps produce a smooth movement even when motor units are firing at frequencies below their tetanic fusion rate. Tremor may develop if the discharges of many motor units become synchronized. It might be helpful, therefore, to consider some of the situations in which synchronization of motor unit discharges does occur.

Synchronization is relatively uncommon under normal conditions, but is increased by factors such as fatigue, anxiety, excess alcohol intake, and hypermetabolic states. It is interesting to note that all of these are factors which can give rise to enhanced physiological tremor. Increased synchronization also occurs in situations where muscles are required to regularly produce large, brief forces (as in weight lifting) and it can be accentuated by isometric training of a muscle (Milner-Brown, Stein and Lee, 1975). While synchronization is probably not necessary for very fine physiological tremor, it is an important factor with larger amplitude oscillations. Freund and Dietz (1978) differentiate between short-term synchronization which may contribute to physiological tremor and long-term synchronization which is required to generate larger amplitude pathological tremors. Other studies have shown a positive correlation between the degree of synchronization and the amount and amplitude of physiological tremor (Dietz *et al.*, 1976). However, there is no convincing evidence that any of these factors which normally increase synchronization are involved in the generation of the common type 2 essential tremor.

Reciprocal firing versus co-activation

The synchronized firing of motor units, which occurs with tremor, may be manifested as alternating bursts of activity in opposing muscle groups or as co-activation of agonist–antagonist pairs.

It has been suggested that the pattern of muscle activation may help differentiate parkinsonian tremor from essential tremor (Shahani and Young, 1976), but this is no longer considered to be a useful diagnostic point (Larsen and Calne, 1983; Geraghty, Jankovic and Zetusky, 1985). The author's observations include patients with parkinsonian tremor who show obvious co-activation, sometimes switching to an alternating pattern, and patients with essential tremor in whom agonist and antagonist muscles are activated in a reciprocal manner (Lee, R. G. and Stein, R. B. 1980, unpublished observations). Indeed, the ability to switch from a reciprocal to a co-activation pattern of muscle activation appears to be a feature of some natural movements. This switcning is possibly controlled in some manner by the cerebellum (Smith, 1981).

Central versus reflex oscillations

There has been considerable discussion as to whether the oscillators which are responsible for driving sustained tremor are located in the central nervous system or in peripheral reflex loops. The stretch reflex is a feedback loop which has many of the features of a servo system. A characteristic property of such a system is a tendency to develop oscillations if the gain is increased beyond certain levels or if appropriate delays are introduced into the feedback pathways. There is evidence to suggest that physiological tremor results from instability of the servo mechanism associated with the spinal reflex loop (Lippold, 1970; Joyce and Rack, 1974). On the other hand, it seems more likely that parkinsonian tremor is driven by central oscillators, possibly involving the basal ganglia and thalamocortical feedback loops.

Where does essential tremor fit into this scheme? To answer this question a group of patients were investigated with essential tremor, using mechanical perturbations to determine the extent to which the pattern and timing of the oscillation can be reset by modifying feedback in the reflex loop (Lee and Stein, 1981). The technique for doing this is shown in *Figure 21.1*. Tremor was recorded at the wrist joint and the frequency and pattern of the tremor was determined by measuring EMG bursts from the forearm muscles. A torque motor was used to introduce randomly timed perturbations at the wrist joint, and the EMG following the perturbations was analysed to determine the extent to which the timing of the bursts differed from the predicted time of occurrence, had the perturbation not occurred. These values were plotted as a function of the time within the tremor cycle at which the perturbation occurred (T in *Figure 21.1*). A 'resetting index' was obtained by calculating the slope of the straight line fitted to these data points for several tremor cycles following the perturbation. With complete resetting of tremor there should be a perfect linear relationship with a slope of 1.0. If the perturbation has no effect on the timing of the tremor bursts, the resetting index should be zero.

For the 11 patients with essential tremor studied by this method the resetting index was 0.64 ± 0.14 (s.e.). For 13 patients with parkinsonian tremor the comparable values were 0.16 ± 0.19. Only two parkinsonian patients had resetting indices greater than 0.2. These results suggest that essential tremor is much more responsive than parkinsonian tremor to perturbations occurring within peripheral reflex loops, although in a study using similar methods Teravainen *et al.* (1979) demonstrated resetting of tremor in the majority of parkinsonian patients investigated. Using a somewhat different approach, Marsden, Obeso and Rothwell (1983) found that essential tremor was relatively resistant to resetting by peripheral stimuli. Although physiological tremor was not looked at in this study, the previous work of Lippold (1970) and Joyce and Rack (1974) would suggest that the resetting index for physiological tremor should be close to 1.0.

Figure 21.1 Tremor recording from a patient with essential tremor. The three tracings from top downward represent: movement at the wrist joint, unrectified EMG recorded with surface electrodes over the wrist flexors, and the same EMG activity after rectification and repeated digital smoothing. A sudden extensor torque was applied at the wrist at the point indicated by the vertical line in the centre of the illustration. Solid vertical lines on the bottom channel indicate the peaks of EMG bursts prior to the stimulus and the predicted time for subsequent bursts based on calculation of the mean interburst interval during the pre-stimulus period. Dashed lines represent actual times of tremor bursts following the stimulus, and the horizontal arrows indicate the deviation between predicted and actual times of tremor bursts. The hatched area (T) indicates the time within the tremor cycle at which the stimulus occurred. (Reproduced with permission from Lee and Stein, 1981)

Another method for determining the effect of perturbing stimuli on the pattern of tremor is illustrated in *Figure 21.2*. Using the time of the mechanical perturbation as a reference point, a number of two-second epochs of tremor recording were averaged. Since the stimulus occurred at random times within the tremor cycle, averaging tended to cancel out the tremor bursts during the

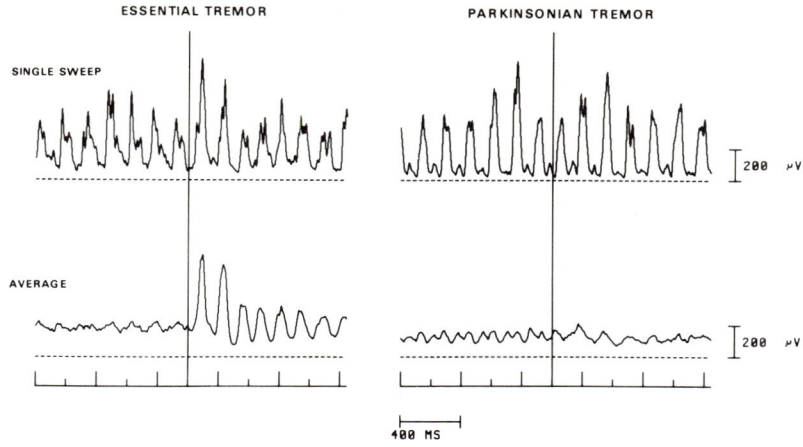

Figure 21.2 Effect of mechanical perturbations on essential tremor and parkinsonian tremor. Top traces show single two-second epochs of EMG activity from the wrist flexors. Bottom traces are averages of 50 such epochs using the onset of perturbation (indicated by the vertical line) as a reference point. The oscillations during the post-stimulus period in the averaged recording from the essential tremor patient (left) indicate that the tremor cycle has become time-locked to the stimulus. In the parkinsonian patient (right), averaging results in cancellation of tremor bursts during both pre-stimulus and post-stimulus periods. (Reproduced with permission from Lee and Stein, 1981)

pre-stimulus period. In the patient with parkinsonian tremor there is little evidence of tremor in the averaged post-stimulus recording, indicating that the tremor pattern has not been altered. However, in the patient with essential tremor the appearance of clear tremor bursts in the post-stimulus period suggests that the tremor has been reset and has become time-locked to the stimulus.

These differences between essential tremor and parkinsonian tremor can also be demonstrated by converting the tremor bursts to a row of points and displaying a number of sequential epochs in a raster format (*Figure 21.3*). The data points can then be shifted to determine whether the post-stimulus timing is related to the perturbation or to the established pattern of tremor during the pre-stimulus period. The results again demonstrate a greater tendency for essential tremor to be reset by external perturbations.

An attempt to summarize schematically the results of these investigations is represented in *Figure 21.4*. Three interconnecting feedback loops are illustrated: the spinal reflex loop, the olivocerebellorubral loop, and the thalamocortical system which includes extensive connections with the basal ganglia. It is proposed that physiological tremor and parkinsonian tremor occur as a result of oscillations in the spinal loop and in the thalamocortical loop, respectively. The origin of essential tremor is unknown but there is some evidence to suggest that it is at least partially due to oscillations occurring in the olivocerebellorubral system (*see below* and Lamarre, 1984). External perturbations would be expected to have the greatest effect on oscillations within the spinal loop and lesser effects on oscillations occurring at higher levels within the central nervous system. It might be predicted that the olivocerebellorubral system is more directly accessible to synchronizing

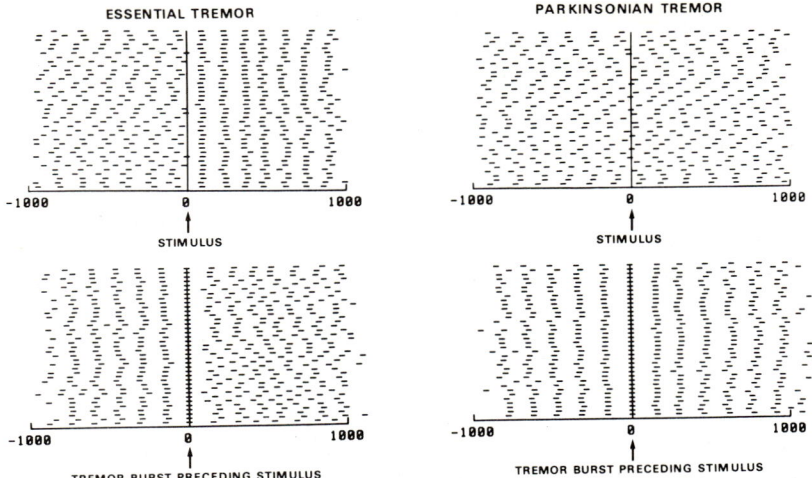

Figure 21.3 Raster displays showing the effect of mechanical perturbations on tremor pattern in essential tremor (left) and parkinsonian tremor (right). Each row of horizontal dashes represents the peaks of EMG bursts during a single two-second epoch. In the top displays the points are aligned on the mechanical stimulus; in the bottom displays the points are rearranged so that the vertical line represents the peak time of the EMG burst immediately preceding the stimulus. Resetting of the tremor pattern can be seen in the patient with essential tremor, but not in the parkinsonian patient. (Reproduced with permission from Lee and Stein, 1981)

Figure 21.4 Schematic representation of mechanisms proposed for different forms of tremor. Three interconnecting loops or neural circuits are shown, each of which is potentially capable of developing abnormal oscillations giving rise to tremor. The resetting capability of external perturbations, represented by the large arrows, is greatest for physiological tremor and least for parkinsonian tremor. (Reproduced with permission from Lee and Stein, 1981)

peripheral inputs than the thalamocortical system and the basal ganglia. The intermediate values for resetting indices obtained from patients with essential tremor would be consistent with this scheme.

PHARMACOLOGICAL CONSIDERATIONS

The pharmacology of essential tremor will be discussed in detail in the following chapter. However, observations that a number of drugs, particularly propranolol, can effectively suppress essential tremor have opened new lines of enquiry concerning the underlying mechanisms responsible for the tremor, and these will be considered briefly here.

Because physiological tremor is accentuated by factors such as fear, anxiety, and hyperthyroidism, it has long been suspected that adrenergic mechanisms contribute in some way to the generation of this type of tremor. This question has been investigated in detail by Marsden and his colleagues (1967). They confirmed that intravenous adrenaline increases the amplitude of physiological tremor in the fingers. Furthermore, they demonstrated that this effect is mediated by peripheral β-adrenoreceptors lying within the forearm. Localized intra-arterial injection of adrenaline into the forearm has the same effect on finger tremor as intravenous adrenaline, and the tremogenic effect of adrenaline can be blocked locally by intra-arterial administration of propranolol.

Similar studies have been carried out on patients with essential tremor in an attempt to identify the site at which propranolol exerts its anti-tremor effect. Young, Growdon and Shahani (1975) reported that intra-arterial propranolol had no effect on spontaneous essential tremor. This was taken as evidence that propranolol suppresses essential tremor by acting at some site within the central nervous system, a view which seemed to be supported by the observations of Young, Growdon and Shahani (1975) that oral propranolol did not become effective for 24–48 hours after initiation of treatment, a time which might be compatible with build-up of adequate drug levels in the central nervous system. However, other investigators report that essential tremor is suppressed following a single oral dose of propranolol (Morgan, Hewer and Cooper, 1973; Calzetti et al., 1983), an observation which seems to be more compatible with a peripheral site of action.

Other studies comparing the effects of several different β-adrenoreceptor blocking drugs also suggest that the tremolytic effect is mediated in the periphery, possibly due to blockade of $β_2$-adrenoreceptors in skeletal muscle (Jefferson, Jenner and Marsden, 1979a; Wilson, Marshall and Richens, 1984). Sotalol, a β blocker which crosses the blood–brain barrier only with considerable difficulty, is just as effective as propranolol in suppressing essential tremor. On the other hand, atenolol, a cardioselective β blocker, is less effective than either propranolol or sotalol, although it is better than a placebo.

$β_2$-Adrenoreceptors are located on both intrafusal and extrafusal fibres within skeletal muscle, and the tremolytic effect of β blocking drugs could be mediated at either of these sites (see Wilson, Marshall and Richens, 1984). Activation of these receptors on the intrafusal fibres of the muscle spindle would result in an increase of the gain within the stretch reflex loop. Whether this occurs in essential tremor is unknown, but it is an interesting possibility considering the other evidence referred to previously which suggests that oscillations wihtin spinal reflex loops make some contribution to essential tremor.

Since essential tremor is accentuated by adrenaline and suppressed by β-adrenoreceptor blocking drugs, it is tempting to speculate that the basic mechanism underlying essential tremor is some abnormality of β-receptors either in skeletal muscle or elsewhere. However, one must be cautious in extrapolating the results of pharmacological studies and, at present, there is very little evidence to indicate any generalized defect in β-adrenoreceptors which might be responsible for essential tremor (Kilfeather et al., 1984). In fact, it is still possible that the tremolytic effect of propranolol may be due to some non-specific action, such as membrane stabilization, rather than β-receptor blockade.

The role of peripheral adrenoreceptors becomes even less clear when we consider the effects of alcohol and other drugs on essential tremor. It is well known that even small doses of ethanol have a markedly beneficial effect on many patients with essential tremor. The site at which alcohol exerts this effect is unknown, but it would seem most likely to be somewhere in the central nervous system (Growdon, Shahani and Young, 1975). Phenobarbital has been used in the past to treat essential tremor and, more recently, primidone has also been shown to be effective, even in some patients who do not respond to propranolol (Findley, Calzetti and Cleaves, 1984). Whatever effect these drugs have on essential tremor is also most likely mediated in the central nervous system.

The obvious effects which excessive alcohol ingestion have on cerebellar function might suggest that smaller amounts of alcohol benefit essential tremor by acting at some point within the cerebellar system. The possibility that abnormal oscillations within the olivocerebellorubral loop may contribute to essential tremor has already been discussed above.

HARMALINE-INDUCED TREMOR AND THE INFERIOR OLIVE

Although there are no spontaneous tremors in laboratory animals which can serve as a satisfactory model of essential tremor, experimental tremors can be produced by using a combination of selective central nervous system lesions and tremogenic drugs. The most widely studied drug of this group is harmaline. Lamarre (1984) described three distinct types of tremor which occur following administration of harmaline to monkeys (*Table 21.3*). In intact monkeys harmaline produces a low amplitude 8–12 Hz tremor which has some similarity to physiological tremor in humans. When harmaline is given to monkeys with lesions in the dentate nucleus or ventral tegmentum of the midbrain the resulting tremors occur at slower frequencies and are of greater amplitude. Lamarre proposes that these forms of

Table 21.3 Experimental tremors in monkeys produced by administration of harmaline in conjunction with brain lesions

Frequency (Hz)	Site of lesion	System involved	Corresponding human tremor
8–12	None	Olivocerebellar	Physiological tremor
6–8	Dentate nucleus	Olivocerebellar	Essential tremor
3–6	Midbrain tegmentum	Thalamocortical	Parkinsonian tremor

After Lamarre, 1984.

harmaline tremor could be considered as models for essential tremor and parkinsonian tremor. He also suggested that the first two types of harmaline-induced tremor occur as a result of oscillations within the olivocerebellar system; type 3 harmaline tremor is more likely to be related to oscillations in thalamocortical loops.

The tremogenic effects of harmaline appear to be mediated through the inferior olive. The 8–12 Hz harmaline tremor in intact monkeys and a slightly slower tremor in decerebrated cats are associated with repetitive firing of neurones in the inferior olive (De Montigny and Lamarre, 1973; Lamarre, 1984). This results in rhythmical activation of Purkinje cells which, in turn, is capable of synchronizing activity of spinal motoneurones, probably via vestibulospinal and reticulospinal pathways (*see* Figure 21.5).

Figure 21.5 Extracellular recordings from neurones in olivary nuclei and other brainstem nuclei following administration of harmaline in a decerebrated, paralysed cat. Rhythmic discharges at frequencies of 6–8 Hz are seen in (*a*) medial excessory olive, (*b*) dorsal accessory olive, (*c*) fastigial nucleus, (*d*) gigantocellular reticular nucleus, (*e*) ventral lateral vestibular nucleus, and (*f*) paramedian reticular nucleus. (Reproduced with permission from De Montigny and Lamarre, 1973)

The harmaline-induced repetitive bursting in the inferior olive persists following curarization or dorsal root section (Llinas and Volkind, 1973), indicating that it is a centrally originating oscillation not dependent on feedback in peripheral reflex loops. Also, destruction of the inferior olive abolishes harmaline tremor (Llinas, 1984). These observations have stimulated considerable interest in the possibility that the inferior olive may be involved in the generation of physiological tremor and possibly essential tremor in humans (Llinas, 1984). A unique feature of the inferior olive is the occurrence of electrical coupling between neurones, probably related to the presence of gap junctions. This could be the basis for the synchronized oscillations which occur in this structure.

434 The pathophysiology of essential tremor

Recordings *in vitro* from brainstem slice preparations have identified the cellular mechanisms underlying the oscillatory activity of the inferior olive (Llinas and Yarom, 1981). Each discharge of an inferior olivary neurone is followed by a depolarization–hyperpolarization sequence resulting from rapid and complex changes in conductances for calcium and potassium. The prolonged after-hyperpolarization is terminated by a period of rebound excitation, and abrupt return of the membrane potential to baseline (*Figure 21.6*). The duration of the hyperpolarization is modulated by the amount of calcium which enters the dendrites during the calcium action potential. Thus, calcium entry determines the

Figure 21.6 Intracellular recordings from a guinea-pig brainstem slice showing the mechanisms responsible for oscillations in the inferior olive. In (*a*) and (*b*) an action potential from an inferior olivary neurone is displayed at two different sweep speeds. The initial spike is followed by a period of depolarization and then a prolonged after-hyperpolarization, the duration of which depends on the amount of calcium entering the dendrites during the calcium action potential. In (*c*) and (*d*) tetrodotoxin has been used to prevent sodium spikes. The after-hyperpolarization is terminated by rebound excitation (arrows) due to activation of a calcium-dependent action potential. (Reproduced with permission from Llinas, 1984)

cycle time of the oscillator. Application of harmaline to the brainstem slice preparation causes further hyperpolarization of inferior olivary neurones and an exaggerated rebound response (Llinas, 1984). Harmaline also causes the resting membrane potential of inferior olivary neurones to oscillate in a sinusoidal manner at frequencies in the 5–10 Hz range.

What does this tell us about the pathogenesis of essential tremor? Could some factor which enhances the natural tendency for synchronized oscillations in the inferior olive be responsible for essential tremor? This is an attractive hypothesis, but so far direct evidence to support it is lacking. As mentioned previously, the limited number of pathological studies on patients with essential tremor have failed to demonstrate any consistent pathology in the inferior olive or at any other site within the central nervous system. Furthermore, other neurological disorders which are sometimes associated with essential tremor are not characterized by any pathological changes in the inferior olive. In fact, the only clinical condition which does correlate with an abnormality in the inferior olive is palatal myoclonus. This results from a lesion involving the central tegmental tract which forms part of the connection between the red nucleus and the inferior olive. Lesions of this pathway are associated with hypertrophy of the inferior olive, possibly due to deafferentation of this structure. Although palatal myoclonus is a rhythmical disorder, it bears little resemblance to essential tremor and occurs at a much slower frequency, around 2 Hz.

CONCLUSIONS

As stated at the outset, the cause of essential tremor is unknown and there is still much uncertainty regarding the exact site of the abnormality which is responsible for this common form of tremor. It is probably overly simplistic to consider that any single structure in either the central or peripheral nervous systems acts as an oscillator to produce the synchronized discharges of motor units which result in essential tremor. However, the experimental work reviewed above supports the concept that the inferior olive and the olivocerebellorubral loop contribute in some manner to the generation of essential tremor. Further studies on animal models and human patients are required to define more precisely the exact mechanism. We do know that the spinal stretch reflex loop is capable of developing oscillations, and the observations that essential tremor can be reset by perturbing stretch reflexes suggest that oscillations at this level may be a contributing mechanism. Possibly, some abnormality in the olivocerebellorubral system releases normal damping influences to allow oscillations to occur within the stretch reflex loop.

There are still many unanswered questions including the relationship of essential tremor to physiological tremor, the role of adrenergic mechanisms, the site at which alcohol acts to suppress essential tremor, and the manner in which the genetic abnormality is expressed in familial cases.

References

BARBEAU, A. and POURCHER, E. (1982) New data on the genetics of Parkinson's disease. *Canadian Journal of Neurological Sciences*, **9**, 53–66

BAXTER, D. W. and LAL, S. (1979) Essential tremor and dystonic syndromes. In *The Extrapyramidal System and Its Disorders*. Eds. L. J. Poirier, T. L. Sourkes and P. J. Bedard. *Advances in Neurology*, Vol. 24, pp. 373–377. New York: Raven Press

CALZETTI, S., FINDLEY, L. J., GRESTY, M. A., PERUCCA, E. and RICHENS, A. (1983) Effect of a single oral dose of propranolol on essential tremor. A double-blind controlled study. *Annals of Neurology,* **13,** 165–171

COUCH, J. R. (1976) Dystonia and tremor in spasmodic torticollis. *Advances in Neurology,* **14,** 245–256

DE MONTIGNY, C. and LAMARRE, Y. (1973) Rhythmic activity induced by harmaline in the olivo-cerebello-bulbar system of the cat. *Brain Research,* **53,** 81–95

DIETZ, V., BISCHOFBERGER, E., WITA, C. and FREUND, H. J. (1976) Correlation between discharges of two simultaneously recorded motor units and physiological tremor. *Electroencephalography and Clinical Neurophysiology,* **40,** 97–105

FINDLEY, L. J., CALZETTI, S. and CLEEVES, L. (1984) Primidone in essential tremor. In *Movement Disorders: Tremor.* Eds. L. J. Findley and R. Capildeo, pp. 271–282. New York: Oxford University Press

FREUND, H. J. and DIETZ, V. (1978) The relationship between physiological and pathological tremor. In *Physiological Tremor, Pathological Tremors and Clonus.* Ed. J. E. Desmedt. *Progress in Clinical Neurophysiology,* Vol. 5, pp. 66–89. Basel: Karger

GEOFFROY, B., BARBEAU, A., BRETON, G. et al. (1976) Clinical description and roentgenologic evaluation of patients with Friedreich's ataxia. *Canadian Journal of Neurological Sciences,* **3,** 279–286

GERAGHTY, J. J., JANKOVIC, J. and ZETUSKY, W. J. (1985) Association between essential tremor and Parkinson's disease. *Annals of Neurology,* **17,** 329–333

GROWDON, J. H., SHAHANI, B. T. and YOUNG, R. R. (1975) The effect of alcohol on essential tremor. *Neurology,* **25,** 259–262

HERSOVITS, D. and BLACKWOOD, W. (1969) Essential (familial, hereditary) tremor. A case report. *Journal of Neurology, Neurosurgery and Psychiatry,* **32,** 509–511

JEFFERSON, D., JENNER, P. and MARSDEN, C. D. (1979a) Beta-adrenoreceptor antagonists in essential tremor. *Journal of Neurology, Neurosurgery and Psychiatry,* **42,** 904–909

JEFFERSON, D., JENNER, P. and MARSDEN, C. D. (1979b) Relationship between plasma propranolol concentration and relief of essential tremor. *Journal of Neurology, Neurosurgery and Psychiatry,* **42,** 831–837

JOYCE, G. C. and RACK, P. M. H. (1974) The effects of load and force on tremor at the normal human elbow joint. *Journal of Physiology,* **240,** 375–396

KILFEATHER, S., MASSARELLA, A., TURNER, P. and FINDLEY, L. J. (1984) Beta-adrenoceptor involvement in tremor production; possible defects in essential tremor. In *Movement Disorders: Tremor.* Eds. L. J. Findley and R. Capildeo, pp. 225–244. New York: Oxford University Press

KORTEN, J. J., NOTERNAMS, S. L. H., FRENKEN, C. W. G. M., GABREELS, F. J. M. and JOOSTEN, E. M. G. (1974) Familial essential myoclonus. *Brain,* **97,** 131–138

LAMARRE, Y. (1984) Animal models of physiological, essential and parkinsonian-like tremors. In *Movement Disorders: Tremor.* Eds. L. J. Findley and R. Capildeo, pp. 183–194. New York: Oxford University Press

LAPRESLE, J. (1979) Rhythmic palatal myoclonus and the dentato-olivary pathway. *Journal of Neurology,* **220,** 223–230

LARSEN, T. A. and CALNE, D. B. (1983) Essential tremor. *Clinical Neuropharmacology,* **6,** 185–286

LARSSON, T. and SJOGREN, T. (1960) Essential tremor. A clinical and genetic population study. *Acta Psychiatrica Neurologica Scandinavica,* **36** (Suppl. 144), 1–176

LEE, R. G. and STEIN, R. G. (1981) Resetting of tremor by mechanical perturbations; a comparison of essential tremor and parkinsonian tremor. *Annals of Neurology,* **10,** 523–531

LIPPOLD, O. C. J. (1970) Oscillation in the stretch reflex arc and the origin of the rhythmical 8–12 C/S component of physiological tremor. *Journal of Physiology,* **206,** 359–382

LLINAS, R. R. (1984) Rebound excitation as the physiological basis for tremor: a biophysical study of the oscillatory properties of mammalian central neurons *in vitro.* In *Movement Disorders: Tremor.* Eds. L. J. Findley and R. Capildeo, pp. 165–182. New York: Oxford University Press

LLINAS, R. and VOLKIND, R. A. (1973) The olivo-cerebello system: functional properties as revealed by harmaline induced tremor. *Experimental Brain Research,* **18,** 69–87

LLINAS, R. and YAROM, Y. (1981) Electrophysiology of mammalian inferior olivary neurons *in vitro.* Different types of voltage-dependent ionic conductances. *Journal of Physiology,* **315,** 549–567

MARSDEN, C. D. (1984) Origins of normal and pathological tremor. In *Movement Disorders: Tremor.* Eds. L. J. Findley and R. Capildeo, pp. 37–84. New York: Oxford University Press

MARSDEN, C. D., FOLEY, T. H., OWEN, D. A. L. and McALLISTER, R. G. (1967) Peripheral beta-adrenergic receptors concerned with tremor. *Clinical Sciences,* **33,** 53–65

MARSDEN, C. D., OBESO, J. and ROTHWELL, J. C. (1983) Benign essential tremor is not a single entity. In *Current Concepts in Parkinson's Disease.* Ed. M. D. Yahr, pp. 31–46. Amsterdam: Excerpta Medica

MILNER-BROWN, H. S., STEIN, R. B. and LEE, P. G. (1975) Synchronization of human motor units, possible roles of exercise and supraspinal reflexes. *Electroencephalography and Clinical Neurophysiology,* **38,** 245–254

MORGAN, M. H., HEWER, R. L. and COOPER, R. (1973) Effect of the beta-adrenergic blocking agent propranolol on essential tremor. *Journal of Neurology, Neurosurgery and Psychiatry,* **36,** 618–624

POIRIER, L. J., BOUVIER, G., BEDARD, P., BOUCHER, R., LAROCHELLE, L., OLIVER, A. and SINGH, P. (1969) Essai sur les circuits neuronaux impliques us dans le tremblement postural et l'hypokinesie. *Revue Neurologique (Paris),* **120,** 15–40

RAUTAKORPI, I., TAKALA, J., MARTTILLA, R. J., SIEVERS, K. and RINNE, U. K. (1982) Essential tremor in a Finnish population. *Acta Neurologica Scandinavica,* **66,** 58–67

SAID, G., BATHIEN, N. and CESARO, T. (1982) Peripheral neuropathies and tremor. *Neurology,* **32,** 480–485

SHAHANI, B. T. and YOUNG, R. R. (1976) Physiological and pharmacological aids in the differential diagnosis of tremor. *Journal of Neurology, Neurosurgery and Psychiatry,* **39,** 772–783

SMITH, A. M. (1981) The coactivation of antagonist muscles. *Canadian Journal of Physiology and Pharmacology,* **59,** 733–747

STEIN, R. B. and LEE, R. G. (1981) Tremor and clonus. In *Handbook of Physiology, Section I, Volume II; Motor Control.* Ed. V. B. Brooks, pp. 325–343. American Physiological Society

STILES, R. N. and POZOS, S. (1976) A mechanical–reflex oscillator hypothesis for parkinsonian hand tremor. *Journal of Applied Physiology,* **40,** 990–998

TERAVAINEN, H., EVARTS, E. and CALNE, D. (1979) Effects of kinesthetic inputs and parkinsonian tremor. In *Advances in Neurology.* Eds. L. J. Piorier, T. L. Sourkes and P. J. Bedard, Vol. 24, pp. 161–173. New York: Raven Press

VILIS, T. and HORE, J. (1977) Effects of changes in mechanical state of limb on cerebellar intention tremor. *Journal of Neurophysiology,* **40,** 1214–1224

WILSON, J. F., MARSHALL, R. W. and RICHENS, A. (1984) Essential tremor: treatment with beta-adrenoceptor blocking drugs. In *Movement Disorders: Tremor.* Eds. L. J. Findley and R. Capildeo, pp. 245–260. New York: Oxford University Press

YANAGISAWA, N., GOTO, A. and NARABAYASHI, H. (1972) Familial dystonia musculorum deformans and tremor. *Journal of Neurological Sciences,* **16,** 125–136

YOUNG, R. R., GROWDON, J. H. and SHAHANI, B. T. (1975) Beta-adrenergic mechanisms in action tremor. *New England Journal of Medicine,* **293,** 950–953

22
The pharmacology of essential tremor
Leslie J. Findley

INTRODUCTION

Essential (benign, familial) tremor is a common disorder of movement. It is usually manifested as a postural tremor of hands and arms, often involving the head. Other body parts, however, can be affected, including the chin, voice, eyelids, and mouth. Although commonly seen in clinical practice, only a small proportion of affected individuals come to the attention of the clinician (Rautakorpi, 1978). It is perhaps unfortunate that this condition is often given the prefix 'benign' as, once developed, it is a life-long affliction which can cause embarrassment and functional incapacity. The main clinical features and natural history of this disorder have been described in a number of extensive reviews (Critchley, 1949, 1972; Marshall, 1962; Murray, 1981a,b; Larsen and Calne, 1983; Findley, 1985).

The aetiology and pathology of essential tremor is unknown. There have been very few reported neuropathological studies (Herskovits and Blackwood, 1969). It is possible that modern techniques for studying structure of the nervous system (nuclear magnetic resonance) and its metabolism (positron emission tomography) may reveal some clues as to the underlying pathophysiology.

Classical essential tremor is a distal, postural tremor of upper limbs which attenuates during movement, becoming more obvious at the end of goal-directed movement. It can be unilateral at onset, but once established is usually bilateral, although invariably asymmetrical, being maximal in the outstretched hands in the vertical plane. The waveform of essential tremor is normally sinusoidal, though in some patients rotational and horizontal movements produce a more complex pattern. Tremor is usually only evident in posture or on action. When the amplitude is large, however, and particularly in the elderly, tremor will be seen with the affected limb supported, i.e. an apparent rest tremor. Rigidity in the tremulous limb, brought out by movement of the opposite limb and similar on palpation to cogwheel rigidity, is common in uncomplicated essential tremor (Salisachs, 1978). This feature with the addition of a 'rest' component to the tremor and the asymmetry may cause difficulties in distinguishing essential tremor from the tremulous phenomena of Parkinson's disease (Salisachs and Findley, 1984).

The prevalence of essential tremor in the United Kingdom is not precisely known, as the necessary epidemiological studies have not been carried out. Sevitt

(1974) gives some indication of how common the disorder is by estimating that there were 80 000 consultations per year in the United Kingdom and 1.4 million for senile tremor (i.e. essential tremor in an elderly population). Community studies in Finland (Rautakorpi, 1978), Sweden (Larsson and Sjogren, 1960), the United States (Rajput, Beard and Kurland, 1982) and Papua New Guinea (Hornabrook and Nagurney, 1976), have cited prevalence rates between 0.4 and 5.6% of the population. The differences in prevalence probably reflect many factors, including the different epidemiological techniques used in these surveys. It is clear, however, that essential tremor is more common than Parkinson's disease, the other common cause of tremor in an elderly population. Although these two disorders have features in common, they are generally considered to be unrelated (Marttila, Rautakorpi and Rinne, 1984; Findley and Cleeves, 1985a). However, a recent study has shown an increased incidence of tremor in the relatives of patients with Parkinson's disease (Lang, Kierens and Blair, 1985).

The diagnosis of essential tremor depends on the presentation of an uncomplicated tremulous disorder in the absence of any underlying progressive neurological disorder. Although it is commonly seen in the elderly it can commence at any age, usually progressing slowly in terms of severity during life and often becoming exacerbated in the senium (Critchley, 1949), when the patient may first present to the medical practitioner. Essential tremor is usually described as monosymptomatic, but it can be associated with other movement disorders such as torticollis, dystonia and other dyskinesias (Couch, 1976; Baxter and Lal, 1979; Martinelli and Gabellini, 1982). There is an increased incidence of vascular disease in patients with essential tremor (Rajput, Beard and Kurland, 1982; Rautakorpi, Marttila and Rinne, 1984). It is considered to be dominantly inherited with variable penetrance and, in our own series, approximately 30% of patients give a family history.

CLASSIFICATION OF ESSENTIAL TREMOR

Most physiological and pharmacological research in essential tremor has concentrated on the upper limbs. It is important to note this, as it is clear that tremor in different parts of the body exhibits differing responsiveness to drugs (Findley, Calzetti and Cleeves, 1985; Koller, Graner and Micoh, 1985), which may imply differing underlying mechanisms controlling tremor.

Essential tremor is no longer considered to be a homogenous disorder, though no satisfactory method of classification exists. Frequency of hand tremor is usually quoted as lying between 6 and 12 Hz (Marshall, 1962), corresponding to the frequency of physiological tremor in age-matched control subjects. In common with other workers, the author and his colleagues have frequently found, in the more symptomatic patients, lower frequency of tremor than physiological controls and an inverse relationship between frequency and amplitude (Findley and Gresty, 1981; Larsen and Calne, 1983). On frequency analysis we observed two dominant groups; one with frequencies between 7 and 11 Hz, which we interpret to be enhancement of physiological tremor, and another with frequencies below 6.5 Hz of larger amplitude and of separate origin to physiological tremor (Findley and Gresty, 1981).

The most practical current method of classifying essential tremor is on the basis of whether tremor predominantly arises from oscillations around peripheral reflexes and thus is entrainable by external perturbations of equal power, or whether the tremor is derived from a higher level within the central nervous system (CNS) and is relatively uninfluenced by peripheral manipulations (Marsden, Obeso and Rothwell, 1983). The former has been designated type I essential tremor, and is inseparable, in terms of its behavioural characteristics, from enhanced physiological tremor. The latter, of lower frequency and higher amplitude, is designated type II essential tremor. This is the type that most commonly presents to the physician, though no epidemiological studies have been attempted using this form of classification. In view of the known differential responsiveness to drugs of tremors arising at different anatomical sites (Findley, Calzette and Cleeves, 1985; Koller, Graner and Micoh, 1985) and with different underlying mechanisms (Findley and Gresty, 1981), drug trials for the management of essential tremor must employ carefully defined patient groups. Marsden, Obeso and Rothwell (1983) also define types III and IV essential tremor. However, the separation of these groups seems somewhat arbitrary, i.e. based on whether there is a separate movement disorder in association with essential tremor, or whether the tremor is generalized and of extremely large amplitude.

The differentiation of essential tremor in terms of pharmacological responsiveness has been attempted. Findley *et al.* (1981) and Calzetti *et al.* (1983b) have

Figure 22.1 Baseline tremor amplitude (cm displacement) plotted against change in tremor amplitude after propranolol (cm) on log scale. Arrow signifies patient showing increment in tremor amplitude after propranolol. (From Calzetti *et al.*, 1983b, courtesy of the Editor and Publishers, *Annals of Neurology*)

shown that patients with tremor of lower amplitude, and therefore higher frequency, were relatively unresponsive to β-adrenoceptor blockade by propranolol (*Figure 22.1*). It was proposed that these patients be termed 'primary' enhanced physiological tremor to distinguish them from patients with 'secondary' enhanced physiological tremor such as seen in anxiety states and after catecholamine infusions, which would have been completely suppressed by peripheral β-adrenoceptor blockade (Marsden et al., 1967).

ASPECTS OF CLINICAL TRIALS

Until the 1970s, with the advent of β-adrenoceptor antagonists and other drugs which could effectively suppress tremor, the treatment of essential tremor was largely based on anecdotal clinical reports. Subsequently, large numbers of clinical trials have been undertaken to evaluate the efficacy of drugs in the management of essential tremor and it has become apparent that a number of factors must be taken into account in order to obtain valid and reliable results.

The amplitude of essential tremor can fluctuate as a result of a large number of external and internal factors, all of which must be controlled. These include level of arousal, time of day, other medication, external stresses (adaptation to the laboratory), nicotine, caffeine and alcohol. If all these are controlled for, within a single period of recording, significant fluctuations in tremor amplitude are not usually seen.

Considerable placebo effects can be observed in the drug treatment of essential tremor. In trials over the last five years, the mean placebo responses have varied between 12 and 27% against baseline values of tremor amplitude. Clearly, therefore, therapeutic trials must be placebo controlled.

Over the last hundred years, methods of objectively measuring tremor in terms of frequency and amplitude have become progressively sophisticated (Brumlik and Yap, 1970). Currently, accelerometry with spectral analysis of average epochs of tremor is a popular and accurate technique to quantitate tremor (Gresty and Findley, 1984). Whilst the objective techniques are clearly important when measuring response to a drug, other parameters must also be considered and evaluated in order to obtain an idea of the drug's overall efficacy in controlling the patient's symptoms. It is possible to show a pharmacological response in terms of objective reduction in tremor amplitude without affecting measures of performance and patient's self-rating (Findley and Cleeves, 1985b). Thus all trials must include validated tests of performance and dexterity (writing, construction, drawing etc.) and, in addition, some index of the patient's function in his own environment. Theoretically, in this respect it would be most appropriate to record tremor over long time periods during the patient's normal activities (Ackmann et al., 1977). This approach is technologically and logistically difficult for routine clinical trials. Reliance must therefore be made on patient's self-rating and, where possible, assessment by a relative or close associate. These types of assessment are perhaps best measured on visual analogue scales.

Clinical trials to date have considered single dose responses or the response of tremor over a period of weeks or, more rarely, months. There have been no clinical trials or prospective follow-up studies to assess whether responses are maintained in the long-term. Prospective longer-term studies are therefore necessary to establish the long-term efficacy of drugs currently used to treat essential tremor.

PHARMACOLOGICAL MANAGEMENT OF ESSENTIAL TREMOR

There is, as yet, no completely satisfactory treatment for essential tremor. Fortunately, many patients who seek medical opinion are not sufficiently disabled to require long-term drug therapy. Some patients require only reassurance that their tremor is not part of a serious progressive neurological disease, such as Parkinson's disease. A few patients with disabling (large amplitude) tremor, particularly if it is predominantly unilateral, can be treated effectively by stereotaxis, thalamotomy being the method of choice (Ohye et al., 1981; Andrew, 1984).

Traditionally, treatment of essential tremor relied upon the use of sedatives and minor tranquillizers. In general, the effect of these drugs on tremor is non-specific and relates to the degree of sedation achieved. Benzodiazepines, by reducing anxiety, will help prevent adrenergic enhancement of ongoing tremor and thus may be of use in patients with chronic anxiety states in association with essential tremor. In a recent single study clonazepam, at a dose of 1–4 mg daily, was found to suppress low frequency, predominantly action tremor, in 12 patients who were considered to have a variant of essential tremor (Biary, 1984). A further study, however, of clonazepam in essential tremor has shown it to be ineffective with a high incidence of side-effects (Thompson et al., 1984). This latter study would concur with our own experience with the use of this drug in the management of essential tremor. There has been renewed interest in phenobarbitone; recent trials have shown that this 'old' drug is effective in attenuating tremor magnitude (*see below*) (Baruzzi et al., 1983; Findley and Cleeves, 1985b).

A large number of drugs have in the past been recommended. The muscle relaxant mephenesin was claimed to be effective, but formal trials were never undertaken (Kelly, 1965; Critchley, 1972). Baclofen, a centrally acting muscle relaxant, was demonstrated to be effective in some patients with postural tremor, indistinguishable from essential tremor, in association with peripheral neuropathy (Findley and Gresty, 1981). It was postulated that tremor in peripheral neuropathy was 'driven' by high levels of descending facilitation in the presence of peripheral weakness and that this was inhibited by baclofen. Antiparkinsonian drugs, such as anticholinergics and levodopa, are ineffective in essential tremor (Critchley, 1972; Sevitt, 1974) and may exacerbate tremor (Barbeau, 1969; Lapresle, Rondot and Said, 1974). Amantadine can exacerbate tremor but has been reported as offering some benefit (Critchley, 1972; Manyam, 1981). L-Tryptophan with pyridoxine is ineffective in essential tremor (Morris et al., 1972).

Alcohol

Many patients with essential tremor comment that small quantitites of alcohol can rapidly attenuate the severity of their tremor (Critchley, 1949, 1972; Davis and Kunkle, 1951; Ashenhurst, 1973; Sutherland, Edwards and Eadie, 1975). Out of 121 consecutive patients with essential tremor studied in the author's laboratory, 36 (42%) specifically noted that alcohol reduced tremor. It has been shown that 10–15 minutes after a single oral dose of 45 ml of 80% proof vodka, tremor was attenuated and remained so for some hours with rebound tremor as the blood alcohol level fell (Young, Growdon and Shahani, 1975). Injections of alcohol directly into the brachial artery do not attenuate essential tremor and, therefore, the site of action of alcohol for its beneficial effect in essential tremor is argued to be within the central nervous system (CNS). In this respect, it is noteworthy that in the 10 patients from the above series of 121 whose tremor was classified as type I, i.e. dependent on peripheral reflexes (Marsden, Obeso and Rothwell, 1983), none had noted any beneficial effect from alcohol. It should be emphasized that the action of alcohol in essential tremor is non-specific as it has been shown to be effective in controlling other movement disorders including spasmodic torticollis (Biary and Koller, 1985), essential myoclonus (Mahloudji and Pikielny, 1967; Korten et al., 1974), dystonic myoclonus (Quinn and Marsden, 1984) and post-anoxic myoclonus (Fahn, 1979).

The mechanism of action of alcohol in essential tremor is not known. Spasmodic torticollis, essential tremor and essential myoclonus may affect the same patient, which suggests a common underlying pathophysiology in these disorders (Biary and Koller, 1985). The effect on essential tremor may be specific to ethyl alcohol as some other alcohols have been found to be ineffective (P. LeWitt, 1985, personal communication).

Ethyl alcohol in any of its forms is, in general, impractical therapy owing to the risks of development of tolerance and addiction. Reports have suggested a higher use of alcohol and an increased incidence of alcoholism in patients with essential tremor (Massey and Paulsen, 1978; Nasrallah, Schroeder and Petty, 1982). A recent prospective study has shown that the prevalence of pathological drinking in patients with essential tremor is not significantly different from other tremulous disorders or chronic neurological disease without tremor (Koller, 1983).

β-Adrenoceptor blockade

β-Adrenoceptor antagonists, in particular propranolol, are now the drugs of first choice in the management of essential tremor. After their introduction in the 1960s, it soon became apparent that drugs like propranolol could effectively suppress the enhancement of physiological tremor produced by adrenaline and that this was by way of an effect on peripheral β receptors (Owen and Marsden, 1965; Marsden et al., 1967). As anxiety and adrenaline could exacerbate parkinsonian tremor (Barcroft, Peterson and Schwab, 1952; Constas, 1962), the early studies suggested propranolol could be effective in reducing the tremor of Parkinson's disease, in particular the exacerbations of tremor produced by adrenergic stimulation (Owen and Marsden, 1965; Strang, 1965; Vas, 1966).

Marshall (1968) first suggested the use of β-adrenoceptor blocking drugs in essential tremor and, independently, Sevitt (1971) and Winkler and Young (1971) reported the beneficial effect of propranolol on essential tremor. Over the next five years a large number of clinical trials were undertaken which demonstrated that propranolol could be effective in attenuating essential tremor (Gilligan, 1972; Gilligan, Veale and Wodak, 1972; Murray, 1972, 1976; Pakkenberg, 1972; Barbeau, 1973; Dupont, Hansen and Dalby, 1973; Morgan, Hewer and Cooper, 1973; Sevitt, 1974; Winkler and Young, 1974; Tolosa and Loewenson, 1975; Young, Growdon and Shahani, 1975; McClure and Davis, 1976; Teravainen, Fogelholm and Larsen, 1976). Since these early studies, no β-adrenoceptor antagonist has been shown to be superior to propranolol. There is, however, continuing debate as to the precise property or site of action of propranolol, which confers its efficacy in essential tremor.

β-Adrenoceptor antagonists differ in certain important properties, the major being cardioselectivity, lipid solubility, membrane stabilizing activity and intrinsic sympathomimetic activity. A summary of these properties in drugs commonly investigated for their efficacy in essential tremor is summarized in Table 22.1. Interpretation of current information firmly supports the contention that *the activity of propranolol in the control of essential tremor is largely by way of the peripheral β_2 receptor, though effects within the CNS or effects at the β_1 receptor site have not been conclusively excluded.*

Table 22.1 Properties of some β-adrenoceptor blocking drugs and their effect on essential tremor

Drug	Receptors blocked β_1	β_2	Lipid* solubility	Membrane stabilizing activity	Metabolism (%)	Half-life (h)	Effect on essential tremor
Propranolol	+	+	20.2	+	>95	2–3	+++
Timolol	+	+	1.2	+/−	50	4–6	+++
Pindolol	+	+	0.8	+	60	3–4	−
Sotalol	+	+	0.04	−	0	8–13	+++
Atenolol	+	+/−	0.02	+/−	<10	6–9	+
Metoprolol	+	+/−	1.0	+	85	3–4	+/−

* Partition coefficient, *n*-octanol/buffer, pH 7.4, 37°C.
Based on data in Wilson, Marshall and Richens, 1984.

Lands *et al.* (1967) first subdivided the β-adrenoceptors into two types, the β_1 receptor associated with the heart and the β_2 receptor occurring in the bronchus, blood vessels and peripheral sites including muscles (Bowman and Nott, 1969; Marsden and Meadows, 1970; Rodger and Bowman, 1983) and muscle spindles (Calma and Kidd, 1962; Smith, 1963; Paintal, 1964). Peripheral tremorgenic β_2 receptors located on the plasma membrane of extrafusal fibres act to shorten the twitch duration of muscle producing a reduction in fusion of incomplete tetanic contractions (Marsden and Meadows, 1970), and those on the muscle spindles act to produce enhanced physiological tremor by increasing the gain in the peripheral reflex loop (Young and Hagbarth, 1980). Propranolol itself fails to affect the tendon-jerk reflexes (Phillips, Richens and Shand, 1973), so the functions of these receptors in the normal subject are not clear. It is well established that the infusion of catecholamines produces exacerbation of tremors by way of their effect on peripheral β_2 receptors (Marsden and Meadows, 1970; Perucca, Pickles and Richens, 1981; Arnold *et al.*, 1982). What has not been proven is that these receptors are the locus of the tremorlytic action of propranolol in unenhanced essential tremor. In this respect it should be noted that propranolol will block isoprenaline-enhanced physiological tremor within one minute (Young, Growden and Shahani, 1975), whereas the latency of effect of unenhanced essential tremor is much greater, suggesting a subset of β_2 adrenoceptors in a less accessible peripheral compartment (Abila *et al.*, 1983; 1985a). It is interesting to note that electron microscopic studies of the capillaries in muscle spindles (Miyoshi, Kennedy and

Yoon, 1979) have shown that they have similarities with the capillaries in brain and peripheral nervous system. It has been proposed that a blood–tissue barrier, similar to the blood–brain barrier, may exist in the spindles. This may account for a pharmacologically less accessible subset of β_2 receptors.

β-Adrenoceptor subtypes in essential tremor

Studies of the effect of β-adrenoceptor antagonists on essential tremor have been constructed to dissect out the relative importance of β_1 and β_2 receptors in the attenuation of essential tremor. These studies have examined the effects of cardioselective agents such as atenolol and metoprolol in comparison to propranolol or other non-selective β-adrenoceptor antagonists. In these studies β-blockers are dosed in such a way that the β_1 activity on the heart is identical, so that any difference in potency can be attributed to a β_2 effect. The problems of such trials have been recently highlighted in an excellent review on β-adrenoceptor blocking drugs in essential tremor (Wilson, Marshall and Richens, 1984). It is difficult to separate cardiac β_1 activity from secondary cardiac effects due to variable β_2 activity in the blood vessels themselves. The usual methods adopted in such trials to estimate β_1 blocking activity, such as the differences between supine and standing heart rate, Valsava's manoeuvre or glyceryl trinitrate stimulation, have all been questioned (McDevitt, 1977). Cardiac stimulation based on maximal exercise would be a preferred technique to assess the β_1 effects of drugs, but this has obvious limitations in elderly patients with essential tremor. Abila et al. (1983) have suggested initial comparative studies of β-adrenoceptor antagonists in healthy volunteers in order to determine the relative potency of β-blockers in antagonizing the increase in heart rate produced by maximal exercise. As yet few studies have adopted this approach.

Of the studies to date, two cardioselective agents have been most commonly used, atenolol and metoprolol. All studies have shown that atenolol is less potent than propranolol, timolol and sotalol when given at doses giving equivalent β_1 effects on the heart (Jefferson, Jenner and Marsden, 1979a; Larsen and Teravainen, 1981; Leigh et al., 1981). An intravenous study has shown atenolol to be superior to placebo but less effective than the non-selective drugs (Abila et al., 1983). It is concluded from this data that the anti-tremor effect is by way of the β_2 subtype. Comparative studies using the cardioselective agent metoprolol are somewhat confusing. Uncontrolled trials claimed a beneficial effect in essential tremor (Britt and Peters, 1979; Ljung, 1979; Riley and Pleet, 1979; Newman and Jacobs, 1980; Turnbull and Shaw, 1980). The first single dose controlled trial of metoprolol showed equipotency with propranolol (Calzetti et al., 1981a); however, chronic dosing showed metoprolol to be ineffective (Leigh et al., 1981; Calzetti et al., 1982). It should be emphasized that studies with metoprolol are complicated by the fact that at doses between 100 and 150 mg daily, cardioselectivity is lost (Jefferson and Marsden, 1980; Ljung, 1980).

The consensus overview is that the β_2 adrenoceptor is the site of major importance in the control of essential tremor with β-adrenoceptor blocking drugs, but β_1 or other sites may be involved. The most recent support for this has come from studies with novel β_2 selective adrenoceptor antagonists. Cleeves and Findley (1984), using single oral doses of the β_2 selective antagonist LI 32-468 (4-(3-*tert*-butylamino-2-hydroxypropoxy)spiro[cyclohexan-1,2-indan]-1-one hydrogen malonate), demonstrated that a 2 mg dose was equipotent with 120 mg of propranolol. This drug is highly water soluble, without membrane stabilizing effect, and at 2 mg doses, devoid of measurable β_1 adrenoceptor effects. In a separate study another β_2 selective antagonist, ICI 118-551, was shown to be effective in suppressing essential tremor (Huttenen, Teravainen and Larsen, 1984). These results support the contention that the beneficial effects of non-selective β-adrenoceptor antagonists is mediated by the β_2 receptor site.

The enhancement of physiological tremor by stimulation of the peripheral β_2 receptors and the suppression of essential tremor by inhibiting these receptors has raised the question as to whether these receptors are involved in the genesis of essential tremor. *In vivo* studies of adrenergic β_2-adrenoceptor sensitivity in essential tremor have concluded that no major abnormality exists (Teravainen and Larsen, 1984). *In vitro* studies using the circulating lymphocyte β_2-adrenoceptor model have also shown no significant differences between normal control subjects and patients with type I and type II essential tremor (Kilfeather et al., 1984). In addition a hyperadrenergic state does not exist in patients with classical essential tremor (type II). A single study has shown raised levels of adrenaline in ten patients with essential tremor. However, the levels were still within the physiological range and the types of tremor examined were not defined (Warren et al., 1984).

Lipid solubility of β-adrenoceptor antagonists

The importance of the ease of CNS penetration and the efficacy of action of β-adrenoceptor antagonists in essential tremor has been investigated by comparative studies of lipid-soluble drugs which will readily penetrate the blood–brain barrier and the more water-soluble drugs which penetrate the CNS at a reduced rate and in reduced amounts (*Table 22.1*). Atenolol (water soluble) achieves much lower central levels compared to propranolol or metoprolol, which are more lipid soluble (Van Zwieten and Timmermans, 1979; Neil-Dwyer et al., 1981; Taylor et al., 1981). However, water-soluble compounds do penetrate in reduced amounts, reaching one-tenth of the concentration of lipid-soluble compounds. Lipid solubility may not only have relevance to penetration of the CNS, as the possibility exists of a blood–tissue barrier rendering some peripheral β_2 receptor sites inaccessible to water-soluble drugs (Abila et al., 1985a).

Studies comparing non-cardioselective agents with different lipid solubilities, such as propranolol and sotalol, have shown the drugs to be equally potent (Jefferson, Jenner and Marsden, 1979a). Comparative studies with metoprolol and atenolol have shown that metoprolol, the more lipid-soluble drug, was less effective in long-term use (Larsen and Teravainen, 1981; Leigh et al., 1983). Cleeves and Findley (1984) showed that LI 32-468, a hydrophilic compound, was equipotent with propranolol.

Young, Growdon and Shahani (1975) found propranol ineffective when given intravenously and, when taken orally, 24 hours was required for an effect to be seen. This was argued to show the necessity of CNS accumulation for drug effect. However, subsequent studies (McAllister et al., 1977; Abila et al., 1983) have shown a significant effect with intravenous propranolol. Furthermore, Morgan, Hewer and Cooper (1973) and, more recently, Calzetti et al. (1983b), have demonstrated that single doses of propranolol do have significant effect on tremor. These studies confirm that CNS accumulation is not necessary for the attenuation of essential tremor, though it cannot be excluded that effects of the drug at central receptor sites may confer additional therapeutic effect.

Membrane-stabilizing activity of β-adrenoceptor antagonists

Propranolol possesses membrane stabilizing properties, which could be contributing to its therapeutic effect in essential tremor. Other, non-cardioselective agents, such as sotalol and timolol, which have respectively no or little membrane-stabilizing activity, have significant effects in essential tremor (*Table 22.1*) (Rangel-Guerra, 1974; Rinne and Kaitaniemi, 1974). In a comparative study, sotalol and propranolol have been shown to be equipotent (Jefferson, Jenner and Marsden, 1979a). LI 32-468, at a dose which has no membrane-stabilizing effect, i.e. 2 mg, was also equipotent with propranolol (Cleeves and Findley, 1984).

Studies with the *d*-isomer of propranolol, which is virtually devoid of β-adrenoceptor blocking effect, but with similar membrane-stabilizing activity, has yielded conflicting results. Recent studies suggest *d*-propranolol is ineffective in essential tremor (Teravainen and Larsen, 1981; Calzetti and Findley, 1984).

Intrinsic sympathomimetic activity of β-adrenoceptor antagonists

Pindolol, a non-cardioselective drug, with a profile of activity similar to propranolol but with intrinsic sympathomimetic activity, is not effective in the control of essential tremor and, indeed, produced an exacerbation of tremor (Teravainen, Larsen and Fogelholm, 1977).

THE USE OF PROPRANOLOL IN THE MANAGEMENT OF ESSENTIAL TREMOR

Calzetti *et al.* (1983b) confirmed that a single oral dose of 120 mg propranolol could significantly reduce the amplitude of essential tremor (overall mean reduction 43%). There was great variability in response, in terms of tremor reduction, between patients, and a positive correlation between pre-treatment amplitude and response and hence a negative correlation with frequency. Patients with tremors of higher amplitude, and therefore lower frequency, responded best. This response characteristic held for chronic use of the drug (*Figure 22.1*).

The fact that propranolol is effective as a single oral dose opens up therapeutic possibilities. Patients who need not, or do not want to, take drugs on a regular basis, and whose tremor becomes more symptomatic during specific predictable activities, can be given a single oral dose and may expect attenuation of tremor for 1–3 hours after dosing. For example, the business executive with essential tremor who finds his tremor a nuisance during board meetings or when speaking in public, may find intermittent dosing with propranolol convenient and beneficial in these situations. It should be emphasized that, in addition to suppressing the intrinsic tremor, propranolol will also prevent exacerbation of tremor due to peripheral adrenergic drive at those times of stress and tension. In practice, patients who may benefit from this form of treatment should try small doses of propranolol and build up the dose until a satisfactory therapeutic response is achieved. The author has found 80–120 mg is required.

Anecdotally, the author has had the opportunity of treating, with single doses of propranolol, golfers with essential tremor who find that their performance is adversely affected by exacerbation of their tremor through anxiety and stress for the first two or three holes of any game. This raises the interesting question as to whether such use of drugs could be considered as legitimate in the context of sporting events, or whether it would be considered as iatrogenic drug 'abuse' to improve performance?

In the more usual continuous dosing regime a daily dose of 120 mg propranolol was not found to be superior to placebo, though 240 mg daily was shown to be effective (mean reduction in tremor amplitude 45%, *Figure 22.2*) (Calzetti *et al.*, 1983a). Divided daily doses (three times daily regime) between 120 and 240 mg are usually recommended and it has even been suggested that doses up to 800 mg are worth trying (McAllister *et al.*, 1977). A single recent study has shown that long-acting propranolol, given once daily, had similar efficacy to propranolol given in divided doses and was preferred by 87% of patients (Koller, 1985).

Figure 22.2 Reduction in tremor magnitude compared to placebo after propranolol (120 mg and 240 mg daily), metoprolol (150 mg and 300 mg daily), primidone (up to 750 mg daily) and phenobarbitone (120 mg daily) in different groups of essential tremor patients studied in the same laboratory using similar experimental protocol and procedures. (* Indicates statistical significance, $P<0.01$)

A finding which is universal to all the studies of propranolol in essential tremor is the great variability of responses between patients, and in every study there are always some patients who do not respond at all. Calzetti *et al.* (1983a) showed that patients with larger amplitude and lower frequency tremor responded best. However, in a recent study, Sabra and Hallett (1984) found that higher amplitude, lower frequency tremors due to alternating muscle activity did not respond to propranolol. In addition to the variability in response, it should be stressed that patients rarely have tremor amplitude suppressed to normal physiological levels. This is not surprising when it is considered that propranolol is acting predominantly at a peripheral receptor site and not, as we understand it, at the primary origin of tremor.

Measurement of drug levels is not helpful as no correlation between plasma level of propranolol (after oral administration) and tremorlytic effect has been found (Jefferson, Jenner and Marsden, 1979b; Calzetti et al., 1981a; Sorensen et al., 1981; Calzetti et al., 1983a).

As previously discussed, no long-term studies have been undertaken to ascertain whether patients maintain their response to propranolol over months or years. Recently, we have had the opportunity of withdrawing propranolol (240 mg daily) in two patients with essential tremor who had been on treatment for one year. A rebound exacerbation of tremor was recorded between three and four days of abrupt withdrawal, followed by a return to tremor amplitude comparable to those measured whilst on treatment. Thus, some patients may not maintain their original response to propranolol and this is an argument for continuous review of patients on long-term therapy and perhaps for periodic withdrawal of the drug.

Propranolol must be avoided in patients with congestive cardiac failure, atrioventricular heart block, and asthma, and should be used with caution in patients with diabetes mellitus. It seems well tolerated in patients with essential tremor: in a recent study of prolonged administration of 240 mg daily, five out of 16 patients complained of side-effects, mainly in the form of tiredness and headache. Two of these five patients complained of breathlessness on propranolol. The commonest complaint is of non-specific fatigue and weakness. Stone (1979) found that 30% of patients with full β-blockade complained of weakness of the legs and difficulty making extra effort. The subject of drug-induced fatigue is reviewed in an editorial in *Lancet* (Editorial, 1980), and its precise mechanism with β-blocking drugs is not understood. Clearly, where possible, β-blocking drugs should be avoided in patients who, for pleasure or for work, indulge in vigorous physical exercise.

In recommending a drug for long-term use in patients who have a normal life expectancy, the possibility of long-term side-effects are of considerable concern. *In vitro* studies have shown that propranolol has a profound effect on platelet aggregation (Winther Hansen et al., 1982) and fibrinolysis (Winther Hansen, 1985, personal communication), producing theoretical risk of increased thrombo-embolic complications in chronically treated patients. In the large numbers of trials which have been carried out with propranolol in many different disorders, it would appear to be a safe drug for long-term use. However, in the Norwegian Multicentre study of timolol in patients surviving myocardial infarction, there was an increased number of patients with thrombotic or embolic disease on treatment than on placebo (Norwegian Multicentre Study Group, 1981). It is not known whether this difference is significant; however, it behoves all physicians treating patients with long-term β-blocking drugs to be aware of this possible risk and that all future large studies of β-blocking drugs should look specifically and prospectively at this problem.

α-Adrenoceptor blockade

The α-adrenergic blocking drug thymoxamine, in single intravenous doses, has been shown to reduce essential tremor (Mai and Olsen, 1981; Abila et al., 1985b) but to have no effect on parkinsonian tremor (Mai and Olsen, 1981). As there are no peripheral tremorgenic α receptors (Marsden et al., 1967), the effect of thymoxamine is argued to be centrally determined and, from studies in animals and man, it is proposed that its action is by way of inhibition of central (spinal cord or higher level) noradrenergic facilitation of the γ loop servo-mechanism of the stretch reflex arc (Phillips, Richens and Shand, 1973; White and Richens, 1974; Mai, 1981). The duration of attenuation of essential tremor by intravenous thymoxamine is brief, which reflects the plasma half-life of 2.5 minutes (Griffin et al., 1972).

In the most recent study of the effect of intravenous thymoxamine on tremors of different origins (Abila et al., 1985b), it has been shown that, although essential tremor was attenuated, physiological tremor and isoprenaline-induced tremor was enhanced. The mechanisms for this are not known. The effect of increased ballistocardiac impulse, due to thymoxamine-induced tachycardia contributing to the enhancement of physiological and isoprenaline-induced tremor, was discounted as no change in tremor was detected following a similar degree of tachycardia induced by sublingual glyceryl trinitrate. Furthermore, it has been shown that the ballistocardiac impulse probably contributes less than 10% to normal physiological tremor (Marsden et al., 1969). Other peripheral mechanisms of α-adrenoreceptor blockade, such as vasodilatation in skeletal muscles and the blocking of α-adrenoreceptors on motor nerve terminals, were considered unrelated to any change in tremor amplitude. Abila et al. (1985b) considered that the most likely cause of the tremor-enhancing effect of thymoxamine was exerted within the CNS, although the exact mechanism is not clear. These authors emphasize that essential tremor and physiological tremor have different pathophysiological mechanisms, and that isoprenaline-induced tremor is not a good pharmacological model of essential tremor.

The beneficial effects of intravenous thymoxamine raise the possibility of using α-adrenoreceptor blockers in the management of essential tremor. Thymoxamine is poorly absorbed; therefore, other orally active α blockers or, perhaps more logically, combined α and β blockers may be effective in controlling essential tremor. Clinical trials of oral α-adrenoreceptor blockers are needed.

Primidone

Many clinical neurologists have found primidone effective in suppressing essential tremor. The first clinical trial was by O'Brien, Upton and Toseland (1981) and was in the form of an open, prospective clinical study in 20 patients. In 12 patients the response was described as 'good to dramatic'. A further open study (Chakrabarti and Pearce, 1981) also found the drug effective. Subsequent double-blind, controlled studies have demonstrated that primidone can be an effective drug in the control of essential tremor (Findley and Calzetti, 1982; Findley, Calzetti and Cleeves, 1985).

In the most recent study (Findley, Calzetti and Cleeves, 1985), primidone was given to 22 patients with moderate to severe essential tremor, starting at 62.5 mg daily and building up to a maximum dose of 750 mg daily (250 mg three times daily) by daily increments of 62.5 mg. Owing to unacceptable side-effects, only 16 patients were able to complete the study. Of these patients, four were unable to tolerate the maximum dose of primidone. Primidone was found to be significantly superior to placebo in reducing hand tremor, calculated as either absolute change in tremor magnitude or as percentage change against placebo levels. The mean percentage reduction was 55.9, ranging from an increase in tremor of 14.4 to a decrease of

98.6. The response seen in these patients was at least equal to that achieved with propranolol at a dose of 240 mg daily (Calzetti et al., 1983a; Figure 22.2). This objectively measured response was supported by statistically significant improvements on clinical assessment, patient's self assessment and manual performance tests. Furthermore, two patients with moderately severe essential tremor had tremor suppressed to within the physiological range, with a concomitant change in frequency (Figure 22.3). This we interpreted as being total suppression of the essential tremor, thus allowing physiological tremor at a separate and higher frequency to manifest itself. Serum primidone levels ranged from 18 to 100 µmol/l (median 48 µmol/l) and serum phenobarbitone from 5 to 87 µmol/l (median 55 µmol/l). There was no correlation between absolute or percentage reduction in tremor and either serum primidone or phenobarbitone concentration. It should be emphasized that nine patients who completed the study had tremor of the head in addition to hands. Primidone had no significant effect on head tremor whilst significantly reducing hand tremor in those patients. This differential reponse may suggest differences in underlying pathophysiological mechanisms in tremors of different parts of the body.

Figure 22.3 Average spectrum of hand tremor under placebo (*a*) and (*b*). Placebo spectrum shows large magnitude tremor (frequency 4.6 Hz; magnitude 108 milli-g root mean square (rms), where g = acceleration of gravity = 981 cm/s^2). On primidone, spectrum (*b*) has an entirely different appearance (frequency 9.5 Hz; magnitude 1.92 milli-g rms) NB The scale of axis of (*b*) is 1/50th that of (*a*). Spectrum (*b*) also shows significant smaller peak at 4.6 Hz. The magnitude of both peaks is within the magnitude of asymptomatic physiological tremor. (From Calzetti and Findley, 1984, courtesy of the Editor and Publishers, Macmillan Press)

The mode of action of primidone in essential tremor is not known. In view of its anticonvulsant effect within the CNS, and its ability, in some patients, to completely suppress essential tremor, its site of action in essential tremor is assumed to be entirely central. It is well absorbed from the gastrointestinal tract with peak serum levels within 3–5 hours. Twenty-five per cent remains as primidone, whilst the rest is converted into two active metabolites: approximately 50% to phenylethylmalonamide with a half-life of 24–48 hours, and approximately 5% to phenobarbitone with a half-life of 120 hours. Phenobarbital accumulates during chronic administration and requires three weeks to reach steady-state plasma levels. In the original study of O'Brien, Upton and Toseland (1981), as a result of phenylethylmalonamide substitution during withdrawal of primidone, it was suggested that the beneficial effect of primidone was achieved by way of phenylethylmalonamide. Subsequently, a double-blind, controlled study of phenylethylmalonamide in essential tremor has shown the drug to be both inert and ineffective in control of tremor (Calzetti et al., 1981b). Derived phenobarbitone will certainly have some effect on essential tremor (see below); however, there is evidence to suggest that primidone itself is contributing to the therapeutic response (Findley and Cleeves, 1985b).

A high incidence of side-effects has been found with use of primidone in essential tremor. In the largest study, 5 out of 22 patients exhibited acute toxic effects with the first 62.5 mg dose, consisting of nausea, ataxia and vomiting severe enough to force the patient to bed (Findley, Calzetti and Cleeves, 1985). The cause of these early toxic effects is not clear. The latency of onset precludes significant metabolism of primidone to have occurred. It has been suggested that such side-effects are due to delayed breakdown of primidone owing to the absence of hepatic enzyme induction in patients previously unexposed to anticonvulsant drugs (Feely, 1981). Primidone, when given to epileptic patients who had previously received other anticonvulsants, had a much lower incidence of acute toxicity (Feely, 1977). It seems likely that primidone itself is responsible for this acute toxicity as neither phenylethylmalonamide (Calzetti et al., 1981b) nor phenobarbitone (Baruzzi et al., 1983; Findley and Cleeves, 1985b) produced acute toxic adverse reactions when given to patients with essential tremor.

Primidone can be a very useful drug in the control of essential tremor. As with propranolol, there are no long-term studies to confirm whether any initial response is maintained. In terms of avoiding the initial side-effects, it has been suggested that pre-treatment with an hepatic enzyme inducing drug, such as phenobarbitone, may be worthwhile (Feely, 1981). In addition, we have found that commencing treatment with very small doses, i.e. 62.5 mg daily, and a slow incremental regime, building up to 250 mg three times daily over a period of three or four weeks, may avoid these side-effects. Patients must be warned of acute, early side-effects and, particularly in the elderly, it is worth admitting to hospital for a few days to start treatment. In addition to the acute, immediate side-effects, patients should be warned of similar, though invariably less severe, dose-related side-effects which may occur with drug increments.

There seems no clear indication from the limited evidence that is available as to what features of essential tremor, i.e. amplitude or frequency, dictate whether an individual patient will respond. From clinical observation, there is the suggestion that higher amplitude hand tremor, previously unresponsive to propranolol, may respond to primidone. Furthermore, a number of patients who have responded moderately to propranolol have shown further improvement with the addition of primidone to propranolol.

Phenobarbitone

There has been renewed interest in the use of phenobarbitone in the control of essential tremor. This drug has been used widely in the control of tremor and other movement disorders throughout most of this century, though few formal clinical trials have been carried out. Baruzzi et al. (1983) measured the effects of phenobarbitone and propranolol in essential tremor. On objective measurement of tremor and patient's self-assessment, the two drugs were equally effective and significantly superior to placebo in reducing the amplitude of tremor. On clinical evaluation, only propranolol was significantly better than placebo, and on tests of manual skill neither drug was effective. In a more recent study (Findley and Cleeves, 1985b), phenobarbitone (60 mg twice daily) produced a significant reduction (mean 52.6%) (*Figure 22.2*) in tremor amplitude compared to placebo. In this study, phenobarbitone was also significantly better than placebo on clinical assessment, but not on patient's self-assessment or tests of motor performance. As in a previous study of primidone conducted in the same laboratory beneficial effects were seen on all methods of assessment, it is suggested that primidone may give additional benefit to that obtained from phenobarbitone alone (Findley, Calzetti and Cleeves, 1985). Clearly, direct comparative studies between phenobarbitone and primidone are required.

As with primidone, the mode of action of phenobarbitone in essential tremor is not known, but is presumed to be within the CNS. It has been suggested that the effectiveness of phenobarbitone is related to the degree of central sedation achieved. This cannot be entirely discounted. However, in the most recent study (Findley and Cleeves, 1985b), the treatment period was long enough for tolerance to sedation to develop and the drug levels achieved were generally less than those reported to produce psychomotor slowing (Reynolds and Travers, 1974). It is interesting also to note in this series of patients that more complained of sedation on placebo (four patients) than on phenobarbitone (three patients), and in only one patient was the level of sedation persistent and unacceptable.

CONCLUSIONS

As yet there is no entirely satisfactory drug for the control of essential tremor. Alcohol, non-specific sedatives and tranquillizers are not practical forms of treatment.

β-Adrenoceptor blocking drugs, in particular propranolol, are the drugs of first choice. Their mode of action is predominantly by way of the peripheral $β_2$-adrenoceptor. Longer-term clinical trials are needed to establish whether initial responses to β-blocking drugs are maintained.

α-Adrenoceptor blocking drugs, administered intravenously, will effectively suppress essential tremor and their action is mediated centrally. Clinical trials are required of oral α-adrenoceptor blocking drugs with suitable pharmacological profiles.

Primidone and phenobarbitone can be effective in the control of essential tremor. Primidone is likely to have a therapeutic effect in addition to derived phenobarbitone. Primidone and β-adrenoceptor blocking drugs may have additive therapeutic effects. Long-term clinical trials are necessary to establish the long-term efficacy of these drugs.

The development of the perfect drug to control essential tremor, unless by serendipity, must await a more complete understanding of the central mechanisms generating classical essential tremor.

References

ABILA, B., MARSHALL, R. W., WILSON, J. F. and RICHENS, A. (1983) Do beta-adrenoceptor blockers have peripheral or central effects in essential tremor? *British Journal of Clinical Pharmacology*, **16**, 210

ABILA, B., WILSON, J. F., MARSHALL, R. W. and RICHENS, A. (1985a) The tremorlytic action of beta-blockers in essential tremor, physiological and isoprenaline-induced tremor is mediated by beta-adrenoceptors located in a deep peripheral compartment. *British Journal of Clinical Pharmacology* (in press)

ABILA, B., WILSON, J. F., MARSHALL, R. W. and RICHENS, A. (1985b) Differential effects of alpha-adrenoceptor blockade on essential, physiological and isoprenaline-induced tremor: evidence for a central origin of essential tremor. *Journal of Neurology, Neurosurgery and Psychiatry* (in press)

ACKMANN, J. J., SANCES, A., LARSON, S. J. and BAKER, J. B. (1977) *IEEE Transactions on Biomedical Engineering*, BME-24, 49–56

ANDREW, J. (1984) Surgical treatment of tremor. In *Movement Disorders: Tremor*. Eds. L. J. Findley and R. Capildeo, pp. 339–352. London: Macmillan

ARNOLD, J. M. O., JOHNSTON, G. D., HARRON, D. W. G., SHANKS, R. G. and McDEVITT, D. G. (1982) The effect of ICI 118-551 on isoprenaline-induced beta adrenoceptor responses in man. *British Journal of Clinical Pharmacology*, **15**, 133–134

ASHENHURST, E. M. (1973) The nature of essential tremor. *Canadian Medical Association Journal*, **109**, 876–878

BARBEAU, A. (1969) L-Dopa therapy in Parkinson's disease: a critical review of nine years' experience. *Canadian Medical Association Journal*, **101**, 791–800

BARBEAU, A. (1973) Traitement du tremblement essentiel familial par le propranolol. *Union Medicale du Canada*, **102**, 899–902

BARCROFT, H., PETERSON, E. and SCHWAB, R. S. (1952) Actions of adrenaline and noradrenaline on the tremor of Parkinson's disease. *Neurology*, **2**, 154–160

BARUZZI, A., PROCACCIANTI, G., MARTINELLI, P., RIVA, R., DENOTH, F., MONTANARO, N. and LUGARESI, E. (1983) Phenobarbital and propranolol in essential tremor: a double blind controlled clinical trial. *Neurology*, **33**, 296–300

BAXTER, D. W. and LAL, S. (1979) Essential tremor and dystonic syndromes. In *Extrapyramidal System and its Disorders*. Eds. L. J. Poirier, T. L. Sourkes and P. J. Bedard. *Advances in Neurology*, Vol. 24, pp. 373–377. New York: Raven Press

BIARY, N. (1984) Essential intentional tremor: a variant form of essential tremor and successful treatment with clonazepam. *Neurology*, **34** (Suppl. 1), 128

BIARY, N. and KOLLER, W. (1985) Effect of alcohol on dystonia. *Neurology*, **35**, 239–240

BOWMAN, W. C. and NOTT, M. W. (1969) Actions of sympathomimetic amines and their antagonists on skeletal muscle. *Pharmacological Reviews*, **21**, 27–72

BRITT, C. W. and PETERS, B. H. (1979) Metoprolol for essential tremor. *New England Journal of Medicine*, **301**, 331

BRUMLIK, J. and YAPP, C. B. (1970) *Normal Tremor: A Comparative Study*. Springfield, Illinois: Charles C. Thomas

CALMA, I. and KIDD, G. L. (1962) The effect of adrenaline on muscle spindles in cat. *Archives Italiennes de Biologie*, **100**, 381–393

CALZETTI, S. and FINDLEY, L. J. (1984) D,L-Propranolol and D-propranolol in essential tremor. In *Movement Disorders: Tremor*. Eds. L. J. Findley and R. Capildeo, pp. 261–269. London: Macmillan

CALZETTI, S., FINDLEY, L. J., GRESTY, M. A., PERUCCA, E. and RICHENS, A. (1981a) Metoprolol and propranolol in essential tremor: a double-blind, controlled study. *Journal of Neurology, Neurosurgery and Psychiatry*, **44**, 814–819

CALZETTI, S., FINDLEY, L. J., GRESTY, M. A., PERUCCA, E. and RICHENS, A. (1983a) Effect of a single oral dose of propranolol on essential tremor: a double blind controlled study. *Annals of Neurology*, **13**, 165–171

CALZETTI, S., FINDLEY, L. J., PERUCCA, E. and RICHENS, A. (1982) Controlled study of metoprolol and propranolol during prolonged administration in patients with essential tremor. *Journal of Neurology, Neurosurgery and Psychiatry*, **45**, 893–897

CALZETTI, S., FINDLEY, L. J., PERUCCA, E. and RICHENS, A. (1983b) The response of essential tremor to propranolol: evaluation of clinical variables governing its efficacy on prolonged administration. *Journal of Neurology, Neurosurgery and Psychiatry*, **46**, 393–398

CALZETTI, S., FINDLEY, L. J., PISANI, F. and RICHENS, A. (1981b) Phenylethylmalonamide in essential tremor: a double blind controlled study. *Journal of Neurology, Neurosurgery and Psychiatry*, **44**, 932–934

CHAKRABARTI, A. and PEARCE, J. M. S. (1981) Essential tremor: response to primidone. *Journal of Neurology, Neurosurgery and Psychiatry*, **44**, 650

CLEEVES, L. A. and FINDLEY, L. J. (1984) Beta-adrenoreceptor mechanisms in essential tremor: a comparative single dose study of the effect of a non-selective and a beta-2 selective adrenoreceptor antagonist. *Journal of Neurology, Neurosurgery and Psychiatry*, **47**, 976–982

CONSTAS, C. (1962) The effects of adrenaline, noradrenaline and isoprenaline on Parkinsonian tremor. *Journal of Neurology, Neurosurgery and Psychiatry*, **25**, 116–121

COUCH, J. R. (1976) Dystonia and tremor in spasmodic torticollis. In *Dystonia*, Eds. R. Eldridge and S. Fahn. *Advances in Neurology*, Vol. 14, pp. 245–258. New York: Raven Press

CRITCHLEY, E. (1972) Clinical manifestations of essential tremor. *Journal of Neurology, Neurosurgery and Psychiatry*, **35**, 365–372

CRITCHLEY, M. (1949) Observations on essential (heredofamilial) tremor. *Brain*, **72**, 113–139

DAVIS, C. H. and KUNKLE, E. C. (1951) Benign essential (heredofamilial) tremor. *Archives of Internal Medicine*, **87**, 808–816

DUPONT, E., HANSEN, H. J. and DALBY, M. A. (1973) Treatment of benign essential tremor with propranolol. *Acta Neurologica Scandinavica*, **49**, 75–84

EDITORIAL (1980) Fatigue as an unwanted side effect of drugs. *Lancet*, **i**, 1285–1286

FAHN, S. (1979) Post-hypoxic action myoclonus: review of the literature and report of two new cases with responses to valproate and estrogen. In *Cerebral Hypoxia and its Consequences*, Eds. S. Fahn, J. N. Davis and L. P. Rowland. *Advances in Neurology*, Vol. 26, pp. 49–84. New York: Raven Press

FEELY, M. (1977) *MD Thesis*, National University of Ireland

FEELY, M. (1981) Benign familial tremor treated with primidone. *British Medical Journal*, **282**, 740–741

FINDLEY, L. J. (1985) The pharmacological management of essential tremor. *Clinical Neuropharmacology* (in press)

FINDLEY, L. J. and CALZETTI, S. (1982) Double-blind controlled study of primidone in essential tremor: preliminary results. *British Medical Journal*, **285**, 608–609

FINDLEY, L. J., CALZETTI, S. and CLEEVES, L. (1985) Primidone in essential tremor of the hands and head: a double blind controlled clinical study. *Journal of Neurology, Neurosurgery and Psychiatry*, **48**, 911–915

FINDLEY, L. J., CALZETTI, S., GRESTY, M. A. and PAUL, E. A. (1981) Amplitude of benign essential tremor and response to propranolol. *Lancet*, **ii**, 479–480

FINDLEY, L. J. and CLEEVES, L. (1985a) The relation of essential tremor to Parkinson's disease. *Journal of Neurology, Neurosurgery and Psychiatry*, **48**, 192

FINDLEY, L. J. and CLEEVES, L. (1985b) Phenobarbital in essential tremor. *Neurology*, **35**, 1784–1787

FINDLEY, L. J. and GRESTY, M. A. (1981) Tremor. *British Journal of Hospital Medicine*, **26**, 16–43

GILLIGAN, B. S. (1972) Propranolol in essential tremor. *Lancet*, **ii**, 980

GILLIGAN, B. S., VEALE, J. L. and WODAK, J. (1972) Propranolol in the treatment of tremor. *Medical Journal of Australia*, **1**, 320–322

GRESTY, M. A. and FINDLEY, L. J. (1984) Definition, analysis and genesis of tremor. In *Movement Disorders: Tremor*, Eds. L. J. Findley and R. Capildeo, pp. 15–26. London: Macmillan

GRIFFIN, J. P., KAMBUROFF, P. L., PRIME, F. J. and ARBAB, A. G. (1972) Thymoxamine and airway obstruction. *Lancet*, **i**, 1288

HERSKOVITS, E. and BLACKWOOD, W. (1969) Essential (familial, hereditary) tremor: a case report. *Journal of Neurology, Neurosurgery and Psychiatry*, **32**, 509–511

HORNABROOK, R. W. and NAGURNEY, J. T. (1976) Essential tremor in Papua New Guinea. *Brain*, **99**, 659–672

HUTTUNEN, J., TERAVAINEN, H. and LARSEN, T. A. (1984) Beta adrenoreceptor antagonists in essential tremor. *Lancet*, **i**, 857

JEFFERSON, D., JENNER, P. and MARSDEN, C. D. (1979a) Beta-adrenoreceptor antagonists in essential tremor. *Journal of Neurology, Neurosurgery and Psychiatry*, **42**, 904–909

JEFFERSON, D., JENNER, P. and MARSDEN, C. D. (1979b) Relationship between plasma propranolol concentration and relief of essential tremor. *Journal of Neurology, Neurosurgery and Psychiatry*, **42**, 831–837

JEFFERSON, D. and MARSDEN, C. D. (1980) Metoprolol in essential tremor. *Lancet*, **i**, 427

KELLY, R. (1965) Tremor. In *Encyclopaedia of General Practice*, Eds. G. F. Abercrombie and R. M. S. McConaghey, pp. 210–216. London: Butterworths

KILFEATHER, S. A., MASARELLA, A., TURNER, P. and FINDLEY, L. J. (1984) Beta-adrenoceptor involvement in tremor production: possible defects in essential tremor. In *Movement Disorders: Tremor*, Eds. L. J. Findley and R. Capildeo, pp. 225–244. London: Macmillan

KOLLER, W. C. (1983) Alcoholism in essential tremor. *Neurology (Cleveland)*, **33**, 1074–1076

KOLLER, W. C. (1985) Long-acting propranolol in essential tremor. *Neurology*, **35**, 108–110

KOLLER, W., GRANER, D. and MICOCH, A. (1985) Essential voice tremor: treatment with propranolol. *Neurology*, **35**, 106–108

KORTEN, J. J., NOTERMANS, S. L. H., FRENKEN, C. W. G. M., GARBELS, F. J. M. and JOOSTEN, E. M. G. (1974) Familial essential myoclonus. *Brain*, **97**, 131–138
LANDS, A. M., ARNOLD, A., McAULIFF, J. P., LUDUENA, F. P. and BROWN, T. G. (1967) Differentiation of receptor systems activated by sympathomimetic amines. *Nature*, **214**, 597–598
LANG, A. C., KIERANS, C. and BLAIR, R. D. G. (1985) Family history of tremor in Parkinson's disease compared to controls and patients with idiopathic dystonia. In *Advances in Neurology*. New York: Raven Press (in press)
LAPRESLE, J., RONDOT, P. and SAID, G. (1974) Tremblement idiopathique de repos, d'attitude et d'action. *Revue Neurologique (Paris)*, **130**, 343–348
LARSEN, T. A. and CALNE, D. B. (1983) Essential tremor. *Clinical Neuropharmacology*, **6**, 185–206
LARSEN, T. A. and TERAVAINEN, H. (1981) Beta-blockers in essential tremor. *Lancet*, **ii**, 533
LARSSON, T. and SJOGREN, T. (1960) Essential tremor. A clinical and genetic population study. *Acta Psychiatrica et Neurologica Scandinavica*, **36** (Suppl. 144), 1–176
LEIGH, P. N., JEFFERSON, D., TWOMEY, A. and MARSDEN, C. D. (1983) Beta-adrenoreceptor mechanisms in essential tremor; a double blind placebo controlled trial of metoprolol, sotalol and atenolol. *Journal of Neurology, Neurosurgery and Psychiatry*, **46**, 710–715
LEIGH, P. N., MARSDEN, C. D., TWOMEY, A. and JEFFERSON, D. (1981) Beta-adrenoceptor antagonists and essential tremor. *Lancet*, **i**, 1106
LJUNG, O. (1979) Treatment of essential tremor with metoprolol. *New England Journal of Medicine*, **301**, 1005
LJUNG, O. (1980) Metoprolol in essential tremor. *Lancet*, **i**, 1032
McALLISTER, R. G., MARKESBERY, W. R., WARE, R. W. and HOWELL, S. M. (1977) Suppression of essential tremor by propranolol: correlation of effect with drug plasma levels and intensity of beta-adrenergic blockade. *Annals of Neurology*, **1**, 160–166
McCLURE C. G. and DAVIS, J. N. (1976) The effect of D-propranolol on action tremors. *Transactions of the American Neurological Association*, **101**, 269–270
McDEVITT, D. J. (1977) The assessment of beta-adrenoceptor blocking drugs in man. *British Journal of Clinical Pharmacology*, **4**, 413–425
MAHLOUDJI, M. and PIKIELNY, R. T. (1967) Hereditary essential myoclonus. *Brain*, **90**, 669–674
MAI, J. (1981) Adrenergic influences on spasticity. *Acta Neurologica Scandinavica*, **63** (Suppl. 85)
MAI, J. and OLSEN, R. B. (1981) Depression of essential tremor by alpha-adrenergic blockade. *Journal of Neurology, Neurosurgery and Psychiatry*, **44**, 1171
MANYAM, B. V. (1981) Amantadine in essential tremor. *Annals of Neurology*, **9**, 198–199
MARSDEN, C. D., FOLEY, T. H., OWEN, D. A. L. and McALLISTER, R. C. (1967) Peripheral beta-adrenoceptors associated with tremor. *Clinical Science*, **33**, 53–65
MARSDEN, C. D. and MEADOWS, J. C. (1970) The effect of adrenaline on the contraction of human muscle. *Journal of Physiology*, **207**, 429–448
MARSDEN, C. D., MEADOWS, J. C., LANGE, G. W. and WATSON, R. S. (1969) The role of the ballistocardiac impulse in the genesis of physiological tremor. *Brain*, **92**, 647–662
MARSDEN, C. D., OBESO, J. and ROTHWELL, J. C. (1983) Benign essential tremor is not a single entity. In *Current Concepts in Parkinson's Disease*. Ed. M. D. Yahr, pp. 31–36. Amsterdam: Excerpta Medica
MARSHALL, J. (1962) Observations on essential tremor. *Journal of Neurology, Neurosurgery and Psychiatry*, **25**, 122–125
MARSHALL, J. (1968) Tremor. In *Handbook of Clinical Neurology*, Eds. P. J. Vinken and G. W. Bruyn, Vol. 6, pp. 809–825. Amsterdam: North Holland Publishing Company
MARTINELLI, P. and GABELLINI, A. S. (1982) Essential tremor and buccolinguofacial dyskinesias. *Acta Neurologica Scandinavica*, **66**, 705–708
MARTTILA, R. J., RAUTAKORPI, I. and RINNE, U. K. (1984) The relation of essential tremor to Parkinson's disease. *Journal of Neurology, Neurosurgery and Psychiatry*, **47**, 734–735
MASSEY, E. W. and PAULSEN, G. W. (1978) Cause and effect in "alcohol tremor". *American Journal of Psychology*, **135**, 1572
MIYOSHI, T., KENNEDY, W. R. and YOON, K. S. (1979) Morphometric comparisons of capillaries in muscle spindles, nerve and muscle. *Archives of Neurology*, **36**, 547–552
MORGAN, M. H., HEWER, R. L. and COOPER, R. (1973) Effect of the beta-adrenergic blocking agent propranolol on essential tremor. *Journal of Neurology, Neurosurgery and Psychiatry*, **36**, 618–624
MORRIS, C. E., PRANGE, A. J., HALL, C. D. and WEISS, E. A. (1972) Inefficacy of tryptophan/pyridoxine in essential tremor. *Lancet*, **ii**, 165–166
MURRAY, T. J. (1972) Treatment of essential tremor with propranolol. *Canadian Medical Association Journal*, **107**, 984–986
MURRAY, T. J. (1976) Long term therapy of essential tremor with propranolol. *Canadian Medical Association Journal*, **115**, 892–894

MURRAY, T. J. (1981a) Essential tremor. *Canadian Medical Association Journal,* **124,** 1559–1565
MURRAY, T. J. (1981b) Essential tremor. In *Disorders of Movement,* Ed. A. Barbeau, pp. 151–170. Lancaster: MTP Press
NASRALLAH, H. A., SCHROEDER, D. and PETTY, F. (1982) Alcoholism secondary to essential tremor. *Journal of Clinical Psychiatry,* **43,** 163–164
NEIL-DWYER, G., BARTLETT, J., McAINSH, J. and CRUICKSHANK, J. M. (1981) Beta-adrenoceptor blockers and the blood–brain barrier. *British Journal of Clinical Pharmacology,* **11,** 549–553
NEWMAN, R. P. and JACOBS, L. (1980) Metoprolol in essential tremor. *Archives of Neurology,* **37,** 596–597
NORWEGIAN MULTICENTRE STUDY GROUP (1981) *New England Journal of Medicine,* **304,** 802–807
O'BRIEN, M. D., UPTON, A. R. and TOSELAND, P. A. (1981) Benign familial tremor treated with primidone. *British Medical Journal,* **282,** 178–180
OHYE, C., HIRAI, T., MIYAZAKI, M., SHIBAZAKI, T. and NAKAJIMA, H. (1981) Vim thalamotomy for the treatment of various kinds of tremor. *Applied Neurophysiology,* **45,** 275–280
OWEN, D. A. L. and MARSDEN, C. D. (1965) The effect of adrenergic beta-blockade on Parkinsonian tremor. *Lancet,* **ii,** 1259–1262
PAINTAL, A. S. (1964) Effects of drugs on vertebrate mechanoreceptors. *Pharmacological Reviews,* **16,** 341–380
PAKKENBERG, H. (1972) Propranolol in essential tremor. *Lancet,* **i,** 633
PERUCCA, E., PICKLES, H. and RICHENS, A. (1981) Effect of atenolol, metoprolol and propranolol on isoproterenol-induced tremor and tachycardia in normal subjects. *Clinical Pharmacology and Therapeutics,* **29,** 425–433
PHILLIPS, S. J., RICHENS, A. and SHAND, D. G. (1973) Adrenergic control of tendon-jerk reflexes in man. *British Journal of Pharmacology,* **47,** 595–605
QUINN, N. P. and MARSDEN, C. D. (1984) Dominantly inherited myoclonus dystonia with dramatic response to alcohol. *Neurology (Cleveland),* **34** (Suppl. 1), 236
RAJPUT, A. H., BEARD, K. P. O. M. and KURLAND, L. T. (1982) An epidemiologic survey of essential tremor in Rochester MN. *Neurology,* **32,** 128–134
RANGEL-GUERRA, R. (1974) Treatment of benign essential tremor with a beta-adrenergic blocking agent (sotalol). In *Advances in Beta-adrenergic Blocking Therapy – Sotolol. International Congress Series 341,* Ed. A. G. Snart, pp. V62–66. Amsterdam: Excerpta Medica
RAUTAKORPI, I. (1978) Essential tremor. An epidemiological, clinical and genetic study. *Research Report,* No. 12, Department of Neurology, University of Turku, Finland
RAUTAKORPI, I., MARTILLA, R. J. and RINNE, U. K. (1984) Epidemiology of essential tremor. In *Movement Disorders: Tremor,* Eds. L. J. Findley and R. Capildeo, pp. 211–218. London: Macmillan
REYNOLDS, E. H. and TRAVERS, R. D. (1974) Serum anticonvulsant concentration in epileptic patients with mental symptoms: A preliminary report. *British Journal of Psychiatry,* **124,** 440–445
RILEY, T. and PLEET, A. B. (1979) Metoprolol tartrate for essential tremor. *New England Journal of Medicine,* **301,** 663
RINNE, U. K. and KAITANIEMI, P. (1974) Sotolol in the treatment of essential tremor. In *Advances in Beta-adrenergic Blocking Therapy – Sotolol. International Congress Series 341,* Ed. A. G. Snart, pp. V56–61. Amsterdam: Excerpta Medica
RODGER, I. W. and BOWMAN, W. C. (1983) Adrenoceptors in skeletal muscle. In *Adrenoceptors and Catecholamine Action – Part B,* Ed. G. Kunos, pp. 123–155. New York: Wiley and Sons
SABRA, A. F. and HALLETT, M. (1984) Action tremor with alternating activity in antagonist muscles. *Neurology (Cleveland),* **34,** 151–156
SALISACHS, P. (1978) Dos signos clinicos no conocidos del tremblor esencial. *Medicina Clinica (Barcelona),* **70,** 120–121
SALISACHS, P. and FINDLEY, L. J. (1984) Problems in the differential diagnosis of essential tremor. In *Movement Disorders: Tremor,* Eds. L. J. Findley and R. Capildeo, pp. 219–224. London: Macmillan
SEVITT, I. (1971) The effect of adrenergic beta-receptor blocking drugs on tremor. *Practitioner,* **207,** 677–678
SEVITT, I. (1974) A comparison of propranolol and benzhexol in essential tremor. *Practitioner,* **213,** 91
SMITH, C. M. (1963) Neuromuscular pharmacology, drugs and muscle spindles. *Annual Review of Pharmacology,* **3,** 223–242
SORENSEN, P. S., PAULSON, O. B., STEINESS, E. and JANSEN, E. C. (1981) Essential tremor treated with propranolol: lack of correlation between clinical effect and plasma propranolol levels. *Annals of Neurology,* **9,** 53–57
STONE, R. (1979) Proximal myopathy during beta blockade. *British Medical Journal,* **2,** 1583
STRANG, R. R. (1965) Clinical trial with beta-receptor antagonist (propranolol) in parkinsonism. *Journal of Neurology, Neurosurgery and Psychiatry,* **28,** 404–406

SUTHERLAND, J. M., EDWARDS, V. E. and EADIE, M. J. (1975) Essential (hereditary or senile) tremor. *Medical Journal of Australia*, **2**, 44–47

TAYLOR, E. A., JEFFERSON, D., CARROLL, J. D. and TURNER, P. (1981) Cerebrospinal fluid concentrations of propranolol, pindolol and atenolol in man: evidence for central actions of beta-adrenoceptor antagonists. *British Journal of Clinical Pharmacology*, **12**, 549–559

TERAVAINEN, H., FOGELHOLM, R. and LARSEN, A. (1976) Effect of propranolol in essential tremor. *Neurology*, **26**, 27–30

TERAVAINEN, H. and LARSEN, T. A. (1981) Beta-blockers in the treatment of benign essential tremor. In *Proceeding of the Twelfth World Congress of Neurology* (Kyoto, Japan), *International Congress Series 548*, Abstract No 130, pp. 41–42. Amsterdam: Excerpta Medica

TERAVAINEN, H. and LARSEN, T. A. (1984) Adrenergic beta-receptor sensitivity in essential tremor. *Journal of Neurology, Neurosurgery and Psychiatry*, **47**, 1216–1218

TERAVAINEN, H., LARSEN, A. and FOGELHOLM, R. (1977) Comparison between the effects of pindolol and propranolol on essential tremor. *Neurology*, **27**, 439–442

THOMPSON, C., LANG, A., PARKES, J. D. and MARSDEN, C. D. (1984) A double blind trial of clonazepam in benign essential tremor. *Clinical Neuropharmacology*, **7**, 83–88

TOLOSA, E. S. and LOEWENSON, R. B. (1975) Essential tremor: treatment with propranolol. *Neurology (Minneapolis)*, **25**, 1041–1044

TURNBULL, D. M. and SHAW, D. A. (1980) Metoprolol in essential tremor. *Lancet*, **i**, 95

VAN ZWIETEN, P. A. and TIMMERMANS, P. B. M. W. M. (1979) Comparison between the acute hemodynamic effects and brain penetration of atenolol and metoprolol. *Journal of Cardiovascular Pharmacology*, **1**, 85–96

VAS, C. J. (1966) Propranolol in parkinsonian tremor. *Lancet*, **i**, 182–183

WARREN, J. B., O'BRIEN, M., DALTON, N. and TURNER, C. T. (1984) Sympathetic activity in benign familial tremor. *Lancet*, **i**, 461–462

WHITE, C. B. and RICHENS, A. (1974) Alpha-adrenoceptor blocking drugs, pressor responses to noradrenaline and the ankle jerk in man. *British Journal of Clinical Pharmacology*, **1**, 223–227

WILSON, J. F., MARSHALL, R. W. and RICHENS, A. (1984) Essential tremor: treatment with beta-adrenoceptor blocking drugs. In *Movement Disorders: Tremor*, Eds. L. J. Findley and R. Capildeo, pp. 245–260. London: Macmillan

WINKLER, G. F. and YOUNG, R. R. (1971) The control of essential tremor by propranolol. *Transactions of the American Neurological Association*, **96**, 66–68

WINKLER, G. F. and YOUNG, R. R. (1974) Efficacy of chronic propranolol therapy in action tremors of the familial, senile or essential varieties. *New England Journal of Medicine*, **290**, 984–988

WINTHER HANSEN, K., KLYSNER, R., GEISLER, A., BJERRE KNUDSON, J., GLAZER, S. and GORMSEN, J. (1982) Platelet aggregation and beta-blockers. *Lancet*, **i**, 224–225

YOUNG, R. R., GROWDON, J. H. and SHAHANI, B. T. (1975) Beta-adrenergic mechanisms in essential tremor. *New England Journal of Medicine*, **293**, 950–953

YOUNG, R. R. and HAGBARTH, K. E. (1980) Physiological tremor enhanced by manoeuvres affecting the segmental stretch reflex. *Journal of Neurology, Neurosurgery and Psychiatry*, **43**, 248–256

Index

The following abbreviations have been used in this index only where the terms do not appear as main terms:
OPCA: olivopontocerebellar atrophy, 251–252; PSP: progressive supranuclear palsy

L-AAAD activity, 237–239
Acanthocytosis, 306
Acetylcholinesterase marker, 195–196
Achilles tendon lengthening for dystonia, 360–361
Adrenergic system, role in essential tremor, 431
α-Adrenoceptor blockers for essential tremor, 449–450
β-Adrenoceptor blockers,
  for essential tremor, 431–432, 441, 443–447
  intrinsic sympathomimetic activity, 447
  lipid solubility, 446
  membrane-stabilizing activity, 447
  properties, 444
  types, 444
Age-specific data,
  in essential tremor, 28
  in Huntington's disease, 48–49
  in Parkinson's disease, 24–25, 85
Aggression in Gilles de la Tourette syndrome, 416
  tics and, 408
Akathisia,
  differential diagnosis of, 386
  tardive, 308
Akinesia, role of dopaminergic deficiency in, 182
Alcohol,
  for dystonia, 367

Alcohol (*cont.*)
  for essential tremor, 432, 442–443
  sensitivity, 310
Alzheimer's disease
  brainstem lesions in, 131
  cholinergic deficiency in, 148–149, 198–201
  cognitive tests, 277
  intellectual deterioration in, 198–201
  Lewy body disease and, 132
  neuropathology, 280
  noradrenergic system deficiency in, 143–145
  Parkinson's disease and, 149–155
  senile parkinsonism and, 130
  serotinergic system deficiency in, 145
  see also Parkinsonism
Amantidine therapy in PSP, 283
Amino acid competition,
  levodopa transport and, 236, 238
  in OPCA, 263
Amitriptyline therapy in PSP, 284
Amyotrophic lateral sclerosis, 27
Animal mode for Parkinson's disease, 77–78
Ansotomy for dystonia, 369
Anti-cholinergic drugs,
  for dystonia, 360, 363–364, 376
  memory and, 196–197
  for PSP, 283–284
  in tardive dyskinesia, 309
Anti-convulsant-induced dystonia, 359

459

Index

Anti-dopaminergic drugs for dystonia, 360, 364–365, 376
Anti-psychotic drug-induced dystonia, 359
Anxiety,
  in Gilles de la Tourette syndrome, 415
  in Wilson's disease, 295–296
Arteriosclerotic parkinsonism, 135
Ataxia in OPCA, 251–252
Atenolol in essential tremor, 444, 445, 446
Auditory evoked responses in OPCA, 261–262

Baclofen,
  for dystonia, 360, 366–367
  for essential tremor, 442
  for Huntington's disease, 307
  for OPCA, 262
Ballism,
  in dystonia, 328
  imaging techniques in, 14
Basal ganglia calcification, 353
Basalis nucleus of Meynert, degeneration in parkinsonism, 146–149, 152–154
Behavioural disturbance,
  in Gilles de la Tourette syndrome, 412
  tics and, 392
  modification technique for dystonia, 361
Bender Gestalt test, 409–410
Benzodiazepines for essential tremor, 442
  for tardive dyskinesia, 360
  for dystonia, 367
Blepharospasm,
  surgery for, 371
  therapy for, 367, 368, 375
Blood analysis in dystonia, 353
Blood–brain barrier, levodopa and, 236–237
Botulinum toxin for dystonia, 367–368, 371–372, 374–375
Braces for dystonia, 362
Bradyphrenia from levodopa therapy, 186
Brain,
  analysis in dementia, 150
  biochemistry of,
    in Parkinson's disease, 213–216
    in tic patients, 394–396
  lesions of,
    in essential tremor, 424–425
    in tics, 389
    in torsion dystonia, 314–318
    in Wilson's disease, 290
  levels of dopamine after levodopa therapy, 241–245
  morphology of normal, 8
  pathology of, in PSP, 278–283
Brain scan techniques, 4–13

Brain surgery for dystonia, 368–371
Brainstem,
  auditory evoked responses in OPCA, 261–262
  lesions in parkinsonism, 131, 172
British anti-Lewisite in Wilson's disease, 289, 300
Bromocriptine therapy,
  for Parkinson's disease, 67
  for PSP, 283–284
Bromospiperone studies in Parkinson's disease, 10

Carbamazepine for dystonia, 367
Carbidopa effects on levodopa pharmacokinetics, 240–241
Carbon monoxide/disulphide encephalopathy, 137
Catechol-O-methyltransferase activity, 232, 239
Caudate atrophy in Huntington's disease, 11
Cerebral blood flow measurement, 5, 6
  in Parkinson's disease, 9
Cerebral cord incision for dystonia, 369
  stimulation in dystonia, 373
Cerebral cortex,
  cholinergic deficiency, intellectual impairment and, 196–198
  cholinergic markers in, 194–196
  levels of peptides in Parkinson's disease, 209
  somatostatin deficiency in, 209
Cerebral oxygen metabolism measurement, 5, 6
  in Parkinson's disease, 9
Cerebral surgery for dystonia, 368–369
Ceruleocortical deficiency in parkinsonism, 188
Ceruloplasmin deficiency in Wilson's disease, 289, 297, 298
Chemopallidectomy for dystonia, 369–370
Chemothalamotomy for dystonia, 370
Cholecystokinin-8 deficiency in Parkinson's disease, 205–207
Choline therapy in Alzheimer's disease, 200
Choline acetyltransferase,
  levels of,
    in Lewy body disease, 132
    in PSP, 281–282
  marker for, 193, 194–195
Cholinergic system,
  degeneration of,
    in parkinsonism, 146–149, 192–201
    in PSP, 281–282
    in tic patients, 399

Cholinergic system (*cont.*)
    effects of anti-cholinergics on, 364
Chorea, 305
    in Huntington's disease, 50
Chorioathetosis, paroxysmal kinesiogenic,
    genetic factors in, 46
Chromosomal location of defective genes,
    35–43
    in dystonia, 45–48
Cingular cortex involvement in tic
    behaviour, 419–420
Clonazepam,
    for essential tremor, 442
    for tics, 399
Clonidine,
    for dystonia, 367
    for tics, 397
CNS lesions causing essential tremor, 424
Cognitive disorders,
    in Gilles de la Tourette syndrome, 409–
        411
    in parkinsonism, role of dopaminergic
        deficiency in, 182–183
    in Parkinson's disease, 192, 194–201, 278
    in PSP, 277
Computed tomography, 4
    in dystonia, 11–12, 353
    in Huntington's disease, 10–11, 307
    in OPCA, 261, 264–265
    in Parkinson's disease, 8
    in PSP, 283
    in Wilson's disease, 299
Copper toxicity *see* Wilson's disease
Coprolalia, 385–386
Cortex *see* Cerebral cortex
Corticospinal tract lesions in dystonia, 320
Cryothalamotomy for dystonia, 370
Cyanide encephalopathy, 137

Decarboxylase inhibitor effect on levodopa
    therapy, 240–241
Decarboxylation of levodopa, 237–239
Delerium from levodopa therapy, 186
Dementia,
    in Alzheimer's disease, 198–201
    morphological basis of, 149–155
    in Parkinson's disease, 75, 198–201
        cortical cholinergic deficiency and, 196–
            198
    progressive myoclonic, 310
    in PSP, 276–277
    senile parkinsonism and, 130
    serotinergic system degeneration in, 145
    in Wilson's disease, 295
    see also Parkinsonism

Dementia of Guam, 27
Dementia–Parkinson complex, 133
Dementia pugilistica, 135–137
Denervation, peripheral, for dystonia, 372–
    373
2-[^{14}C] Deoxyglucose metabolism, 5–6
Deprenyl for Parkinson's disease, 69–70, 97
Depression,
    in Gilles de la Tourette syndrome, 411,
        415
    in MPTP-induced Parkinson's disease,
        75–76
Diazepam for dystonia, 359
Diet effects on levodopa transport, 236
    in OPCA, 263
    tic abatement and, 399
Dihydroxyphenylserine in OPCA, 262
2,3-Dimercaptopropanol in Wilson's
    disease, 289, 300
Diphenhydramine for dystonia, 359
DNA studies, 38–41, 44
    in dystonia, 48
    in Lesch–Nyhan syndrome, 54–57
Dopamine,
    agonists for dystonia, 364–365
    antagonists of,
        for dystonia, 260, 265, 366, 376
        for tics, 396
    metabolism of, 231–233, 241–243
    receptors for, 233
        hypersensitivity in tic patients, 395
        in Parkinson's disease, 176–180
    role in tics, 397
Dopaminergic system,
    deficiency in parkinsonism, 138–140, 167–
        186
    in Parkinson's disease, 213–216
        peptide deficiency and, 210–213
    in PSP, 281
Dorsal motor vagus nucleus in Parkinson's
    disease, 147
Dorsalis raphe nucleus degeneration in
    parkinsonism, 145–146
Drug-induced dystonia, 349, 350, 359
Drug-induced parkinsonism, 137
Dynorphin,
    deficiency in Parkinson's disease, 208–209
    levels in tic patients, 395
Dysarthria,
    following brain surgery, 371
    in Wilson's disease, 292–293
Dyskinesia,
    from levodopa therapy, 77, 78, 184
    management of, 68–69
    paroxysmal, 336

Dyskinesia (cont.)
  problems in, 305–312
  tardive, 308–309
    differential diagnosis of, 307
    treatment, 360
Dystonia,
  aetiology of, 337–339
  age at onset of, 337, 346–347
  diphasic, 360
  distribution, 339–343
  diurnal, 336–337
  drug-induced, see Drug-induced dystonia
  essential tremor and, 425
  focal, 340, 343–344, 347, 374–375
  'formes frustes', 345
  generalized, 341–342, 343–344, 347, 376–377
  genetic studies, 45–48
  idiopathic, 337–347
  imaging techniques in, 11–13
  multifocal, 342
  musculorum deformans, 332–333, 344–345
  myoclonic, 346
  onset and progression, 346–347
  in Parkinson's disease, 350
  paroxysmal, 336
  peak-dose, 360
  in PSP, 276
  psychiatric-induced, 351
  segmental, 340–341, 343–344, 347, 376–377
  tardive, 309, 350, 360
  tics and, 336
  torsion,
    classification, 337–345
    clinical features, 345–347
    definitions, 333–337, 344, 345
    epidemiology of, 29
    investigations, 351–353
    pathological anatomy, 314–318
    physiology, 318–328
    symptomatic, 347–351
    treatment of, 359–377
      pharmacological, 362–372, 375
      physical and behavioural, 361–362
      surgical, 368
  in Wilson's disease, 293–294

EEG,
  in PSP, 283
  in tics, 387–389
Electromyography,
  in dystonia,
    active, 322–323

Electromyography (cont.)
  in dystonia (cont.)
    ballistic movement, 328–329
    rest, 320–321
    stretch reflexes, 323–324
  in OPCA, 262
  in tremor, 427–429
Endocrine disorders in Parkinson's disease, role of dopaminergic system deficiency in, 183
Environmental factors in Parkinson's disease, 26, 79–82
Enzyme activity in brain, in Parkinson's disease, 169, 212
Epidemiological studies, 17–30
  in Parkinson's disease, 92
Epilepsy,
  in myoclonus, 309–310
  startle, 311
Ethanol see Alcohol
Ethopropazine for dystonia, 376
Extraspinal peripheral denervation for dystonia, 372–373

Fahn–Marsden rating scale, 351
Family examination for genetic factors, 33–34, 41–42
  see also Genetic aspects
[^{18}F]Fluoro-2-deoxyglucose metabolism, 6
  in dystonia, 12–13
  in Parkinson's disease, 9–10
6-[^{18}F]Fluoro-L-dopa metabolism, 6
Fluphenazine for tics, 396
Freezing in Parkinson's disease, 188

G8 linkage in Huntington's disease, 306
GABAergic system deficiency,
  in Parkinson's disease, 201–204
  in tic patients, 399
Gamma-aminobutyric acid levels in PSP, 282
Gamma-vinyl-GABA for dystonia, 367
Gastric emptying, levodopa absorption and, 235
Genetic factors, 33–58
  chromosomal location of defective genes, 35–43
  in dystonia, 45–48
    torsion, 338–339
  in essential tremor, 425
  family examinations, 33–34, 41–42
  in Gilles de la Tourette syndrome, 57–58, 412
  in Huntington's disease, 50–52, 306
  inheritance modes, 34–35

Genetic factors (*cont.*)
  in Lesch–Nyhan syndrome, 53–57
  markers for disease, 44
  nature of defective genes, 43–44
  in OPCA, 226–229
  in Parkinson's disease, 16, 58–59
  in tics, 390
  in Wilson's disease, 289
Gilles de la Tourette syndrome, 383–400, 406–420
  genetic factors in, 57–58
  hospital studies, 414–417
  intellectual performance and, 409–411
  obsessive–compulsive neurosis, 412–413
  psychopathology of, 407, 411–420
  see also Tics
Glucose metabolism measurement, 5–6
  in Huntington's disease, 11
  in Parkinson's disease, 9
  in PSP, 277
L-Glutamate decarboxylase activity in Parkinson's disease, 201–204
Glutamate dehydrogenase deficiency in OPCA, 255–256
  genetics of, 258–259
Glutamatergic activity in Huntington's disease, 307
Glutamatic acid level in PSP, 282

H-reflex studies, 324–325
Hallervorden–Spatz disease, dystonia in, 13
Hallucinations from levodopa therapy, 186
Haloperidol for tics, 396, 414
Harmaline-induced tremor, 432–435
Hemidystonia, 342, 349, 376
Hemiplegia from brain surgery, 368–369
HLA linkage in OPCA, 256
Homovanillic acid levels,
  in Lesch–Nyhan syndrome, 393
  in Parkinson's disease, 168–169, 174–176
  in PSP, 281
  in tic patients, 394
Huntington's disease,
  clinical features of, 49–50
  diagnosis, 306–307
  epidemiology of, 29
  genetic factors, 50–52, 306
  imaging techniques, 10–11
  pathology, 49
  prevalence and age at onset, 48–49
  therapy, 307–308
Hyperactivity, differential diagnosis, 392
Hyperekplexia, 311
  differential diagnosis, 384
Hypnotherapy for dystonia, 361

Hypotension, orthostatic, 132
Hypothalamic activity deficiency in
    Parkinson's disease, 171–172, 212
  noradrenaline levels, 188–189
Hypoxanthine guanine phosphoribosyltransferase deficiency, 52
  genetic location, 54–57

ICI 118–551 for essential tremor, 446
Imaging techniques, 4–13
Intellectual impairment *see* Cognitive disorders
Intestinal absorption of levodopa, 235–236

Jerks, differential diagnosis, 384, 385
Joseph disease, 133, 255, 257

Kayser–Fleischer rings, 296–297
Klazomania, 394

Lafora's body disease, 310
Learned behaviour studies, 8
Lecithin therapy in Alzheimer's disease, 200
Leigh's disease, dystonia in, 13
Lesch–Nyhan syndrome, 393
  clinical features of, 52–57
  genetic factors, 53–57
Leucine activity in OPCA, 263
Leucine-enkephalin deficiency in Parkinson's disease, 208–209
Levodopa,
  absorption of, 235–236
  biotransformation, 237–240
  decarboxylation, 237–239
  distribution, 234, 236–237
  excretion, 239–240
  metabolism, 231–232, 234, 237, 240
  O-methylation, 239
  pharmacokinetics, 231–245
    cerebral, 241–245
    extracerebral, 234–241
  transport, 234
Levodopa-induced dystonia, 360
Levodopa therapy,
  effects of decarboxylase inhibitors on, 240–241
  for dystonia, 337, 364–365, 376
  for Parkinson's disease,
    adverse reactions to dopaminergic system deficiency and, 184–186
    continuous infusion, 68
    failure to respond to, 245
    fluctuations in response to, 68–69, 184–186, 244–245

Levodopa therapy (*cont.*)
  for Parkinson's disease (*cont.*)
    GABAergic system and, 204
    measured by PET, 9
    prognosis and, 96–97
    starting, 66–67, 76
    wearing-off effect, 77, 244–245
    withdrawal, 69
  in PSP, 283–284
Lewy body disease, 70
  development of, 79
  diffuse, 130–132
  in vascular parkinsonism, 135
LI 32-468 for essential tremor, 445–446
Linkage analysis in genetics, 36–41
Lipid solubility of drugs for tremor, 446
Lisuride,
  for Parkinson's disease, 68
  for PSP, 283
Lithium for dystonia, 366
Liver changes in Wilson's disease, 290, 297
Locus ceruleus changes in parkinsonism, 144, 188
Lod scores in genetic studies, 42–43

Machado–Joseph disease, 133
Magnetic resonance imaging, 5
  in dystonia, 11–12
  in Huntington's disease, 10–11
  in OPCA, 264–265
  in Parkinson's disease, 8
  in Wilson's disease, 299
Manganese encephalopathy, 137
Memory,
  anti-cholinergic drugs and, 196–197
  in PSP, 277
Mephesin for essential tremor, 442
Mesocorticolimbic system degeneration in Parkinson's disease, 170–171
Methionine-enkephalin deficiency in Parkinson's disease, 207–208
3-Methoxy-4-hydroxyphenylethylene glycol levels in tic patients, 397
Methylphenidate for dystonia, 357
1-Methyl-4-phenyl-1,2,3,6-tetrahydropyridine *see* MPTP
1-Methyl-4-propionoxypiperidine (MPP),
  metabolism, 82–83, 85
  synthesis, 73
Methysergide therapy in PSP, 284
3-*N*-Methylspiperone tracer studies, 7–8
Metoprolol for essential tremor, 444, 445, 446
Micrographia, 81

Monoamine oxidase activity, 232
  inhibitors, MPTP metabolism and, 83
  therapy in Parkinson's disease, 86
Morbidity data in Parkinson's disease, 20–21
Mortality data in Parkinson's disease, 19–20
Motor symptom abnormalities,
  in parkinsonism, role of dopaminergic deficiency in, 182
  in Parkinson's disease,
    role of cholinergic system deficiency in, 193–194
    role of serotinergic system deficiency in, 192
  in torsion dystonia, 313–330
  in Wilson's disease, 291–294
  see also Athetosis; Ballism; Chorea; Dyskinesia; Dystonia; Myoclonus; Tics; Tremor
Motor unit,
  central versus reflex oscillations of, 427–431
  reciprocal firing versus coordination, 426–427
  synchronization, 426
Movements, involuntary,
  in dystonia, 320–321
  in Gilles de la Tourette syndrome, 418
  from levodopa therapy, 184
  in Wilson's disease, 293
  see also Motor symptom abnormalities
MPTP, 73–87
  historical review, 73–75
  mechanism of action, 82–85
  Parkinson's disease and, 26–27
  toxicity studies, 69, 70
MPTP-induced parkinsonism, 75–77, 137–138
  motor lesions in, 182
  peptide levels and, 210
Multiple system atrophy, 132, 254–255, 265
Muscarinic receptor markers, 195, 196
Muscle reflexes in dystonia, 323–328
Myoclonic dystonia, 346
Myoclonus, 309–310
  differential diagnosis, 384
  palatal, 435
  sleep, 310–311
  startle, 311–312

Nausea and vomiting from levodopa therapy, 184
Neuroacanthocytosis, 306, 392
Neuro-epidemiology, 17–30
Neurofibrillary tangles,
  in Alzheimer's disease, 280

Index 465

Neurofibrillary tangles (*cont.*)
  in dementia, 150
  in post-encephalitic parkinsonism, 135–136
  in PSP, 134–135, 278–280
Neuro-imaging *see* Computed tomography; Magnetic resonance imaging; Position emission tomography
Neuroleptics, Parkinson's disease and, 27
Neurological abnormalities,
  in tics, 383–400
  in Wilson's disease, 291–294
Neurological tests in PSP, 283
Neuromediators in hypothalamus in Parkinson's disease, 212
Neuropeptide deficiency in Parkinson's disease, 204–213
Neurosis, obsessive–compulsive, in tic patients, 412–413
Neurotensin receptor changes in Parkinson's disease, 210
Neurotoxins, environmental, Parkinson's disease and, 79–82
Neurotransmitters,
  in Alzheimer's disease, in cerebral cortex, 200
  in Huntington's disease, changes in, 50
  in Parkinson's disease,
    biochemistry of, 166–215
    in cerebral cortex, 200
    in substantia nigra, 211
    systems, 213
  in tic patients, 395
Nigrostriatal system deficiency,
  dopamine receptor hypersensitivity and, 177–180
  motor lesions and, 182
  in Parkinson's disease, 167–169, 174–175, 213–216
  in PSP, 281
Noradrenaline, role in tics, 397
Noradrenergic system deficiency in parkinsonism, 143–145, 186–190

Obsessive–compulsive neurosis,
  in Gilles de la Tourette syndrome, 412–413, 415–417, 418–419
  in tic patients, 408
Ocular abnormalities in Wilson's disease, 294
Oculomotor dysfunction in OPCA, 259–260, 264
Olivocerebellar system, tremor and, 433–435

Olivopontocerebellar atrophy (OPCA), 132, 249–271
  classification, 249–251
  clinical aspects, 251–252
  clinical definition, 263–265
  clinical entity, 270–271
  clinical features, 253
  genetic aspects, 256–259
  glutamate dehydrogenase deficiency, 255–256
  multiple system atrophy and, 254–255
  neuro-imaging, 260–261
  neurophysiology, 261–262
  oculomotor dysfunction, 259–260, 264
  parkinsonism and, 262–264
  pathological entity, 269–270
  terminology, 269–271
  therapy, 262–263
Olivocerebellorubral system, essential tremor and, 429
Ophthalmoplegia, supranuclear, in PSP, 274, 275–276
Orthopaedic therapy for dystonia, 360

Pallidonigral degeneration, 80
Palsy, progressive supranuclear (PSP), 70–71, 133, 272–285
  cardinal features, 275–278
  clinical signs, 273–275
  course, 284–285
  diagnostic investigations, 283
  differentiation, 263–265
  management, 283–284
  neuropathology, 277–283
  oculomotor dysfunction in, 259–264
  pathology and neurochemistry, 214–215
Paraventricular nucleus in Parkinson's disease, 147
Parkinson–dementia complex, 133
Parkinsonism,
  L-AAAD brain activity in, 241–242
  brain weight in, 150–151
  cerebellar, 252–254, 264
  cholinergic system degeneration in, 146–159, 192–201
  dopaminergic system deficiency in, 138–140, 167–186, 181–186
  MPTP-induced *see* MPTP-induced parkinsonism
  noradrenergic system deficiency in, 143–145, 186–190
  peptidergic system deficiency, 149
  post-encephalitic, 131, 135
  post-traumatic, 135–137

Parkinsonism (*cont.*)
  senile, 130
    brainstem lesions in, 131
    serotinergic system deficiency in, 145, 190–192
  symptomatic, 138
  toxic, 137–138
  tremor and, 427–429
  vascular, 131, 135
Parkinsonism–dementia of Guam, epidemiology of, 27
Parkinson's disease,
  aetiology of, 92–93
  age-specific factor, 24–25, 85
  Alzheimer's disease and, 150–155
  analytical studies, 25–27
  animal model for, 77–78
  biochemistry of neurotransmitters in, 166–215
  brain biochemistry, 213–215
  brainstem lesions in, 131
  cholinergic system deficiency in, 146–149, 192–201
  classification, 155–156
  cognitive disorders in, 192, 194–201, 278
  dopaminergic system deficiency, 138–140, 167–186, 213–216
  dystonia and, 350
  environmental neurotoxins and, 79–82
  epidemiology, 18–27, 92
  GABAergic system deficiency in, 201–204
  genetic factors, 58–59
  historical aspects, 91–96
  imaging techniques, 8–10
  incidence data, 20–21
  Lewy body disease and, 132
  mortality data, 19–20
  motor system deficiencies in, 192, 193–194
  MPTP-induced, 73–87
  neuropeptide deficiency in, 204–213
  neurotransmitter systems in, 166–216, 213
  noradrenergic system deficiency in, 143–145, 186–190
  oculomotor dysfunction in, 259
  pathobiochemistry, morphological basis for, 138–149
  prevalence data, 21–25
  prognosis, 91–97
  risk factors, 25–27
  serotoninergic system deficiency in, 145, 190–201
  subcortical nuclei degeneration, 147
  symptoms, 92–93
  therapy,
    for cause, 69–70
    for dyskinesia, 68–69

Parkinson's disease (*cont.*)
  therapy (*cont.*)
    for fluctuations, 68–69
    levodopa *see* Levodopa
    monoamine oxidase I in, 86
    new dopamine agonists in, 68
    new trials in, 97
    starting, 66–67
  transplants for, 69
  tremor and, 425
  see also Parkinsonism
Pathobiochemistry in Parkinson's disease, morphological basis for, 138–149
Penicillamine in Wilson's disease, 289, 300
Peptidergic system deficiency in parkinsonism, 149
Pergolide,
  for Parkinson's disease, 68
  for PSP, 283
Personality factor in Parkinson's disease, 26
Pesticide risk of Parkinson's disease, 27, 82
Pharmacokinetics of levodopa, 231–245
  cerebral, 241–245
  extracerebral, 234–241
Phenobarbital for essential tremor, 432
Phenobarbitone for essential tremor, 442, 452–453
Phenylethylmalonamide for essential tremor, 452
Phobias, tics and, 408
Phthalazinol in OPCA, 262
Physostigmine in OPCA, 262
Pimozide,
  for dystonia, 366
  for tics, 396
Pindolol for essential tremor, 444, 447
Pneumoencephalography in OPCA, 260–261
Positron emission tomography, 5–8
  in dystonia, 11–13
  in Huntington's disease, 11, 307
  in MPTP-induced parkinsonism, 86
  in Parkinson's disease, 9–10
Post-encephalitic parkinsonism, 131, 135
Primidone for essential tremor, 432, 450–452
Progressive supranuclear palsy (PSP) *see* Palsy, progressive supranuclear
Propranolol,
  in essential tremor, 431–432, 441, 443, 446–449
  in OPCA, 262
Pseudobulbar palsy in PSP, 276
Psychiatric disturbance,
  in Wilson's disease, 295–296
  dystonia induced by, 351

Psychopathology of tics, 406–420
Psychotherapy, supportive, in dystonia, 361–362

Race-specific data,
  in dystonia, 47–48, 338
  in Huntington's disease, 29
  in Parkinson's disease, 23–24
Radiopharmaceutical studies, 7–8
Ramsay Hunt syndrome, 309–310
Reciprocal inhibition of antagonist muscles, 324–328
Relaxation techniques in dystonia, 361
Restless leg syndrome, 310–311
Restriction fragment length polymorphism studies, 39–41
Rett's syndrome, 393
Rhizotomy for torticollis, 372
Risk factors in Parkinson's disease, 25–27
Risus sardonicus in Wilson's disease, 293
Rorchach projective test, 408

Schizophrenia relapse, 308
Scopolamine for dystonia, 363
Self-hypnosis in dystonia, 261
  mutilation in Lesch-Nyhan syndrome, 53
Senile *see under* Parkinsonism
Senile dementia of Alzheimer type (SDAT),
  brainstem lesions in, 131
  see also Alzheimer's disease
Sensory biofeedback,
  for dystonia, 361
  disorders in Parkinson's disease by, role of dopaminergic system deficiency in, 183
  'tricks' of, 346, 362
Serotinergic system deficiency,
  in parkinsonism, 145, 190–192
  in tic patients, 399
Shy–Drager syndrome, 132, 255
  genetics, 257–258
Sleep,
  disturbances in OPCA, 261
  in PSP, 283
  periodic movements of, 309–310
  tic persistence during, 387–388
Smoking factors in Parkinson's disease, 26
Somatostatin deficiency in Parkinson's disease, 208–209
Sotalol for essential tremor, 444, 446, 447
Spinal cord,
  dopamine levels in Parkinson's disease, 172
  morphology, normal, 8
  noradrenaline levels, 188

^{3}[H]Spiperone levels,
  as marker for dopamine receptors, 179
  in PSP, 281
Startle syndromes, 311–312, 383
  differential diagnosis, 384
Steele–Richardson–Olszewski syndrome *see* Palsy, progressive supranuclear
Stereotactic surgery for dystonia, 369–370
Stress-induced tics, 386, 413
Stretch reflexes in dystonia, 323–324
Striatal dopamine receptor hypersensitivity, 176, 177–180
  dopaminergic compensation, 180–181
  levodopa levels, 234, 241–243
Striatonigral degeneration, 132
  in multiple system atrophy, 254–255
  genetics of, 157–158
Striopallidum changes in parkinsonism, 142
Substance P deficiency in Parkinson's disease, 207
Substantia nigra,
  deficiency in,
    of cholecystokinin-8, 206
    of methionine-enkephalin, 207–208
    of substance P, 207
  hyperactivity in dopaminergic neurones, 176
  lesions of,
    in parkinsonism, 138–140
    in Parkinson's disease, 75, 80, 167–169, 173–174
  MPTP uptake by, 83–85
  neurochemistry in Parkinson's disease, 211
Supranuclear palsy, progressive *see* Palsy, progressive supranuclear
Supra-optic nucleus degeneration in Parkinson's disease, 147

Target mapping in genetic studies, 43–44
Tetrabenazine,
  for dystonia, 366
  for tics, 396–397
Thalamic surgery for dystonia, 369–370, 376
Thalamotomy for tics, 399
Thymoxamine for essential tremor, 449–450
Tics,
  botulinum toxin for, 368, 371–372, 375
  classification, 393
  differential diagnosis, 386, 391–394
  dystonic, 336
  neurology, 383–400
  neuropharmacology and management, 394–400

Tics (*cont.*)
  phenomenology and pathophysiology, 385–391
  psychopathology, 406–420
Torsion dystonia *see under* Dystonia
Torticollis, 318, 346
  behavioural modification in, 361
  drugs for, 375
  sensory tricks in, 362
  surgery for, 371, 372, 375
Tourettism, acquired, 392
Transplants for Parkinson's disease, 70
Trauma causing parkinsonism, 135–137
Tremor,
  CNS site lesions causing, 424
  essential,
    classification, 423, 439–441
    definition, 438
    epidemiology of, 27–28
    pathophysiology, 423–435
    pharmacology, 431–432, 438–453
    prevalence, 438–439
  in Wilson's disease, 294
Triethylene tetramine in Wilson's disease, 300–301
Trihexyphenidyl for dystonia, 363–364, 366, 376
Tyrosine-hydroxylase immunoreactive neurones degeneration, 140–141, 171, 189

Vascular parkinsonism, 131, 135
Verbal task dysfunction,
  in Gilles de la Tourette syndrome, 409
  in PSP, 277

Westphal–Edinger nucleus in Parkinson's disease, 147, 149
Wide Range Achievement test, 410
Wilson's disease, 288–301
  biochemistry, 289–294
  clinical manifestations, 291
  diagnosis, 294–299
  dystonia in, 13
  epidemiology of, 29
  genetics and prevalence, 289
  pathology, 290
  treatment, 299–301, 359
WISC test, 410
Wolf–Hirschhorn syndrome, genetic factors in, 52
Writer's cramp, 322
  therapy, 375

Yellow star thistle toxicity, 80

Zinc therapy in Wilson's disease, 300